Brody's Human Pharmacology

Molecular to Clinical

FOURTH EDITION

WITH 284 ILLUSTRATIONS

Brody's Human Pharmacology

Molecular to Clinical

Editors

Kenneth P. Minneman, PhD
Charles Howard Candler Professor of Pharmacology,
Department of Pharmacology,
Emory University School of Medicine,
Atlanta, Georgia

Lynn Wecker, PhD
Distinguished Research Professor and Chair,
Department of Pharmacology and Therapeutics,
University of South Florida College of Medicine,
Tampa, Florida

Consulting Editors

Joseph Larner, MD, PhD
Professor Emeritus and Chair,
Department of Pharmacology,
University of Virginia School of Medicine,
Charlottesville, Virginia

Theodore M. Brody, PhD
Emeritus Professor and Chair,
Department of Pharmacology and Toxicology,
Michigan State University College of Human Medicine,
East Lansing, Michigan

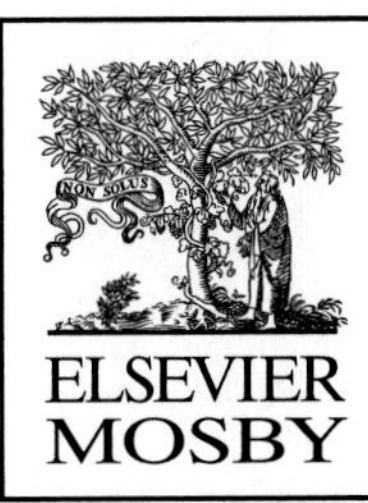

ELSEVIER
MOSBY

The Curtis Center
170 S Independence Mall W 300E
Philadelphia, Pennsylvania 19106

BRODY'S HUMAN PHARMACOLOGY ISBN 0-323-03286-9

NOTICE

Pharmacology is an ever-changing field. Standard safety precautions must be followed, but as new research and clinical experience broaden our knowledge, changes in treatment and drug therapy may become necessary or appropriate. Readers are advised to check the most current product information provided by the manufacturer of each drug to be administered to verify the recommended dose, the method and duration of administration, and contraindications. It is the responsibility of the licensed prescriber, relying on experience and knowledge of the patient, to determine dosages and the best treatment for each individual patient. Neither the publisher nor the author assumes any liability for any injury and/or damage to persons or property arising from this publication.

Previous editions copyrighted 1991, 1994, 1998

International Standard Book Number 0-323-03286-9

Acquisitions Editor: Alexandra Stibbe
Developmental Editor: Shirley Kuhn

Printed in China

Last digit is the print number: 9 8 7 6 5 4 3 2 1

Dedicated to our families
Jeff, Rebecca, and Jenny Minneman
Jonathan Tigue and Sarah Rachel Wecker-Tigue

Kenneth P. Minneman
Lynn Wecker

Contributors

Barrie Ashby, PhD
Professor, Department of Pharmacology,
Temple University School of Medicine,
Philadelphia, Pennsylvania

Rosemary R. Berardi, PhD
Professor of Pharmacy, Clinical Specialist in Gastrointestinal and Liver Diseases, Department of Pharmacy,
University of Michigan College of Pharmacy,
Ann Arbor, Michigan

Dale L. Birkle, PhD
Scientific Review Administrator,
National Center for Complementary and Alternative Medicine,
National Institutes of Health,
Department of Health and Human Services,
Bethesda, Maryland

Henry M. Blumberg, MD
Professor, Department of Medicine,
Program Director, Division of Infectious Diseases
Emory University School of Medicine;
Hospital Epidemiologist,
Grady Memorial Hospital,
Atlanta, Georgia

Steven L. Brody, MD
Associate Professor of Medicine, Department of Internal Medicine,
Washington University School of Medicine,
St. Louis, Missouri

Theodore M. Brody, PhD
Emeritus Professor and Chair, Department of Pharmacology and Toxicology,
Michigan State University College of Human Medicine,
East Lansing, Michigan

David B. Bylund, PhD
Professor, Department of Pharmacology,
University of Nebraska Medical Center,
Omaha, Nebraska

Glenn Catalano, MD
Associate Professor and Director of Medical Student Education, Department of Psychiatry and Behavioral Medicine,
University of South Florida College of Medicine;
Medical Director of Psychiatry, Department of Psychiatry,
Tampa General Hospital,
Tampa, Florida

George P. Chrousos, MD
Professor of Pediatrics and Physiology,
Georgetown University Medical School,
Washington, DC;
Chief, Pediatric and Reproductive Endocrinology Branch,
National Institutes of Health Clinical Center,
Bethesda, Maryland

James B. Chung, MD, PhD
Associate Professor, Department of Clinical Research and Development,
Pfizer, Inc.,
Ann Arbor, Michigan

Lynn M. Crespo, PhD
Assistant Professor, Department of Pharmacology and Therapeutics,
University of South Florida College of Medicine,
Tampa, Florida

Richard C. Dart, MD, PhD
Director, Rocky Mountain Poison and Drug Center;
Professor of Surgery, Pharmacy and Medicine,
University of Colorado Health Sciences Center,
Denver, Colordado

Richard A. Deitrich, PhD
Professor, Department of Pharmacology,
University of Colorado Health Sciences Center,
Denver, Colorado;
Fellow, Institute for Behavioral Genetics,
University of Colorado at Boulder,
Boulder, Colorado

Frederick J. Ehlert, PhD
Professor, Department of Pharmacology,
College of Medicine,
University of California, Irvine,
Irvine, California

William S. Evans, MD
Professor of Internal Medicine and Obstetrics & Gynecology, Department of Internal Medicine,
University of Virginia School of Medicine,
Charlottesville, Virginia

William P. Fay, MD
Associate Professor, Department of Internal Medicine,
University of Michigan Medical School,
Ann Arbor, Michigan

Peter S. Fischbach, MD
Assistant Professor, Department of Pediatrics and Communicable Diseases,
University of Michigan Medical School,
Ann Arbor, Michigan

Lawrence J. Fischer, PhD
Professor of Pharmacology and Toxicology;
Director, Center for Integrative Toxicology,
Michigan State University College of Human Medicine,
East Lansing, Michigan

Michael K. Fritsch, MD, PhD
Assistant Professor, Department of Pathology and Laboratory Medicine,
University of Wisconsin College of Medicine,
Madison, Wisconsin

James C. Garrison, PhD
Professor and Chair, Department of Pharmacology,
University of Virginia School of Medicine,
Charlottesville, Virginia

William T. Gerthoffer, PhD
Professor, Department of Pharmacology,
University of Nevada School of Medicine,
Reno, Nevada

Frank J. Gordon, PhD
Associate Professor, Department of Pharmacology,
Emory University School of Medicine
Atlanta, Georgia

Carolyn V. Gould, MD
Senior Associate in Medicine, Department of Medicine,
Division of Infectious Diseases,
Emory University School of Medicine;
Associate Hospital Epidemiologist,
Department of Medicine,
Emory Crawford Long Hospital,
Atlanta, Georgia

William W. Grosh, MD
Associate Professor of Internal Medicine, Department of Internal Medicine, Hematology, and Oncology,
University of Virginia School of Medicine,
Charlottesville, Virginia

Daniel H. Havlichek, JR., MD
Associate Professor, Departments of Medicine and Microbiology,
Chief, Division of Infectious Diseases,
Michigan State University College of Human Medicine,
East Lansing, Michigan

Erik L. Hewlett, MD
Professor, Department of Medicine and Pharmacology,
University of Virginia School of Medicine;
Attending Physician, Department of Internal Medicine,
University of Virginia Hospital,
Charlottesville, Virginia

Paul F. Hollenberg, PhD
Maurice H. Seevers Collegiate Professor and Chair, Department of Pharmacology,
University of Michigan Medical School,
Ann Arbor, Michigan

Stephen G. Holtzman, PhD
Professor, Department of Pharmacology,
Emory University School of Medicine,
Atlanta, Georgia

Kambiz Kalantarinia, MD
Assistant Professor of Medicine, Division of Nephrology,
University of Virginia School of Medicine,
Charlottesville, Virginia

Thomas T. Kawabata, PhD
Research Fellow, Department of Safety Sciences,
Pfizer Global Research and Development,
Groton, Connecticut

Mark D. King, MD, MS
Assistant Professor of Medicine, Department of Medicine,
Division of Infectious Diseases,
Emory University School of Medicine;
Director of the Antimicrobial Utilization Program and Assistant Hospital Epidemiologist, Department of Hospital Epidemiology,
Grady Health System,
Atlanta, Georgia

Wende M. Kozlow, MD
Fellow, Department of Internal Medicine,
Division of Endocrinology and Metabolism,
University of Virginia School of Medicine,
Charlottesville, Virginia

James M. Larner, MD
Associate Professor of Radiation Oncology and Internal Medicine (Hem/Onc), Department of Radiation Oncology,
University of Virginia School of Medicine,
Charlottesville, Virginia

John C. Lawrence, JR., PhD
Professor of Pharmacology and Medicine, Department of Pharmacology,
University of Virginia School of Medicine,
Charlottesville, Virginia

Benedict R. Lucchesi, MD, PhD
Professor, Department of Pharmacology,
University of Michigan Medical School,
Ann Arbor, Michigan

Jeffery R. Martens, PhD
Assistant Professor, Department of Pharmacology,
University of Michigan Medical School,
Ann Arbor, Michigan

Kenneth P. Minneman, PhD
Charles Howard Candler Professor of Pharmacology, Department of Pharmacology,
Emory University School of Medicine,
Atlanta, Georgia

B.F. Mitchell, MD, FRCSC
Professor, Department of Obstetrics and Gynecology,
University of Alberta;
Department of Obstetrics and Gynecology,
Royal Alexandra Hospital,
Edmonton, Canada

Dave Morgan, PhD
Professor, Department of Pharmacology and Therapeutics,
University of South Florida College of Medicine,
Tampa, Florida

Fern E. Murdoch, PhD
Scientist, Department of Pathology and Laboratory Medicine,
University of Wisconsin College of Medicine,
Madison, Wisconsin

Mark D. Okusa, MD
Associate Professor of Medicine and Attending Physician, Department of Internal Medicine,
University of Virginia School of Medicine,
Charlottesville, Virginia

John D. Palmer, PhD, MD
Professor Emeritus, Department of Pharmacology,
University of Arizona College of Medicine;
Attending Physician, Department of Internal Medicine,
Southern Arizona Veterans Administration Health Care System,
Tucson, Arizona

Christopher H. Parsons, MD
Fellow, Department of Medicine–Infectious Diseases,
University of Virginia School of Medicine,
Charlottesville, Virginia

Richard D. Pearson, MD
Professor, Departments of Medicine and Pathology,
University of Virginia School of Medicine,
Charlottesville, Virginia

Susan M. Ray, MD
Associate Professor, Department of Medicine,
Division of Infectious Diseases,
Emory University School of Medicine;
Associate Hospital Epidemiologist,
Grady Health System,
Atlanta, Georgia

Melvyn Rubenfire, MD
Professor of Internal Medicine, Department of Cardiovascular Medicine,
University of Michigan Medical School,
Ann Arbor, Michigan

Margaret A. Shupnik, PhD
Professor, Department of Internal Medicine,
Division of Endocrinology and Metabolism,
University of Virginia School of Medicine,
Charlottesville, Virginia

I. Glenn Sipes, PhD
Professor and Chair, Department of Pharmacology,
College of Medicine,
University of Arizona,
Tucson, Arizona

Helmy M. Siragy, MD, FACP, FAHA
Professor, Deparment of Medicine,
University of Virginia School of Medicine;
Attending Physician, Department of Medicine,
University of Virginia Hospital;
Charlottesville, Virginia

Andrew A. Somogyi, PhD
Professor, Department of Clinical and Experimental Pharmacology,
University of Adelaide;
Professor, Clinical Pharmacology Unit,
Royal Adelaide Hospital,
Adelaide, Australia

Stephen W. Spaulding, MD, CM
Professor, Department of Medicine, Physiology, and Biophysics,
University of Buffalo, State University of New York;
Associate Chief of Staff for Research and Development, Department of Medical Research,
VA Western New York Healthcare System,
Buffalo, New York

Gary E. Stein, PhD
Professor of Medicine and Pharmacology,
Director, Clinical Antiinfectives Research, Department of Medicine,
Michigan State University College of Human Medicine,
East Lansing, Michigan

James P. Steinberg, MD
Professor of Medicine, Department of Medicine,
Division of Infectious Diseases,
Emory University School of Medicine;
Associate Chief of Medicine and Hospital Epidemiologist,
Emory Crawford Long Hospital,
Atlanta, Georgia

Paula H. Stern, PhD
Professor and Vice-Chair, Department of Molecular Pharmacology and Biological Chemistry,
Northwestern University Feinberg School of Medicine,
Chicago, Illinois

Gary R. Strichartz, PhD
Professor of Anesthesia and Pharmacology, Department of Biological Chemistry and Molecular Pharmacology,
Harvard Medical School;
Director, Pain Research Center,
Department of Anesthesiology, Perioperative and Pain Medication,
Brigham and Women's Hospital,
Boston, Massachusetts

Janet L. Stringer, MD, PhD
Associate Professor, Department of Pharmacology and Neuroscience,
Baylor College of Medicine,
Houston, Texas

Yung-Fong Sung, MD, FACA
Professor, Department of Anesthesiology,
Emory University School of Medicine;
Medical Director and Chief, Anesthesiology,
Ambulatory Surgery Center,
The Emory Clinic,
Atlanta, Georgia

John R. Traynor, PhD
Associate Professor, Department of Pharmacology,
University of Michigan Medical School,
Ann Arbor, Michigan

R. Clinton Webb, PhD
Robert B. Greenblatt Professor and Chairperson, Department of Physiology,
Medical College of Georgia,
Augusta, Georgia

Lynn Wecker, PhD
Distinguished Research Professor and Chair, Department of Pharmacology and Therapeutics,
University of South Florida College of Medicine,
Tampa, Florida

David Westfall, PhD
Dean, College of Science;
Foundation Professor of Pharmacology,
University of Nevada School of Medicine,
Reno, Nevada

Stephen J. Winters, MD

Professor, Department of Medicine and Biochemistry/Molecular Biology,
Chief, Division of Endocrinology, Metabolism, and Diabetes,
University of Louisville Health Sciences Center,
Louisville, Kentucky

Brian Wispelwey, MS, MD

Professor, Department of Medicine,
University of Virginia School of Medicine,
Charlottesville, Virginia

Gordon M. Wotton, MD

Fellow, Department of Internal Medicine,
Division of Endocrinology and Metabolism,
University of Virginia School of Medicine,
Charlottesville, Virginia

Preface

This fourth edition of *Brody's Human Pharmacology: Molecular to Clinical* has been altered substantially to assist health professional students learn the most up-to-date and relevant pharmacological information. As the number and classes of drugs and sources of information in pharmacology continue to proliferate at an astonishing rate, it has become increasingly difficult for students to identify the concepts required for a basic understanding of pharmacology. An important goal of this book has been to assist the student by presenting the most relevant information in a clear and concise manner, excluding material more suitable for advanced training in particular subspecialities. The text focuses on prototypical drugs to illustrate basic mechanisms and uses boxes and tables to emphasize key points and relevant clinical information. Multicolored illustrations depict key concepts, mechanisms, and important structural formulas. This book is designed for teaching and learning and is not intended to be an all-inclusive reference work.

The information is provided in eight parts, each of which contains an overview of the topics covered within each section. As with previous editions, we have focused on the relationship between the mechanisms of action of drugs at the cellular/molecular level and their effects on the patient. Each chapter dealing with specific drug types has a consistent structure, as in the prior edition, with sections titled:

- Therapeutic Overview
- Mechanisms of Action
- Pharmacokinetics
- Relation of Mechanisms of Action to Clinical Response
- Side Effects, Clinical Problems and Toxicity
- New Horizons

Standard color-coded boxes include Major Drugs, Abbreviations, Therapeutic Overview, Clinical Problems, and Trade Names. In combination with over 300 color figures demonstrating critical concepts, this orderly structure should help students focus on learning the critical information associated with each class of drugs.

The fourth edition includes contributions from 26 new experts and new chapters on Herbals and Natural Products (Chapter 7) and Eating Disorders and Obesity (Chapter 26) because of their emerging importance in modern medicine. To help emphasize key concepts, the overall number of chapters has been reduced by consolidating several chapters in the prior edition and by eliminating material appropriate for more specialized texts. All chapters contain Self-Assessment Questions at the end of the chapter, and the answers are provided in the back of the book. We hope these questions help students evaluate their understanding of the material presented in each chapter and point to sections where further review might be helpful.

Chapters have been authored by experts in a particular area and edited for consistency of coverage and style. Content was selected to emphasize the immediate needs of medical and other health professional students within the framework of a traditional lecture-based course, an innovative organ systems approach, or a problem-based learning curriculum. To increase the consistency in the level of coverage for each chapter, but to avoid as much redundancy as possible, many of the chapters submitted were revised and extensively reformatted by the editors before production.

The multicolor figures that help explain key concepts will be available for download from the Elsevier web site for use in preparing electronic teaching materials. There will also be a Question Bank on the web site containing the questions printed in the chapters as well as others, along with the answers and short explanations of why they are correct. This should be helpful to both teachers and students evaluating their progress in understanding the material covered and in preparing examinations.

We hope that the content revisions, the focus on key concepts, the consistent organization, and the new figures make this new edition even more user-friendly and helpful to students and teachers alike.

KENNETH P. MINNEMAN
LYNN WECKER

Contents

PART IV

Drugs affecting the brain and behavior

PART V

Drugs affecting endocrine systems

PART VI

Antineoplastic drugs

PART VII

Drugs that kill invading organisms

PART VIII

Special topics

PART I

General principles

THIS SECTION EXPLAINS THE basic concepts that are critical for learning how drugs are used in prevention and treatment of disease. The principles discussed in this section are essential for understanding the use of all the different drug classes described in the remainder of the book. Chapter 1 provides key definitions of important terms in pharmacology and a basic knowledge of the most important concepts. Chapter 2 describes drug targets, called **receptors**, and how drugs interact with these targets to cause functional responses. The relationship between drug concentration and biological effect can often be inferred from these interactions and is discussed extensively. Chapter 3 explains the dynamics of the absorption of drugs, their distribution to various body sites, their metabolism into active and inactive compounds, and their routes of elimination. These issues are fundamental to an understanding of the biological effects of any drug. Clinical pharmacokinetics and dosing schedules and how they are impacted at the extremes of age are described in Chapter 4. These include temporal relationships between plasma concentrations of drugs and their pharmacological effects, including the concepts of half-life, steady-state, clearance, and bioavailability. Chapter 5 considers novel molecular therapeutic approaches that are emerging because of the revolution in biology and medicine that has occurred recently. These include gene therapy, other nucleic acid-based therapies, the use of specific antibodies, and strategies for targeted drug delivery. Chapter 6 describes how drugs are developed, regulated, and marketed, and provides a summary of the enormous hurdles involved in the development of novel, therapeutically useful compounds. The principles of prescription writing are also described. Finally, Chapter 7 discusses the increasingly widespread use of dietary and herbal supplements, what we know and do not know about these products, and their potential to impact conventional drug therapy and medical interventions.

CHAPTER 1

Introduction and definitions

Theodore M. Brody

Therapeutic importance of drugs

Both physicians and patients acknowledge the fundamental importance of drug treatment as one of the primary means used for prevention and alleviation of disease. Billions of prescriptions are written each year in the United States for more than 1600 active ingredients available in 40,000 different preparations or forms of delivery. In addition, over 100,000 over-the-counter preparations (OTCs) can be found on pharmacy and supermarket shelves. Although all prescription drugs are federally certified for safety and efficacy, OTC products can vary from those with a single, effective ingredient to others containing multiple compounds, many of questionable usefulness. Thousands of herbal supplements and food additives are also available, often without regulatory control.

The medical practitioner has the unenviable task of selecting the appropriate drug or drugs from this "therapeutic jungle." The degree of difficulty in drug selection varies from physician to physician, depending on the medical specialty and nature of the patient population. Generally, specialists concerned with a particular organ system (e.g., heart and circulation) use a limited number of drugs and have substantial experience with drug selection, dosing schedules, and side effects. Conversely, family physicians treating more diverse patient populations are continuously challenged by the enormous pool of drugs available. Physicians who treat the elderly, who suffer from multiple diseases and often take many different classes of drugs simultaneously, must be particularly aware of drug interactions. Both prescription and OTC medicines are now part of daily life, and the quality of life is often influenced by the choices made.

The drug revolution

Prior to World War II, drugs were usually partially purified ingredients of plant or animal origin. Although some advances in drug discovery occurred during those years, less than 5% of currently available drugs are found in pharmacology texts published in the 1940s. The salicylates, barbiturates, digitalis, quinine, nitrites, morphine, codeine, heparin, and insulin were mainstays of therapy. Ether was the principal anesthetic agent; organic mercurial compounds were used as diuretics, and reserpine was used to treat high blood pressure. Sulfa drugs served as the primary antimicrobial agents.

Several factors were responsible for the impressive rise in the number of medicines available after World War II:

1. Development and increased production of penicillin, which was discovered earlier but whose potential was not fully implemented until later, and which stimulated a subsequent intensive search for new antimicrobials.

2. The large number of former servicemen training in the biological and physical sciences and the subsequent growth in graduate and postdoctoral programs in pharmacology.
3. Expansion in both number and size of U.S. medical schools and increased funding of the National Institutes of Health.
4. European pharmaceutical companies, which had generally been the source of new drugs, established successful subsidiaries in the United States, which discovered many new compounds.
5. Studies on how cells communicate with each other opened up new approaches to drug discovery.

Federal regulations have also been critical for new drug development. Several tragedies fueled more extensive efforts by pharmaceutical firms to evaluate toxicity prior to drug marketing. One example was the use of diethylene glycol (a component of antifreeze) as a solvent for sulfanilamide, resulting in more than 100 deaths in the United States. More tragic was the widespread use of the drug thalidomide. Prescribed as a sedative hypnotic for pregnant women, thalidomide caused deaths and fetal abnormalities in thousands of infants before its teratogenicity was recognized. The U.S. Food and Drug Administration, which earlier mandated that manufacturers demonstrate drug safety, instituted new regulations requiring demonstration of drug effectiveness and more extensive animal and human safety testing prior to approval of new drugs (see Chapter 6).

Animal models of disease are still used in drug discovery, but many companies now rely heavily on new molecular technology to synthesize and screen thousands of compounds in short periods of time. In addition, rational drug design by molecular modeling has been facilitated by increased computing power and three-dimensional imaging. Molecules present in minute quantities in the body can now be produced in large amounts through gene cloning and expression. In fact, sequencing of the human genome has provided a bewildering number of potential targets for new medicines, making it difficult for pharmaceutical companies to know where to focus new efforts.

Table 1-1 Definitions

Term	Definition
Pharmacology	The study of drugs in its broadest sense, including interactions between drugs and body constituents at any level of organization.
Pharmacodynamics	What the drug does to the body; includes mechanisms of action of drugs at physiological, biochemical, and molecular levels.
Pharmacokinetics	What the body does to the drug; how drug concentrations in body fluids and tissues vary with time and intensity of response.
Pharmacogenetics	The relationship of genetic factors to variations in drug responsiveness.
Receptor	Specific macromolecule that is the target for drug binding; initial "site of action" of a drug.
Therapeutic index	Also called "margin of safety." Ratio between the dose of drug causing undesirable effects and the dose causing the desired therapeutic response.
Toxicology	Study of poisons, their effects, their antidotes, and drug overdoses.
Proprietary name	Brand or trade name of a drug that is the patented property of the drug manufacturer; drugs of identical composition may have many different proprietary names.
Generic name	Internationally recognized, nonproprietary name of a drug. There is only a single generic name for each drug.

Scope of pharmacology

Pharmacology is the study of drugs in its broadest sense. The explosion of knowledge in pharmacology is such that no future physician is likely to be able to know even a fraction of all available knowledge and will increasingly rely on new databases and search technologies. Several specific areas, however, will remain essential for rational prescribing of drugs.

Pharmacodynamics

Pharmacodynamics is what the drug does to the body, ideally including the molecular mechanism(s) by which a drug acts. Most drugs interact with proteins, such as receptors or enzymes, to control changes in physiological function of particular organs, thus altering pathology or abnormal physiology to benefit the patient.

Although physicians can observe the obvious functional effects of drug administration, the need to know its mechanism of action is less well recognized. With most drugs, observed effects provide little insight into the molecular events occurring following drug administration. Figure 1-1 shows the cascade of events that occur following administration of digitalis, a drug used to treat congestive heart failure.

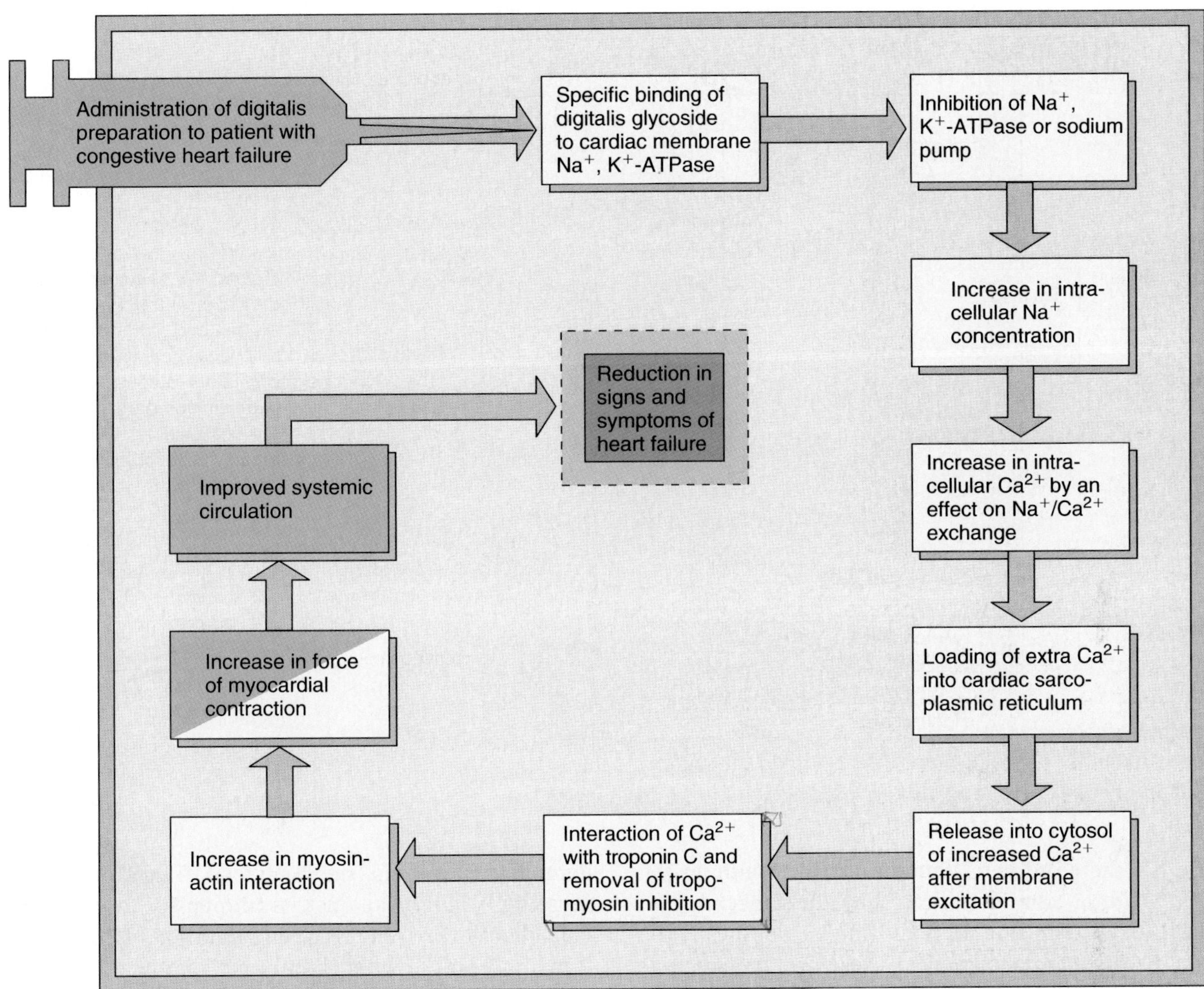

Figure 1-1 Putative mechanism of action of the cardiac glycosides.

Digitalis selectively binds to and inhibits the heart's sarcolemmal Na^+ pump. Normally, the primary action of the Na^+ pump is to exchange three intracellular Na^+ ions for two extracellular K^+ ions, both of which move against their concentration gradients. This results in one net positive charge (Na^+) moving from inside the cardiac cell to the outside, against an electrical potential, with the energy supplied by hydrolysis of ATP. The Na^+,K^+-ATPase, which hydrolyzes ATP in the presence of Na^+ and K^+, is known as the Na^+ pump. The rise in intracellular Na^+ concentration as a result of pump inhibition by digitalis reduces Ca^{++} efflux coupled to Na^+ influx, thereby increasing Ca^{++} loading of the sarcoplasmic reticulum of the cardiac cell and enhancing sarcoplasmic reticulum Ca^{++} release. This augments Ca^{++} transients, leading to an increase in force of contraction of the heart, enhancing perfusion, and reducing edema (see Fig. 1-1).

Moderate inhibition of the Na^+ pump results in the therapeutic effects of digitalis, whereas an excessive reduction produces cardiac arrhythmias resulting from Ca^{++} overload. Because the positive inotropic effect of digitalis and its arrhythmogenic action are both caused by pump inhibition and enhanced Ca^{++} loading, the therapeutic and toxic mechanisms cannot be easily separated but are merely dependent on drug concentration. The small **therapeutic index**, or margin of safety, of digitalis is an inherent property of this class of drugs.

Pharmacokinetics

Pharmacokinetics is what the body does to the drug. For almost all drugs, the magnitude of the pharmacological effect depends on its concentration at its site of action. Factors that influence rates of delivery, distribution, and disappearance of drug to and from its site of

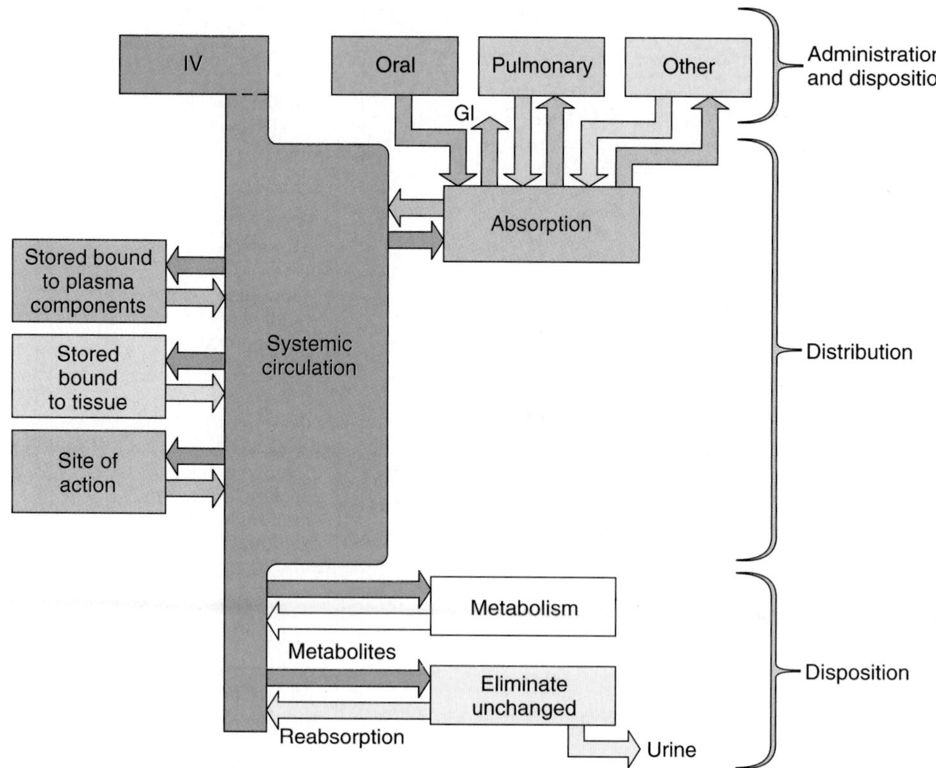

Figure 1-2 Factors influencing drug concentration at its site of action and at different times following administration. The circulatory system is the major pathway for drug delivery to its site of action. Possible entry routes and distribution and disposition sites are also shown.

action are therefore very important in determining the success of drug administration. How the concentration of drug varies with time in body fluids or tissues is the substance of pharmacokinetics. These factors, summarized in Figure 1-2, are discussed more extensively in Chapters 3 and 4.

Pharmacogenetics

Pharmacogenetics is the area of pharmacology concerned with unusual responses to drugs caused by genetic differences between individuals. Such responses are different from toxic or side effects of drugs that are generally similar in most people, or those that result from specific allergies. Pharmacogenetic differences are usually caused by an inherited defect resulting in variability in drug metabolism and may produce either a diminished or enhanced response. This topic is discussed more extensively in Chapters 3 and 4.

Toxicology

Toxicology is the study of poisons. Drugs, which are usually foreign substances, can become poisons and produce undesirable or toxic effects when taken in large enough doses. Thus, the beneficial effects of any drug must be balanced against its propensity to do harm—a consideration of the risk/benefit ratio. In some situations, use of a drug known to produce significant adverse effects may be justified, if there are few alternatives. However, such drugs should obviously not be used to treat trivial clinical problems.

In this book, the pharmacodynamic and pharmacokinetic effects of drugs are followed by descriptions of their side effects, clinical problems, and toxicity. **Signs** of toxicity are objective measurements usually made by the physician, including laboratory findings. **Symptoms** are subjective events described by the patient. Chapter 56 provides additional information on toxicology and treatment of poisons.

Factors in drug therapy

In addition to knowledge of the principles of pharmacology, many other factors are important in maximizing the beneficial effects of drugs. These include:

- Maintaining a positive, supportive relationship with the patient.

- Avoiding drug interactions by obtaining a careful drug history, including the patient's use of OTCs and herbal supplements.
- Monitoring changes in the patient's condition and changing the medicine or modifying its dosage, if necessary.
- In drug failure, ensuring patient compliance.
- Providing adequate information to the patient about the anticipated actions of the drug and its potential adverse effects.

Drug nomenclature

An important aspect of drug therapy that often confounds both prescriber and patient is drug nomenclature. Serious errors in patient management can occur, if this issue is not well understood.

A drug has three kinds of names:

1. The chemical name is often long and extremely complex. This name is of interest to chemists but of little concern to clinical pharmacologists or medical professionals.
2. The generic, or nonproprietary, name is one selected and recognized internationally and is used throughout this book. A drug has only one generic name. Generic names, for example, atorvastatin and pravastatin, often indicate that they are members of a class of drugs (statins) having the same mechanism of action, in this case treating hyperlipidemias and lowering cholesterol.
3. The proprietary name (brand, or trade name) is the patented exclusive property of the drug manufacturer. Trade names are often not helpful in identifying the pharmacological action or class of drug (for example, trade names for atorvastatin and pravastatin are Lipitor and Pravachol). However, trade names are often designed to be shorter and easier to remember than generic names. In some instances, there may be as many as a dozen or more trade names for a single drug, marketed by different companies. Trade names in this book are used for recognition purposes only. Generic preparations of drugs become available when proprietary patents expire, as discussed in Chapter 6. Generic and proprietary drugs are both subject to government regulation but are not always completely equivalent due to potential differences in bioavailability.

Using generic drug names is less likely to result in prescribing error and can give the pharmacist the option of substituting a cheaper generic version, if available. In addition, trade names can sometimes be similar, yet refer to drugs with entirely different pharmacodynamic actions, increasing the hazard of prescribing error. Generic drugs are generally less expensive than brand-name drugs, which may contribute to lower health care costs.

Potency and efficacy

Potency and **efficacy** are important terms that are frequently confused. Although often used interchangeably, they have very different meanings.

Potency refers to the amount of drug necessary to elicit a response. Thus, a drug that optimally lowers blood pressure at a 1-mg dose is said to be more potent than a drug with a similar action at a 10-mg dose. However, potency is not always the most critical factor in selection of a drug, if side effects produced by less potent drugs are tolerable.

Efficacy, or effectiveness, of a drug is its ability to produce the maximal desired response and is much more important in determining whether a drug will be clinically useful. For example, no dose of codeine can produce the same degree of pain relief as morphine, despite the fact that they act through the same mu opioid receptors. Morphine is therefore more efficacious. In choosing a drug, efficacy is much more important than potency because, if a drug does not produce a desired outcome, its potency is irrelevant. On the other hand, if drugs have similar efficacies, the most potent one is often the most desirable. These concepts are discussed further in Chapter 2.

Self-assessment questions

1. The term that describes what a drug does to the body and, particularly, its mechanism of action is called:
   a. Efficacy.
   b. Pharmacodynamics.
   c. Pharmacokinetics.
   d. Pharmacogenetics.
   e. None of the above.

2. The proprietary name of a drug:
   a. Is the exclusive property of the manufacturer.
   b. Indicates that the drug is unique in its pharmacology from any other proprietary drug.
   c. Is also called the trade name.
   d. Is characterized by both *a* and *c*.
   e. Is characterized by *a*, *b*, and *c*.

3. The term concerned with how the drug concentration in the body varies with time is called:

a. Pharmacodynamics.
b. Pharmacokinetics.
c. Laboratory findings.
d. Pharmacognosy.
e. Pharmacogenomics.

4. Difficulty in determining drug selection and dosing schedule for an individual patient may be attributable to:

a. Patient-to-patient variability in drug response.
b. Change in disease state of the patient.
c. Variability in drug disposition.
d. *a* and *c* only.
e. *a*, *b*, and *c*.

CHAPTER 2

Receptors and concentration-response relationships

Kenneth P. Minneman
James C. Garrison

Sites of drug action

For most drugs, the site of action is a specific macromolecule, generally termed a **receptor** or a **drug target,** which may be a membrane protein, a cytoplasmic or extracellular enzyme, or a nucleic acid. A drug may show organ or tissue selectivity because of selective tissue expression of the drug target. For example, the action of the proton pump inhibitor esomeprazole occurs specifically in the parietal cells that line the gastric pits of the stomach because that is where its target, the K^+/H^+ ATPase, is expressed. Although the actions of a few drug types, such as osmotic diuretics (see Chapter 13), may not involve receptors as they are usually defined, the concept of receptors as sites of drug action is critical to understanding pharmacology.

Receptors (i.e., drug targets) fall into many classes, but two types predominate:

- Molecules, such as enzymes and DNA, which are essential to a cell's normal biological function or replication, and
- Biological molecules that have evolved specifically for intercellular communication.

The former molecules could be considered **generalized** and the latter **specialized** receptors. Generalized receptors can include biological molecules with any function, including enzymes, lipids, or nucleic acids. The earlier example of the parietal cell K^+/H^+ ATPase is an example of this type of drug target. Specialized receptors include molecules like ion channels and proteins in the plasma membrane, designed to detect chemical signals and initiate a cellular response via activation of signal transduction pathways. The biological function of these molecules is to respond to neurotransmitters, hormones, cytokines, and autocoids and convey information to the cell, resulting in an altered cellular response. These types of receptors are the primary targets of the majority of drugs in clinical use.

The concept of receptors was first proposed more than a century ago by a German chemist, Paul Ehrlich, who was trying to develop specific drugs to treat parasitic infections. He proposed the idea of specific "side chains" on cells that would specifically interact with a drug, based on mutually complementary structures. Each cell would have particular characteristics that would allow it to recognize particular molecules. He proposed that a drug binds to a receptor much like a key fits into a lock. This **lock and key hypothesis** is still relevant to how we understand receptors today. It emphasizes the idea that the drug and receptor must be

Abbreviations

cAMP	cyclic adenosine monophosphate
GABA	γ-aminobutyric acid
GPCR	G-protein–coupled receptor
β-ARK	β-adrenergic receptor kinase

structurally complementary in order to recognize each other and initiate an effect.

The specificity of such interaction raises the concept of molecular recognition. Drug receptors or targets must have molecular domains that are spatially and energetically favorable for binding specific drug molecules. That most receptors are proteins is not surprising, because proteins undergo folding to form three-dimensional structures that could easily be envisioned to be complementary to the structures of drug molecules. Enzymes are also reasonably common drug targets, although they fall under the generalized receptor class discussed earlier.

The vast majority of drugs are small molecules with molecular weights below 500 to 800. These molecules interact with their protein targets via a number of different chemical bonds. A short summary of the principal types of chemical bonds is shown in Figure 2-1. These bond types apply to the interactions between drugs and classical receptors. Covalent bonds require considerable energy to break and are classified as irreversible when formed in drug-receptor interactions. Ionic bonds are also strong but may be reversed by a change in pH. Most drug- receptor interactions involve multiple weak bonds.

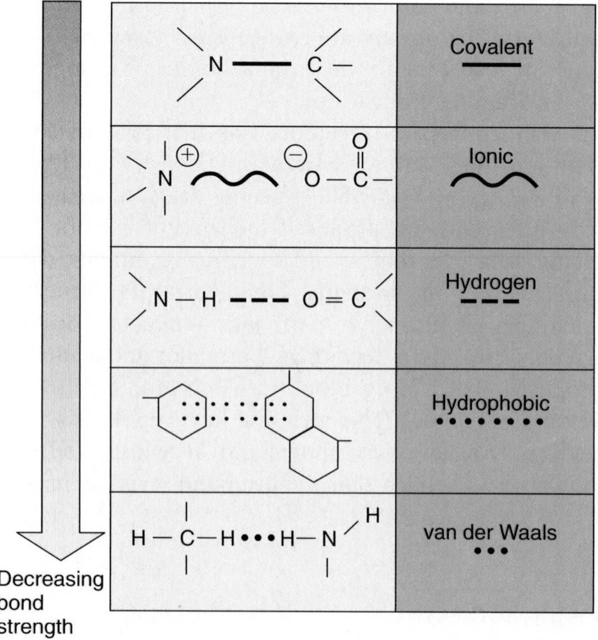

Figure 2-1 Types of chemical bonds and attractive forces between molecules that are pertinent to the interaction of drugs with their active sites.

Agonists and antagonists

Molecules that bind to receptors may have two major effects on the conformation of the receptor molecule. **Agonists** will bind to the receptor and activate it, like a key will fit into a lock and turn it. Activation of the receptor by agonist binding initiates a conformational change in the receptor and activation of one or more downstream signaling pathways. An example of the action of an agonist is provided by the effect of acetylcholine on the nicotinic acetylcholine receptor at the neuromuscular junction. When acetylcholine binds to its binding sites on the external surface of this receptor, the channel opens and allows Na^+ to flow down its electrochemical gradient and depolarize the muscle cell.

Antagonists are drugs that bind to the receptor but do not have the unique structural features necessary to activate it. In the lock and key analogy, antagonists can fit in the lock but cannot open it. Like agonists, antagonists fit into a specific binding site within their receptors but lack the right structural features to initiate the conformational change leading to receptor activation. However, since they occupy the binding site of the receptor, antagonists **inhibit activation** by agonists. An example of molecules that are antagonists is the class of neuromuscular blocking drugs used in the operating room to relax skeletal muscles during surgery. These drugs are analogs of **curare,** the active molecule in plant extracts used as arrow poisons by Native South Americans and studied by early European explorers. Curare is an antagonist at nicotinic cholinergic receptors at the neuromuscular junction and blocks the ability of acetylcholine or other agonists to activate this receptor. This blockade inhibits muscle depolarization and causes paralysis of skeletal muscle, including the diaphragm and intercostal muscles needed for respiration. A number of modern analogs of curare are available and used routinely during general anesthesia for relaxing muscle tone in patients undergoing surgery (see Chapter 29).

A third, but less common, class of drugs that interact with receptors are **allosteric modulators.** These compounds bind to a separate site on the receptor from that which normally binds agonist, called an **allosteric site.** Occupation of this site can either increase or decrease the response to the natural agonist, depending on whether it is a positive or negative modulator. Because they bind to different sites, interactions between agonists and allosteric modulators are not competitive.

Receptors

Receptors have now become the focus for investigation of the mechanisms by which drugs act. With the sequencing of the human genome, the structures and varieties of most receptors have now been identified. This advance has revealed many new receptors that could be potential drug targets for further pharmaceutical development. The major features of receptors are summarized schematically in Figure 2-2 and are also described in Box 2-1 and Table 2-1. There are three major concepts that are illuminated by the concept of drug receptors.

The first is the **quantitative relationship** between drug concentration and the subsequent physiological response. This is determined primarily by the **affinity** of the drug for the receptor, which is a measure of the binding constant of the drug for the receptor protein. A high affinity means that a low concentration of drug is needed to occupy the receptor sites, whereas a low affinity means that much higher concentrations of drug are needed. The concentration-response curve is also influenced by the **number of receptors** available for binding. When there are more receptors, there can be a greater response. However, this is not always the case, as will be discussed later in this chapter.

The second key concept is that receptors and their distribution in the tissues of the body are responsible for the **specificity** of drug action. The size, shape, and charge of a receptor determines its affinity for binding any of the vast array of chemically different hormones, neurotransmitters, or drug molecules it may encounter. If the structure of the drug changes even slightly, the type of receptor the drug binds to will also often change. Drug binding to receptors often exhibits **stereoselectivity**, where stereoisomers of a drug that are chemically identical, but have different orientations around a single bond, can have very different affinities. For example,

Box 2-1 Features of receptors

Protein: Lipoprotein, glycoprotein with one or more subunits.
Molecular weights of 45-200 kilodaltons.
Different tissue distributions.
Drug binding is usually reversible and stereoselective.
Specificity of binding not absolute, leading to nonspecific effects.
Receptors are saturable because of their finite number.
Agonist activation results in signal transduction.
May require more than one drug molecule to activate receptor.
Magnitude of signal depends on degree of binding.
Signal can be amplified by intracellular mechanisms.
Drugs can enhance, diminish, or block signal generation or transmission.
Can be upregulated or downregulated.

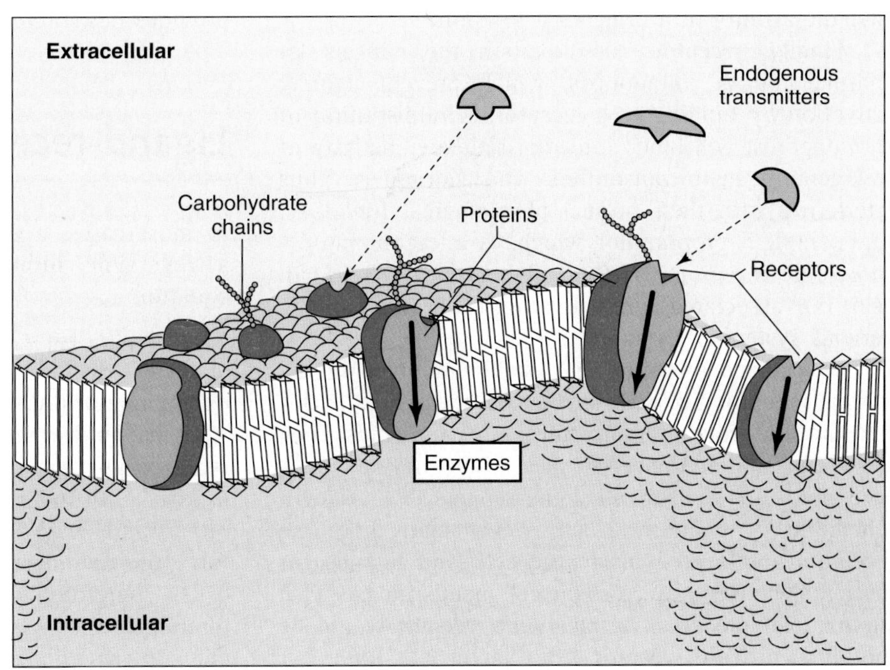

Figure 2-2 Proteins embedded in cell membranes generally extend further on both the extracellular and intracellular sides. Attached to the proteins on the extracellular side are carbohydrate (glycosylation) chains. Also shown on the extracellular side of some of the proteins are receptor sites to which endogenous transmitter compounds bind. Arrows indicate the direction of communication to the other side of the membrane.

Table 2-1 Examples of specialized receptors

Type	Subtype	Endogenous Ligand
LIGAND-GATED CHANNELS		
Acetylcholine	Nicotinic	Acetylcholine
GABA	A	GABA
Glutamate	NMDA, kainate, AMPA	Glutamate or aspartate
G-PROTEIN–COUPLED RECEPTORS		
ACTH	—	ACTH
Acetylcholine	Muscarinic	Acetylcholine
Adrenergic	α_1, α_2, β	Epinephrine and norepinephrine
GABA	B	GABA
Glucagon	—	Glucagon
Glutamate	Metabotropic	Glutamate
Opioid	μ, κ, δ	Enkephalins
Serotonin	5-$HT_{1\text{-}7}$	5-HT
Dopamine	$D_{1\text{-}5}$	Dopamine
Adenosine	A_1, A_{2a}, A_{2b}, A_3	Adenosine
Histamine	H_1, H_2, H_3, H_4	Histamine
TYROSINE KINASE RECEPTORS		
Insulin	—	Insulin
NGF	—	NGF
EGF	—	EGF
NUCLEAR HORMONE RECEPTORS		
Estrogen	α, β	Estrogen
Glucocorticoid	Type 1	Glucocorticoid, mineralocorticoid
	Type 2	Glucocorticoid
Androgens	—	Testosterone

GABA, γ-Aminobutyric acid; *ACTH*, adrenocorticotrophic hormone; *NGF*, nerve growth factor; *EGF*, epidermal growth factor.

the L-isomer of narcotic analgesics is about 1000 times more potent than the D-isomer, which is essentially inactive (see Chapter 31). The presence or absence of a single hydroxyl group, methyl group, and other apparently minor structural changes can also dramatically alter the affinity of a drug for a receptor.

Finally, receptors also explain the concept of pharmacological antagonists, which prevent agonist activation by binding to a receptor. Administration of an antagonist will block tonic or stimulated activity of endogenous neurotransmitters and hormones, thus interfering with their normal physiological functions. An example is propranolol, which, by antagonizing β_1-adrenergic receptors, prevents the normal increase in heart rate associated with activation of the sympathetic nervous system (see Chapter 10).

Specialized receptors are usually involved in the normal regulation of cell function by hormones, neurotransmitters, growth factors, steroids, or autocoids. They are often found on the cell surface, where they are easily accessible to hydrophilic messengers, as shown schematically in Figure 2-3. However, many hormone receptors are located inside the cell, and ligands for these molecules easily cross the cell membrane (see Part V). An example of an intracellular receptor would be the glucocorticoid receptor (see Chapter 33). Table 2-1 contains a selected list of receptors that are important in the actions of several therapeutically useful drugs. For most receptor types, it is now clear that there are multiple distinct subtypes that can cause similar or distinct responses. This diversity of receptors and responses provides new targets for drug development.

Ligand-receptor interactions

In most cases, a drug (D) binds to a receptor (R) in a **reversible bimolecular reaction** as described in equation 1:

$$D + R \rightleftharpoons DR \rightleftharpoons DR^* \rightarrow\rightarrow\rightarrow\rightarrow\rightarrow \text{Response} \quad (1)$$

Occupancy of the receptor by the drug may or may not alter its conformation. Antagonists can bind to the receptor and occupy its binding site and, therefore, participate only in the first equilibrium. Agonists, on the other hand, have the appropriate structural features to force the bound receptor into an active conformation (DR*). Therefore, agonists participate in both equilibria, binding to the receptor and initiating a conformational change. This conformational change leads to a series of

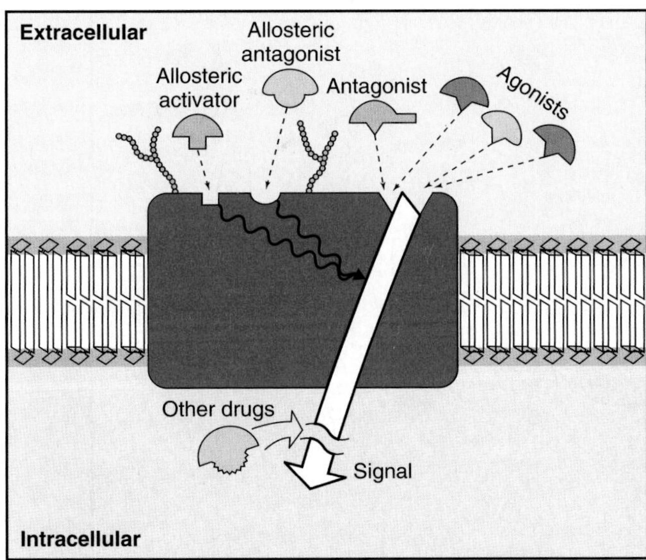

Figure 2-3 Major features of receptors. These include embedding in a membrane, glycosylated chains on the extracellular side, binding sites on the extracellular side for an endogenous transmitter (dark blue symbols) with two molecules sometimes needing to be bound (as shown here) to activate the transmembrane receptor. Drugs can use many sites on the receptor: (1) The agonist and antagonist compete with the endogenous transmitter for binding sites; (2) allosteric agonists or antagonists enhance or block the signal, respectively, by binding to allosteric sites that influence (wavy line) signal transmission; and (3) other drugs can block signal transmission within the membrane or at intracellular signal reception points.

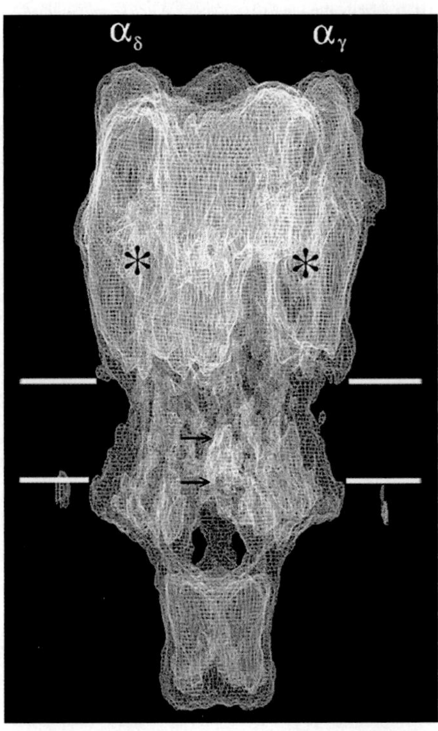

Figure 2-4 Crystal structure of the nicotinic acetylcholine receptor. Binding sites for acetylcholine are shown as asterisks, with the gating portions shown with arrows. (From Unwin N. *Philos Trans R Soc Lond B Biol Sci* 2000; 355:1813-1829.)

events causing a cellular response. It is important to remember that the DR complex is usually reversible for both agonists and antagonists.

Receptor superfamilies

There are four major superfamilies of receptors that are involved in signal transduction, which are the targets of clinically useful drugs. These include ligand-gated ion channels, G-protein–coupled receptors, receptor tyrosine kinases, and nuclear hormone receptors.

Ligand-gated ion channels are most important in the brain, peripheral nervous system, excitable tissues, such as the heart, and the neuromuscular junction. They include nicotinic cholinergic receptors (Fig. 2-4) at the neuromuscular junction and many of the GABA and glutamate receptors in the brain. These receptors are responsible for fast synaptic transmission, where release of a transmitter causes an electrical effect on the post-synaptic neuron by opening a specific ion channel and leading to a change in membrane potential. Ligand-gated channels are complex proteins composed of multiple subunits; for example, nicotinic cholinergic receptors have five subunits. Nicotinic receptors expressed in different sites in the body have different combinations of these subunits. For example, the nicotinic receptor in the neuromuscular junction has five different subunits (2α, β, δ, and γ), and the receptor in the autonomic ganglia contains only three different subunits (2α and 3β). Although the responses to acetylcholine and ion gating properties of these two channels are nearly identical, they can be antagonized by different drugs. This property allows selective blockade of the neuromuscular channel with drugs that have no effects on the channel in autonomic ganglia (see Chapter 29). Channels often have multiple binding sites for neurotransmitters, and nicotinic cholinergic receptors have two binding sites for acetylcholine: one on each α subunit in the channel. Channels may also have binding sites for allosteric modulators, which bind to separate sites on the protein from the transmitter and increase or decrease the ability of the transmitter to open the channel. The most important class of allosteric modulators is represented by the benzodiazepines, which are used extensively for treatment of anxiety and sleep disorders (see Chapter 24). These drugs all interact with

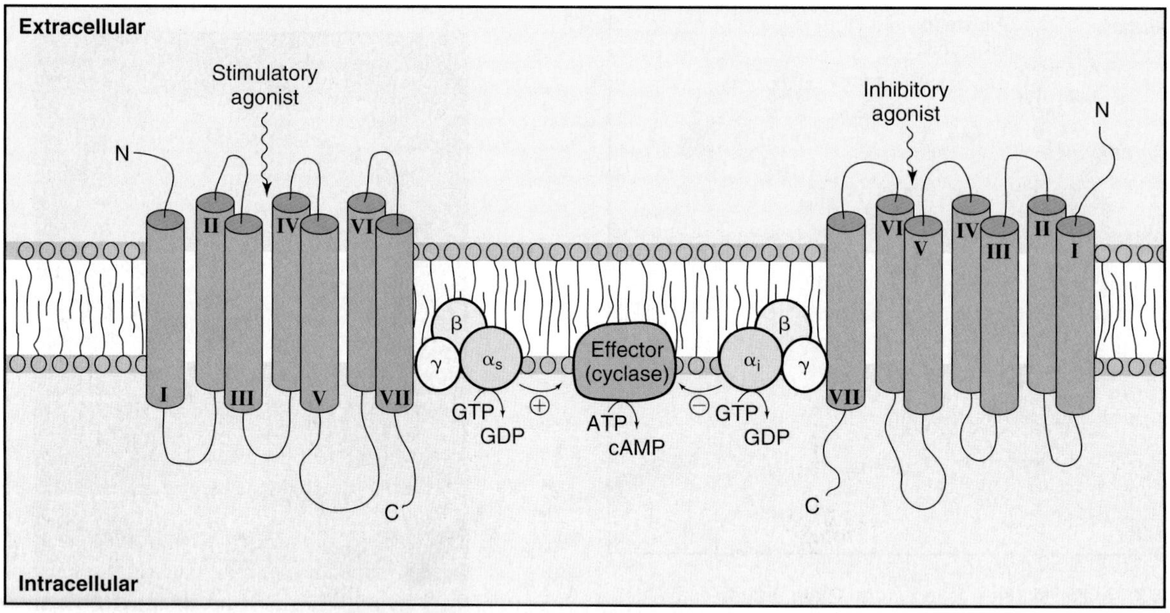

Figure 2-5 Structure of G-protein–coupled receptors and signaling molecules involved in regulation of adenylate cyclase. Binding of the ligand to the stimulatory receptor, *(left)* produces a conformation change that is transmitted to the α subunit of G_s. This activates G_s by exchanging bound GDP with GTP to give active α_s. G_s dissociates, with active α_s activating the adenylyl cyclase. The $\beta\gamma$ subunits are released and freed for other signaling functions. Activation of an inhibitory receptor, *(right)* causes GDP–GTP exchange on the α_i subunit, which can inhibit the adenylyl cyclase.

receptors for the inhibitory neurotransmitter GABA. Benzodiazepines bind selectively to $GABA_A$ receptors, which are ligand-gated chloride channels. Binding of the benzodiazepine has no effect on channel opening but dramatically increases the ability of GABA to open the channel.

G-protein–coupled receptors (GPCRs) are probably the most important class of receptors in pharmacology because a majority of currently marketed drugs target this receptor superfamily. GPCRs are much simpler than ligand-gated ion channels, being usually composed of a single subunit that contains seven transmembrane spanning domains. They are thought to have a single binding site, and as yet there are only a few allosteric modulators for this class of receptors. GPCRs activate signals not by binding to and opening channels, but by a conformational change that activates a large family of G-proteins to regulate signaling pathways (Fig. 2-5). These events regulate a host of important cellular functions (Box 2-2). GPCRs are the largest protein family in the human genome, accounting for around 2% of all human genes. About half of these are olfactory receptors for detecting odorants; most of the remaining GPCRs respond to neurotransmitters, hormones, autocoids, and cytokines. These latter receptors are targets for a large group of therapeutically important drugs.

Receptor tyrosine kinases contain an extracellular ligand binding domain, one transmembrane spanning segment, and an intracellular tyrosine kinase domain. Binding of a ligand to the extracellular domain causes dimerization of the receptor and stimulates a tyrosine kinase activity within the intracellular domain. The best examples of these receptors are the growth factor receptors, such as epidermal growth factor or nerve growth factor receptors (Fig. 2-6). When growth factors bind to these receptors, they cause tyrosine phosphorylation of the receptor and/or other proteins, which leads to activation of a large number of cellular pathways. **Cytokine receptors** are part of this subfamily because they are structurally very similar. However, instead of intrinsic enzymatic activity within the receptor molecule, they have docking sites where tyrosine kinase enzymes bind (Fig. 2-7). These receptors are activated by a variety of molecules, such as erythropoietin, interleukins, and growth hormone. Tyrosine kinase receptors are an increasingly important target for drugs to treat neoplastic diseases, where cell growth is uncontrolled (see Chapter 42).

Nuclear hormone receptors are found in the cytosol, and, unlike the other receptor superfamilies that are activated on the cell surface, these receptors bind their ligand in the cytoplasm and translocate to the nucleus. Intracellular receptors respond to highly

Box 2-2 G-protein–coupled receptor signaling

Agonist binding to G-protein–coupled receptors activates heterotrimeric G-proteins to activate effector molecules, such as enzymes and channels. These G-proteins are located at the inner surface of the plasma membrane and consist of α, β, and γ subunits. The α subunit is a key component because:

- It interacts specifically with receptors.
- Upon activation, it exchanges bound GDP for GTP, undergoes a conformational change releasing the βγ subunits, and interacts with effectors.
- It has an intrinsic ability to hydrolyze bound GTP, which is activated by regulatory proteins that aid in turning off the signal.
- αGDP binds to and sequesters the βγ subunit. βγ subunits exist as dimers and can also activate certain effectors. Activated αGTP interacts directly with effectors, such as adenylyl cyclase (see Fig. 2-5) to regulate their activity and raise the concentration of a second messenger (see later).

Genes for 17 different G α subunits have been identified, which can be grouped into four families. Although there is great structural homology between α subunits, each protein has unique regions that impart specificity to its interactions with receptors and effectors. The C-terminal region displays the most variability and interacts with receptors. Generally, members within a family have similar functional properties. The four families are:

- G_s, which activates adenylyl cyclase.
- G_i, which inhibits adenylate cyclase. This family also includes G_o, which regulates ion channels, and G_t, which couples rhodopsin to a phosphodiesterase in the visual system.
- G_q, which activates phospholipase C-β.
- $G_{12/13}$, which activates small G proteins, such as *Rho*.

The β and γ subunits of G-proteins form a tightly associated functional unit and are also characterized by multiple genes. There are 7 β and 12 γ subunits known. When βγ is released from the α subunit by GTP binding, βγ subunits also regulate effectors, such as ion channels, and enzymes, such as adenylyl cyclase or phospholipase C-β. βγ also activates muscarinic K^+ channels in cardiac and neural cells and is an important inhibitor of L and N type Ca^{2+} channels in neurons.

Activation of many G-proteins raises the level of "second messengers" in target cells. A second messenger is a small molecule, such as cyclic AMP, Ca^{2+} or K^+ ions, inositol trisphosphate, or diacylglycerol. These often activate protein kinases that produce responses by phosphorylating other regulatory proteins. Cyclic AMP activates a cyclic AMP-dependent protein kinase; inositol trisphosphate (by releasing Ca^{2+}) activates many Ca^{2+} and calmodulin-dependent protein kinases, and diacylglycerol activates protein kinase C. This phosphorylation leads to either activation or inactivation of downstream pathways, and produces the characteristic response of the cells to receptor activation.

hydrophobic compounds that easily cross cell membranes, including various classes of **steroids**, but there are also nuclear receptors for compounds, such as retinoic acid. These receptors are usually ligand-activated transcription factors that, when bound by ligand, dimerize, enter the nucleus, and bind directly to specific DNA recognition sequences and increase or decrease transcription of particular genes (Fig. 2-8).

Currently, the two most important receptor superfamilies in mammals are the ligand-gated ion channels and the GPCRs. They are the most numerous, they are on the cell surface where they are most easily accessible to synthetic drugs, and they are important in regulating pathways involved in disease. Many currently available drugs act through one of these two families. Major exceptions are the nuclear hormone receptors, which are the targets for a number of drugs acting on metabolic pathways, and the endocrine system (see Part V).

Other targets

In contrast to the four classes of specialized receptors that have been honed by evolution to provide the selectivity and specificity required for intercellular communication, there are also intracellular enzymes that provide drug targets with excellent specificity. Two notable examples include esomeprazole, which inhibits the parietal cell H^+/K^+ ATPase and is very useful for treatment of gastric hyperacidity (see Chapter 55), and imatinib mesylate, which inhibits the abl tryrosine kinase and is useful in the treatment of leukemias (see Chapter 42). Neither the H^+/K^+ ATPase nor the abl tyrosine kinase are specialized receptors for transmembrane signaling, but both are central to control of a primary function in the cells in which they are expressed. Thus, both of these drugs act with excellent specificity.

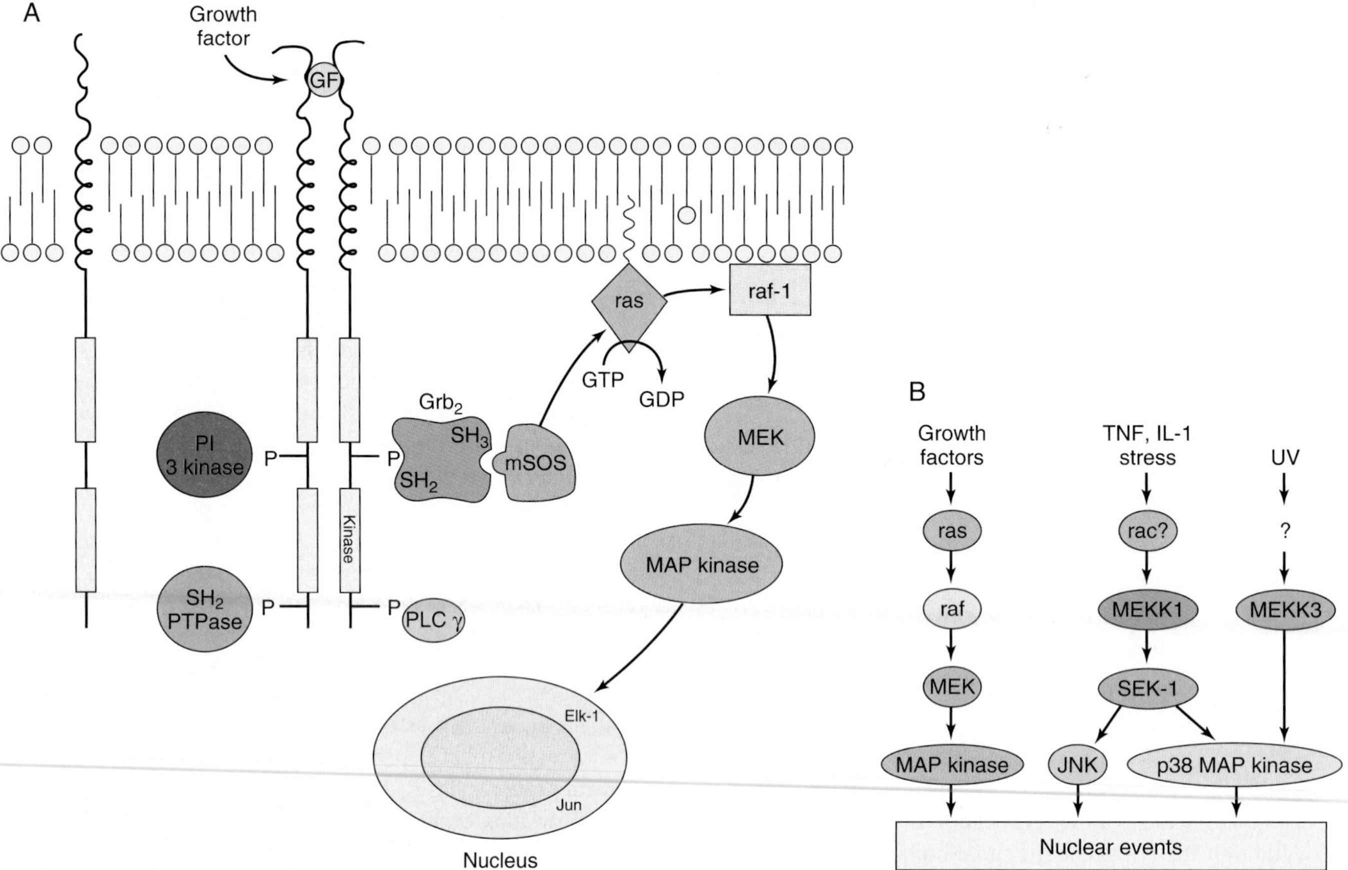

Figure 2-6 Pathways used by growth factors, stressors, and ultraviolet radiation to regulate cell function. **A,** Example of the mechanism used by growth factors *(GF)* to activate mitogen-activated protein kinases *(MAP kinase).* Binding of the GF induces dimerization of the receptor, thereby activating its kinase, which leads to phosphorylation of the receptor *(–P)* on tyrosine residues. This creates binding sites for SH_2 domains of multiple signaling proteins (*PI 3 kinase, Grb_2, PLC γ,* and an SH_2-containing tyrosine phosphatase *[SH_2 PTPase]* are shown). The interaction between Grb_2 and the mSos protein activates ras, leading to activation of the MAP kinase cascade. **B,** The similarity of the protein kinase cascades used by growth factors, stressors, and ultraviolet radiation, leading to the activation of MAP kinase and two related kinases, the Jun N-terminal kinase *(JNK)* and p38 MAP kinase; *rac,* a low molecular weight G-protein in the ras superfamily; *MEKK1* and *MEKK3,* two MEK kinases analogous in function to raf-1 but with differing substrate specificities; *SEK-1,* a kinase analogous to MEK that phosphorylates and activates JNK.

Receptor classification

For each type of hormone, neurotransmitter, growth factor, or autocoid there is at least one specific receptor. Although it was first thought that there was a single receptor for each messenger, it is now clear that in most cases there is a **family** of receptors with multiple subtypes. Some of these families are quite large. For example, there are 14 known receptors responding specifically to serotonin, 9 responding to epinephrine and norepinephrine, about 15 for acetylcholine, and 25 to 30 for glutamate. Although the evolutionary pressure leading to the continued existence of so many receptors is not understood, it is clear that there can be complexity, redundancy, and/or multiplicity in the effects of a single agonist. Therefore, understanding the tissue distribution and biology of these different receptor isoforms is an important goal that will allow developing specific drugs for each novel target. This strategy will provide opportunities for obtaining specific therapeutic responses without unwanted side effects.

Receptors are commonly named after the natural agonist that activates them. For example, acetylcholine acts through cholinergic receptors, epinephrine (adrenaline) and norepinephrine (noradrenaline) act through adrenergic receptors, and serotonin acts through serotonergic receptors. Receptor activation is very specific, and there is little cross-reactivity between natural compounds and other receptors. For instance, acetylcholine

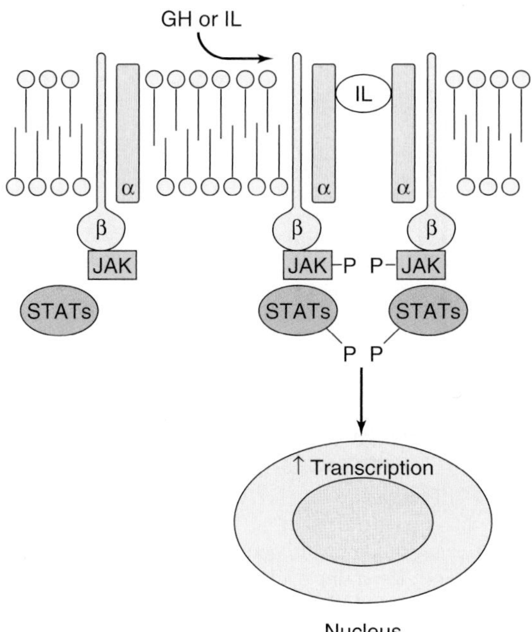

Figure 2-7 The pathways used by growth hormone, interferons, and cytokines to regulate nuclear events. The two isoforms of the receptor, α and β are shown, with the Janus kinase *(JAK)* bound to the β form. The cytoplasmic signal transducers and activators of transcription *(STAT)* proteins are shown as ovals. Activation of the receptor by growth hormone *(GH)* or cytokines, such as interleukins *(IL)*, leads to dimerization and phosphorylation of the JAK and STAT proteins on tyrosine residues. The STAT proteins translocate to the nucleus and activate transcription of certain genes.

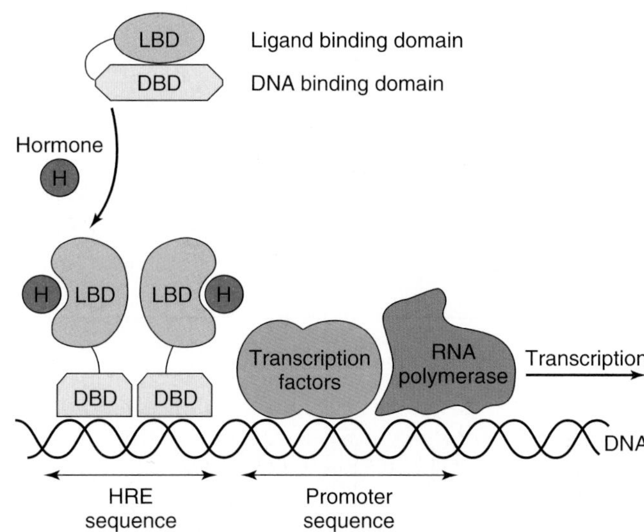

Figure 2-8 Members of the steroid receptor family bind to DNA at the hormone response element *(HRE)* and facilitate (or inhibit) formation of active transcription complexes at the promoter. Binding of the hormone *(H)* to the ligand-binding domain *(LBD)* causes translocation of the protein to the nucleus, dimerization, and the formation of a complex of proteins with the DNA-binding domain *(DBD)* binding to the HRE and activating the promoter.

binds only to cholinergic receptors and does not bind to adrenergic receptors or members of other receptor families. This is true for essentially all transmitters and hormones. However, a transmitter like dopamine (the immediate precursor of norepinephrine) has its own family of dopaminergic receptors, yet is less specific than acetylcholine. Because of its structural similarity to norepinephrine, dopamine does bind with low affinity to adrenergic receptors and is used clinically to stimulate β_1-adrenergic receptor in cardiac failure (see Chapter 10).

As mentioned previously, each receptor family usually contains multiple subtypes. These are usually characterized pharmacologically by the use of **selective agonists** and/or **antagonists.** For example, there are two major subfamilies of cholinergic receptors, nicotinic and muscarinic. Nicotinic cholinergic receptors are selectively activated by the agonist nicotine and are selectively blocked by drugs like curare. Muscarinic cholinergic receptors are selectively activated by the agonist muscarine and are selectively blocked by the antagonist atropine (see Chapter 9). Nicotine and curare have essentially no effect on muscarinic cholinergic receptors, and muscarine and atropine have essentially no effect on nicotinic cholinergic receptors. Both the nicotinic and muscarinic cholinergic receptor subfamilies consist of multiple subtypes, which are discussed further in Chapters 8, 9, and 29. Similarly, complex populations of receptors exist for most other neurotransmitters and will be discussed in the appropriate chapters.

The situation is complicated because multiple receptor subtypes for one transmitter can coexist on a single cell, raising the possibility that one transmitter can deliver multiple messages to the same cell. These messages may be opposing, complementary, or independent. For example, various combinations of adrenergic receptors can be present on the same cell. The β_1-adrenergic subtype activates adenylate cyclase through a G-protein (G_s). Because the α_2-adrenergic subtype inhibits adenylate cyclase through a different G-protein (G_i), mutually antagonistic signals will be generated by the presence of both subtypes in response to the same neurotransmitter, norepinephrine. In a like manner, additive signals can be generated by the presence of the β_2-adrenergic subtype, which also activates adenylate cyclase through G_s, or independent signals can be generated by the presence of the α_1-adrenergic subtype, which activates phospholipase C (Fig. 2-9). Overall, the response of a cell to a single transmitter (or a drug that mimics a neurotransmitter) depends on the types and relative proportions of receptor subtypes present in the membrane of the cell.

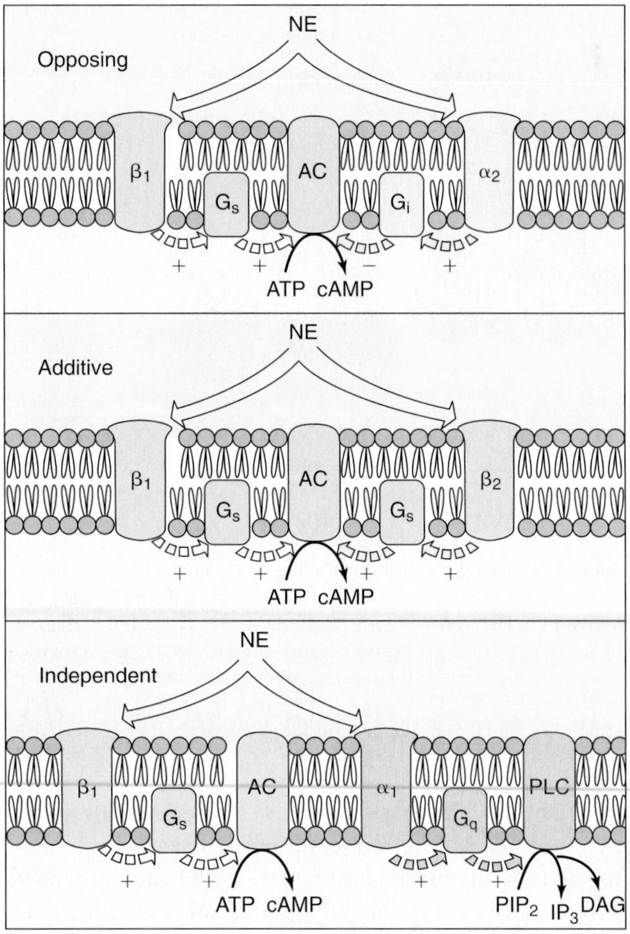

Figure 2-9 Activation of multiple receptors by a single transmitter: effects on signal transduction. Coactivation of more than one receptor subtype for norepinephrine can result in second-messenger responses, which are opposing, additive, or independent. G-proteins shown for stimulatory *(G_s)*, inhibitory *(G_i)*, and phospholipase *(G_q)*. *NE,* Norepinephrine; *AC,* adenylate cyclase; *ATP,* adenosine triphosphate; *cAMP,* cyclic adenosine monophosphate; *PLC,* phospholipase C; *PIP_2,* phosphatidylinositol 4,5-bisphosphate; *IP_3,* inositol 1,4,5-trisphosphate; *DAG,* 1,2-diacylglycerol.

Concentration-response relationships

Binding of a drug to a receptor is a reversible bimolecular interaction, as described earlier in equation 1. This equation follows the **law of mass action,** which states that at equilibrium the product of the active masses on one side of the equation divided by the product of active masses on the other side of the equation is a constant. Therefore, concentrations of both drug and receptor are important in determining the extent of receptor occupation and subsequent tissue response.

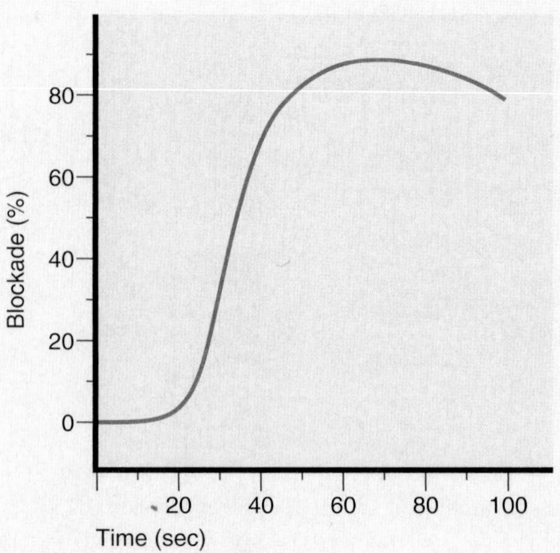

Figure 2-10 Magnitude of the neuromuscular blockade produced by succinylcholine after a single intravenous injection and monitored by recording the force of thumb jerk on repeated electrical stimulation of the ulnar nerve.

Quantification of the amount of drug necessary to produce a given response is referred to as a **concentration–response** relationship. Practically, one rarely knows the concentration of drug at the active site, so it is usually necessary to work with dose-response relationships. The dose of a drug is simply the amount administered (e.g., 10 mg), whereas the concentration is the amount per unit volume (e.g., mg/ml, etc.). To achieve similar concentrations in patients, it is often necessary to adjust the dose based on patient size, weight, and other factors (see Chapter 4).

Concentrations of drugs are influenced by how rapidly they are absorbed and how they are distributed, which will be discussed in Chapter 3. Dose-response curves are usually assumed to be at **equilibrium,** or steady-state, when the rate of drug influx equals the rate of drug efflux, although this is an ideal that is not often achieved in practice.

Once the drug reaches its receptors, many responses are **graded;** that is, they vary from minimum to maximum response. Figure 2-10 illustrates the actions of the neuromuscular blocking agent succinylcholine. Succinylcholine acts by binding to nicotinic acetylcholine receptors on skeletal muscle and depolarizing the membrane to prevent further depolarization by acetylcholine, as described further in Chapter 29. The response is defined as the percent blockade of neuromuscular transmission, determined from the force of contraction of the thumb muscle following repeated electrical stimulation of the ulnar nerve. The magnitude of the response increases continuously with increasing drug concentrations, caused by progressive increases in receptor occupancy and blockade. Most concentration- and dose-response curves are plotted on log scales rather than linear scales to make it easier to compare drug potencies (Fig. 2-11). When examining two drugs with large differences in affinity, using a log scale makes it easier to compare their concentration response curves (Fig. 2-11). The log scale will give an S-shaped curve, as shown.

Quantal responses are all-or-none responses to a drug. For example, following administration of a hypnotic drug, a patient is either asleep or not. Construction of dose-response curves for quantal responses requires the use of populations of subjects who are characterized by interindividual variability. A few subjects demonstrate an initial response at a low dose, most subjects demonstrate an initial response at an intermediate dose, and a few subjects demonstrate an initial response at a high dose (Fig. 2-12, *A*), resulting in a bell-shaped "Gaussian" distribution of sensitivity. Quantal dose-response curves are often plotted in a cumulative manner, comparing the dose of drug on the x-axis with the cumulative percentage of subjects responding to that dose on the y-axis (Fig. 2-12, *B*).

Occupation of a receptor by a drug is derived from the mass action law (equation 1) and is

$$\frac{[DR]}{[R_T]} = \frac{[D]}{[D] + K_D} \quad (2)$$

where R_T represents the total number of receptors and K_D is the equilibrium dissociation constant (or affinity constant) of the drug for the receptor. Therefore, the proportion of drug bound, relative to the maximum proportion that could be bound, is equal to the concentration of drug divided by the concentration of drug plus its affinity constant. It is important to note that $[DR]/[R_T]$ describes the proportion of receptors bound, or **fractional occupancy.** It ranges from zero when no drug is bound, to one when all receptors are occupied by drug. This equation can be used to calculate what *proportion* (not actual number) of receptors will be occupied at a particular concentration of drug. This equation demonstrates that fractional occupancy depends only on the concentration of drug and its affinity constant but not total receptor number.

The K_D value is a **fixed parameter** describing the affinity of a drug for the receptor binding site. From equation 2, it is clear that K_D represents the concentration of drug at which half of the receptors are occupied, because when K_D equals [D], half of the receptors are occupied. Therefore, drugs with a high K_D (low affinity) will require a high concentration for occupancy, whereas drugs with a low K_D (high affinity) require lower concentrations. K_D is also equal to the ratio of the rate of dissociation of the [DR] complex to its rate of formation. Thus, the K_D of a drug is a reflection of structural affinity of the drug and its receptor, that is, how quickly the drug binds to the receptor and how long it stays bound. Every drug/receptor combination will be characterized by a characteristic K_D, although they can differ by many orders of magnitude. For example, glutamate has approximately millimolar affinity for its

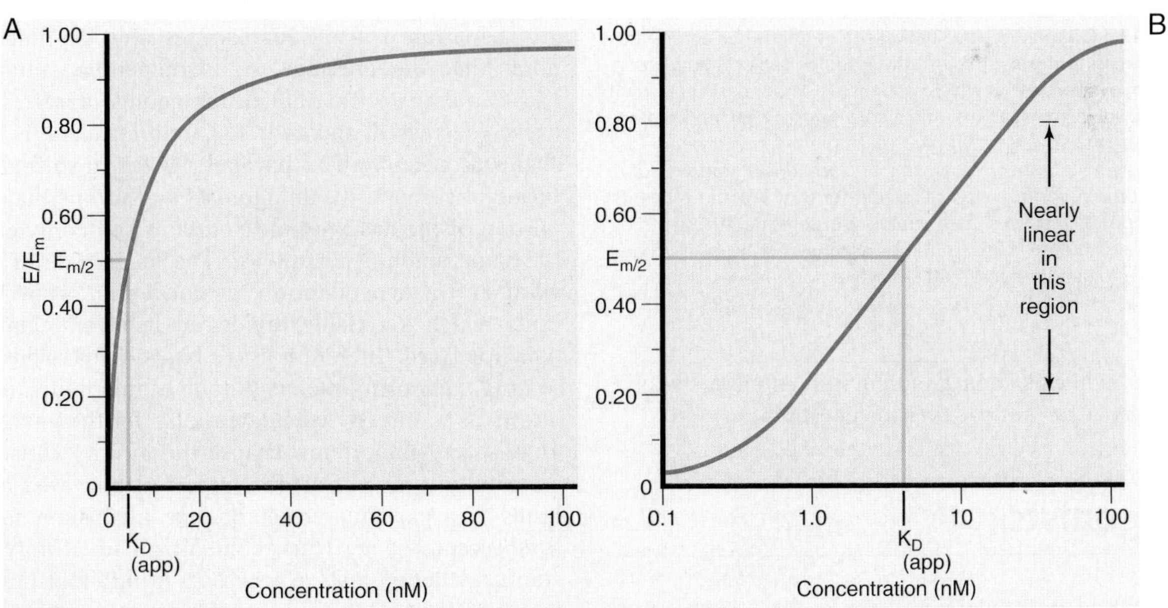

Figure 2-11 Concentration-response curve for receptor occupancy. **A,** Arithmetic scale. **B,** Logarithmic concentration scale. K_D (app) is the concentration of drug occupying half of the available receptor pool.

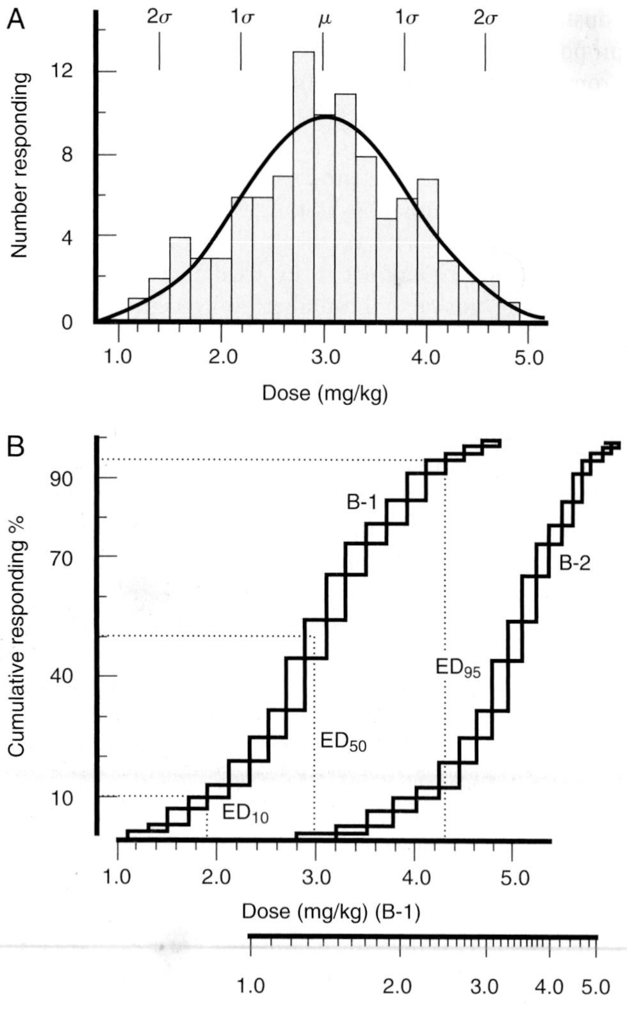

Figure 2-12 Quantal effects. Typical set of data after administration of increasing doses of drug to a group of subjects and observation of minimum dose at which each subject responds. Data shown are for 100 subjects. Mean (μ) (and median) dose is 3.0 mg/kg; standard deviation (σ) is 0.8 mg/kg. **A,** Results plotted as histogram (*bar graph*) showing number responding at each dose; smooth curve is normal distribution function calculated for μ of 3.0 and σ of 0.8. **B,** Data from **A** replotted as a cumulative percentage responding versus dose with dose shown in B-1 on arithmetic scale (as in **A**) and in B-2 on a logarithmic scale. ED (effective dose) values are shown for doses at which 10%, 50%, or 95% of subjects respond.

receptors, whereas some β-adrenergic antagonists have nanomolar affinities for their receptors.

Antagonists

There are two major classes of antagonists. Most antagonists are **competitive** antagonists. These drugs compete with agonists for the same binding site on a given receptor. If the receptor is occupied by a competitive antagonist, then agonist binding to the receptor is reduced. Likewise, if the receptor is bound by an agonist, antagonist binding will be diminished. When present alone, each drug will occupy the receptors in a concentration-dependent manner as described in equation 2. However, when both drugs are present and competing for the same binding site, the equation describing agonist occupancy is as follows:

$$\frac{[DR]}{[R_T]} = \frac{[D]}{[D] + K_D(1 + [B]/K_B)} \qquad (3)$$

where D represents agonist, B represents antagonist, and K_D and K_B their relative affinity constants. This equation demonstrates that in the presence of a competitive antagonist, the apparent affinity (K_D) of the agonist [D] for the receptor is altered by the factor $1 + [B]/K_B$. As the concentration of the antagonist increases, the decrease in apparent affinity for the agonist also increases. As a result, more agonist is required to cause an effect. Therefore, a competitive antagonist reduces the response to the agonist. However, if the concentration of the agonist is increased, it can overcome the receptor blockade caused by the competitive antagonist. In other words, blockade by competitive antagonists is **surmountable** by increasing the concentration of agonist. With two drugs competing for the same binding site, the drug with the higher concentration relative to its affinity constant will dominate. It is important to remember that the key factor is the ratio of the drug concentration **relative** to its affinity constant, not simply drug concentration.

Equation 3 also demonstrates the very important point that the presence of a competitive antagonist causes a shift to the right in the agonist dose-response curve (decreased apparent K_D), but no change in the shape of the curve. This **parallel rightward shift** is diagnostic of competitive antagonists and means that every portion of the dose-response curve is shifted by exactly the same amount (Fig. 2-13). The magnitude of rightward shift is dependent on the concentration of antagonist, which is variable, divided by its affinity constant, which is fixed. Therefore, if we know the concentration of drug, measuring the magnitude of the rightward shift allows us to directly calculate the K_B for the antagonist. This is very important because the affinity constant is essentially a molecular description of how well a drug binds to a particular receptor and is constant for any drug/receptor pair. Thus, comparison of affinity constants for antagonists at receptors in different tissues is the best way to determine whether they are the same or different, making antagonists extremely useful in subclassifying receptors.

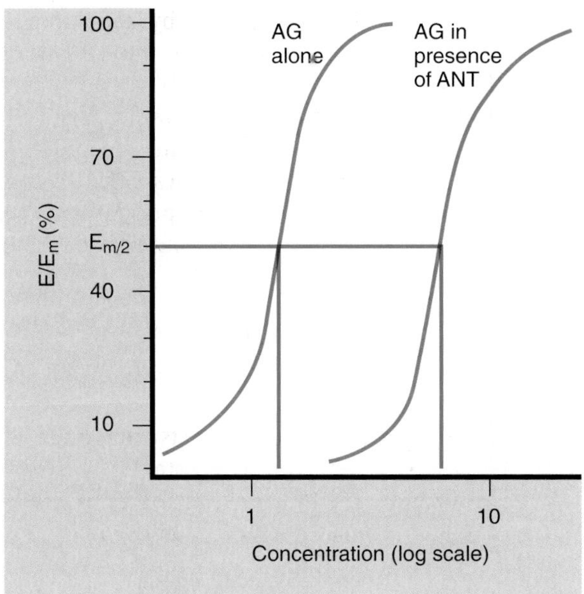

Figure 2-13 Competitive antagonism; both the agonist *(AG)* and the antagonist *(ANT)* compete and bind reversibly to the same receptor site. The presence of the competitive antagonist causes a parallel shift to the right in the concentration-response curve for the agonist.

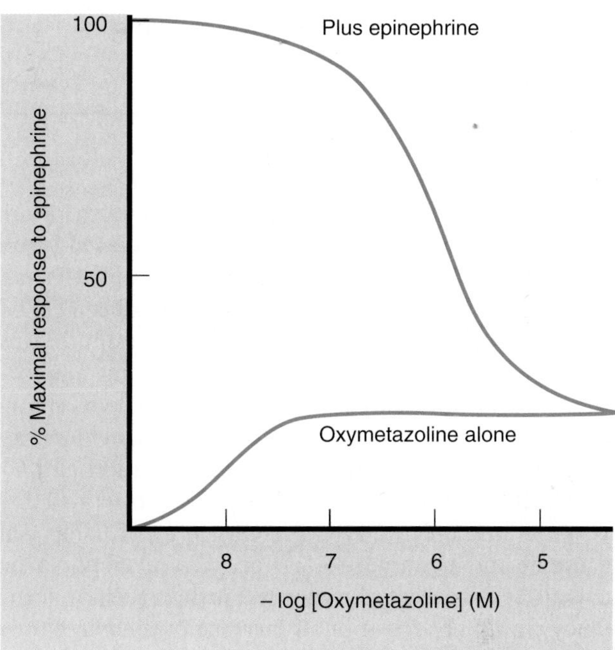

Figure 2-14 Partial agonists, such as the nasal decongestant oxymetazoline, give maximal responses that are lower than those of full agonists, such as epinephrine, in vascular smooth muscle. At high enough concentrations of oxymetazoline, the effect of epinephrine is reduced to the level of activity of oxymetazoline alone.

The second, less common, type of antagonist is the **noncompetitive** antagonist. There are a number of different noncompetitive antagonists, but most drugs in this class are **irreversible alkylating** agents. An example of this class of drug is phenoxybenzamine, a drug that acts predominantly on α_1-adrenergic receptors and is used to mitigate the effects of catecholamines secreted by adrenal tumors (see Chapter 10). Drugs of this class contain highly reactive groups, and when they bind to receptors they form covalent bonds, occupying the binding site in an essentially irreversible, nonsurmountable manner. Since they decrease the number of available receptors, noncompetitive antagonists will usually decrease the maximum response to an agonist without affecting its EC_{50} (concentration causing half-maximal effect). An advantage of a noncompetitive antagonist is its long lasting effect. Since the drug binds a receptor irreversibly, the drug effect lasts until new receptors are synthesized.

Partial agonists

As discussed previously, agonists can participate in both equilibria shown in equation 1, binding to and activating receptors to cause a conformational change. **Partial agonists** have a dual activity, that is, they act partially as agonists and partially as antagonists. When bound to their receptors, partial agonists are only partly able to shift the receptor to its activated conformational state. **Efficacy** is the proportion of receptors that are forced into their active conformation when occupied by a particular drug. It is used to describe the maximal effect of partial agonists in causing a receptor conformational change and can range from 0 to 1. Drugs with a full efficacy are called “full agonists,” drugs with some efficacy are “partial agonists,” whereas drugs with zero efficacy are “antagonists.”

Partial agonists can also partially inhibit the response to full agonists acting at the same receptor type (Fig. 2-14). If both full and partial agonists are present, as the concentration of partial agonist is increased, more receptors will be occupied by the partial agonist. This will cause a decrease in response, because some of the receptors will no longer be activated. At very high concentrations of partial agonist relative to its affinity constant, all of the receptors will be occupied by partial agonist, and the full agonist becomes essentially irrelevant. Therefore, a diagnostic feature of a partial agonist is that it inhibits the action of a full agonist down to the level of its own maximal effect.

Signal amplification—spare receptors

In some cases, the response elicited by a drug is proportional to the fraction of receptors occupied. More commonly, a maximal response can be achieved when only a small fraction of receptors are occupied by an agonist. This phenomenon defines what has been called spare receptors, or a receptor reserve. The reason for this behavior is that there are several intervening amplification steps downstream from the initial receptor-triggering event. If there were a 1 : 1 stochiometry between G-protein–coupled receptor activation and G-protein stimulation, for example, the existence of 10,000 receptors and only 1000 G-proteins in a particular cell would result in only 10% of receptors needing to be activated to cause a full response. Further receptor occupancy would not result in an increase in the magnitude of response. When the signaling pathways involve amplification steps, the EC_{50} for an agonist may be much lower than the concentration needed to cause half maximal receptor occupation (K_D).

Spare receptors are important in all-or-none responses, where it is especially important that activation does not fail (for example, the neuromuscular junction or the heart). The presence of spare receptors **shifts the agonist dose-response curve to the left** of the K_D for binding of agonist to receptor, and the degree of shift is proportional to the proportion of spare receptors (Fig. 2-15). Thus, spare receptors make a tissue more sensitive to an agonist without changing its affinity for the receptor. Because the existence of spare receptors is fairly common, the EC_{50} for an agonist is usually not equal to its K_D. For example, the β_1-adrenergic receptor has the same chemical and physical properties in every tissue in which it is expressed. However, the EC_{50} for a particular drug in activating responses mediated by this receptor can vary by orders of magnitude in different tissues, depending on the degree of receptor reserve.

This means that if an agonist has a different EC_{50} in two different tissues, one cannot conclude that the receptors in one tissue are different from the receptors in the other tissue, because there is no predictable relationship between EC_{50} and K_D for a particular agonist/receptor combination. Spare receptors are also responsible for **tissue specific actions** of agonists. Since the presence of spare receptors increases the potency of an agonist, tissues with a high proportion of spare receptors will respond to agonists at lower concentrations, even if they contain exactly the same receptor subtypes.

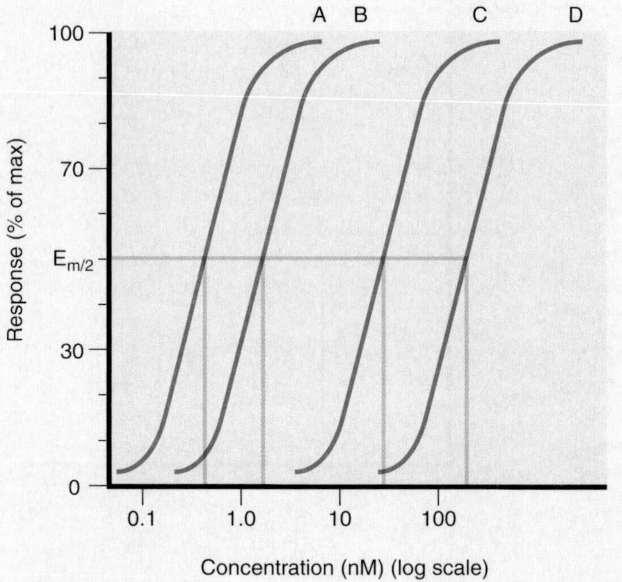

Figure 2-15 Logarithmic concentration–response curves for a single agonist acting on the same receptor subtype in tissues with different proportions of spare receptors (*A*, *B*, *C*, and *D*) and eliciting muscle contraction in vitro. Note that all tissues show the same maximum response to drug (intrinsic activity). The agonist shows its highest potency (lowest EC_{50}) at the tissue with greatest proportion of spare receptors (*A*), and its lowest potency at the tissue with the lowest proportion of spare receptors (*D*).

Spare receptors also complicate the analysis of partial agonists. If a drug is a partial agonist in one tissue, it may be a full agonist in another tissue, which has a higher proportion of spare receptors. In the GPCR example described previously, where only 10% of the receptors must be activated to cause a full response, a weak partial agonist may activate this 10% and appear to be a full agonist. Because of this problem, a different term, **intrinsic activity**, is used to describe the ability of a tissue to respond to agonist stimulation. Efficacy, which is the ability of the agonist to cause the receptor to assume an active conformation, is like K_D in that both are constant for a given drug/receptor pair. It is an intrinsic property that depends on the structural complementarity of the drug and the receptor molecules. Intrinsic activity, however, is highly context dependent. It varies in different tissues because of the presence of different proportions of spare receptors and downstream amplification mechanisms. A drug can be a partial agonist in efficacy, but a full agonist in intrinsic activity when spare receptors are present.

Receptor desensitization and supersensitivity

The response of any cell to hormones or neurotransmitters is tightly regulated and can vary depending on the other stimuli impinging on the cell. Very often, the number of receptors in the membrane of a cell or responsiveness of the receptors themselves is regulated. One hormone can **sensitize** a cell to the effects of another hormone and, more commonly, when a cell is continuously exposed to stimulation by a transmitter or hormone, it may become **desensitized.** An example of this phenomenon is the loss of the ability of inhaled β_2-adrenergic agonists to dilate the bronchi of asthmatic patients following repeated use of the drug (see Chapter 34). A hormone or agonist can affect the way a cell responds to itself (homologous effects) or how it responds to other hormones (heterologous effects). As an example of the latter phenomenon, exposure of a cell to estrogen sensitizes many cells to the effects of progesterone.

Changes in receptor binding affinity and signaling efficiency often occur rapidly. Receptor phosphorylation of serines, threonines, or tyrosines is a common mechanism of regulating responsiveness. Phosphorylation can rapidly change affinity or signaling efficiency and can also target a receptor for internalization and degradation.

The mechanisms involved in homologous and heterologous desensitization of β_2-adrenergic receptors are well understood (Fig. 2-16). Receptor phosphorylation on serine-threonine residues by three different protein kinases plays a role in the loss of responsiveness. These include β-adrenergic receptor kinase (β-ARK), cAMP-dependent protein kinase, and protein kinase C. Phosphorylation of the β-adrenergic receptor inhibits its ability to interact with G-proteins and subsequently leads to its sequestration or internalization in a compartment where it cannot interact with extracellular hormone. β-ARK is particularly important in homologous desensitization. It is capable only of phosphorylating the active, agonist-bound form of the receptor.

Other protein kinases, such as cAMP-dependent protein kinase, may also prefer the agonist-bound form of the receptor but not to the same extent as β-ARK. Although β-ARK was originally described as a kinase specific for the β-adrenergic receptor, its specificity is not unique, in that a large family of related protein kinases has been discovered. Between them, they can phosphorylate many different G-protein–coupled receptors in their agonist-bound state. Phosphorylation inhibits the ability of the receptor to interact with G

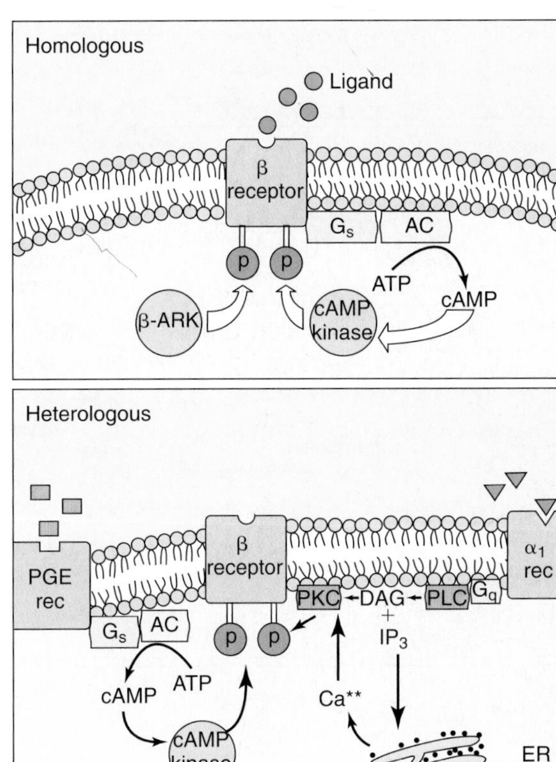

Figure 2-16 Phosphorylation is important in receptor desensitization. Pathways of stimulation of β-adrenergic receptor kinase (*β-ARK*), cAMP-dependent protein kinase in homologous desensitization, and cAMP-dependent protein kinase and protein kinase C (*PKC*) in heterologous desensitization by α_1-adrenergic receptor (*α_1 rec*) and prostaglandin PGE receptor (*PGE rec*). *AC,* Adenylate cyclase; *DAG,* diacylglycerol; *ER,* endoplasmic reticulum; *G,* G-protein; *IP_3,* inositol trisphosphate; *p,* phosphorylated state; *PLC,* phospholipase C.

proteins and subsequently leads to its sequestration or internalization in a compartment where it cannot interact with extracellular hormone.

In the absence of hormone, most receptors are not localized to particular regions of the cell membrane. When a hormone binds, receptors rapidly migrate to coated pits. These are specialized invaginations of the membrane surrounded by an electron-dense cage formed by the protein clathrin. Here receptor-mediated endocytosis occurs. Segments of membranes within coated pits rapidly pinch off to form intracellular vesicles rich in receptor-ligand complexes (Fig. 2-17). Vesicles then fuse with tubular-reticular structures. In most cases, dissociated hormone is incorporated into vesicles that fuse with lysosomes, with the hormone then degraded by lysosomal enzymes. Dissociated receptor recirculates to the cell surface. However, a fraction of internalized hormone may also be recirculated to the cell surface along with receptor, and then released. This

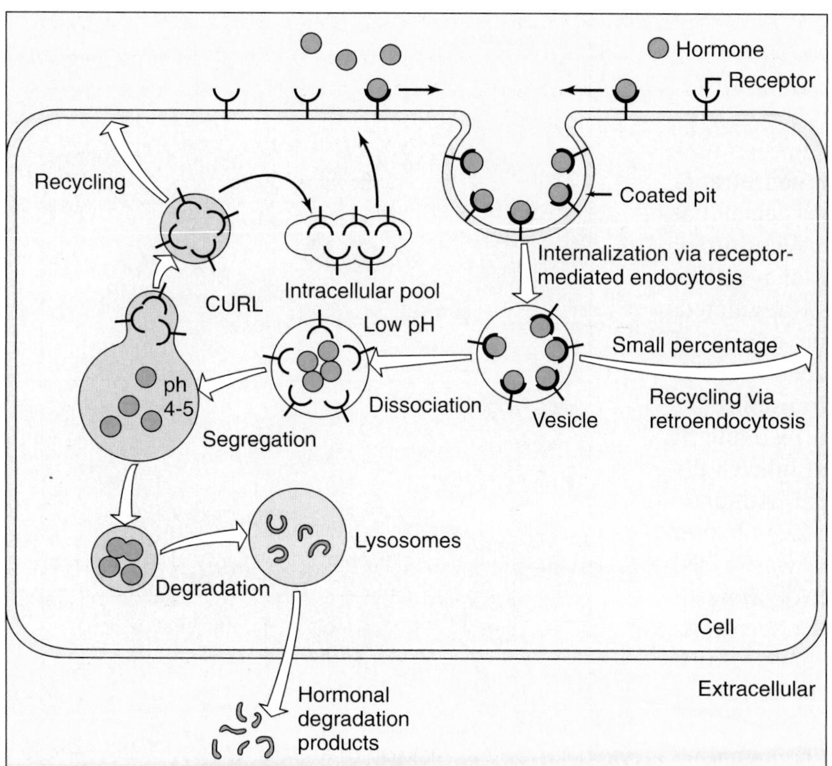

Figure 2-17 Pathways of receptor internalization and recycling. *CURL,* Compartment of uncoupling of receptor and ligand.

process is termed *retroendocytosis*. Free receptors may recirculate to the cell surface or may temporarily be sequestered in an intracellular membrane compartment. Alternatively, receptor may be transported to lysosomes, where it is also degraded. The latter two cases result in a net decrease in cell receptor number.

Finally, it is important to realize that the number of receptors in the plasma membrane of cells is not static (Fig. 2-18). Receptor number may be increased or decreased under the influence of hormonal mechanisms. Altered receptor number attributable to internalization or degradation has an intermediate time course, whereas an altered rate of receptor synthesis occurs even more slowly. Receptors may also be upregulated, and this phenomenon can result in receptor supersensitivity. Upregulation can occur after exposure of the receptor to an antagonist, or inhibition of transmitter synthesis, or release. In addition, other hormones can increase receptor number. For example, excessive production of thyroid hormone can increase the synthesis of β-adrenergic receptors in cardiac tissue, leading to some of the signs and symptoms of Graves' disease (see Chapter 37). Thus, the number of cell-surface receptors, and thereby hormone sensitivity, can be continuously regulated. This property of receptor biology can be

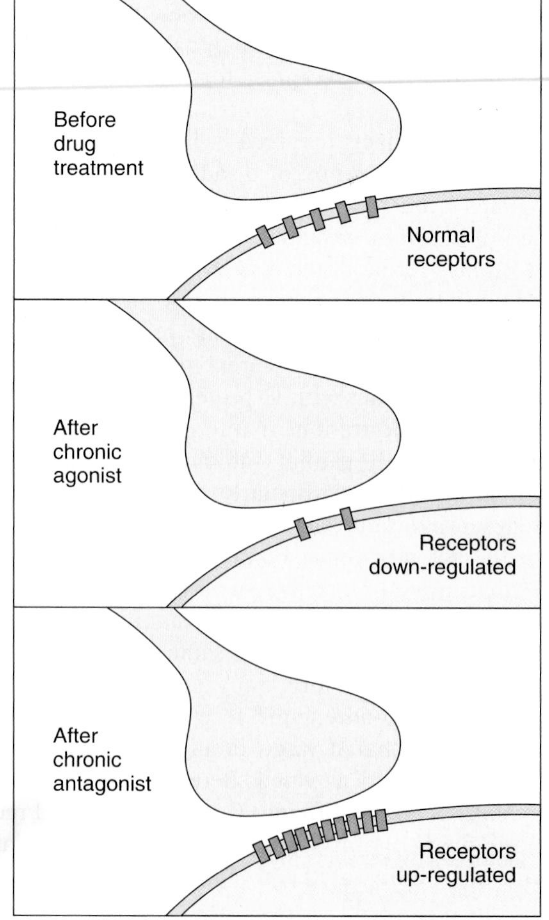

Figure 2-18 Long-term treatment with agonists or antagonists can alter postsynaptic receptor density or responsiveness.

exploited therapeutically. For example, during the third trimester of pregnancy, under the influence of nuclear hormones, the number of β_2-adrenergic receptors on uterine smooth muscle is dramatically increased allowing the use of selective β_2-adrenergic agonists, like terbutaline, to delay premature labor (see Chapter 10).

FURTHER READING

Domene C, Haider S, Sansom MS. Ion channel structures: a review of recent progress. *Curr Opin Drug Discov Dev* 2003; 6:611-619.

Kenakin T. Drug efficacy at G protein-coupled receptors. *Annu Rev Pharmacol Toxicol* 2002; 42:349-379.

Pratt WB, Taylor P. Principles of Drug Action: The Basis for Pharmacology. 3rd ed. Edinburgh, Churchill Livingstone, 1990.

Self-assessment questions

1. Binding of a drug to a receptor generally:

a. Involves covalent binding between receptor and drug.
b. Involves more than one type of weak bond between drug and receptor.
c. Requires long-lasting stable bonds between drug and receptor.
d. Has a similar affinity for the several stereoisomers of the drug.
e. Is characterized by high K_D values.

2. Long or continuous exposure of a receptor to an agent that is an antagonist can:

a. Result in a phenomenon called supersensitivity.
b. Desensitize the receptor.
c. Produce tachyphylaxis.
d. Cause downregulation of the receptor.
e. *b* and *c* are correct.

3. Which of the following is *not* a feature of receptors?

a. By acting on receptors, drugs can enhance, diminish, or block generation or transmission of signals.
b. The K_D of drug binding to receptors is generally in the range of 1 to 100 micromolar.
c. Specificity of drug binding to receptors is not absolute.
d. It may require more than one drug molecule to bind to a receptor and elicit a response.
e. Receptors are frequently glycosylated.

4. Hormone signaling can occur by:

a. Tyrosine phosphorylation.
b. Receptor association with G-proteins.
c. Formation of second messengers, such as cAMP.
d. Mobilization of Ca^{2+} from endoplasmic reticulum.
e. All are correct.

5. When added to an intestinal smooth muscle in a tissue bath, two different drugs both cause relaxation of the muscle but with different EC_{50} values. Based on this information, which of the following statements are true?

a. The two drugs have similar chemical structures.
b. The two drugs have different potencies in causing relaxation.
c. Both drugs activate the same receptor in the muscle.
d. Both drugs are directly-acting agonists.
e. The maximum relaxation caused by the two different drugs will be similar.

6. The affinity constant of a drug for a receptor (K_D) is:

a. The concentration of drug that occupies half of the available receptor sites.
b. The ratio of the reverse to forward rate constants for the drug-receptor interaction.
c. Important in determining fractional occupancy of the receptor by the drug.
d. Characterized by all of the above.
e. Characterized by *a* and *b* only.

CHAPTER 3

Absorption, distribution, metabolism, and elimination

Paul F. Hollenberg

What happens to drugs

In nearly all cases drugs must traverse membranes to reach their site of action. The ease by which a compound crosses membranes is key to assessing rates and extent of absorption and distribution throughout multiple compartments of the body. This chapter considers factors for assessing how specific drugs cross membranes and what variables are most important.

Drugs are transported throughout the circulatory system and, except for a few targeting techniques, end up at tissues and organs where their presence is beneficial and also in some areas where their presence may be detrimental. Because of the potential importance of this problem, special mention is made in this chapter about drug distribution to the brain.

The principal routes by which drugs disappear from the body are by elimination of unchanged drug or by metabolism to other active or inactive compounds, subject to further elimination or metabolism. Mechanisms of elimination and the principal pathways involved in drug metabolism are also described.

Absorption and distribution

Transport of drugs across membranes

Drugs administered orally, intramuscularly, or subcutaneously must cross membranes to be absorbed and enter the systemic circulation. Not all agents need to enter the systemic circulation, but even drugs given orally to treat gastrointestinal (GI) tract infections, stomach acidity, and other diseases within the GI tract often cross membranes and are absorbed into the general circulation. Drugs administered by intravenous injection must also cross capillary membranes to leave the systemic circulation and reach extracellular and intracellular sites of action. Even materials directed against platelets or other blood-borne elements must cross membranes. Renal elimination also requires the drugs or metabolites to traverse membranes.

Membranes are composed of a lipid bilayer and are strongly hydrophobic. However, most drugs must have some affinity for water (i.e., hydrophilicity) or they cannot dissolve and be transported by blood and other body fluids to their sites of action.

Abbreviations

CL_h	hepatic clearance
CL_r	renal clearance
CSF	cerebrospinal fluid
GI	gastrointestinal
NAD(P)	nicotinamide adenine dinucleotide (phosphate)
pH	logarithm of the reciprocal of the hydrogen ion concentration
pK_a	logarithm of the reciprocal of the dissociation constant
UDP	uridine diphosphate
V_{max}	maximum rate of reaction

Several factors that favor the ability of a drug to cross membranes are listed in Box 3-1. Compounds that are ionized or in which the electronic distribution is distorted so that there is a separation of positive and negative charge imparting polarity are not compatible with the uncharged nonpolar lipid environment. Also, the ordered lipid membrane does not allow for existence of aqueous pores large enough (>0.4 nm diameter) to allow passage of most drugs (generally >1 nm diameter). Thus, only molecules with low molecular weights can normally pass through membranes. Large molecular weight proteins, for example, cannot pass through many membranes by simply dissolving in the membrane and diffusing to the other side, as do lower molecular weight lipophilic compounds. With proteins, active transport using carrier molecules is often required to accomplish transmembrane transport. Most high molecular weight polypeptides and proteins cannot be administered orally because there are no mechanisms for their absorption from the GI tract, even if they could survive the high acidity of the stomach or the proteolytic enzymes present there.

Generally, drugs that have high lipid solubility cross membranes better than those with low lipid solubility. This is exemplified in Figure 3-1 for three different barbiturates. The oil/water equilibrium partition coefficient is a measure of lipid solubility, or hydrophobicity. Drug is added to a mixture of equal volumes of oil and water, and the mixture is agitated to promote solubilization of the compound in each phase. When equilibrium is attained, the phases are separated and assayed for drug. The ratio of the concentration in the two phases is the partition coefficient. Therefore, the larger the partition coefficient, the greater the lipid solubility. Figure 3-1 shows that absorption across the stomach wall is greater for the barbiturate with the largest lipid solubility.

Many drugs are weak acids or bases and take up or release a hydrogen ion. Within some ranges of pH, these drugs will be ionized; in other pH ranges the compounds will be uncharged. The uncharged form of a drug is lipid soluble and crosses biological membranes readily. In the barbiturate example, the compounds were selected so that the pK_a (the logarithm of the reciprocal of the dissociation constant) of each drug was very similar. Otherwise, the differences in absorption could have been caused by varying degrees of ionization of the three compounds. As shown below, study of the pH influence helps to predict the distribution of a drug between body compartments that differ in pH.

Box 3-1 Characteristics of drug molecules that favor drug transport across membranes

Uncharged	Low molecular weight
Nonpolar	High lipid solubility

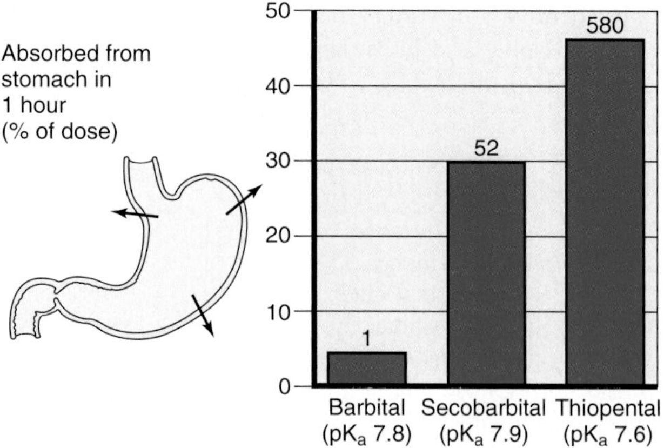

Figure 3-1 Increased lipid solubility influences the amount of drug absorbed from the stomach for three different barbiturates. The number above each column is the oil/water equilibrium partition coefficient. The compounds have roughly equivalent pK_a values and so the degree of ionization is similar for all three drugs.

Influence of pH on drug absorption and distribution

Passive diffusion of a drug that is a weak electrolyte is generally a function of the pK_a of the drug and the pH of the two compartments, because only the uncharged form of the drug can diffuse across membranes. The pH values of the major body fluids are shown in Table 3-1. The range is from pH 1 to pH 8. To predict how a drug will be distributed with gastric juice at pH 1.0 on one side of the membrane and blood at pH 7.4 on the other side, the degree of dissociation of the drug at each pH value is determined.

An acid is defined as a compound that can dissociate and release a hydrogen ion, whereas a base can take up a hydrogen ion. By this definition, RCOOH and RNH_3^+ are acids and $RCOO^-$ and RNH_2 are bases. The equilibrium dissociation expression and the equilibrium

Table 3-1 pH of selected body fluids

Fluids	pH
Gastric juice	1.0-3.0
Small intestine: Duodenum	5.0-6.0
Small intestine: Ileum	8
Large intestine	8
Plasma	7.4
Cerebrospinal fluid	7.3
Urine	4.0-8.0

dissociation constant (K_a) can be described for an acid HA or BH^+ and a base A^- or B, as shown below. The convention for K_a requires that the acid appear on the left and the base appear on the right of the dissociation equation:

$$HA \rightleftharpoons A^- + H^+ \qquad K_a = \frac{[A^-][H^+]}{[HA]} \qquad (1)$$

$$BH^+ \rightleftharpoons B + H^+ \qquad K_a = \frac{[B][H^+]}{[BH^+]} \qquad (2)$$

Taking the negative log of both sides gives

$$-\log K_a = -\log[H^+] - \log\frac{[A^-]}{[HA]} \qquad (3)$$

$$-\log K_a = -\log[H^+] - \log\frac{[B]}{[BH^+]} \qquad (4)$$

By definition the negative log of $[H^+]$ is pH and the negative log of K_a is pK_a. Therefore, equations 3 and 4 can be simplified and rearranged to give

$$pH = pK_a + \log\frac{[A^-]}{[HA]} \qquad (5)$$

$$pH = pK_a + \log\frac{[B]}{[BH^+]} \qquad (6)$$

Equations 5 and 6 are the acid and base forms, respectively, of the Henderson-Hasselbalch equation and they can be used to calculate the pH of the solution when the pK_a and the ratios of $[A^-]/[HA]$ or $[B]/[BH^+]$ are known. In pharmacology it is often of interest to calculate the ratios of $[A^-]/[HA]$ or $[B]/[BH^+]$ when the pH and the pK_a are known. For this calculation, equations 5 and 6 are rearranged to equations 7 and 8:

$$pH - pK_a = \log\frac{[A^-]}{[HA]} \qquad (7)$$

$$pH - pK_a = \log\frac{[B]}{[BH^+]} \qquad (8)$$

The results are plotted in Figure 3-2 to show the fraction of the nonionized (HA or B) forms. The pK_a is the pH when the drug is 50% dissociated. Applying equations 7 and 8 to an acidic drug with a pK_a of 6.0 enables one to calculate the degree of ionization for this drug in the stomach or blood (assume the blood pH is 7.0 for ease of calculation), as follows:

Stomach: 1.0 − 6.0 = log Y; log Y = −5, or Y = 10^{-5}; Y = $[A^-]$ / [HA] = 0.00001; if [HA] is 1.0, then $[A^-]$ is 0.00001 and the compound is ionized very little.

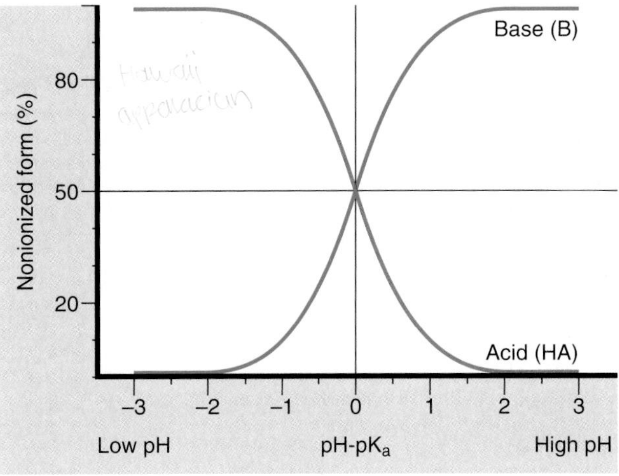

Figure 3-2 Degree of acidic or basic drug in nonionized (uncharged) form (HA, acid; B, base) at different pH values, with pH expressed relative to the drug pK_a.

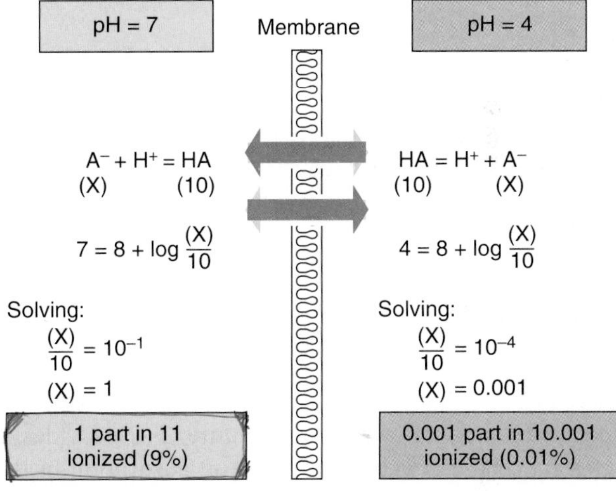

Figure 3-3 Equilibrium distribution of drug when pH is 4 on one side and 7 on the other side of membrane for an acid drug with a pK_a of 8.0. Nonionized form, HA, of the drug can readily cross the membrane. Thus, HA has the same concentration on both sides of the membrane. The concentration of nonionized drug is arbitrarily set at 10 μg/ml, and the expressions are solved to determine the concentration of ionized species at equilibrium.

Blood: 7.0 − 6.0 = log Y; log Y = +1, or Y = 10^{+1}; Y = $[A^-]$ / [HA] = 10.0; if [HA] is 1.0, then $[A^-]$ is 10.0 and the compound is ionized considerably.

Thus, the drug is ionized little in stomach but appreciably in blood and should cross readily in the stomach-to-plasma direction but hardly at all in the reverse direction.

Another example is shown in Figure 3-3 for a basic drug. This approach is particularly useful for predicting whether drugs can be absorbed in the stomach, the

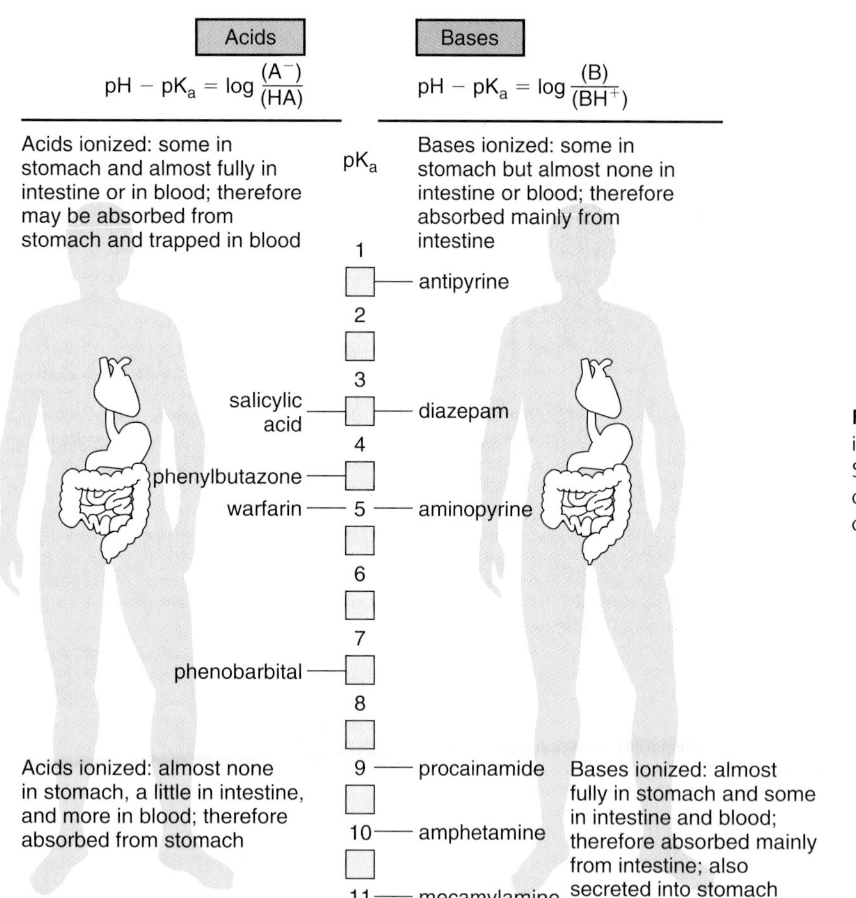

Figure 3-4 Summary of pH effect on degree of ionization of several acidic and basic drugs. Statements refer to compounds with extremes of pK_a values and allow prediction of where drugs with various pK_as will be absorbed.

upper intestine, or not at all. Figure 3-4 provides a summary of the effects of pH on drug absorption in the GI tract for several acidic and basic drugs. It also assists in predicting which drugs will undergo tubular reabsorption, as discussed later.

Most drugs are transported across membranes by simple passive diffusion. The concentration gradient across the membrane is the driving force that establishes the rate of diffusion from high to low concentrations. Other mechanisms, including active transport, facilitated diffusion, or pinocytosis, also exist. Active transport involves specific carrier molecules in the membrane that bind to and carry the drug across the lipid bilayer. Because there are a finite number of carrier molecules, they exhibit classical saturation kinetics. Drugs may also compete with a specific carrier molecule for transport, which can lead to drug-drug interactions that modify the time and intensity of action of a given drug. An active transport system may concentrate a drug on one side of a membrane, because cellular energy is used to drive transport, with no dependence on a concentration gradient. The primary active drug transport systems are present in renal tubule cells, biliary tract, blood-brain barrier, and the GI tract.

Distribution to special organs and tissues

The rate of blood flow determines the maximum amount of drug that can be delivered per minute to specific organs and tissues at a given plasma concentration. Tissues that are well perfused can receive a large quantity of drug, provided the drug can cross the membranes or other barriers present. Similarly, tissues, such as fat that are poorly perfused, receive drug at a slower rate, so the concentration of drug in fat may still be increasing long after the concentration in plasma has started to decrease.

Two compartments of special importance are the brain and the fetus. Many drugs do not readily enter brain. Capillaries in brain differ structurally from those in other tissues, with the result that a barrier exists between blood within brain capillaries and the

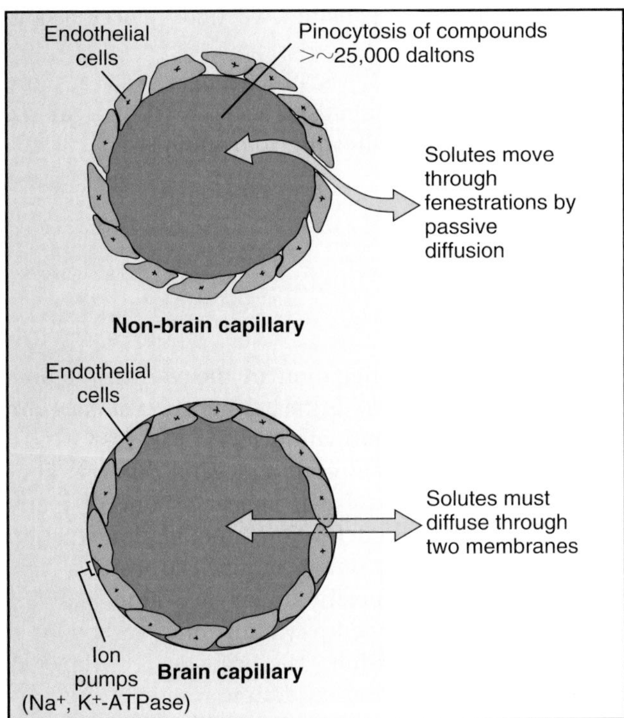

Figure 3-5 Structural differences between non-brain and brain capillaries. In brain capillaries, lack of openings between endothelial cells in capillary wall requires drugs and other solutes to pass through two membranes to move from blood to tissue or the reverse. Ion pumps are mainly on the outer membrane of the brain endothelial cells and maintain a concentration difference between the two fluid regions.

extracellular fluid in brain tissue. This **blood-brain barrier** hinders transport of drugs and other materials from blood into brain tissue. The blood-brain barrier is found throughout brain and spinal cord at all regions central to the arachnoid membrane, except for the floor of the hypothalamus and the area postrema. Structural differences between brain and non-brain capillaries and how these differences influence blood-brain transport of solutes are shown schematically in Figure 3-5. Non-brain capillaries have fenestrations (openings) between the endothelial cells through which solutes move readily by passive diffusion, with compounds having molecular weights greater than about 25,000 daltons undergoing transport by pinocytosis. In brain capillaries, tight junctions are present because there are no fenestrations, and pinocytosis is greatly reduced. Special transport systems are available at brain capillaries for glucose, amino acids, amines, purines, nucleosides, and organic acids; all other materials must cross two endothelial membranes plus the endothelial cytoplasm to move from capillary blood to tissue extracellular fluid. Thus, the main route of drug entry into central nervous system (CNS) tissue is by passive diffusion across membranes, restricting the available compounds used to treat brain disorders. At the same time, the potential deleterious effects of many compounds on the CNS are not realized, because the blood-brain barrier acts as a safety buffer. Generally, only highly lipid-soluble drugs cross the blood-brain barrier, and thus for these drugs no blood-brain barrier exists. In infants and the elderly, the blood-brain barrier may be compromised and drugs diffuse into brain.

An alternative approach for drug delivery to brain is by intrathecal injection into the subarachnoid space and the CSF using lumbar puncture. However, injection into subarachnoid space can be difficult to perform safely because of the small volume of this region and the proximity to easily damaged nerves. In addition, drug distribution within the CSF and across the CSF-brain barrier can be slow and show much variability; however, for some drugs there may be no alternate route.

Metabolism and elimination of drugs

The term **elimination** refers to the removal of drug from the body without chemical changes. For some drugs this is the only route of disappearance; for most drugs only some of the dose is removed unchanged. Elimination occurs primarily by renal mechanisms into the urine, and to a lesser extent by mixing with bile salts for solubilization followed by transport into the intestinal tract. However, in many cases there is reabsorption from the intestine, and highly volatile or gaseous agents may be excreted by the lungs. The terms **metabolism** and **biotransformation** refer to the disappearance of a drug when it is changed chemically into another compound, called a **metabolite.** Some drugs are administered as inactive "**prodrugs,**" which must be metabolized into a pharmacologically active form. Although drug metabolism occurs for many drugs primarily in the liver, almost all tissues and organs, especially the lung, can also carry out varying degrees of metabolism. A few drugs become essentially irreversibly bound to tissues and are metabolized or otherwise removed over long periods of time. Finally, drugs may be excreted in feces, exhaled through the lung, or secreted through sweat or salivary glands.

Metabolism of drugs

Drug metabolism involves the alteration of the chemical structure of the drug by an enzyme. When drugs are metabolized, the change generally involves conversion

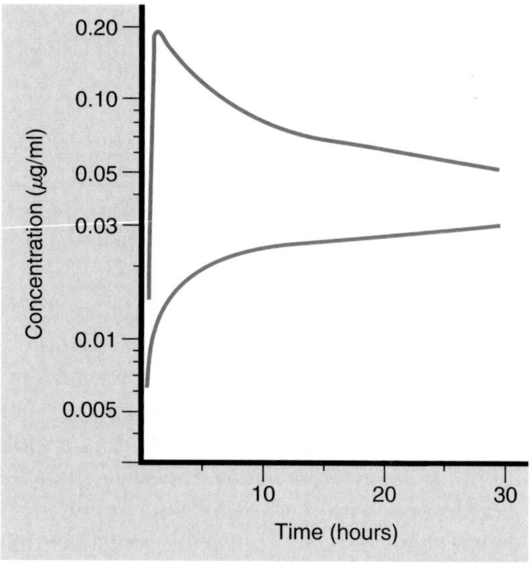

Figure 3-6 Plasma concentration of diazepam *(red line)* and its main metabolite, desmethyldiazepam, *(blue line)* after a single oral dose of 10 mg of diazepam in humans.

of a nonpolar, lipid-soluble compound to a more polar form that is more water soluble and can be more readily excreted in the urine. Some drugs are administered as prodrugs in an inactive or less active form to promote absorption, to overcome potential destruction by stomach acidity, to minimize exposure to highly reactive chemical species, or to allow for selective generation of pharmacologically active metabolites at specific target sites in vivo. In this case, drug-metabolizing systems convert the prodrug into a more active species following absorption. In some cases, drugs administered as the active species are metabolized to products that are also "active" and produce pharmacological effects similar to or different from those generated by the parent drug. An example is diazepam (Fig. 3-6), an antianxiety compound that is demethylated to an active metabolite. The half-life of the parent drug is about 30 hours; the half-life of the metabolite averages about 70 hours. Thus, the effect of the metabolite is present long after the parent drug disappears. Here, the magnitude of the pharmacological effect is much less for metabolite than for parent drug, but, in general, the lingering presence of active metabolites makes control of the intensity of pharmacological effect more difficult. With diazepam, the therapeutic index (ratio of toxic to therapeutic dose) is large enough so that precise control is not required.

For most drugs, metabolism takes place primarily in liver, catalyzed by microsomal and, in some cases, nonmicrosomal enzyme systems. However, considerable levels of drug-metabolizing enzymes are found in other tissues, including lung, kidney, GI tract, placenta, and GI tract bacteria.

Although many types of chemical reactions are observed in drug metabolism, most reactions can be categorized into the following four groups:

- Oxidation
- Conjugation
- Reduction
- Hydrolysis

Oxidation and conjugation are the two most important and are discussed further. Simpler examples are given for reduction and hydrolysis.

Oxidation can take place at several different sites on a drug molecule and can appear as one of many chemical reactions. By definition, an oxidation reaction requires the transfer of one or more electrons to a final electron acceptor. Typically, an oxygen atom may be inserted, resulting in hydroxylation of a carbon or a nitrogen atom, oxidation, N- or O-dealkylation, or deamination. Many drug-oxidation reactions are catalyzed by the cytochrome P450-dependent mixed-function oxidase system. The overall reaction can be summarized as:

$$\mathrm{DH} + \mathrm{NAD(P)H} + \mathrm{H^+} + \mathrm{O_2}$$
$$= \mathrm{DOH} + \mathrm{NAD(P)^+} + \mathrm{H_2O}$$

where DH is the drug, NADH or NADPH is a reduced nicotinamide adenine dinucleotide cofactor, and NAD or NADP is an oxidized cofactor. In this reaction molecular oxygen serves as the final electron acceptor.

In most cells, the **cytochrome P450s** are associated with the endoplasmic reticulum. More than 50 isoforms of human P450 exist, with various substrate specificities and different mechanisms regulating their expression. This plethora of enzyme systems provides the body with the ability to metabolize large numbers of different drugs. The common feature of P450 substrates is their lipid solubility. Most lipophilic drugs and environmental chemicals are substrates for one or more forms of P450. During the catalytic reaction, the heme iron in the enzyme undergoes a cycle that begins in the ferric oxidation state, when the drug binds to cytochrome P450. The heme iron undergoes reduction to the ferrous state, binds oxygen, and the molecular oxygen bound to the active site is reduced to a reactive form that inserts one oxygen atom into the drug substrate with the other oxygen being reduced to water, with the eventual regeneration of the ferric state of the heme iron. Free radical or iron-radical groups are formed at one or more parts of the cycle. The reaction cycle is summarized in Figure 3-7. The cytochrome

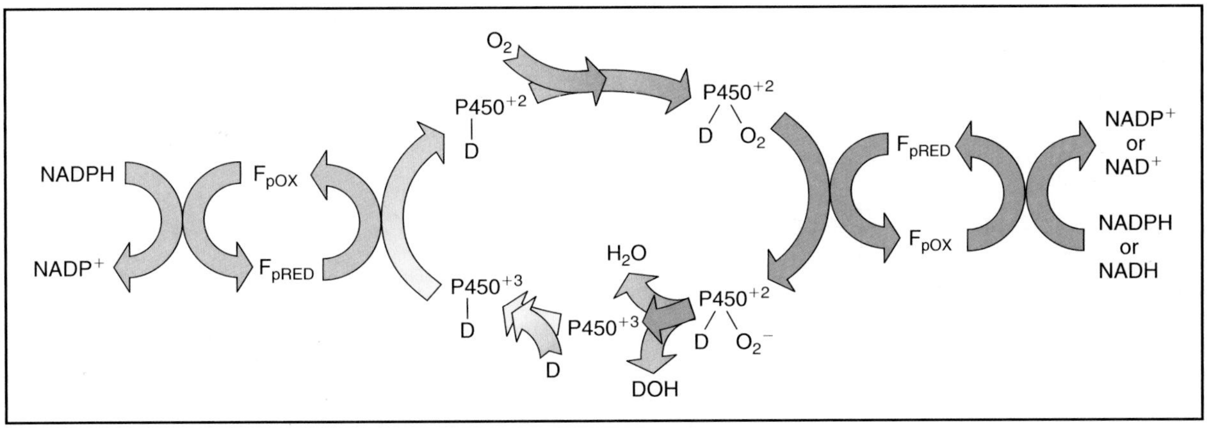

Figure 3-7 Simplified model of cytochrome P450 mixed-function oxidase reaction sequence. *D* is the drug undergoing oxidation to produce *DOH*. Molecular oxygen serves as the final electron acceptor. Flavin protein cofactor (F_p) systems are involved at several sites. The iron of the cytochrome P450 is involved in binding oxygen and electron transfer with changes in valence state.

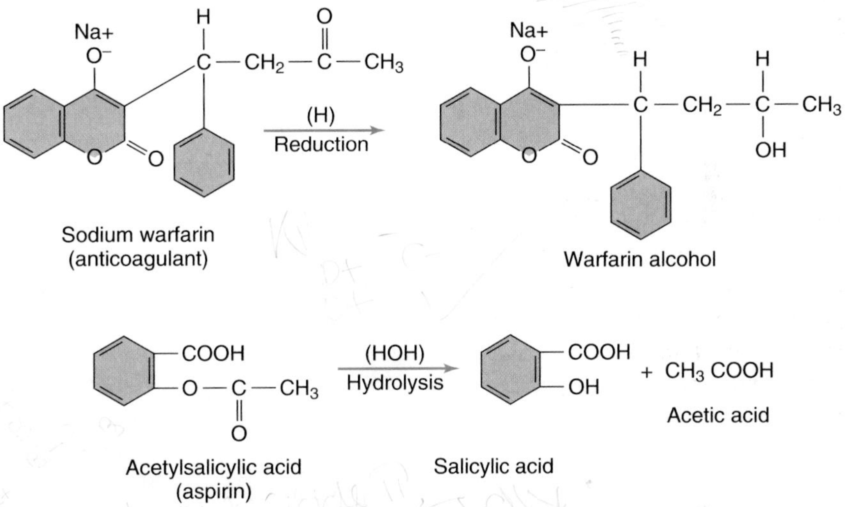

Figure 3-8 Representative reduction and hydrolysis reactions for metabolism of drugs.

P450-dependent mixed-function oxidases are very complex systems of enzymes in which detailed mechanistic studies are leading to important molecular insights that will play a role in drug design. Because metabolism by the cytochrome P450 route may lead to the generation of highly reactive free radical groups, this must be considered in drug design to minimize the possible formation of reactive and potentially toxic drug metabolites.

Typical metabolic reactions involving reduction and hydrolysis of drugs are shown in Figure 3-8. Oxidations, reductions, and hydrolytic reactions are commonly referred to as **Phase I** reactions.

Conjugation, the second class of reactions to drug metabolism, involves coupling the drug molecule to an endogenous substituent group so that the resulting product will have greater water solubility or other modifications that lead to enhanced renal or biliary elimination. Conjugation reactions, like other metabolic processes, are catalyzed by **Phase II** drug-metabolizing enzymes. In addition, the groups that are being coupled need to be "activated" by transfer of energy from high energy phosphate compounds. For example, glucuronic acid can be conjugated by the enzyme UDP-glucuronosyl transferase to compounds of the general types ROH, RCOOH, RNH_2, or RSH, where R represents the remainder of the drug molecule. However, glucuronic acid must first be activated by the reaction of glucose-1-phosphate with uridine triphosphate to form UDP-glucose followed by oxidation to activated UDP-glucuronic acid. The reaction sequence is shown in Figure 3-9 for the formation of the ROH glucuronide of salicylic acid. Another glucuronide could be formed through conjugation with the RCOOH group. Many drugs, as well as endogenous materials, including bilirubin, thyroxine, and steroids, also undergo conjugation

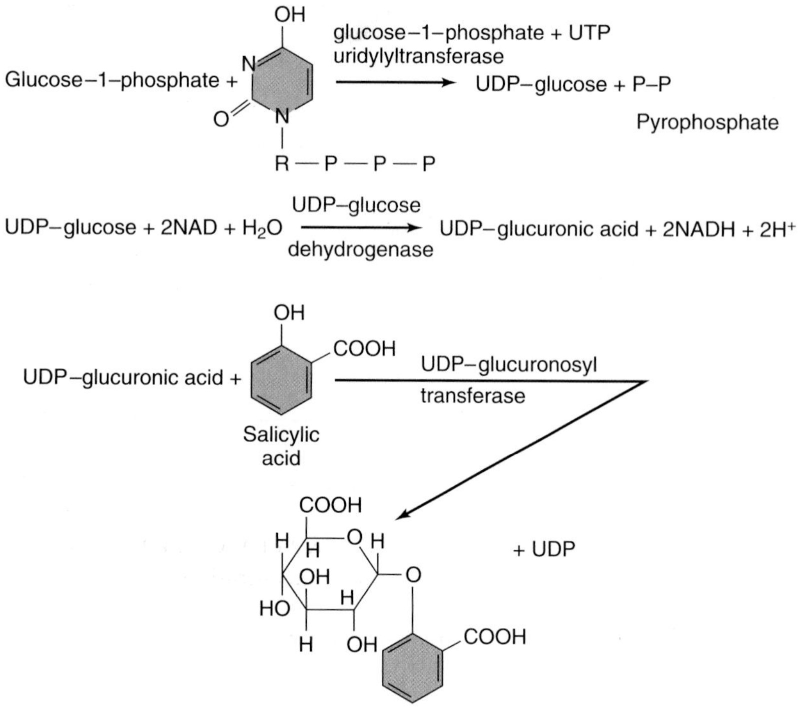

Glucose–1–phosphate + [UTP structure: OH, N, O, N, R—P—P—P] —glucose–1–phosphate + UTP uridylyltransferase→ UDP–glucose + P–P (Pyrophosphate)

UDP–glucose + 2NAD + H_2O —UDP–glucose dehydrogenase→ UDP–glucuronic acid + 2NADH + $2H^+$

UDP–glucuronic acid + Salicylic acid —UDP–glucuronosyl transferase→ salicyl phenolic glucuronide + UDP

Figure 3-9 Sequence of reactions for conjugation of salicylic acid to form salicyl phenolic glucuronide. *P*, Phosphate. The glucuronic acid must first be activated, with glucose-1-phosphate coupling with high-energy UTP to UDP-glucose followed by oxidation to UDP-glucuronic acid before conjugation can occur.

with activated glucuronic acid in the presence of UDP-glucuronosyl transferase. In addition to glucuronate, conjugation may occur also with activated glycine, acetate, sulfate, and other groups besides glucuronate, leading to drug conjugates that will be readily excreted.

Factors regulating rates of drug metabolism The chemical reactions involved in drug metabolism are catalyzed by enzymes. Because these enzymes obey Michaelis-Menten kinetics, the rates of drug metabolism can be approximated by the relationship:

$$v = \frac{V_{max}(S)}{K_m + (S)} \qquad (9)$$

where:

v = rate of reaction

V_{max} = maximum rate of reaction

(S) = concentration of drug

K_m = Michaelis constant

V_{max} is directly proportional to the concentration of the enzyme. If a change occurs in the concentration of enzyme, there should be a similar change in rate of metabolism. Because different drugs may be substrates for the same metabolizing enzyme, they can competitively inhibit each other's metabolism. However, this is usually not a significant problem, because the capacity of the metabolizing system is large, and drugs are usually present in concentrations less than their K_m.

Many drugs, environmental chemicals, air pollutants, and components of cigarette smoke stimulate the synthesis of higher concentrations of drug-metabolizing enzymes. This process, termed **enzyme induction,** may elevate the level of hepatic drug-metabolizing enzymes. In most cases, the inducers are also substrates for the enzymes they induce. However, the induction is generally nonspecific and may result in increases in metabolism of a variety of substrates. For example, phenobarbital and the highly reactive air pollutant 3,4-benzo[a]pyrene can increase the rate of oxidation of the CNS muscle relaxant zoxazolamine in animals (Fig. 3-10). Because cigarette smoke contains compounds that can promote induction, chronic smokers have considerably higher levels of some hepatic and lung drug-metabolizing enzymes. Induction of P450 by polycyclic aromatic hydrocarbons in smoke causes female smokers to have lower circulating estrogen than nonsmokers.

For nearly all drugs, the normal therapeutic range of concentrations is much smaller than the K_m. Thus, hepatic or other drug-metabolizing enzymes are operating at concentration levels far below saturation, where equation 9 reduces to a first-order reaction. Thus, drug metabolism typically follows first-order kinetics. An exception is the metabolism of salicylic acid, in which enzyme saturation can occur at elevated drug concen-

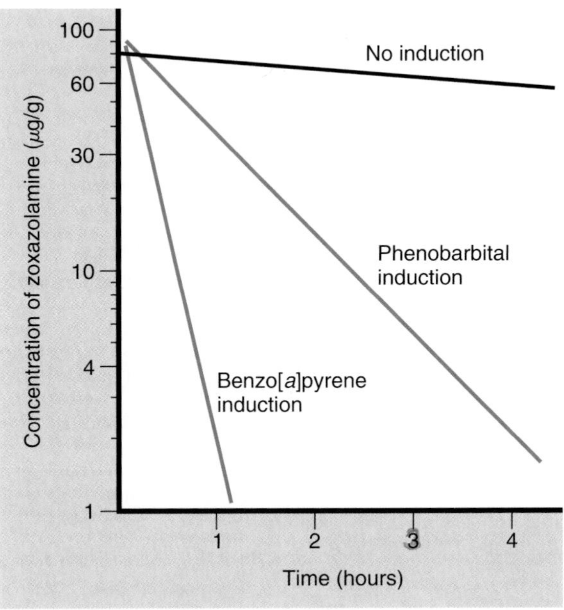

Figure 3-10 Example of enzyme induction. Zoxazolamine administered by intraperitoneal injection to rats. For induction studies, phenobarbital or 3,4-benzo[a]pyrene was injected twice daily for 4 days before injection of zoxazolamine.

trations. Aspirin (acetylsalicylic acid) is used extensively for treatment of inflammatory diseases, with the optimum therapeutic concentration only slightly below the concentration where signs of toxicity appear. Aspirin is hydrolyzed to salicylic acid, which in turn has several routes of metabolism before elimination (Fig. 3-11). Two pathways are subject to saturation in humans:

- Conjugation with glycine to form salicyluric acid
- Conjugation with glucuronic acid to form the salicyl phenolic glucuronide

For enzyme saturation, the kinetics become zero order, and the rate of reaction becomes constant at V_{max}. This is consistent with equation 9 when (S) is much larger than K_m. Saturation of drug-metabolizing enzymes has a pronounced influence on drug-plateau concentrations. With zero-order kinetics, elimination rates no longer depend on dose or blood concentration.

Hepatic and biliary clearance

Hepatic clearance, $(CL)_h$, can be defined as:

$$\frac{\text{rate of drug removal by the liver}}{\text{concentration of drug in portal vein}} \quad (10)$$

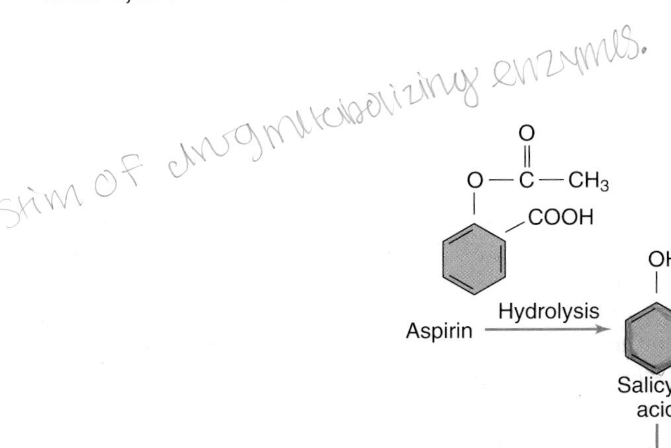

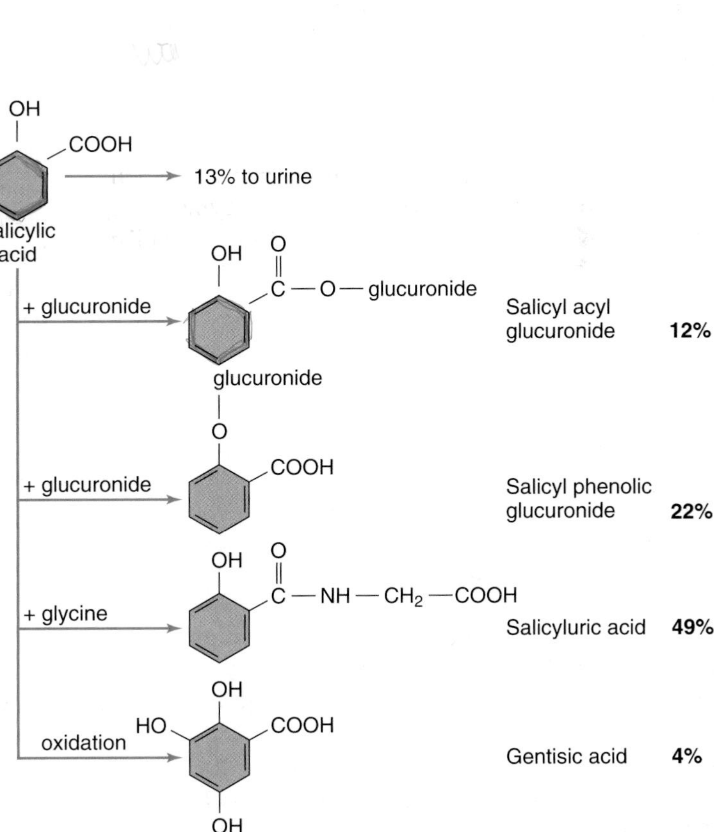

Figure 3-11 Disposition of the primary metabolite of aspirin, salicylic acid, at a single dose of 4 grams (54 mg/kg of body weight) in a healthy adult. The percentage values refer to the dose. Oxidation produces a mixture of *ortho* and *para* (relative to original OH group) isomers.

It is the apparent volume of plasma that is cleared of drug by the liver per unit time and has the units of volume/time. Biliary clearance can be similarly defined, with the bile flow rate times the drug concentration in bile a measure of the rate of biliary removal. Direct measurement of hepatic or biliary clearance in humans is not practical because of the difficulty and risk in obtaining appropriate blood samples. The concept of hepatic and biliary clearance is included here to emphasize that the concept of clearance can be applied to any body region or organ system.

A complicating result of biliary elimination of a drug sometimes occurs when the drug is reabsorbed from the GI tract and returned to the systemic circulation. This is termed **enterohepatic cycling** and can result in a measurable increase in the plasma concentration of drug several half-lives after the drug originally was administered and will delay its eventual disposition.

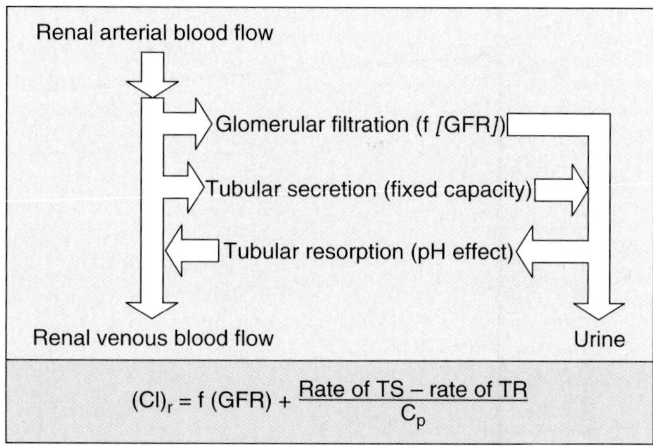

Figure 3-12 Summary of renal clearance $(CL)_r$ mechanisms. C_p, Renal arterial blood concentration of drug; *f*, fraction of drug in plasma not bound; *GFR*, glomerular filtration rate of drug; *TR*, tubular reabsorption of drug; *TS*, tubular secretion of drug.

Renal elimination of drugs

The removal of drug by the renal route is another process included in "total body clearance," or the sum of removal by all routes. The same general definition of clearance can be applied to the renal route to define **renal clearance,** $(Cl)_r$, as the volume of plasma that needs to be cleared per unit time to account for the rate of drug removal that takes place in the kidneys. This can be expressed in equation form as:

$$(Cl)_r = \frac{\text{rate of drug removal by the kidneys}}{\text{concentration of drug in renal artery}} \quad \textbf{(11)}$$

For a drug, such as the antibiotic cephalexin, that is removed entirely by renal elimination, renal clearance and total body clearance are equal. In this example, renal clearance can be determined from plasma data if one plots the log plasma concentration of cephalexin versus time after intravenous injection.

The mechanisms by which the renal clearance of drugs takes place (glomerular filtration, tubular secretion, and tubular reabsorption) are the same as those responsible for the renal elimination of endogenous substances (Fig. 3-12).

Molecules smaller than those of about 15Å readily pass through the glomeruli, with approximately 125 ml of plasma cleared each minute in a healthy adult. Because this figure is independent of the plasma concentration, removal by glomerular filtration (mg/min) shows a linear increase with increasing plasma drug concentrations in the renal artery. The glomerular filtration rate of 125 ml/min represents less than 20% of the total renal plasma flow of 650 to 750 ml/min, indicating that only a small fraction of the total renal plasma flow is cleared of drug on each pass through the kidneys. Because albumin and other plasma proteins normally do not pass through the glomeruli, drug molecules that are bound to these proteins are retained. Inulin and creatinine can be used to assess glomerular filtration capability in individual patients because these materials show very little binding to plasma proteins and do not undergo appreciable tubular secretion or reabsorption.

Tubular secretion, a second mechanism for renal clearance, is an active process that occurs in the proximal tubule, with independent and relatively nonspecific carrier systems for secretion of acids and bases. Compounds that are secreted usually also undergo glomerular filtration, and so renal clearance is the sum of both routes. Tubular secretion involves active transport by carriers, and because there are a limited number of carriers, the process can become saturated. The volume of plasma that can be cleared per unit time by tubular secretion varies with the concentration of drug in plasma. This is in contrast to glomerular filtration, where the volume filtered per unit time is independent of plasma concentration. At very low plasma concentrations, tubular secretion can operate at its maximum rate of clearing approximately 650 ml/min. If the concentration of drug in arterial plasma is 4 ng/ml, clearing 650 ml/min removes 2600 ng each minute. If the concentration of the same drug increases to 200 ng/ml and tubular secretion is saturated at 4 ng/ml, the tubules will still remove only 2600 ng/min by secretion, and so the clearance by tubular secretion falls to 13 ml/min. If drug disappearance studies show that the renal clearance is considerably greater than 125 ml/min, tubular secretion must be involved because glomerular filtration cannot exceed that rate. Tubular secretion removes bound and free drug because tubular transit time can be sufficiently long, such that dissociation from plasma proteins can take place.

The third mechanism affecting renal clearance is reabsorption of filtered or secreted drug from the tubules back into the venous blood of the nephrons. Although this process may be either active or passive, for most drugs it occurs by passive diffusion. Drugs that are readily reabsorbed are characterized by high lipid solubility or by a significant fraction in a nonionized form at urine pH and in the ionized form at plasma pH. For example, salicylic acid (pK_a of 3.0) is about 99.99% ionized at pH 7.4 (Equation 7) but only about 90% ionized at pH 4.0. Thus, some reabsorption of salicylic acid could be expected from acidic urine. In drug overdose, the manipulation of urine pH is sometimes used to prevent reabsorption. Ammonium chloride administration leads to acidification of the urine; sodium bicarbonate administration leads to alkalinization of the urine. Some additional examples are given in Box 3-2.

Modified renal function and drug elimination Renal clearance of drugs may be less in neonates, geriatric patients, and those with improperly functioning kidneys. The effects of patient age on renal clearance of drugs is discussed in Chapter 4.

The following situation is typical:

- It is desirable to use a particular drug in a patient.
- The drug is disposed of primarily by renal elimination.
- The patient's renal function is compromised.

The problem is whether a safe dosing schedule can be developed in this patient. In many cases the problem can be solved. However, it is essential that the extent of renal function is known. Creatinine clearance is the standard clinical determination used to obtain an approximate measure of renal function. Creatinine is used routinely instead of inulin clearance because the assay and methodology with inulin are more difficult. To determine the rate of urinary excretion of creatinine, urine is collected over a known period (often 24 hours) and pooled, its volume is measured, and urine is assayed for creatinine. At the midpoint of the urine collection period, a serum sample is obtained and assayed for creatinine. Creatinine clearance is calculated by dividing the rate of urinary excretion of creatinine (mg/min) by the serum concentration of creatinine (mg/ml), resulting in units of ml/min.

Determination of creatinine clearance gives a measure of glomerular filtration. In addition, the relationship between the rate constant for renal elimination of unchanged drug and creatinine clearance must be demonstrated. For the usual case of first-order renal elimination, that relationship is linear, and so a creatinine clearance of 50% of normal means that renal elimination of this drug would be expected to operate at 50%, and the rate of drug input should be reduced accordingly. For example, a drug administered 100 mg every 6 hours (400 mg in 24 hours) to a patient with normal creatinine clearance could be given 40 mg every 12 hours (80 mg in 24 hours), if the creatinine clearance decreased to only 20% of normal. It is assumed that other pathways for disappearance of this drug retain normal function.

Clearance is considered further in Chapter 4.

Box 3-2 Effect of urine pH on renal clearance for drugs that undergo tubular resorption

Bases Cleared Rapidly by Making Urine More Acidic	Acids Cleared Rapidly by Making Urine More Alkaline
Amphetamine	Acetazolamide
Chloroquine	Nitrofurantoin
Imipramine	Phenobarbital
Levorphanol	Probenecid
Mecamylamine	Salicylates
Quinine	Sulfathiazole

Pharmacogenetics

Variation in drug responses in different people can result from genetic differences in drug disposition. The study of this phenomenon is called **pharmacogenetics.** Differences in drug disposition are inherited in a way similar to inborn errors of metabolism but with major differences. Patients with pharmacogenetic abnormalities may lead normal lives and never encounter difficulties unless challenged with the drug capable of producing the aberrant response. A nutrient or its metabolite is not involved; rather, the problem is abnormal drug disposition. Pharmacogenetic differences result in either enhancement or reduction in intensity of the drug response, with its duration of action lengthened or shortened.

A plot of the plasma drug concentration curve in a population of patients receiving the same drug dosage results in a normal bell-shaped curve. However, if a genetic factor or factors are involved, the population

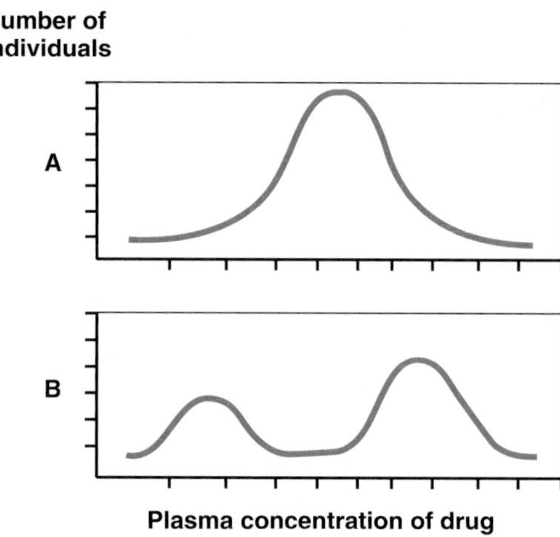

Figure 3-13 **A,** Frequency distribution curve shows the normal variability in plasma concentrations when a fixed dose of drug X is administered to a large population of patients. **B,** Frequency distribution curve under the same conditions with drug Y, indicating a bimodal curve typical of a pharmacogenetic alteration.

distribution curve is bimodal (or sometimes multimodal)—an indication of separate populations, one drug sensitive and one less drug sensitive (Fig. 3-13).

Genetic differences in enzyme activity associated with biotransformation of specific drugs is often responsible for differences in pharmacogenetics. An example is acetylation polymorphism. *N*-Acetylation of aromatic amines and hydrazines is one of several reactions for drug and chemical detoxification. Primary sites for acetylation are the liver and GI mucosa. Differences in *N*-acetylation were originally recognized in tuberculosis patients treated with isoniazid, a drug metabolized principally by this mechanism. By determining the plasma concentration at a specific time after a fixed dose of isoniazid, patients could be classified as slow or rapid acetylators, indicating that *N*-acetylating activity is distributed bimodally. Acetylation polymorphisms are now known to influence the metabolism of many drugs and chemicals (Box 3-3), in addition to isoniazid. This phenomenon varies widely with race and geographical distribution; 45% of whites and African-Americans in the United States are slow acetylators, whereas 10% of Asians are slow acetylators.

Consequently, acetylation polymorphism has important clinical and toxicological significance. The acetylation phenotype modulates metabolism of drugs with free amino groups, such as sulfonamides, hydralazine, procainamide, dapsone, and others. The metabolism of carcinogenic aromatic amines, such as benzidine and β-naphthylamine is also altered. Affected too are drugs, such as sulfasalazine, clonazepam, and nitrazepam—compounds lacking a free amino group initially but with one introduced during metabolic biotransformation. Slow acetylation is responsible for peripheral neuropathy in patients treated with isoniazid, for lupus erythematosus during procainamide and hydralazine treatment, for hemolytic anemia during sulfasalazine treatment, and for urinary bladder cancer after environmental exposure to benzidine.

Box 3-3 Some drugs and chemicals that undergo *N*-acetylation

Isoniazid	Nitrazepam
Hydralazine	Aminoglutethimide
Procainamide	β-Naphthylamine
Dapsone	Benzidine
Sulfonamides	Phenelzine
Clonazepam	

A cholinesterase (termed *pseudocholinesterase* or *butyrylcholinesterase*) is another drug-metabolizing enzyme found to be genetically altered in plasma and liver. This enzyme catalyzes the hydrolysis of succinylcholine, used as a muscle relaxant during surgery. Some patients hydrolyze a standard dose of succinylcholine more slowly, resulting in prolonged muscle relaxation and an ensuing apnea. These patients have an atypical plasma cholinesterase with an abnormally long duration of drug action resulting from reduced affinity of the aberrant enzyme for succinylcholine. The atypical enzyme gene has a ubiquitous distribution with an allele frequency of approximately 2% in many populations but is rare to undetectable in Africans, Filipinos, Eskimos, and Japanese. An enzyme variant several times more active than the normal enzyme has been reported that results in resistance to normal doses of succinylcholine.

Genetic differences among cytochrome P450s are implicated in differences in clearance of several drug classes. An example is seen in patients treated with the antihypertensive debrisoquine, which is normally hydroxylated to an inactive product in liver. Liver biopsy studies established that patients who were poor metabolizers of debrisoquine were deficient in cytochrome P450 activity, resulting from an ineffective binding of substrate to enzyme. Impaired metabolism of several other drugs is now considered to result from an aberrant or deficient cytochrome P450. These include dextromethorphan, phenytoin, nortriptyline, phenformin, and metoprolol.

Drugs can induce hemolytic anemia in patients genetically deficient in red blood cell glucose-6-phosphate dehydrogenase (Box 3-4). This enzyme, part

Box 3-4 Drugs capable of inducing hemolytic anemia in glucose-6-phosphate–deficient patients

Chloramphenicol
Chloroquine
Nitrofuran derivatives
p-Aminosalicylic acid
Primaquine
Sulfonamides
Vitamin K analogs

of the red blood cell hexose monophosphate shunt, is a primary source of reduced NADPH, a cofactor for glutathione reductase. Hemolysis of red blood cells results from the cell's inability to maintain sufficient reduced glutathione critical for maintaining reduced protein sulfhydryl groups. The oxidized state of glutathione promotes enzyme denaturation and erythrocyte membrane instability. Many glucose-6-phosphate dehydrogenase variants have been identified, and it is estimated that more than 200 million people worldwide have a variant enzyme.

These specific examples emphasize the importance of considering genetic variation in evaluating abnormal responses to drugs in patients.

Summary

Understanding the major routes of disposition of a drug and the factors that influence the functionality and capacity of each route can aid profoundly in the safe and effective use of drugs, especially in patients in whom the state of the disease has compromised one or more of the main drug disposition routes.

FURTHER READING

Freeman BD, McLeod HL. Challenges of implementing pharmacogenetics in the critical care environment. *Nat Rev Drug Discov* 2004; 3:88-93.

Guengerich FP. Cytochromes P450, drugs, and diseases. *Mol Interv* 2003; 3:194-204.

Self-assessment questions

1. Cell membranes are composed of:
   a. Phospholipids.
   b. Receptor proteins.
   c. DNA.
   d. *a* and *b*.
   e. All of the above are correct.

2. All of the following tend to lower the plasma concentration of a drug *except:*
   a. Metabolic biotransformation.
   b. Renal tubular reabsorption.
   c. Binding to plasma proteins.
   d. Renal secretion.
   e. Biliary excretion.

3. What is the approximate percentage of a weak acid (pK_a 5.4) in the nonionized form in plasma having a pH of 7.4?
   a. 99%
   b. 90%
   c. 10%
   d. 1%
   e. 0.1%

4. Passive diffusion of a drug across a lipid membrane is enhanced if:
   a. It is highly polar.
   b. It contains a quaternary nitrogen.
   c. A substantial gradient exists between extracellular and intracellular concentrations.
   d. The drug is water soluble and very lipid soluble.
   e. *c* and *d* are correct.

5. Drug oxidations frequently involve all of the following *except:*
   a. Cytochrome P450 proteins.
   b. NADH or NADPH cofactors.
   c. Liver endoplasmic reticulum.
   d. Esterases.
   e. Molecular oxygen.

6. Conjugation reactions:
   a. Occur with weak acids but not weak bases.
   b. Do not require the presence of drug-metabolizing enzymes.
   c. Need activation by high energy phosphate compounds.
   d. Can involve amino acids.
   e. *c* and *d* are correct.

CHAPTER 4

Clinical pharmacokinetics and issues in therapeutics

Andrew A. Somogyi

Drug concentrations

When planning drug therapy for a patient, deciding on the choice of drug and its dosing schedule are obviously essential. To make such decisions, an observable pharmacological effect is usually selected, and the dosing rate manipulated until this effect is observed. With some drugs this approach works quite well. For example, blood pressure can be monitored in a hypertensive patient (Fig. 4-1, *drug A*) and the dose of drug modified until blood pressure is reduced to the desired level. However, for other drugs, this approach is more problematic, usually due to the lack of an easily observable effect, a narrow **therapeutic index** (ratio of therapeutic to toxic dose), or changes in the condition of the patient that require modification of dosing rate.

For example, when an antibiotic with a low therapeutic index is used to treat a severe infection (Fig. 4-1, *drug B*), it can be difficult to quantify therapeutic progress because a visible effect is not immediately apparent. Because of its narrow therapeutic index, care must be taken so that the drug concentration does not become too high and cause toxicity. Similarly, if the desired effect is not easily visualized due to other considerations, such as inflammation in an internal organ, this approach is also problematic (Fig. 4-1, *drug C*). Finally, changes in the condition of the patient can also necessitate adjustments in dose rates. For example, if a drug is eliminated through the kidneys, changes in renal function will be important. Without an observable effect that is easily monitored (as with drugs B and C), it is not always clear that such adjustments are beneficial.

An alternative approach is to define a target drug concentration in blood, rather than an observable effect. The **plasma concentration** of a drug is usually chosen for simplicity and can be very useful in achieving therapeutic responses while minimizing undesirable side effects. This chapter will concentrate on factors controlling drug plasma concentration, how it changes with different routes and schedules of drug administration, and how drug input rates and dosing schedules can be rationally developed, or modified, to achieve plasma concentrations associated with beneficial therapeutic effects.

In most clinical situations, it is important to maintain an appropriate response for prolonged periods. This requires that the plasma concentration of drug must be maintained over the same period. Multiple doses or

Abbreviations

AUC	area under the drug plasma concentration–time curve
C_{ss}	steady state concentration
CL	clearance
CL_p	plasma clearance
F	bioavailability
$t_{1/2}$	half-life
T	dosing interval
V_d	apparent volume of distribution

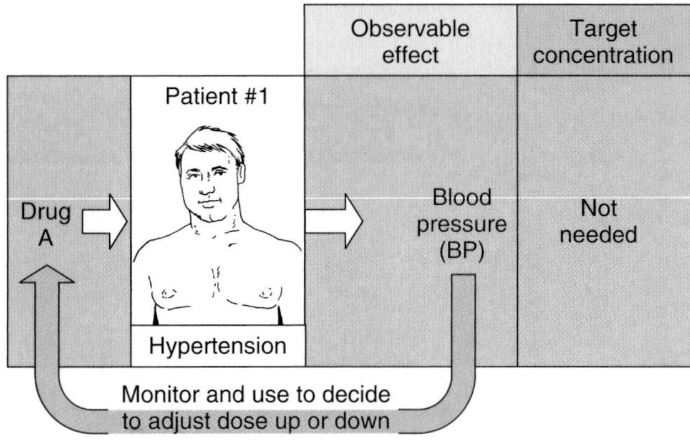

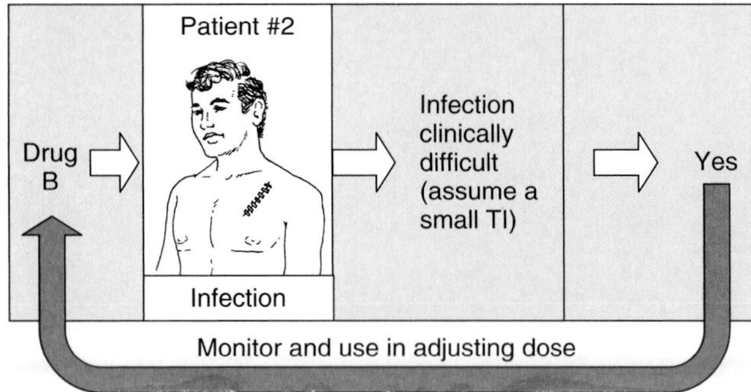

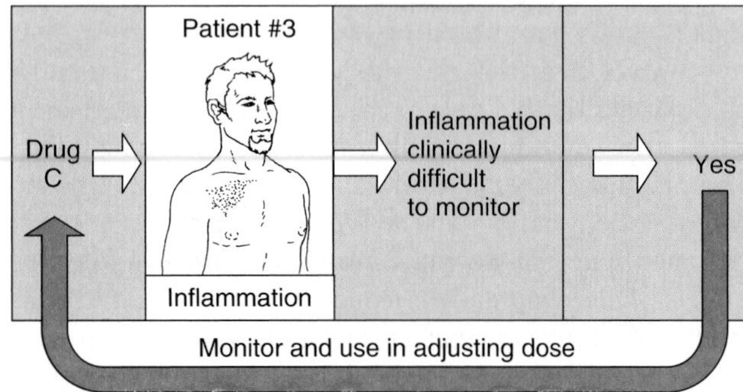

Figure 4-1 Concept of target plasma concentration of drug as an alternative to observable effect for determining whether drug input rate is sufficient or must be modified. *TI*, Therapeutic index. For a discussion of target concentration, see the text.

continuous administration is usually required, with dose size and frequency of administration constituting the **dosing schedule** or dosing regimen. In providing instructions for treatment of a patient, the choice of drug, the dosing schedule, and the mode and route of administration must be specified. Pharmacokinetic considerations have a major role in establishing the dosing schedule, or in adjusting an existing schedule, to increase effectiveness of the drug or to reduce symptoms of toxicity.

Before addressing how to design or adjust a dosing schedule, several key pharmacokinetic parameters and principles must be described. For clarity, a single acute dose of drug is presented here and used in a later part of this chapter for the design or modification of multiple dosing regimens. The relevant pharmacokinetic concepts and parameters can be developed either intuitively or mathematically and used in the rational design of dosing schedules. The emphasis in this chapter is to combine both approaches to stress general principles and parameters and provide sufficient background for understanding their general importance.

Box 4-1 Main routes of drug administration

Per os, by mouth

Oral (swallowed)
Sublingual (under the tongue)
Buccal (in the cheek pouch)

Injection

IV (intravenous)
IM (intramuscular)
SC (subcutaneous)
IA (intraarterial)
Intrathecal (into subarachnoid space)

Pulmonary

Rectal

Topical

Routes of administration

Major routes of administration are divided into (1) **enteral,** drugs entering the body via the gastrointestinal (GI) tract and (2) **parenteral,** drugs entering the body by injection. Specific examples are given in Box 4-1. The oral route is most popular because it is most convenient. However, poor absorption in the GI tract, first-pass metabolism in the liver, delays in stomach emptying, degradation by stomach acidity, or complexation with food may preclude oral administration. Intramuscular (IM) and subcutaneous (SC) routes bypass these problems. In many cases, absorption into the blood is rapid for drugs given IM and only slightly slower after SC administration. The advantage of the intravenous (IV) route is a very rapid onset of action and a controlled rate of administration; however, this is countered by the disadvantages of possible infection, coagulation problems, and a greater incidence of allergic reactions. Also, most injected drugs, especially when given IV, require trained personnel.

Dose adjustment for size of patient

The average male adult weighs approximately 70 kg and has a body surface area of 1.7 m^2. The dose of drug is sometimes scaled to give a constant mg/kg of body weight for persons of different sizes. For some drugs, especially with children, such scaling works better when based on body surface area, because this correlates better with cardiac output and glomerular filtration rate. Because it is easily measured, body weight is favored by most clinicians. Since therapeutic plasma concentrations of many drugs can cover a considerable range without evidence of toxicity, only in certain cases are significant dose adjustments required for patient size.

Single doses

Single-dose IV injection and plasma concentration

If a drug is injected as a single bolus over 5 to 30 seconds into a vein and blood samples are taken periodically and analyzed for the drug, the results appear as in Figure 4-2, *A*. The concentration will be greatest shortly after injection, when distribution of drug in the circulatory system has come to equilibrium. This initial mixing of drug and blood (red blood cells and plasma) is essentially complete after several passes through the heart. Drug leaves the plasma by several processes:

- Distribution across membranes to tissue or other body fluids
- Excretion of unchanged drug by renal or biliary routes
- Metabolism to other active or inactive compounds
- Exhalation through the lungs, if the drug is volatile

Some of the drug in plasma is bound to proteins or other plasma constituents; this binding occurs very rapidly and usually renders the bound portion of the drug inactive. Similarly, a considerable fraction of the injected dose may pass through capillary walls and bind to extravascular tissue, also rendering this fraction of drug inactive. The values of drug concentration plotted on the vertical scale in Figure 4-2 represent the sum of unbound drug and bound drug. Note that the concentration-time profile shows continuous curvature.

The data in Figure 4-2, *A*, are often more useful, if concentrations are plotted on a logarithmic scale (Fig. 4-2, *B*), resulting in the terminal data points (after 1 hour) lying on a straight line. The section marked "1" represents the **distribution phase** (sometimes called **alpha phase**), wherein the main process is distribution of drug across membranes and into body regions that are not well perfused. Section "2" (**beta phase** or **elimination**) is primarily influenced by elimination of the drug, which causes the gradual decrease in plasma concentration. In many clinical situations, the duration of the distribution phase is very short compared with that of the elimination phase.

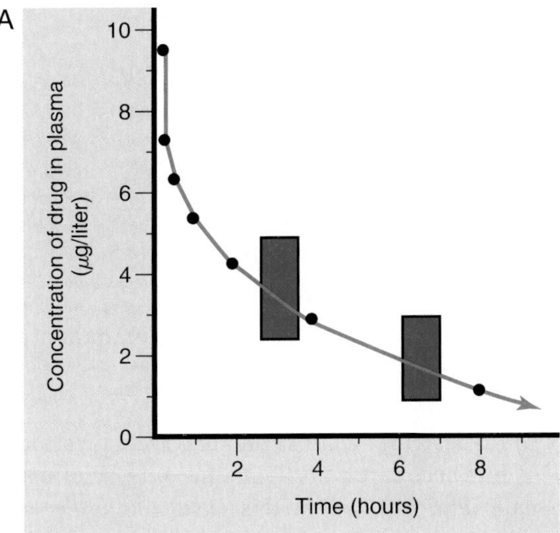

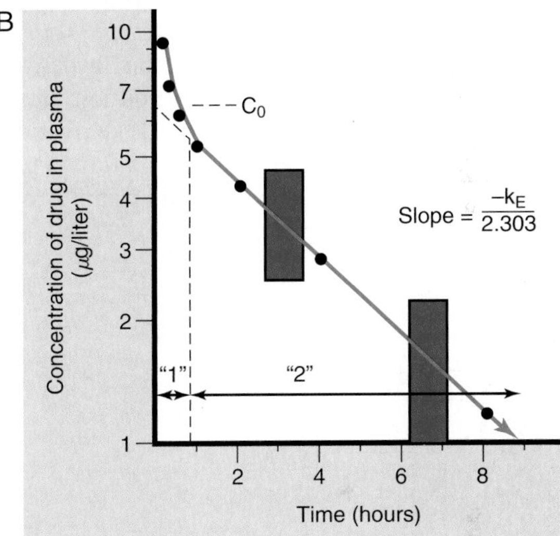

Figure 4-2 Plasma concentration of drug as a function of time after IV injection of a single bolus over 5 to 30 seconds. **A,** Arithmetic plot. **B,** Same data with concentrations plotted on a logarithmic scale. The 1 represents the distribution (or α) phase, and 2 represents the elimination (or β) phase. Fractional decrease in concentration is constant for a fixed time interval during the straight-line portion of **B,** shown here as an 18.6% decrease for any 1-hour period (*shaded areas*).

If the distribution phase in Figure 4-2, *A* or *B*, is neglected, the equation of the line is

$$C(t) = C_0 e^{-k_E t} \quad (1)$$

where:

$C(t)$ = Concentration of drug in the plasma at any time

C_0 = Concentration at time zero

e = Base for natural logarithms

k_E = First-order rate constant for the elimination phase

t = Time

Equation 1 describes a curve on an arithmetic scale (Fig. 4-2, *A*) but becomes a straight line on a semilogarithmic scale (Fig. 4-2, *B*). In this case, the slope will be $-k_E/2.3$, and the y-intercept is log C_0. A characteristic of this type of curve is that *a constant fraction of drug dose remaining in the body is eliminated per unit time.*

When elimination is rapid, the error in describing C(t) becomes appreciable if the distribution phase is omitted. Although the mathematical derivation is beyond the scope of this text, such a situation is plotted in Figure 4-3 to emphasize the importance of the distribution phase. For most drugs, distribution occurs much more rapidly than elimination, and therefore the distribution term becomes zero after only a small portion of the dose is eliminated. By back extrapolation of the linear postdistribution data, the value of C_0 can be obtained, whereas k_E can be determined from the slope. The concentration component responsible for the distribution phase (shaded area in Fig. 4-3) is obtained as the difference between the actual concentration and the extrapolated elimination line. This difference can be used to calculate the rate constant for distribution (k_d) and the extrapolated time zero-concentration component for the distribution phase (C^d_0). However, this complexity is often ignored because C(t) for many drugs can be described adequately in terms of the monoexponential equation 1. Therefore, the rest of this chapter deals only with the postdistribution phase kinetics described by equation 1.

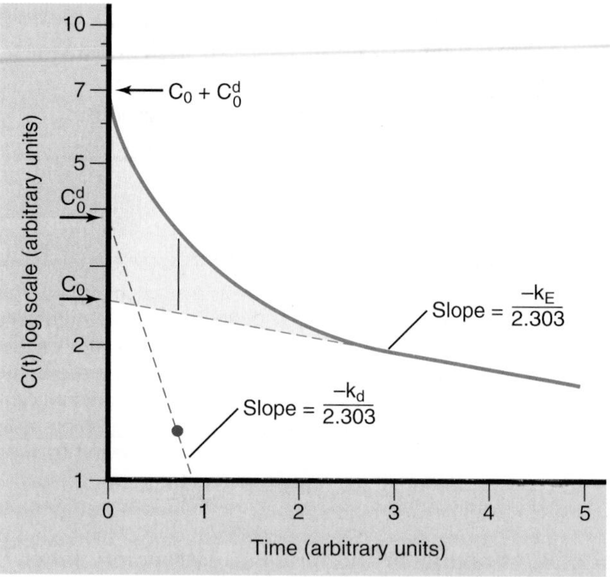

Figure 4-3 Semilogarithmic plot of plasma concentration of drug versus time where the distribution phase is included. Solid line represents an equation (not shown) governing distribution and elimination, which can be obtained using one of many available computer programs. This equation can also be obtained by graphical means in which extrapolation of the linear portion of the data (elimination phase) is used to obtain C_0 and k_E. The differences between the data points and the red dotted extrapolated line in the distribution phase (vertical line at 0.65 time units and plotted as 1.3 concentration units shaded area) are plotted (blue dotted line) and extrapolated linearly to obtain C^d_0 and k_d.

Single oral dose and plasma concentration

The plot of C(t) versus time after oral administration is different from that after IV injection only during the drug absorption phase, assuming equal bioavailability. The two plots become identical for the postabsorption or elimination phase. A typical plot of plasma concentration versus time after oral administration is shown in Figure 4-4. Initially, there is no drug in the plasma because the preparation must be swallowed, undergo dissolution if administered as a tablet, await stomach emptying, and be absorbed, mainly in the small intestine. As the plasma concentration of drug increases due to rapid absorption, the rate of elimination also increases, because elimination is usually a **first-order process**, where rate increases with increasing drug concentration. The peak concentration is reached when the rates of absorption and elimination are equal.

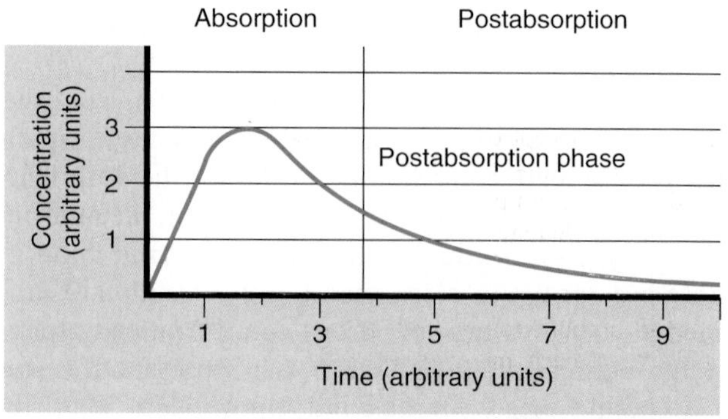

Figure 4-4 Typical profile for plasma concentration of drug versus time after oral administration and with a rate constant for drug absorption of at least 10 times larger than that for drug elimination.

Calculation of pharmacokinetic parameters

As shown in Figures 4-2 and 4-4, the concentration-time profile of a drug in plasma is different after IV and oral administration. The shape of the area under the concentration-time curve (AUC) is determined by several factors, including dose magnitude, route of administration, elimination capacity, and single or multiple dosing. Experimentally, the information derived from such profiles allows derivation of the important pharmacokinetic parameters—**clearance, volume of distribution, bioavailability,** and **half-life.** These terms are used to calculate drug dosing regimens.

Clearance

Drug clearance (CL) is defined as the volume of blood cleared of drug per unit time (e.g., ml/min) and describes the efficiency of elimination of a drug from the body. Clearance is an *independent* pharmacokinetic parameter; it does not depend on the volume of distribution, half-life, or bioavailability, and is the most important pharmacokinetic parameter to know about any drug. It can be considered to be the volume of blood from which all drug molecules must be removed each minute to achieve such a rate of removal (Fig. 4-5). Chapter 3 contains descriptions of the mechanisms of clearance by renal, hepatic, and other organs. Total body clearance is the sum of all of these and is constant for a particular drug in a specific patient, assuming no change in patient status.

The plot of plasma C(t) versus time (Fig. 4-2) shows the concentration of drug decreasing with time. The corresponding elimination rate (e.g., mg/min) represents the quantity of drug being removed. The rate of removal is assumed to follow first-order kinetics, and total body clearance can be defined as follows,

$$CL_p = \frac{\text{rate of elimination of drug (mg/min)}}{\text{plasma concentration of drug (mg/ml)}} \qquad \textbf{(2)}$$

where CL_p indicates total body removal from plasma (p).

Clinical utility of clearance Clearance is the parameter that determines the maintenance dose rate required to achieve the target plasma concentration at steady state.

$$\underset{\text{(mg/h)}}{\text{Maintenance dose rate}} = \underset{\text{(mg/L)}}{\text{target concentration}} \times \underset{\text{(L/h)}}{\text{clearance}} \qquad \textbf{(3)}$$

So for a given maintenance dose rate, steady state drug concentration is inversely proportional to clearance.

Volume of distribution

The actual volume in which drug molecules are distributed within the body cannot be measured. However, an apparent volume of distribution (V_d) can be obtained and is of some clinical utility. V_d is defined as the proportionality factor between the concentration of drug in blood or plasma and the total amount of drug in the body. Although it is a hypothetical term with no actual physical meaning, it can serve as an indicator of drug binding to plasma proteins or other tissue constituents. V_d can be calculated from the time zero concentration (C_0) after IV injection and the dose (D).

$$C_0 = D/V_d \qquad \textbf{(4)}$$

If C_0 is in mg/L and D in mg, then V_d would be in liters. In some cases it is meaningful to compare the apparent V_d with typical body water volumes. The following

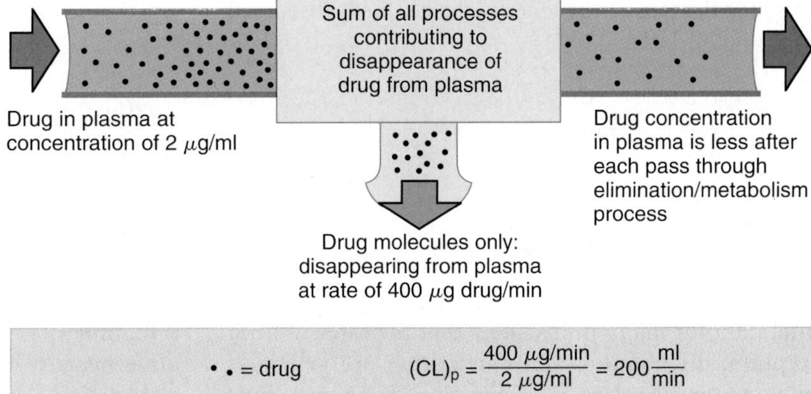

Figure 4-5 Concept of total body clearance of drug from plasma. Only some drug molecules disappear from plasma on each pass of blood through kidneys, liver, or other sites, contributing to drug disappearance (elimination). In this example, it required 200 ml of plasma to account for the amount of drug disappearance each minute (400 μg/min) at the concentration of 2 μg/ml. Total body clearance is thus 200 ml/min.

volumes in liters and percentage of body weight apply to adult humans:

Body Weight	Body Water (%)	Volume (approx. liters)
Plasma	4	3
Extracellular	20	15
Total body	60	45

Experimental values of V_d vary from 5 to 10 liters for drugs, such as warfarin and furosemide, to 15,000 to 40,000 liters for chloroquine and loratadine in a 70-kg adult. How can one have apparent V_d values grossly in excess of the total body volume? This usually occurs as a result of different degrees of protein and tissue binding of drugs and using plasma as the sole sampling source for determination of V_d (Fig. 4-6). For a drug, such as warfarin, that is 99% bound to plasma albumin at therapeutic concentrations, nearly all the initial dose is in the plasma, and so a plot of log plasma C(t) versus time, when extrapolated back to time zero, gives a large value for C_0 (for bound plus unbound drug). Using a rearranged equation 4, $V_d = D/C_0$, the resulting value of V_d is small (usually 2-10 L). At the other extreme is a drug, such as chloroquine, which binds strongly to tissue sites but weakly to plasma proteins. Most of the initial dose is at tissue sites, thereby resulting in very small concentrations in plasma samples. In this case, a plot of log plasma C(t) vs. time will give a small value for C_0 that can result in apparent V_d values greatly in excess of total body volume.

V_d can serve as a guide in determining whether a drug is bound primarily to plasma or tissue sites or distributed primarily in plasma or extracellular spaces. V_d is also an *independent* pharmacokinetic parameter and does not depend on clearance, half-life, or bioavailability.

Clinical utility of V_d In some clinical situations it is important to achieve the target drug concentration (C_{ss}) instantaneously. A loading dose is often used, and V_d determines the size of the loading dose. This is discussed in more detail later.

$$\underset{(mg)}{\text{Loading dose}} = \underset{(mg/L)}{C_{ss}} \times \underset{(L)}{V_d} \qquad (5)$$

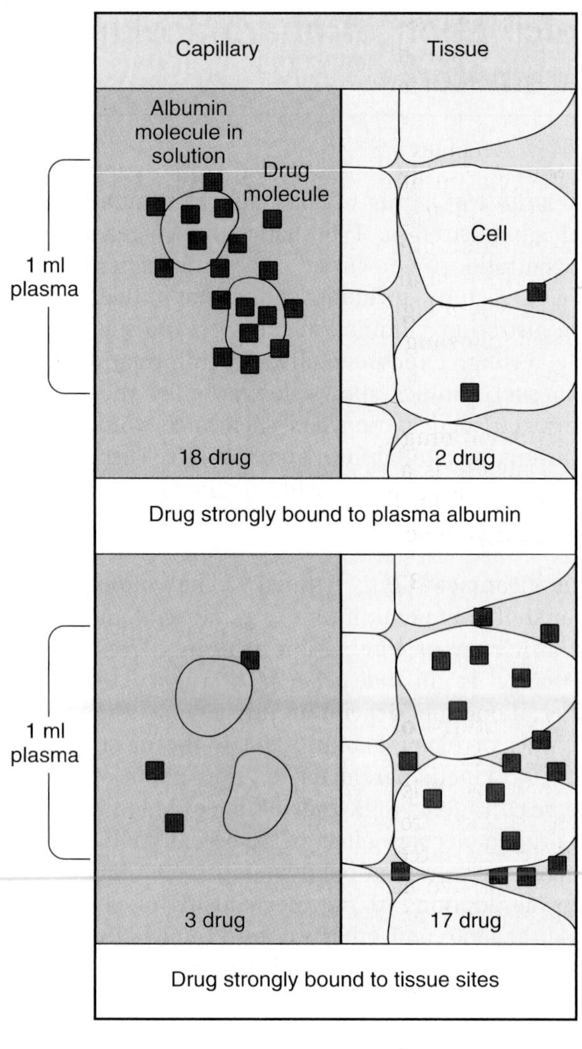

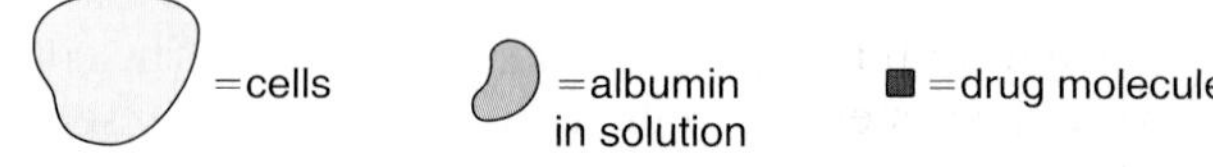

Figure 4-6 Influence of drug binding to plasma protein versus tissue sites on apparent volume of distribution. Numbers represent relative quantity of drug in 1 ml of plasma as compared with adjacent tissue. Only the plasma is sampled to determine V_d, and the albumin-bound drug is included in this sample.

Half-life

Equation 1 for C(t) was given earlier without explanation of its derivation or functional meaning. Experimental data for many drugs show that the rates of drug absorption, distribution, and elimination are generally directly proportional to concentration. Such processes follow **first-order kinetics** because the rate varies with the first power of the concentration. This is shown quantitatively

$$(dC(t)/dt) = -k_E C(t) \qquad (6)$$

where dC(t)/dt is the rate of change of drug concentration, and k_E is the **elimination rate constant.** It is negative because the concentration is being decreased by elimination.

Rate processes can also occur through **zero-order kinetics**, where the rate is independent of concentration. Two prominent examples are the metabolism of ethanol and phenytoin. Under such conditions the process becomes saturated, and the rate of metabolism is independent of drug concentration.

Half-life ($t_{1/2}$) is defined as the time it takes for the concentration of drug to decrease by half. The value of $t_{1/2}$ can be read directly from a graph of log C(t) versus t, as shown in Figure 4-2. Note that half-life can be calculated following any route of administration (e.g., oral or subcutaneous). Values of $t_{1/2}$ for the elimination phase range in practice from several minutes to days or longer for different drugs.

Half-life is a *dependent* pharmacokinetic parameter derived from the independent parameters of clearance and volume of distribution.

$$t_{1/2} = (0.693 \times V_d)/CL \qquad (7)$$

Changes in the half-life of a drug can be due to a change in clearance, V_d, or both.

Clinical utility of half-life Half-life determines how long it takes to reach steady state after multiple dosing or when dosage is altered and how long it takes to eliminate the drug from the body when dosing is ended. It is generally agreed that steady state is achieved after dosages of five half-lives. When dosing is terminated, most of the drug will have been eliminated after five half-lives (but could still exist as metabolites with longer half-lives).

Bioavailability and first-pass effect

Bioavailability (F) is defined as the fraction of the drug reaching the systemic circulation following administration. When a drug is administered by IV injection, the entire dose enters the circulation and F is 100%. However, this is not true for most drugs administered by other routes, especially drugs given orally.

$$F = \frac{(AUC)_{oral}}{(AUC)_{IV}} \times \frac{dose_{IV}}{dose_{oral}} \qquad (8)$$

Physical or chemical processes that account for reduced bioavailability include poor solubility, incomplete absorption in the GI tract, metabolism in the enterocytes lining the intestinal wall, efflux transport out of enterocytes back into the intestinal lumen, and rapid metabolism during the first pass of the drug through the liver. Values of F can be determined by comparing the area under the curves (AUC) for oral and IV doses. In interpreting bioavailability, clearance is assumed to be independent of the route of administration. For drugs in which absorption from the GI tract is not always 100%, the drug formulations must now pass a stringent bioavailability test to verify that bioavailability is constant, within certain limits, among lots, and between generic formulations.

Low bioavailability can also result when the drug is well absorbed from the GI tract, but metabolism is high during its transit from the splanchnic capillary beds through the liver and into the systemic circulation. The drug concentration in the plasma is at its highest level during this "**first pass**" through the liver. Therefore, drugs that are metabolized by the liver may encounter a very significant reduction in their plasma concentration during this first pass. For example, the first-pass effect of lidocaine is so large that this drug is not administered orally. Some drugs that show high first-pass effects include, but are not limited to, felodipine and propranolol (antihypertensives), isoproterenol (bronchodilator), methylphenidate (CNS stimulant), morphine and propoxyphene (analgesics), sumatriptan (antimigraine), and venlafaxine (antidepressant).

In summary, there are two calculations that need to be performed on plasma concentration-time data: the area under the curve (AUC) and the terminal slope. These two calculations can then be used to calculate clearance, volume of distribution, half-life, and bioavailability.

Binding of drug to plasma constituents

The degree of binding of a drug to plasma constituents is important because it helps in interpreting the mechanisms of clearance and volume of distribution. The free drug concentration is referred to as the unbound fraction. Some drugs, such as caffeine, have high unbound fractions (0.9), whereas other drugs, such as warfarin, have low unbound fractions (0.01).

The rates of drug disappearance and the concentration of free drug available to the site of action are altered substantially, if a significant portion of the drug is plasma bound. Clinical tests for plasma drug concentrations are based on the total (bound plus unbound) concentration of drug and do not provide information about protein binding. A knowledge of the free drug concentration in plasma would be clinically useful because only the free drug is available to interact at its receptor(s) but is only rarely available.

The binding of drugs to plasma or serum constituents involves primarily albumin, α_1-acid glycoprotein, or lipoprotein (Table 4-1). Serum albumin is the most abundant protein in human plasma. It is synthesized in the liver at roughly 140 mg/kg of body weight/day under normal conditions, but this can change dramatically in certain disease states. Many acidic drugs bind strongly to albumin, but because of the normally high concentration of plasma albumin,

Table 4-1 Drugs that bind appreciably to serum or plasma constituents

Bind Primarily to Albumin	Bind Primarily to α_1-Acid Glycoprotein	Bind Primarily to Lipoproteins
Barbiturates	Alprenolol	Amphotericin B
Benzodiazepines	Bupivacaine†	Cyclosporin
Bilirubin*	Dipyridamole	Tacrolimus
Digitoxin	Disopyramide	
Fatty acids*	Etidocaine	
Penicillins	Imipramine	
Phenylbutazone	Lidocaine‡	
Phenytoin	Methadone	
Probenecid	Prazosin	
Streptomycin	Propranolol	
Sulfonamides	Quinidine	
Tetracycline	Sirolimus	
Tolbutamide	Verapamil	
Valproic acid		
Warfarin		

*May be displaced by drugs in some disease states.
†In Japan the drug name is bupivacain.
‡In the UK the drug name is lignocaine.

drug binding does not saturate all the sites. Basic drugs bind primarily to α_1-acid glycoprotein, which is present in plasma at much lower concentrations than albumin but varies more widely between and within people due to disease. Less is known about drug binding to lipoproteins, although this is also often altered during disease.

Multiple or prolonged dosing

As mentioned earlier, most drugs require administration over a prolonged period to achieve the desired therapeutic effect. The two principal modes of administration employed to achieve such a prolonged effectiveness are continuous IV infusion or discrete multiple doses on a designated dosing schedule. The basic objective is to increase the plasma concentration of drug until a steady state is reached that produces the desired therapeutic effect with little or no toxicity. This steady state concentration is then maintained for minutes, hours, days, weeks, or longer, as required by the situation. Pharmacokinetic considerations for designing or adjusting continuous infusion or discrete multiple dosing schedules are described later.

Continuous intravenous infusion

Continuous intravenous infusion of a drug is used when it is necessary to obtain a rapid onset of action and

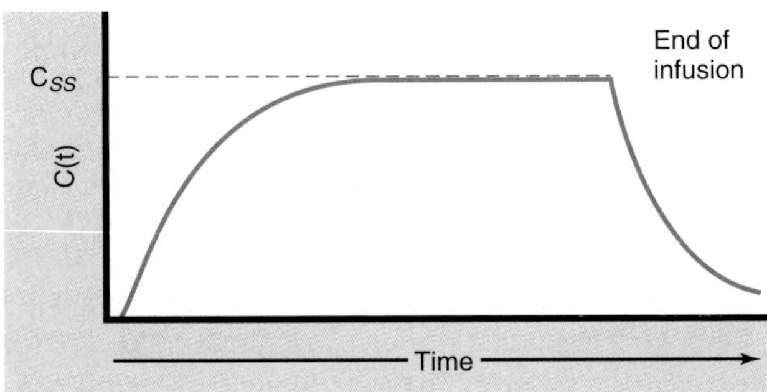

Figure 4-7 Typical profile showing drug plasma concentrations with time for continuous IV injection (called infusion) at a constant rate and without a loading dose. C_{ss} is the concentration at plateau, or steady state, where rate of drug input equals rate of drug elimination. At termination of infusion, decay in the concentration will be the same as for any acute IV injection with C_o being equal to C_{ss}.

maintain this action for an extended period under controlled conditions. This usually occurs in a hospital or emergency setting.

During continuous infusion, the drug is administered at a fixed rate. The plasma concentration of drug gradually increases and then plateaus at a concentration where the rate of infusion equals the rate of elimination. A typical plasma concentration profile is shown in Figure 4-7. The plateau is also called the steady state concentration (C_{ss}). Key points are:

- At steady state the rate of drug input must equal the rate of drug disappearance.
- The input rate is the infusion rate (mg/min).
- Conversion of the steady state concentration (mg/L) to the disappearance rate (mg/min) requires a knowledge of clearance (L/min).
- Thus, at steady state one calculates the maintenance dose rate = target concentration × clearance (Equation 3).

The plateau concentration is influenced by the infusion rate and the total body clearance. Of these factors, only the infusion rate can be easily modified. For example, if the plateau concentration is 2 ng/ml with an infusion rate of 16 μg/hr, and it is determined that the concentration is too high, such that 1.5 ng/ml would be better, this concentration can be achieved by decreasing the infusion rate by 25% to 12 μg/hr, which should give a 25% decrease in the plateau concentration. The length of time necessary to achieve the new plateau concentration is discussed later.

Dosing schedule

Discrete multiple dosing is usually specified so that the size of the dose and T (the time between doses) are fixed.

Two considerations are important in selecting T. Smaller intervals result in minimal fluctuations in plasma drug concentration; however, the interval must be a relatively standard number of hours to ensure patient compliance. In addition, for oral dosing the quantity must be compatible with the size of available preparations. Thus, an oral dosing schedule of 28 mg every 2.8 hours is impractical, because the drug is probably not available as a 28-mg tablet, and taking a tablet every 2.8 hours is completely impractical. More practical dosing intervals for patient compliance are every 6, 8, 12, or 24 hours.

The plasma concentration of drug versus time is shown in Figure 4-8 for multiple dosing by repeated IV injections. In *panel A,* T is selected so that all drug from the previous dose disappears before the next dose is injected and there is no accumulation of drug, and no plateau or steady state is reached. If a plateau concentration is desired, T must be short enough so that some drug from the previous dose is still present when the next dose is administered. In this way the plasma concentration gradually increases until the drug lost by elimination during T is equal to the dose of drug added at the start of T. When this is achieved, the mean concentration for each time period has plateaued. This stepwise accumulation is illustrated by *panel B* in Figure 4-8, where a plot of plasma drug concentration versus time for multiple IV injections is shown, with T roughly equivalent to the half-life of drug elimination. The average rate (over a dose interval) of drug input is constant at D/T. The amount of drug eliminated is small during the first T but increases with drug concentration during subsequent intervals, until the average rate of elimination and the average rate of input are equal. That is, the dose is eliminated during T. For significant accumulation, T must be at least as short as the half-life and preferably shorter.

At the plateau, the mean concentration of drug (C_{ss}) is equal to the input dose rate divided by the clearance, just as for continuous infusion.

$$\text{mean } C_{ss} = (D/T)/CL_p \quad \textbf{(9)}$$

This equation illustrates that the size of the dose or the duration of T can be changed to modify the mean plateau concentration of drug during multiple dosing regimens.

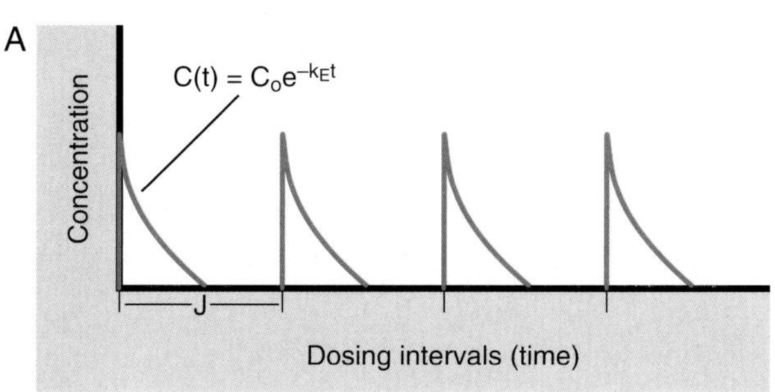

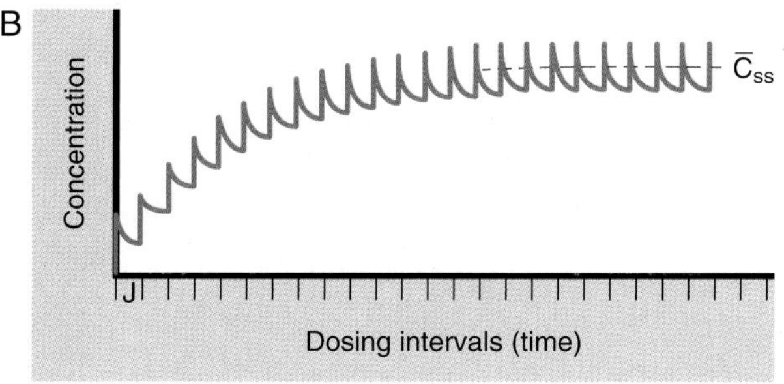

Figure 4-8 Discrete multiple-dosing profile of plasma concentration of drug given by IV injections with the same dose given each time. **A,** T is long enough so that each dose completely disappears before administration of the next dose. **B,** T is much shorter so that drug from previous injection is present prior to administration of the next dose. Accumulation results, with C_{ss} representing the mean concentration of drug at plateau level, where the mean rate of drug input equals the mean rate of drug elimination for each T. No loading dose is shown.

Loading dose

If all of the multiple doses are the same size, the term **maintenance dose** is used. In certain clinical situations, however, a more rapid onset of action is required, which can be achieved by giving a much larger, or **loading dose,** before starting the smaller maintenance dose regimen. A single IV loading dose (bolus) is often used before starting a continuous IV infusion, or a parenteral or oral loading dose may be used at the start of discrete multiple dosing. Ideally, the loading dose is calculated to raise the plasma drug concentration immediately to the plateau target concentration (see equation 5), and the maintenance doses are designed to maintain the same plateau concentration. Multiplying the plateau concentration by the apparent volume of distribution results in a value for the loading dose (see equation 5). However, the uncertainty in V_d for individual patients usually leads to administration of a more conservative loading dose to prevent overshooting the plateau and encountering toxic concentrations. This is particularly important with drugs with a narrow therapeutic index.

Duration of time to steady state

For a continuous IV infusion or a series of discrete multiple doses, the time to reach the plateau concentration or to move from one plateau concentration to another depends only on the half-life of the drug. After one half-life, 50% of plateau steady state concentration is achieved. In practice, steady state occurs when 95% of the plateau steady state concentration has been achieved, which occurs after five half-lives. In summary, clearance determines the steady state concentrations and half-life determines when steady state has been achieved.

Practical example

A patient has received the cardiac drug digoxin orally at 0.25 mg (one tablet/day) for several weeks, and symptoms of toxicity have recently appeared. A blood sample was taken and assayed to give a plasma concentration of 3.2 ng/ml (in the toxic range). For therapeutic reasons, you do not want to drop the plasma concentration too low, but decide to try reducing it to 1.6 ng/ml. What new dosing schedule should be used and how long will it take to reach the new plateau?

The once-a-day dosing interval is convenient; so you now specify 0.125 mg/day (one-half tablet/day); a 50% reduction in the plateau level requires a 50% decrease in dose. There are two options for reaching the lower plateau: (1) Immediately switch to the 0.125 mg/day dosing rate and achieve the 1.6 ng/ml concentration in approximately five half-lives (you do not know what the half-life for digoxin is in your patient), or (2) stop the digoxin dosing for an unknown number of days until the concentration reaches 1.6 ng/ml, and then begin again at a dosing schedule of 0.125 mg/day. The second procedure undoubtedly will be more rapid, but you must determine how many days to wait. You decide to stop all digoxin dosing, wait 24 hours from the previous 3.2 ng/ml sample, and get another blood sample. The concentration now has decreased to 2.7 ng/ml or by about one-sixth in a day. From equation 1, the fractional decrease each day should remain constant. Therefore, a decrease of one-sixth of the remaining concentration each day should result in 2.25 ng/ml after day 2, 1.85 ng/ml after day 3, and 1.55 ng/ml after day 4. Therefore, by withholding drug for a total of 4 days, you can reduce the plasma concentration to 1.6 ng/ml. Because the half-life is calculated to be 3.8 days in this patient, switching to the 0.125 mg/day dosing rate without withholding drug would have required 15 to 19 days to reach the 1.6 ng/ml concentration.

Clearance and elimination

Elimination refers to the removal of drug from the body. There are two processes involved in drug elimination, as discussed in Chapter 3. Metabolism, in which there is conversion of the drug to another chemical species, and excretion, in which there is loss of the chemically unchanged form of the drug. The two principal organs of elimination are the liver and kidneys. The liver is mainly concerned with metabolism but has a minor role in excretion of some drugs into the bile. The kidney is mainly involved in drug excretion.

Determination of relative importance of metabolism and renal excretion to drug elimination

The relative importance of the two elimination pathways is often determined by giving a dose (IV) of drug, collecting all urine over five half-lives, measuring how much unchanged drug is present in urine (the rest is assumed to have been metabolized), and expressing this as a fraction of the dose. This is called the fraction excreted unchanged and can vary from less than 5% (essentially all the drug is metabolized, for example, amiodarone) to greater than 90% (essentially none of the drug is metabolized, for example, gentamicin). The fraction of the dose metabolized is one minus the fraction excreted unchanged.

Total body clearance of a drug is simply the sum of clearances across the organs of elimination, usually kidney and liver.

$$\text{Total clearance} = \text{renal clearance} + \text{hepatic clearance} + (\text{other minor clearances}) \quad (10)$$

That is, individual organ clearances are additive so that renal clearance can be calculated by multiplying the fraction excreted unchanged by total clearance; therefore, nonrenal (usually inferred to be hepatic) clearance is calculated as total clearance minus renal clearance.

Physiological concepts of clearance and bioavailability

As discussed earlier, clearance is the most important pharmacokinetic parameter, because it controls the steady state concentration of a drug.

Clearance by the liver

Having determined that a drug is mainly cleared by hepatic mechanisms (metabolism) and having calculated a value for hepatic clearance, it is important to relate this to the functions (blood flow, enzyme activity) of liver. For example, if hepatic clearance of a drug is calculated to be 1000 ml/min and liver blood flow is 1500 ml/min, it does not mean that 1000 ml of blood going through liver is totally cleared of drug and the other 500 ml/min is not cleared of drug. It means that 1000/1500 (i.e., two-thirds) of the drug in blood entering liver is irreversibly removed (usually metabolized) by liver in one pass. The two-thirds refers to the hepatic extraction ratio (E), which is the fraction of the unbound dose of drug entering the liver from blood that is irreversibly eliminated (metabolized) during one pass through the liver.

$$\text{Extraction ratio (E)} = \frac{\text{rate of elimination}}{\text{rate of entry}} \quad \textbf{(11)}$$

Note that E can range from zero (no extraction) to 1.0 (complete extraction). If Q is liver blood flow, then clearance by the liver can be described by the following equation.

$$CL = Q \times E \quad \textbf{(12)}$$

Thus, clearance of a drug by any eliminating organ is a function of blood flow rate (rate of delivery) to the organ and the extraction ratio (efficiency of drug removal). It should now be clear that clearance of any drug cannot exceed the blood flow rate to its eliminating organ. In the case of drugs metabolized by liver, the maximum hepatic clearance value is about 1.5 L/min. For kidney, the maximum renal clearance value is 1.2 L/min (kidney blood flow).

For drugs cleared by the liver, hepatic clearance and bioavailability can be described in terms of three important physiologically-based determinants: liver blood flow (Q), unbound fraction in plasma, and liver drug metabolizing activity.

Most hepatically eliminated drugs are classified as being either low or high (hepatic) clearance. This makes it possible to predict the influence of altered liver function or drug interactions on plasma concentrations and pharmacological response. For example, metabolism of a drug is often reduced in patients with liver disease, or when a second drug inhibits its metabolic enzyme. For a high clearance drug, this results in no change in the plasma concentration-time profile after IV dosing, because blood flow is the sole determinant of clearance (whereas plasma and tissue binding are determinants of V_d). However, when the drug is administered orally, a decrease in metabolism will result in a small reduction in E, and therefore a large increase in bioavailability, resulting in substantially increased plasma concentrations. For a low hepatic clearance drug, a decrease in metabolism will cause increased concentrations after IV dosing, because metabolism is a determinant of clearance. There will be no change in bioavailability, however, because that is already close to 100%. On the other hand, concentrations after oral dosing will be raised because clearance has decreased. The outcome of this scenario is that for a low clearance drug, both oral and IV dose may need to be reduced to avoid toxicity, but for a high clearance drug, only oral dose may need adjustment (Fig. 4-9).

In summary, it is important to know which drugs are eliminated via renal or hepatic mechanisms. If the latter, then it is important to characterize the drug as being of low or high clearance. If low, enzyme activity and binding are determinants of clearance, and bioavailability is unchanged. If high, liver blood flow is the sole determinant of clearance, and blood flow, binding, and enzyme activity all impact on bioavailability. From these parameters, it is then often possible to predict the effect of disease (e.g., liver, cardiac) and administration of other drugs on the resultant pharma-

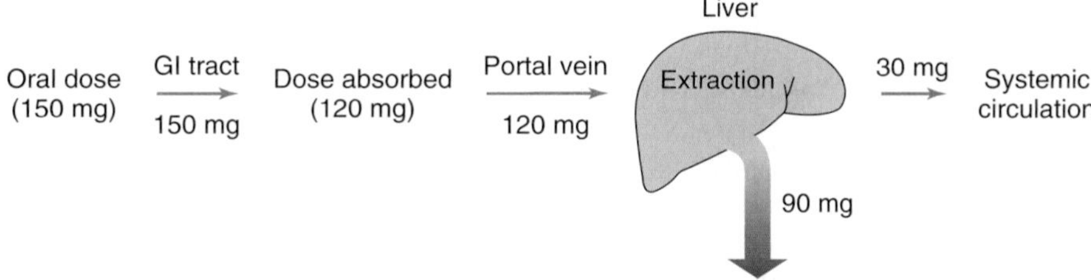

Figure 4-9 Determinants of oral bioavailability: 150 mg of drug is swallowed, enters the lumen of the GI tract, and 120 mg is absorbed (30 mg is lost due to one or a combination of mechanisms) and enters the portal vein, which drains into the liver. The hepatic extraction ratio is 0.75, and the fraction escaping this first pass loss is 0.25. Bioavailability is the fraction of the absorbed dose (0.8) entering the portal vein multiplied by the fraction escaping first-pass metabolism (0.25). In this example, bioavailability is 20% (or 30 mg/150 mg). (Adapted from Birkett DJ. Pharmacokinetics made easy. Sydney, McGraw-Hill, 2002.)

cokinetics of the drug, which helps in designing a rational dosage regimen.

Drug use at the extremes of age

Pharmacokinetic, pharmacodynamic, and pharmacological responses differ between young adults and infants and between young adults and the elderly. These differences are due to the many physiological changes that occur during the normal life span, but especially at the extremes, the infant and the elderly (Fig. 4-10).

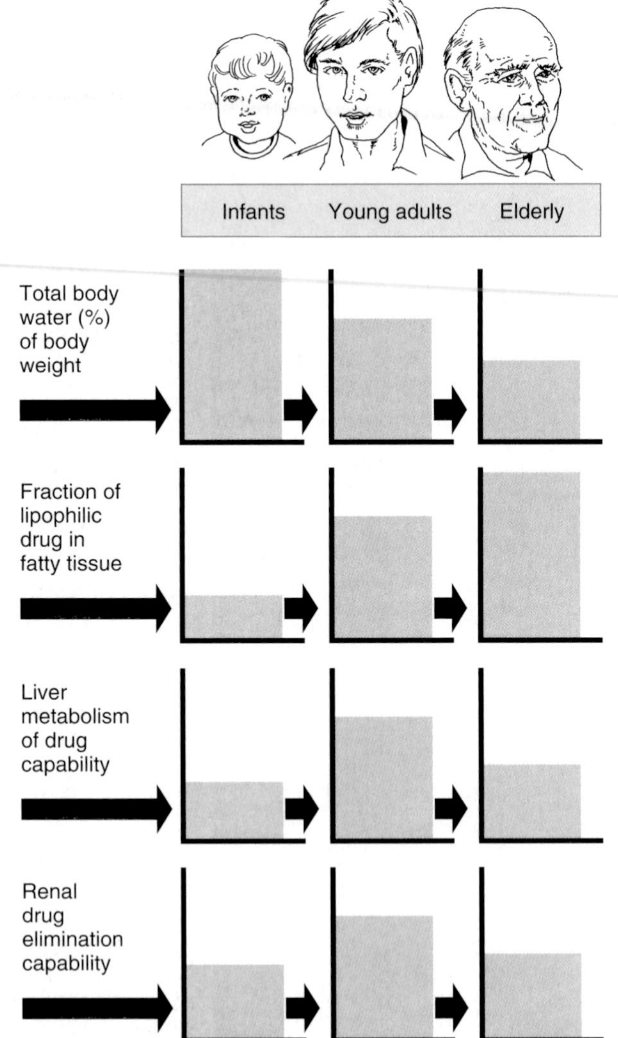

Figure 4-10 Areas of boxes indicate relative size or capability of function at each age.

Drug dosing in neonates

The limited understanding of the clinical pharmacology of specific drugs in pediatric patients predisposes this population to problems in the course of drug treatment, particularly in younger children, such as newborns. The absence of specific FDA requirements for pediatric studies and the resulting reliance on pharmacological and efficacy data derived primarily from adults to determine doses for use of drugs in children invites for suboptimal drug therapy. The problems of establishing efficacy and dosing guidelines for infants is further complicated by the fact that the pharmacokinetics of many drugs change appreciably as an infant ages from birth (sometimes prematurely) to several months after birth. The dose-response relationships of some drugs may change markedly during the first few weeks after birth.

The physiological changes that occur during the first month include higher than normal gastric pH, prolonged gastric emptying (compounded by gastroesophageal reflux, respiratory distress syndrome, and congenital heart disease), lower adipose tissue and higher total body water content, decreased plasma albumin, drug metabolizing activity, glomerular filtration, and tubular secretion. These result in decreased drug clearance and oral absorption and increased volume of distribution for water soluble drugs but decreased volume of distribution for lipid soluble drugs. Because of these dramatic and continuously changing parameters, dosing in neonates (<1 year) requires the advice of specialists.

Because of the often compromised cardiac output and peripheral perfusion of seriously ill infants, IV drug administration is generally used to ensure adequate systemic delivery of the agent. The potential problems with such treatment can be serious, and to minimize such problems requires the dilution and timed administration of small dosage volumes, the maintenance of fluid balance, and consideration of the effect of the specific drug administration technique on resultant serum concentrations.

Certain drugs pose particular difficulties when used in neonates or during the perinatal period because of the unique characteristics of their distribution or elimination in patients in this age group or because of the unusual side effects they may cause. These drugs include the antibiotics, digoxin, methylxanthines, and indomethacin. These issues are covered later in the chapters discussing these drugs.

Drug dosing in aged patients

The rational use of drugs by the elderly population (>65 years) is a challenge for both patient and prescriber. Compared with young adults, the elderly have an

Box 4-2 Factors contributing to altered drug effects in the elderly

Altered drug absorption and disposition

Decreased gastric acid
Decreased lean body mass
Increased percentage of body fat
Decreased liver mass and blood flow
Reduced renal function

Altered response to drug

Altered receptor and/or postreceptor properties
Impaired sensitivity of homeostatic mechanisms
Common diseases: diabetes, arthritis, hypertension, coronary artery disease, cancer, glaucoma

Social and economic factors

Inadequate nutrition
Multiple-drug therapy
Noncompliance

increased incidence of chronic illness and multiple diseases, take more drugs (prescription and over the counter) and drug combinations, and have more adverse drug reactions. Inadequate nutrition, decreased financial resources, and poor adherence to medication schedules may also contribute to inadequate drug therapy. These factors are compounded by the decline in physiological functions as part of the normal aging process, leading to altered drug disposition and sensitivity (Box 4-2). The elderly can have a different and more variable response to drugs compared to young adults. Drug selection and decisions about dosage in the elderly are largely based on trial and error, anecdotal data, and clinical impression. Following selection of the most appropriate drug, the dosing schedule should be "start low, go slow."

Pharmacokinetic changes with aging

Physiological changes

Several physiological functions decline beginning between 30 and 45 years of age and have important influences on pharmacokinetics. Of course, such changes are highly individualized, and some elderly people show little changes compared to population means. Cardiac output decreases about 1% a year beginning at 30 years of age, and in the elderly is associated with a redistribution of blood flow favoring the brain, heart, and kidney, and a reduction in hepatic blood flow. The percent of lean body mass also declines with age, whereas total body water decreases by 10% to 15% between 20 and 80 years of age. Plasma albumin concentrations are also lower in the elderly, particularly in the chronically ill or poorly nourished. Concentrations of α_1-acid glycoprotein increase, but do so more sharply in response to acute illness than simply aging. Glomerular filtration rate and effective renal plasma flow decline steadily with advancing age, although the serum creatinine concentration does not, due to the smaller lean body mass. The tubular secretory capacity declines in parallel with the glomerular filtration rate.

Drug absorption

Several physiological alterations in gastrointestinal (GI) function have been reported to occur with aging, although there is little clinically significant alteration in drug absorption in the elderly. One exception is a threefold increase in the bioavailability of levodopa, stemming from the reduced activity of dopa decarboxylase in the stomach wall.

Drug distribution

The reduced lean body mass, reduced total body water content, increased fat, and decreased plasma albumin concentration in the elderly can contribute to significant alterations in drug distribution, depending on the physiochemical properties of individual drugs. Lipid-soluble drugs, such as diazepam and lidocaine, have a larger V_d in the elderly, whereas water-soluble drugs, such as acetaminophen and ethanol, have a smaller V_d. Digoxin also has a lower V_d in the elderly, and therefore loading doses must be reduced. There are slightly lower plasma albumin concentrations in healthy elderly patients, whereas the hospitalized or poorly nourished elderly patient may have decreases of 10% to 20%.

Drug metabolism

The decline in the ability of the elderly to metabolize most drugs is relatively small and difficult to predict. In general, Phase I metabolic reactions decrease slightly with aging, whereas conjugation reactions, such as glucuronidation, are not greatly affected. The effects of cigarette smoking, diet, and alcohol consumption may be more important than physiological hepatic changes. For example, decreased dietary protein intake or reduction in cigarette smoking may lead to decreased liver microsomal enzyme activity. Whereas hepatic enzyme inhibition by drugs is similar in the elderly compared with young adults, the response to enzyme inducers (cigarette smoke, drugs, etc.) is more variable.

Hepatic clearance and first-pass metabolism

For drugs with a high hepatic clearance, the age-related decline in total liver blood flow of about 40% results in a similar reduction in total body clearance. The effect on first-pass hepatic extraction (and hence bioavailability) is complicated by potential alterations in other physiological variables, such as protein binding and enzyme activity. In healthy elderly subjects, first-pass metabolism and bioavailability are generally not markedly altered. However, on chronic oral dosing, the higher plasma concentrations often observed in the elderly are due to reduced Phase I metabolism, irrespective of whether the drug has a high or low hepatic clearance.

Renal clearance

Consistent with the physiological decline in renal function that occurs with aging, the rate of elimination of drugs excreted by the kidney is reduced. Such drugs include aminoglycosides, lithium carbonate, metformin, allopurinol (due to its active metabolite), and digoxin. To prevent drug toxicity, renal function must be estimated and downward adjustments in dosage made accordingly. Although there are no absolute guidelines, two general principles apply. First, most elderly patients do not have "normal" renal function even though serum creatinine appears "normal." Second, most elderly patients require adjustments in dosage for drugs (or drugs with active metabolites) eliminated primarily by the kidneys.

The decreased rate of elimination of inhalation anesthetics, resulting from declining **pulmonary function** with aging, is another important consideration for elderly patients receiving general anesthesia.

Drug response changes associated with aging

Changes in drug responses in the elderly have been less studied than have pharmacokinetic changes. In general, an enhanced response can be expected (Table 4-2), and a reduced dosage schedule is recommended to prevent serious side effects for many drugs. Reduced responses to some drugs, such as the β-adrenergic receptor agonist isoproterenol, do occur, however, through nonpharmacokinetic mechanisms, such as age-related changes in receptors and postreceptor signaling mechanisms, changes in homeostatic control, and disease-induced changes.

Table 4-2 Altered drug responses in the elderly

Drugs	Direction of Change
Barbiturates	Increased
Benzodiazepines	Increased
Morphine	Increased
Pentazocine	Increased
Anticoagulants	Increased
Isoproterenol	Decreased
Tolbutamide	Decreased
Furosemide	Decreased

Changes in receptors and postreceptor mechanisms

Age-related changes may occur at receptor and postreceptor levels. Mechanisms include changes in receptor density or affinity, alteration in signaling pathways, alteration in biochemical responses, such as glycogenolysis, or mechanical effects, such as vascular relaxation.

The function of the β-adrenergic receptor system is reduced in the elderly (see Table 4-2). The sensitivity of the heart to adrenergic agonists is decreased in elderly subjects, and a higher dose of isoproterenol is required to cause a 25-beat/min increase in heart rate. However, α-adrenergic receptor function is not usually changed in the elderly.

There is an increased CNS sensitivity to many drugs in elderly patients. The increased response to benzodiazepines can lead to increased sedation, confusion, gait disturbances, and other adverse effects that cannot be explained on pharmacokinetic grounds alone. Psychotropic drugs are associated with more adverse effects (delirium, sedation, confusion) in elderly compared to young adults, and tricyclic antidepressants also cause more confusion, seizures, and enhanced anticholinergic effects. Opioids, such as morphine, can cause more constipation, confusion, nausea and vomiting, and respiratory depression in elderly patients.

Impaired homeostatic mechanisms

Aging is often associated with decreased activity of aortic and carotid body chemoreceptors, reduced baroreceptor reflexes, impaired thermoregulation, inappropriate response of blood glucose and insulin to glucose, and altered neurological control of bowel and bladder. All of these may contribute to drug toxicity. The decreased baroreflex sensitivity may lead to an increased risk of orthostatic (postural) hypotension. This is a common problem in elderly patients taking some of the phenothiazines and antidepressants (those with significant α_1-adrenergic antagonist properties), nitrates,

Table 4-3 Drug-disease interactions

Drug	Disease
Ibuprofen, other NSAIDs	Gastrointestinal tract hemorrhage, increased blood pressure, renal impairment
Digoxin	Dysrhythmias
Levothyroxine	Coronary artery disease
Prednisone, other glucocorticoids	Peptic ulcer disease
Verapamil, diltiazem	Congestive heart failure
Propranolol, other β-adrenergic antagonists	Congestive heart failure, chronic obstructive pulmonary disease

diuretics, and some antihypertensives, such as prazosin and α-methyldopa. Multiple mechanisms are implicated in the impaired thermoregulation seen in many elderly people and include an absence of shivering, failure of metabolic rate to rise, poor vasoconstriction, and insensitivity to a low body temperature. Chlorpromazine and many other psychoactive drugs may cause hypothermia, and alcohol tends to augment this effect.

Disease-induced changes

It is common for elderly patients to have multiple chronic diseases, such as diabetes, glaucoma, hypertension, coronary artery disease, and arthritis. The presence of multiple diseases leads to the use of multiple medications, an increased frequency of drug-drug interactions (see later), and adverse drug reactions (Table 4-3). Moreover, a disease may increase the risk of adverse drug reactions or preclude the use of the otherwise most effective or safest drug for treatment of another problem. For example, anticholinergic drugs may cause urinary retention in men with enlarged prostate glands or precipitate glaucoma, and drug-induced hypotension may cause ischemic events in patients with vascular disease.

Guidelines for drug prescribing in the elderly

In summary, many drugs exhibit more narrow therapeutic indices when used in the elderly. The impact of the physiological changes that occur with aging alter the pharmacokinetics and pharmacodynamics of drugs and predispose the elderly to adverse drug effects. This is amplified by their reduced physiological compensatory capacity. Practical considerations when prescribing for the elderly include: (1) Use nonpharmacological approaches when possible; (2) use the lowest possible dose and the smallest dose increment ("start low, go slow"); (3) use the smallest number of medications; (4) regularly review drug treatments and potential interactions; and (5) recognize that any new symptoms may be due to the drugs prescribed and not to the aging process.

Drug interactions

Many patients take several drugs simultaneously, and many elderly patients receive as many as 12 drugs concurrently, resulting in many opportunities for drug interactions, often through the pharmacokinetic mechanisms discussed previously.

A drug interaction refers to a change in magnitude or duration of the pharmacological response of one drug because of the presence of another drug. Drug interactions can cause either more rapid elimination or slower elimination, with plasma concentrations increasing or decreasing above or below minimum effective values. There are many mechanisms by which drugs interact, including acceleration or inhibition of metabolism; displacement of plasma protein binding; impaired absorption; altered renal clearance; modifications in receptors; and changes in electrolyte balance, body fluid pH, or rates of protein synthesis. Many drug interactions are well documented in the literature, and prescribing of multiple drugs should take these potential interactions into account.

Summary

Pharmacokinetics provides a firm basis for design of dosing regimens and characterization of the kinetics of drug disposition, although many parameters must be taken into account for such rational design, particularly at the extremes of age. The major points include the following:

- Clearance
- Bioavailability and first-pass metabolism
- Half-life
- Effects of plasma protein binding
- Concept of the apparent volume of distribution

- Exponential disposition of drug (first-order decline) in which a constant fraction of drug is disposed of per unit time
- Concept that the rates of drug input and elimination are equal at the steady state or plateau concentrations
- How to modify a dosing regimen to achieve a desired change in plateau concentration
- Concept that the time to reach plateau depends only on the elimination half-life of the drug, and the plateau concentration is determined by clearance
- The use of a loading dose to accelerate the onset of the desired therapeutic effect
- Requirement for special expertise in determining drug dosage in neonates
- Changes in pharmacodynamic and pharmacokinetic parameters associated with aging
- Simultaneous administration of multiple drugs can alter their disposition and bioavailability

FURTHER READING

Rowland M, Tozer TN. Clinical Pharmacokinetics, 3rd ed. Philadelphia, Lea & Febiger, 1995.

Birkett DJ. Pharmacokinetics Made Easy. Sydney, McGraw-Hill, 2002.

Mangoni AA, Jackson SHD. Age-related changes in pharmacokinetics and pharmacodynamics: basic principles and practical applications. *Br J Clin Pharmacol* 2003; 57:6-14.

Kearns GL, Abdel-Rahman S, Alander SW, et al. Developmental pharmacology–drug disposition, action, and therapy in infants and children. *N Engl J Med* 2003; 349:1157-1167.

Wilkinson GR. Clearance approaches in pharmacology. *Pharmacol Rev* 1987; 39:1.

Self-assessment questions

1. The half-life of a drug:

a. Is an independent pharmacokinetic parameter.
b. Depends on clearance.
c. Depends on the volume of distribution.
d. Must be known to calculate the loading dose.
e. *b* and *c* only are true.

2. Drug clearance is:

a. The volume of blood cleared of drug per unit time.
b. Dependent on the volume of distribution.
c. Dependent on half-life.
d. Dependent on bioavailability.
e. Characterized by all of the above.

3. Which of the following statements concerning the binding of drugs to plasma proteins is/are correct?

a. The rates of drug disappearance and the concentration of free drug available to the site of action are altered substantially, if a significant portion of the drug is bound.
b. Many acidic drugs bind strongly to albumin.
c. Many basic drugs bind strongly to α_1-acid glycoprotein.
d. Induction of metabolic enzymes by another drug can cause significant changes in the free concentration of a second drug.
e. All of the above are true.

4. Altered pharmacokinetics of a drug in the elderly may be attributable to:

a. Decreased total body fat.
b. Increased total body water content.
c. Increased gastric acid secretion.
d. Decreased glomerular filtration rate.
e. Increased plasma albumin concentrations.

5. The hepatic drug metabolism reaction most likely *not* to be decreased in the elderly is:

a. *N*-Demethylation.
b. Hydroxylation.
c. Sulfoxidation.
d. Glucuronidation.
e. Deesterification.

CHAPTER 5

Gene therapy and emerging molecular therapies

Steven L. Brody

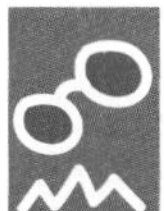

Therapeutic overview

Advances in understanding molecular mechanisms of disease and manipulating genetic material, protein receptors, and antibodies provide new approaches for treatment of human diseases. Emerging therapeutic reagents include not only novel **antibody** and **protein** therapies, but **nucleic acid-based molecules**, including complete genes, (deoxyribonucleic acid; DNA), complementary DNA (cDNA), RNA, and oligonucleotides. Together with **cell therapies** and targeted approaches for protein and nucleic acid **delivery,** these reagents and strategies for administration are conceptualized within the broad borders of gene therapy and the emerging field of molecular medicine. Gene therapy was originally conceived as a treatment for monogenic (Mendelian) disease by complementation of a mutant gene with a normal (wild type) gene. However, gene therapy also includes treatment of acquired human disease by delivery of DNA encoding a therapeutic protein, or introducing a fragment of nucleic acid to interrupt the messenger RNA (mRNA) of a pathogenic protein. A key component of the use of nucleic acids are the spectrum of strategies used to focus therapies on specific organs and/or deliver genes to specific cells. **Targeting** is achieved through genetically engineered viruses, receptor-ligand interactions, and antibodies. Therefore, these gene-based reagents and the vehicles used to delivery them represent a novel form of "gene as drug." This chapter presents a discussion of these molecular therapies.

Although gene therapy is in preliminary stages, more than 600 clinical trials worldwide have been completed or are in progress, using different genes and transfer strategies. Their primary goal is to determine the **safety** of gene transfer and to detect evidence of gene transfer and expression. To date, only a handful of trials have resulted in significant therapeutic effects attributable to gene transfer. However, the rapid rate of improvement in gene transfer vectors and a greater understanding of the pharmacology and toxicology of gene transfer suggest that this will improve rapidly. Gene therapy has several potential advantages over drug therapy in that delivery of a functional gene: (1) can replace a mutant gene that results in disease,

Abbreviations

ADA	adenosine deaminase
cDNA	complementary DNA
CF	cystic fibrosis
CFTR	cystic fibrosis transmembrane conductance regulator
DNA	deoxyribonucleic acid
HIV	human immunodeficiency virus
HS-TK	herpes simplex virus thymidine kinase
mRNA	messenger RNA
RNA	ribonucleic acid
RNAi	RNA interference
SCID	severe combined immunodeficiency disease
siRNA	short interfering RNA
VEGF	vascular endothelial growth factor

(2) can result in continuous production of a therapeutic protein with a short half-life that would otherwise require frequent dosing, (3) can be targeted to a specific site or cell type to avoid potentially toxic systemic therapy, and (4) can improve patient compliance.

Basic molecular mechanisms of gene transfer

The phases of nucleic acid delivery, gene expression, action of the newly produced protein, and consideration of adverse effects of gene delivery vectors and gene products are analogous to issues in conventional drug therapy. Development of molecular therapy using nucleic acid begins with the identification and cloning of a gene. The choice of DNA sequence to be transferred is typically a cDNA sequence containing its **entire protein coding sequence,** but may include introns, nuclear localization, or protein secretion signals. In addition, DNA must also contain transcriptional regulatory sequences, a transcription start site, and RNA polyadenylation sequence to transcribe and stabilize mRNA. These DNA sequences are linked into a single unit that is inserted (subcloned) into a circularized piece of DNA called a **plasmid.** Plasmids contain genetic sequences that allow replication within bacteria so that large quantities of DNA can be produced and purified. The plasmid containing the therapeutic DNA can be delivered to target cells using one of the many vehicles ("**vectors**") for gene transfer (see later). Intracellular transfer of most full-length human genes and associated regulatory elements (that may be over 100 kilobases) is theoretically optimal but limited by current technology.

Basic concepts of gene transfer and gene expression (Fig. 5-1) are similar, regardless of the vehicle used to carry genetic material to the target cell. After DNA-vector administration, the vehicle carrying DNA enters the cell by passing through the cell membrane or by active uptake via a specific receptor. The DNA is then taken into the nucleus where it can be processed. The host cell supplies enzymes necessary for **transcription** of the DNA into messenger RNA (mRNA) and **translation** of the mRNA into protein within the cytoplasm. The protein functions intracellularly or extracellularly to replace a hereditary deficient or defective protein, or to provide a therapeutic function. The protein may: (1) function intracellularly, such as adenosine deaminase (ADA) used to correct the mutation in lymphocytes responsible for one form of the severe combined immunodeficiency disease (SCID) syndrome; (2) replace a cell membrane protein, such as the cystic fibrosis (CF) transmembrane conductance regulator chloride channel (CFTR) mutant in CF; or (3) introduce a secreted protein, such as factor VIII that is deficient in hemophilia.

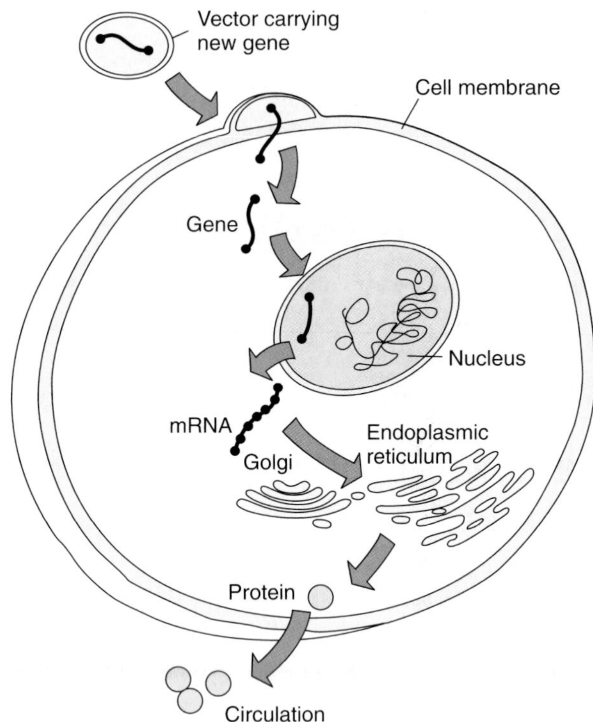

Figure 5-1 Generalized cellular schema of gene transfer. A vector carrying an exogenous gene coding for a secreted protein is taken up by a target cell and transferred to the nucleus, where the DNA is transcribed to mRNA. The mRNA travels to the endoplasmic reticulum, where it is translated to protein. The therapeutic protein is then secreted into the circulation.

Successful gene transfer (also called **transfection**) and expression are evaluated by measuring RNA, protein, and, importantly, function in the target cell. In contrast to traditional pharmacological approaches, the goal of this therapy is alteration of the **genotype** of the cell, rather than altering the phenotype of cell function only.

Molecular mechanisms of mRNA interruption Nucleic acids can also be delivered into the cell to interrupt specific mRNA translation and subsequent protein production. The two general classes of nucleic acids, using independent mechanisms to silence genes through binding and triggering destruction of targeted mRNA, are **antisense** and **RNA interference** (RNAi) (Fig. 5-2). Antisense oligonucleotides are 12 to 28 nucleotide, single-strand sequences, that are chemically modified to enhance their half-life. Binding of these oligonucleotides to a complementary mRNA sequence results in cleavage of the targeted mRNA by endogenous RNaseH, an endoribonuclease that specifically recognizes RNA-DNA heteroduplexes. The cleaved mRNA and oligonucleotide is degraded, and protein translation is reduced. However, a high abundance of oligonucleotides are required for efficient antisense silencing. Larger

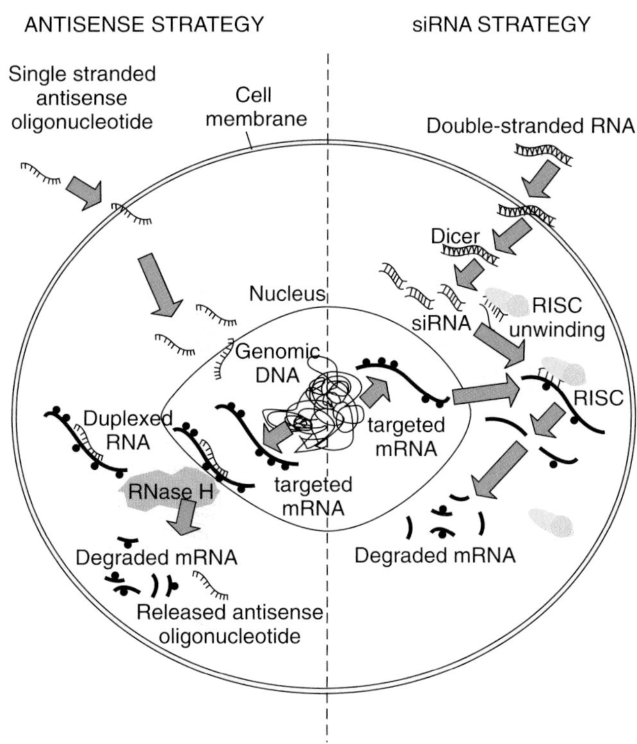

Figure 5-2 Mechanisms of RNA interruption. *Left,* Antisense mechanism. Antisense oligonucleotide enters cell and binds complementary mRNA sequence in the nucleus and cytoplasm. The oligonucleotide-RNA duplex is recognized and degraded by RNase H. *Right,* RNA interference mechanism. Double-strand RNA is chopped by the enzyme Dicer into 21 to 25 nucleotide siRNAs. siRNA is incorporated into a nuclease complex called the RNA-induced silencing complex *(RISC)* that unwinds the double-strand RNA. Complementation of the siRNA antisense strand sequence and the target mRNA result in nuclease enzyme binding and cleavage.

oligonucleotides can also be engineered as a **ribozyme** to bind and directly cleave mRNA, and then repeat this process without self degradation. Over 50 different antisense oligonucleotides and ribozymes are in clinical trials, primarily directed toward oncogenic genes and infectious virus RNAs.

A recently developed **mRNA silencing system** is RNAi that takes advantage of endogenous RNA regulatory pathways (Fig. 5-2). Large, double-stranded RNA sequences designed to target endogenous mRNA enter the cell and are cut into short interfering RNA (siRNA) by the dicer enzyme. Alternatively, synthetic siRNA may be delivered to the cell directly. In either case, the double-strand siRNA molecules are bound by a group of proteins called the RNA-induced silencing complex (RISC). The RISC proteins activate unwinding of the siRNA to single-strand RNA that then binds a specific mRNA molecule. The RISC cuts the mRNA in the region paired with the antisense siRNA sequence, and the cleaved mRNA is degraded to prevent protein translation. Clinical trials are in development using RNAi.

Box 5-1 Prerequisites for gene therapy

Disease identification
Gene cloning
Gene mutation identification
Establish the relationship of mutation to pathophysiology
Gene transfer target cell identification
Detection of gene expression and protein function
Gene transfer efficacy and safety testing systems
Production of a biologically pure reagent

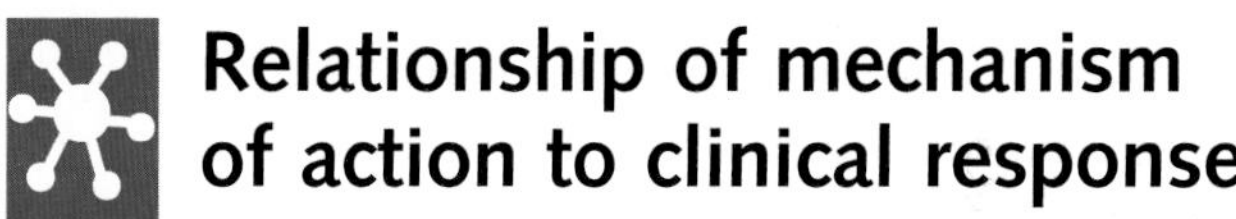

Relationship of mechanism of action to clinical response

Prerequisites for human gene therapy

Application of gene transfer principles to gene therapy requires several critical steps. Prerequisites are shown in Box 5-1. First, a candidate disease for gene therapy must be selected. Typically, this is a disease not successfully treated by currently available therapies. Second, the genetic basis of the disease must be determined, by cloning the gene either by identifying the gene that encodes for that protein or by locating the mutant gene, using classical genetic studies. Third, the pathophysiology of the disease must be known so that the cellular site of normal and abnormal gene expression can be ascertained to target the therapy. A corollary is that the magnitude and duration of exogenous gene expression likely to ameliorate the disease should be estimated. Fourth, tools for detection of gene expression must be in hand, including methods for detection of RNA, protein, and protein function. Fifth, preclinical in vitro and in vivo systems for testing efficacy of gene transfer must be developed. This usually mandates that an animal model of disease be available. With few exceptions, these steps are developed in the laboratory before considering a strategy for clinical gene therapy. Finally, pharmaceutical grade nucleic acid or virus vector must be produced free of biological and chemical contaminants.

Principles of clinical gene therapy The basic concepts and principles of gene delivery also guide the development of strategies for gene therapy. However, no single approach can be used for all diseases, and many

Box 5-2 Variables in design of gene therapy strategies

Disease

Monogenic
Polygenic
Cancer
Infectious

Gene delivery

Ex vivo/cell-based
In vivo

Nucleic acid

Genomic DNA
cDNA
Antisense
Ribozyme
siRNA

Vector

Nonviral
Molecular conjugate
Viral

Administration

Single/repeat
Local/systemic

variables, listed in Box 5-2, must be considered when designing a therapeutic strategy. The biological basis and clinical features dictate the strategic variables used for the appropriate therapeutic outcome.

Gene therapy as gene addition Gene therapy as currently conceived is gene addition therapy, whereby exogenous DNA delivered to a cell complements a mutant DNA. Gene repair therapy, whereby the mutant gene is directly corrected, using techniques of homologous recombination, is technically feasible and would be more definitive. Unfortunately, current methods of homologous recombination result in very low efficiency of gene repair.

DNA and RNA targeting and delivery

How therapeutic DNA is transferred to a specific target cell depends on the biology of the target cell and the vector. Targeting mechanisms are shown in Box 5-3, and different features of these approaches can be used in combination. The procedure of gene transfer can take place in cells removed from the body (ex vivo), then reintroduced into the patient or by direct delivery of DNA or RNA to the patient (in vivo).

Box 5-3 Mechanisms for targeting gene therapy

Ex vivo delivery (cell-mediated)
In vivo directed injection
mRNA sequence-specific
Receptor-mediated delivery
Antibody-mediated delivery
Promoter-specific gene expression

Ex vivo delivery Cells genetically altered by ex vivo gene transfer must be capable of removal, survival outside the body, and reimplantation. Examples of ex vivo cells targeted for gene transfer include lymphocytes, hepatocytes, tumor cells, myocytes, fibroblasts, and bone marrow cells. One valuable strategy of ex vivo transfer is to isolate bone marrow hematopoietic stem cells for gene transfer ($CD34^+$ cells). These stem cells have a long life and the potential to pass on the transferred gene to progeny. An alternative approach to gene targeting, particularly feasible for secreted proteins having a systemic effect, such as a clotting factor (for hemophilia) or insulin (for diabetes), is to use human cells as depots for gene product delivery. In this strategy, cells such as autologous skin fibroblasts, muscle cells, or bone marrow cells, can be transfected with a selected DNA ex vivo and, subsequently, produce the desired therapeutic-specific protein. The cells can then be implanted (e.g., subcutaneously or intramuscularly) where they function as "protein factories," secreting a gene product into the circulation. This approach is used for gene therapy of hemophilia by transfection of autologous skin fibroblasts that were reinjected. A variation in anticancer gene therapy trials is the use of a patient's own tumor cells modified to secrete a cytokine (e.g., interleukin-4), implanted subcutaneously, in an attempt to enhance a systemic immune response.

In vivo delivery Often, in vivo gene delivery is the only feasible strategy. Examples of in vivo targets for gene therapy include brain, lung, liver, muscle, blood vessels, and tumors. Intravenous injection of DNA and oligonucleotides can result in broad distribution to multiple tissues, with concentrations often highest in the liver and kidney. Thus, for efficient in vivo delivery, gene vectors are often directed to a cell population through sophisticated interventional techniques often used in clinical medicine. For example, in vivo transfer to a specific organ may be achieved through catheterization of that organ, by surgical approaches, or by fiberoptic-guided methods. Therefore, specificity of cell targeting to achieve cell-specific gene expression also depends on the technical aspects of the in vivo delivery system.

Bone marrow cells as vehicles for organ repair and gene therapy Autologous bone marrow cells can function as vehicles for gene delivery and have also been demonstrated to traffic to injured organs and acquire the phenotype of an injured organ cell. Using animal models, bone marrow cells have been harvested, genetically modified by gene addition, re-injected into the donor, and observed to express the **transgene** (inserted gene) in cells of various organs. This suggests the possibility that stem cells can be used for expression of a normal gene in an organ or cell previously thought to be genetically modified only by in vivo therapy. For example, experimental models have suggested that stem cells trafficking to the lung can transdifferentiate or proliferate to generate epithelial cells expressing a gene inserted in the stem cell.

Receptor- and antibody-mediated targeting Cellular targeting can also be accomplished through receptor-mediated gene transfer. In these delivery systems, therapeutic DNA is linked to a ligand specific for a cell surface receptor or to an antibody (or antibody fragment) directed toward a specific cell surface protein. These strategies facilitate internalization of DNA through receptor-mediated endocytosis or other pathways. Alternatively, gene expression may be targeted by providing a cell type–specific promoter gene sequence driving the delivered DNA. This strategy uses transcriptional regulatory sequences to permit gene expression only in cells containing appropriate transactivating factors that bind the promoter.

Quantification of gene expression The pharmacokinetics of gene therapy can be determined by the magnitude and duration of gene expression. Following delivery of DNA, gene expression must be quantified by determining amount of DNA reaching the target cell, amounts of RNA and protein produced, and functionality of the protein produced. Magnitude and duration of gene expression depends on the disease to be treated. To treat some diseases, it may be necessary to produce a minimal amount of functional protein but in a large number of cells. Alternatively, to treat other diseases, larger amounts of protein must be secreted to reach a large number of cells within an organ or systemically. The magnitude of expression is typically determined by the half-life of the protein, therapeutic goal, efficacy of gene transfer, and potency of the gene promoter used to direct gene expression.

Duration of gene expression varies with the type of vector used (see later). Most nonviral and viral systems result in only transient (days to months) expression. This may be desirable for gene therapy not associated with hereditary diseases, such as cancer or infectious diseases. Alternatively, gene transfer may be repeated, potentially in a titratable fashion, so that benefits of transient expression are achieved. Persistent gene expression is usually associated with integration of the transferred gene into host cell genome and is possible only with a few viral-based gene transfer systems. Long-term expression (>1 year) has been achieved with current gene transfer systems employing ex vivo transfer of hematopoietic cells by a retrovirus vector. Regardless of the system used, the life span of the cell targeted for gene transfer is also an important factor in duration of gene expression. The viability of cells targeted with DNA using viral vectors may be decreased due to host destruction as a response to a foreign invader, resulting in only transient gene expression.

Evaluation of toxicity of the gene therapy system Toxicity of gene therapy may result from some of the many components of the gene therapy system (e.g., the DNA, the transcribed protein, or the viral/nonviral vehicle). Assessment of balance between safety and efficacy is similar to that applied to standard drug use. Gene transfer vectors utilizing viral genomes may produce several additional proteins, induce a host immune response, have oncogenic properties, or expose caregivers or family members to shed virus. Immunological response to gene transfer vectors (especially virus-based systems) has been a critical factor in causing toxicity and limiting the duration of gene expression. Gene product toxicity is an additional issue, even if the gene is normally expressed in healthy humans. This may occur because, following gene transfer, expression is often much higher than normal endogenous levels and concentrated within a localized population of cells, perturbing normal homeostasis. For example, transfer of the CF gene is potentially harmful, inducing high expression of the CFTR protein and over-expressing many copies of a chloride channel in cells having carefully balanced salt and water channel expression. The integration of foreign DNA in a sensitive site of the genome has also been shown to induce oncogenesis in animals and human trials. Like all experimental therapies, patients treated with gene therapy may be willing to tolerate adverse effects, if diseases are not treatable by currently available therapies.

Ethical issues The scientific goal of current gene therapy is directed at introducing genes into somatic cells only and not into germ cells containing inherited genetic material. Although it is technically possible to transfer DNA through the germ line (often done in experimental animals), application of these technologies to humans has profound social and ethical implications. Ethical considerations include: (1) the choice of disease; (2) attributes to be altered, for example, genetic defects that result in aberrant behaviors; and (3) cosmetic concerns. Human gene therapy trials are tightly regulated and reviewed at local institutions by Biosafety Committees and Human Investigation Review Boards (IRBs) and require informed consent from participants. As with any biological agent administered to humans, newly developed gene therapy vectors must be approved for use by the Food and Drug Administration.

Vehicles for gene transfer

DNA and vector-based methods used to introduce DNA or RNA into mammalian cells and the advantages and disadvantages of different systems are listed in Box 5-4 and Table 5-1. Therapeutic DNA transfected into cells by nonviral means is subcloned into a plasmid so that large quantities of plasmid DNA can be produced and purified. Plasmids can carry large pieces of DNA (over 20 kilobases) so that proteins with large coding sequences can be accommodated. Traditional methods for in vitro gene transfer are purified plasmid DNA delivered to cell lines by microinjection, coprecipitation of DNA with calcium phosphate, and transient electrical current to enhance permeability for DNA entry (electroporation). Although these techniques are often satisfactory experimentally, they generally result in DNA transfer to far less than 1% of primary culture cells, are difficult to use in vivo, and therefore have limited therapeutic use. More efficient vehicles have been developed for gene transfer, making in vivo gene delivery possible. Vehicles for DNA delivery include various plasmid- and virus-based vector systems (Box 5-4). Viral vectors are designed to use specific receptors and entry functions specific to particular cell types, then utilize the host genome for transcription and translation. Viral vectors rarely use the wild-type virus, but rather a genetically engineered virus that minimizes cytotoxicity and replication, but retains the ability to enter and express a specific gene within the cell. The most widely studied vehicles for gene transfer are: (1) genetically engineered viruses that carry nucleic acid into cells, (2) liposomes mixed with DNA, and (3) DNA transferred alone by direct injection ("naked DNA"). Virtually all viruses have been considered as potential vehicles for introducing genes. Those commonly used in clinical trials include mouse Maloney retroviruses, adenoviruses, adeno-associated viruses, lentiviruses, herpes simplex virus, and vaccinia virus.

Box 5-4 Vectors for gene therapy

Plasmid-based vectors

Plasmid
Plasmid with liposome
Plasmid linked to ligand/receptor
Plasmid linked to antibody
Plasmid linked to nanoparticles

Virus-based vectors

Retrovirus
Adenovirus
Adeno-associated virus
Lentivirus
Herpes simplex virus

Plasmid-based vehicles

Plasmid DNA Plasmid DNA alone enters cells but with low efficiency. However, delivery of DNA under pressure (using a "gene gun") has been shown to transfect

Table 5-1 Comparison of commonly used vectors for gene transfer

Vehicle	Advantages	Disadvantages
NONVIRAL		
Naked DNA	Ease of production No DNA size limitation	Low efficiency Transient expression
Liposome-DNA	Ease of production No DNA size limitation Low immune reaction	Low efficiency Transient expression
VIRAL		
Retrovirus	Ease of production Efficient DNA transfer Stable expression Low immune reaction	Transfer to dividing cells only Random DNA integration DNA transfer size limited
Adenovirus	Ease of production Efficient DNA transfer Transfer to nondividing cells	Host immune reaction Transient expression DNA transfer size limited
Adeno-associated	Prolonged expression Transfer to nondividing cells	Difficult production Limited insert size

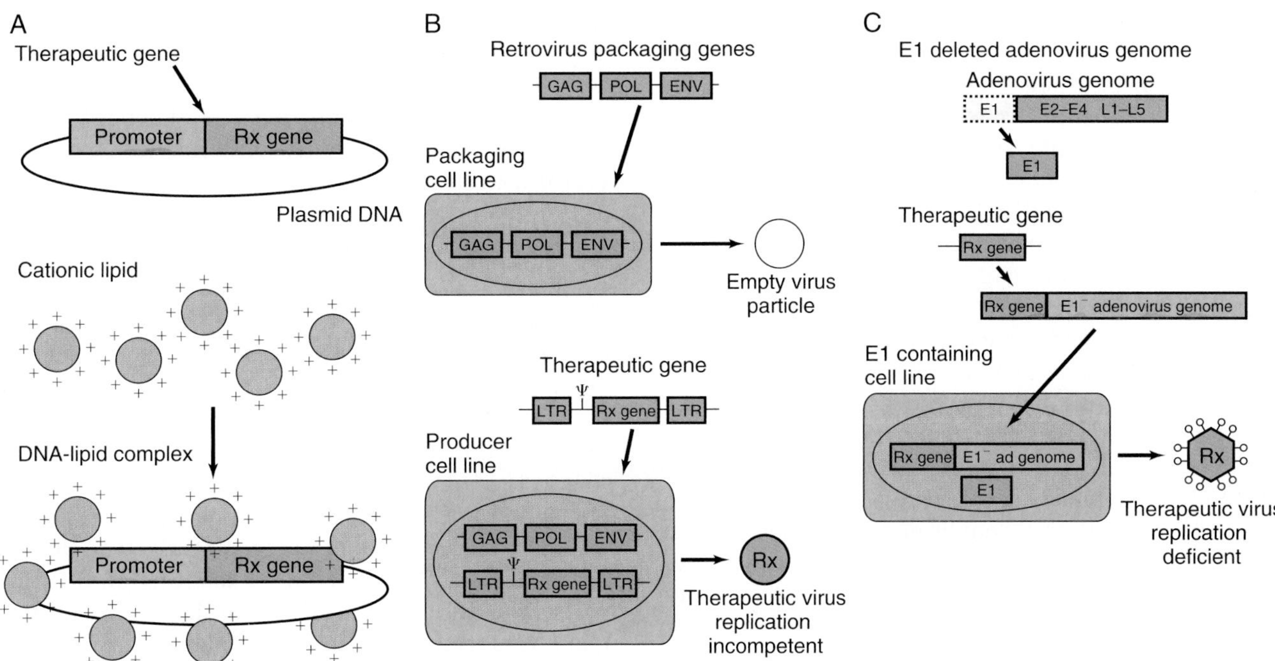

Figure 5-3 Construction of commonly used vehicles for gene transfer. **A,** Liposomes for gene transfer. Plasmid DNA containing a gene or cDNA coding for a therapeutic protein is combined with cationic lipids to form a lipid-DNA complex that facilitates gene transfer. **B,** Retrovirus vector for gene transfer. A modified murine retrovirus vector gene transfer system is composed of a packaging cell line containing retrovirus genes *gag*, *pol*, and *env* that produce empty viral envelopes. The therapeutic gene (*Rx* gene) is inserted into a retrovirus vector containing promoter sequences (long terminal repeat, LTR), and a packaging sequence (ψ) that is subsequently transfected into a packaging cell to make a producer cell. This cell permits production of infectious but nonreplicating virus for gene transfer. **C,** Adenovirus vector for gene transfer. The early gene *E1* is deleted from the adenovirus genome and replaced with the therapeutic gene (*Rx* gene). The newly constructed DNA is then transfected into a cell line that contains the *E1* gene so that infectious, replication deficient adenovirus is produced for gene transfer.

muscle cells. This has the advantage of simplicity and essentially no toxicity. DNA has been condensed and linked to ligands to form molecular conjugates, permitting cell entry by receptor-mediated endocytosis. Efficiency of DNA transfection is good in vitro but poor in vivo. The chemical binding of DNA to nanoparticles may enhance gene delivery, though clinical trials have not yet been developed.

Liposomes Liposomes are lipid molecular aggregates that bind to DNA, antisense oligonucleotides, or siRNA to facilitate cell entry (Fig. 5-3, *A*). Cell entry occurs by fusion with the cell membrane or by endocytosis. Liposome formulations have been developed containing monolayers, bilayers, or multilayers and possess charged (e.g., cationic lipids) or neutral surfaces. Transfection efficiency is variable, and the specific lipid type must be matched to that of the target cell to maximize gene transfer. Nucleic acid-lipid complexes have been combined with selected antibodies or receptor-specific ligands to further enhance cell targeting.

Advantages of DNA-liposome complexes are that large DNA sequences in plasmids can be used and that large scale production and purification is simple. Toxicity of liposomes in vivo is less problematic, because proteins are not transferred. However, gene transfer using liposomes is relatively inefficient compared to virus-based vectors. Therefore large amounts of DNA-lipid complexes may be required, potentially increasing toxicity. Liposomes have been used successfully for gene transfer in humans, and improvements in lipid composition to enhance transfection efficiency and decrease toxicity are in progress.

Virus-based vehicles

Retroviruses Recombinant retrovirus vectors are among the most widely used gene transfer vehicles. They have the advantage of integrating a therapeutic gene into the target cell genome. Production of a retrovirus vector that can carry nonviral (therapeutic) genes and is not capable of replication is a two-step process similar to that used to produce vectors from many different viruses (Fig. 5-3, *B*). First, a cell line containing the genes necessary for creating viral envelopes and viral replication must be created by transferring the retrovirus genes gag, pol, and env to a cell. This "packaging" cell line does not contain the psi (ψ) sequence necessary for inserting the genes into the envelope and hence produces empty retrovirus "packages" that do not contain the therapeutic gene. Second, the packaging cell line is modified to contain other retrovirus sequences with a therapeutic gene (up to 9 kilobases in length) and a psi encapsidation sequence, permitting the therapeutic gene (but not the gag, pol, and env genes) to be inserted into the retrovirus envelope. This "producer" cell line creates and secretes viral particles containing the therapeutic gene that can enter a host cell, but, in the absence of gag and pol, cannot replicate to make new virus. Thereby a replication incompetent retrovirus is produced, collected from the cell media, and used in vitro or in vivo to deliver a gene to a target. After entering the target cell, integration of the therapeutic gene into the host genome is required for expression. Such integration is advantageous, if a sustained therapeutic effect is desired, but can only occur in dividing cells. Therefore, this technique is particularly useful for ex vivo therapies. Retroviruses integrate DNA into the host genome randomly, potentially resulting in interruption of host DNA (insertional mutagenesis) or a silencing of transferred DNA expression.

Adenovirus Gene transfer vectors derived from adenoviruses have the major advantage of high efficiency delivery to nondividing cells and high virus production, making them attractive for in vivo gene delivery. Adenovirus is a double-stranded DNA virus whose genome consists of early genes (E1-E4) that code for regulatory proteins necessary for replication, and late genes (L1-L5) coding for structural proteins. To produce an adenovirus vector for gene transfer (Fig. 5-3C), the immediate early gene E1, responsible for replication but not infection, is deleted and replaced with the therapeutic gene (up to 7 kilobases). The E1 deficient therapeutic adenovirus only grows in cells expressing the E1 gene (serving much the same function as the retrovirus producer cells), generating adenoviruses used for gene transfer. Adenovirus infection occurs through a defined receptor and functions within the nucleus without integration into the host cell genome. Expression of the therapeutic DNA transferred by adenovirus vectors is transient (often less than 1 month). Although adenovirus vectors are highly efficient for transfer of genes to cells in vivo, some limitations prevent their more extensive use. Expression of viral proteins in infected cells can trigger a cellular immune response resulting in adverse clinical symptoms, precluding long-term expression of the transferred gene and repeat administration. Because adenovirus results in transient expression, after initial immune sensitization, repeat dosing may result in even briefer expression due to immune destruction of vector-containing cells. Newer adenovirus vectors developed by removal of genes known to contribute to an immune response are currently under evaluation.

Other virus-based vectors Adeno-associated and herpes simplex virus-based vectors have been approved for human use. Adeno-associated virus is a human single-stranded DNA parvovirus that integrates DNA into target cell genomes of cells not actively dividing. The adeno-associated virus vector system is similar to the retrovirus vector system, relying on a packaging cell line but also requiring wild-type adenovirus as a "helper" to complete viral production in vitro. Disadvantages of the adenovirus-associated vector system include a minimal size of the therapeutic gene that can be carried (<4.5 kilobases) and a low titer of virus particles produced. Lentivirus can be used to infect nonreplicating cells and can be produced in high titer. Herpes simplex derived vectors can be used to enhance gene delivery to neurons.

Side effects, clinical problems, and toxicity

Clinical gene therapy studies

Over 600 clinical gene therapy trials using various strategies for treatment of hereditary and acquired diseases are underway with many other protocols in development. Clinical trials fall into such general categories as genetic diseases, cancer, infectious diseases, and other multifactorial acquired diseases, such as arthritis or vascular disease. Monogenic hereditary diseases currently under trial include immunodeficiency SCID syndrome and a variant of chronic granulomatous disease, Gaucher disease, hemophilia, hereditary emphysema (α-1 antitrypsin deficiency), hereditary hypercholesterolemia (due to low density lipoprotein receptor gene mutation), muscular dystrophy, and CF (Table 5-2). Over half of the current trials are cancer therapies. Many gene-based molecular therapies are in Phase II or Phase III clinical trials. Problems related to inefficient gene delivery, limited gene expression, and, in rare cases, serious toxicity have been identified. To date, only one reagent, an antisense oligonucleotide for the treatment of infectious retinitis, has received FDA approval. Therapeutic issues related to different strategies for disease treatment are discussed later.

Table 5-2 Some current protocols for gene therapy

Disease	Gene	Vector	Strategy and Target Cell
GENETIC			
SCID	ADA	RV	Ex vivo: Lymphocytes, CD34+, bone marrow
CF	CFTR	Ad, L + P, AAV	In vivo: Lung epithelial
Hypercholesterolemia	LDL receptor	RV	Ex vivo: Hepatocytes
Hemophilia	Factors VIII, IX	RV, AAV, EP	In vivo, ex vivo: Fibroblasts
Gaucher's disease	Glucocerebrosidase	RV	Ex vivo: Monocytes, CD34+, bone marrow
α-1 Antitrypsin deficiency	α-1 Antitrypsin	L + P, Ad	In vivo: Lung epithelial
CANCER			
Melanoma	TNF, IL-2	RV	Ex vivo: TIL
	GM-CSF	RV	Ex vivo: Melanoma
	HLA-B7	L + P	In vivo: Melanoma
Renal cell	IL-4	RV	Ex vivo: Fibroblasts + tumor
Glioblastoma	HS-TK	RV producers	In vivo: Tumor cells
Lung	P53	RV	In vivo: Tumor cells
Breast	c-myc/c-fos antisense	RV	In vivo: Tumor cells
Breast, ovarian	MDR	RV	Ex vivo: Bone marrow, CD34+
INFECTION			
HIV	HIV gp 120	RV	In vivo: Myocyte
	HIV TAT antisense	RV	Ex vivo: CD 4 T cell
	HIV RNA ribozyme	RV	Ex vivo: CD 4 T cell
OTHER			
Rheumatoid arthritis	IRAP	RV	In vivo: Synovial
Peripheral vascular disease	VEGF	Plasmid, Ad, L + P	In vivo: Endothelial

SCID, Severe combined immunodeficiency disease; *ADA*, adenosine deaminase; *CF*, cystic fibrosis; *CFTR*, cystic fibrosis transmembrane conductance regulator; *RV*, retrovirus; *Ad*, adenovirus; *AAV*, adeno-associated virus; *L + P*, liposomes with plasmid; *EP*, electroporation; *TNF*, tumor necrosis factor; *IL-2*, interleukin-2; *TIL*, tumor-infiltrating lymphocytes; *GM-CSF*, granulocyte macrophage colony–stimulating factor; *HLA-B7*, histocompatibility locus antigen class I-B7; *IL-4*, interleukin-4; *HS-TK*, herpes simplex virus-thymidine kinase; *MDR*, multiple drug resistance; *HIV*, human immunodeficiency virus; *IRAP*, interleukin-2 receptor antagonist; *VEGF*, vascular endothelial growth factor.

Ex vivo trials The first human gene therapy trial used ex vivo gene transfer for therapy of a rare form of SCID syndrome due to ADA deficiency. In this protocol, T lymphocytes, known to be the critical functional site of a deficient ADA enzyme, were removed from blood and infected ex vivo with a retrovirus vector containing normal ADA cDNA. The genetically modified lymphocytes were reinfused, functioned normally in vivo, and led to an improved clinical status in treated individuals. Unfortunately, two children with fatal X-linked SCID that were treated with hematopoietic stem cells transduced ex vivo with an ADA retrovirus vector had a marked therapeutic response for several years but later developed a leukemia-like syndrome. This syndrome is thought to occur when the retrovirus genome in progeny T cells inserted in a site of the host genome and resulted in expression of an oncogenic protein. This finding underscores the complexity of studying the toxicity of these therapies. Another example of ex vivo gene transfer in clinical trial is treatment of hemophilia (factor VIII deficiency). In one protocol, skin fibroblasts were harvested, and the number of these cells expanded in vitro. These cells were then genetically complemented with a normal factor VIII gene using electroporation. After injecting the genetically altered cells into patients the plasma levels of factor VIII transiently increased, and bleeding episodes were diminished. Adverse effects were not described in these trials.

In vivo trials In vivo gene therapy for treatment of pulmonary manifestations of CF was the first in vivo gene delivery trial. To date, results of 29 such trials have been published. CF, the most common monogenic disease in Caucasians, is caused by a mutation in the CFTR chloride channel that results in disturbed salt and water regulation, abnormal mucus and unremitting infection in the airway. Lung cells cannot be removed, modified ex vivo, and reimplanted, thus in vivo delivery of a normal CFTR cDNA in bronchial airway epithelial cells to complement the mutant gene was attempted. Many studies have demonstrated that gene transfer can be achieved, but only in small numbers of cells. Genetically modifying CF airway epithelial cells to achieve a therapeutic response represents challenges shared in several diseases. First, the airway mounts a marked immunological response to foreign agents, limiting some viral gene

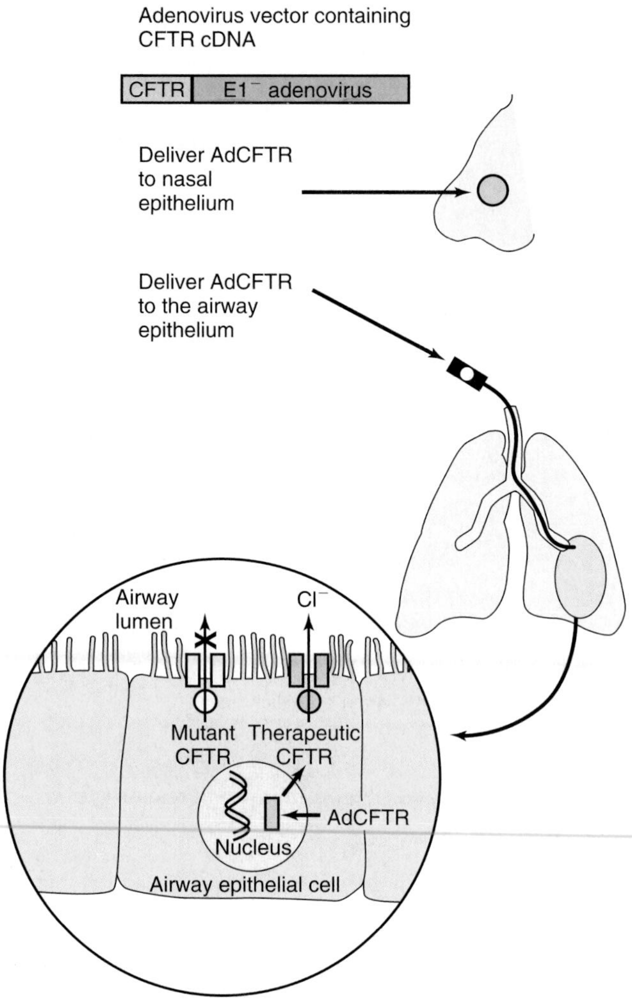

Adenovirus vector containing CFTR cDNA

CFTR | E1⁻ adenovirus

Deliver AdCFTR to nasal epithelium

Deliver AdCFTR to the airway epithelium

Airway lumen

Cl⁻

Mutant CFTR

Therapeutic CFTR

AdCFTR

Nucleus

Airway epithelial cell

Figure 5-4 Protocol for evaluation of gene therapy for cystic fibrosis. An *E1⁻* deleted adenovirus containing the CF transmembrane conductance regulator *(CFTR)* cDNA is delivered to the nasal and/or lung epithelium *(AdCFTR)*. Delivery to cells in the nose allows ready access for evaluation. Delivery to the lung is facilitated by a flexible fiberoptic bronchoscope. The detail from the lung diagrams the complementation of the mutant CFTR with a functional CFTR protein expressed in the cell membrane, moving chloride ions out of the epithelial cell into the airway.

transfer systems, and repeat administration. Second, airway epithelial cells do not rapidly divide; thus vectors such as retroviruses cannot provide the necessary transfection efficiency. Third, receptors for many virus vectors (e.g., retrovirus, adenovirus) are on the basolateral aspect of cells and cannot be directly accessed. Finally, the presence of abnormal airways, infection and inflammation, and increased mucus in the CF lung impair efficient gene delivery. Current protocols for CF are focused on adeno-associated virus and nonvirus DNA-liposome delivery (Fig. 5-4). Other in vivo protocols using delivery of adenovirus carrying

Box 5-5 Strategies for cancer gene therapy

Immunomodulation-cancer vaccine
- Lymphocyte-mediated
- Dendritic cell-activated
- Tumor antigen-mediated

Toxicity/prodrug (suicide gene)
Mutation complementation
Oncogene antisense
Tumor suppressor complementation
Anti-angiogenesis
Multidrug resistance protection

cDNA to treat inherited metabolic diseases and lysosomal storage diseases have also been performed. In one trial, injection of high dose of adenovirus vector into the liver of a patient resulted in a fatal inflammatory response, diminishing enthusiasm for in vivo use of the current adenovirus vector systems.

Gene therapy for cancer

Cancer cells are the most extensively evaluated target for gene therapy because many malignancies are unresponsive to conventional therapy and rapidly fatal. In contrast to hereditary diseases, cancer-related gene therapy is not exclusively directed toward correction of genetic mutations but also uses gene delivery to target a therapeutic biological agent to the cancer cell. Several highly creative therapeutic approaches developed for gene therapy for cancer (Box 5-5) include: (1) addition of a wild-type tumor suppressor gene to complement a mutant tumor suppressor gene; (2) antisense RNA strategies to "turn-off" expression of an oncogene; (3) transfer of a gene to enhance immunogenicity of the tumor by expression of an immunomodulating gene or cytokine gene in the tumor; (4) transfer of a gene coding for a "prodrug" to the tumor, leading to tumor-specific cell killing by production of a toxic metabolite; (5) inhibition of tumor angiogenesis; and (6) chemoprotective genes transferred to save patients' hematopoietic cells from chemotherapy-induced toxicity.

Carcinogenesis gene regulation Genetic manipulation by wild type complementation of mutant tumor suppressor genes, inhibition of oncogenesis and anti-apoptotic genes are in clinical trials. Mutation of the tumor suppressor P53 gene induces carcinogenesis, such mutations are commonly found in tumors, and when complemented with a normal wild type P53, can halt cell growth. P53 gene addition has been used in many different solid organ cancer therapy protocols. This requires that P53 be transferred to a high percentage of tumor cells, and thus adenovirus vectors have been used. Other genes are identified in carcinogenesis and maintenance of the malignant cell phenotype, including those of the ras family. Antisense oligonucleotides directed toward H-ras have been evaluated in phase I and II clinical trials for cancer. Oligonucleotides have also been used to attempt to decrease expression of anti-apoptotic proteins in leukemia, melanoma, lung, breast, and prostate cancer. The best studied is the use of antisense oligonucleotides to the anti-apoptosis gene Bcl-2, but to date, a significant survival benefit has not been observed. Protocols using Bcl-2 antisense oligonucleotides as an adjuvant with chemotherapy are in progress.

Cancer immunotherapies Enhancement of an immunological response to tumor cells is a long sought goal, and hundreds of nucleic acid based or genetically modified cell trials have been completed or are in progress based on a vaccine response. One approach is to deliver in vivo genes that will express HLA-B7 (histocompatibility locus antigen class I-B7) and β-2 microglobulin to melanoma, colon, and lung tumors. These are costimulatory molecules necessary for activation of T lymphocytes, resulting in generation of a T lymphocyte-dependent immune response. Delivery of these genes complexed with liposomes to metastatic tumors demonstrates biological evidence of an antitumor T cell response but has not yet reproducibly resulted in a clinical response. An alternative approach is to modify the tumor with a gene for a cytokine to induce a local antitumor response generalizing to a systemic response, termed a cancer "vaccine" trial. In over 75 trials, tumor cells (from cancer of lung, colon, brain, breast, kidney, prostate, or melanoma) are genetically modified with genes expressing a cytokine, such as interleukin-2, interleukin-4, interleukin-12, interferon-γ, or granulocyte-macrophage colony stimulating factor. These genes are typically delivered to tumor cells ex vivo by retrovirus or adenovirus vectors, and then the cells are reimplanted into the patient, or, in other protocols, delivered in vivo with adenovirus vectors or liposomes. Although an immunological response was demonstrated, only a few clinical responses were noted. A variant of the vaccine trial is to generate a selected population of tumor-infiltrating lymphocytes capable of mounting a tumor-specific response. The tumor-infiltrating lymphocytes are isolated and modified to express interleukin or other cytokine genes ex vivo and then reinfused.

Pro-drug/suicide gene therapies An ingenious antitumor strategy is to deliver a gene coding for a nontoxic "prodrug" that when metabolized generates a toxic agent that will kill the cell, a so-called suicide gene. The most widely used gene for this strategy is the herpes simplex thymidine kinase gene (HS-TK) that selectively metabolizes the antiviral agent ganciclovir to produce a toxic metabolite that kills the cell expressing the gene. In addition, by diffusion, it can kill surrounding cells by a "bystander" effect. Retrovirus or adenovirus vectors have been used to deliver the HS-TK gene for treatment of mesothelioma, metastatic breast, and metastatic ovarian carcinomas. In vivo or ex vivo strategies have been used to express HS-TK in tumor cells in brain, prostate, or mesothelioma. This has been used to treat brain tumors, such as glioblastomas (Fig. 5-5) and incorporates use of a retrovirus that will only transfer genes into dividing cells of the brain tumor and not to normal brain cells that do not divide. After retrovirus producer cells are injected (and continue to secrete the HS-TK vector), and as tumor cells divide, systemic ganciclovir is administered, leading to tumor cell death. Because producer cells also express HS-TK, they also are killed by ganciclovir, providing a fail-safe mechanism to prevent adverse effects of producer cells. As with other gene therapy trials, results remain inconclusive.

Gene therapy for infectious disease

Chronic infectious diseases with persistent virus expression, including HIV, hepatitis B, and hepatitis C, represent targets for nucleic acid-based therapies to block virus production or enhance immune responses. Many approaches have been used for gene therapy of HIV infection; such as enhancing the immune response to HIV and providing gene products that suppress virus replication. One approach is to use a retrovirus to transfer the HIV gp160 envelope protein gene as a vaccine to enhance virus-specific immune responses following injection into muscle. Vaccine-type gene transfer trials may be less successful in individuals who are already immunologically impaired by HIV infection. Another approach to decrease HIV replication is to modify CD4 T cells ex vivo to express proteins that interfere with the function of the HIV TAT or REV transcription factors. These protocols depend on persistent gene expression and long-term survival of genetically modified HIV-infected cells infused into the patient. Several hundred individuals have been involved in these trials, and the protocols appear to be safe, however, sufficient data are not yet available to judge clinical efficacy.

Multifactorial diseases

Many diseases without complex genetics and environmental interactions can be amenable to molecular therapies by identification of therapeutics. Vascular diseases due to thrombosis and atherosclerosis have been studied following the delivery of genes coding for angiogenic

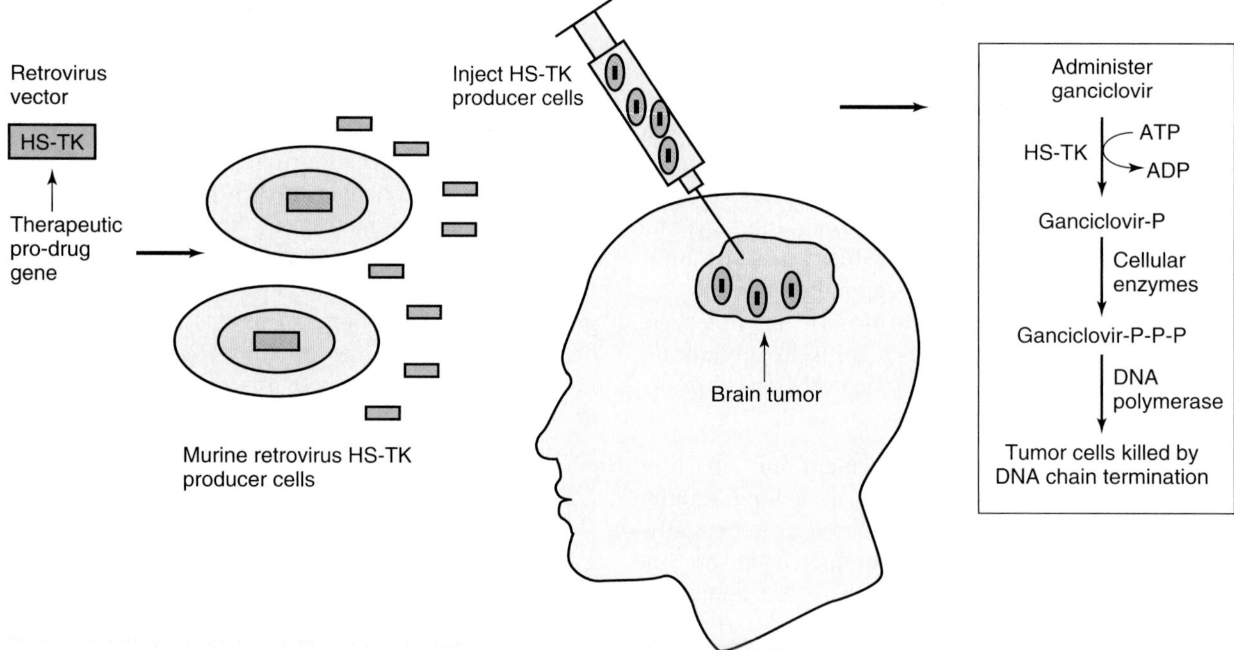

Figure 5-5 Strategy for prodrug gene therapy for brain cancer. A retrovirus vector containing the gene for HS-TK is constructed and transfected into a murine packaging cell line. The producer cells produce retrovirus containing HS-TK. The HS-TK is injected into the brain tumor, where the producer cells reside within the tumor, continuously releasing HS-TK retrovirus that can transfer the HS-TK gene only to cells that are dividing (i.e., tumor cells). The patient is then administered intravenously the nucleoside analog ganciclovir, which is an excellent substrate for HS-TK. In the presence of HS-TK, ganciclovir is phosphorylated to produce a highly phosphorylated nucleotide that interferes with DNA replication and causes cell death.

growth factors. Delivery of genes for vascular endothelial growth factor (VEGF) has been used to successfully stimulate vascular proliferation in coronary artery disease and peripheral vascular disease. Although used in a limited number of people, VEGF has shown promise for induction of angiogenesis and relief of symptoms.

Inflammatory diseases, such as inflammatory bowel disease, arthritis, asthma, and skin diseases, have been studied as candidates for delivery of genes that encode anti-inflammatory or immunomodulatory cytokines. In some trials, antisense oligonucleotides designed to silence expression of pro-inflammatory cytokines are under investigation.

New horizons

Continued progress in the understanding of molecular mechanisms of disease will lead to the development of novel genetic-based therapies. Broad application of in vivo gene transfer for treatment of human inherited or acquired diseases will require development of new viral or nonviral systems or a substantial improvement of existing systems. Critical issues being evaluated are immunological responses of gene transfer vectors, regulation of gene expression, and persistence of expression. High efficiency approaches for repair of mutation, rather than addition to mutant genes, using homologous recombination is also being actively pursued. Tailoring therapies to humans with specific genetic mutations or polymorphisms is a related area for future investigation. The application of basic principles of drug therapy continues to guide evaluation of novel gene therapy strategies.

FURTHER READING

Dean NM, Bennett CF. Antisense oligonucleotide-based therapeutics for cancer. *Oncogene* 2003; 22:9087-9096.

Noguchi P. Risks and benefits of gene therapy. *N Engl J Med* 2003; 348:193-194.

Ratko TA, Cummings JP, Blebea J, Matuszewski KA. Clinical gene therapy for non-malignant disease. *Am J Med* 2003; 115:560-569.

Ribas A, Butterfield LH, Glaspy JA, Economou JS. Current developments in cancer vaccines and cellular immunotherapy. *J Clin Oncol* 2003; 21:2415-2432.

Thomas CE, Ehrhardt A, Kay MA. Progress and problems with the use of viral vectors for gene therapy. *Nat Rev Genet* 2003; 4:346-358.

Self-assessment questions

1. The most common current strategy for human gene therapy of monogenic (Mendelian) disease is:
   a. Repair the mutant gene in the cell.
   b. Repair the mutant RNA in the cell.
   c. Repair the mutant protein in the cell.
   d. Add a nonmutant gene to the cell to complement the mutant gene.
   e. Add nonmutant RNA to the cell to interrupt the mutant gene expression.

2. Current concepts for successful human gene therapy dictate that:
   a. After gene transfer, expression of the transferred gene must be undetectable.
   b. After gene transfer, immune response to the vector should be monitored.
   c. After successful gene transfer, life-threatening toxic effects are expected to occur.
   d. Gene transfer to germ cells is essential.
   e. Gene transfer to somatic cells is not important.

3. Vectors for gene transfer in clinical trials include the following *except:*
   a. Recombinant plasmids.
   b. Recombinant plasmids mixed with phospholipids.
   c. Genetically engineered murine leukemia virus.
   d. Genetically engineered human adenovirus.
   e. Genetically engineered adeno-associated virus.

4. Mechanisms of gene silencing using mRNA antisense oligonucleotides for gene therapy include:
   a. Oligonucleotide binding to mutant DNA to block the function of DNA.
   b. Degradation of mutant proteins.
   c. Complementary pairing of the oligonucleotide and mRNA.
   d. Permanent blockade of targeted gene expression.
   e. Production of new mRNA sequence by a virus vector.

CHAPTER 6

Regulated drug development and usage

Gary E. Stein

Therapeutic overview

The discovery, development, and clinical introduction of new drugs is a process involving close cooperation between researchers, medical practitioners, the pharmaceutical industry, and the U.S. Food and Drug Administration (FDA). The drug development process begins with the synthesis or isolation of a new compound with biological activity and potential therapeutic use. This entity must then pass through preclinical, clinical, and regulatory review stages before becoming available as a therapeutically safe and effective drug. Similar governmental agencies regulate the development and distribution of drugs in other countries.

The FDA authority over drug review and approval began with the Federal Pure Food and Drug Act of 1906. This first drug law established **standards for drug strength and purity.** This legislation was followed by the Federal Food, Drug and Cosmetic Act of 1938, which prohibited the marketing of new drugs, unless they were adequately tested and **shown to be safe** under the conditions indicated on their labels. The 1938 act was amended by Congress in 1962 to state that pharmaceutical manufacturers must also provide scientific proof that new products are **efficacious and safe** before marketing them. The amendment also required that the FDA be notified before the testing of drugs in humans. More recent legislation includes controls on the manufacture and prescribing of **habit-forming drugs** (Comprehensive Drug Abuse Prevention and Control Act, 1970), drug development for treating **rare diseases** (Orphan Drug Act, 1983), new drug applications for **generic** drug products (Drug Price Competition and Patent Restoration Act, 1984), and incentives for **pediatric** drug testing (Best Pharmaceuticals for Children Act, 2002).

Other regulations that have been passed are relevant to drug use and aimed at reducing health care costs from unnecessary, inappropriate, and unmonitored prescription drug use. These regulations required all states receiving Medicaid dollars to submit a plan to carry out prospective and retrospective drug utilization reviews and to counsel Medicaid patients on drug use to the Health Care Finance Administration for approval (Federal Omnibus Budget Reconciliation Act of 1990, activated in 1993).

Abbreviations

DEA	Drug Enforcement Administration
FDA	Food and Drug Administration
IND	Investigational New Drug
IRB	Institutional Review Board
NDA	New Drug Application
NIH	National Institutes of Health
PMS	postmarketing surveillance

Clinical testing and introduction of new drugs

Potential new drugs or biological products must first be tested in animals for their acute and chronic toxicity, influence on reproductive performance, carcinogenic and mutagenic potential, and safe dosing range. Early research and preclinical testing often takes 5 to 8 years and costs millions of dollars. Long-term safety testing in animals continues during subsequent trials in humans.

After successful preclinical pharmacological and toxicological studies, the sponsor files an **Investigational New Drug** (IND) application with the FDA. In addition to animal data, the IND contains protocols for clinical testing in humans. Approximately 2000 INDs are received each year by the FDA. If the IND passes FDA review, clinical trials in humans are initiated. These studies are generally conducted in three phases:

Phase 1: Conducted on a small number of normal volunteers to determine safe dosage range and pharmacokinetic parameters

Phase 2: Conducted on several hundred patients with specific diseases to determine short-term safety and effectiveness of the drug

Phase 3: Conducted on several thousand patients with specific diseases to determine overall risk-benefit relationships

These studies provide the basis for *drug labeling.* The completion of these clinical studies may take 3 to 10 years and costs more than $300 million. Only one out of every five drugs that enter clinical trials receives FDA approval. When that one drug is marketed, it often represents an average $800 million investment because the pharmaceutical company must pay for the thousands of failed drugs that did not meet approval (Fig. 6-1). The patent protection (17 years) of new drugs may be increased on some drugs, based upon delays in FDA approval (Patent Term Restoration Act, 1984). Extensions in patent life may also occur for products that provide pediatric studies to support pediatric labeling (Best Pharmaceuticals for Children Act, 2002).

Before initiating a study of an investigational drug in humans, an investigator must also obtain approval from the local Institutional Review Board (IRB) of the hospital, university, or other institution where the planned study will be conducted. The IRB is responsible for ensuring the ethical acceptability of the proposed research and approves, requires modification, or disapproves the research protocol. To approve a clinical research study, the IRB must determine that the research

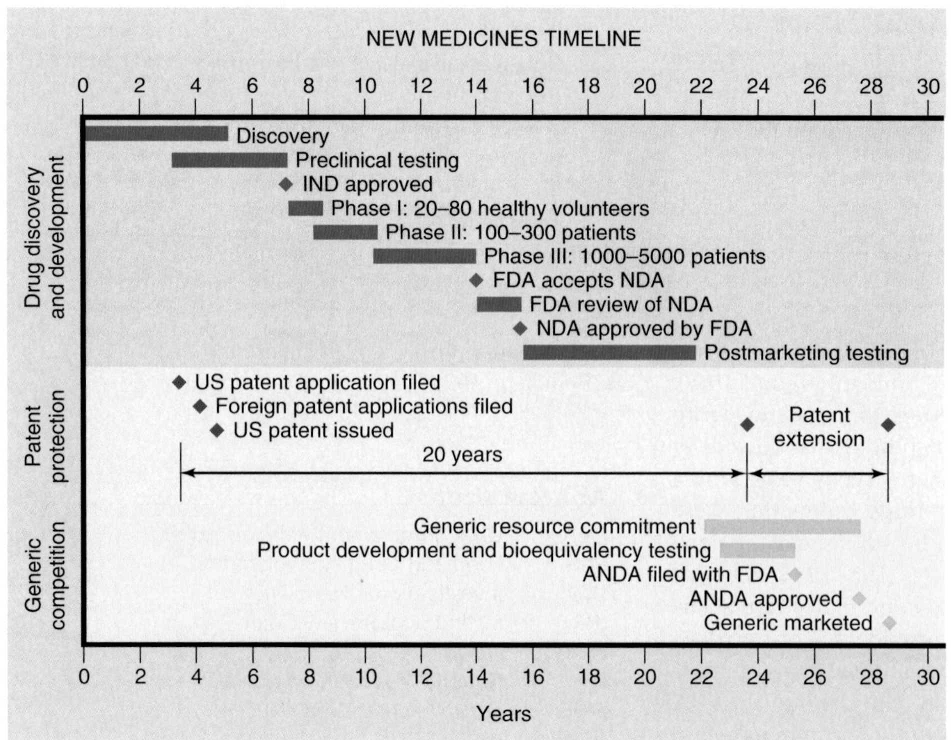

Figure 6-1 Stages of new drug development and the approval process, patent protection, and generic competition.

design and procedures are sound and that the risk to subjects is minimized. In addition, the IRB must also approve the informed consent document that must be signed by each prospective subject or the subject's legally authorized representative. IRB approval is usually valid for 1 year.

The basic elements of informed consent include: (1) explanation of the purposes and procedures of the research; (2) description of foreseeable risks; (3) description of expected benefits; (4) statement of available alternative procedures or courses of treatment; (5) statement on confidentiality of records; (6) explanation of compensation or available medical treatments, if injury occurs; (7) description of whom to contact about the research and the subject's rights and the procedure to follow in the event of injury to the subject; and (8) statement that participation is voluntary and refusal to participate does not involve penalty to the subject.

If suitable preclinical and clinical findings demonstrate efficacy with minimal toxicity, the sponsors can submit a **New Drug Application** (NDA) to the FDA (see Fig. 6-1). In approving an NDA, the FDA ensures the drug's safety and effectiveness for each use. Usually, the sponsor and the FDA review the data and negotiate on the detailed information to accompany the drug for its use. This includes contraindications, precautions, side effects, dosages, routes of administration, and frequency of administration. The NDA approval process usually takes 1 to 2 years, with drugs having the greatest potential benefit given priority. Drug applications are now identified and placed into specific categories under a new FDA classification system (Table 6-1). Postapproval research may be requested by the FDA as a condition of new drug approval. Such research may be used to speed drug approval, uncover unexpected adverse drug reactions, and define the incidence of known drug reactions under actual clinical use.

After NDA approval, the manufacturer promotes the new drug for the approved uses described on the label. During the post-NDA approval or marketing period (**Phase 4**) the safety of the new drug must be monitored during clinical use. The label information does not include all conditions in which a released drug is safe and effective. *It should be noted that the FDA does not restrict use of approved drugs to those conditions described on the label; the physician is allowed to determine its most appropriate use.* However, from both an ethical and liability standpoint, there should be compelling scientific evidence before a drug is used for an unapproved indication. Examples are β-adrenergic receptor blocking drugs, which often are used interchangeably for various indications, though not all have identical FDA-approved indications (Table 6-2).

Early clinical testing of new drugs does not provide an absolute assurance of safety, as evidenced by later discoveries of rare adverse effects after drugs are used clinically and, thus, much larger patient populations are exposed. In some instances, released drugs are withdrawn from the market after toxic or fatal adverse effects are discovered during large-scale clinical use. There are also instances in which a new drug is not found to be efficacious for a specific indication until it is in large-scale clinical use in selected patient populations. The goal of **postmarketing surveillance** (PMS) is also to define the true side effect profile of a new drug.

New safety information obtained during large-scale clinical testing is used to update the current NDA and make changes in the drug label. Side effect profiles in patients with multiple diseases are often incomplete during early studies, and such information is vitally

Table 6-1 FDA drug classification system

Designation	Meaning
AA	Drugs for AIDS or complications related to AIDS
P	Priority
S	Standard
O	Orphan

Table 6-2 Varied FDA approved uses of several β-adrenergic receptor antagonists

Label Indications	Acebutolol	Atenolol	Labetalol	Metoprolol	Nadolol	Propranolol	Carvedilol
Hypertension	X	X	X	X	X	X	X
Congestive heart failure	—	—	—	X	—	—	X
Angina	—	X	—	X	X	X	—
Dysrhythmia	X	—	—	—	—	X	—
Postmyocardial infarction	—	X	—	X	—	X	—
Pheochromocytoma	—	—	—	—	—	X	—
Hypertrophic subaortic stenosis	—	—	—	—	—	X	—
Essential tremor	—	—	—	—	—	X	—
Migraine prophylaxis	—	—	—	—	—	X	—

important for improving subsequent use. Reporting of rare and unexpected side effects not listed on the drug label is an important responsibility for prescribers; such information is supplied to the FDA on the **Drug Experience Form** (FDA form 1639). Med Watch is a voluntary reporting program initiated by the FDA to encourage and facilitate monitoring by pharmacists and other health professionals of adverse effects and problems with medications, medical devices, and other products regulated by the FDA. Any adverse effects or suspect problems may be reported on FDA form 3500.

Several sources of information are available to the physicians concerning the safety of new drugs. These include the Medical Letter on Drugs and Therapeutics, Facts and Comparisons, AMA Drug Evaluations, and the Physician's Desk Reference (PDR), a compilation of FDA-approved drug package inserts.

Orphan drugs, pediatric drug testing, and treatment INDs

There is little economical incentive for pharmaceutical manufacturers to develop and file an IND or NDA for new drugs that may benefit only a small number of patients with **rare diseases,** defined in the United States as fewer than 200,000 people. The Orphan Drug Act of 1983 provides special incentives, such as tax advantages and marketing exclusiveness, to compensate companies for the developmental costs of such agents. The National Institutes of Health (NIH) also participates in the development of orphan drugs. More than 300 drugs have been given orphan status, including human growth hormone, erythropoietin, and α_1-antitrypsin.

Most drugs are studied, approved, and labeled for use in adults. At present, fewer than 25% of all drug labels include **pediatric** information. Young children often metabolize drugs at different rates than adults (see Chapter 4), and therefore testing is needed to clarify which doses work best in children. These studies would also help define the types of adverse reactions that are likely to occur. Current legislation allows for incentives to drug manufacturers for pediatric testing and provides funding to the NIH for research on drugs for which additional pediatric studies are needed (e.g., heparin, furosemide, dopamine).

The FDA has also established guidelines to help make promising investigational drugs available for the treatment of patients with **immediate life-threatening diseases,** such as AIDS. These drugs receive highest priority at all stages of the drug review process. The Treatment IND application enables patients not qualified for participation in ongoing studies to be treated with investigational drugs outside controlled clinical trials. The FDA generally considers Treatment INDs for drugs in later stages of clinical testing. The initial criteria include the following:

- The drug is intended to treat a serious life-threatening disease (such as AIDS).
- There is no comparable or satisfactory alternative to treat the disease.
- The drug is under investigation in a controlled clinical trial under an IND.
- The sponsor is actively pursuing marketing approval of the investigational drug.

When no Treatment IND is in effect for an investigational drug, a physician may obtain the drug for *"compassionate use."* In such cases, the physician submits a Treatment IND to the FDA requesting authorization to use an investigational drug for that purpose.

Prescription writing

Prescriptions are written by the prescriber to instruct the pharmacist to dispense a specific medication for a specific patient. These include precompounded medications (prepared by the pharmaceutical manufacturer) and extemporaneously prepared medications. It is vitally important that a prescription communicate clearly to the pharmacist the exact medication needed and how this medication is to be used by the patient. Patient compliance is often related to the clarity of the directions on the prescription, and terms, such as "take as directed," should be avoided. Equally important is the necessity for clarity when using proprietary drug names because of their similarities. In these instances the physician should designate the generic name, as well as the brand name, to avoid confusion.

Prescriptions contain the following elements to facilitate interpretation by the pharmacist (Fig. 6-2):

- Physician's name, address, and office telephone number
- Date
- Patient's name and address
- Superscription (Rx how drug is to be taken)
- Inscription (name and dosage of drug)
- Subscription (directions to the pharmacist)
- Signature or transcription (directions to the patient)
- Refill and safety cap information
- Prescriber's (physician's) signature
- DEA number of physician required for controlled substances

Prescriber's Name, Address, and Telephone Number	
Date ________ Patient ____________	
Address ________________________	
Rx	
Drug name and strength Quantity to be dispensed Patient instructions	
Refill _____ times	Dr. Signature ___________
No safety cap ☐	DEA No. ___________

Figure 6-2 Typical prescription form.

Because both apothecary and metric systems are in use, it is important that prescribers become familiar with conversion units. Following are commonly used apothecary weights and measures and their metric equivalents:

2.2 pounds (lb) = 1 kilogram (kg)

1 grain (gr) = 65 milligrams (mg)

1 fluid ounce (oz) = 30 milliliters (ml)

1 tablespoonful (tbsp) = 15 ml

1 teaspoonful (tsp) = 5 ml

20 drops (gtt) = 1 ml

Patient instructions ("signature") on a prescription are sometimes written using Latin abbreviations as a short cut for prescribers, giving concise directions to the pharmacist on how and when a patient should take the medication. Although instructions written in English are preferred, some common Latin abbreviations are as follows:

po: by mouth

ac: before meals

pc: after meals

qd: every day

b.i.d.: twice a day

t.i.d.: three times a day

q.i.d.: four times a day

hs: at bedtime

prn: as needed

c̄: with

s̄: without

ss: one-half

Table 6-3 Controlled substances

Schedule	Symbol	Abuse Potential	Example
I	C-I	High; no accepted medical use in the United States	Heroin
II	C-II	High	Morphine
III	C-III	Moderate	Glutethimide
IV	C-IV	Lower	Diazepam
V	C-V	Lowest	Diphenoxylate

Additional instructions may be added to the prescription to instruct the pharmacist to place an additional label on the prescription container (e.g., Take with Food). When a prescriber intends to use a drug for an unauthorized indication, or when two drugs have been prescribed that may cause a clinically significant drug interaction, the prescriber should communicate to the patient and pharmacist that this is indeed the intended therapy.

In the United States, many drugs require a prescription from a licensed practitioner (e.g., physician, dentist, veterinarian, podiatrist) before they can be dispensed by a pharmacist. In addition, use of specific drugs, called **schedule drugs**, with potential for abuse, are further restricted by the FDA, and special requirements must be met when these drugs are prescribed. These controlled drugs (Table 6-3) are classified according to their potential for abuse and include opioids, stimulants, and depressants. Schedule I drugs have a high abuse potential and no currently accepted medical use in the United States. Schedule II drugs also have a high potential for abuse, but they also have an accepted medical use. In addition, Schedule II drugs may not be refilled or prescribed by telephone. Other schedule drugs (III to IV) have a five-refill maximum, and the prescription is invalid 6 months from the date of issue. An exception to these regulations are drugs in Schedule V, which may be dispensed without a prescription, if the patient is at least 18 years old, the drug is distributed by a pharmacist, and only a limited quantity of the drug is purchased (refer to the Controlled Substance Act of 1970).

Many prescribed proprietary (brand-name) drugs are available from multiple pharmaceutical manufacturers under a brand-name, or trade name, or as less costly nonproprietary (**generic** name) preparations after their patent protection has expired. Pharmacists receiving prescriptions for brand-name products may dispense an equivalent generic drug (except as noted later) without prescriber approval and pass on the savings to the patient. Some states have mandatory substitution laws, and the brand-name product is dispensed only when "Dispense as Written" (D.A.W.) is stated on the prescription. Although generic products are considered to be pharmaceutically equivalent to brand-name counterparts, some may not be therapeutically equivalent, because bioavailability can be less stringently controlled.

Generic products tested by the FDA and determined to be therapeutic equivalents are listed by the FDA in Approved Drug Products with Therapeutic Equivalence Evaluations (Orange Book). These products contain the same active ingredients as their brand-name counterparts and also meet bioequivalence standards within certain tolerances. The FDA recommends the substitution of only those products listed as therapeutically equivalent (A-rated products). Not all generic drugs listed in the Orange Book are therapeutic equivalents of the brand-name products. Brand-name products, such as Lanoxin (digoxin), Dilantin (phenytoin), Premarin (conjugated estrogens), and Theo-Dur (slow-release theophylline), contain either unique chemicals (Premarin) or exhibit bioavailability characteristics that differ from those of generic products. Therefore, these should not be substituted without a physician's approval. In addition, there are drugs with narrow therapeutic ranges (e.g., warfarin and carbamazepine), where small changes in bioavailability can lead to increased adverse effects or decreased therapeutic efficacy. For a patient who is having difficulty maintaining therapeutic range of a given drug, it may not be appropriate to substitute a pharmaceutically equivalent product, even if it is rated therapeutically equivalent.

New horizons

Recently the FDA has suggested four initiatives for streamlining the drug approval process. These include the use of outside expert reviewers to reduce the backlog of new applications awaiting approval, elimination of duplicate animal testing, institution of a parallel-track policy to increase patient access to treatment for those who cannot participate in controlled studies, and introduction of the use of surrogate markers (e.g., $CD4^+$ cell count for new drugs to treat HIV infection) for evaluating the efficacy of new drugs.

As noted earlier, the FDA has also instituted a program called Med Watch to encourage and facilitate the reporting of serious adverse events and product problems.

FURTHER READING

Ascione FJ, Kirking DM, Gaither CA, et al. Historical overview of generic medication policy. *J Am Pharm Assoc* 2001; 41:567.

Health G, Colburn WA. An evolution of drug development and clinical pharmacology during the 20th century. *J Clin Pharmacol* 2000; 40:918.

Kaitin KI. The prescription drug user act of 1992 and the new drug development process. *Am J Ther* 1997; 4:167.

Self-assessment questions

1. A proprietary (brand-name) drug cannot be prescribed if:
- a. The FDA has not approved the use for which you are prescribing it.
- b. A generic form of the drug is available.
- c. The drug has a very high abuse potential.
- d. None of the above restricts prescribing a brand-name drug.

2. Phase I studies are important to:
- a. Reveal the adverse and toxic effects of a new drug in people.
- b. Determine the efficacy of a new drug in a specific disease.
- c. Determine a safe dosage range of a new drug in humans.
- d. Indicate the effectiveness of a new drug in animal models of disease.

3. Which of the following controlled drug schedules contains drugs that have no accepted medical use in the United States?
- a. Schedule I
- b. Schedule II
- c. Schedule III
- d. Schedule IV
- e. Schedule V

4. The Latin abbreviation q.i.d. on a prescription means that the drug is to be taken:
- a. Twice a day.
- b. Four times a day.
- c. Whenever needed.
- d. Every day.
- e. Every other day.

5. How many milligrams are contained in five grains of aspirin?
- a. 30 mg
- b. 80 mg
- c. 130 mg
- d. 325 mg
- e. 500 mg

CHAPTER 7

Herbals and natural products

Dale L. Birkle

Therapeutic overview

Since prehistoric times, humans have used plants as medicines. Of the 520 new prescription drugs approved between 1983 and 1994, 39% were natural products or derived from plants or animals, with 60% to 80% of antimicrobials and anticancer drugs obtained from such products. Over millions of years, plants have developed the capacity to synthesize a diverse array of chemicals, which attract or repel other organisms, serve as photocollectors or protectants, and/or respond to environmental challenges. For example, **phytochemicals** can assist plants in resisting pathogens, make them unpalatable, aid in collecting light energy, protect plants from photooxidation, or help dissipate excess light energy as heat. With the advent of modern scientific medicine, phytochemicals have been refined, or altered, to produce a share of the modern pharmacopoeia. Despite the increasing availability of many potent and selective drugs, there remains an increasing interest in folk remedies, including herbal medicines.

Herbal medicine is the most commonly employed form of **alternative medicine.** Alternative medicine refers to those practices other than the conventional medicine practiced and taught in Western medical institutions. In a 1998 survey, alternative medicine visits surpassed visits to conventional health care providers, with the highest rates of use in middle-aged (35-64 years old) people. In 1997, out-of-pocket expenses for alternative therapies were estimated at $27 billion, which was more than similar costs for conventional physician services.

The reasons for such common use of alternative therapies are varied. These include dissatisfaction with conventional medicine, the view that alternative therapies are empowering because of more patient control, and the perception that alternative therapies are more compatible with personal values or ethical beliefs. Predictors for use of alternative therapies include a higher educational level, poorer health status, holistic orientation to health, having had a transformational experience changing one's world view, and patients with chronic health conditions, such as diabetes, chronic pain, or cancer, which have not responded to conventional treatment. Even though the use of alternative therapies is common, it is rarely exclusive; only 4.4% of respondents in a 1997 survey relied primarily on alternative therapies. It should be emphasized that most people using alternative medicine do not report such use to their physicians or other conventional medical providers.

The biologically based alternative therapies include the use of botanicals (e.g., herbs, Box 7-1) and supple-

Abbreviations

DHEA	dehydroepiandrosterone
DSHEA	Dietary Supplement Health and Education Act
FDA	Food and Drug Administration
HIV	human immunodeficiency virus

Box 7-1 Major botanical preparations

Bulk herbs are raw or dried, essentially unprocessed plants or plant parts (leaves, roots, stems, flowers).
Oils are concentrates of the fat-soluble components of herbs.
Essential oils are the distillates of the volatile components of herbs.
Tablets or ***capsules*** are prepared from powdered herbs with the intent of providing a fixed, easily administered dose.
Teas are hot or cold water extractions of herbs. Teas are traditionally brewed 1-2 minutes.
Infusions are aqueous extracts of herbs that are steeped at least 20-30 minutes.
Decoctions are prepared by extracting plant material for 10-20 minutes in boiling water.
Tinctures are alcohol extracts that are usually mixed with water for oral administration.
Poultices or ***plasters*** are bulk herbs, moistened and prepared in a form suitable for applying to the skin.

ments (e.g., amino acids, vitamins, minerals), sometimes referred to as **orthomolecular medicine**. This is the practice of preventing and treating disease by providing optimal amounts of endogenous chemicals. In the orthomolecular view, providing vitamins, amino acids, trace elements, or fatty acids in amounts sufficient to correct abnormal physiological or biochemical abnormalities will be useful in preventing or treating particular diseases. The most commonly used botanicals and supplements are shown in Box 7-2.

The **Dietary Supplement Health and Education Act** (DSHEA), passed by the United States Congress in 1994, defines a dietary supplement as a product intended to supplement the diet, that contains a vitamin, mineral, amino acid, herb, or other botanical product intended for ingestion in the form of a capsule, powder, or extract. Dietary supplement products must bear an ingredient label that includes the name and quantity of each ingredient or the total quantity of all ingredients (excluding inert ingredients) in a blend. Labeling of products containing herbal and botanical ingredients must state the part of the plant from which the ingredient is derived.

Federal regulations provide for the use of various types of statements on the **label** of dietary supplements, but claims cannot be made about the use of a dietary supplement to diagnose, prevent, mitigate, treat, or cure a specific disease without sufficient clinical evidence. For example, a product may not carry the claim "cures diabetes" or "treats cancer," unless that claim is supported by clear evidence. Some health claims can be made, if the product has been so approved. For example, the claim that calcium may reduce the risk of osteoporosis has been approved by the Food and Drug Administration (FDA). Products can make claims about classical nutrient deficiency diseases, provided the statements disclose the prevalence of the disease in the United States. In addition, manufacturers may describe a supplement's effects on "structure or function" of the body or the "well-being" achieved by consuming the dietary ingredient. To use these claims, manufacturers must have substantiation that the statements are truthful and not misleading.

Box 7-2 Most commonly used dietary supplements

Echinacea—to treat colds
Ginseng—to boost energy, to treat type II diabetes
Gingko biloba—to improve memory
Garlic—to treat hypertension and high cholesterol
Glucosamine—to treat osteoarthritis
St. John's wort—to treat depression
Peppermint—to treat nausea and vomiting (pregnancy, chemotherapy)
Omega-3 fatty acids—for heart health and to treat inflammation and depression
Ginger—to treat nausea and vomiting (pregnancy, chemotherapy)
Soy—to treat symptoms of menopause

Mechanisms of actions

Like any other drug or chemical, the components of herbal medicines are presumed to exert their effects on physiological or biological systems. One major difference is that herbs contain large numbers of chemicals, which may interact synergistically or antagonistically. Some herbal remedies consist of mixtures of several herbs, so that the number of chemicals in a single preparation can reach into the hundreds or thousands. The complex nature of herbal medicines creates a major challenge to determining their mechanisms of action, and in only a few cases is there strong clinical evidence for efficacy (Box 7-3).

Antioxidant effects

Oxidation of DNA, proteins, carbohydrates, and lipids by reactive oxygen species has been implicated in normal aging and a number of different diseases,

Box 7-3 Levels of clinical evidence for efficacy of dietary supplements (from strongest to weakest)

Randomized controlled clinical trials: Participants are assigned by chance to separate groups for the comparison of different treatments. These trials can be "double-blinded" or "nonblinded." Double-blinded trials have a stronger study design because expectations are not a factor in determining outcome.

- **Double-blinded:** None of the participants know which groups are receiving the therapy under study or the comparison treatment. Comparison treatments can be no treatment, placebo treatment, and/or a different treatment, for example, standard of care.
- **Nonblinded:** The researcher(s) and the study participants know what treatment is being given. This design must be used when characteristics of the treatment cannot be disguised (e.g., massage therapy).

Nonrandomized controlled clinical trials: Participants are assigned to a treatment or control group, based on criteria that are known to the researcher, such as birth date, chart number, or day of clinic appointment. This type of study design is weaker because the composition of the treatment and control groups may not be equivalent.

Case series: Studies that describe results from a group or series of patients who were given the treatment that is being investigated. These studies are weaker because there is no control group. Different types of case series, in descending order of strength, are as follows:

- **Population-based, consecutive case series:** The study population is defined and is either the entire population of interest or a representative random sample of the population. The study subjects receive treatment in the order in which they are identified by the researcher.
- **Consecutive case series:** Studies describing a series of patients who were not limited to a specific population and who received treatment in the same order in which they were identified by the researcher.
- **Nonconsecutive case series:** Studies describing a series of patients who were not limited to a specific population and who do not represent a consecutive series of patients identified and treated by the researcher.

Best case reports: The study population consists of only the patients who benefited from the treatment under study. There is no control group, and patients who did not benefit from the treatment are not included. A best case report of one patient is an anecdote.

Box 7-4 Herbs commonly used as antioxidants

Tea
Garlic
Milk thistle (Silymarin)
Soy (isoflavones)
Ginkgo biloba
Red grape
Green vegetables, carrots, tomatoes
Vitamin E
Vitamin C
Red clover

including arthritis, cancer, and Alzheimer's disease. Oxidative stress occurs when there is an imbalance between **free radical** generation (by the action of reactive oxygen species) and endogenous antioxidants in cells and tissues. Reactive oxygen species are produced by some toxins, ultraviolet light, normal biochemical pathways (e.g., nitric oxide synthase), and pathological events in cells (e.g., free radicals that escaped from the mitochondrial complex). Endogenous antioxidants include reduced glutathione and the enzymes superoxide dismutase, catalase, and glutathione peroxidase. Many plants contain antioxidants (Box 7-4), including several typically used as food, and some vitamins also function as antioxidants. However, there is little high-level clinical evidence that supplementation with dietary antioxidants will ameliorate or prevent any disease. On the other hand, there is a wealth of scientific evidence for the free radical scavenging ability of many plant-derived antioxidants; thus the interest in this mechanism of action remains strong.

Immunomodulation

Some herbal medicines are thought to act by modulation of immune function. This modulation can be indirect, via antioxidant effects, or direct, via effects on immune cells. In general, herbal remedies are thought to enhance immune function by removing **toxins** from the body (a common concept in herbalism).

The herbal approach to immunomodulation is holistic and focuses on boosting liver function and cleansing the blood (Box 7-5). In the herbal philosophy, detoxification by the liver has a crucial role in health and in regulating immune function. Again, there is a dearth of clinical evidence for the efficacy of any herbal medicine in altering the course of disease, but some evidence in animal models and cell cultures suggests possible effects on immune function.

Box 7-5 Herbs commonly used for immunomodulation

Milk thistle	Elderberry
Dandelion	Astragalus root
Echinacea	Licorice
Cleavers	Olive leaf
Marigold	Cat's claw
Beet root juice	Thunder God vine

Table 7-1 Herbs proposed to act on the central nervous system

Sedatives	Stimulants
Kava	Lobelia
Valerian	Coffee
Skull cap	Tea
Passion flower	Tobacco
Lavender	Ginseng
Antiemetics	**Analgesics**
Black horehound	Cayenne
Lemon balm	White willow bark
Cayenne	Feverfew
Clove	Jamaican dogwood
Dill	St John's wort
Lavender	Ginseng
Meadowsweet	Corydalis (Corydalis yanhusuo)
Ginger	

Box 7-6 Herbs commonly used for hormonal problems

Menopausal symptoms

Vasomotor instability (hot flashes)
Soy, black cohosh, evening primrose, dong quai (angelica)
Mood disorders
St John's wort, valerian
Loss of libido, vaginal dryness, dyspareunia
Chasteberry (vitex)
Ginseng
Wild yam
Raspberry leaves

Androgen deficiency

Saw palmetto
Tongkat Ali (Eurycoma longifolia)
Tribulus Terrestris
Yohimbe bark
Pygeum
DHEA

Actions on neurotransmission

Many plants contain compounds that are used or abused for their psychoactive qualities, usually for sedative, stimulant, or analgesic purposes. These include coffee (caffeine), tobacco (nicotine), coca (cocaine), opium poppy (opiates), marijuana (cannabinoids), and peyote (mescaline). Ethnobotanical studies of shamanism in native populations have revealed many other hallucinogenic plants. A variety of herbal products are now also commonly used for sedative, stimulant, analgesic, and antiemetic effects (Table 7-1).

Plants contain many compounds that may act on neurotransmitter receptors in the central and peripheral nervous system. Plants also contain compounds that can interfere with uptake of neurotransmitters (prolonging their action), stimulate or block their release, or alter their enzymatic degradation. Many of these compounds have been isolated and modified to produce drugs in common use today. The classic examples are the opiate narcotics found in the opium poppy. Compounds from the opium poppy have been modified chemically to yield products with increased specificity in terms of opiate receptor subtype and ability to activate or block individual receptor subtypes.

Hormonal actions

Some herbs contain compounds that mimic or block the actions of hormones, notably **estrogen.** Currently used products include highly concentrated extracts of phytochemicals, synthetic derivatives, and even steroids like dehydroepiandrosterone (DHEA) and androstenedione, which are classified as dietary supplements because they are produced from plant precursor sterols (Box 7-6).

Phytoestrogens can be classified into three groups. **Isoflavones** are plant sterol molecules found in soy and other legumes. **Lignins** are a constituent of the cell wall of plants and become bioavailable as a result of the effect of intestinal bacteria on grains. The highest amounts are found in the husk of seeds used to produce oils, especially flaxseed. **Coumestans** are found in high concentrations in red clover, sunflower seeds, and bean sprouts. The plant lignan and isoflavonoid glycosides become hormone-like compounds with weak estrogenic and antioxidant activity after modification by intestinal flora. These compounds exert measurable effects on circulating gonadotropins and sex steroids, suggesting they have biological activity. High isoflavone intake may depress luteinizing hormone levels and secondarily depress estrogen production. Phytoestrogens can also act on intracellular enzymes, protein synthesis, growth factors, cellular proliferation, differentiation, and angiogenesis. Bean foods provide large amounts of fiber, and fiber modifies the level of sex hormones by increasing gastrointestinal motility. Fiber also alters bile acid metabolism and partially interrupts the enterohepatic circulation, causing increased estrogen excretion by decreasing the rate of estrogen reuptake.

Other botanicals have been proposed to modify hormonal balance in men. Saw palmetto contains steroid-like compounds that may antagonize the actions of testosterone and is suggested for treatment of benign prostatic hyperplasia and prostate cancer. Tribulus and Tongkat Ali are thought to enhance testosterone production through stimulation of luteinizing hormone production. Yohimbe contains yohimbine, an antagonist at α_2-adrenergic receptors known to increase norepinephrine release by blocking inhibitory presynaptic autoreceptors, thus enhancing sympathetic activity (see Chapter 10). Synthetic yohimbine is regulated as a drug and prescribed for erectile dysfunction, whereas yohimbe bark is sold as a dietary supplement. Pygeum may interfere with testosterone production by inhibition of 5-α-reductase and aromatase and is used for treating benign prostatic hyperplasia. DHEA is a naturally occurring adrenal hormone that is a precursor of estrogen and testosterone. Levels of DHEA decline with aging, so it is often used as a supplement to restore those levels toward more "youthful" values.

Anticancer effects

There are several approaches to herbal therapy of cancer (Box 7-7). Some herbal products have been suggested to prevent cancer by stimulating the immune system or by their antioxidant effects. Others are thought to act by direct toxic effects on neoplastic cells; for example, by inhibition of topoisomerases, inhibition of polyamine synthesis, or stimulation of apoptosis pathways. Other postulated mechanisms include blockage of angiogenesis (e.g., shark cartilage) and reversal of multidrug resistance pumps (e.g., flavonoids).

Herbs are also used to treat either the symptoms of cancer or the adverse effects of conventional chemotherapy and radiation treatments.

Several potent conventional cancer treatments (see Chapter 42) are derived from plants and other natural products. These include taxol from Pacific yew and the vinca alkaloids (vincristine, vinblastine) from Madagascar periwinkle.

Many cancer patients take large doses of vitamins and antioxidants with the belief that it may boost immune function and prevent further neoplastic transformation. Patients believe that, at worst, these supplements can do no harm. However, current research indicates this may be incorrect. Because conventional cancer therapy frequently depends on oxidative mechanisms, it is possible that the use of antioxidants could interfere with this treatment. Also, recent evidence suggests that apoptosis of cancer cells is increased by reactive oxygen species, and antioxidants can slow or block this process. The American Institute for Cancer Research has concluded that supplementation with individual

Box 7-7 Common uses of dietary supplements

Treatment of cancer

Antioxidant micronutrients (vitamin E, vitamin C, beta-carotene, selenium)
Immunomodulatory herbs (see above)
Soy protein
Polyunsaturated fatty acids

Increased athletic performance (ergogenics)

Antioxidants
Amino acids (arginine, lysine, aspartate, glutamine)
Caffeine
Carbohydrates
Creatine
DHEA
Glucosamine
Glycerol
HMB (β-hydroxy-β-methylbutyrate, a branched chain metabolite of leucine)
Ornithine
Protein
Pycnogenol
D-ribose
Sodium bicarbonate

Other uses

Glucosamine/chondroitin for osteoarthritis
Melatonin for insomnia
Acidophilus (probiotics) for lactose intolerance and the gastrointestinal side effects of antibiotics
Lutein for retina health
Grapeseed (antioxidant effects)
Cranberry for urinary tract infections
Lycopene as an antioxidant
Bitter melon (momordica), ginseng, and gymnema for diabetes

or combined antioxidants above levels established by the Institute of Medicine's Dietary Reference Intakes cannot be recommended as either safe or effective. Patients undergoing either chemotherapy or radiation therapy should be advised not to exceed the upper limits for vitamin and mineral supplements and to avoid dietary supplements that contain high levels of antioxidants.

Ergogenics

Ergogenics are substances that increase energy production, use, or recovery. Many products claim to give athletes a competitive edge through an ergogenic effect (see Box 7-7). Surveys have shown that three-fourths of college athletes and 100% of body builders take supplements for this purpose. There are a handful of supplements on the market that have been shown to be effective in high quality clinical studies.

Oral **creatine** supplementation can increase muscle phosphocreatine stores by 6% to 8%, leading to faster regeneration of adenosine triphosphate. Elevated levels of muscle creatine also buffer lactic acid produced during exercise, delaying muscle fatigue and soreness.

Caffeine increases contractility of skeletal and cardiac muscle and stimulates fat metabolism, thereby sparing muscle glycogen stores. It is also a central nervous system stimulant, which can aid in activities that require concentration. However, ergogenic doses of caffeine (250-500 mg) may cause restlessness, nervousness, insomnia, tremors, hyperesthesia, and diuresis.

Protein and amino acid supplements are used by some athletes to enhance muscle repair and growth. Athletes in training have increased protein needs, and inadequate protein intake causes a negative nitrogen balance, which slows muscle growth and causes fatigue.

Carbohydrates, specifically muscle glycogen, are the body's main source of rapidly available energy. Loading, or increasing the carbohydrate content of the diet for several days before an athletic event, has been suggested as a means to prolong exercise endurance. A meal prior to exercise will ensure that muscle and liver glycogen stores are maximized. Studies investigating ingestion of food 2 to 4 hours prior to exercise have shown a positive effect, regardless of the "glycemic index" of the foods ingested. Replenishment with carbohydrate-containing fluids during an endurance event may also help delay fatigue. Eating a mixture of carbohydrates and protein within 2 hours after exercise has also been associated with benefits, including replenishment of depleted muscle and liver glycogen stores and decreased muscle catabolism.

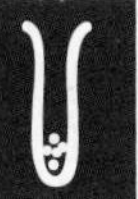

Pharmacokinetics

In most cases, it is not possible to determine the pharmacokinetics of herbal products due to their complex nature. When the active components are unknown, it is difficult to select the key components to follow in a pharmacokinetic study.

An important issue that needs additional investigation is the interaction of herbal products with other drugs. Drug-herb interactions can occur at the level of absorption, distribution, metabolism, or excretion (see Chapter 3), but metabolic interactions have received the most attention. These interactions go in both directions, with drugs either interfering with or enhancing the effects of herbs, and herbs or other supplements either interfering with or enhancing the effects (and side effects) of drugs.

Drugs, such as cholestyramine, colestipol, and sucralfate, may bind to certain herbs, forming an insoluble complex, and decrease absorption of both substances. Absorption of herbs may also be adversely affected by drugs that change the pH of the stomach. Antacids, H_2-histamine receptor antagonists and proton pump inhibitors (see Chapter 55), such as cimetidine and omeprazole, are used to neutralize, decrease, or inhibit secretion of stomach acid for treatment of ulcers or gastroesophageal reflux. With decreased stomach acid, herbs may not be broken down properly, leading to poor absorption in the intestines. Drugs that affect gastrointestinal motility may also affect herb absorption. Slower motility would mean the herbs stay in the intestines longer, thus increasing absorption. Metoclopramide and cisapride can increase gastrointestinal motility and decrease absorption of herbs. Haloperidol and some opiate narcotics decrease gastrointestinal motility and may increase absorption of herbs.

Many herbs induce the cytochrome P450 system (see Chapter 3), although the specific herbal components that induce P450s may be different from those responsible for therapeutic efficacy. Induction of P450s leads to increased metabolism of other concomitantly administered drugs that are metabolized through the same pathways.

Conversely, drugs that inhibit cytochrome P450s can increase the accumulation of herbs. Examples of drugs that inhibit liver metabolism include, but are not limited to, cimetidine, erythromycin, ethanol, and antifungal drugs, such as fluconazole, itraconazole, and ketoconazole (see Chapter 50).

Drug-food interactions are numerous and often overlooked. These interactions occur most often with diuretics, antibiotics, anticoagulants, antihypertensives, thyroid drugs, antiretrovirals, and antidepressants. For example, grapefruit is a potent inhibitor of specific cytochrome P450s (see Chapter 3). Some common drugs metabolized by these enzymes are cyclosporin, estrogens, benzodiazepines, HIV protease inhibitors, and simvastatin. Grapefruit juice can increase peak serum concentrations of some of these drugs as much as tenfold, and the effects can last as long as 24 hours.

Broccoli, cabbage, and related cruciferous vegetables can induce CYP1A2, whereas carrots can inhibit the enzyme. Drugs metabolized by CYP1A2 include warfarin, theophylline, and clozapine.

Foods that contain vitamin K, such as brussel sprouts, asparagus, avocado, and liver, can interfere with the actions of anticoagulants by direct action on the clotting cascade. Green tea contains vitamin K and can reduce the efficacy of warfarin.

Flavonoids, present in hops (beer), soybeans, and many herbs, can also inhibit certain P450s. Garlic inhibits CYP2E1, whose substrates include the general anesthetics halothane and methoxyflurane.

An herb-drug interaction that has received much media attention is the induction of CYP3A4 by St. John's wort, commonly ingested to treat depression. CYP3A4 is involved in metabolism of more than half of all prescribed drugs, including anti-retrovirals used to treat HIV infection and oral contraceptives, making this a very important source of potential herb-drug interactions.

Side effects, clinical problems, and toxicity

Difficulties in identifying side effects of herbs also arise because the identity of herbal ingredients is largely unknown, most reports are anecdotal, and effects may be attributed to herbs simply because there is no other obvious cause.

Because of the complex nature of herbal products, the potential for side effects would be expected to be large. However, a central tenet of herbalism is that complex composition minimizes side effects due to the presence of chemicals that exert the desired effect and other chemicals that antagonize side effects. However, these tenets have not been tested in controlled studies. In addition, the potency of an herbal product may be very low, when compared to typical drugs that are administered in the milligram or even microgram range.

Concurrent use of herbs and drugs with similar therapeutic actions creates the risk of **pharmacodynamic interactions**. The highest risk of clinically significant interactions occurs between herbs and drugs with sympathomimetic, cardiovascular, diuretic, anticoagulant, and antidiabetic effects. Some herbs contain salicylates and coumarins, which have antiplatelet activity that may potentiate prescribed anticoagulants. Ginger and ginseng have direct antiplatelet activity and can potentiate anticoagulant therapy and alter bleeding time. Licorice, consumed as an herbal remedy or as candy, raises blood pressure and should be avoided by people with hypertension. Hawthorn, a cardiotonic herb, may potentiate the actions of digoxin. St. John's wort may potentiate the actions of antidepressants, such as serotonin and norepinephrine reuptake inhibitors and monoamine oxidase inhibitors.

Provisions in DSHEA state that the manufacturer is responsible for ensuring that its dietary supplement products are safe before they are marketed. Unlike drug products that must be proven safe and effective for their intended use before marketing (see Chapter 6), there are no provisions in the law for the FDA to "approve" dietary supplements for safety or effectiveness before they reach the consumer. Also, unlike drugs, manufacturers and distributors of dietary supplements are not currently required by law to record, investigate, or forward to government agencies any reports they receive of injuries or illnesses that may be related to the use of their products. Under DSHEA, once the product is marketed, the FDA has the responsibility for showing that a dietary supplement is "unsafe" before it can take action to restrict its use or remove it from the marketplace.

The pharmacological actions of herbal products can give rise to serious **safety concerns**. Ephedra was used for many years for weight loss, as a stimulant, and to improve athletic performance. It was frequently mixed with caffeine, caffeine-containing herbs, or other herbs. Ephedra represented an interesting aspect of the current regulatory framework for herbs, because it contains ephedrine and other ephedrine-like compounds that, when prepared synthetically, are regulated as drugs. For example, low doses of ephedrine, an effective decongestant, were present in numerous over-the-counter cold remedies. The potential adverse effects of ephedrine were well known and include stroke, cardiac arrhythmias, and hyperthermia, caused by its sympathomimetic actions. Because there is no system for reporting adverse events that occur after ingestion of a dietary supplement, the incidence of these events linked to ephedra is not well established. However, evidence began to accumulate and reanalysis of the few clinical studies of ephedra, in conjunction with the untimely death of a well-known athlete, led the FDA to conclude that ephedra was unsafe, and it was removed from the market in 2004.

A second safety issue is that of **contaminants.** Because herbs are agricultural products or wild-crafted (i.e., gathered in the wild), they can be contaminated with pesticides, herbicides, and soil contaminants, such as heavy metals, fungi, and bacteria. In addition, contaminants can be introduced through the manufacturing process, such as solvents used for extraction. The liver toxicity of kava appears to be related to acetone extraction. Whether residual acetone is responsible for this toxicity, or whether acetone extracts additional chemicals from the bulk plant material that are not normally present in the teas made by native populations that use kava, remains to be determined. However, it is clear that some people who used a commercially available kava extract suffered liver damage, which led the FDA to ban acetone-extracted kava preparations.

A third safety issue is **adulteration.** Unscrupulous herb dealers and manufacturers of herbal remedies have been known to add pharmaceuticals to their products. Some complex herbal mixtures have been found to contain indomethacin, warfarin, and diethylstilbestrol. Because these pharmaceuticals could account for any therapeutic effect, it can be impossible to determine whether the herbal components of a remedy possess any efficacy. If the presence of pharmaceuticals is confirmed, the herbal product would be banned from the market.

A fourth safety issue is **misidentification.** A pharmacologically active herb may be only one species of a large genus of plants. Proper identification of the species can often be difficult. One example of this is ginseng. American ginseng is highly sought after for its tonic effects, but the collection of wild American ginseng is strictly controlled to avert decimation of the species. There are other ginseng varieties that, according to herbalists, are much less efficacious but could appear as American ginseng in the marketplace. There are essentially no guarantees that the plants identified on the label of an herbal remedy are actually the plants present.

Finally, herbs are natural products, and the chemistry of the plant is determined by growing conditions, including seed stock. This can lead to considerable variation in the chemical composition of any given batch of herbs (Fig. 7-1). There are no "standards" or methods of certification that are accepted across the industry. When the active ingredients are not known, it is obviously impossible to standardize preparations to achieve a reproducible pharmacological effect. Not only does this make the clinical use of herbs difficult, but it is also a major impediment to research in this area.

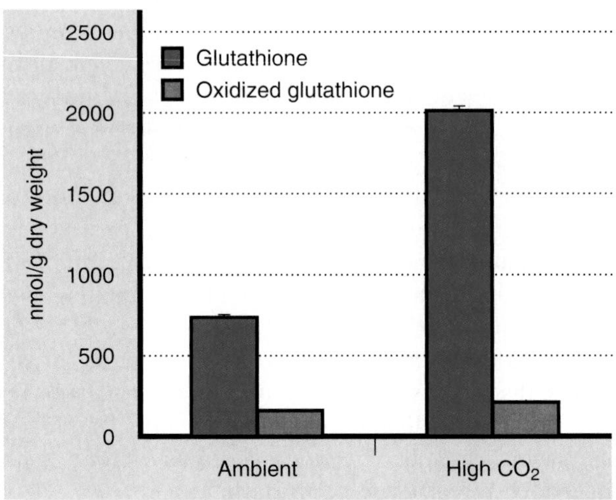

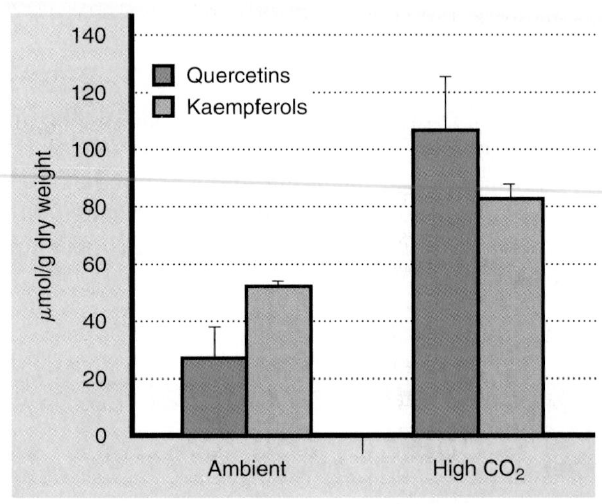

Figure 7-1 Relative concentrations of active ingredients in plants are known to be affected by environmental conditions. In this illustration, growing strawberries in a high CO_2 environment increased the content of the endogenous antioxidants, glutathione, and flavonoids. Adapted from Wang et al. *J Agric Food Chem* 2003; 51:4315-4320.

New horizons

Centuries of use have created the impression that herbal remedies are both safe and effective. The challenge to science is to provide controlled, clinical evidence for

Box 7-8 Important considerations in using herbals and natural products

- Labeling an herbal supplement as "natural" does not mean it is safe or without any harmful effects.
- Herbal supplements contain pharmacologically active chemicals. Therefore, they can cause medical problems, if not used correctly or if taken in large amounts.
- Women who are pregnant or nursing, children, the elderly, and people with liver or renal insufficiency should be especially cautious about using herbal supplements.
- It is important to consider other drugs taken with an herbal supplement, because some herbal supplements interact with medications.
- In the United States, herbal and other dietary supplements do not have to meet the same standards as drugs and over-the-counter medications for proof of safety, effectiveness, and what the FDA calls "good manufacturing practices."
- The active ingredient(s) in many herbs and herbal supplements are not known. There may be dozens, even hundreds, of such compounds in a single herbal supplement preparation.
- Published analyses of herbal supplements have found differences between what is listed on the label and what is in the bottle. Also, the word "standardized" on a product label is no guarantee of higher product quality, because in the United States there is no legal definition of "standardized" (or "certified" or "verified") for supplements.
- Some herbal supplements have been found to be contaminated with metals, unlabeled prescription drugs, microorganisms, or other substances.

these claims. In a typically reductionist fashion, Western science has approached the study of herbs via a drug development model. Once an effect has been established, bioassay-directed fractionation of the plant extract can lead to isolation of a single active chemical. However, it is also of interest to investigate the more holistic philosophy, which requires development of research strategies for the study of highly complex systems. These might include complex mixtures of herbs, or a complex, individually tailored treatment plan using several different herbs at different times in conjunction with dietary changes. Research is also needed to determine potential mechanisms of action and to more rationally guide design of clinical trials. The concept of detoxification, with consequent increases in well-being and ability to ward off disease, is central to herbal medicine but has not been well studied by Western scientists. Safety concerns about herbal medicines require well-designed toxicological and pharmacokinetic studies and may lead to more restrictive approval and marketing requirements and more stringent monitoring of adverse effects (Box 7-8). Herbal medicine is practiced by several types of alternative medicine providers, including doctors of traditional Chinese medicine, naturopaths, homeopaths, and Ayurvedic physicians (the traditional medicine of India). An expanding trend in health care is the concept of complementary medicine, where such therapies are combined with conventional Western approaches. More research is needed to determine the advantages (or disadvantages) of these combined, integrated approaches, because this trend is being driven by patient demand as well as evidence for improvements in health care and outcomes.

FURTHER READING

Information on herbal medicine from the National Library of Medicine (MedLine Plus), available online at http://www.nlm.nih.gov/medlineplus/herbalmedicine.html

National Center for Complementary and Alternative Medicine, available online at http://www.nccam.nih.gov/

Searchable herb database from Memorial Sloan Kettering Cancer Center, available online at http://www.mskcc.org/mskcc/html/11570.cfm

Self-assessment questions

1. The strongest type of evidence for efficacy comes from:
   a. Case reports.
   b. Randomized, controlled experiments.
   c. Case-controlled comparisons.
   d. Personal experience.

2. Herbal products are regulated by:
   a. USP.
   b. DSHEA.
   c. NCCAM.
   d. NAFTA.

3. An herb commonly used to increase immune function is:

a. Kava.
b. Cayenne.
c. Echinacea.
d. Ginger.

4. An herb commonly used to treat mild depression is:

a. Milk thistle.
b. Marigold.
c. Licorice.
d. St. John's wort.

5. Herbal products can make certain claims on their labels. For a hypothetical product, which statement is *not* allowed?

a. This product will improve the function of the female reproductive system.
b. This product will reverse a deficiency in calcium.
c. This product will cure cancer.
d. This product will give you increased energy.

6. Herbal products are more likely to be used by:

a. Middle-aged compared to older people.
b. Adolescents compared to the elderly.
c. High-school graduates compared to college graduates.
d. People with acute pain compared to people with cancer.

PART II

Drugs affecting the autonomic nervous system

THE HUMAN NERVOUS SYSTEM is the most complex of all body systems and is responsible for processing and transmitting information throughout the organism. The nervous system can be divided into the **peripheral nervous system (PNS)** and the **central nervous system (CNS)** (Fig. II-1). The PNS is subdivided into the **autonomic nervous system (ANS)** that controls automatic functioning, like breathing and heart rate, and the **somatic nervous system** that sends information to the CNS and skeletal muscles. The CNS is comprised of the **brain** and **spinal cord** and integrates and controls all bodily functions as well as thought processes. All these systems are interconnected and work together.

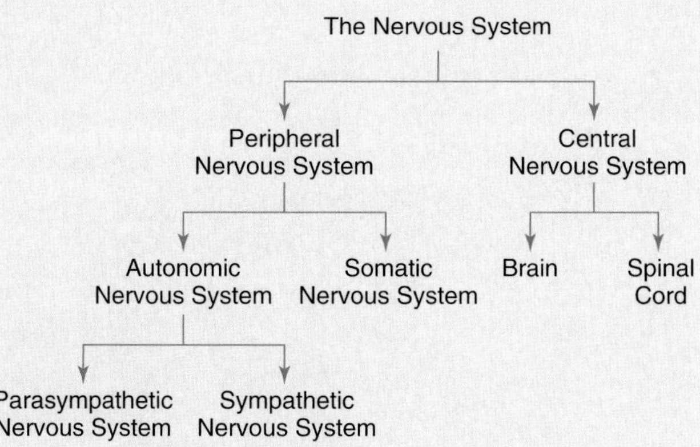

Figure II-1 Divisions of the nervous system.

The ANS innervates the heart, blood vessels, visceral organs, glands, and virtually all other organs that contain at least some smooth muscle. It controls key visceral processes, including cardiac output, blood flow to specific organs, glandular secretions, waste removal, and sexual activity. Regulation of the functions of these organs occurs in a manner that is generally not under conscious control, which is why the ANS is often referred to as the "involuntary" nervous system. Although the ANS innervates most bodily structures, it does not innervate skeletal muscle fibers, which are under the voluntary control of higher centers in the CNS. Nerves that control skeletal muscles are called somatic nerves and are functionally and anatomically different from autonomic nerves.

The ANS is divided both functionally and anatomically into the **sympathetic** and **parasympathetic** systems. Stimulation of the sympathetic system expends energy and leads to "flight, fright, or fight" responses characterized by increased heart rate, blood pressure, and respiration; increased blood flow to skeletal muscles; and mydriasis. In contrast, stimulation of the parasympathetic system conserves energy ("rest and digest") and leads to responses characterized by decreased heart rate, blood pressure, and respiration; increased secretions; and miosis.

Drugs may affect autonomic function indirectly through actions on the CNS, directly through actions on autonomic nerve fibers innervating specific organs, or directly on synapses between nerves and the innervated organ. Part II deals with the effects of drugs on the ANS.

Drug actions in the CNS and on somatic nerves are described in Part IV. Chapter 8 describes basic aspects of synaptic transmission and the ANS, with an emphasis on functional responses and sites of drug action. Chapter 9 covers the parasympathetic division of the ANS and autonomic ganglia, both of which utilize **acetylcholine (ACh)** as their endogenous neurotransmitter. Chapter 10 covers the sympathetic division of the ANS, which usually utilizes **norepinephrine (NE)** as its endogenous neurotransmitter.

CHAPTER 8

Introduction to the autonomic nervous system

David B. Bylund

Divisions of the autonomic nervous system

The two major divisions of the autonomic nervous system (ANS), the **parasympathetic** and **sympathetic** systems, function in parallel to maintain homeostasis by regulating bodily functions. Although these divisions differ both anatomically and functionally, they also share some commonalities. The outflow of both divisions from the spinal cord consists of two neuron relays named after their anatomical location relative to the **autonomic ganglia,** or relay centers. **Preganglionic neurons** have their cell bodies in the spinal cord and their nerve terminals at autonomic ganglia, where they relay information to cell bodies of postganglionic neurons. **Postganglionic neurons** send their axons directly to effector organs (heart, blood vessels, visceral organs, and glands), where they relay information to these cells; these synapses are often referred to as **neuroeffector junctions.** Thus, the preganglionic fibers of both the sympathetic and parasympathetic systems synapse with postganglionic fibers at autonomic ganglia. However, the location of the ganglia differs for the two systems, with parasympathetic ganglia located close to the organ innervated and most sympathetic ganglia located near the spinal cord. Due to the different ganglionic locations, the length of the preganglionic fibers relative to the postganglionic fibers also differs. Both sympathetic and parasympathetic preganglionic neurons release **acetylcholine (ACh)** as the neurotransmitter at ganglia. However, parasympathetic postganglionic neurons release ACh to relay their information at the neuroeffector junction, whereas most sympathetic postganglionic fibers release **norepinephrine** (NE, also called **noradrenaline).** Parasympathetic and sympathetic neurons are defined anatomically, with parasympathetic neurons arising from the cranial and sacral regions of the spinal cord and sympathetic neurons arising from thoracic and lumbar regions. They are not defined by the neurotransmitter released, and sympathetic fibers that innervate some sweat glands release ACh rather than NE. An anatomical representation of the sympathetic and parasympathetic systems is shown in Figure 8-1, and the commonalities and

Abbreviations

ACh	acetylcholine
AChE	acetylcholinesterase
ANS	autonomic nervous system
ATP	adenosine triphosphate
cAMP	cyclic adenosine monophosphate
CNS	central nervous system
COMT	catechol-O-methyltransferase
DA	dopamine
DOPA	dihydroxyphenylalanine
Epi	epinephrine
GI	gastrointestinal
MAO	monoamine oxidase
NE	norepinephrine
PNS	peripheral nervous system

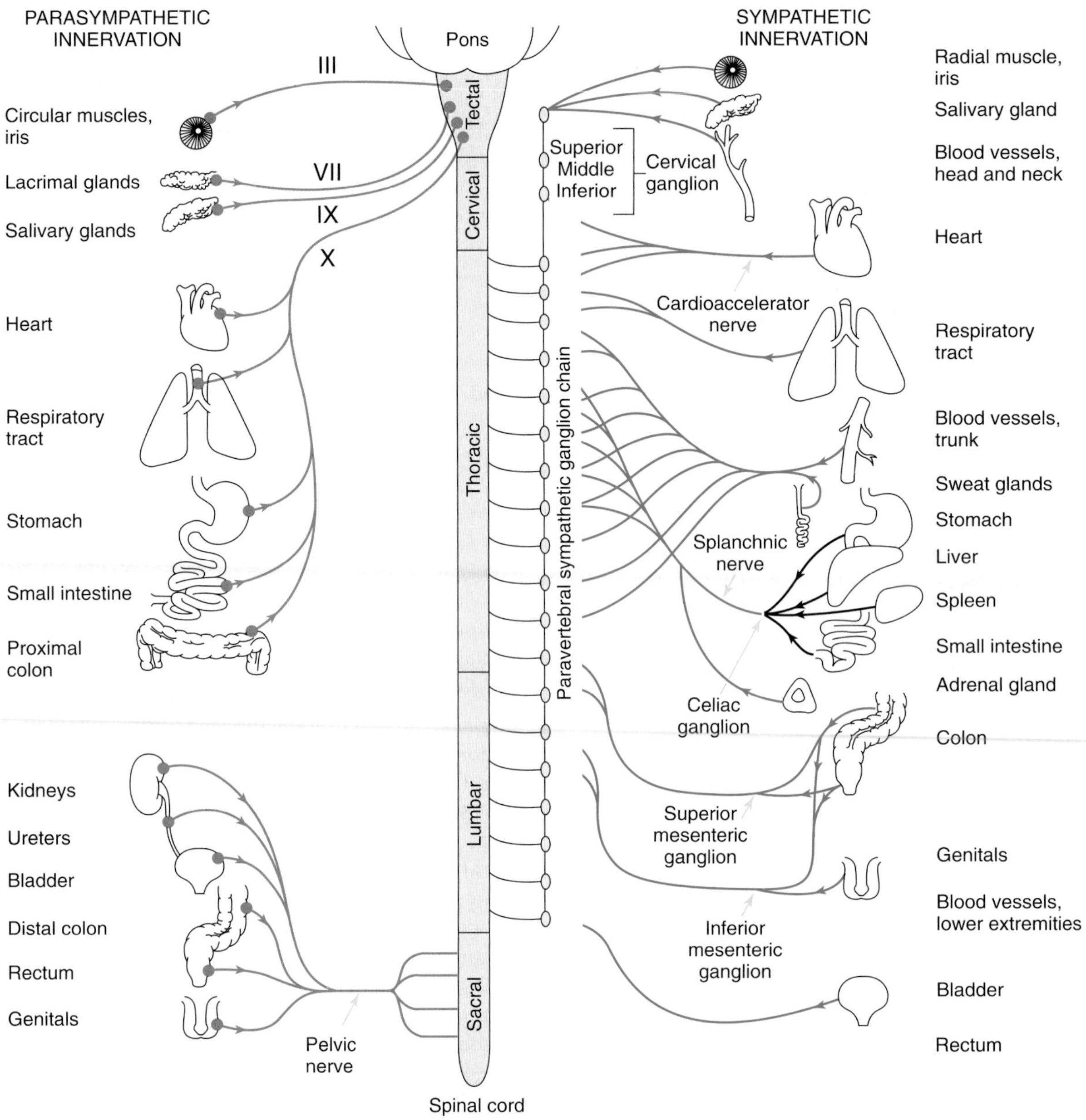

Figure 8-1 Schema of the autonomic nervous system depicting the functional innervation of peripheral effector organs and the anatomical origin of peripheral autonomic nerves from the spinal cord. The Roman numerals on nerves originating in the tectal region of the brainstem refer to the cranial nerves that provide parasympathetic outflow to the effector organs of the head, neck, and trunk.

differences between the systems are summarized in Table 8-1.

The **enteric nervous system** is often considered to be a third division of the ANS. This system is composed of a meshwork of fibers innervating the gastrointestinal (GI) tract, pancreas, and gall bladder. The enteric nervous system releases a variety of different neurotransmitters and is independent of **central nervous system (CNS)** control. Although components of the enteric system are innervated by parasympathetic preganglionic fibers, local control appears to dominate its function.

Although the ANS is considered to be an efferent system, almost all peripheral nerves (both autonomic and somatic) have afferent sensory fibers that provide feedback to the brain. These visceral afferent fibers are unmyelinated and have their cell bodies in the dorsal root ganglia of the spinal nerves and in cranial nerve ganglia. These sensory neurons and nerve fibers function as a feedback system to autonomic efferent control

Table 8-1 Comparison of the components of the autonomic nervous system (ANS)

	Parasympathetic Nervous System		Sympathetic Nervous System	
	Preganglionic Neuron	**Postganglionic Neuron**	**Preganglionic Neuron**	**Postganglionic Neuron**
Synaptic location	ganglia located near organ innervated	synapses at organ innervated	ganglia located near spinal cord	synapses at organ innervated
Neuron length	long	short	short-medium	medium-long
Neurotransmitter	ACh	ACh	ACh	NE*

*Postganglionic sympathetic neurons to some sweat glands release ACh.

centers in the CNS mediating sensation and vasomotor, respiratory, and viscerosomatic outflow.

Parasympathetic nervous system

Cell bodies giving rise to preganglionic parasympathetic nerves exit the spinal cord at the cranial and sacral levels (see Fig. 8-1). The cranial (tectobulbar) portion of the parasympathetic outflow innervates structures in the head, neck, thorax, and abdomen. The sacral division of the parasympathetic nervous system forms the pelvic nerve and innervates the remainder of the intestines and the pelvic viscera, including the bladder and reproductive organs.

The preganglionic neurons of the parasympathetic nervous system are myelinated and very long, such that parasympathetic ganglia are located in, or near, the effector organs. Consequently, postganglionic parasympathetic neurons, which are generally unmyelinated, are short.

Sympathetic nervous system

Cell bodies for preganglionic sympathetic neurons originate in the intermediolateral cell column of the spinal cord at the thoracic and lumbar levels (see Fig. 8-1). Relatively short preganglionic, usually myelinated, neurons project to the sympathetic ganglia outside the spinal vertebrae. These 22 segmentally arranged ganglia consist of two chains located bilaterally, with respect to the spinal cord, often called the paravertebral chain. Postganglionic sympathetic neurons are generally unmyelinated and send long postganglionic fibers to their effector organs. Most preganglionic sympathetic neurons synapse in the paravertebral sympathetic ganglia. Several, however, are prevertebral and lie near the bony vertebral column in the abdomen and pelvis (celiac, superior and inferior mesenteric, and aorticorenal), while a few (cervical ganglia and ganglia connected to urinary bladder and rectum) lie near the organs innervated.

The adrenal medulla is also a part of the sympathetic nervous system. It contains chromaffin cells that are embryologically and anatomically similar to sympathetic ganglia. Chromaffin cells are innervated by typical preganglionic sympathetic nerves and synthesize and secrete **epinephrine (Epi,** also called **adrenaline)** into the blood, analogous to postganglionic sympathetic neurons, which release NE.

Autonomic regulation of peripheral organs

Most organs of the body are innervated by both parasympathetic and sympathetic nerves. Generally, these two branches of the ANS stimulate opposing responses in effector organs. However, there are some exceptions where the two systems cause similar responses. There is generally a balance between sympathetic and parasympathetic effects on most organs, such that inhibition of one often leads to an increase in the response mediated by the other. Some organs, such as the vasculature and spleen, receive only one type of innervation, which, in these cases, is sympathetic.

One sympathetic preganglionic neuron may ramify and ultimately synapse with many postganglionic sympathetic neurons, leading to diffuse responses. By contrast, parasympathetic preganglionic neurons generally form only single synapses with postganglionic neurons, resulting in more discrete and localized responses. This anatomical distinction has profound physiological significance. Activation of sympathetic outflow, triggered by anger, fear, or stress, causes a state of activation characteristic of the "fight, flight, or fright" response. Heart rate is accelerated, blood pressure is increased, perfusion to skeletal muscle is augmented as blood flow is redirected from the skin and splanchnic region, the blood glucose concentration is elevated, bronchioles and pupils are dilated, and piloerection occurs. In contrast, activation of parasympathetic outflow is associated with conservation of energy and maintenance of function during periods of lesser activity. Activation of parasympathetic outflow reduces heart rate and blood pressure, activates GI movements, and results in emptying of the urinary bladder and rectum. Furthermore, lacrimal, salivary, and mucous cells are activated, and the smooth muscle of the bronchial tree is contracted. Although the parasympathetic nervous system is essential for life, the sympathetic nervous system is not. Animals completely deprived of their sympathetic nervous system can survive in a controlled environment but have difficulty responding to stressful conditions.

Neurotransmission and neurotransmitters in the autonomic nervous system

Neurotransmission

Neurotransmission is the process of effective transfer and integration of information in the nervous system. **Neurotransmitters** are endogenous substances released from **nerve terminals,** which act on **receptors** present on the membrane of **postsynaptic cells.** It is the interaction of the released neurotransmitter with the receptor that produces a functional change in the cell (Fig. 8-2).

Depolarization of a presynaptic nerve terminal leads to release of a neurotransmitter into the extracellular fluid between the presynaptic and postsynaptic cells **(the synaptic cleft).** Calcium provides the essential link between depolarization and transmitter release. When a nerve terminal is depolarized, there is a large influx of calcium caused by opening of voltage-dependent calcium channels in the membrane. This influx promotes fusion of transmitter-containing **synaptic vesicles** with the plasma membrane resulting in **exocytosis** of the vesicular content of neurotransmitter. Following exocytosis, the voltage-dependent calcium channels inactivate rapidly, and the intracellular calcium concentration returns to normal by sequestration into intracellular compartments and active extrusion from the cell. The steps linking the arrival of an action potential to neurotransmitter release are summarized in Figure 8-3.

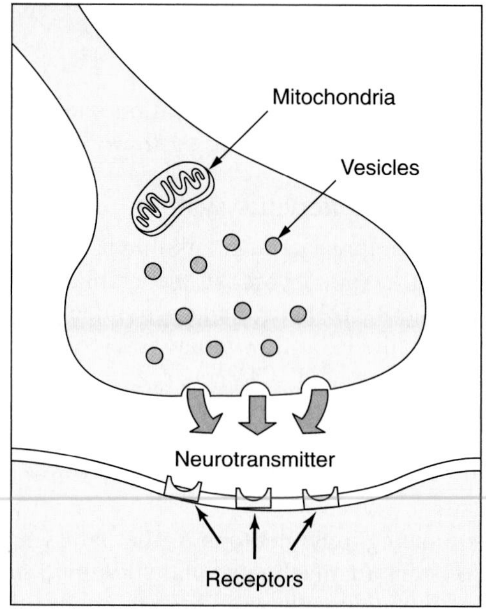

Figure 8-2 The process of chemical neurotransmission. Neurotransmitter molecules are released from synaptic vesicles within the nerve terminal into the synaptic cleft, where they diffuse to the postjunctional side and interact with their receptors.

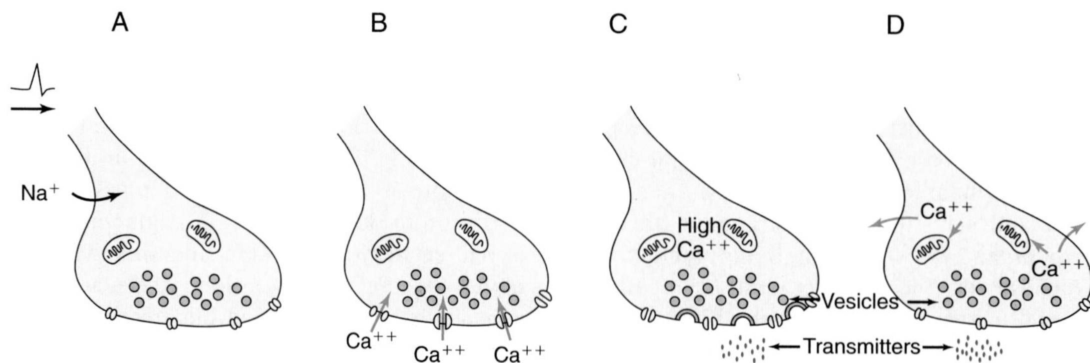

Figure 8-3 Sequence of events linking nerve terminal depolarization to release of neurotransmitter. **A,** The action potential arrives at the nerve terminal and depolarizes the membrane. **B,** Voltage-gated calcium channels open, allowing the influx of calcium down its concentration gradient. **C,** The increased intracellular calcium concentration promotes the fusion of transmitter-containing synaptic vesicles with the plasma membrane, resulting in exocytosis of the vesicular contents. **D,** The calcium channels rapidly inactivate, and the intracellular calcium concentration is returned to normal by both sequestration into mitochondria and active extrusion from the cell.

It is important to understand that voltage-dependent calcium channels in nerve terminals differ from those in other tissues. The calcium channel antagonists are an important class of drugs that block voltage-dependent calcium channels in cardiac and smooth muscle (see Chapter 12). However, there are distinct subtypes of these channels that can be distinguished by their electrical and pharmacological properties. The calcium-channel antagonists block the channels most often found in cardiac and smooth muscle (L type) and have no effect on most of the voltage-dependent calcium channels found in nerve terminals (N type). This is fortunate because if calcium-channel antagonists also blocked neurotransmitter release, their toxicity would undoubtedly prevent them from being useful therapeutically.

Following release, the neurotransmitter diffuses across the synaptic cleft to interact with specific receptors on the dendrites and cell body of the postganglionic neuron or on cells of the effector organ to deliver its message. The postsynaptic cell must then respond in an appropriate fashion to the received message. Thus, the nerve terminal has mechanisms for storing and releasing neurotransmitters in response to depolarization, and the postsynaptic cell has receptors for detecting the presence and identity of different neurotransmitters and initiating appropriate changes in physiology or metabolism. Nerve terminals also have efficient mechanisms for the degradation and reutilization **(reuptake)** of neurotransmitters to ensure the rapid termination of arriving messages. These processes, neurotransmitter synthesis, storage, release, reuptake, and degradation represent the sites of action of many drugs.

Neurotransmission at autonomic ganglia and neuroeffector junctions is illustrated in Figure 8-4. In both sympathetic and parasympathetic ganglia, preganglionic stimulation leads to the release of ACh, which activates postjunctional **nicotinic acetylcholine receptors** on postganglionic neurons to increase ion permeability, resulting in generation of an action potential that is propagated down the postganglionic nerve. When the action potential reaches the neuroeffector junction, either ACh or NE is released to activate **muscarinic cholinergic** or **adrenergic receptors,** respectively, on cells of the effector organ to produce an appropriate response. Receptors are discussed in greater detail later in this chapter and in Chapters 2, 9, and 10.

Neurotransmitter synthesis, storage, and inactivation

Acetylcholine ACh is synthesized in cholinergic nerve terminals by acetylation of choline, a process catalyzed by the enzyme choline acetyltransferase. As shown in Figure 8-5, acetyl coenzyme A is provided by mitochondria and serves as the acetyl donor, whereas choline is provided by both high-affinity uptake pumps after ACh hydrolysis and phospholipid hydrolysis within the neuron.

Following synthesis, ACh is stored in vesicles in cholinergic nerve terminals, where it is released upon depolarization to interact with its receptors. The action of ACh is terminated by the enzyme **acetylcholinesterase (AChE),** which rapidly hydrolyzes ACh into acetic acid and choline. Acetic acid diffuses from the synaptic cleft, whereas the majority of the choline is taken back up into the nerve terminal by the high-affinity choline uptake transporter. Once inside the nerve terminal, choline can be reused for the synthesis of ACh.

Norepinephrine and epinephrine NE is synthesized in adrenergic nerve terminals by a series of enzymatic reactions beginning with the precursor tyrosine, as depicted in Figure 8-6. As is evident from this schematic, the catecholamine neurotransmitter **dopamine (DA)** serves as an intermediate in this pathway. The reactions are depicted chemically in Figure 8-7. The first step involves hydroxylation of tyrosine in the meta position by **tyrosine hydroxylase** to form the catechol derivative DOPA. Tyrosine hydroxylase is rate-limiting in the biosynthesis of all catecholamines (NE, Epi, and DA), and this step takes place in the cytoplasm of postganglionic sympathetic nerve terminals. DOPA is subsequently decarboxylated by l-aromatic amino acid decarboxylase to form DA, also in the cytoplasm. DA is actively accumulated by storage vesicles in the sympathetic nerve terminals, as depicted in Figure 8-6. A hydroxyl group is added by dopamine-β-hydroxylase inside the vesicle to make NE. NE is retained in the vesicle in association with ATP until released by arrival of an action potential. Dopamine-β-hydroxylase is the last enzyme in the biosynthesis of NE in postganglionic sympathetic neurons, which release only NE.

In contrast, NE and Epi coexist in the adrenal medulla, and Epi is also found in neurons in the CNS. The synthesis of Epi from NE occurs through phenethanolamine-*N*-methyltransferase, which methylates NE that has diffused out of the storage granules into the cytoplasm. Cytoplasmic Epi is stored in granules until released. In adult humans, Epi constitutes approximately 80% of the catecholamines in the adrenal medulla, with NE making up the remainder.

The action of NE is terminated by a combination of neuronal reuptake into the sympathetic nerve terminal by an energy-dependent pump **(uptake$_1$)** and

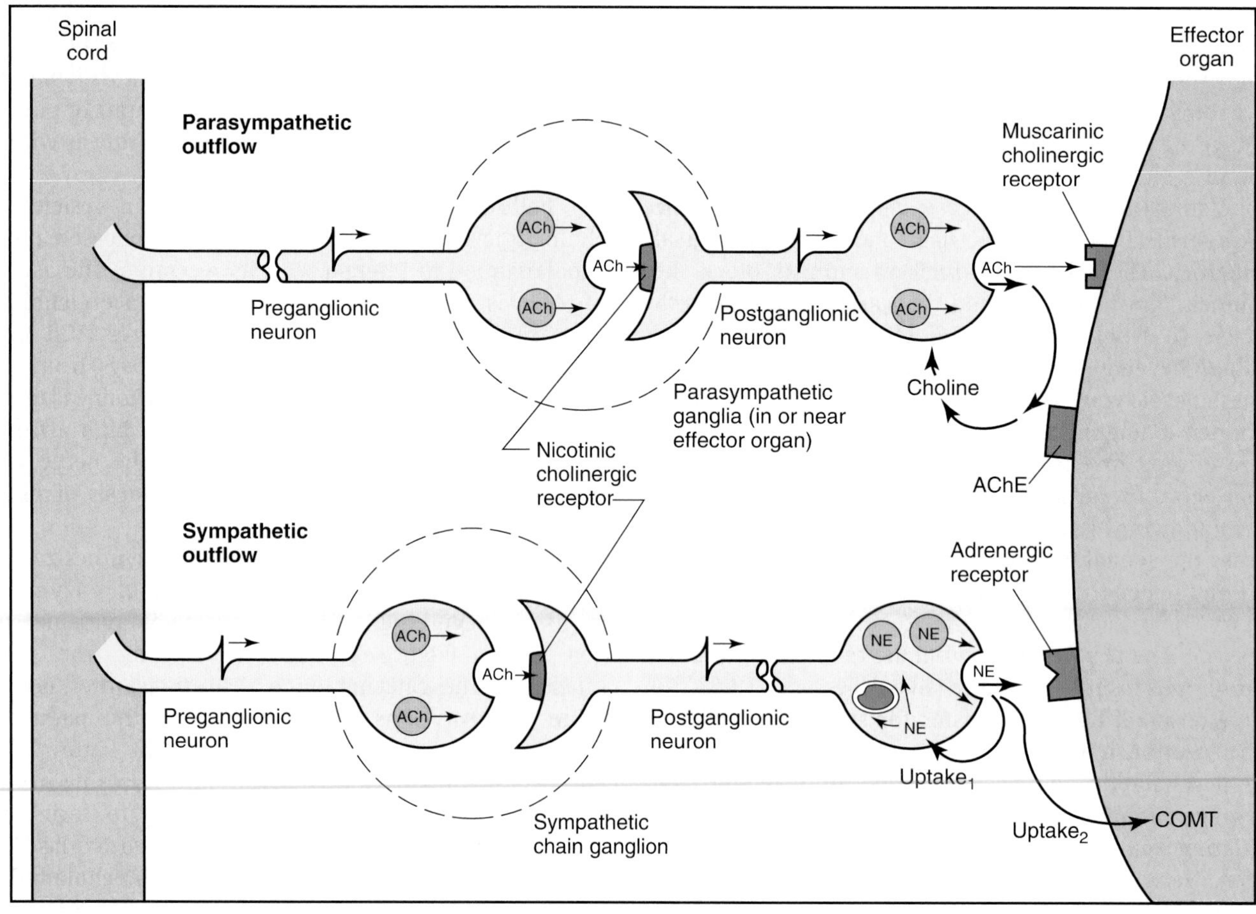

Figure 8-4 Neurochemical transmission in the parasympathetic and sympathetic divisions of the ANS. Upon the arrival of an action potential at the preganglionic nerve terminal, the neurotransmitter ACh is released by both parasympathetic and sympathetic ganglia. ACh diffuses across the synaptic cleft to interact with nicotinic cholinergic receptors on postganglionic neurons (often referred to as ganglionic receptors). This interaction results in the generation and propagation of action potentials down postganglionic neurons to elicit the release of neurotransmitter at the postganglionic nerve terminal (neuroeffector junction). The neurotransmitter released from postganglionic parasympathetic nerves is ACh, which diffuses across the synaptic cleft and activates muscarinic cholinergic receptors on the effector organ. The liberated ACh is rapidly metabolized by AChE to acetic acid and choline, the latter which is taken up into the parasympathetic nerve terminal and used to resynthesize ACh. At the postganglionic sympathetic neuroeffector junction, the neurotransmitter released is NE, which diffuses across the neuroeffector junction to stimulate adrenergic receptors and elicit the end-organ response. Most of the liberated NE is taken back up into the sympathetic nerve terminal (uptake$_1$) and is either stored in vesicles or metabolized by MAO located in the mitochondria. A smaller amount of the liberated NE may diffuse away and be accumulated by extraneuronal cells (uptake$_2$), after which it may be metabolized by COMT.

diffusion and uptake by an extraneuronal process **(uptake$_2$)**, as depicted in Figure 8-4. NE that is taken back up into sympathetic nerves may be oxidatively deaminated by the enzyme **monoamine oxidase (MAO)** present in the mitochondria of the nerve terminal, or it may be sequestered in vesicles for subsequent release. NE that diffuses to the extraneuronal uptake site may be inactivated by the enzyme **catechol-*O*-methyltransferase (COMT).** The metabolism of NE and Epi by MAO and COMT is depicted in Figure 8-8. Numerous inactive metabolites are formed and the levels of these inactive metabolites in blood and urine have been used previously, but incorrectly, as an index of catecholamine metabolism in the brain.

Neurotransmitter receptors in the autonomic nervous system

ACh and NE use different receptors to mediate their end-organ responses, and each neurotransmitter may interact with many distinct receptor subtypes (see Chapter 2). The many receptor subtypes are currently classified by pharmacological studies using selective agonists and antagonists as well as by their amino acid sequences. It should be emphasized that the end-organ response is as much a function of the type of receptor present as of the neurotransmitter involved. Classification of cholin-

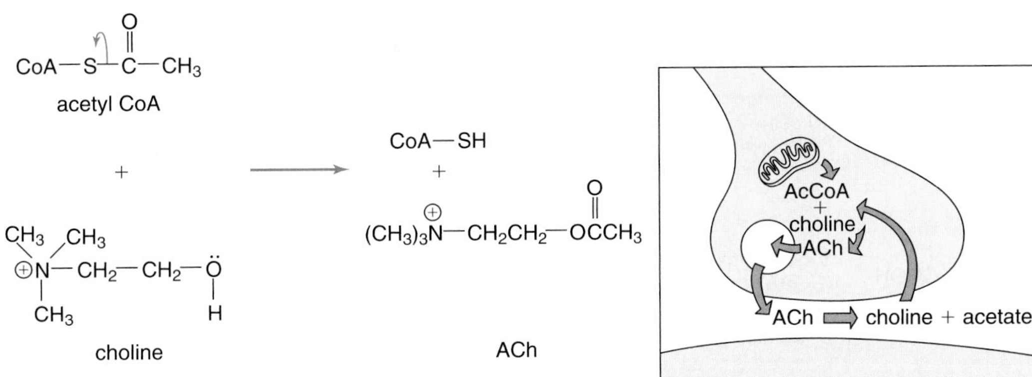

Figure 8-5 Synthesis, storage, and inactivation of ACh. ACh is synthesized in cholinergic nerve terminals through the acetylation of choline, a process catalyzed by the enzyme choline acetyltransferase. Acetyl coenzyme A (*AcCoA*) is provided by mitochondria and serves as the acetyl donor, whereas the choline comes from the cytoplasm and is provided by both high-affinity choline uptake and phospholipid hydrolysis within the neurons. Following the release of ACh and its interaction with its receptors, it is hydrolyzed by AChE to acetate and choline, the latter of which is taken back up into the nerve terminal and reutilized for ACh synthesis.

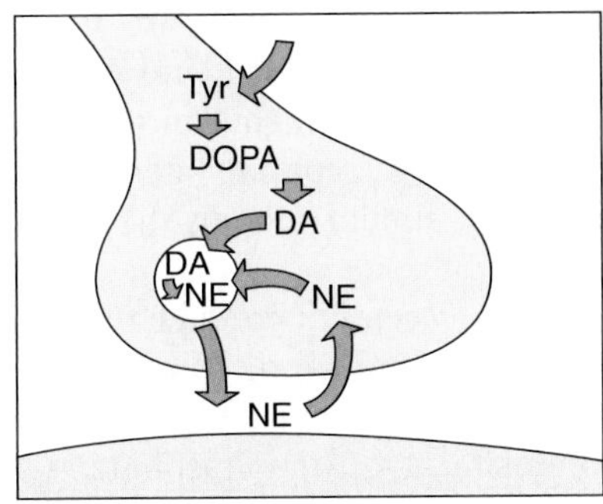

Figure 8-6 Synthesis, storage, and termination of the action of NE. NE is synthesized in adrenergic nerve terminals by a sequence of reactions beginning with the conversion of tyrosine to DOPA and DOPA to DA in the cytoplasm. DA is taken up by storage vesicles in sympathetic nerve terminals, where it is converted to NE. Following the release of NE and its interaction with its receptors, the action of NE is terminated by neuronal reuptake into the nerve terminal.

ergic and adrenergic receptor subtypes is presented in Figure 8-9.

Cholinergic receptors

ACh produces different effects at various sites throughout the body, often resulting from differences in the cholinergic receptors involved. The actions of ACh are mimicked in certain organs by the plant alkaloid nicotine, whereas the response to ACh in other organs is more closely mimicked by the plant alkaloid muscarine. Thus, responses to exogenous ACh or activation of the parasympathetic nervous system are described as being mediated by **nicotinic** or **muscarinic** cholinergic receptors. Nicotinic receptors are ligand-gated ion channels, which, when activated by ACh, allow influx of sodium and calcium. In contrast, muscarinic receptors are G-protein-coupled receptors which, when activated by ACh, activate G-proteins to induce downstream effects. These actions are illustrated schematically in Figure 8-10.

The primary actions of ACh at both parasympathetic and sympathetic ganglia are mediated by activation of ganglionic nicotinic cholinergic receptors. These receptors are similar structurally and functionally to the nicotinic cholinergic receptors in the CNS and on immune cells but differ from the nicotinic cholinergic receptors in skeletal muscle at the neuromuscular junction. These different types of nicotinic receptors can be selectively stimulated or blocked by different agonists and antagonists. Drugs affecting ganglionic nicotinic receptors are discussed in Chapter 9, and agents that affect skeletal muscle nicotinic receptors are discussed in Chapter 29.

The receptors mediating responses to ACh at parasympathetic neuroeffector junctions are muscarinic. Muscarinic cholinergic receptors are currently divided into five subtypes (M_1 to M_5), based on both their pharmacological specificities and their amino acid sequences. Activation of M_1, M_3, and M_5 receptors leads to activation of G_q and phospholipase C mediated generation of diacylglycerol and inositol-1,4,5-trisphosphate. Activation of M_2 and M_4 receptors leads to inhibition of adenylyl cyclase through G_i and a decrease in intracellular cAMP.

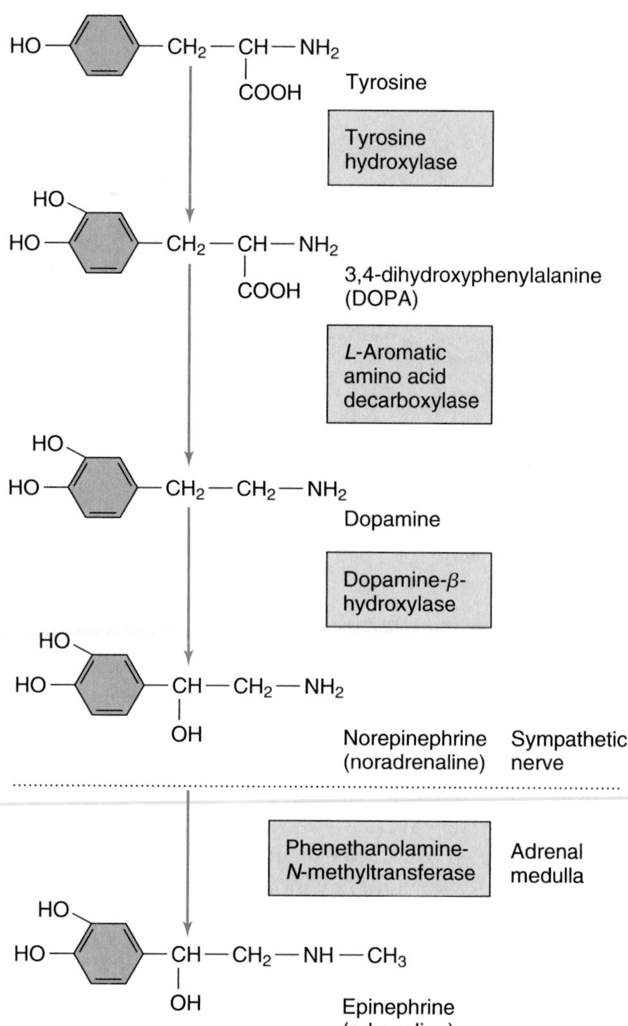

Figure 8-7 Steps in the enzymatic biosynthesis of the catecholamines DA, NE, and Epi. The enzymes involved in each catalytic step are enclosed in boxes. The first three enzymatic steps occur in postganglionic sympathetic nerve terminals, leading to the synthesis of NE, and all four enzymatic steps occur in the adrenal medulla, resulting in the synthesis of Epi.

In general, M_1 receptors are located in autonomic ganglia (where they modulate effects of nicotinic receptor activation), M_2 receptors are located in the heart, and M_3 receptors are located in many glands and smooth muscles. The locations of the M_4 and M_5 receptors are less certain, although all five muscarinic receptor subtypes are found in the CNS. Drugs affecting muscarinic receptors are discussed in Chapter 9.

Adrenergic receptors

Comparing the effects of several agonists on different tissues in 1948, Ahlquist provided the first evidence that NE and Epi could activate more than one type of adrenergic receptor. The rank order of potency for activation of responses in a number of tissues was Epi > NE > isoproterenol, whereas the rank order of potency in other tissues was isoproterenol > Epi > NE. These results suggested the existence of two types of adrenergic receptors, which were termed α and β. The existence of these distinct subtypes was later confirmed by development of selective antagonists.

Subsequent studies have shown that there are many more adrenergic receptor subtypes (see Fig. 8-9). There are three β-adrenergic receptor subtypes (β_1, β_2, and β_3), and selective agonists and antagonists have been developed with different potencies at these receptors. Stimulation of each β-adrenergic receptor subtype leads to activation of G_s, an increase in cAMP, and activation of cAMP-dependent protein kinase and phosphorylation of various intracellular proteins.

Pharmacological studies further subdivided α-adrenergic receptors into two major types, α_1 and α_2, each of which is now known to comprise three additional subtypes (see Fig. 8-9). Cloning and comparison of the genes for the adrenergic receptors have confirmed this classification scheme. There are a total of nine adrenergic receptors, subdivided into three subfamilies (α_1, α_2, and β), each of which contains three distinct subtypes encoded by separate genes. Amino acid sequences are very similar among the subtypes within a given subfamily.

α_1-Adrenergic receptors produce their effects in the same way as M_1, M_3, and M_5 receptors, by activation of G_q and phospholipase C-mediated generation of diacylglycerol and inositol-1,4,5-trisphosphate. α_2-Adrenergic receptors usually produce their effects in the same way as M_2 and M_4 receptors, by inhibiting adenylyl cyclase through G_i and decreasing intracellular cAMP. However, α_2-adrenergic receptors may also use other mechanisms of signal transduction. For example, in blood vessels, effects of α_2-receptor activation are mediated by activation of a membrane calcium channel, resulting in influx of calcium.

Prejunctional autoreceptors

Although the adrenergic receptors mediating the actions of NE at sympathetic neuroeffector junctions are located postsynaptically on the organ innervated, prejunctional α_2-adrenergic receptors have been identified on both adrenergic and cholinergic nerve terminals. Activation of these receptors by released NE or by administered α_2-adrenergic receptor agonists decreases further release of neurotransmitter. This presynaptic inhibitory "autoreceptor" mechanism may be involved in the normal regulation of neurotransmitter release because

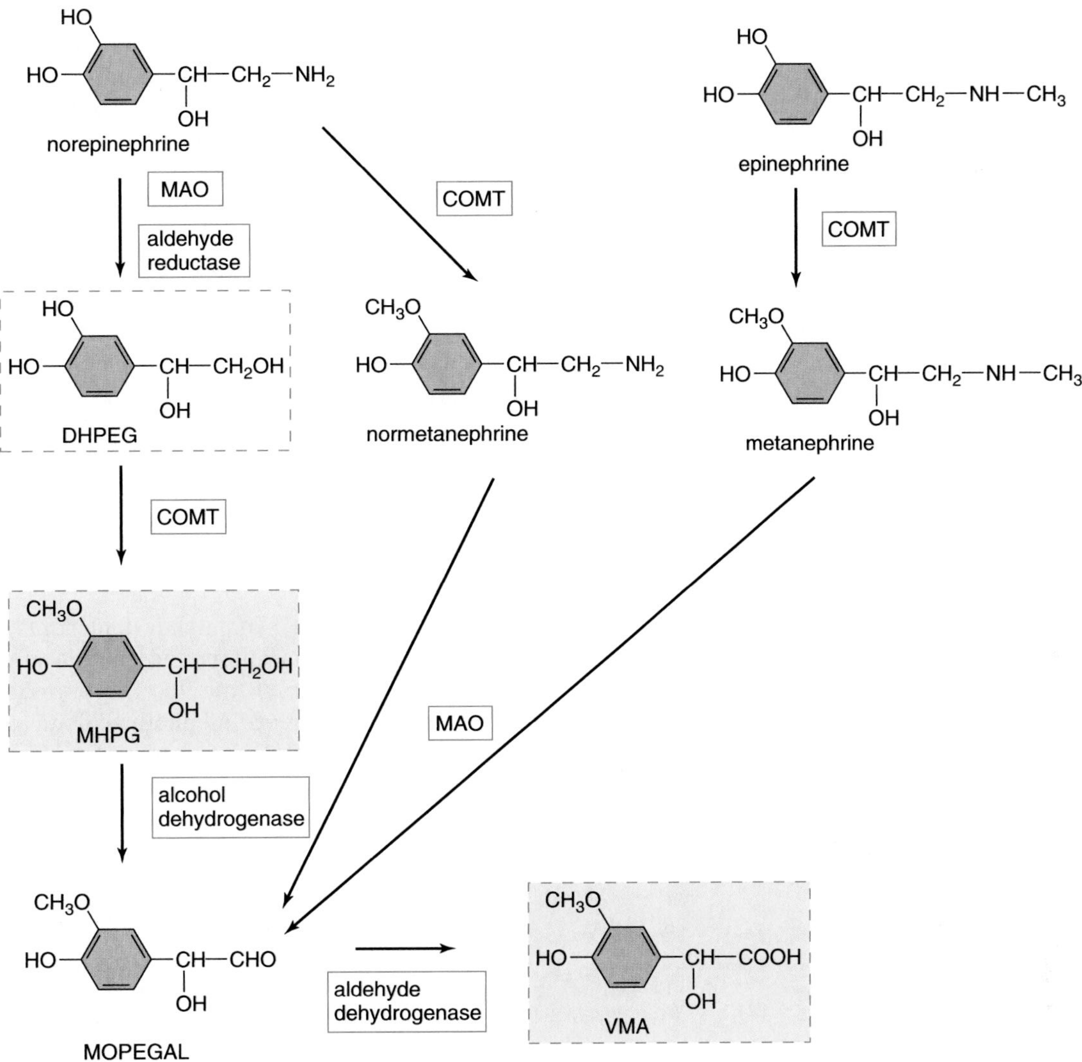

Figure 8-8 Main pathways of metabolism of norepinephrine and epinephrine. The major pathway of norepinephrine is on the left. NE is metabolized to 3,4-dihydroxyphenylethylene glycol (*DHPEG*) by the sequential actions of monoamine oxidase (*MAO*), and aldehyde reductase DHPEG is converted to 3-methoxy-4-hydroxyphenylethylene glycol (MHPG) by catechol-O-methyltransferase (*COMT*). The sequential actions of alcohol dehydrogenase and aldehyde dehydrogenase lead to subsequent conversion to 3-methoxy-4-hydroxyphenylglycolaldehyde (*MOPEGAL*; a short-lived intermediate) and formation of 3-methoxy-4-hydroxymandelic acid (*VMA*) in the liver. Released NE is metabolized to normetanephrine and then to VMA as indicated. Similarly, epinephrine is metabolized to VMA through metanephrine.

blockade of prejunctional α_2-receptors leads to enhanced NE release. Presynaptic α_2-receptors also exist on most cholinergic nerve terminals, and when these receptors are activated, release of ACh is inhibited. The prejunctional α_2-receptors on cholinergic nerves may be activated by administered α_2-receptor agonists, or by NE released from postganglionic sympathetic neurons synapsing near parasympathetic nerve terminals.

Functional responses mediated by the autonomic nervous system

Many organs receive both cholinergic and adrenergic innervation, and responses in these organs represent a complex interplay between the parasympathetic and sympathetic nervous systems. Often an organ is under the predominant control of a single division of the ANS, although both components are usually present and can influence any given response. Organs innervated by both sympathetic and parasympathetic nerves include the heart, eye, bronchial tree, GI tract, urinary bladder, and reproductive organs. Some structures, such as blood vessels, the spleen, and piloerector muscles, receive only a single type of innervation, generally sympathetic. The responses to nerve stimulation in each organ are mediated by the particular muscarinic cholinergic or adrenergic receptors present.

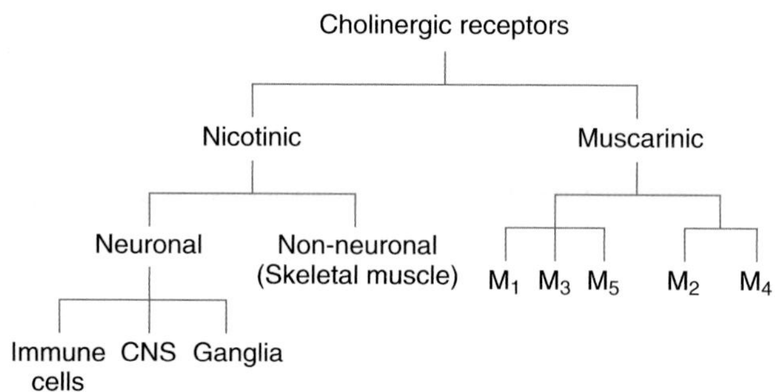

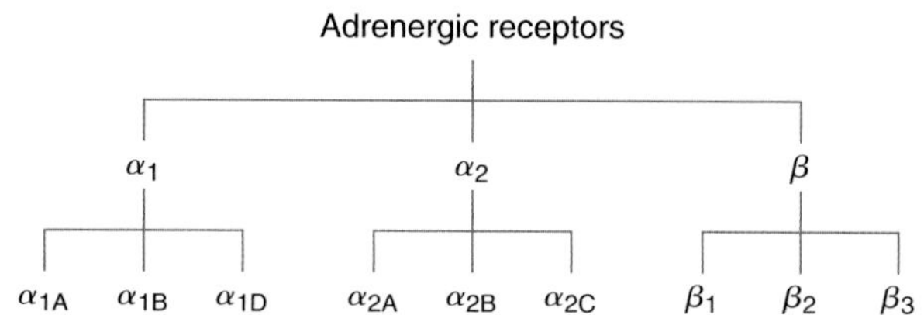

Figure 8-9 Classification of cholinergic and adrenergic receptor types and subtypes.

The responses to parasympathetic and sympathetic stimulation that occur in many important organs of the body are presented in Table 8-2. In most instances, sympathetic and parasympathetic nerves mediate physiologically opposing effects. Thus, if one system inhibits a certain function, the other enhances it. The responses presented in Table 8-2 represent only those responses mediated by nerve stimulation, that is, they represent responses only in innervated organs. Autonomic receptors are also found at sites lacking nerve innervation. For example, although vascular smooth muscle generally has no parasympathetic innervation, it often expresses muscarinic cholinergic receptors. Although these receptors are functional and mediate responses to exogenously administered drugs, they probably play little or no normal physiological role.

Drugs acting on autonomic nerves and receptors

Drugs that alter the sympathetic and parasympathetic nervous systems and autonomic ganglia are discussed in detail in Chapters 9 and 10. This introduction will briefly review the types of pharmacological interventions possible (Table 8-3) and provide a few examples of drugs that act by different mechanisms.

Ganglionic blockers Drugs that block autonomic ganglia interfere with the transmission of nerve impulses from preganglionic nerve terminals to the cell bodies of postganglionic neurons. Because the neurotransmitter (ACh) and receptor (nicotinic) are identical in sympathetic and parasympathetic ganglia, ganglionic blockers inhibit both divisions of the ANS equally. However, the end-organ response may show a predominant adrenergic or cholinergic effect because one

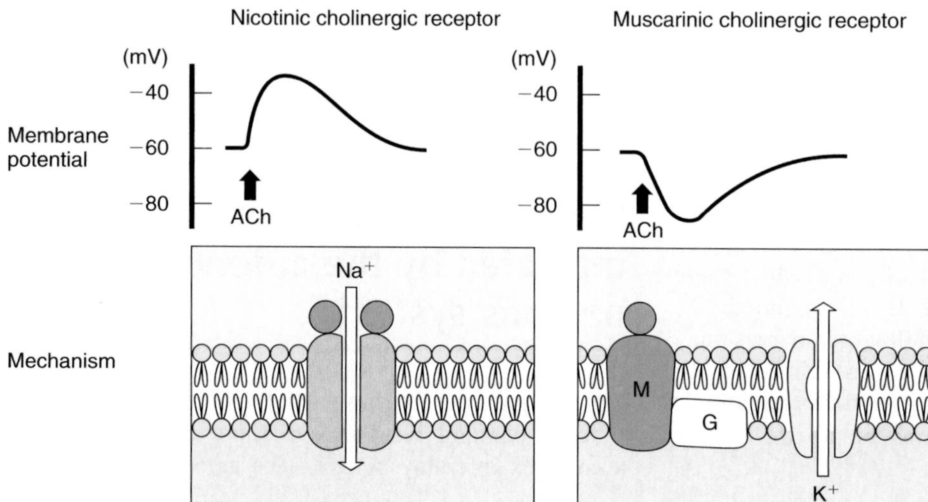

Figure 8-10 Activation of different cholinergic receptors by ACh can cause opposite effects on the membrane potential. Activation of the nicotinic cholinergic receptor *(left)* opens a ligand-gated channel to allow sodium to enter and depolarize the cell. Activation of the muscarinic cholinergic receptor *(right)* activates a G-protein, which in turn can open a potassium channel, leading to potassium efflux and hyperpolarization.

Table 8-2 Responses elicited in effector organs by stimulation of sympathetic and parasympathetic nerves

Effector Organ	Sympathetic (Adrenergic) Response		Parasympathetic (Cholinergic) Response		Dominant Response
	Response	Receptor	Response	Receptor	
Heart					
Rate of contraction	Increase	β_1	Decrease	M_2	C
Force of contraction	Increase	β_1	Decrease	M_2	C
Blood vessels					
Arteries (most)	Vasoconstriction	α_1 (α_2)	—	—	A
Skeletal muscle	Vasodilation	β_2	—	—	A
Veins	Vasoconstriction	α_2 (α_1)	—	—	A
Bronchial tree	Bronchodilation	β_2	Bronchoconstriction	M_3	C
Splenic capsule	Contraction	α_1	—	—	A
Uterus	Contraction	α_1	Variable	—	A
Vas deferens	Contraction	α_1	—	—	A
Gastrointestinal tract	Relaxation	α_2	Contraction	M_3	C
Eye					
Radial muscle, iris	Contraction (mydriasis)	α_1	—	—	A
Circular muscle, iris	—	—	Contraction (miosis)	M_3	C
Ciliary muscle	Relaxation	β_2	Contraction (accommodation)	M_3	C
Kidney	Renin secretion	β_1	—	—	A
Urinary bladder					
Detrusor	Relaxation	β_2	Contraction	M_3	C
Trigone and sphincter	Contraction	α_1	Relaxation	M_3	A, C
Ureter	Contraction	α_1	—	—	A
Insulin release from pancreas	Decrease	α_2	—	—	A
Fat cells	Lipolysis	β_1 (β_3)	—	—	A
Liver glycogenolysis	Increase	α_1 (β_2)	—	—	A
Hair follicles, smooth muscle	Contraction (piloerection)	α_1	—	—	A
Nasal secretion	Decrease	α_1 (α_2)	Increase	—	C
Salivary glands	Increase secretion	α_1	Increase secretion	—	C
Sweat glands	Increase secretion	α_1	Increase secretion	—	C

A, Adrenergic; C, cholinergic.

system is generally dominant in a given organ (see Table 8-4). Therefore, interruption of ganglionic transmission selectively eliminates the dominant component, leading to a response characteristic of the less dominant component. For example, in the heart, the cholinergic system generally dominates at the level of the sinoatrial (SA) node. When a ganglionic blocker is administered, its greatest effect is on this cholinergic component, resulting in an apparent adrenergic effect (tachycardia). The classic ganglionic blockers are hexamethonium and mecamylamine, but due to their many actions, they have limited clinical use.

Drugs that inhibit neurotransmitter synthesis Several enzymes are necessary for the biosynthesis of NE and Epi from tyrosine (see Fig. 8-7). Tyrosine hydroxylase, the rate-limiting enzyme, is inhibited by α-methyltyrosine. The next enzyme, l-aromatic amino-acid decarboxylase, is inhibited by carbidopa and α-methyldopa. α-Methyldopa is also a substrate for the decarboxylase, which converts it to α-methyl-NE, a selective α_2-adrenergic receptor agonist. Fusaric acid is a selective inhibitor of dopamine-β-hydroxylase and significantly reduces NE concentrations. In the adrenal medulla, phenethanolamine-*N*-methyltransferase catalyzes formation of Epi and can be inhibited by agents, such as 2,3-dichloro-α-methylbenzylamine.

ACh is synthesized by acetylation of choline through the action choline acetyltransferase (see Fig. 8-5). Although no potent and specific inhibitors of choline acetyltransferase are available, the biosynthesis of ACh can be indirectly inhibited with the experimental drug hemicholinium-3, which blocks the high-affinity choline transport system that provides choline to the

Table 8-3 Mechanisms of action of pharmacological compounds affecting the ANS

Action	Mechanism(s) of Action	Example
Ganglionic blockade	Interferes with transmission of nerve impulses between preganglionic and postganglionic neurons	Hexamethonium Mecamylamine
Inhibits neurotransmitter synthesis	Inhibits enzyme involved in NE biosynthesis	α-Methyltyrosine (inhibits tyrosine hydroxylase)
	Inhibits availability of choline for ACh synthesis	Hemicholinium-3
Inhibits neurotransmitter release	Interferes with adrenergic transmission	Guanethidine
	Interferes with cholinergic transmission	Botulinum toxin
Promotes neurotransmitter release	Activates ganglionic nicotinic receptors	Nicotine
	Releases NE from cytoplasmic stores	Tyramine Amphetamine
	Releases ACh from storage vesicles	Black widow spider venom (latrotoxins)
Inhibits neurotransmitter storage	Blocks vesicular NE uptake	Reserpine
	Blocks vesicular ACh uptake	Vesamicol
Inhibits neuronal reuptake	Blocks NE reuptake pump	Imipramine
Inhibits neurotransmitter metabolism	Inhibits NE catabolism	Pargyline (inhibits MAO) Tolcapone (inhibits COMT)
	Inhibits ACh hydrolysis	Physostigmine (inhibits AChE)
Stimulates autonomic receptors	Stimulates adrenergic receptors	Phenylephrine (α_1) Clonidine (α_2) Isoproterenol (β) Dobutamine (β_1) Terbutaline (β_2)
	Stimulates cholinergic receptors	Muscarine (muscarinic) Bethanechol (muscarinic) Nicotine (nicotinic)
Blocks autonomic receptors	Blocks adrenergic receptors	Phentolamine (α_1 and α_2) Prazosin (α_1) Yohimbine (α_2) Propranolol (β_1 and β_2)
	Blocks cholinergic receptors	Atropine (muscarinic) Trimethaphan (nicotinic)

Table 8-4 Effects of ganglionic blockade on major organ systems

Organ System	Predominant Tone	Effect of Ganglionic Blockade
Cardiovascular System		
Atria; SA node	Parasympathetic	Tachycardia
Ventricle	Sympathetic	Reduced force of contraction
Blood vessels	Sympathetic	Vasodilation; decreased venous return; hypotension
Eye		
Ciliary muscle	Parasympathetic	Focused for far vision
Iris	Parasympathetic	Mydriasis
Glands		
Sweat	Sympathetic	Decreased sweat
Salivary	Parasympathetic	Dry mouth
Gastrointestinal Tract		
Smooth muscle	Parasympathetic	Decreased contractions; constipation
Secretions	Parasympathetic	Decreased gastric and pancreatic secretions

nerve terminal. This results in considerable depletion of ACh in cholinergic neurons.

Drugs that inhibit neurotransmitter release The exocytotic release of NE from postganglionic sympathetic nerve terminals is inhibited by bretylium and guanethidine. These compounds are classified as adrenergic neuronal blocking agents.

Release of ACh is inhibited by botulinum toxin, which prevents exocytotic release of ACh from all types of cholinergic nerve fibers. Because of the essential role of the cholinergic nervous system (particularly in controlling the muscles of respiration), this toxin is lethal when administered systemically.

Drugs that promote neurotransmitter release Two processes can promote release of NE from postganglionic sympathetic nerve terminals. At sympathetic ganglia, nicotine activates nicotinic cholinergic receptors, which generates action potentials causing NE release. In the second process, tyramine, ephedrine, or amphetamine act indirectly to cause an increase in release of NE. These drugs enter the sympathetic nerve terminal and displace NE, which diffuses through the neuronal membrane into the synaptic cleft by a process that does not involve calcium or exocytosis.

The release of ACh from postganglionic cholinergic nerve terminals can also be evoked by activation of ganglionic nicotinic cholinergic receptors by nicotine. In addition, black widow spider venom contains latrotoxins, which have been shown to promote the exocytotic release of ACh.

Drugs that interfere with neurotransmitter storage Both ACh and NE are taken up into storage vesicles by specific energy-dependent pumps located in the vesicle membrane. These pumps transport the neurotransmitter from the cytoplasm into the vesicle. The uptake of NE into vesicles is inhibited by reserpine, thereby decreasing the amount of NE available for release, and can lead to complete depletion of catecholamines from postganglionic sympathetic nerve terminals. The compound vesamicol prevents the packing of ACh into storage vesicles, but this compound has no known therapeutic function.

Drugs that affect the duration of action of neurotransmitter After the exocytotic release of NE from postganglionic sympathetic nerve terminals, most of the released catecholamine is actively reaccumulated in the nerve terminal by uptake$_1$. Agents, such as imipramine and cocaine, block this uptake pump, thereby increasing synaptic concentrations of NE and enhancing adrenergic neurotransmission. Although reuptake of NE is the primary mechanism terminating its action, there are also enzymes that metabolize the catecholamines (see Fig. 8-8). MAO is inhibited by pargyline, and COMT is inhibited by tolcapone. Inhibition of these enzymes results in higher concentrations of NE in peripheral tissues but does not enhance responses of neuroeffector organs to sympathetic nerve stimulation.

The action of ACh at synapses is terminated by the action of AChE. AChE is inhibited by numerous compounds, including physostigmine and other drugs, which enhance the magnitude and duration of effects elicited by stimulation of cholinergic neurons (see Chapter 9).

Drugs that stimulate autonomic receptors NE activates all subtypes of adrenergic receptors, although it is less potent at β_2-receptors. Epi, however, activates all adrenergic receptor subtypes with a similar potency. Phenylephrine is a selective α_1-receptor agonist, and clonidine is a selective α_2-receptor agonist. Isoproterenol is equally effective at stimulating all β-adrenergic receptor subtypes but does not stimulate α_1- or α_2-receptors. Dobutamine is a selective β_1-receptor agonist, whereas terbutaline is a selective β_2-receptor agonist.

ACh activates all subtypes of both muscarinic and nicotinic cholinergic receptors. Muscarinic cholinergic receptors are selectively stimulated by the alkaloid muscarine or by synthetic agonists such as bethanechol, whereas nicotinic cholinergic receptors are selectively stimulated by the alkaloid nicotine.

Drugs that block autonomic receptors The prototypical α-adrenergic blocker phentolamine is an antagonist at both α_1- and α_2-adrenergic receptors. Prazosin blocks α_1-receptors, and yohimbine blocks α_2-receptors with relatively high selectivity. Prototypical β-adrenergic receptor antagonists such as propranolol, block both β_1- and β_2-adrenergic receptors More selective β-adrenergic receptor antagonists have been developed for the treatment of a variety of cardiovascular disorders and include metoprolol, a relatively selective β_1-adrenergic receptor antagonist.

Most effector organs of the ANS that contain muscarinic cholinergic receptors are blocked in a competitive manner by atropine. Nicotinic cholinergic receptors in autonomic ganglia are selectively inhibited by trimethaphan.

New horizons

With the sequencing of the human genome essentially complete, a major focus of research currently centers on defining polymorphisms in proteins involved in autonomic processes (enzymes, receptors, transporters). A polymorphism is a variability in DNA sequence that occurs with an allele frequency of greater than 1% in the population, whereas a mutation occurs with a frequency of less than 1%. For example, the gene encoding the human β_1 adrenergic receptor has 18 single nucleotide polymorphisms, 17 within the coding exon, with 7 leading to amino acid substitutions. The substitutions of most interest are glycine for serine at amino acid 49 and arginine for glycine at 389. The latter variant shows a gain of function phenotype, with enhanced coupling to G_s and cAMP formation. The other consistently reported alteration is an enhanced susceptibility to agonist-promoted down-regulation of the glycine-49 genotype.

Because the ANS plays a pathophysiological role in many diseases of peripheral organs, including the heart, kidney, GI tract, and reproductive system, the ability to selectively regulate autonomic function to these organs continues to be a major objective.

FURTHER READING

Eisenhofer G, Irwin J, Kopin IJ, et al. Catecholamine metabolism: A contemporary view with implications for physiology and medicine. *Pharmacol Rev* 2004; 56:331-349.

Guimaraes S, Moura D. Vascular adrenoceptors: An update. *Pharmacol Rev* 2001; 53:319-356.

Small KM, McGraw DW, Liggett SB. Pharmacology and physiology of human adrenergic receptor polymorphisms. *Annu Rev Pharmacol Toxicol* 2003; 43:381-411.

Wess J. Novel insights into muscarinic acetylcholine receptor function using gene targeting technology. *Trends Pharmacol Sci* 2003; 24:414-420.

Self-assessment questions

1. Which of the following is not a characteristic of the parasympathetic nervous system?

a. ACh is the neurotransmitter at parasympathetic ganglia.
b. ACh is the neurotransmitter for postganglionic neurotransmission.
c. The postganglionic neurons are long and unmyelinated.
d. Cell bodies for preganglionic neurons originating in the brainstem and sacral region of the spinal cord.
e. It is essential for life.

2. The sympathetic nervous system is characterized by all of the following except:

a. Cell bodies for preganglionic sympathetic neurons originate in the brain.
b. The neurotransmitter for preganglionic sympathetic neurons is ACh.
c. Postganglionic sympathetic neurons are long.
d. Postganglionic sympathetic nerve terminals have an active uptake process for NE called the NE transporter.
e. Nicotinic cholinergic receptors are present at the paravertebral ganglia.

3. Which of the following autonomic receptors results in the activation of adenylate cyclase as the major component of its signal transduction process?

a. Nicotinic
b. Muscarinic
c. α_1-Adrenergic receptor
d. α_2-Adrenergic receptor
e. β_1-Adrenergic receptor

4. Stimulation of prejunctional or presynaptic α_2-adrenergic receptors on postganglionic sympathetic neurons causes the following:

a. Inhibition of ACh release.
b. Stimulation of Epi release.
c. Stimulation of NE release.
d. Inhibition of NE release.
e. Has no effect on neurotransmitter release.

5. Which of the following signal transduction processes can be used by muscarinic cholinergic receptors?

a. Inhibition of adenylate cyclase
b. Stimulation of adenylate cyclase
c. Activation of phospholipase C
d. Stimulation of a sodium-hydrogen exchange system
e. *a* and *c*

6. Activation of the parasympathetic nervous system results in which of the following responses?

a. An increase in heart rate
b. Vasoconstriction
c. Bronchoconstriction
d. Renin secretion
e. Relaxation of the GI tract

CHAPTER 9

Drugs affecting the parasympathetic nervous system and autonomic ganglia

Frederick J. Ehlert

Major Drugs

- Muscarinic agonists
- Cholinesterase (ChE) inhibitors
- Muscarinic antagonists
- Nicotinic agonists
- Ganglionic nicotinic antagonists

Therapeutic overview

The parasympathetic nervous system has a trophotropic function to conserve energy. Stimulation of this system leads to decreased heart rate, blood pressure and respiration, increased secretions, and miosis. Postganglionic parasympathetic nerves release **acetylcholine (ACh)**, which activates **muscarinic cholinergic receptors** on exocrine glands, smooth muscle, and cardiac muscle to produce parasympathetic responses. ACh is also released from some postganglionic sympathetic nerves, where it stimulates muscarinic receptors located on sweat glands and some blood vessels. Both parasympathetic and sympathetic ganglia use ACh as the neurotransmitter, as do the skeletal neuromuscular junction and innervation to the adrenal medulla. The receptors that mediate these responses of ACh are **nicotinic cholinergic receptors.** ACh is also released from neurons throughout the central nervous system (CNS), where it can act on both muscarinic and nicotinic receptors.

Drugs affecting the parasympathetic nervous system mimic, antagonize, or prolong the actions of ACh at muscarinic receptors. Drugs that mimic or prolong the actions of ACh at muscarinic receptors are termed **parasympathomimetics** or **cholinomimetics** and are used to reduce intraocular pressure in glaucoma and to increase the motility of the gastrointestinal (GI) and urinary tracts. Drugs that antagonize the actions of ACh at muscarinic receptors are termed **parasympatholytics, cholinolytics,** or **muscarinic antagonists** and are used to treat motion sickness, relieve some of the symptoms of Parkinson's disease (see Chapter 21), dilate the pupils for ocular examination, reduce motility of the GI and urinary tracts, dilate the airways of the lung in patients with chronic obstructive pulmonary disease (COPD), and reduce acid secretion in individuals with peptic ulcer disease.

Drugs affecting autonomic ganglia either mimic or antagonize the actions of ACh at nicotinic cholinergic receptors. Drugs that antagonize the actions of ACh at ganglionic nicotinic receptors are used to treat hypertensive emergencies. Drugs that antagonize the actions

Abbreviations

AcCoA	acetyl coenzyme A
ACh	acetylcholine
AChE	acetylcholinesterase
ChAT	choline acetyltransferase
ChE	cholinesterase, butyrylcholinesterase
CNS	central nervous system
COPD	chronic obstructive pulmonary disease
EPSP	excitatory postsynaptic potential
GI	gastrointestinal
2-PAM	pralidoxime
PNS	peripheral nervous system

of ACh at nicotinic receptors at the neuromuscular junction are termed **neuromuscular blocking agents** and are used to relax skeletal muscle (see Chapter 29).

The Therapeutic Overview box presents a summary of the classes and primary uses of compounds that affect the parasympathetic nervous system and autonomic ganglia.

THERAPEUTIC OVERVIEW

Muscarinic agonists

Glaucoma
Postoperative ileus, congenital megacolon, and urinary retention

Cholinesterase (ChE) inhibitors

Glaucoma
Postoperative ileus, congenital megacolon, urinary retention
Diagnosis and treatment of myasthenia gravis
Reversal of neuromuscular blockade following surgery
Alzheimer's disease

Muscarinic antagonists

Motion sickness
Examination of the retina and measurement of refraction; inflammatory uveitis
Excessive motility of GI and urinary tract; urinary incontinence; irritable bowel syndrome
Chronic obstructive pulmonary disease
Parkinson's disease

Ganglionic blockers

Hypertensive emergencies

Mechanisms of action

The biochemistry and physiology of the autonomic nervous system, including a discussion of muscarinic and nicotinic cholinergic receptors are presented in Chapter 8. Detailed information on receptors and signaling pathways are discussed in Chapter 2. This section covers topics that pertain specifically to cholinergic neurotransmission and its modulation by drugs.

Cholinergic transmission

The neurochemical steps that mediate cholinergic neurotransmission are summarized in Figure 9-1. ACh is synthesized from **choline** and **acetyl coenzyme A** (AcCoA) by the enzyme **choline acetyltransferase** (ChAT). Inhibitors of ChAT have little or no effect on ACh concentrations, and ChAT is not rate-limiting in production of ACh. AcCoA used for formation of ACh is synthesized in mitochondria from its immediate precursor, pyruvate, and is transported out of mitochondria and into the cytoplasm.

The majority of the choline used for ACh synthesis is provided to the cytoplasm by a high-affinity, sodium-dependent choline transporter; a small amount of choline is also generated from the hydrolysis of phospholipids within the neuron. The choline transporter provides choline from the extracellular fluid, which is ultimately derived from both the extraneuronal catabolism of ACh and the blood. Choline exists in the circulation primarily in an esterified form as phosphatidylcholine (lecithin) and, to a much lesser extent, as free choline. Circulating phosphatidylcholine is derived from both dietary sources and from hepatic methylation of phosphatidylethanolamine.

Once formed in the cytosol, ACh is transported actively into synaptic vesicles by the vesicular ACh transporter. The arrival of an action potential at the nerve terminal causes an influx of Ca^{2+}, triggering the release of ACh from storage vesicles. The toxin from *Clostridium botulinum* (**botulinum toxin**) prevents the release of ACh from synaptic vesicles and blocks cholinergic neurotransmission. This mechanism underlies the clinical and cosmetic use of botulinum toxin in conditions that involve involuntary skeletal muscle activity or increased muscle tone, including strabismus, blepharospasm, hemifacial spasm, and facial wrinkles. Following release from the nerve terminal, ACh elicits cellular responses by activating postsynaptic muscarinic or nicotinic receptors. Muscarinic receptors are also located presynaptically where they inhibit further neurotransmitter release. The effects of ACh are rapidly terminated by the enzyme **acetylcholinesterase** (**AChE**), which hydrolyzes ACh to acetate and choline. Choline is then transported back into nerve terminals by the high-affinity choline transporter and used for resynthesis of ACh.

Drugs can modify the activity of parasympathetic neurons by increasing or decreasing cholinergic neurotransmission. Parasympathomimetics may mimic cholinergic transmission by acting directly on postsynaptic receptors (e.g., bethanechol) or by prolonging the action of released ACh (e.g., physostigmine); these sites of action are depicted in green circles in Figure

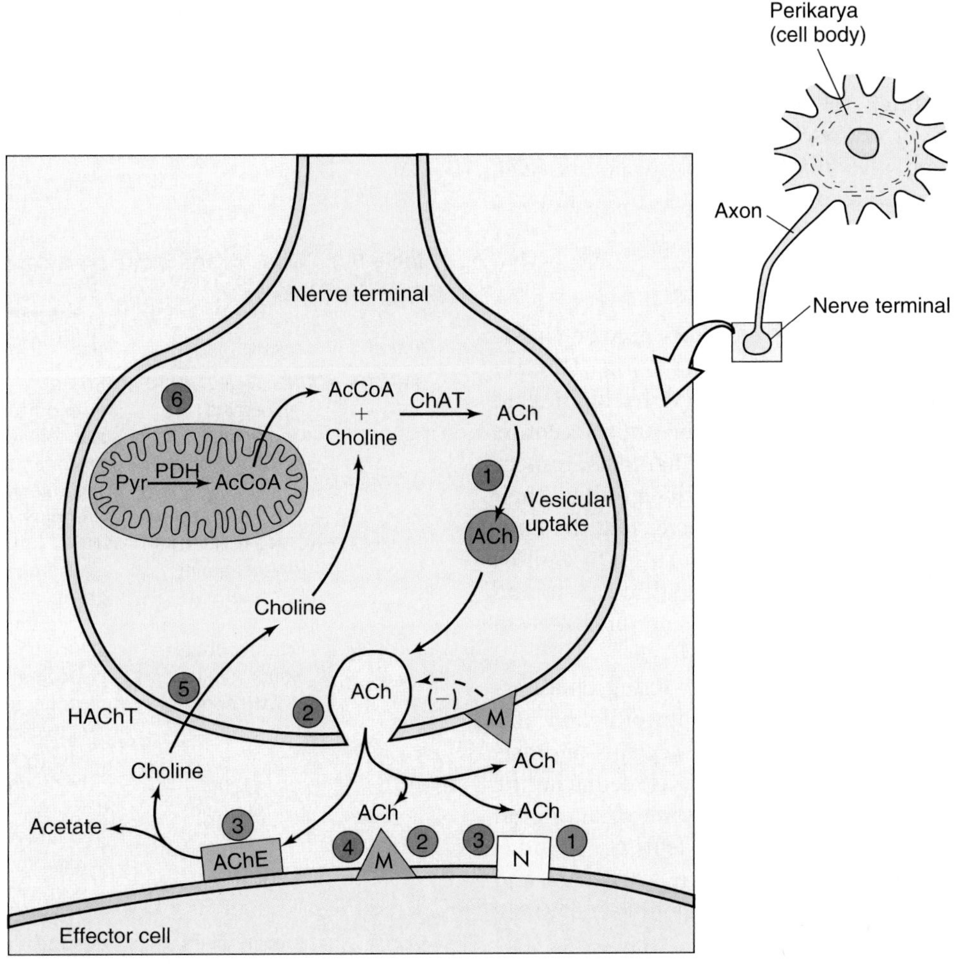

Figure 9-1 Cholinergic neurotransmission and its perturbation by drugs. Acetylcholine *(ACh)* is synthesized from choline and acetyl coenzyme A (AcCoA) by the enzyme choline acetyltransferase *(ChAT)*. Choline gains access to the cytosol by active transport from the extracellular fluid via the high-affinity choline transporter *(HAChT)*. AcCoA is synthesized in mitochondria from pyruvate *(Pyr)* by the enzyme pyruvate dehydrogenase *(PDH)*. AcCoA is transported out of the mitochondria for the synthesis of ACh. ACh is transported into synaptic vesicles by a vesicular ACh transporter. The arrival of an action potential at the nerve terminal causes the synaptic vesicles to fuse with the nerve membrane, followed by the exocytotic release of ACh. Upon release, ACh can activate postjunctional muscarinic *(M)* or nicotinic *(N)* receptors, as well as presynaptic muscarinic receptors *(M)*; stimulation of the latter inhibits the release of ACh. The actions of ACh are rapidly terminated by acetylcholinesterase *(AChE)*, which hydrolyzes ACh into choline and acetate. The choline can be transported back into the nerve terminal for the synthesis of new ACh. Sites at which drugs act to enhance cholinergic transmission are identified by numbers in green circles; sites at which drugs act to inhibit transmission are identified by numbers in red circles.

Drugs that enhance cholinergic transmission:
1. Nicotinic agonists (e.g., nicotine)
2. Muscarinic agonists (e.g., bethanechol)
3. Cholinesterase inhibitor (e.g., physostigmine)

Drugs that inhibit cholinergic transmission:
1. Inhibitors of vesicular storage (e.g., vesamicol)
2. Inhibitors of release (e.g., botulinum toxin)
3. Nicotinic antagonists (e.g., trimethaphan)
4. Muscarinic antagonists (e.g., atropine)
5. Inhibitors of high-affinity choline transport (e.g., hemicholinium)
6. Inhibitors of pyruvate dehydrogenase (e.g., bromopyruvate)

9-1. Drugs that inhibit cholinergic transmission can inhibit the availability of precursor for ACh (e.g., bromopyruvate), the high affinity transport of choline (e.g., hemicholinium), the vesicular transport of ACh (e.g., vesamicol), or the release of ACh (e.g., botulinum toxin). Drugs can also directly block receptors (e.g., trimethaphan, atropine). All these sites of action are depicted in red circles in Figure 9-1.

Activation of cholinergic receptors

Drugs that activate cholinergic receptors may be classified as either directly or indirectly acting. Directly acting compounds produce their effects by binding to and activating either muscarinic or nicotinic receptors and are termed *muscarinic* or *nicotinic* **agonists**, respectively. Indirectly acting cholinomimetics produce their effects by inhibiting AChE, thereby increasing the concentration and prolonging the action of ACh at cholinergic synapses. The directly and indirectly acting cholinomimetics and their clinical uses are presented in Table 9-1.

The structures of several directly-acting cholinergic agonists are shown in Figure 9-2. Introduction of a methyl group in the β position of ACh yields agonists selective for muscarinic receptors, such as methacholine and bethanechol. In addition, substitution of an amino group for the terminal methyl group yields corresponding carbamic acid ester derivatives (i.e., carbachol and bethanechol), which make these compounds relatively resistant to hydrolysis by AChE.

Muscarinic agonists Muscarinic receptors mediate cellular responses by interacting with heterotrimeric G proteins to affect ionic conductances and the cytosolic concentration of second messengers, as discussed in Chapters 2 and 8. Five subtypes of muscarinic receptors (M_1 to M_5) have been identified, and most tissues express a mixture of subtypes. The distribution of these receptors throughout the body, their signaling properties, and their physiological responses are discussed in Chapter 8.

Table 9-1 Directly and indirectly acting cholinomimetic drugs and their uses

Action	Agent	Use
DIRECTLY ACTING (MUSCARINIC AGONISTS)		
	Pilocarpine	glaucoma
	Carbachol	glaucoma
	Bethanechol	postoperative ileus, congenital megacolon, urinary retention
INDIRECTLY ACTING (ChE INHIBITORS)*		
	Physostigmine	glaucoma
	Decamerium	glaucoma, treatment of myasthenia gravis
	Echothiophate	glaucoma
	Isoflurophate	glaucoma
	Neostigmine	postoperative ileus, congenital megacolon, urinary retention, reversal of neuromuscular blockade
	Edrophonium	diagnosis of myasthenia gravis, reversal of neuromuscular blockade, supraventricular tachyarrhythmias
	Ambenonium	treatment of myasthenia gravis
	Pyridostigmine	reversal of neuromuscular blockade

*ChE inhibitors used for Alzheimer's disease are listed in Chapter 21.

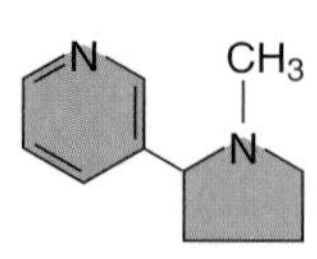

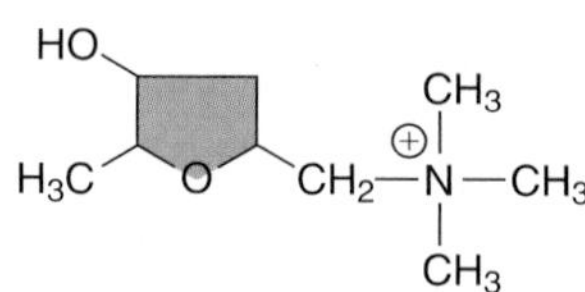

Figure 9-2 Structures of some directly acting cholinergic agonists.

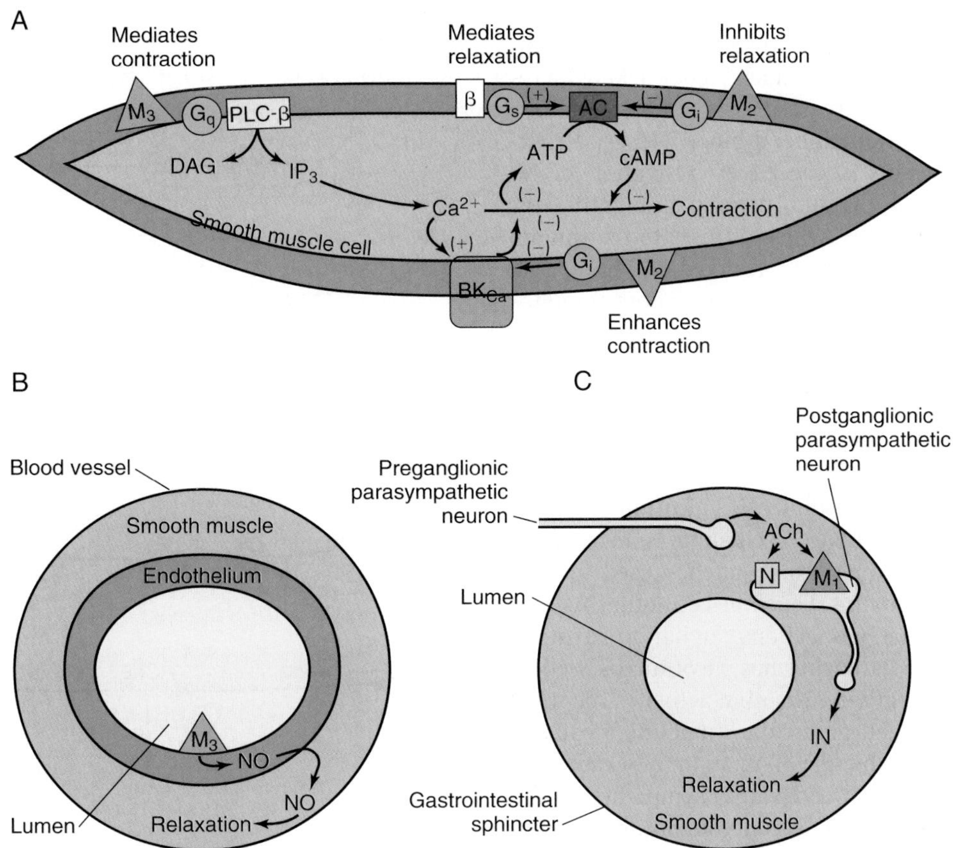

Figure 9-3 Muscarinic receptor–mediated contraction and relaxation in different types of smooth muscle. **A,** Most smooth muscle cells express M_2 and M_3 receptors. Activation of M_3 receptors elicits contraction through stimulation of phospholipase C-β *(PLC-β),* which cleaves phosphatidylinositol-4,5-bisphosphate into diacylglycerol *(DAG)* and inositol-1,4,5-trisphosphate *(IP_3).* The IP_3 mobilizes Ca^{2+} and triggers contraction. β-adrenergic receptor activation (β) stimulates adenylyl cyclase *(AC)* to generate cyclic AMP *(cAMP),* which causes the relaxation of smooth muscle. M_2 receptors inhibit AC to prevent the relaxant effects on stimulation of the β-adrenergic receptor. **B,** Most peripheral blood vessels express M_3 receptors on the endothelium, which trigger the synthesis of nitric oxide *(NO).* The NO diffuses into the smooth muscle, where it mediates relaxation through the production of cyclic guanosine monophosphate. **C,** Activation of M_1 receptors and nicotinic receptors *(N)* in parasympathetic ganglia causes the release of an inhibitory neurotransmitter *(IN)* from postganglionic neurons in gastrointestinal sphincters. This inhibitory neurotransmitter is usually ATP, NO, or VIP and causes the sphincter smooth muscle to relax.

Most agonists used clinically are not selective for muscarinic receptor subtypes.

When activated by an agonist, M_1, M_3, and M_5 receptors interact with G_q proteins to activate phospholipase C leading to increased phosphoinositide hydrolysis and the release of intracellular Ca^{2+}. This signaling pathway mediates the contraction of smooth muscle and the secretion of substances from various exocrine glands following the activation of M_3 receptors, as depicted in Figure 9-3, *A*. In contrast, M_2 and M_4 receptors interact with G_i to inhibit adenylyl cyclase. In smooth muscle cells, activation of M_2 receptors promotes contraction by opposing the actions of β-adrenergic receptor activation, which leads to smooth muscle relaxation (Fig. 9-3, *A*). In the myocardium, the activation of M_2 receptors decreases the force of contraction (negative inotropic effect) and heart rate (negative chronotropic effect). Thus, M_2 receptor activation in the heart opposes the increased force of contraction elicited by activation of β_1-adrenergic receptors. M_2 and M_4 receptors also interact with G_o, mediating a presynaptic inhibition of neurotransmitter release.

Most, but not all, peripheral effects of muscarinic agonists resemble those elicited by the activation of parasympathetic nerves (see Chapter 8). These effects include: (1) constriction of the iris sphincter; (2) contraction of the ciliary muscle resulting in accommodation of the lens; (3) constriction of the airways; (4) an increase in GI motility; (5) contraction of the bladder reservoir and relaxation of its outlet; (6) a decrease in heart rate; and (7) an increase in secretions of sweat glands, salivary glands, lacrimal glands, and glands of the trachea and GI mucosa. Although the ventricular myocardium and most peripheral blood vessels lack cholinergic innervation, they express muscarinic receptors. When activated by exogenously administered agonists, these receptors decrease the force of contraction in the heart and dilate peripheral blood vessels. Relaxation of blood vessels is caused by activation of M_3 receptors on the endothelium, thereby stimulating the production of nitric oxide, which diffuses to the smooth muscle, causing relaxation, as depicted in Figure 9-3, *B*. Muscarinic agonists also activate receptors throughout the CNS, and muscarinic receptors in the brain play an important role in learning, memory, control of posture, and temperature regulation. Excessive activation of central muscarinic receptors causes tremor, convulsions, and hypothermia.

Nicotinic agonists The prototypic nicotinic agonist, nicotine, is found in tobacco, cigarette smoke, some insecticides, and in transdermal patches used to ease withdrawal from smoking. Lobeline is another natural nicotinic agonist that has actions similar to nicotine. The cholinomimetic carbachol has nicotinic as well as muscarinic agonist activity. Nicotine activates nicotinic receptors at the neuromuscular junction, causing contraction followed by depolarization blockade and paralysis. Nicotine also activates sympathetic and parasympathetic ganglia. As a consequence, due to differences in the predominant tone of autonomic systems (see Chapter 8), its effects on the cardiovascular system are primarily sympathetic, whereas its effects on the GI tract are primarily parasympathetic. Nicotine elevates blood pressure and heart rate, with the latter opposed by reflex bradycardia. The sympathetic effects of nicotine are reinforced by stimulation of nicotinic receptors at the adrenal medulla leading to release of catecholamines. Nicotine also stimulates the GI and urinary tracts, causing diarrhea and urination. Nicotine readily enters the brain, and increasing doses cause alertness, vomiting, tremors, convulsions, and, ultimately, coma.

Cholinesterase inhibitors

Two types of cholinesterases are expressed in the body, AChE and butyrylcholinesterase (ChE, also called plasmaChE or pseudoChE), each having different distributions and substrate specificities. AChE is located at synapses throughout the nervous system and is responsible for terminating the action of ACh. ChE is located at nonneuronal sites, including plasma and liver, and is responsible for the metabolism of certain drugs, including ester-type local anesthetics and succinylcholine. Most inhibitors of AChE used clinically do not discriminate between the two types of ChE.

The mechanism involved in hydrolysis of ACh provides the biochemical basis by which the actions of ChE inhibitors can be understood (Fig. 9-4). AChE is a member of the serine hydrolase family of enzymes that contain a catalytic triad–serine, glutamate, and histidine–at the active site. The substrate-binding domain on AChE also contains a glutamate and an aromatic tryptophan that interact with the charged ammonium group of ACh. When ACh binds to AChE, the ester moiety undergoes a nucleophilic attack by the serine of the catalytic triad, resulting in hydrolysis of ACh and

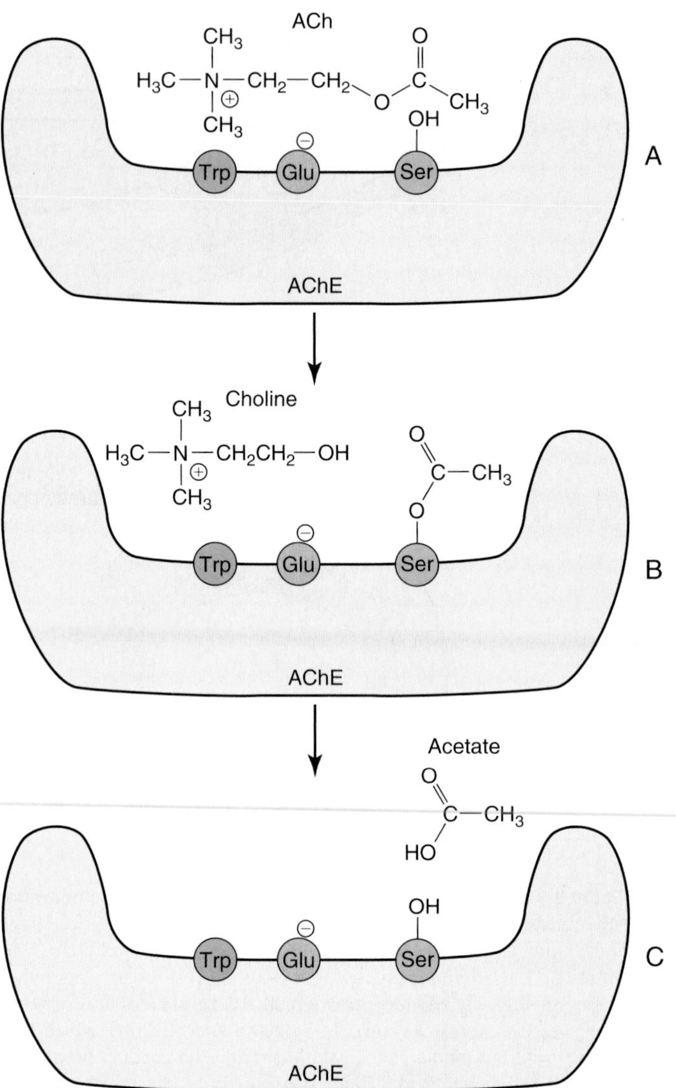

Figure 9-4 Hydrolysis of acetylcholine (ACh) by acetylcholinesterase *(AChE)*. The tryptophan 86 *(Trp)*, glutamate 202 *(Glu)*, and serine 203 *(Ser)* residues of the enzyme are shown. **A,** ACh is attracted to the substrate-binding site of AChE by the interaction of its quaternary ammonium group with a tryptophan residue on the enzyme and the interaction of the ester group with the serine residue. **B,** ACh is hydrolyzed, yielding choline and the acetylated enzyme complex. **C,** The acetylated enzyme complex rapidly hydrolyzes to yield acetate and the free enzyme.

acetylation of serine. The acetylated serine is then rapidly hydrolyzed, thereby regenerating free enzyme. This enzymatic reaction is one of the fastest known; approximately 10^4 molecules of ACh are hydrolyzed per second by a single AChE molecule.

ChE inhibitors are divided into two main types, **reversible** and **irreversible.** Reversible inhibitors are further subdivided into competitive enzyme inhibitors and substrate inhibitors. A competitive inhibitor, such as edrophonium, binds reversibly to the substrate-binding domain of AChE. The duration of action is determined in part by the way in which the inhibitor binds. Edrophonium binds weakly and has a rapid renal clearance, resulting in a brief duration of action (approximately 10 minutes). Ambenonium binds more tightly and has a longer duration of action (3 to 4 hours).

Substrate inhibitors, such as physostigmine and neostigmine, are hydrolyzed by AChE but at a relatively slow rate. These inhibitors are usually carbamic acid ester derivatives, sometimes referred to as carbamate inhibitors. The insecticide carbaryl is one example. When the carbamate binds to AChE, it is cleaved, yielding a free amino alcohol and a carbamylated enzyme (Fig. 9-5).

However, unlike the acetylated enzyme produced by hydrolysis of ACh, which is deacetylated within seconds, the carbamylated enzyme is more stable, with a half-life of approximately 30 minutes. This contributes to the moderate duration of action of carbamates *in vivo* (typically 3 to 4 hours).

Irreversible ChE inhibitors phosphorylate the serine in the active site of AChE (Fig. 9-6). These compounds are alkyl phosphate molecules and include the toxic nerve gases sarin, soman, and tabun; the insecticides parathion and malathion; and the therapeutic agents echothiophate and isoflurophate. Collectively these compounds are termed **organophosphorus** ChE inhibitors. The phosphorylated enzyme formed with these compounds is extremely stable, unlike that formed from the hydrolysis of ACh. Dephosphorylation of the phosphorylated enzyme takes hours, if it occurs at all. In the case of secondary (isoflurophate) and tertiary (soman) alkyl-substituted phosphates, the phosphorylated enzyme is so stable that it is not dephosphorylated, and new enzyme molecules must be synthesized for enzyme activity to recover. Many organophosphorus ChE inhibitors also irreversibly phosphorylate and inactivate other serine hydrolases, including trypsin and chymotrypsin.

ChE inhibitors amplify the effects of ACh at all sites throughout the nervous system. Thus, ChE inhibitors indirectly activate nicotinic receptors at the neuromuscular junction and at sympathetic and parasympathetic ganglia. In skeletal muscle, low doses of ChE inhibitors increase the force of contraction, intermediate doses elicit muscle fasciculations and fibrillations, and high doses cause depolarization blockade and muscle paralysis. ChE inhibitors indirectly activate muscarinic receptors at all postjunctional sites in the parasympathetic nervous system and sweat glands. In GI smooth muscle, ChE inhibitors increase motility by prolonging the action of ACh at muscarinic receptors on smooth muscle. ChE

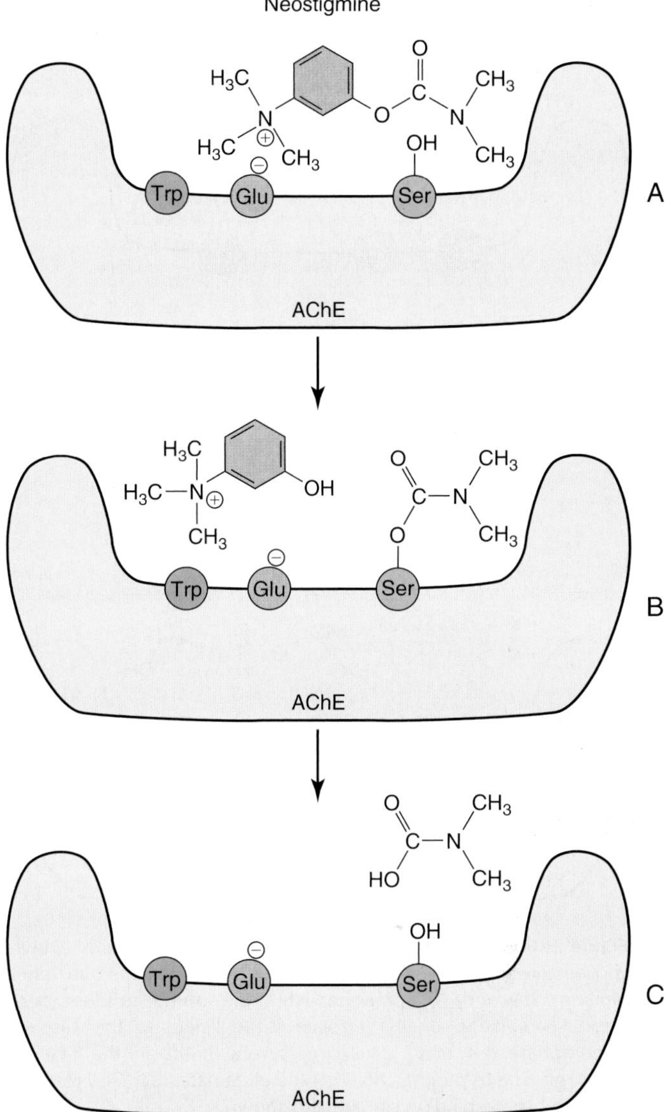

Figure 9-5 The interaction of neostigmine with acetylcholinesterase *(AChE)*. The tryptophan 86 *(Trp)*, glutamate 202 *(Glu)*, and serine 203 *(Ser)* residues of the enzyme are shown. **A,** Neostigmine is attracted to the substrate-binding site of AChE. **B,** Neostigmine is hydrolyzed, yielding an alcohol and the carbamylated enzyme complex. **C,** The carbamylated enzyme complex undergoes hydrolysis to yield a carbamic acid derivative and the free enzyme.

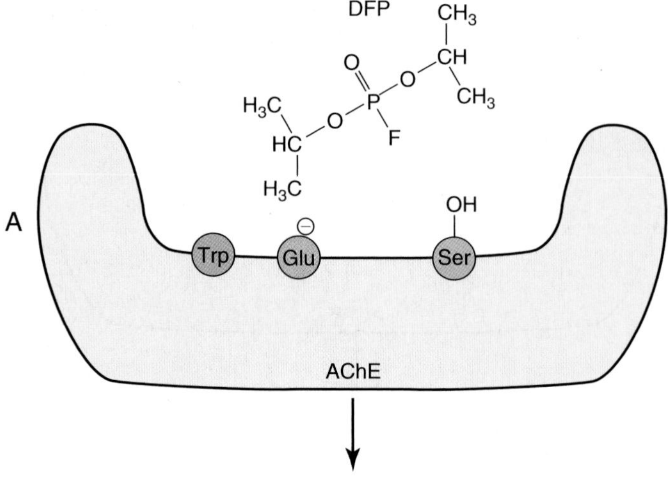

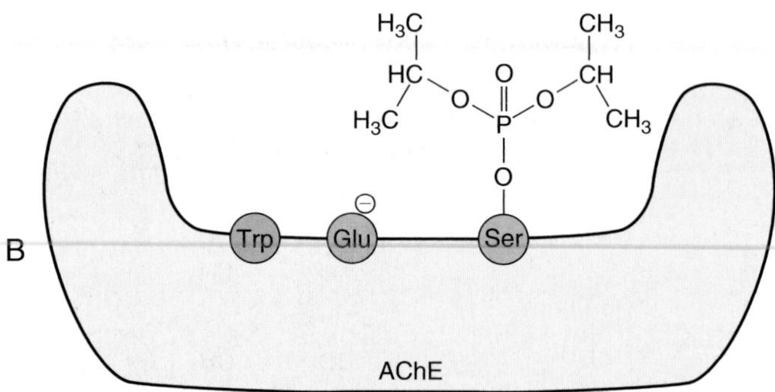

Figure 9-6 The interaction of isoflurophate *(DFP)* with acetylcholinesterase *(AChE)*. **A,** Isofluorophate diffuses to the substrate-binding site and, **B,** phosphorylates the serine residue *(Ser)*. Dephosphorylation of the enzyme is negligible in the case of isoflurophate but may occur over several hours in the case of paraoxon. The tryptophan 86 *(Trp)* and glutamate 202 *(Glu)* residues of the substrate-binding site are also shown.

inhibitors also relax sphincters by enhancing neurotransmission through parasympathetic ganglia, causing the release of a noncholinergic inhibitory neurotransmitter that directly relaxes sphincter smooth muscle (see Fig. 9-3, C).

The effects of ChE inhibitors on the cardiovascular system are complicated by opposing effects resulting from the activation of both sympathetic and parasympathetic ganglia. Because the effects of the parasympathetic system predominate in the heart, ChE inhibitors decrease heart rate and cardiac output but have little effect on ventricular contraction. Moderate doses of ChE inhibitors have little effect on blood pressure because few blood vessels receive cholinergic innervation, but high doses decrease blood pressure. Most organophosphorus ChE inhibitors and tertiary amine carbamate inhibitors readily penetrate the blood-brain barrier and indirectly activate central nicotinic and muscarinic receptors.

Table 9-2 Muscarinic antagonists and their uses*

Agent	Use
TERTIARY AMINES	
Atropine	Treatment of anti-ChE poisoning
Scopolamine	Treatment of motion sickness
Homatropine	Mydriatic and cycloplegic; for mild uveitis
Dicyclomine	Alleviates GI spasms, pylorospasm, and biliary distention
Oxybutynin	Treatment of urinary incontinence
Oxyphencyclimine	Antisecretory agent for peptic ulcer
Cyclopentolate	Mydriatic and cycloplegic
Tropicamide	Mydriatic and cycloplegic
Benztropine	Treatment of Parkinson's disease
Trihexyphenidyl	Treatment of Parkinson's disease
Pirenzepine	Antisecretory agent for peptic ulcer
QUATERNARY AMMONIUM DERIVATIVES	
Methylatropine	Mydriatic, cycloplegic and antispasmodic
Methylscopolamine	Antisecretory agent for peptic ulcer, antispasmodic
Ipratropium	Aerosol for COPD
Glycopyrrolate	Antisecretory agent for peptic ulcer, antispasmodic
Tolterodine	Treatment of urinary incontinence
Propantheline	Antispasmodic
Clidinium	Antispasmodic
Tiotropium	Aerosol for COPD

*Muscarinic antagonists used for Parkinson's disease are also listed in Chapter 21.

Blockade of cholinergic receptors

Cholinergic receptor blockers are classified as **muscarinic** or **nicotinic antagonists.**

Muscarinic antagonists Muscarinic antagonists block muscarinic receptors competitively. Because the effects of these drugs resemble those of agents that block postganglionic parasympathetic nerves, these agents are sometimes referred to as **parasympatholytics.** Included in this group are the naturally occurring belladonna alkaloids atropine and scopolamine.* Muscarinic antagonists and their clinical uses are presented in Table 9-2. Most antagonists used clinically are not selective for different muscarinic receptor subtypes. An exception is pirenzepine, which is used in Europe to treat peptic ulcers and has selectivity for M_1 receptors.

*In the UK the drug name is hyoscine.

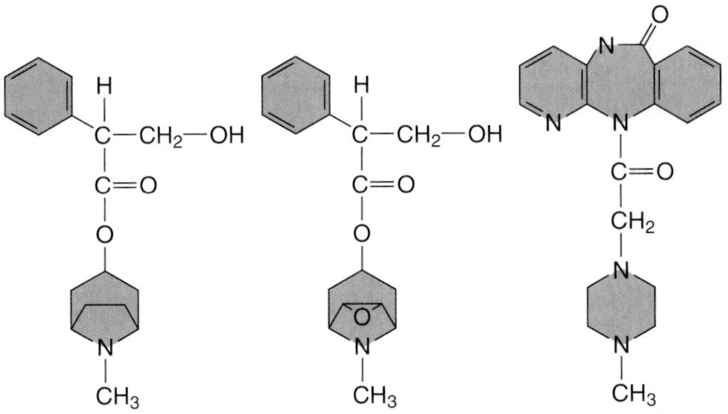

Figure 9-7 The structures of some muscarinic antagonists.

The structures of several muscarinic antagonists are shown in Figure 9-7. The prototypical compound is atropine, which has been used for a long time to define muscarinic responses. Scopolamine differs from atropine by the addition of an epoxide group that reduces the base strength and enables it to penetrate into the brain more readily than atropine. Other drugs, including some antihistamines, tricyclic antidepressants, and antipsychotics, are structurally similar to the muscarinic antagonists and have prominent antimuscarinic side effects. The anticholinergic effects of these compounds are discussed in chapters specifically dealing with these compounds.

The effects of muscarinic antagonists can be understood by a knowledge of the distribution of muscarinic receptors throughout the body, as discussed in Chapter 8. For example, in the anterior segment of the eye, muscarinic antagonists relax the iris sphincter and ciliary muscle, causing pupillary dilation (mydriasis) and a paralysis of the accommodation reflex (cycloplegia), resulting in blurred vision. Muscarinic antagonists also relax nonvascular smooth muscle, including that in the lung airways, the GI tract, and the urinary bladder. Muscarinic antagonists inhibit the secretion of substances from various exocrine glands, including sweat, salivary, lacrimal, and mucosal glands of the trachea and GI tract. In moderate to high doses, muscarinic antagonists block the effects of ACh on the heart, resulting in an increased heart rate. Muscarinic antagonists that reach the brain (e.g., atropine and scopolamine) interfere with short-term memory and, in moderately high doses, cause delirium, excitement, agitation, and toxic psychosis.

Atropine and other muscarinic antagonists produce moderately selective effects after systemic administration. Low doses of atropine cause dry mouth, whereas high doses cause tachycardia and blockade of acid secretion by gastric parietal cells. These selective actions are attributed to the differential release of ACh at various synapses and junctions. Atropine antagonizes the effects of ACh more readily at sites where less neurotransmitter is released (e.g., salivary glands) than at sites where more is released (e.g., sinoatrial node).

Ganglionic blocking agents Neurotransmission in sympathetic and parasympathetic ganglia and in the adrenal medulla is mediated primarily by ganglionic nicotinic cholinergic receptors. Nicotinic transmission triggers a fast excitatory postsynaptic potential (EPSP) in postganglionic neurons, which is caused by the flow of cations through the nicotinic receptor ion channel. The nicotinic receptors in ganglia are different from the nicotinic receptors at the neuromuscular junction. Hexamethonium, mecamylamine, and trimethaphan selectively antagonize ganglionic nicotinic receptors, causing a blockade of both sympathetic and parasympathetic neurotransmission. These ganglionic blockers cause hypotension (orthostatic and postural), paralysis of the smooth muscles of the anterior chamber of the eye, and a decrease in GI and genitourinary tract functions.

Muscarinic receptors also contribute to cholinergic responses in autonomic ganglia, although they have a less important role than nicotinic receptors. Some postganglionic neurons contain M_1 muscarinic receptors that mediate a slow EPSP that increases the excitability of the postganglionic neurons. Pirenzepine selectively antagonizes the M_1 receptor–induced slow EPSP, and antagonism of this current in the parasympathetic ganglia of the stomach wall is thought to be the mechanism by which pirenzepine blocks gastric acid secretion.

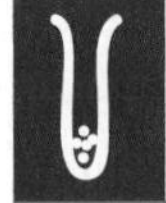

Pharmacokinetics

As indicated, many clinically used drugs that modify cholinergic function lack selectivity for receptor subtypes. Nevertheless, a degree of selectivity can be achieved *in vivo,* depending on the route of administration and tissue distribution of the drug. An important structural feature to keep in mind is whether a compound is or is not **charged,** because tertiary amines, unlike quaternary ammonium compounds, readily penetrate the brain (see Chapter 3).

Cholinomimetics

The rapid hydrolysis of ACh limits its clinical utility. Among the ChE-resistant muscarinic agonists, lipid solubility is important in influencing absorption and distribution. Quaternary ammonium agonists (e.g., bethanechol) do not penetrate into the brain and are poorly absorbed orally. Consequently, oral administration confines their action to the GI tract, making them useful for enhancing GI motility.

The tertiary amines pilocarpine and physostigmine are well absorbed from the GI tract and penetrate readily into the CNS. They are administered topically in the eye to treat glaucoma. Pilocarpine is available in a reservoir-type diffusional device (Ocusert), which is placed behind the lower eyelid to deliver the drug at a constant rate for up to 1 week. Pilocarpine is also used to stimulate salivary secretion in patients after laryngeal surgery.

Highly lipophilic organophosphorus ChE inhibitors are well absorbed from the GI tract, lung, eye, and skin, making these compounds extremely dangerous and accounting for their use as nerve gases. The carbamate insecticides are not highly absorbed transdermally. The organophosphorus insecticides malathion and parathion are prodrugs, that is, they are inactive but can be metabolized to the active ChE inhibitors, paraoxon and malaoxon. Malathion is relatively safe in mammals because it is hydrolyzed rapidly by plasma carboxylesterases. This detoxification occurs much more rapidly in birds and mammals than in insects. Malathion is available outside the United States in the form of a lotion or shampoo for the treatment of head lice.

Cholinergic blocking drugs

The lipophilicity and degree of ionization of cholinergic antagonists also influences their absorption and distribution. Quaternary ammonium antagonists are poorly absorbed from the GI tract and do not penetrate readily into the CNS. The passage of these agents across the blood-brain barrier is strongly influenced by their degree of ionization, even among the tertiary amines. Although atropine and scopolamine have a similar affinity for muscarinic receptors, scopolamine is approximately 10-fold more potent at producing central effects. This is attributed to its weaker base strength (pK_a, 7.53) relative to atropine (pK_a, 9.65). Consequently, a greater fraction of scopolamine is present in an unionized form at physiological pH relative to atropine (see Chapter 3). The relatively low pK_a of scopolamine facilitates its absorption through the skin, making the transdermal route of administration of the free base feasible. The M_1-selective antagonist pirenzepine contains three tertiary amine groups, with a resultant high degree of ionization, thereby preventing its entry into brain.

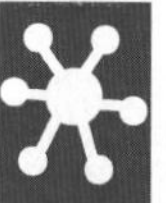

Relation of mechanisms of action to clinical response

Central nervous system

Scopolamine is effective for preventing motion sickness through an inhibitory effect on the vestibular apparatus. Scopolamine base is available in a transdermal patch that is placed behind the ear and delivers scopolamine for approximately 3 days. When administered in this fashion, scopolamine is effective against motion sickness without causing substantial anticholinergic side effects. It is more effective when administered prophylactically.

Both muscarinic agonists and antagonists are used in treatment of several neurodegenerative disorders. Muscarinic antagonists, such as trihexyphenidyl and benztropine, are used for Parkinson's disease with some benefit, and centrally acting ChE inhibitors have been noted to improve the cognitive deficits in Alzheimer's disease without halting the underlying progression of the disease. These agents and uses are discussed in Chapter 21.

Ophthalmology

When left unchecked, high intraocular pressure (glaucoma) damages the optic nerve and retina, resulting in blindness. Usually, glaucoma is caused by impaired drainage of aqueous humor produced by the ciliary epithelium in the posterior chamber of the eye. Normally, aqueous humor flows into the anterior chamber by first passing between the lens and iris and then out through the pupil (Fig. 9-8, *A*). It leaves the anterior chamber by flowing through the fenestrated trabecular meshwork and into Schlemm's canal, which lies at the vertex of the angle formed by the intersection of the cornea and the iris. This region is known as the ocular angle. In primary angle-closure glaucoma, pressure from the posterior chamber pushes the iris forward, closing the ocular angle and preventing the drainage of aqueous humor (Fig. 9-8, *B*). People with narrow angles are predisposed to closed-angle glaucoma. In primary open-angle glaucoma, the ocular angle remains open, but abnormalities in the trabecular meshwork cause the outflow of aqueous humor to be impeded. In secondary glaucoma, inflammation, trauma, or various ocular diseases can cause intraocular pressure to increase.

Glaucoma is treated with directly- and indirectly-acting cholinergic agonists. Open-angle glaucoma is also treated with carbonic anhydrase inhibitors, β-blockers, and epinephrine.* When applied topically to

*In the UK the drug name is adrenaline.

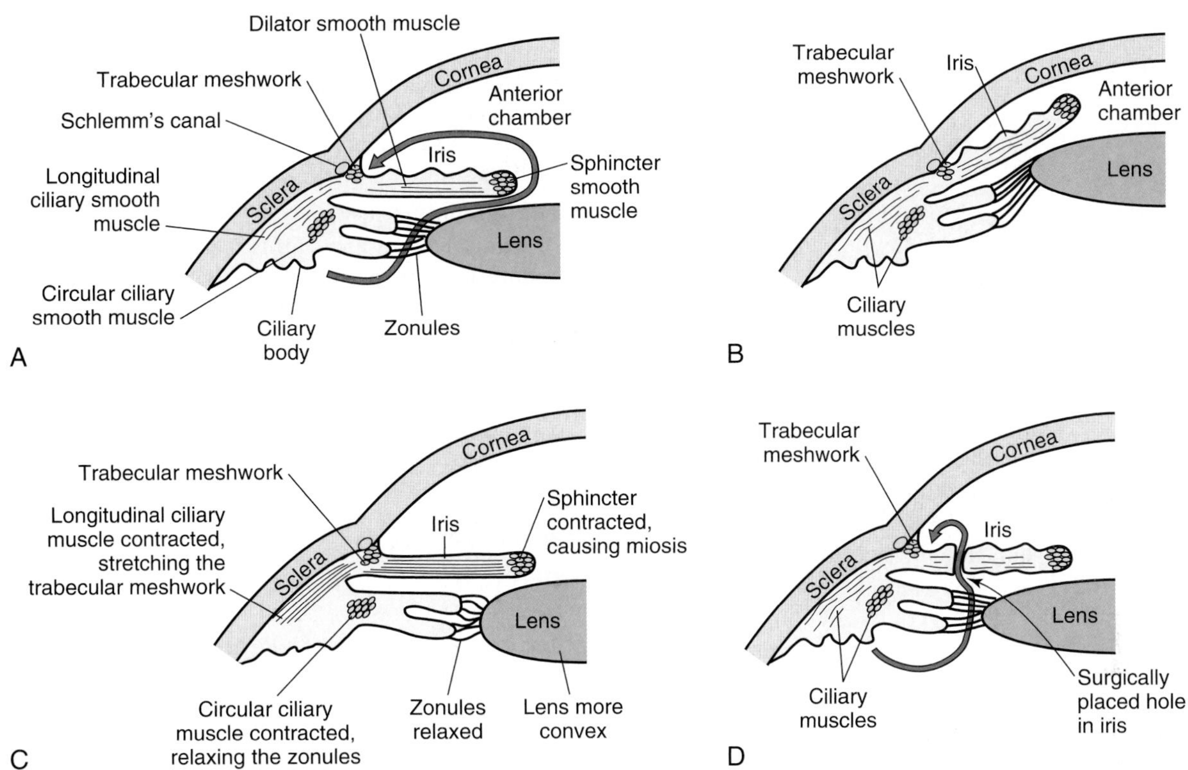

Figure 9-8 The anterior chamber of the eye and the pharmacological and surgical measures used to treat glaucoma. **A,** The flow of aqueous humor (*arrow*) from the ciliary body to the trabecular meshwork. **B,** In angle-closure glaucoma, pressure from the posterior chamber pushes the iris against the trabecular meshwork, closing the ocular angle and preventing the drainage of aqueous humor. **C,** Cholinomimetics constrict the iris sphincter, thereby opening up the ocular angle and causing a decrease in intraocular pressure in closed-angle glaucoma. Cholinomimetics also elicit contraction of the longitudinal and circular ciliary muscles. Contraction of the longitudinal ciliary muscle stretches open the trabecular meshwork and facilitates the drainage of aqueous humor, particularly in open-angle glaucoma. The circular ciliary muscle forms a sphincter-like ring around the lens, into which the zonules are attached. Constriction of the circular muscle relaxes the tension on the zonules and allows the lens to relax into a more convex shape, which increases its refractive power and enables near vision. **D,** The surgical treatment of closed-angle glaucoma entails the placement of a hole in the peripheral iris, either surgically or with a laser. The procedure provides a pathway for drainage of aqueous humor (*arrow*) and thus reduces intra-ocular pressure.

the eye, cholinomimetics constrict the pupil, contract the ciliary muscles, and decrease intraocular pressure. In open-angle glaucoma, the contraction of the longitudinal ciliary muscle decreases intraocular pressure by stretching the trabecular meshwork and opening its tubules. In closed-angle glaucoma, pupillary constriction lowers the intraocular pressure by pulling the iris away from the trabeculum and opening the angle (see Fig. 9-8, *C*). Closed-angle glaucoma is a medical emergency that is corrected surgically by placing a hole in the peripheral portion of the iris to release pressure in the posterior chamber (see Fig. 9-8, *D*). Cholinomimetics are used acutely to treat closed-angle glaucoma until surgery can be performed. Occasionally, patients with closed-angle glaucoma exhibit a paradoxical increase in intraocular pressure in response to cholinomimetics because constriction of the pupil causes the iris to be pressed against the lens, thereby blocking the flow of aqueous humor into the anterior chamber. Cholinomimetics are also used to treat a variety of noninflammatory secondary glaucomas.

Among the cholinomimetics, pilocarpine is most commonly used. Because its duration of action is approximately 6 hours, it must be administered topically approximately four times a day. Pilocarpine can also be delivered in a reservoir as described. Although pilocarpine can cause local irritation, it is tolerated better than other cholinomimetics. Other short-acting cholinomimetics used in the treatment of glaucoma are carbachol and physostigmine. The long-acting organophosphorus ChE inhibitors—demecarium, echothiophate, and isoflurophate—are sometimes used to treat glaucoma; however, these agents cause cataracts if used long term. Consequently, they are used only in aphakic patients (i.e., those lacking a lens) or in those cases in which other agents are ineffective.

Muscarinic antagonists dilate the pupil and relax the ciliary muscle, making them useful for examination

Table 9-3 Pharmacokinetic parameters for muscarinic antagonists used for refraction

Antagonist	Duration of Cycloplegia	Duration of Mydriasis
Atropine	6-12 days	7-10 days
Scopolamine	3-7 days	3-7 days
Homatropine	1-3 days	1-3 days
Cyclopentolate	6 hr-1 day	1 day
Tropicamide	6 hr	6 hr

of the retina and measurement of refractive errors of the lens, which often requires complete paralysis of the ciliary muscle. Choice of a mydriatic depends on its effectiveness and duration of action. Young children have a powerful accommodation reflex, requiring a highly potent and long-acting mydriatic, such as atropine to cause complete blockade (cycloplegia). In contrast, shorter-acting agents, such as tropicamide, are used in older children and adults. The muscarinic antagonists used in ophthalmology for refraction and their durations of action, are given in Table 9-3.

Muscarinic antagonists are also used in the treatment of inflammatory uveitis and its associated glaucoma. Although the mechanism is not completely understood, they reduce the pain and photophobia associated with inflammation by paralyzing the eye muscles. Muscarinic antagonists are also useful for breaking adhesions (synechiae) between the lens and iris that may be produced by inflammation. When treating uveitis, it is desirable to achieve a continuous relaxation of the eye muscles. Consequently, the long-acting agents atropine and scopolamine are frequently used.

Gastrointestinal and urinary tracts

The muscarinic agonist bethanechol and the ChE inhibitor neostigmine are used to treat urinary retention and decreased stomach and bowel motility when there is no obstruction (e.g., postoperatively) and to treat congenital megacolon. When administered orally, these drugs primarily affect the GI tract.

Muscarinic antagonists are used to treat conditions characterized by excessive motility of the GI and urinary tracts. Oxybutynin and tolterodine are frequently used in treatment of urge incontinence and overactive bladder, whereas clidinium, dicyclomine, and propantheline are often used in irritable bowel syndrome. The latter two antagonists are also sometimes used in treatment of urinary incontinence. Clidinium and propantheline are quaternary ammonium compounds; consequently, their actions are limited to the peripheral nervous system (PNS). Tolterodine is selective for the bladder and exhibits little inhibitory effect on salivation and GI motility. Its inhibitory effect on the bladder is due in part to an active major metabolite, which exhibits slightly greater antimuscarinic potency than tolterodine itself.

Nonselective muscarinic antagonists were occasionally used to inhibit gastric acid secretion in peptic ulcer disease but have now been supplanted by the histamine antagonists and proton pump inhibitors (see Chapter 54). Pirenzepine, a selective M_1 antagonist, which causes fewer side effects, is used in Europe to treat peptic ulcer disease and is undergoing clinical trials in the United States.

Respiratory tract

COPD is characterized by a persistent narrowing of the airways and excessive vagal tone contributing to bronchoconstriction. Muscarinic antagonists are useful in the treatment of COPD. The quaternary antagonists ipratropium and tiotropium are administered using an inhaler (see Chapter 34). Because systemic absorption of these compounds by the lung is poor, their antimuscarinic effects are usually confined to the lung. Tiotropium has a much longer duration of action than ipratropium, but both ipratropium and tiotropium have little or no inhibitory effect on mucociliary clearance, unlike most other muscarinic antagonists (e.g., atropine), which typically inhibit this function.

Myasthenia gravis

Myasthenia gravis is an autoimmune disease characterized by skeletal muscle weakness. Many people afflicted with this disorder have circulating autoantibodies against the nicotinic cholinergic receptor at the neuromuscular junction. The ability of ChE inhibitors to amplify the effects of neuronally released ACh makes these drugs useful for restoring muscle strength in myasthenic patients. ChE inhibitors are used alone in mild cases and in combination with corticosteroids in more severe cases. Corticosteroids and other immunosuppressive drugs are commonly used; the condition is also treated surgically by thymectomy.

The reversible ChE inhibitors, including pyridostigmine, neostigmine, and ambenonium, are often used because these are all quaternary ammonium compounds, limiting their pharmacological effects to the PNS. These agents can also enhance neurotransmission at muscarinic receptors throughout the parasympathetic nervous system. Consequently, they frequently elicit GI side effects, including abdominal cramping and diarrhea. The effects of these agents last for 2 to 6 hours. Thus, they must be administered frequently. The use of an organophosphorus ChE inhibitor might appear beneficial because it can provide a long-lasting enhancement of neuromuscular transmission. However, frequent dose adjustments of the ChE inhibitor are necessary in patients with myasthenia gravis, making the use of irreversible agents inappropriate. In addition, an excess of an organophosphorus ChE inhibitor could cause a long-lasting paralysis of muscle resulting from desensitization and depolarization blockade.

The short-acting ChE inhibitor edrophonium is useful for the diagnosis of myasthenia gravis. Affected patients show a brief improvement in strength after administration of edrophonium, whereas patients with other muscular diseases do not. Muscle strength can suddenly deteriorate during therapy with ChE inhibitors as a consequence of insufficient ChE inhibition (myasthenic crisis) or too much ChE inhibition, resulting in depolarization blockade (cholinergic crisis). Edrophonium is used to distinguish between these two conditions. A resulting improvement in strength is diagnostic of a myasthenic crisis; no response or a worsening indicates a cholinergic crisis.

Hypertensive emergencies

Ganglionic blockers were developed initially for the treatment of hypertension, but better agents are now available (see Chapter 12). Because blockade of both sympathetic and parasympathetic ganglia causes numerous side effects, ganglionic blockers are used only for treatment of hypertensive emergencies that occur during surgery or with an aortic aneurysm. Because of its quaternary ammonium structure, trimethaphan, which is used clinically, has effects only on the PNS. In addition, it selectively blocks nicotinic receptors at autonomic ganglia and not at the neuromuscular junction. Mecamylamine, a second drug, is rarely used and has both central and peripheral effects.

Miscellaneous uses of cholinesterase inhibitors

ChE inhibitors are also used to rapidly reverse the neuromuscular blockade induced for some surgeries. Neuromuscular blocking agents are often administered as adjuncts during general anesthesia, and it is sometimes useful to rapidly reverse neuromuscular blockade following surgery. The short-acting ChE inhibitors, such as edrophonium, neostigmine, and pyridostigmine, are used to amplify the effects of ACh and restore function at the neuromuscular junction; atropine is often used in combination with the ChE inhibitor to counteract the muscarinic effects of ChE inhibition.

Side effects, clinical problems, and toxicity

Clinical problems are summarized in the Clinical Problems box.

CLINICAL PROBLEMS

Cholinomimetics

Excessive parasympathetic activity: decreased blood pressure, bronchoconstriction, salivation, miosis, sweating, gastrointestinal discomfort.

Contraindicated in patients with asthma, chronic obstructive pulmonary disease, peptic ulcer, obstruction of the urinary or gastrointestinal tract.

Muscarinic antagonists

Urinary retention, constipation, tachycardia, dry mouth, mydriasis, inhibition of sweating, toxic psychosis.

Contraindicated in patients with atony of the bowel, urinary retention, or prostatic hypertrophy.

Ophthalmological use contraindicated in the elderly and in patients with narrow angles.

Ganglionic blockers

Lack of selectivity makes drugs difficult to use.

Muscarinic agonists

The side effects of muscarinic agonists are an extension of their parasympathomimetic actions and include miosis, blurred vision, lacrimation, excessive salivation and bronchial secretions, sweating, bronchoconstriction, bradycardia, abdominal cramping, increased gastric acid secretion, diarrhea, and polyuria. Muscarinic agonists that can penetrate into the brain also cause tremor, hypothermia, and convulsions. Although most peripheral blood vessels lack cholinergic innervation, they have endothelial muscarinic receptors that trigger vasodilation and a decrease in blood pressure. Similarly, cardiac ventricles receive little parasympathetic innervation, yet they contain muscarinic receptors that decrease the force of contraction. If given in sufficient doses or administered parenterally, muscarinic agonists can trigger acute circulatory failure with cardiac arrest. Atropine antagonizes all of these effects and is a useful antidote to poisoning with muscarinic agonists.

Muscarinic agonists are contraindicated in patients with diseases that make them susceptible to parasympathetic stimulation. The bronchoconstriction induced by muscarinic agonists can have disastrous consequences in patients with asthma or COPD. Similarly, they are contraindicated in patients with peptic ulcer disease because they stimulate gastric acid secretion. Muscarinic agonists are also contraindicated in patients with an obstruction in the GI or urinary tract because the stimulatory effect exacerbates the blockage, causing pressure to build up that may lead to perforation.

Mushrooms of the genera *Inocybe* and *Clitocybe* contain appreciable amounts of muscarine, which can cause rapid-type mushroom poisoning. Signs and symptoms occur within 30 to 60 minutes after ingestion of the mushrooms and are similar to the peripheral muscarinic effects described earlier. Atropine is administered as an antidote.

Cholinesterase inhibitors

The side effects of the ChE inhibitors are similar to those of the muscarinic agonists but also include toxic effects at the neuromuscular junction. For quaternary ammonium compounds, the cholinergic symptoms are confined to the PNS. Organophosphorus ChE inhibitors are particularly dangerous because they are readily absorbed through the skin, lungs, and conjunctiva. They are used as insecticides and can be dangerous to agricultural workers. They are contraindicated in patients with asthma, COPD, peptic ulcer disease, or GI or urinary tract obstruction for the same reasons that muscarinic agonists are contraindicated in these patients.

People accidentally exposed to organophosphorus insecticides experience miosis, blurred vision, profuse salivation, sweating, bronchoconstriction, difficulty breathing, bradycardia, abdominal cramping, diarrhea, polyuria, tremor, and muscle fasciculations that can progress to convulsions. With increased exposure, blood pressure decreases and skeletal muscles weaken as a result of depolarization blockade at the neuromuscular junction, causing paralysis of the diaphragm and respiratory failure, exacerbated by increased bronchial secretions and pulmonary edema. Death usually results from respiratory failure.

AntiChE poisoning is diagnosed on the basis of the signs and symptoms and the patient's history. Diagnosis can be verified by a plasma or erythrocyte ChE determination, if time permits. Atropine is used to reverse the effects of ACh at muscarinic synapses and must be continually administered as long as ChE is inhibited. In certain instances, the compound pralidoxime (2-PAM) may be used to reactivate the ChE and treat the neuromuscular side effects of organophosphorus antiChE poisoning. 2-PAM is a site-directed nucleophile that reacts with the phosphorylated-ChE complex to regenerate the free enzyme. However, 2-PAM must be administered as soon as possible after ChE is phosphorylated because, if the phosphate group on the enzyme loses an alkyl or alkyloxy group, a process referred to as aging, it becomes resistant to reactivation by 2-PAM. 2-PAM is ineffective against the toxicity caused by carbamate inhibitors. Diazepam is used to treat the seizures caused by ChE inhibitors. Supportive therapy is also useful, including airway maintenance and oxygen administration.

Muscarinic antagonists

The side effects associated with the use of muscarinic antagonists can be attributed to blockade of muscarinic receptors throughout the CNS and PNS. These agents cause mydriasis, cycloplegia, blurred vision, dry mouth, tachycardia, urinary retention, cutaneous vasodilation, and paralysis of the stomach and intestines with constipation. In low doses, muscarinic antagonists that enter the brain interfere with memory and are sedating; sedation is a prominent side effect of scopolamine. However, in moderate to high doses, centrally active muscarinic antagonists cause excitation, hallucinations, delirium, stupor, toxic psychosis, and convulsions, which can be followed by respiratory depression and death.

The ophthalmological use of muscarinic antagonists is contraindicated in the elderly and in patients with inherently narrow angles. In such patients, topical application of muscarinic antagonists to the eye can trigger acute angle-closure glaucoma. Muscarinic antagonists are also contraindicated in patients with bowel atony, urinary retention, or prostatic hypertrophy. They are also contraindicated in patients receiving other drugs with prominent anticholinergic side effects.

Nicotine

Nicotine poisoning results from the ingestion of tobacco products or exposure to nicotine-containing insecticides. The pharmacological response is complex (see earlier discussion) because nicotine stimulates nicotinic receptors at sympathetic and parasympathetic ganglia, at the neuromuscular junction, and in the brain. Moreover, nicotine stimulates the neuromuscular junction but can produce a blockade, with muscle weakness, paralysis of the diaphragm, and respiratory failure. Signs and symptoms of acute nicotine intoxication include nausea, vomiting, salivation, diarrhea, perturbed vision, mental confusion, tremors and convulsions, followed by depression and coma. The actions of nicotine on the cardiovascular system include an initial increase in blood pressure, followed by a decrease, weak pulse, and variable heart rate. Treatment of toxicity after oral ingestion includes gastric lavage or inducement of vomiting with syrup of ipecac. Support of respiration and maintenance of blood pressure are also important.

New horizons

Some muscarinic antagonists are known to exhibit tissue selectivity in their ability to block muscarinic agonist-induced contractions of isolated smooth muscle organs. These observations suggest that it may be possible to develop bladder selective antagonists for the treatment of urinary incontinence and intestinal selective antagonists for the treatment of irritable bowel syndrome. Moreover, it is now clear that both M_2 and M_3 muscarinic receptors contribute differentially to ACh-mediated contraction in various peripheral smooth muscles. The development of antagonists selective for M_2 and M_3 receptors may be another means of developing tissue selective antagonists.

Identification of new nicotinic receptor subtypes in the brain may lead to the development of novel, subtype-selective agonists of use in the treatment of smoking withdrawal. Such agents may lack many of the side effects of nicotine currently used for this purpose.

TRADE NAMES

In addition to generic and fixed-combination preparations, the following trade-named materials are some of the important compounds available in the United States.

Cholinomimetic agonists

Acetylcholine chloride (Miochol)
Bethanechol (Myotonachol, Urecholine)
Carbachol chloride (Miostat)
Methacholine chloride (Provocholine)
Pilocarpine HCl (Akarpine, Isopto Carpine, Ocusert, Pilagan, Pilocar, Salagen)

Cholinesterase inhibitors

Demecarium bromide (Humorsol)
Donepezil (Aricept)
Echothiophate iodide (Phospholine Iodide)
Edrophonium chloride (Enlon, Reversol, Tensilon)
Galantamine (Reminyl)
Isoflurophate (Floropryl)
Neostigmine bromide (Prostigmin)
Physostigmine salicylate (Antilirium)
Pyridostigmine bromide (Mestinon, Regonol)
Rivastigmine (Exelon)
Tacrine (Cognex)

Muscarinic antagonists

Atropine sulfate (Isopto, Atropine)
Benztropine mesylate (Cogentin)
Biperiden HCl (Akineton)
Clidinium bromide (Quarzan)
Glycopyrrolate (Robinul)
Homatropine HBr (Isopto Homatropine)
Ipratropium bromide (Atrovent)
Methscopolamine bromide (Pamine)
Procyclidine (Kemadrin)
Propantheline bromide (Pro-Banthine)
Scopolamine HBr (Hyoscine, Transderm-Scop)
Tiotropium (Spiriva)
Tolterodine (Detrol)
Tridihexethyl chloride (Pathilon)
Trihexyphenidyl HCl (Artane)

Ganglionic blocking drugs

Mecamylamine HCl (Inversine)
Trimethaphan camsylate (Arfonad)

Phosphorylated ChE reactivator

Pralidoxime chloride (Protopam)

FURTHER READING

Coulson FR, Fryer AD. Muscarinic acetylcholine receptors and airway diseases. *Pharmacol Ther* 2003; 98:59-69.

Eglen RM, Choppin A, Watson N. Therapeutic opportunities from muscarinic receptor research. *Trends Pharmacol Sci* 2001; 22:409-414.

Lang B, Vincent A. Autoantibodies to ion channels at the neuromuscular junction. *Autoimmunity* 2003; 2:94-100.

Self-assessment questions

1. A 60-year-old man complains of difficulty reading in artificial light. Lenticular opacities are diagnosed, and he undergoes cataract removal. After surgery, ACh chloride (Miochol) is administered to:

a. Relax the circular muscle of the iris.
b. Ensure complete miosis.
c. Decrease lacrimal secretion (tearing).
d. Decrease the flow of aqueous humor.
e. All of the above.

2. An elderly woman is found to exhibit elevated intraocular pressure, and open-angle glaucoma is diagnosed. Her physician prescribes pilocarpine (Isopto Carpine) every 6 hours. The anticipated effect of pilocarpine eyedrops would be to:

a. Relax the ciliary muscles.
b. Improve accommodation.
c. Relax the sphincter muscle of the iris.
d. Inhibit the production of aqueous humor by the ciliary epithelium.
e. Contract the longitudinal ciliary muscle, and pull on the trabecular meshwork to relieve pressure.

3. An agricultural worker is accidentally sprayed with an insecticide. He complains of a tightness in the chest and difficulty with vision. In the hospital emergency room he is found to have pinpoint pupils and to be profusely salivating. It is assumed he has been exposed to an anticholinesterase. The most appropriate medication for treating his condition would be:

a. Atropine sulfate.
b. Physostigmine (Isopto-Eserine).
c. Edrophonium (Tensilon).
d. Propantheline (Pro-Banthine).
e. Atropine plus pralidoxime.

4. If anticholinesterase poisoning goes untreated, the expected cause of death would be:

a. Hypertension.
b. Hypotension.
c. Congestive heart failure.
d. Respiratory failure.
e. *b* and *c*.

5. The most toxic substance known that affects the cholinergic nervous system is an exotoxin secreted by the anaerobe *Clostridium botulinum*. There are several forms of botulinum toxin, all of which are highly toxic after they are ingested in contaminated food. The toxin produces respiratory paralysis by:

a. Blocking nicotinic receptors.
b. Blocking release of ACh from nerve endings.
c. Blocking peristalsis.
d. Causing circulatory collapse.
e. Stimulating the vagal nerve.

6. Bethanechol is administered subcutaneously to a patient with postoperative abdominal distention and gastric atony. The subcutaneous route of administration is chosen over the oral route because gastric retention is complete and there is no passage of gastric contents into the duodenum. Which of the following effects might be observed after the subcutaneous administration of bethanechol?

a. Skeletal muscle twitching
b. Decrease in heart rate
c. Peripheral vasodilatation
d. Constriction in the airways of the lung
e. *b*, *c*, and *d*

CHAPTER 10

Drugs affecting the sympathetic nervous system

Kenneth P. Minneman

Major Drugs

- Nonselective adrenergic agonists
- α-Adrenergic agonists
- β-Adrenergic agonists
- Indirectly acting sympathomimetics
- Nonselective adrenergic antagonists
- α-Adrenergic antagonists
- β-Adrenergic antagonists
- Indirectly acting sympatholytics
- Agents that reduce central sympathetic outflow

Therapeutic overview

The sympathetic nervous system is an energy-expending system that has an ergotrophic function. Stimulation of this system leads to the "flight, fright, or fight" response characterized by increased heart rate, blood pressure and respiration, an increased blood flow to skeletal muscles, and mydriasis. Almost all postganglionic sympathetic neurons release norepinephrine (NE) as their neurotransmitter to alter the activity of the effector organs. A minor exception is the small number of anatomically sympathetic neurons projecting to sweat glands and a few blood vessels that release acetylcholine. NE released from sympathetic neurons activates **adrenergic receptors** on exocrine glands, smooth muscle, and cardiac muscle to produce sympathetic responses.

Activation of sympathetic outflow also causes secretion of epinephrine (Epi) and NE into the blood from the adrenal medulla. Epi and NE are catecholamines, and outside the United States are called adrenaline and noradrenaline, respectively, from which the adjectives "adrenergic" and "noradrenergic" are derived.

Drugs that facilitate or mimic the actions of the sympathetic nervous system are called **sympathomimetics** or **adrenergic agonists.** Sympathomimetics constrict most arterioles and veins and can be used locally to reduce bleeding, slow diffusion of drugs such as local anesthetics, decongest mucous membranes, and reduce formation of aqueous humor to lower intraocular pressure in glaucoma. Systemic administration of sympathomimetics increases peripheral vascular resistance and mean arterial blood pressure and can increase blood pressure in hypotensive states, including neurogenic shock. By increasing blood pressure, sympathomimetics cause a reflex slowing of heart rate, which can be used to treat paroxysmal atrial tachycardia.

Epi and certain other sympathomimetics strongly stimulate cardiac muscle and are used to treat cardiogenic shock. These drugs also relax various nonvascular smooth muscles, including bronchial and uterine smooth muscle, and are useful in treating bronchospasm and delaying delivery during premature labor. Drugs mimicking Epi also contract the radial muscle in the iris, causing pupillary dilation and facilitating eye examinations.

Abbreviations

CNS	central nervous system
COMT	catechol-*O*-methyltransferase
DA	dopamine
Epi	epinephrine
GI	gastrointestinal
MAO	monoamine oxidase
NE	norepinephrine
IP	isoproterenol

Drugs that block or reduce the actions of NE are called **sympatholytics** or **adrenergic antagonists.** Drugs that decrease sympathetic activity at vascular smooth muscle are used to treat essential hypertension and hypertensive emergencies, as well as benign prostatic hyperplasia. Drugs that reduce the actions of NE and Epi on cardiac muscle are used to treat cardiac dysrhythmias, angina pectoris, and other cardiac disorders, such as postmyocardial infarction. These drugs are also used in treating migraines, glaucoma, and essential tremor.

Due to the widespread distribution of sympathetic nerves throughout the body, and the many different types of adrenergic receptors, drugs that modify the actions of sympathetic neurons produce many different clinically important responses. It is also important to keep in mind that as a consequence of the anatomical and functional diversity within the sympathetic nervous system, many drugs affecting this system will also have undesirable side effects.

The Therapeutic Overview box presents a summary of the primary uses of different classes of compounds that affect the sympathetic nervous system.

THERAPEUTIC OVERVIEW

Sympathomimetics

Nasal decongestion
Decrease formation of aqueous humor in glaucoma
Neurogenic shock, cardiogenic shock
Paroxysmal atrial tachycardia
Bronchospasm, asthma
Decrease diffusion of local anesthetics

Sympatholytics

Essential hypertension, hypertensive emergencies
Benign prostatic hyperplasia
Cardiac dysrhythmias, angina pectoris, postmyocardial infarction
Essential tremor
Glaucoma

Mechanisms of action

The biochemistry and physiology of the autonomic nervous system, including a discussion of adrenergic receptors, are discussed in Chapter 8. Detailed information on receptors and signaling pathways involved are presented in Chapter 2. This section covers topics that pertain specifically to noradrenergic neurotransmission and its modulation by drugs.

Noradrenergic transmission

The neurochemical steps that mediate noradrenergic neurotransmission are summarized in Figure 10-1. The first step involves the transport of tyrosine into the neuron followed by its conversion to l-DOPA by the rate-limiting enzyme tyrosine hydroxylase. L-DOPA is rapidly decarboxylated to dopamine (DA) by aromatic l-amino acid decarboxylase, also known as DOPA decarboxylase. In dopaminergic neurons within the central nervous system (CNS), this is the last step in the synthetic process, and DA is released as a neurotransmitter. Noradrenergic neurons in the CNS and peripheral sympathetic nervous system contain an additional enzyme, DA β-hydroxylase, which converts DA to NE. This enzyme is located in synaptic vesicles, so DA must be actively transported into these vesicles before conversion to NE.

When the action potential depolarizes the nerve terminal, voltage-gated calcium channels open, allowing Ca^{2+} to enter the neuron and cause the vesicles to release NE. At the neuroeffector junction, NE binds to various adrenergic receptor subtypes on both the presynaptic and postsynaptic membranes, with different organs containing different receptor subtypes. Activation of α_2-"autoreceptors" on the presynaptic neuronal membrane causes feedback inhibition and reduces further NE release. The signaling mechanisms occurring after adrenergic receptor activation are discussed in Chapter 8.

After NE has activated its receptors, its action is terminated primarily by a high-affinity reuptake system (termed "uptake 1" in Fig. 10-1), which transports it back into the neuron for eventual re-release. A smaller fraction of the NE in the synapse diffuses away from the receptors and can be taken up by a lower affinity extraneuronal process (termed "uptake 2" in Fig. 10-1). Some of the NE taken back into the sympathetic neurons by reuptake can be oxidatively deaminated by **monoamine oxidase (MAO)** on the external mitochondrial membrane. The biologically inactive deaminated metabolites enter the circulation and are excreted in the urine. The NE that is transported into the postjunctional cell is *O*-methylated by **catechol-*O*-methyltransferase (COMT)** to normetanephrine. The high affinity reuptake of NE into presynaptic terminals is the major mechanism that terminates its actions, although COMT and MAO also play important roles in metabolizing circulating NE and Epi and some exogenously administered sympathomimetic amines.

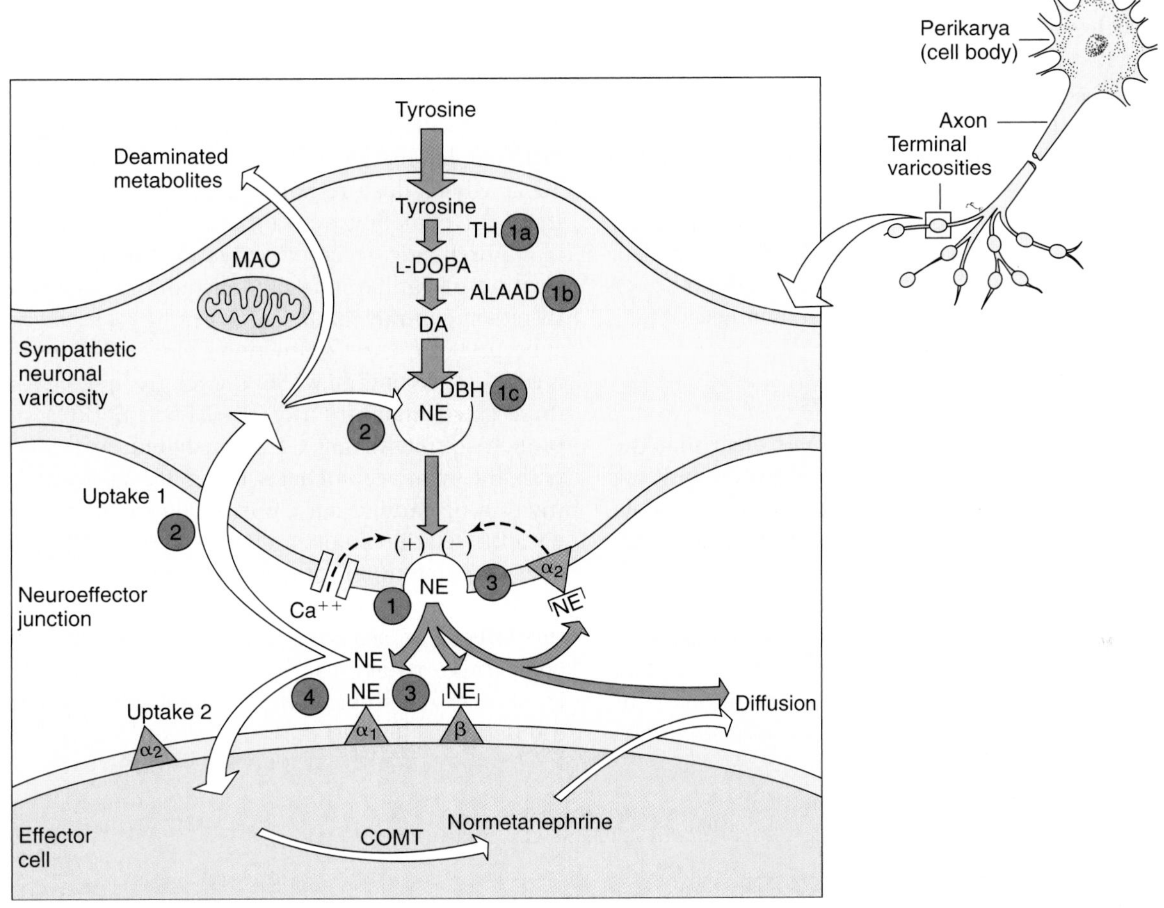

Figure 10-1 Prejunctional and postjunctional sites of action of drugs that modify noradrenergic transmission at a sympathetic neuroeffector junction. L-Tyrosine is actively transported into the neuron, where it is converted to l-DOPA by tyrosine hydroxylase *(TH)* and then to DA by aromatic l-amino acid decarboxylase *(ALAAD)*. DA is actively transported into synaptic vesicles, where it is converted by DA β-hydroxylase *(DBH)* to norepinephrine *(NE)*. The arrival of an action potential at the varicosity causes calcium influx, which promotes exocytotic release of NE. After release, NE can activate postjunctional α_1, α_2, or β-adrenergic receptors or α_2-receptors on the prejunctional membrane. Activation of prejunctional α_2 receptors inhibits further release of NE. The action of NE is terminated by transport back into the neuron by high affinity uptake (*Uptake 1*), where it can be repackaged into synaptic vesicles or metabolized by MAO to inactive products. NE is also removed by diffusion and transport into the postjunctional cell (*Uptake 2*), where it is metabolized to normetanephrine by catechol-*O*-methyltransferase (COMT). Sites at which drugs act to enhance or mimic noradrenergic transmission are identified by numbers in *green circles*; numbers in *red circles* identify sites where drugs block or reduce this process.

Drugs that enhance or mimic noradrenergic transmission:
1. Facilitate release (e.g., amphetamine)
2. Block reuptake (e.g., cocaine)
3. Receptor agonists (e.g., phenylephrine)

Drugs that reduce noradrenergic transmission:
1. Inhibit synthesis (e.g., *1a*, α-methyltyrosine; *1b*, carbidopa; *1c*, disulfiram)
2. Disrupt vesicular storage (e.g., reserpine)
3. Inhibit release (e.g., guanethidine)
4. Receptor antagonists (e.g., phentolamine)

NE is also synthesized in and released from chromaffin cells in the adrenal medulla. These cells usually contain another enzyme, phenylethanolamine-N-methyltransferase, which converts NE to Epi. Chromaffin cells are innervated by sympathetic preganglionic cholinergic neurons and release catecholamines into the blood, where they are transported to various organs to act on adrenergic receptors. Circulating catecholamines, whether administered as drugs or released from the adrenal medulla, are also removed by high affinity uptake into sympathetic nerves or metabolized, as discussed.

Drugs modify the activity of sympathetic neurons by increasing or decreasing the noradrenergic signal (see Fig. 10-1). Sympathomimetics may mimic noradrenergic transmission by acting directly on postsynaptic receptors (e.g., phenylephrine), by facilitating NE release (e.g., amphetamine), or by blocking neuronal reuptake (e.g., cocaine). Sympatholytics reduce noradrenergic transmission by inhibiting synthesis (e.g., α-methyltyrosine), disrupting vesicular storage (e.g., reserpine), inhibiting release (e.g., guanethidine), or directly blocking receptors (e.g., phentolamine).

Activation of adrenergic receptors

Over the last half century it has become clear that the actions of NE and Epi are mediated through multiple adrenergic receptor subtypes (see Chapter 8). We now know that there are nine different subtypes of adrenergic receptors, each encoded by separate genes, which are grouped into three major families (α_1, α_2, β), each containing three different members. Of these, only four (α_1, α_2, β_1, and β_2) are currently important in clinical pharmacology; therefore, they are the major focus of this chapter. Both NE and Epi activate most adrenergic receptors with similar, but not identical, potencies, although NE is much less potent than Epi at the β_2-subtype. Isoproterenol (IP) is a synthetic analog of NE and Epi and selectively activates only β-adrenergic receptors. Differences in the pharmacological profiles of different adrenergic receptors are illustrated in Figure 10-2, where dose-response curves for the actions of these catecholamines on different tissues are depicted.

Adrenergic receptor activation increases the contraction of cardiac muscle and induces smooth muscle to either contract or relax, depending on the receptor subtype(s) present. Contraction of arterial strips is mediated by α_1-receptors, where the relative potencies of the three catecholamines are Epi≥NE>>>IP. Relaxation of bronchial smooth muscle is mediated by β_2-receptors, with the relative potencies being IP>Epi>>>NE. Contraction of cardiac muscle is mediated by β_1-receptors, with the relative potencies being IP>Epi≥NE. The presence of different receptor subtypes in these three tissues is further demonstrated in Figure 10-3 by examining the effects of selective antagonists. Phentolamine, a competitive antagonist at α_1-receptors, causes a parallel shift to the right of the NE-induced contractions of arterial strips (Fig. 10-3, *A*) but does not affect the other

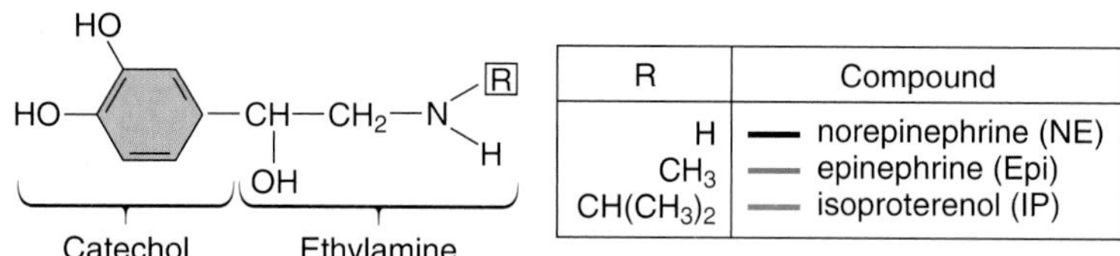

R	Compound
H	norepinephrine (NE)
CH_3	epinephrine (Epi)
$CH(CH_3)_2$	isoproterenol (IP)

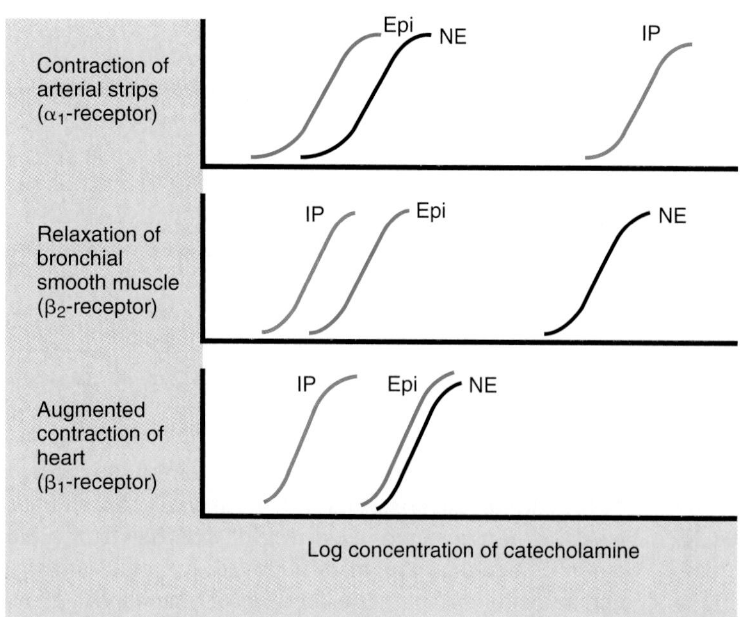

Figure 10-2 Dose-response curves (arbitrary scales) show relative potencies of three catecholamines in experimental muscle preparations. Changes in the force of contraction or relaxation for each muscle is shown after addition of progressively increasing concentrations of each catecholamine.

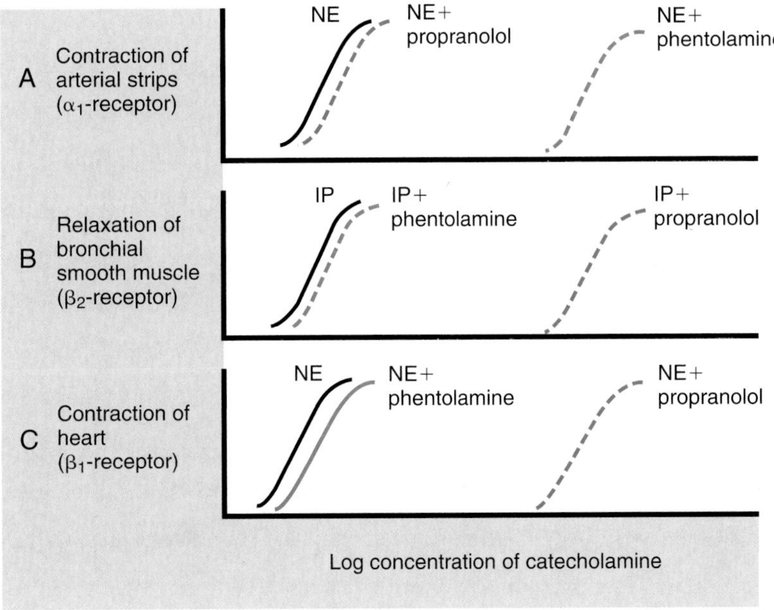

Figure 10-3 Changes in force of contraction or relaxation (arbitrary scale) of different tissues hung in separate tissue baths after addition of increasing concentrations of catecholamine in absence and presence of a fixed concentration of an α-adrenergic (phentolamine) or β-adrenergic (propranolol) receptor blocking drug. *NE,* Norepinephrine; *IP,* isoproterenol.

two responses. Propranolol, a competitive antagonist at both β_1- and β_2-adrenergic receptors, causes a parallel shift to the right of responses mediated by bronchial β_2-receptors (Fig. 10-3, *B*) and cardiac β_1-receptors (Fig. 10-3, *C*), without affecting the α_1-response.

α_2-Adrenergic receptors are found on platelets, in the CNS, and postsynaptically in several other peripheral tissues (blood vessels, pancreas, and enteric cholinergic neurons). As mentioned above, activation of α_2-receptors on the terminals of sympathetic neurons reduces NE release. α_2-Receptors are also found both presynaptically and postsynaptically on neurons in brain, and activation of these receptors reduces central sympathetic outflow.

Directly acting sympathomimetics

Directly acting adrenergic receptor agonists mimic some of the effects of sympathetic nervous system activation by binding to and activating specific receptor subtypes (see *site 3* [green] in Fig. 10-1). For example, as mentioned, IP selectively activates β-receptors, phenylephrine selectively activates α_1-receptors, and clonidine selectively activates α_2-receptors. Similarly, dobutamine and albuterol are relatively specific agonists at β_1- and β_2-receptors, respectively. The structures of some clinically important adrenergic receptor agonists are shown in Figure 10-4.

Indirectly acting sympathomimetics

Indirectly acting sympathomimetics do not activate receptors directly but facilitate the release of NE from sympathetic neurons or block high affinity reuptake. Amphetamine and related drugs produce their sympathomimetic effects by facilitating NE release (see *site 1* [green] in Fig. 10-1); the effects of these drugs in the CNS are described in Chapter 32. On the other hand, cocaine and tricyclic antidepressants, such as desipramine, exert their sympathomimetic effects by blocking high affinity reuptake (see *site 2* [green] in Fig. 10-1). The structure and characteristics of cocaine are discussed in Chapter 32, with similar information for tricyclic antidepressants given in Chapter 23.

Because neuronal reuptake, and not metabolism, is the primary mechanism for terminating the actions of NE and Epi, it is not surprising that drugs that inhibit metabolism of these amines show little or no sympathomimetic actions. On the other hand, inhibitors of MAO (e.g., pargyline) or COMT (e.g., tolcapone) can enhance the actions of other synthetic sympathomimetic amines that are substrates for these enzymes (see Fig. 10-1), with some important toxicological implications. For example, the actions of tyramine, a sympathomimetic amine present in a variety of foods, are greatly enhanced in patients treated with MAO inhibitors (see Chapter 23).

An indirectly acting sympathomimetic amine that releases NE must penetrate the noradrenergic neuron before it can act. Nonpolar, lipid-soluble drugs (e.g., amphetamine) can diffuse across neuronal membranes, whereas polar, water-soluble compounds (e.g., tyramine) must rely on high affinity uptake by the NE transporter. Figure 10-5 illustrates that drugs that reduce or block the effects of tyramine enhance the effects of Epi, which acts directly on the adrenergic receptors. The enhanced effects of Epi in denervated tissues result from both an

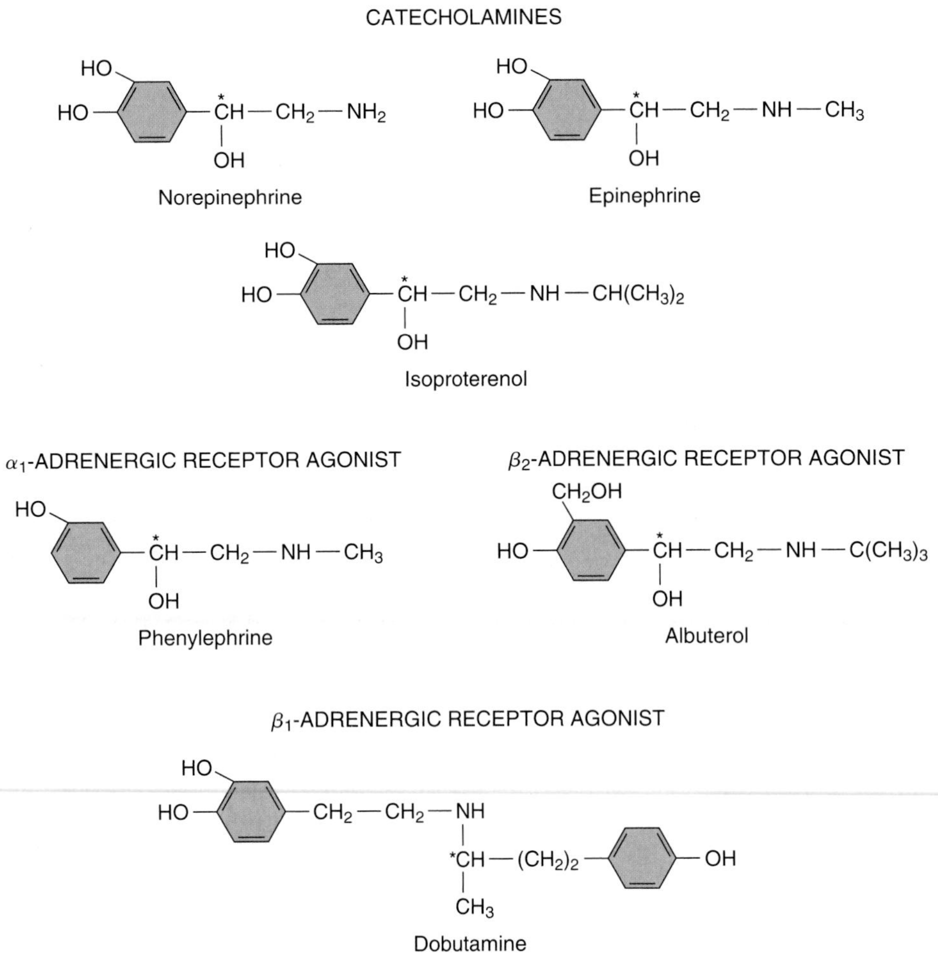

CATECHOLAMINES

Norepinephrine

Epinephrine

Isoproterenol

α_1-ADRENERGIC RECEPTOR AGONIST

Phenylephrine

β_2-ADRENERGIC RECEPTOR AGONIST

Albuterol

β_1-ADRENERGIC RECEPTOR AGONIST

Dobutamine

Figure 10-4 Structures of some directly acting sympathomimetic agonists. Asterisk indicates asymmetrical carbon.

early (2 to 3 days) loss of reuptake sites due to loss of the neuronal membrane, and a later (days to weeks) increase (upregulation) in postjunctional receptors. Cocaine also causes a prompt increase in the response to Epi by blocking the reuptake system, whereas reserpine disrupts amine transport from the cytoplasm into synaptic vesicles not by neuronal membranes. Therefore, reserpine has only small effects on responses to directly acting sympathomimetics.

Sympatholytics

Inhibition of synthesis, storage, or release of NE Catecholamine synthesis can be disrupted at several steps, but effective in vivo blockade is obtained only when tyrosine hydroxylase, the enzyme catalyzing the first and rate-limiting step, is inhibited (see site *1a* in Fig. 10-1). This can be produced clinically with α-methyltyrosine (metyrosine). Several compounds can inhibit other biosynthetic enzymes (e.g., DOPA decarboxylase is inhibited by carbidopa and DA β-hydroxylase is inhibited by disulfiram [see sites *1b* and *1c* in Fig. 10-1]). Although these drugs do not effectively block endogenous catecholamine synthesis when administered, they do have clinical utility by affecting other systems. By virtue of its ability to inhibit peripheral DOPA decarboxylase, carbidopa is used in combination with l-DOPA to increase DA synthesis in the brains of patients with Parkinson's disease (see Chapter 21). Similarly, disulfiram is used in treating chronic alcoholism (see Chapter 25).

Disruption of vesicular storage also modifies noradrenergic transmission (see site *2* [red] in Fig. 10-1). As discussed, reserpine disrupts the ability of the synaptic vesicles to transport and store DA and NE. Inhibition of release can also modulate adrenergic responses (see site *3* [red] in Fig. 10-1). Drugs, such as bretylium and guanethidine, which accumulate in noradrenergic nerve terminals, prevent NE release.

Antagonists There are many antagonists with different subtype-selectivities now available to block adrenergic receptors (see site *4* [red] in Fig. 10-1). The early antagonists blocked α-(phenoxybenzamine) or β-receptors

Pretreatment	Response of effector organ to: Direct sympathomimetic (e.g., epinephrine)	Indirect sympathomimetic (e.g., tyramine)
1. Denervation	Increased	Reduced
2. Reserpine	Slightly increased	Reduced
3. Cocaine	Increased	Reduced

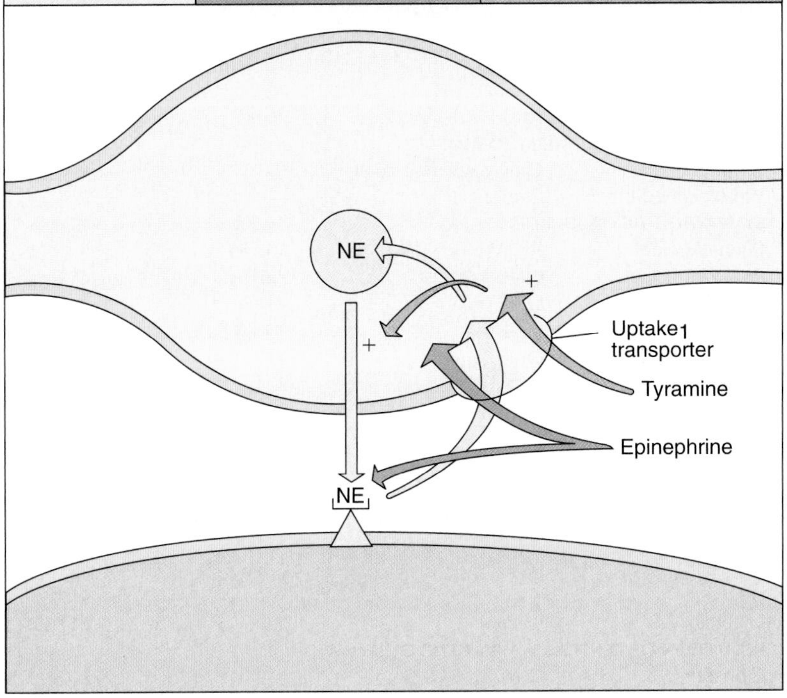

Figure 10-5 Comparison of directly acting and indirectly acting sympathomimetics.

(propranolol), whereas drugs are now available that specifically block α_1-(prazosin), α_2-(yohimbine), or β_1-receptors (metoprolol). These selective antagonists have important therapeutic advantages over the original broad-spectrum adrenergic receptor blockers and are used for various indications, such as the control of blood pressure (see Chapter 12).

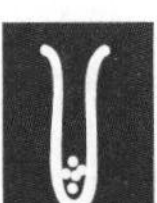

Pharmacokinetics

Detailed pharmacokinetics are not known for many of these drugs in humans. Some known pharmacokinetic parameters for major drugs are summarized in Table 10-1.

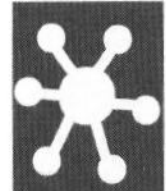

Relation of mechanisms of action to clinical response

Direct and reflex cardiovascular actions of adrenergic agents

The sympathetic nervous system plays an important role in regulating the cardiovascular system; thus, adrenergic drugs have pronounced effects on this system. These drugs alter the rate and force of contraction of the heart and the tone of blood vessels (and, consequently, blood pressure) through activation of adrenergic receptors on cardiac and vascular smooth muscle cells. Compensatory reflex adjustments occur as a result of these responses, and these reflexes must be considered to understand the overall actions of adrenergic drugs on the heart and blood vessels.

Table 10-1 Pharmacokinetic parameters

Drug	Route of Administration	Half-Life (hrs)	Disposition	Remarks
DIRECTLY ACTING SYMPATHOMIMETICS				
Norepinephrine	IV	—	M	
Epinephrine	IV, inhalation, topical	—	M	
Isoproterenol	IV, inhalation	—	M	
Phenylephrine	Oral, topical	—	M	primarily topical
Albuterol	Oral, inhalation	3.6	R (30%), M (50%)	
Terbutaline	IV, oral, inhalation	~6	M (60%), first pass; crosses placenta	
Salmeterol	Inhalation	5.5	M	
Ritodrine	IV, oral	12 (oral)	R (90%)	30% bioavailability (oral)
Dobutamine	IV	2 min	M (main)	
INDIRECTLY ACTING SYMPATHOMIMETICS				
Amphetamine	Oral, exchange resin	—	R	
Pseudoephedrine	Oral	—	R	
SYMPATHOLYTICS: BLOCKERS				
Phentolamine	IV, IM	19 min	R (13%), M	
Prazosin	Oral	2.5	M (main), B	>90% pb
Terazosin	Oral	~12	M	>90% pb
Doxazosin	Oral	10-20	M	
Propranolol	Oral	4	M	
Nadolol	Oral	22	R (90%)	
Pindolol	Oral	3.5 7 (elderly)	M (60%), no first pass R (40%)	40% pb
Atenolol	Oral	6.5	R (90%)	50% absorbed, 10% pb
Metoprolol	IV, oral, inhalation	5	M (90%), first pass (50%) R (50%)	12% pb
Esmolol*	IV	9 min	M (98%), weak met R	
Labetalol	IV, oral	5.5	M (65%), first pass	50% pb
REDUCTION OF CENTRAL SYMPATHETIC OUTFLOW				
Clonidine	Oral†	~12	R (50%)	
Guanabenz	Oral	4-6	M (90%)	

B, Biliary; *first pass*, liver first-pass effect; *inhalation*, inhalation as an aerosol; *M*, metabolism; *pb*, plasma protein bound; *R*, renal, unchanged drug.
*Ester hydrolysis, gives weakly active metabolite.
†Transdermal adhesive patch, 1 week.

Mean arterial blood pressure does not fluctuate widely because of feedback mechanisms that evoke compensatory responses to maintain homeostasis (Fig. 10-6). Baroreceptors are stretch receptors located in the walls of the heart and blood vessels that are activated by distention of the blood vessels. Increased blood pressure increases impulse traffic in afferent baroreceptor neurons that project to vasomotor centers in the medulla. Impulses generated in the baroreceptors inhibit the tonic discharge of sympathetic neurons projecting to the heart and blood vessels and activate vagal fibers projecting to the heart. When phenylephrine, which contracts vascular smooth muscle, is administered, peripheral resistance and blood pressure increase (Fig. 10-7). In turn, this increase in pressure increases afferent baroreceptor neuronal activity, thereby reducing sympathetic nerve activity and increasing vagal nerve activity. Consequently, heart rate decreases (bradycardia). Drugs, such as histamine, which relax vascular smooth muscle, decrease blood pressure, reducing impulse traffic in afferent buffer neurons. Consequently, sympathetic nerve activity increases and vagal nerve activity decreases, resulting in an increased heart rate (tachycardia).

In summary, drugs causing vasoconstriction secondarily cause reflex slowing of the heart, whereas drugs causing vasodilation produce reflex tachycardia. Thus, the actions of adrenergic drugs on the cardiovascular system include both the direct actions of the drug on effector organs and compensatory reflex actions.

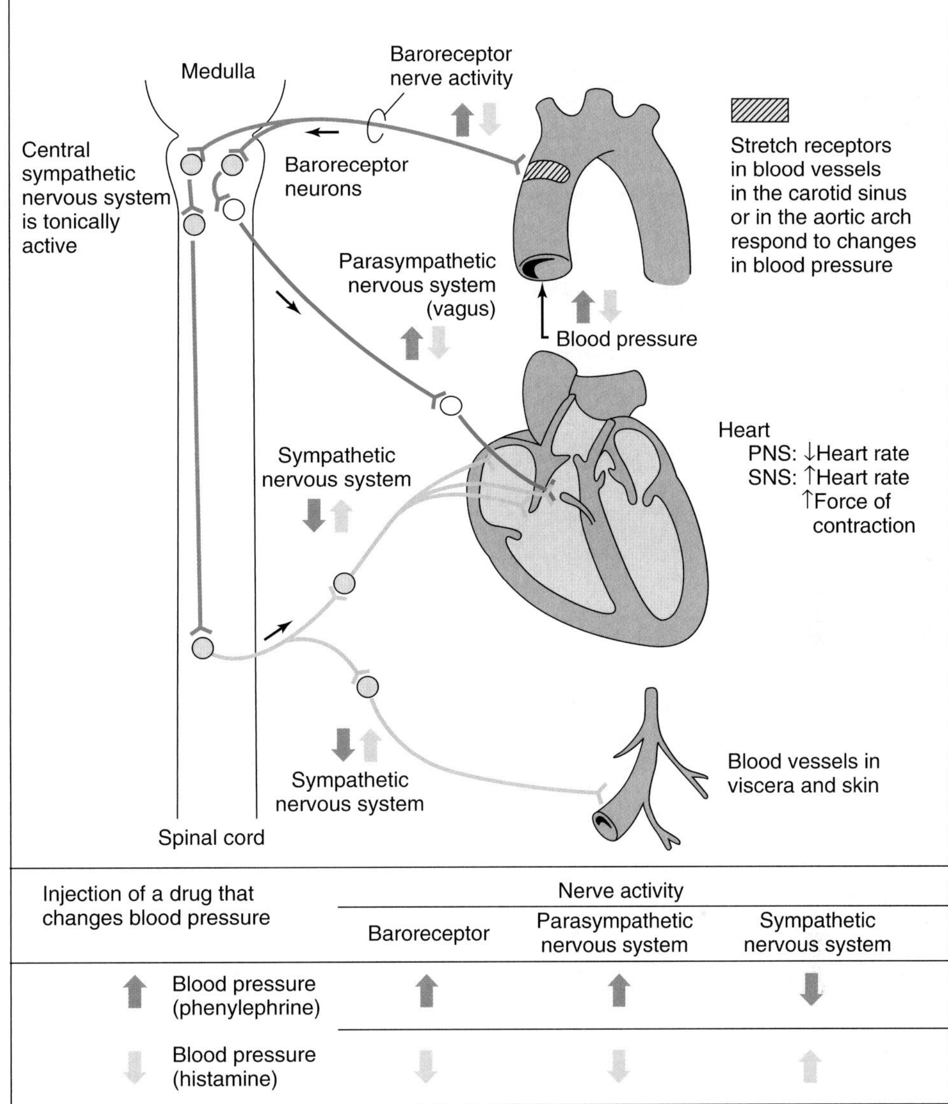

Injection of a drug that changes blood pressure	Nerve activity		
	Baroreceptor	Parasympathetic nervous system	Sympathetic nervous system
↑ Blood pressure (phenylephrine)	↑	↑	↓
↓ Blood pressure (histamine)	↓	↓	↑

Figure 10-6 Baroreceptor control of blood pressure and heart rate. *SNS*, Sympathetic nervous system; *PNS*, parasympathetic nervous system.

Directly acting sympathomimetics

Epi is the prototype of directly acting sympathomimetic drugs because it activates all known adrenergic receptor subtypes. The effects of directly acting sympathomimetic drugs on selected tissues and organ systems are discussed in this section. Epi is discussed first, and the properties of more selective sympathomimetics are then compared with those of the prototype.

Cardiac muscle By activating cardiac β_1-adrenergic receptors, Epi alters the strength, rate, and rhythm of cardiac contractions; these actions may be either desirable or dangerous. Epi increases the force of contraction (positive inotropic effect) by activating β_1-receptors on myocardial cells and increases the rate of contraction (positive chronotropic effect) by activating β_1-receptors on pacemaker cells in the sinoatrial node. Epi also accelerates the rate of myocardial relaxation so that systole is shortened relatively more than diastole. Thus, while Epi is exerting its effects, the fraction of time spent in diastole is increased, which allows for increased filling of the heart. The combination of an increased diastolic filling time, more forceful ejection of blood, and increased rates of contraction and relaxation of the heart result in increased cardiac output. The initial increase in heart rate after administration of Epi may be followed by slowing of the heart (bradycardia) due to reflex activation of the vagus.

Epi also activates conducting tissues, thereby increasing conduction velocity and reducing the

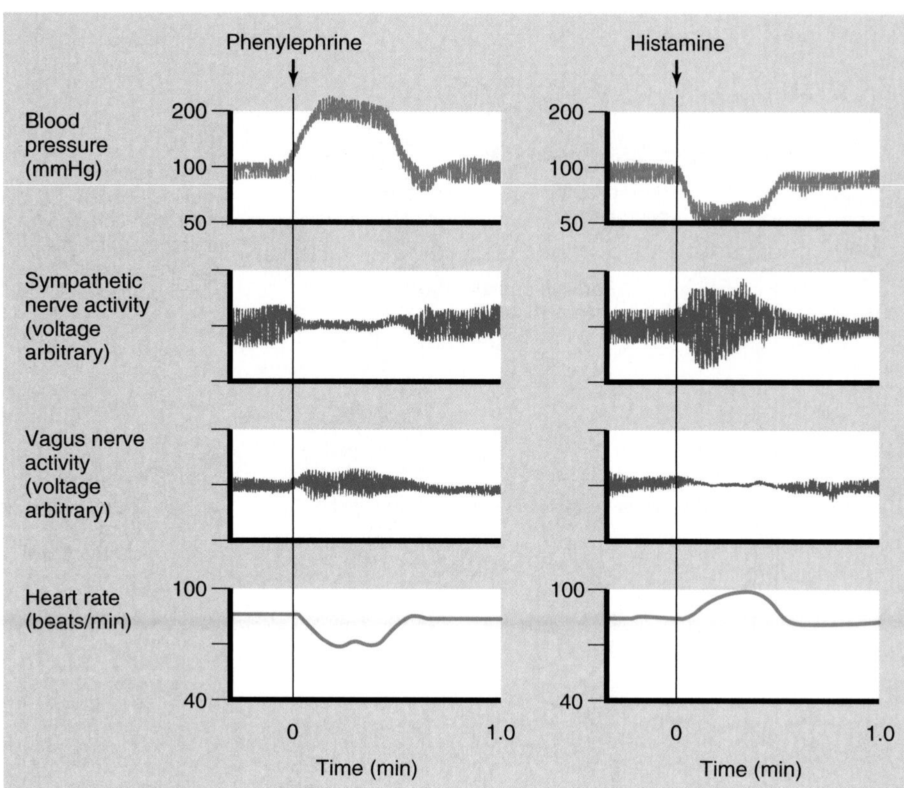

Figure 10-7 Responses to intravenous injections of drugs that cause vasoconstriction (phenylephrine) or vasodilation (histamine) by acting directly on vascular smooth muscle.

refractory period in the atrioventricular node, the bundle of His, Purkinje fibers, and ventricular muscle. These changes, and the activation of latent pacemaker cells, may lead to alterations in the rhythm of the heart. Large doses of Epi may cause tachycardia, premature ventricular systole, and possibly fibrillation; these effects are more likely to occur in hearts that are diseased or have been sensitized by halogenated hydrocarbons (e.g., certain anesthetic agents) (see Chapter 28).

Vascular smooth muscle The effects of Epi on smooth muscle cells in different organs depend on the type of adrenergic receptors present. Vascular smooth muscle is regulated primarily by α_1- or β_2-receptors, depending on the location of the vascular bed. Epi is a powerful vasoconstrictor in some beds; it activates α_1-receptors to cause smooth muscle cells to contract in precapillary resistance vessels (arterioles) in skin, mucosa, kidney, and veins. At low doses, Epi also activates β_2-receptors, causing relaxation of vascular smooth muscle in skeletal muscle, liver, and the gastrointestinal (GI) tract. Thus, Epi increases blood flow in skeletal muscle and some splanchnic beds but reduces flow in skin and kidney.

Systemic administration of Epi alters cerebral and coronary blood flow, but the changes do not result primarily from its direct actions on vascular smooth muscle in the brain. Rather, changes in cerebral blood flow reflect changes in systemic blood pressure, and increased coronary blood flow results from a greater duration of diastole and production of vasodilator metabolites (e.g., adenosine) secondary to the increased work of the heart.

Other smooth muscle Epi is a potent bronchodilator, relaxing bronchial smooth muscle by activating β_2-receptors. It dramatically reduces responses to endogenous bronchoconstrictors and can be lifesaving in acute asthmatic attacks (see Chapter 34). Epi also relaxes smooth muscle in other organs through β_2-receptors. It reduces the frequency and amplitude of GI contractions, decreases the tone and contractions of the pregnant uterus, and relaxes the detrusor muscle of the urinary bladder. However, it causes the smooth muscle of the prostate and splenic capsule and of GI and urinary sphincters to contract by activating α_1-receptors. Epi can foster urinary retention by relaxing the detrusor muscle and contracting the trigone and sphincter of the urinary bladder.

The radial pupillary dilator muscle of the iris contains α_1-receptors and contracts in response to activation of sympathetic neurons, causing mydriasis. Because Epi is a highly polar molecule, it does not penetrate the cornea readily when instilled into the conjunctival sac.

Mydriasis occurs when less polar, more lipid soluble α-adrenergic agonists (e.g., phenylephrine) are applied. If Epi is instilled, however, intraocular pressure is lowered, possibly because the agent reduces formation of aqueous humor by the ciliary bodies, although this mechanism is not well understood.

Because Epi and all other catecholamines are polar and cannot penetrate the blood-brain barrier, systemic administration of these amines has no direct cerebral action. Nevertheless, systemic administration of Epi can cause anxiety, restlessness, and headache, possibly through secondary reflexes.

Metabolic effects Epi exerts many metabolic effects, some of which are secondary to its action on the secretion of insulin and glucagon. The predominant action of Epi on islet cells of the pancreas is inhibition of insulin secretion from pancreatic β cells through activation of α_2-receptors and stimulation of glucagon secretion from pancreatic α cells through activation of β_2-receptors.

The major metabolic effects of Epi are increased circulating concentrations of glucose, lactic acid, and free fatty acids. In humans, these effects are attributable to the activation of β-receptors at liver, skeletal muscle, heart, and adipose cells (Fig. 10-8). β-Adrenergic receptor activation results in G protein-mediated activation of adenylyl cyclase. The resulting increase in cyclic AMP leads to a series of phosphorylation events, culminating in activation of phosphorylase and lipase. Lipase catalyzes breakdown of triglycerides in fat to free fatty acids. The characteristic "calorigenic action" of Epi, which is reflected in a 20% to 30% increase in oxygen consumption, is caused, in part, by the breakdown of triglycerides in brown adipose tissue and subsequent oxidation of the resulting fatty acids. In liver, phosphorylase catalyzes the breakdown of glycogen to glucose. In muscle,

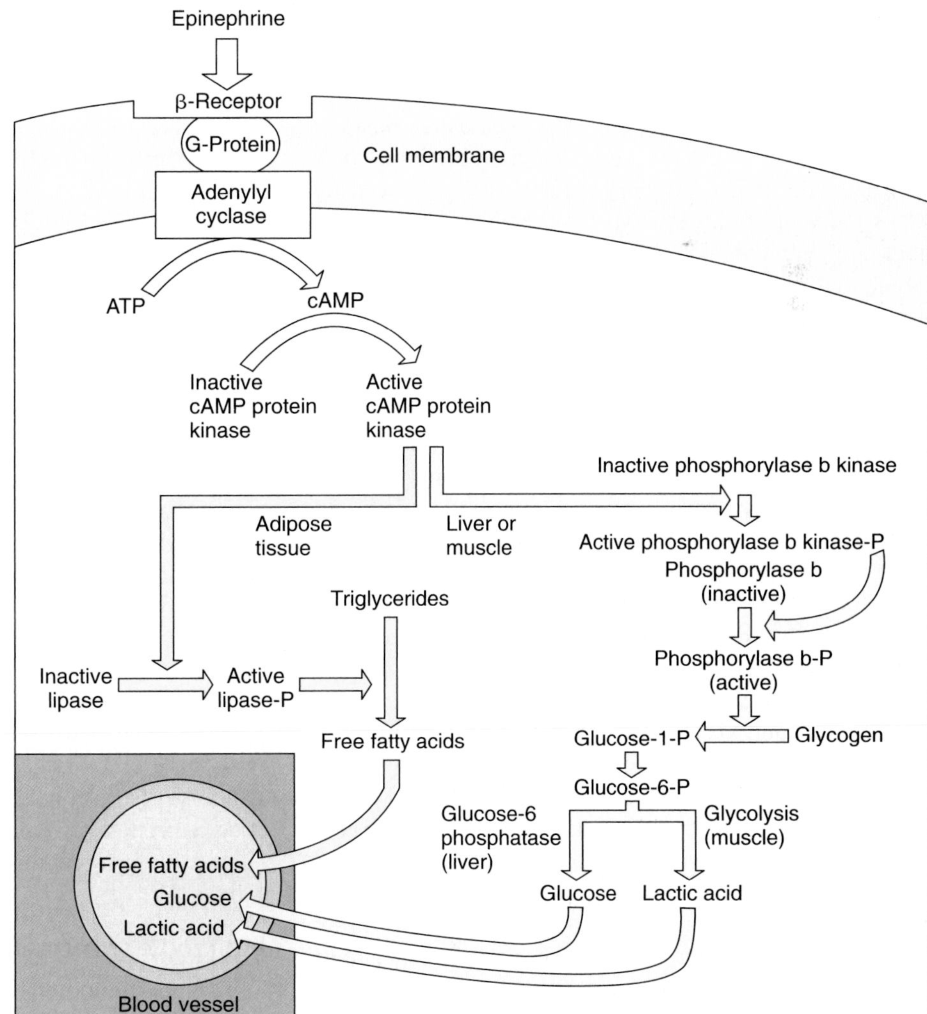

Figure 10-8 Mechanisms by which epinephrine (and other β-adrenergic agonists) exerts metabolic effects in adipose, liver, heart, and skeletal muscle cells.

glycogenolysis and glycolysis produce lactic acid, which is released into the blood. Release of glucose from the liver is accompanied by the efflux of potassium, so that Epi induces hyperglycemia and a brief period of hyperkalemia. The hyperkalemia is followed by a more pronounced hypokalemia, as the potassium released from the liver is taken up by skeletal muscle.

Miscellaneous actions Secretion of sweat from glands located on the palms of the hands and forehead is increased during psychological stress, and this effect is mediated by α_1-receptors. When administered systemically, Epi does not activate these glands, but secretion of sweat in these areas can be induced if Epi is injected locally. Epi, by acting on β_1-receptors, also causes the release of renin from the juxtaglomerular apparatus in the kidney.

Other directly acting sympathomimetics Most clinically useful directly acting sympathomimetics differ from Epi because they selectively activate specific adrenergic receptor subtypes. The properties of some of these compounds are compared with those of Epi below.

NE has a relatively low potency at β_2-receptors; thus, clinically relevant doses of NE stimulate only α- and β_1-adrenergic receptors. NE produces vasoconstriction only in vascular beds, therefore increasing diastolic blood pressure. Because total peripheral resistance increases, the reflex slowing of heart rate produced by NE is more pronounced than that produced by Epi. NE does not usually relax bronchial smooth muscle, and metabolic responses (e.g., hyperglycemia) are much less pronounced than those produced by Epi, because they primarily involve β_2-receptor activation.

Phenylephrine and methoxamine are selective α_1-receptor agonists and differ from NE because they do not activate α_2- or β_1-receptors, and, therefore, do not stimulate the heart. These drugs increase total peripheral resistance by causing vasoconstriction in most vascular beds. Consequently, they produce a reflex slowing of the heart that can be blocked by atropine. These drugs, which are less potent but longer acting than NE, have been used to treat hypotension and shock. Phenylephrine is also used in topical preparations as a mydriatic and nasal decongestant.

IP is a potent agonist at all β-receptor subtypes and differs from Epi because it does not activate α-adrenergic receptors. It reduces total peripheral resistance through β_2-receptors, resulting in a considerable reduction in diastolic blood pressure. It has a strong stimulatory effect on the heart; tachycardia results from a combined direct action on β_1-receptors and a reflex action secondary to the hypotension. Like Epi, it relaxes bronchial smooth muscle and induces metabolic effects. Clinically, IP may be used to relieve bronchoconstriction; however, the cardiac side effects resulting from its β_1-agonist property can be troublesome. Accordingly, β-agonists that are relatively specific for β_2-receptors have been developed.

Metaproterenol, terbutaline, albuterol, bitolterol, salmeterol, and ritodrine are relatively specific agonists at β_2-adrenergic receptors. Because these drugs are less potent at β_1-receptors, they have less tendency to stimulate the heart. Nevertheless, their selectivity for β_2-receptors is not absolute and at higher doses these drugs stimulate the heart directly. These drugs also differ from IP because they are effective orally and have a longer duration of action. Selective β_2-receptor agonists relax vascular smooth muscle in skeletal muscle and smooth muscle in bronchi and uterus. Although the pharmacological properties of all β_2-agonists are similar, ritodrine is marketed as a tocolytic agent; that is, it relaxes uterine smooth muscle and thereby arrests premature labor. All other drugs are marketed for the treatment of bronchospasm and bronchial asthma (see Chapter 34). By activating β_2-receptors, these drugs cause bronchodilation and may inhibit the release of inflammatory and bronchoconstrictor mediators (histamine, leukotrienes, prostaglandins) from mast cells in the lungs. The compounds are most effective when delivered by inhalation, which results in the least systemic adverse effects (tachycardia, skeletal muscle tremor). When used orally, selective β_2-agonists have an advantage over ephedrine (see later discussion) because they lack CNS-stimulant properties.

DA and dobutamine are relatively specific for β_1-receptors and are used to stimulate the heart. DA is an endogenous catecholamine with important actions as a neurotransmitter in the brain (see Chapter 20). When administered by intravenous infusion, DA produces a positive inotropic action on the heart, directly, by stimulating β_1-receptors and, indirectly, by releasing NE. DA relaxes smooth muscle in some vascular beds, specifically in the kidney, increasing glomerular filtration rate, sodium excretion, and urinary output. DA is also administered by intravenous infusion for treatment of shock, resulting from myocardial infarction, trauma, or renal failure.

Dobutamine is a relatively specific β_1-receptor agonist that also increases myocardial contractility without greatly altering total peripheral resistance. It has less effect on heart rate than IP because it does not produce reflex tachycardia. Dobutamine is also administered by intravenous infusion to treat acute cardiac failure.

Indirectly acting sympathomimetics

The sympathomimetic actions of some drugs stem from their ability to cause the release of NE from sympathetic

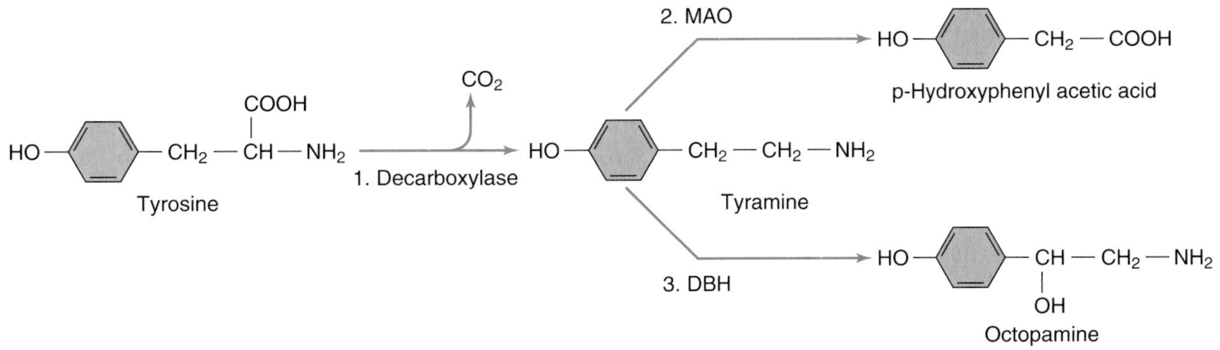

Figure 10-9 Synthesis and metabolism of tyramine. *Reaction 1:* decarboxylation of tyrosine in liver and gastrointestinal tract. *Reaction 2:* oxidative deamination of tyramine by monoamine oxidase *(MAO)* in liver, kidney, and other tissues. *Reaction 3:* β-oxidation of tyramine by DA β-hydroxylase *(DBH)* located in synaptic vesicles within terminal of sympathetic neurons.

neurons or block the neuronal reuptake of NE. Some of these drugs (e.g., amphetamine, cocaine) have noticeable CNS-stimulant actions (see Chapter 32).

Tyramine is present in a variety of foods (e.g., ripened cheese, fermented sausage, wines) and is formed in the liver and GI tract by decarboxylation of tyrosine (Fig. 10-9). However, significant quantities of tyramine are not normally found in blood or tissues because of rapid metabolism by MAO (Fig. 10-9). Injection of tyramine causes its accumulation in synaptic vesicles and the release of NE. Vesicular tyramine is converted to octopamine by DA β-hydroxylase (Fig. 10-9), reducing the ability of the vesicles to store NE. Tolerance to repeated tyramine administration occurs quickly, because newly synthesized octopamine fills the vesicles and is released as a "false transmitter" that does not activate α- or β-receptors (compare *A* and *B* in Fig. 10-10). Similarly, in patients treated long term with an MAO inhibitor, circulating concentrations of tyramine increase (Fig. 10-10, *C*), resulting in less NE release. This leads to a reduction in blood pressure and explains why MAO inhibitors may cause orthostatic hypotension. A more serious adverse effect of MAO inhibitors occurs, if a patient eats food containing tyramine, which can cause the release of NE (Fig. 10-10, *D*) and a severe hypertensive response. Thus, patients treated with MAO inhibitors should avoid eating foods containing tyramine (see Chapter 23).

Amphetamine and ephedrine are related chemically to Epi (Fig. 10-11) but exert their sympathomimetic effects mainly by facilitating release or blocking reuptake of NE. Ephedrine is not metabolized by COMT or MAO, prolonging its duration of action. Ephedrine readily crosses the blood-brain barrier, and thus is effective after oral administration. Ephedrine is a mixture of four isomers: d- and l-ephedrine and d- and l-pseudoephedrine. L-Ephedrine is the most potent, but the racemic mixture is often used, as is D-pseudoephedrine. Ephedrine was widely used as a dietary supplement for its stimulant and appetite-suppressant properties (see Chapter 7) but has now been removed from the market in the United States because of increasing reports of adverse effects.

Pseudoephedrine has fewer central stimulant actions than ephedrine and is widely available as a component of over-the-counter preparations used for relief of upper respiratory tract conditions that accompany the common cold. It is often combined with analgesics, anticholinergics, antihistaminics, and/or caffeine. Pseudoephedrine is thought to act as a decongestant both by indirectly releasing NE and by activating α_1-adrenergic receptors, constricting nasal blood vessels.

Methamphetamine and amphetamine exist as d- and l-optical isomers. On peripheral sympathetic neurons, d- and l-amphetamine are equipotent, but in the CNS, the d-isomer is three to four times more potent than the l-isomer. Amphetamine is used therapeutically only for its central stimulant action (see Chapter 32), and only the d-isomer is employed to minimize peripheral sympathomimetic actions. Amphetamine facilitates the release and blocks the reuptake of NE. However, the central stimulant actions of amphetamine appear to result from its ability to cause release of DA (see Chapter 32). Cocaine is structurally distinct but has similar central stimulant and sympathomimetic actions. It also blocks the neuronal reuptake of NE and DA; however, unlike amphetamine, it does not facilitate neurotransmitter release.

Drugs that block α-adrenergic receptors

The prototype α-adrenergic receptor blocking drug is phentolamine. Phentolamine is a competitive antagonist, meaning that blockade can be surmounted by increasing agonist concentration (Fig. 10-12). Phenoxybenzamine, on the other hand, binds covalently to

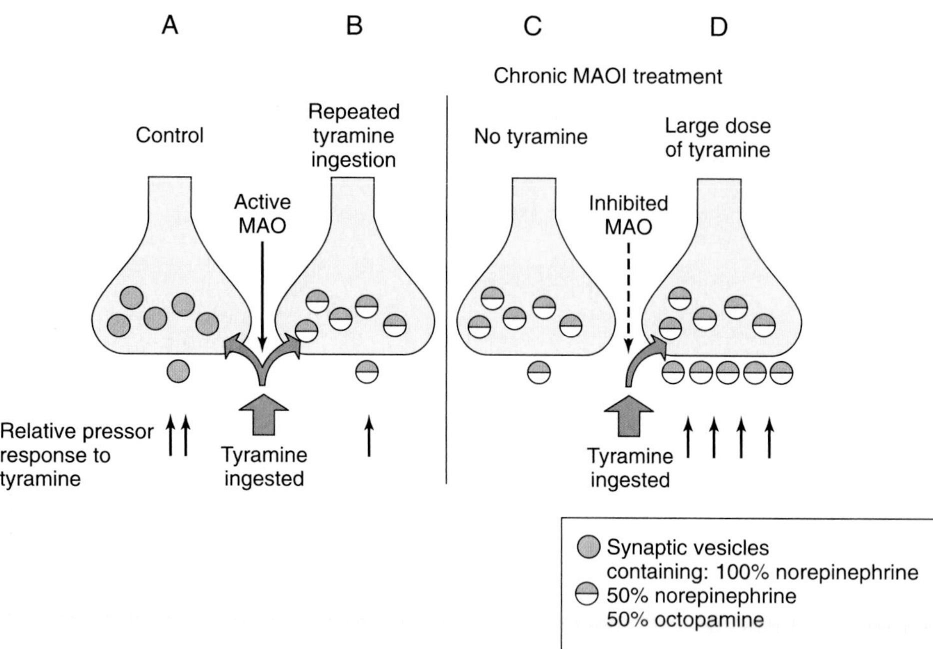

Figure 10-10 **A,** Acute response to ingestion of tyramine; **B,** tolerance to repeated ingestions of tyramine; **C,** long-term treatment with a monoamine oxidase inhibitor *(MAOI);* **D,** effects of tyramine after long-term MAOI pretreatment. The relative increase in blood pressure is denoted by the number of arrows.

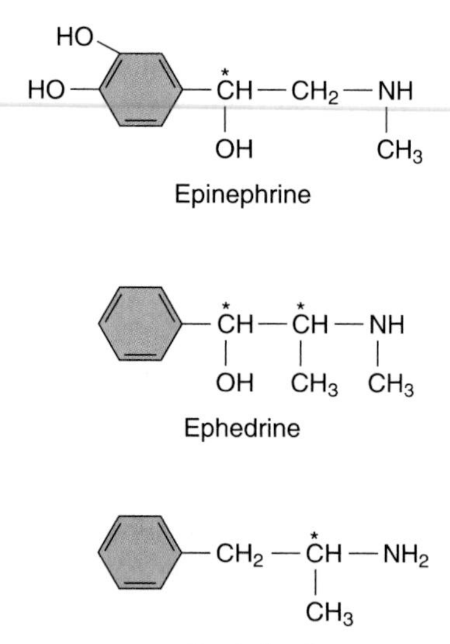

Figure 10-11 Structures of some indirectly acting sympathomimetics compared to epinephrine. Asterisk indicates asymmetrical carbon.

α-receptors and produces an irreversible blockade that cannot be overcome by addition of more agonist (Fig. 10-12).

Phenoxybenzamine and phentolamine have similar affinities for α_1- and α_2-receptors. They cause vasodilation by blocking sympathetic activation of blood vessels, an effect proportional to the degree of sympathetic tone. α-Adrenergic receptor blocking drugs cause only small decreases in recumbent blood pressure but can produce a sharp decrease during the compensatory vasoconstriction that occurs on standing because reflex sympathetic control of capacitance vessels is lost. This can result in orthostatic or postural hypotension accompanied by reflex tachycardia, although tolerance to this effect occurs with repeated use.

The effects of α-adrenergic receptor blockade on mean blood pressure and heart rate in response to NE and Epi are illustrated in Figure 10-13. The intravenous injection of NE and Epi produces a brief increase in blood pressure by activating α_1-receptors in blood vessels. A reflex decrease in sympathetic and increase in vagal tone to the heart occur (see Fig. 10-6), but reflex bradycardia is masked by direct activation of cardiac β_1-receptors. Because of such complex and opposing actions, the effects of these compounds on heart rate can vary. Blockade of α-receptors with phentolamine slightly lowers blood pressure but is accompanied by a reflex increase in heart rate. NE now has little effect on blood pressure and does not cause reflex bradycardia, whereas heart rate is increased by stimulation of cardiac β_1-receptors. When Epi is administered, the former pressor response is converted to a strong depressor response because vasodilatation resulting from β_2-receptor activation is unmasked. Epi now causes pronounced tachycardia by direct activation of cardiac β_1-receptors as well as a reflex tachycardia after the blood pressure decrease. Thus, when α-adrenoceptors are blocked, the actions of Epi resemble those of the pure β-agonist IP.

The tachycardia that occurs after administration of α-blockers is attributable in part to blockade of presynaptic α_2-receptors on sympathetic neurons (Fig. 10-14).

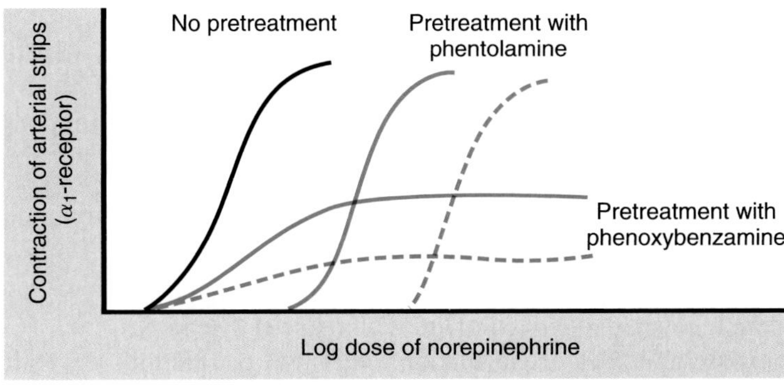

Figure 10-12 Comparison of the effects of a reversible (phentolamine) and an irreversible (phenoxybenzamine) inhibitor of α-adrenergic receptors. Changes in the force of contraction of arterial strips were recorded after addition of increasing concentrations of NE in the absence and in the presence of low and high concentrations of phentolamine and low and high concentrations of phenoxybenzamine. The broken lines are larger doses of the antagonist.

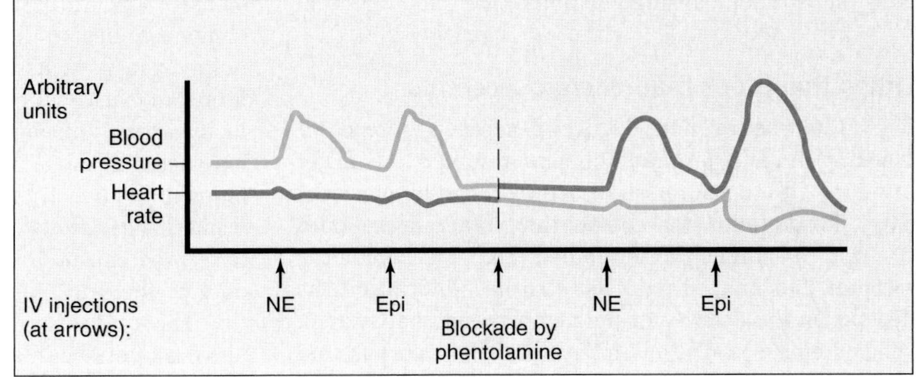

Figure 10-13 Effects of intravenous injections of NE and Epi on mean blood pressure and heart rate before and after blockade of α-adrenergic receptors by phentolamine.

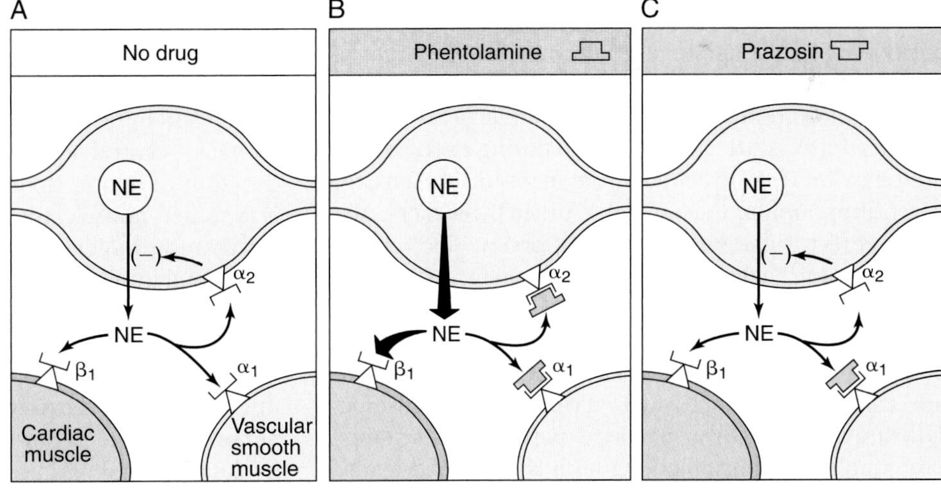

Figure 10-14 Comparison of the actions of phentolamine (α_1- and α_2-antagonist) and prazosin (α_1-antagonist) at noradrenergic neuroeffector junctions in cardiac muscle (β_1-adrenergic receptors) and vascular smooth muscle (α_1-adrenergic receptors).

Activation of these receptors inhibits NE release, and this feedback inhibition is disrupted when α_2-receptors are blocked. This has little consequence when the postsynaptic receptors are α_1 because the α-receptor antagonists mentioned earlier also block these receptors. In the heart, however, the postsynaptic receptors are β_1. Thus, effects of sympathetic activation are enhanced when α_2-receptors are blocked, increasing NE release and enhancing reflex tachycardia (see Fig. 10-14, *B*).

Prazosin, terazosin, doxazosin, tamsulosin, and alfuzosin are selective α_1-adrenergic receptor antagonists with similar pharmacological profiles but some differences in pharmacokinetics. By blocking α_1-receptors in arterioles and veins, these drugs reduce peripheral vascular resistance and lower blood pressure; accordingly, they are used in treating hypertension. Selective α_1-receptor antagonists cause less tachycardia than nonselective α-antagonists because the α_2-receptors, which reduce NE release, are not blocked by these drugs (see Fig. 10-14, *C*). α_1-Adrenergic receptor antagonists also relax smooth muscle in the prostate and bladder neck and, thereby, relieve urinary retention in benign prostatic hyperplasia. Tamsulosin, terazosin, and alfuzosin are commonly prescribed for this condition.

The major side effects of α-adrenergic receptor antagonists are related to a reduced sympathetic tone at α-receptors. These effects include orthostatic hypotension, tachycardia (less common with α_1-selective antagonists), inhibition of ejaculation, and nasal congestion. Other adverse effects are not related to their α-blocking properties; for example, phentolamine stimulates the GI tract, causing abdominal pain and diarrhea.

Drugs that block β-adrenergic receptors

The prototype of nonselective β-adrenergic receptor blocking drugs is propranolol. Newer compounds differ primarily in their duration of action and subtype selectivity. Propranolol is a competitive antagonist at both β_1- and β_2-adrenergic receptors. Like all adrenergic receptor blocking drugs, its pharmacological effects depend on the activity of the sympathoadrenal system. When impulse traffic in the sympathetic neurons and circulating concentrations of NE and Epi are high (e.g., during exercise), the effects of the drugs are more pronounced. The most profound effects of propranolol are on the cardiovascular system. Propranolol blocks the positive chronotropic and inotropic responses to β-adrenergic agonists and to sympathetic activation. It reduces the rate and contractility of the heart at rest, but these effects are more dramatic during exercise. The drug may precipitate acute failure in an uncompensated heart. Propranolol, but not some other β-blockers, also has a direct membrane-stabilizing action (local anesthetic action), which may contribute to its cardiac antiarrhythmic effect.

When administered acutely, propranolol does not greatly affect blood flow because vascular β-receptors are not tonically activated, although compensatory reflexes cause slightly increased peripheral resistance. Propranolol administered long term is an effective antihypertensive agent. How it lowers blood pressure is not completely understood, but it probably results from several actions, including reduced cardiac output, reduced release of renin from the juxtaglomerular apparatus, and possibly some actions in the CNS.

Propranolol also blocks the metabolic actions of β-adrenergic receptor agonists and activation of the sympathoadrenal system. It inhibits increases in plasma free fatty acids and glucose from lipolysis in fat and glycogenolysis in liver, heart, and skeletal muscle. This can pose a problem for diabetics by augmenting insulin-induced hypoglycemia. However, β_1-selective blockers are less likely to augment insulin-induced hypoglycemia. β-Adrenergic receptor–blocking drugs also reduce the premonitory tachycardia associated with insulin-induced hypoglycemia, so diabetic patients taking them must learn to recognize sweating (induced by activation of cholinergic sympathetic neurons) as a symptom of low blood glucose.

Propranolol causes few serious side effects in healthy people but can do so in patients suffering from various diseases; heart failure is the main threat. Propranolol is usually contraindicated in patients with sinus bradycardia, partial heart block, or compensated congestive heart failure. Sudden withdrawal of propranolol from patients who have received this drug long term can cause "withdrawal symptoms," such as angina, tachycardia, and dysrhythmias. Rebound hypertension may occur in such patients taking propranolol to control blood pressure. These withdrawal symptoms probably result from the development of β-receptor supersensitivity and can be minimized by gradually reducing the dose of the drug.

The ability of propranolol to increase airway resistance is of little clinical importance in normal people but can be very hazardous in patients with obstructive pulmonary disease or asthma. β_1-selective antagonists (see later discussion) should be used in these patients, although even these drugs should be used with caution because they are not completely inactive at β_2-receptors.

Nadolol is a nonselective β-receptor blocking drug that is less lipid soluble than propranolol and less likely to cause central effects. It has a significantly longer duration of action than most other β-blockers. Timolol is another nonselective β-blocker administered orally for treating hypertension and angina pectoris or as an ophthalmic preparation for treating glaucoma.

Carteolol, pindolol, and penbutolol are nonselective β-adrenergic receptor–blocking drugs that have modest intrinsic sympathomimetic properties. These drugs cause less slowing of resting heart rate and fewer abnormalities of serum lipid concentrations than other β-blockers, and it has been suggested that they also produce less upregulation of β-receptors. These drugs generally cause less severe withdrawal symptoms and are used to treat hypertension.

Labetalol and carvedilol are competitive antagonists of α_1-, β_1-, and β_2-adrenergic receptors. Consequently, they have hemodynamic effects similar to those of a combination of propranolol (β_1- and β_2-receptor blockade) and prazosin (α_1-receptor blockade). Unfortunately, side effects are also similar to those of both drugs (e.g., orthostatic hypotension, nasal congestion, bronchospasm). However, these drugs are potent antihypertensive agents.

At low doses, acebutolol, atenolol, metoprolol, and esmolol are more selective in blocking β_1-receptors on cardiac muscle than in blocking β_2-receptors on bronchiolar smooth muscle. They are less likely than nonselective β-blockers to increase bronchoconstriction in patients with asthma. These β_1-blockers are useful in treating hypertension and angina pectoris. Esmolol is a β_1-selective antagonist that is rapidly metabolized by esterases in red blood cells and has a very short half-life. It is used for the emergency treatment of sinus tachycardia and atrial flutter or fibrillation.

Drugs that interfere with sympathetic neuronal function

Drugs that disrupt the synthesis, storage, or release of NE or act in the brain to reduce sympathetic neuronal activity have been used primarily in treatment of hypertension; however, they are no longer widely used. Guanethidine is the prototype of this class of drugs, which impairs release of NE from postsynaptic sympathetic neurons. Related drugs include guanadrel and bretylium, as well as reserpine, which depletes sympathetic neurons of stored NE. These drugs reduce sympathetic tone in a relatively nonspecific manner, causing substantial side effects, including reduced blood pressure, heart rate, and cardiac output and increased GI motility and diarrhea. Because of their side effects and the availability of better drugs, these drugs are no longer widely used.

Drugs that reduce central sympathetic outflow

The activity of peripheral sympathetic neurons is regulated in a complex manner by neuronal systems located in the lower brainstem. These central neurons, in turn, are regulated in part by α_2-adrenergic receptors. Drugs, such as clonidine, that activate these receptors reduce the outflow of impulse traffic in peripheral sympathetic neurons without interfering with baroreceptor reflex control. Accordingly, these drugs lower blood pressure in patients with moderate to severe hypertension and produce less orthostatic hypotension than drugs acting in the periphery.

Clonidine is the prototype α_2-adrenergic receptor agonist. Clonidine is lipid soluble and penetrates the blood-brain barrier to activate α_2-receptors in the medulla, resulting in diminished sympathetic outflow. Clonidine lowers blood pressure by reducing total peripheral resistance, heart rate, and cardiac output. It does not interfere with baroreceptor reflexes and does not produce noticeable orthostatic hypotension. However, side effects of clonidine may include dry mouth, sedation, dizziness, nightmares, anxiety, and mental depression. Various signs and symptoms related to sympathetic nervous system overactivity (hypertension, tachycardia, sweating) may occur after withdrawal of long-term clonidine therapy; thus, the dose of clonidine should be reduced gradually. Clonidine is also used to ameliorate signs and symptoms associated with increased activity of the sympathetic nervous system that accompany withdrawal from long-term opioid use.

Guanabenz and guanfacine are other α_2-receptor agonists that act centrally to inhibit sympathetic tone with a relative sparing of cardiovascular reflexes. Guanfacine is longer acting, less likely to reduce cardiac output, and less sedating than clonidine.

Methyldopa is an analog of the catecholamine precursor l-DOPA that is transported into noradrenergic neurons, where it is converted to α-methyl-NE (Fig. 10-15). α-Methyl-NE partially displaces NE in synaptic vesicles, where it is released in place of NE. This compound selectively activates α_2-receptors to cause hypotensive actions, which appear to be attributable to α-methyl-NE in the brain not in the periphery.

Drugs that inhibit catecholamine synthesis

Metyrosine (α-methyltyrosine) inhibits tyrosine hydroxylase in the brain, periphery, and adrenal medulla, thereby reducing tissue stores of DA, NE, and Epi. Metyrosine is used in the management of patients with pheochromocytoma not amenable to surgery. Its most prevalent side effect is sedation.

Carbidopa, a hydrazine derivative of methyldopa, inhibits aromatic l-amino acid decarboxylase. Unlike methyldopa, carbidopa does not penetrate the blood-brain barrier and therefore has no effect in the CNS. Because aromatic l-amino acid decarboxylase is ubiquitous, is present in excess, and does not control the rate-limiting step in catecholamine synthesis, clinical doses of carbidopa have no appreciable effect on the endogenous synthesis of NE in sympathetic neurons. They do, however, reduce the conversion of exogenously administered l-DOPA to DA outside the brain, rendering carbidopa useful for the adjunctive treatment of Parkinson's disease (see Chapter 21).

Side effects, clinical problems, and toxicity

Major clinical problems are summarized in the Clinical Problems box.

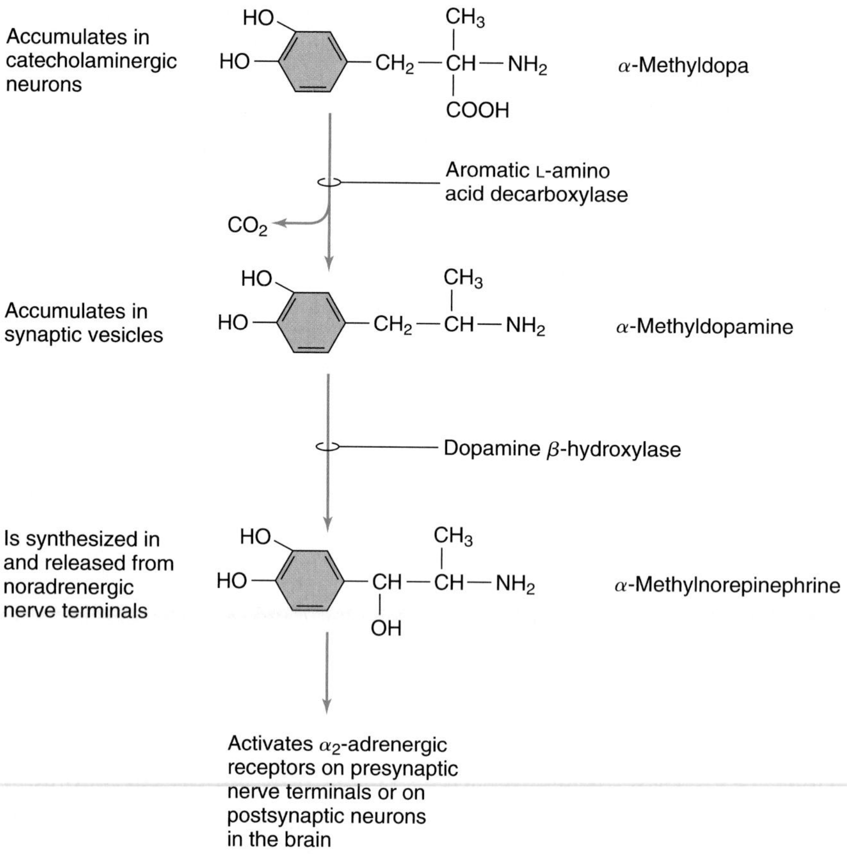

Figure 10-15 Metabolism of α-methyldopa in central noradrenergic nerve terminals.

CLINICAL PROBLEMS

Drugs that interfere with sympathetic nervous system neuronal function

Block NE Release and Storage

- Orthostatic hypotension
- Nasal congestion
- Impaired ejaculation
- Increased GI activity

Decreased Central Sympathetic Outflow

- Sedation
- Endocrine problems
- Sodium and water retention
- Rebound hypertension

Drugs that block adrenergic receptors

α-Adrenergic Receptor Blockers

- Orthostatic hypotension
- Tachycardia
- Nasal congestion
- Impairment of ejaculation
- Sodium and water retention

β-Adrenergic Receptor Blockers

- Heart failure in patients with cardiac disease
- Increased airway resistance
- Fatigue and depression
- Rebound hypertension
- Augmented hypoglycemia

New horizons

The development of selective agonists and antagonists for α_1, α_2, β_1, and β_2 subtypes of adrenergic receptors has led to compounds with fewer and less severe side effects than those used previously. We now know that there are several additional adrenergic receptor subtypes ($\alpha_{1A,B,D}$; $\alpha_{2A,B,C}$; $\beta_{1,2,3}$), and much effort is being expended into developing drugs with specific agonist or antagonist effects at these receptors and determining whether they have therapeutic potential. For example, β_3-receptors are located on brown and, possibly, white adipose cells, where activation promotes fat breakdown and heat generation. It has been suggested that β_3-receptor agonists may be useful in treating obesity. In a similar manner, development of subtype-selective α_1-receptor blockers may be helpful in treating benign prostatic hypertrophy while reducing the risks of orthostatic hypotension, whereas subtype-selective α_2-agonists may be useful centrally acting antihypertensives with fewer side effects.

TRADE NAMES

In addition to generic and fixed-combination preparations, the following trade-named materials are some of the important compounds available in the United States.

Sympathomimetics

Directly acting agonists
- Dopamine (Intropin, Dopastat)
- Epinephrine* (Medihaler, Vaponefrin, EpiPen)
- Isoproterenol† (Isuprel)
- Norepinephrine‡ (Levofed)

α_1-Selective agonists
- Methoxamine (Vasoxyl)
- Phenylephrine (Neo-synephrine)

β_1-Selective agonists
- Dobutamine (Dobutrex)

β_2-Selective agonists
- Albuterol§ (Proventil)
- Bitolterol (Tornalate)
- Metaproterenol (Metaprel, Alupent)
- Ritodrine (Yutopar)
- Salmeterol (Serevent)
- Terbutaline (Brethine)

Nonselective indirectly acting agonists
- D-Amphetamine (Dexedrine)

Sympatholytics

α-Blockers, nonselective
- Phentolamine (Regitine)

α_1-Selective blockers
- Doxazosin (Cardura)
- Prazosin (Minipress)
- Tamsulosin (Flomax)
- Terazosin (Hytrin)

β-Blockers, nonselective
- Carteolol (Cartrol)
- Nadolol (Corgard)
- Pindolol (Visken)
- Propranolol (Inderal)
- Timolol (Blocadren)

β_1-Selective blockers
- Atenolol (Tenormin)
- Betaxolol (Kerlone)
- Esmolol (Brevibloc)
- Metoprolol (Lopressor)

Combined α_1- and β-blockers
- Carvedilol (Coreg)
- Labetalol (Normodyne)

Reduce central sympathetic outflow
- Clonidine (Catapres)
- Guanabenz (Wytensin)
- Guanfacine (Tenex)

*In the UK the drug name is adrenaline.
†In the UK the drug name is isoprenaline.
‡In the UK the drug name is noradrenaline.
§In the UK and Japan the drug name is salbutamol.

FURTHER READING

Blease K, Lewis A, Raymon HK. Emerging treatments for asthma. *Expert Opin Emerg Drugs* 2003; 8:71-81.

Drugs for hypertension. *Med Lett Drugs Ther* 2003; 43:17-22.

Self-assessment questions

1. Metoprolol would be most effective in blocking the ability of Epi to:

a. Reduce secretion of insulin from the pancreas.
b. Increase release of renin from juxtaglomerular apparatus.
c. Increase secretion of glucagon from the pancreas.
d. Produce mydriasis (dilatation of pupil).
e. Increase secretion of saliva.

2. Which of the following drugs is most likely to produce orthostatic hypotension?

a. Propranolol
b. Dobutamine
c. Labetalol
d. Nadolol
e. Methoxamine

3. Which of the following drugs would be most likely to increase airway resistance in a patient with pulmonary obstructive disease?

a. Isoproterenol
b. Atenolol
c. Bitolterol
d. Terbutaline
e. Nadolol

4. Systemic administration of which of the following drugs would most likely cause bradycardia?

a. Dopamine
b. Phentolamine
c. Phenylephrine
d. Prazosin
e. Metaproterenol

5. Terbutaline would be expected to cause all of the following effects *except:*

a. Mydriasis.
b. Reduced pulmonary airway resistance.
c. Tachycardia.
d. Hyperglycemia.
e. Increased blood flow in skeletal muscle.

6. The cardiovascular effects of Epi in a person treated with phentolamine will most closely resemble the responses after the administration of:

a. Phenylephrine.
b. Terbutaline.
c. Isoproterenol.
d. NE.
e. Methoxamine.

PART III

Drugs acting on the cardiovascular system

DYSFUNCTION OF THE CARDIOVASCULAR system is the major cause of death in people living in industrialized nations. In the United States about 50% of deaths are attributed to cardiovascular problems.

Included within functions of the cardiovascular system are:

- Cardiac pumping ability, including the rhythmic nature of the electrical signals, force of contraction, and magnitude of the discharge pressure.
- Integrity of the vasculature, including presence of flow-restricting deposits in the arterial lumen, muscular tone and structural integrity of vessel walls, and pressure drops required to pump blood through vascular beds at rates needed to provide nutrients and remove wastes.
- Blood volume and composition, including water, electrolyte and iron balances, lipid composition, and capabilities for clot formation and lysis.

Many of these functions can be modified therapeutically or prophylactically with drugs. This section describes such drugs, how they act at the molecular level, and their clinical applications.

In considering drugs used to modify the pumping ability of the heart, it is necessary to understand the physiological and biochemical processes that govern cardiac pacing, the force of cardiac and smooth muscle contraction, and blood pressure. The nervous system plays such a large role in the control of blood pressure that the physiology (see Chapter 11) and pharmacology (see Chapter 12) of blood pressure control are discussed in separate chapters. The physiology and pharmacology of cardiac pacing (see Chapter 14) and cardiac contractile force (see Chapter 15) are also described. Another topic that relates to the heart is drugs that relax smooth muscle and provide relief in angina pectoris (see Chapter 16).

Pharmacological intervention to ensure integrity of the vasculature is discussed in Chapter 18 in relation to the reduction of deposits that narrow the arterial lumen and cause atherosclerosis. Pharmacological intervention is also considered, to a lesser extent, in Chapter 17, where the prostaglandins are discussed.

Control of the water volume and electrolyte content of the blood, primarily through renal mechanisms, is discussed in Chapter 13. The section closes with a discussion of the pharmacological approaches for treatment of blood disorders, including clotting, dissolution of clot emboli (especially in conjunction with post-myocardial infarction), and anemia (see Chapter 19).

CHAPTER 11

Regulation of blood pressure by the autonomic nervous system

Frank J. Gordon

Arterial blood pressure is the product of cardiac output and total peripheral resistance to blood flow through the vascular system. Cardiac output is determined by the rate and efficiency of the pumping of the heart. Vascular resistance increases as the viscosity of the blood and the length of blood vessels increases. Resistance to blood flow increases as blood vessel luminal diameter (caliber) decreases, particularly in precapillary arterioles, which represent the major structural determinant of vascular resistance. Cardiac performance and vascular caliber are controlled by several intrinsic regulatory mechanisms. Heart rate is determined by pacemaker cells in the sinoatrial node, and cardiac pumping efficiency is subject to several types of homeostatic regulation. Local regulation of the caliber of most resistance-producing blood vessels is influenced by the intrinsic contractile state of vascular smooth muscle, balanced by the production of vasodilator and vasoconstrictor substances originating from the endothelial cell monolayer lining the vessel lumen.

Superimposed on these control processes intrinsic to the heart and blood vessels are extrinsic factors that affect cardiovascular function. These include the metabolic status of the tissues in which blood vessels are embedded and locally produced and blood-borne vasoactive chemicals (autocrine/paracrine/endocrine regulation). However, overall coordination and integration of organismal cardiovascular function is accomplished primarily by the autonomic nervous system (ANS). Through its sympathetic and parasympathetic limbs, the ANS system has powerful effects on both cardiac performance and blood vessel caliber.

Drugs used to treat hypertension lower blood pressure. Some drugs reduce blood pressure by acting directly on the ANS or the receptors for its neurotransmitters. Because the ANS produces moment-to-moment regulatory adjustments in cardiovascular function, interference with this regulation by antihypertensive drugs can produce undesirable side effects. Other antihypertensive drugs target mechanisms controlling vascular and/or cardiac contractility, endocrine mechanisms, or mechanisms affecting renal conservation of salt and water. When blood pressure is reduced by these drugs, baroreflex-related changes in ANS function are frequently engaged and may counteract the action of many antihypertensive drugs. To understand and appreciate how antihypertensive drugs reduce blood pressure, it is important to review the function of the ANS. Some key features of autonomic control of blood pressure are described in this chapter to facilitate understanding the pharmacology and physiological effects of drugs used to treat hypertension (see Chapter 12).

Abbreviation

ANS	autonomic nervous system

Overview of autonomic cardiovascular regulation

The sympathetic and parasympathetic nerves innervating cardiovascular end organs are tonically active. For this reason, autonomic effects can be modulated by either increasing or decreasing the firing of these nerves. Effects of autonomic nerve activity on the mechanisms that control blood pressure are summarized in Figure 11-1. Parasympathetic effects are mediated by acetylcholine released from postganglionic parasympathetic nerve endings (see Chapter 9). Because of high cholinesterase activity in tissue and blood, no acetylcholine escapes from parasympathetic neuroeffector junctions. In contrast, degradation and/or reuptake of norepinephrine is incomplete. Norepinephrine released from postganglionic sympathetic nerve endings, as well as epinephrine and norepinephrine released into the blood from the adrenal medulla, influence cardiovascular function as circulating neurohormones (see Chapter 10).

Cardiac performance is influenced by both parasympathetic (vagus) and sympathetic effects on the heart. Heart rate is decreased by parasympathetic activity and increased by sympathetic activity at the sinoatrial node, but the parasympathetic effect is usually dominant. Contractile force of the ventricles is little influenced by parasympathetic activity but can be greatly increased by sympathetic activity, including epinephrine and norepinephrine released into the circulation from the adrenal medulla. Increased sympathetic activity reduces vascular caliber by contracting vascular smooth muscle. Although there are parasympathetic influences on a few vascular beds, their contribution to overall vascular resistance is insignificant. Constriction of veins in response to sympathetic activity reduces venous capacitance, thereby increasing venous return to the heart, which augments atrial and ventricular filling, resulting in increased cardiac output. Sympathetically-mediated constriction of arterioles can reduce cardiac output by increasing the resistance against which the heart must pump blood. In addition, elevated sympathetic activity to the kidney increases renin release and subsequent angiotensin II formation, as well as causing sodium and water retention. All of these effects act in concert to elevate arterial blood pressure. Conversely, a reduction of sympathetic activity reduces blood pressure by removing the sympathetic stimulus. The receptors and signaling pathways involved are discussed in Chapter 8.

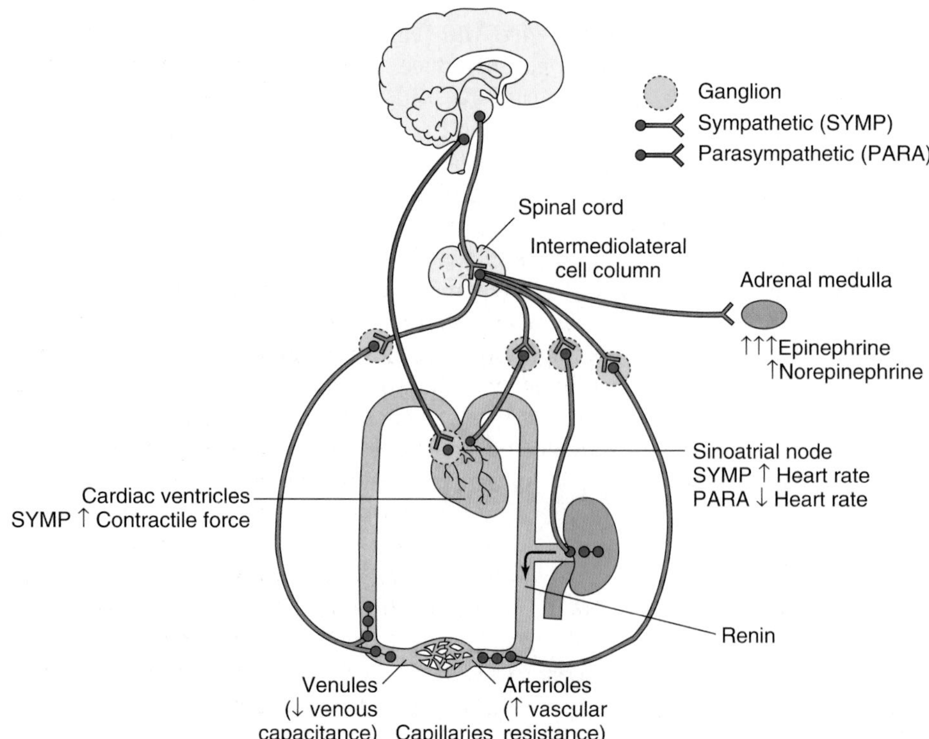

Figure 11-1 Effects of the autonomic nervous system on blood pressure control. Vascular resistance is affected almost exclusively by the sympathetic nervous system, whereas cardiac output is regulated by both sympathetic and parasympathetic influences.

Control of autonomic nerve activity

The organization of autonomic cardiovascular control systems within the central nervous system is summarized in Figure 11-2. The final common (preganglionic) output neurons for cardiovascular control by the parasympathetic nervous system are located principally in the nucleus ambiguus of the brainstem. The preganglionic neurons of the sympathetic nervous system are located in the intermediolateral columns of the thoracolumbar spinal cord. Antecedent to these final output neurons, much of the integration of neural signals contributing to autonomic regulation of cardiovascular function occurs at other sites in the brainstem. These neurons, in turn, receive input from all levels of the central nervous system, some of the more important of which are diagrammed in Figure 11-2.

Origin and regulation of autonomic activity

One of the principal roles of the ANS is to provide adaptive regulation and coordination of blood pressure and flow to various organs of the body in the face of an ever changing internal environment. This is accomplished by neural circuits intrinsic to the central nervous system and as a response to mechanical and humoral signals originating in the periphery. Integration of these signals by the central nervous system produces patterns of autonomic activity that ensure adequate organ perfusion appropriate to such diverse demands as changes in posture, hemorrhage, digestion, and exercise.

Parasympathetic preganglionic neurons that project to the heart via the vagus nerves have low levels of spontaneous firing, and their discharge rate is driven mostly by inputs from various afferents, particularly arterial baroreceptors. Inputs to spinal sympathetic preganglionic neurons originate in the brainstem, pons, and hypothalamus and can be either excitatory or inhibitory. However, the activity of spinal sympathetic

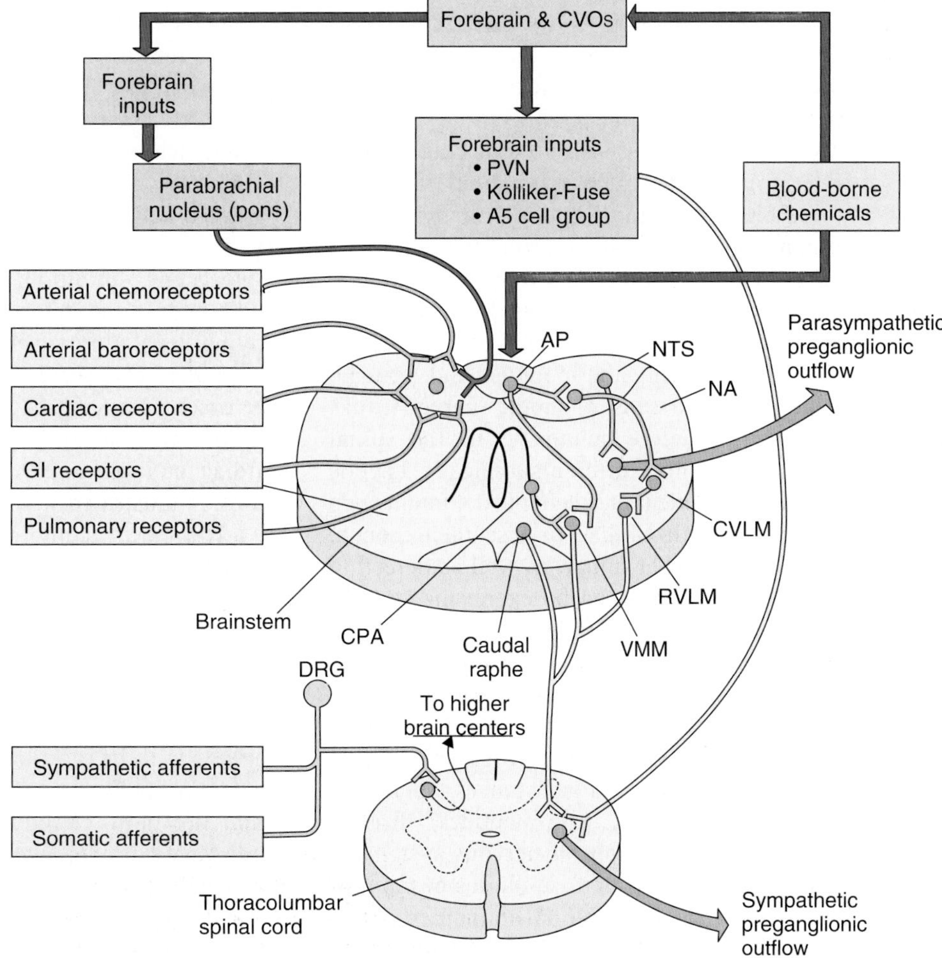

Figure 11-2 Organization of autonomic cardiovascular control systems. Major inputs are in boxes. Many reciprocal connections are not illustrated. *AP,* Area postrema; *CPA,* caudal pressor area; *CVLM,* caudal ventrolateral medulla; *CVO,* circumventricular organs; *DRG,* dorsal root ganglia; *NA,* nucleus ambiguus; *PVN,* paraventricular nucleus; *RVLM,* rostral ventrolateral medulla; *VMM,* ventromedial medulla.

preganglionic neurons regulating cardiovascular function is driven primarily by excitatory neurons located in the rostral ventrolateral medulla.

In addition to intrinsic central nervous system control, the efferent activity of autonomic nerves is powerfully regulated by neural signals arising from the periphery. Activation of visceral sensory afferents projecting to the brain via the vagus nerves generally reduces sympathetic activity and increases parasympathetic activity. These afferents include stretch receptors located in the cardiovascular system, which provide information about arterial pressure (arterial baroreceptors) and cardiac filling (cardiac baroreceptors), as well as stretch receptors and chemosensory receptors in the lungs, which provide information about respiratory mechanics and lung irritants, respectively. Afferents with chemosensory terminals located in the carotid sinus encode blood gas oxygen concentration, send projections to the brain via the glossopharyngeal nerve, and, when activated by hypoxia, hypercapnia, or acidic pH, increase efferent sympathetic nerve activity. All of these afferents make their first central synapse within the nucleus of the tractus solitarius located in the dorsomedial brainstem. Vagal afferents producing sympathoinhibition project primarily to the lateral aspects of the solitary tract nucleus, whereas glossopharyngeal afferents that produce sympathoexcitation project to more medial aspects of this nucleus.

Other visceral mechanosensitive and chemosensitive nerve terminals are located throughout the body. Some of these bipolar neurons, with cell bodies in the dorsal root ganglia, may initially co-mingle their axons within various sympathetic nerve trunks ("sympathetic afferents") before synapsing on cells located in the dorsal horns of the spinal cord. Other sensory afferents do not travel with the sympathetic nerves and, instead, associate with various sensory-motor nerve trunks ("somatic afferents") before synapsing in the spinal dorsal horns. All of these afferents typically encode noxious or painful chemical or mechanical stimuli, such as those associated with cardiac or visceral ischemia, visceral organ distension or injury, as well as detecting the metabolic products produced by exercising skeletal muscle. Activation of these afferents typically produces sympathoexcitation.

In addition to neural signals from the periphery, the brain also detects chemical signals (including drugs, such as digitalis) that circulate in the blood. A wide variety of circulating humoral substances, including catecholamines, indolamines, and peptides, directly contact neurons within the central nervous system by diffusing through the fenestrated capillaries of circumventricular organs that lack a blood-brain barrier (see Fig. 11-2). Activation of circumventricular organ neurons produces integrated autonomic, endocrine, and behavioral responses that can regulate salt and water balance and nutrient homeostasis, in addition to cardiovascular function. The most important of the circumventricular organs for central autonomic control are the area postrema, subfornical organ, and organum vasculosum of the lamina terminalis.

Baroreceptor reflex

The most rapidly acting autonomic control system for regulating blood pressure is the baroreceptor reflex. The principal role of this reflex is to ensure adequate organ perfusion, particularly to the brain and heart, and to promote return of blood to the heart in the face of conditions that lower arterial blood pressure. These might include gravitational pooling of blood, when assuming an upright posture, and instances where blood volume is lost, such as during severe dehydration or hemorrhage. The baroreceptor reflex is also activated when drugs are used to lower blood pressure in patients with cardiovascular disease, and this reflex may profoundly affect both the therapeutic effects and potential side effects that accompany drug therapy.

Minute-to-minute control of arterial blood pressure is achieved when small pressure changes are linked to reflex alterations in autonomic nerve activity. Sensory nerve endings embedded in the wall of the carotid sinus and aortic arch (baroreceptors) are activated by wall stretch when arterial pressure increases. This leads within a few seconds to an increase in vagal (parasympathetic) activity and a reduction in sympathetic activity. Parasympathetic activation slows heart rate, and sympathetic inhibition results in passive vasodilation, thus tending to return arterial pressure toward the original level. Conversely, a decrease in arterial pressure is rapidly countered by increased sympathetic and decreased parasympathetic activity. This results in vasoconstriction and an elevated cardiac rate and force of cardiac contraction. Organization of the baroreceptor reflex is illustrated in Figure 11-3.

The baroreceptor reflex is primarily important in short-term control of blood pressure. When changes in blood pressure persist beyond a few minutes, reflex autonomic responses diminish. This is called baroreflex adaptation and involves both peripheral and central nervous system components. Varying degrees of baroreflex impairment occur with normal aging and in patients with heart failure or hypertension. This impairment may help to explain why some antihypertensive drugs are more effective in hypertensive than in normotensive patients, because lowering of blood pressure by antihypertensive drugs may be less effectively counteracted by baroreflex-mediated sympathetic vasoconstriction in these individuals.

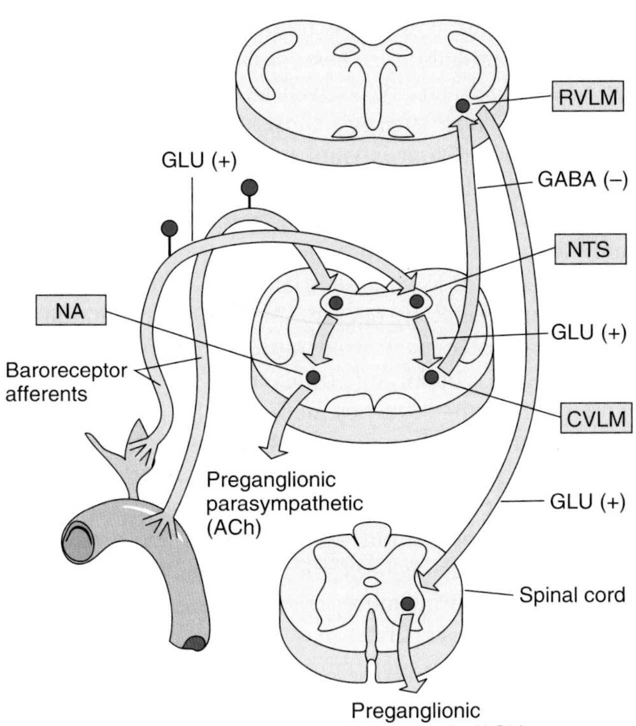

Blood pressure	NORMAL	INCREASED	DECREASED
Baroreceptor afferent activity	NORMAL	↑	↓
Sympathetic activity	NORMAL	↓	↑
Parasympathetic activity	NORMAL	↑	↓

Figure 11-3 Brainstem organization of the baroreceptor reflex and associated neurotransmitters. Primary pathways only are shown. Other afferents and interneurons are omitted. *ACh,* Acetylcholine; *CVLM,* caudal ventrolateral medulla; *GABA,* γ-aminobutyric acid: *GLU,* l-glutamate; *NA,* nucleus ambiguus; *NTS,* nucleus of the solitary tract; *RVLM,* rostral ventrolateral medulla; +, excitatory pathway; –, inhibitory pathway.

The influence of baroreceptors on sympathetic nerve activity can vary greatly in different vascular beds. Some beds, such as the cutaneous vasculature, are largely independent of arterial baroreceptor influence, and contribute little to total peripheral vascular resistance. In contrast, the baroreceptor reflex predominates in controlling sympathetic regulation of vascular caliber in many organs that receive a significant fraction of the cardiac output, such as skeletal muscle and kidney. For this reason, baroreflex regulation of sympathetic vasoconstriction plays an important role in determining total peripheral resistance. In fact, except under some special circumstances (exercise, sleep, and certain behavioral

Table 11-1 Prejunctional modulators of sympathetic neurotransmitter release

Chemical	Source	Receptor	Mechanism	Effect
Norepinephrine	SNT	α_2	↓Ca^{2+}	↓
Neuropeptide Y	SNT	Y_2	↓Ca^{2+}	↓
ATP	SNT	P_3, P_{2x}	↓Ca^{2+}	↓
Epinephrine	Blood	β_2	↑cAMP	↑
Angiotensin II	Blood/PJT	AT_1	↑PLC	↑
Prostanoids	PJT	EP3	↓Ca^{2+}	↓
Adenosine	PJT	P_1	↓Ca^{2+}	↓
Opioids	Blood	μ, κ, δ	↓Ca^{2+}	↓
Acetylcholine	Nerve	M_2	↑cGMP	↓
Dopamine	SNT	D_2	↑K^+	↓
Atrial natriuretic peptide	Blood	?	↑cGMP	↓
Nitric oxide	EC	guanylate cyclase	↑cGMP	↓

cAMP, Cyclic adenosine monophosphate; *cGMP,* cyclic guanosine monophosphate; *EC,* endothelial cell; *PJT,* postjunctional tissue; *PLC,* phospholipase C; *SNT,* sympathetic nerve terminal.

states), baroreceptors are able to override all other inputs affecting autonomic regulation of arterial blood pressure. This may reflect the importance of maintaining a stable systemic blood pressure to ensure adequate organ perfusion under diverse environmental conditions.

Control of neurotransmitter concentrations at the neuroeffector junction

Neurotransmission at parasympathetic and sympathetic neuroeffector junctions is reviewed in Chapters 9 and 10. The electrical activity of postganglionic nerves closely follows the activity of preganglionic neurons. Under physiological conditions, the amount of transmitter that is released, coincident with depolarization of the nerve terminal, is influenced by various chemicals, most of which bind to receptors located on the nerve terminal itself (Table 11-1 and Fig. 11-4). In addition to prejunctional regulation of release, the concentration of neurotransmitter at neuroeffector junctions can be influenced by alterations in transmitter synthesis, storage within the nerve terminal, and removal from the neuroeffector junction by diffusion, metabolism, and reuptake. These latter mechanisms are important targets for therapeutically active drugs. Because of the importance of the sympathetic nervous system in controlling

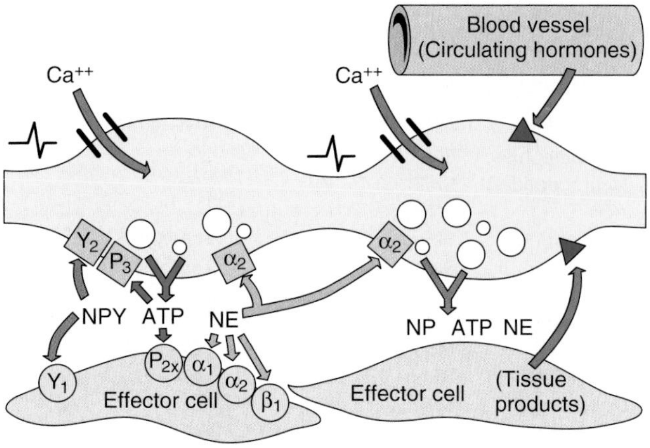

Figure 11-4 Prejunctional regulation at the sympathetic neuroeffector junction. The left varicosity illustrates autoinhibition of neurotransmitter release, including possible "lateral" inhibition (i.e., transmitter from one varicosity inhibiting release from an adjacent varicosity). The right varicosity illustrates prejunctional regulation of transmitter release by tissue and blood-borne chemicals. See Table 11-1 for a list of involved substances. Postjunctional receptors are shown as circles, ○; prejunctional inhibitory autoreceptors are shown as squares, □; prejunctional heteroreceptors are shown as triangles, △.

blood pressure, the prejunctional regulation of norepinephrine secretion is summarized.

Sympathetic neuroeffector junctions

Axons of postganglionic sympathetic neurons branch repeatedly near and within their effector tissues. The smallest branches arborize extensively and exhibit numerous varicosities containing the transmitter norepinephrine. Neuropeptide Y and adenosine triphosphate are co-released with norepinephrine at some sympathetic neuroeffector junctions and exert some cardiovascular actions through specific postjunctional receptors.

Depolarization-induced Ca^{2+} influx into the varicosities is the main stimulus for exocytotic release of neurotransmitters. It is likely that the entire contents of a secretory vesicle are released in response to depolarization. Receptors in nerve terminal membranes can enhance or inhibit norepinephrine secretion when activated by endogenous chemicals. Such prejunctional receptors are called **autoreceptors,** if they are activated by the released transmitter itself and **heteroreceptors,** if activated by other transmitters or hormones. Activation of prejunctional receptors does not affect nerve firing rate or the amount of transmitter released by individual vesicles. Instead, activation of prejunctional receptors appears to modulate the probability that individual vesicles will discharge their contents by exocytosis congruent with depolarization of the nerve terminal. Several signals contribute to modulation of vesicular exocytotic probability. These include altered Ca^{2+}, Na^+, or K^+ channel activity, as well as various second messenger systems, such as those for cyclic adenosine monophosphate and inositol trisphosphate. Figure 11-4 illustrates some of these mechanisms. The probable sources and mechanisms of action for some of these modulators are listed in Table 11-1.

Prejunctional regulation allows for the fine-tuning of neurotransmitter release. Activation of inhibitory autoreceptors by neurotransmitters may function as a physiological brake on transmitter secretion during periods of high-frequency nerve discharge, thus limiting postjunctional responses. Agonists at heteroreceptors facilitating transmitter release (e.g., angiotensin II) amplify the effects of sympathetic nerve depolarization. In contrast, activation of inhibitory heteroreceptors (e.g., adenosine) reduces the probability of vesicular exocytosis and transmitter release. Thus, similar rates of sympathetic nerve firing may produce different effects in different tissues, depending on the local mechanisms regulating the release of neurotransmitter from nerve varicosities.

Autonomic nervous system in hypertension

One of the causes of hypertension is a relative increase in the balance between sympathetic and parasympathetic control over the heart and blood vessels. Increased sympathetic effects can be produced by changes in neural firing rate, catecholamine concentration at the neuroeffector junction, postjunctional receptors, or signal transduction pathways. Although there is support for each of these mechanisms, the first two are probably most important. It is clear that control of sympathetic nerve activity and neurotransmitter concentration at the neuroeffector junction is extremely complex. Some factors that have been postulated to play a causative role in hypertension are listed in Box 11-1. However, regardless of the ultimate cause of sympathetic overactivity in hypertensive patients, drugs that inhibit sympathetically-mediated cardiovascular effects are useful for treating hypertension. In addition, lowering blood pressure in hypertensive patients by drugs acting independently of the ANS engages the baroreceptor reflex, resulting in increased sympathetic activity and decreased parasympathetic activity to the cardiovascular system (see Table 11-1). This may diminish the action of some antihypertensive drugs as well as produce side effects related to sympathetic overactivity,

Box 11-1 Some factors proposed to cause increased sympathetic nervous system activation in hypertension

Elevated sympathetic discharge

Physiological dysfunction

Sleep apnea
Stress
Obesity
Increased central sympathetic outflow
Impaired baroreceptor reflexes

Humoral

Increased plasma insulin
Increased plasma leptin
Increased plasma or tissue angiotensin II
Increased extracellular sodium

Enhanced norepinephrine release

Increased angiotensin II facilitation
Increased β_2-adrenergic receptor facilitation
Decreased neuropeptide Y inhibition

such as palpitations and tachycardia, which often necessitates concomitant administration of a sympathetic antagonist drug to reduce or eliminate these side effects (see Chapter 12).

FURTHER READING

Pang CC. Autonomic control of the venous system in health and disease: effects of drugs. *Pharmacol Ther* 2001; 90:179-230.

Robertson D, Biaggioni I, Burnstock G, Low PA. Primer on the autonomic nervous system. New York, 2004, Elsevier.

Sved AF, Ito S, Sved JC. Brainstem mechanisms of hypertension: role of the rostral ventrolateral medulla. *Curr Hypertens Rep* 2003; 5:262-268.

Self-assessment questions

1. Increased activity of the sympathetic nervous system:

a. Increases heart rate.
b. Increases the force of cardiac contraction.
c. Decreases arteriolar caliber.
d. Increases venous return to the heart.
e. Produces all of the above effects.

2. Sympathetic activity to which of the following vascular beds is influenced the least by arterial baroreflexes?

a. Muscle
b. Skin
c. Kidney
d. Heart
e. Splanchnic viscera

3. Exocytotic release of norepinephrine from postganglionic sympathetic nerve terminals can be promoted or increased by all of the following *except* increased:

a. Intracellular Ca^{2+}.
b. Intracellular Na^{+}.
c. Intracellular cyclic guanosine monophosphate.
d. Extracellular angiotensin II.
e. Intracellular cyclic adenosine monophosphate.

4. A decrease in arterial pressure causes all of the following changes *except:*

a. Decreased baroreceptor afferent activity.
b. Increased sympathetic nerve discharge.
c. Increased heart rate.
d. Increased vagal nerve discharge.
e. Increased release of norepinephrine from postganglionic neurons.

CHAPTER 12

Antihypertensive drugs

Frank J. Gordon

Major Drugs

- Diuretics
- Angiotensin inhibitors
- Adrenergic receptor blockers
- Centrally acting sympatholytics (α_2-adrenergic agonists)
- Peripherally acting sympatholytics
- Ca^{2+}-channel blockers
- Direct vasodilators

Therapeutic overview

Cardiovascular disease is responsible for nearly one-third of all deaths worldwide, and almost 40% of deaths in the United States. Hypertension is perhaps the most prominent risk factor contributing to the prevalence of cardiovascular disease. The risk of death from ischemic heart disease and stroke doubles for every 20 mm Hg increase in systolic blood pressure or 10 mm Hg increase in diastolic blood pressure. The incidence of hypertension, particularly elevated systolic blood pressure, increases with age. Approximately half of all people aged 60 to 69 years old and three-quarters of those more than 70 years old have elevated blood pressure, and the importance of hypertension as a public health problem will increase as the population ages. Preventing hypertension will be a major public health challenge for the twenty-first century.

Although these statistics are daunting, prevention of hypertension and the associated reduction in cardiovascular disease has been remarkably successful over the last 30 years. Principally due to increased detection and treatment of hypertension, age-adjusted death rates from stroke and coronary heart disease have declined approximately 50% since 1972. However, it is also estimated that in the United States, approximately 30% of hypertensive adults are unaware of their condition, more than 40% are not being treated, and adequate control is not achieved in more than two-thirds of patients who are receiving treatment. Clearly, control of hypertension remains an important public health goal.

Hypertension is defined as an elevation of arterial blood pressure above an arbitrarily defined normal value. The seventh report of the Joint National Committee on Prevention, Detection, Evaluation and Treatment of High Blood Pressure classifies hypertension based on both systolic and diastolic blood pressures. Most candidates for antihypertensive drug therapy have a systolic blood pressure above 140 mm Hg and/or a diastolic pressure above 90 mm Hg. The presence of other risk factors (e.g., smoking, hyperlipidemia, target-organ damage) is also an important determinant in the decision to treat patients with drugs. The prevalence of hypertension varies in different subgroups of the population and increases with age. Overall, approximately 20% of all adults in the United States have high blood pressure. A physician in general practice can expect to see 20 to 40 patients with hypertension each week.

A small number (<10%) of people have hypertension traceable to specific causes, such as renal disease or endocrine tumors. However, most patients are simply at the upper end of the normal distribution of blood pressure values for their population group. This most

Abbreviations

ACE	angiotensin-converting enzyme
CNS	central nervous system
CO	cardiac output
TPR	total peripheral resistance

common form of hypertension, with no readily identifiable cause, is called **essential hypertension.** It is usually first diagnosed in middle-aged people but can also be found in children and young adults. Because of its prevalence, it is the disease most often treated with antihypertensive drugs.

Unless its onset is rapid and severe, hypertension does not produce noticeable symptoms. The purpose of treating hypertension is to prevent and/or reduce the severity of diseases, such as atherosclerosis, coronary artery disease, aortic aneurysm, congestive heart failure, stroke, diabetes, and renal and retinal disease. In this regard, many clinical trials have shown that antihypertensive drug therapy reduces the morbidity and mortality associated with these disorders.

THERAPEUTIC OVERVIEW

Hypertension is defined as:

Systolic pressure >140 mm Hg and/or diastolic pressure >90 mm Hg

Hypertension is a major risk factor for:

Atherosclerosis
Coronary artery disease
Congestive heart failure
Diabetes
Insulin resistance
Stroke
Renal disease
Retinal disease

Hypertension therapy

Nonpharmacological
↓ Na^+, ↓ alcohol, ↓ weight, ↓ smoking
Pharmacological: see Major Drugs box

Regulation of blood pressure

Arterial blood pressure is the product of cardiac output (CO) and total peripheral resistance (TPR). Because of the overriding importance of ensuring optimal tissue perfusion throughout the body, systemic blood pressure is redundantly regulated by a variety of physiological control systems (see Chapter 11). When blood pressure is reduced by any means, including antihypertensive drug therapy, one or more of these regulatory mechanisms are usually activated to compensate for decreases in arterial blood pressure (Fig. 12-1).

Renin-angiotensin-aldosterone system

A decrease in arterial pressure induces release of renin from the juxtaglomerular cells of the kidney into the blood. Decreased renal perfusion pressure as well as baroreflex-mediated sympathetic activation of renal β_1-adrenergic receptors causes renin release. Renin cleaves the decapeptide angiotensin I from a circulating glycoprotein, angiotensinogen, which is synthesized mainly in liver. Angiotensin I is converted to the octapeptide angiotensin II by **angiotensin-converting enzyme (ACE)** found in endothelial cell membranes, especially in the lung. **Angiotensin II** constricts blood vessels, enhances sympathetic nervous system activity, and causes renal Na^+ and water retention by direct intrarenal actions and by stimulating the adrenal cortex to release aldosterone.

Sympathetic nervous system

A decrease in blood pressure activates the **baroreceptor reflex** (see Chapter 11), producing increases in sympathetic activity and leading to:

- Increased force and rate of cardiac contraction and enhanced cardiac filling, which combine to elevate CO.
- Constriction of most blood vessels, leading to an increase in TPR and venous return of blood to the heart.
- Release of renin from the kidney.
- Renal retention of salt and water, mediated by sympathetic nerves innervating renal blood vessels and tubules.

Vasopressin system

A decrease in arterial pressure causes a baroreflex-mediated release of vasopressin (antidiuretic hormone) from the neurohypophysis of the pituitary gland, which acts on the renal collecting duct to enhance water retention by the kidney.

Fluid retention by the kidney

A decrease in arterial pressure causes the kidney to excrete less Na^+ and water. This results, in part, from the direct intrarenal hydraulic effect of reduced renal perfusion pressure and, in part, from the mechanisms outlined previously. The resultant expansion of extracellular fluid and plasma volume tends to increase CO and arterial pressure, which can reduce the blood pressure lowering action of many antihypertensive drugs.

The most effective and best-tolerated antihypertensive drug regimens impair the operation of one or more of these physiological mechanisms. In addition,

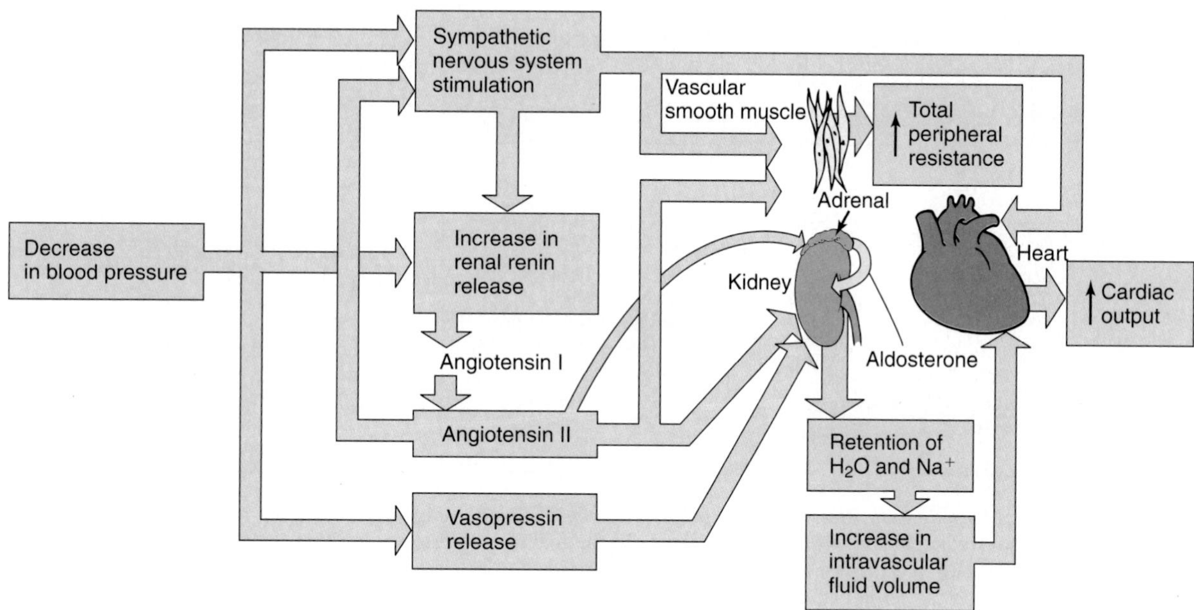

Figure 12-1 Physiological compensatory mechanisms that counteract a decrease in blood pressure.

drug therapy for hypertension must usually be continued for the lifetime of the patient. Major approaches used to reduce elevated blood pressure are summarized in Figure 12-2.

Therapeutic measures

Antihypertensive drugs can be divided into seven classes, based on their sites and/or mechanisms of action (see Major Drugs box and Fig. 12-2). Physiological responses to each drug class are summarized in Table 12-1. The therapeutic goal is to reduce systolic blood pressure below 140/90 mm Hg (Fig. 12-3). This can often be accomplished by targeting a reduction in systolic blood pressure to below 140 mm Hg, which is usually accompanied by a reduction in diastolic pressure below 90 mm Hg. For initial treatment of hypertension, monotherapy with a single drug is advisable. If necessary, drug dose should be gradually increased toward the upper range of its therapeutic effectiveness or until side effects become limiting. Although monotherapy increases patient compliance, nearly two-thirds of patients will require more than one drug to control their blood pressure (see Fig. 12-3). If two or more drugs are used, each should be selected to target distinct physiological mechanisms (see Fig. 12-2). For example, it would be more beneficial to combine a diuretic with a vasodilator than to use two drugs that both reduce smooth muscle contraction. In most instances, a diuretic should be included in any regimen employing two or more antihypertensive drugs. When multiple drugs are used, their actions are usually

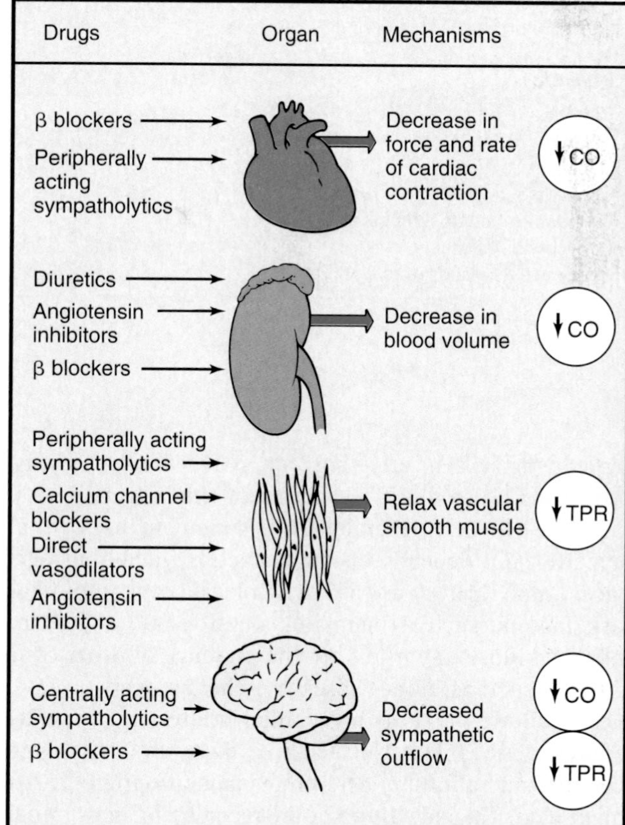

Figure 12-2 Summary of sites and mechanisms by which antihypertensive drugs reduce blood pressure. *CO*, Cardiac output; *TPR*, total peripheral resistance.

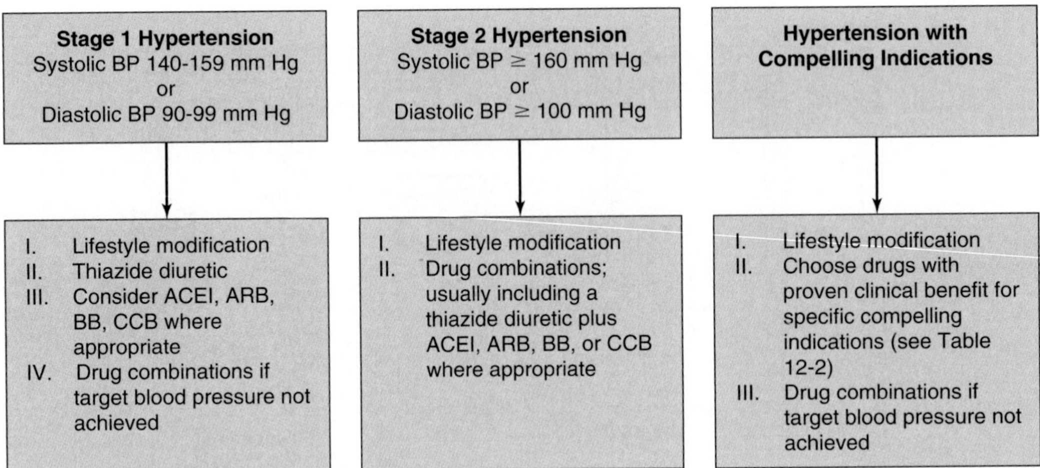

Figure 12-3 Treatment of hypertension. Treatment goal is to reduce systolic blood pressure to less than 140 mm Hg and diastolic blood pressure to less than 90 mm Hg. In patients with diabetes or renal disease goal blood pressure is less than 130/80 mm Hg. *ACEI,* Angiotensin-converting enzyme inhibitor; *ARB,* angiotensin receptor blocker; *BB,* β-blocker; *CCB,* calcium channel blocker. Adapted from Chobanian AV, Bakris GL, Black HR, et al. *Hypertension* 2003; 42:1206-1252.

Table 12-1 Physiological responses to antihypertensive drugs

Drug Class	Plasma Volume	CO	Heart Rate	TPR	Plasma Renin Activity	Sympathetic Nerve Activity
Diuretics	↓	↓	↔ ↑	↓	↑	↔ ↑
Angiotensin inhibitors	↔	↑ ↓ ↔	↔	↓	↑	↔
β-blockers	↔	↓	↓	↑ ↔	↓	↔ ↓
Centrally acting sympatholytics	↑ ↔	↓	↓	↓	↓ ↔	↓
Peripherally acting sympatholytics	↔ ↑	↔ ↓	↔ ↓	↓	↔	↑
Ca^{2+}-channel blockers	↔	↔	↔ ↑	↓	↑ ↔	↔ ↑
Orally active vasodilators	↑	↔ ↑	↑	↓	↑	↑

↑, Increase; ↓, decrease; ↔, no change.

synergistic, often allowing for reduced dose levels, which may also diminish unwanted side effects.

The choice of therapy for a patient with essential hypertension depends on many factors, including age, race, family history of cardiovascular disease, and other risk factors, such as smoking, obesity, and sedentary lifestyle. More important are the presence of other conditions, such as kidney disease, ischemic heart disease, heart failure, previous myocardial infarction or stroke, or diabetes (Table 12-2). Each of these must be given due consideration to determine an appropriate treatment plan. Thiazide diuretics are recommended as initial therapy for uncomplicated hypertension. If a diuretic cannot be used, or if a compelling indication is present (see Table 12-2), substitution of an alternate drug should be considered for monotherapy or used in combination with a diuretic.

Lifestyle modification

There are also several **nonpharmacological** therapies for hypertension (Box 12-1). Adoption of healthy lifestyles may lower blood pressure as much as some drugs. It may also prevent the onset and/or progression of hypertension. Patients differ in their sensitivity to these techniques. For example, maintenance of normal body weight and increased physical activity lowers blood pressure in most sedentary and overweight hypertensive individuals, whereas Na^+ restriction lowers blood pressure mainly in hypertensive people categorized as "salt-sensitive." The major advantage of nonpharmacological therapies is their relative safety, compared with drug therapy. Their principal limitation is the relatively modest reduction in blood pressure they can achieve (5-10 mm Hg) and a lack of compliance by most people.

Table 12-2 Compelling indications for use of individual drug classes

Compelling Indicator	Diuretic	BB	ACEI	ARB	CCB	Aldo ANT
Heart failure	●	●	●	●		●
Angina		●			●	
Postmyocardial infarction		●	●			●
High coronary disease risk	●	●	●		●	
Diabetes	●	●	●	●	●	
Chronic kidney disease			●	●		
Recurrent stroke prevention	●		●			

Indications for which specific classes of antihypertensive drugs have proven clinical benefit. These drugs may be used alone or in combination with a thiazide diuretic. *BB*, β-Blocker; *ACEI*, angiotensin-converting enzyme inhibitor; *ARB*, angiotensin receptor blocker; *CCB*, Ca^{2+} channel blocker; *Aldo ANT*, aldosterone antagonist (see Chapter 15). Adapted from Chobanian AV, Bakris GL, Black HR, et al. *Hypertension* 2003; 42:1206-1252.

Box 12-1 Nonpharmacological therapy of hypertension

- Weight reduction
- Dietary—reduce salt and saturated fat; increase fruits, vegetables, low fat dairy products
- Exercise
- Cessation of smoking
- Decrease in excessive (>30 ml of ethanol per day) alcohol consumption

Box 12-2 Diuretic drugs used to treat hypertension*

Amiloride†	Indapamide
Benzothiadiazides (thiazides)	Metolazone
Bumetanide	Spironolactone
Chlorthalidone	Triamterene†
Eplerenone	
Furosemide‡	

*See Chapter 13.
†Primarily used as adjunctive therapy to prevent K^+ loss caused by other diuretics.
‡In the UK the drug name is frusemide.

For the majority of hypertensive patients, control of hypertension requires drug treatment to achieve an adequate, sustained blood pressure reduction. Nevertheless, lifestyle modification plays a valuable and important role in management of hypertension.

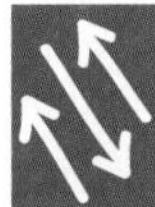

Mechanisms of action

Diuretics

Diuretics cause Na^+ excretion and reduce fluid volume by inhibiting electrolyte transport in the renal tubules. The diuretics can be classified into three broad categories related to their sites and mechanisms of action (see Box 12-2 and Chapter 13). Thiazide diuretics inhibit the $Na^+/K^+/2Cl^-$ cotransporter principally in the distal convoluted tubules and produce a relatively sustained diuresis, natriuresis, and kaliuresis. Thiazide diuretics are most effective in patients with adequate renal function. Loop diuretics inhibit electrolyte transport in the ascending limb of the loop of Henle. They are useful in patients with compromised renal function and in those resistant to the actions of thiazides. Loop diuretics produce a pronounced, although shorter, diuresis than do the thiazides. Both thiazide and loop diuretics can cause K^+ depletion. With chronic administration, this effect is more pronounced with the longer-acting thiazides. K^+-sparing diuretics inhibit Na^+ reabsorption in the collecting duct. Thiazide and loop diuretic-induced hypokalemia can often be alleviated by including one of the K^+-sparing diuretics in the drug regimen. The K^+-sparing diuretics, although producing relatively less diuresis and natriuresis than the thiazide or loop diuretics, can counteract their hypokalemic properties.

Angiotensin inhibitors

The active component of the renin-angiotensin system, angiotensin II, is generated by enzymatic conversion of the decapeptide angiotensin I, as described previously. The enzyme catalyzing this reaction, ACE (or kininase II), is widely distributed in the body, but its highest activity is in the endothelium of the pulmonary vasculature. ACE inhibitors reversibly inhibit this enzyme and reduce blood pressure by inhibiting angiotensin II formation.

The angiotensin receptor blockers reversibly bind to the AT_1 subtype of angiotensin II receptors in blood vessels and other tissues. Blockade of AT_1 receptors reduces the physiological effects of angiotensin II. The angiotensin receptor blockers have antihypertensive actions similar to those of the ACE inhibitors.

Drugs affecting the sympathetic nervous system

Adrenergic receptor antagonists There is wide diversity in the pharmacological profile of clinically useful "β-blockers" (see Chapter 10). Some drugs are antagonists at both β_1- and β_2-adrenergic receptors (propranolol), whereas others are selective for the β_1-receptor subtype (atenolol). Some β-blockers readily penetrate into the CNS (propranolol), whereas others do not (sotalol). Still other β-blockers are partial agonists at β_1 and β_2-receptors (pindolol), whereas others are antagonists at α_1-adrenergic receptors in addition to their action at β-receptors (labetalol, carvedilol). However, the common characteristic of all β-blockers used for treatment of hypertension is their ability to competitively antagonize the effects of norepinephrine and epinephrine on β_1-adrenergic receptors in the heart and renin-secreting cells of the kidney. Clinically useful α_1-adrenergic receptor antagonists lower blood pressure by blocking α_1 receptors on vascular smooth muscle.

Sympatholytics Sympatholytics with central actions decrease blood pressure by reducing the firing rate of sympathetic nerves. This action is mediated principally by activation of α_2-adrenergic receptors in the CNS. Drugs in this class include α-methyldopa, clonidine, guanfacine, and guanabenz.

α-Methyldopa is a prodrug that must be converted in the brain by l-aromatic amino acid decarboxylase and dopamine-β-hydroxylase to α-methylnorepinephrine to exert its effect (see Chapter 10). α-Methylnorepinephrine is a preferential agonist at α_2-adrenergic receptors.

Clonidine, guanfacine, and guanabenz are selective agonists at α_2-adrenergic receptors (see Chapter 10). They readily enter the brain after systemic administration. Their antihypertensive actions are due to activation of central α_2-adrenergic receptors. There is also evidence for "imidazoline" receptors in the brain, which have antihypertensive actions. Newly developed drugs, such as moxonidine and rilmenidine, may lower blood pressure by activation of these receptors. Finally, because these drugs are given peripherally for treatment of hypertension, activation of presynaptic α_2-adrenergic receptors on peripheral sympathetic nerve terminals may inhibit the release of norepinephrine and potentially contribute to their antihypertensive action.

The central site(s) where α_2-agonists act to lower blood pressure have not been completely identified and characterized. Potential sites include the nucleus of the solitary tract and the C1 neurons of the rostral ventrolateral medulla (see Chapter 11).

Sympatholytics with a peripheral action lower blood pressure by interfering with synthesis, storage, and/or release of norepinephrine from sympathetic nerve terminals. α-Methyl-para-tyrosine (metyrosine) inhibits the enzyme tyrosine hydroxylase, which is rate-limiting for synthesis of catecholamines. Guanethidine and guanadrel are charged molecules that do not readily enter the brain. However, they are substrates for the norepinephrine transporter and the vesicular amine transporter and are thus taken up into peripheral noradrenergic nerve terminals and concentrated in synaptic vesicles. These drugs reduce the amount of norepinephrine released by sympathetic nerves, in part, by inhibiting vesicular exocytosis. In addition, norepinephrine is displaced from synaptic vesicles into the cytoplasm of the nerve terminal, where the transmitter is degraded by monoamine oxidase. This reduces the amount of vesicular norepinephrine that can be released by depolarization and causes a long-term depletion of norepinephrine from synaptic vesicles in peripheral sympathetic nerves.

Reserpine is a plant alkaloid that was the first drug to be widely used for treatment of mild to moderate hypertension. Reserpine is lipophilic and binds almost irreversibly to the vesicular amine transporter in peripheral and CNS catecholaminergic and serotonergic nerves. This action prevents accumulation of monoamines into protective synaptic vesicles, and catecholamine and indoleamine neurotransmitters are degraded by intraneuronal monoamine oxidase. This results in long-term depletion of norepinephrine from peripheral sympathetic nerves, accompanied by some reduction in monoaminergic neurotransmitters in the brain.

Ca^{2+}-channel blockers

The primary action of these drugs is to inhibit the inward movement of Ca^{2+} through the L type of voltage-dependent Ca^{2+} channels. Based on their electrophysiological and pharmacological properties, the voltage-dependent Ca^{2+} channels can be divided into different types. The best characterized are L type (long-lasting, large channels), T type (transient, tiny channels), and N types (found in neuronal tissue and resembling neither of the other two in kinetics or inhibitor sensitivity). Only the L type of Ca^{2+} channels, which are enriched in cardiac and vascular muscle, are affected by Ca^{2+} channel blockers, which accounts for the generally low toxicity of these drugs.

The primary modulator of these channels is membrane potential. Under resting conditions, the membrane potential is −30 to −100 mV, depending on cell type, and channels are closed. Free intracellular Ca^{2+} (0.1 μM) is more than 10,000 times lower than extracellular Ca^{2+} (1-1.5 mM). This gradient represents an enormous driving force for Ca^{2+} to enter the cell. It is maintained by a membrane that is largely impermeable to Ca^{2+} and contains active-transport systems that pump Ca^{2+} out of the cell. When the membrane is "resting" at a hyperpolarized membrane potential, Ca^{2+} channels are closed. When the membrane depolarizes, the channels open, and Ca^{2+} enters the cell. This is followed by relatively slow inactivation of the L type Ca^{2+} channels. Channels in the inactivated state are not permeable to Ca^{2+}. They must transition from the inactivated state to the resting conformation before they can open again.

Ca^{2+} channel blocking drugs bind with high affinity only when the channel is in the inactivated state. Because the channel can only transition to the inactivated state after opening and channel opening depends on membrane depolarization, drug binding is said to be "use-dependent." In addition to use-dependence, binding of Ca^{2+} channel blockers is also frequency-dependent. In part, because these drugs are lipid soluble, they dissociate relatively rapidly from their binding sites on the channel. If the time between sequential membrane depolarizations is relatively long, most drugs will dissociate from the channel between depolarizations, resulting in little inhibition of Ca^{2+} flux. However, if the frequency is rapid, the channels will cycle more frequently, drug will bind to, and/or remain bound to the channel, and blockade of the channel will persist. Therefore, inhibition of Ca^{2+} channels will be directly proportional to depolarization rate, that is, it will be frequency-dependent. Verapamil shows much more frequency dependence than does nifedipine. The frequency dependence of diltiazem is intermediate.

Voltage-dependent Ca^{2+} channels play important roles in the excitation-contraction-relaxation cycle (see Chapters 14 and 16). Under resting conditions, when intracellular Ca^{2+} is low, regulatory proteins prevent actin and myosin filaments from interacting with each other and muscle is relaxed. When intracellular Ca^{2+} concentrations increase by influx and/or release from internal stores, Ca^{2+} occupies binding sites on Ca^{2+}-binding regulatory proteins, such as troponin C (in cardiac and skeletal muscle) and calmodulin (in vascular smooth muscle). These proteins then interact with other proteins and enzymes (e.g., troponin I in cardiac and skeletal muscle and myosin light-chain kinase in smooth muscle), facilitating cross-bridge formation between actin and myosin, which underlies contraction. When Ca^{2+} channels inactivate, Ca^{2+} is pumped out of the cell, activation of contractile proteins is reversed, actin dissociates from myosin, and the muscle relaxes.

Direct vasodilators

The directly acting vasodilators are among the most powerful drugs used to lower blood pressure. They may also produce marked compensatory reactions (see Fig. 12-1), including fluid retention and reflex-mediated increases in renin release, heart rate, and contractility. Because of their pronounced antihypertensive action and potential for producing these and other side effects (see Chapter 16), the directly acting vasodilators are usually reserved for treatment of hypertension that is severe and/or refractory to other drugs.

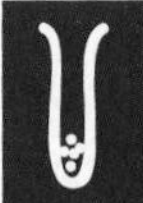

Pharmacokinetics

Pharmacokinetic parameters of selected antihypertensive drugs are summarized in Table 12-3. β-Adrenergic receptor blocking drugs and sympatholytics are discussed in Chapter 10, diuretics in Chapter 13, and directly acting vasodilators in Chapter 16.

ACE inhibitors are given orally and have a rapid onset of action (minutes for captopril and hours for the prodrug enalapril). They are subject to both metabolism and renal excretion. Several drugs in this class require biotransformation to an active compound for activity. The angiotensin receptor blockers are typically greater than 90% bound to plasma proteins. Although there are some differences in plasma half-life and selectivity for the AT_1 angiotensin receptor subtype, these drugs have similar effectiveness as antihypertensive agents.

Verapamil is well absorbed from the gastrointestinal tract, although bioavailability is low because of extensive first-pass metabolism by the liver. Norverapamil, an active metabolite, has a potency approximately 20% to 30% of that of verapamil. Metabolites are excreted in the urine, with an elimination half-life of about 5 hours, which is much longer in patients with hepatic disease.

Absorption of nifedipine is essentially complete. Because of first-pass metabolism by the liver, only 60% to 70% of administered drug reaches the systemic circulation. Nifedipine is metabolized to inactive metabolites in liver, which are excreted in urine. The elimination half-life is approximately 2 hours but is longer in patients with compromised hepatic function.

Diltiazem is well absorbed and also subject to first-pass hepatic metabolism, with low bioavailability. Desacetyl diltiazem is an active metabolite with an activity of approximately 25% to 50% of the parent compound. The elimination half-life of diltiazem is 3.5 hours and longer in patients with liver disease.

Table 12-3 Selected pharmacokinetic parameters

Agent	Plasma Half-Life (hrs)	Disposition	Remarks
Angiotensin-converting enzyme inhibitors			
Captopril	1-2	M (50%), R (50%)	Absorption reduced by food
Enalapril*	11	Active metabolite	
Lisinopril	12-24	R (mainly)	No biotransformation required
Benazepril*	10-11	M, R (90%)	
Fosinopril*	11-12	M (50%)	
Quinapril*	2	M, R (95%)	
Ramipril*	3-17	M, R (60%)	
Angiotensin receptor blockers			
Losartan	2-3	M (90%)	
Valsartan	6	M	Highly selective for AT_1 receptor
Candesartan*	9-12	M, R (26%)	Given as prodrug; low bioavailability
Telmisartan	24	M, F	
Calcium channel blockers			
Verapamil	2-5	Active metabolite	
Nifedipine	2-5	M, R	
Diltiazem	4-6	Weakly active metabolite	

M, Metabolized; *R*, renal elimination; *F*, fecal elimination.
*Metabolized by deesterification to more active compound.

Of the drugs used for the emergency reduction of hypertension, nitroprusside is given by continuous intravenous infusion; full effects occur in seconds, and recovery takes place within a few minutes of terminating the infusion. Diazoxide is usually given in repeated low-dose intravenous injections, with the desired reduction in blood pressure occurring 1 to 5 minutes after dosing. The duration of effect varies from hours to a day. Trimethaphan must be administered by continuous intravenous infusion; a full response occurs in seconds and is greater when the patient is upright. It takes 10 to 60 minutes for blood pressure to recover after trimethaphan infusion.

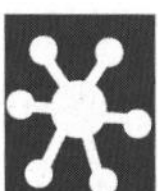

Relation of mechanisms of action to clinical response

Diuretics

A recent large-scale clinical trial (ALLHAT) comparing a thiazide diuretic with a Ca^{2+} channel blocker and an ACE inhibitor found that these latter two drugs were no more effective than the diuretic in lowering blood pressure and reducing adverse cardiovascular events. The diuretics are well tolerated and less costly than many other drugs. They are particularly effective for treating hypertension in African-Americans. These findings are consistent with many previous clinical trials demonstrating the effectiveness of thiazide diuretics in reducing hypertension and associated cardiovascular sequelae. Based upon these results, thiazide diuretics are recommended as initial therapy for treatment of hypertension.

A variety of diuretic drugs are used for the treatment of hypertension (Box 12-2). Initial administration of a diuretic produces a pronounced increase in urinary water and electrolyte excretion and a reduction in extracellular and plasma fluid volume. Reduced plasma volume decreases CO, which lowers arterial pressure. After several days, urinary excretion returns to normal, but blood pressure remains reduced. Plasma volume and CO return to, or nearly to, pretreatment values and TPR declines. The net result of these changes is a long-term lowering of arterial blood pressure.

The precise mechanism(s) responsible for the antihypertensive action of the diuretics are not known, but their renal targets are discussed in Chapter 13. The decline in TPR may initially involve autoregulatory vascular adjustments in response to decreased perfusion; but this would not be expected to remain operative after CO is normalized. Other possible mechanisms include a decreased vascular reactivity to norepinephrine and other endogenous pressor substances, and a decreased "structural" vascular resistance secondary to removal of Na^+ and water from the blood vessel wall. These changes could result directly from the actions of diuretic drugs or indirectly from the generalized loss of Na^+ and water. The latter seems probable because diuretics fail to lower blood pressure in patients who do not exhibit salt and water loss (i.e., nephrectomized patients on hemodialysis). However, the antihypertensive actions of diuretics do not parallel their efficacy in causing fluid loss, except in patients with renal insufficiency.

Finally, some diuretics relax vascular smooth muscle directly but usually only at doses well above the effective diuretic range. An exception is indapamide, which is a vasodilator at normal therapeutic doses, an action probably producing a major portion of its antihypertensive effect.

Angiotensin inhibitors

ACE inhibitors are particularly effective antihypertensive drugs in patients with elevated plasma renin activity and presumably increased circulating levels of angiotensin II. However, ACE inhibitors also lower blood pressure in hypertensive individuals with normal, or even low plasma renin activity. This may be due to ACE inhibition, reduced angiotensin II formation and/or activation of AT_1 receptors at local tissue sites.

In vascular smooth muscle, there is some evidence that inhibition of vascular ACE activity correlates temporally with the hypotensive response to ACE inhibitors. In the kidney, angiotensin II can be produced locally by intrarenal renin and may exert an antinatriuretic and antidiuretic effect. Inhibition of intrarenal angiotensin II formation by ACE inhibitors could lower blood pressure by promoting salt and water excretion in a manner similar to that of diuretics. A third potential site is angiotensin II formed in brain. In experimental animals, CNS administration of angiotensin II increases sympathetic nervous system activity and blood pressure. ACE inhibitors could decrease blood pressure in hypertensive individuals by reducing sympathetic nervous system activity in a manner similar to that of the centrally acting sympatholytics.

ACE inhibitors are particularly useful for treating hypertension associated with other risk factors, like heart failure, postmyocardial infarction, diabetes, kidney disease, and stroke (see Table 12-2).

Angiotensin receptor blockers inhibit angiotensin II binding to AT_1 receptors and reduce its physiological effects. The antihypertensive action of angiotensin receptor blockers are therefore similar to those of the ACE inhibitors, although they may produce fewer side effects.

Drugs affecting the sympathetic nervous system

Many mechanisms have been proposed to account for the antihypertensive action of the β-blockers, but none by itself can account for the blood pressure lowering action of these drugs. Acute and chronic decreases in CO are observed in most studies assessing β-blockers in hypertensive patients. A long-term decrease in CO, which may be accompanied by a transient increase in TPR, appears to be responsible for lowering arterial pressure acutely. In some studies, however, CO is reported to return to normal over a period of days to weeks, whereas TPR declines over the same time period. The decrease in TPR may result from a long-term autoregulatory response to decreased tissue blood flow or to other effects of the drugs. Although an initial decrease in CO is characteristic of most β-blockers, this is not always the case. β-Blockers with partial agonist activity modestly stimulate β-adrenergic receptors (intrinsic sympathomimetic activity), do not appreciably reduce CO, and lower blood pressure primarily by reducing TPR. This may be due, in part, to partial activation of vascular vasodilatory β_2-adrenergic receptors or blockade of presynaptic β-receptors that reduce norepinephrine release.

In addition to these hemodynamic mechanisms, inhibition of sympathetically-evoked renin release contributes significantly to the antihypertensive efficacy of the β-blockers in patients with elevated plasma renin activity. However, pretreatment plasma renin activity is not a good predictor of the clinical response to β-blockade. There is also evidence in humans that β-blockers have a CNS-mediated sympathoinhibitory effect, and studies in animals have shown that administration of β-blockers into the CNS lowers blood pressure at doses that are ineffective when given peripherally. However, some β-blockers, such as sotalol, do not readily penetrate into the brain after oral administration but still retain antihypertensive efficacy.

In addition to their use as primary antihypertensive drugs, β-blockers are often used in combination with other antihypertensive agents, particularly direct vasodilators and α_1-adrenergic receptor antagonists. As blood pressure is reduced, the baroreceptor reflexes become activated and increase sympathetic nerve discharge. Catecholamines can then activate β-adrenergic receptors on the heart and kidney to increase cardiac function (tachycardia, contractility) and renin release, respectively. Because these sympathetic effects can offset the blood pressure lowering action of some drugs, as well as increase cardiac work that increases the potential to produce angina, β-blockers are valuable adjuncts to ameliorate these effects.

Peripherally acting α_1-adrenergic receptor antagonists (prazosin, doxazosin) lower blood pressure primarily by reducing TPR. Because of the propensity toward fluid retention, diuretics are often given in conjunction with the α_1-blockers when used for treatment of hypertension.

The centrally acting sympatholytics reduce sympathetic nerve discharge. They lower blood pressure mainly by reducing TPR with an additional contribution from reduced CO. Baroreceptor reflexes are relatively well maintained. Sympatholytic drugs with actions primarily on peripheral sympathetic nerve terminals reduce TPR and CO consistent with their effects on sympathetic nerves. They produce more marked fluid retention and impairment of baroreceptor reflexes than do the centrally acting drugs.

Ca^{2+} channel blockers

All excitable tissues contain voltage-dependent Ca^{2+} channels and high-affinity, reversible, and stereospecific binding sites for Ca^{2+} channel blockers. However, Ca^{2+} channel blockers do not affect every tissue equally. Some tissues (atrioventricular node) rely primarily on exogenous Ca^{2+} and are more sensitive to these drugs than other tissues (skeletal muscle) that require little or no external Ca^{2+} for function. Moreover, because the resting membrane potential differs in various tissues, the effects of these drugs may also vary. The resting potential of vascular smooth muscle is less hyperpolarized (–30 to –40 mV) than heart muscle (–70 to –90 mV). This may contribute to the vascular selectivity of many Ca^{2+} channel blocking drugs.

Verapamil was the first selective Ca^{2+}-channel inhibitor available for treatment of cardiovascular disorders, including hypertension. Like the dihydropyridines, it relaxes both coronary and peripheral arterioles. However, it is a significantly more potent negative inotropic agent than the dihydropyridines or diltiazem. Verapamil can also depress AV nodal rate and conduction, and for this reason can be used for treatment of supraventricular tachycardias (see Chapter 14). It is also effective for treatment of angina pectoris and hypertension. The reflex increase in adrenergic tone caused by a sudden decrease in blood pressure mitigates but does not overcome its strong direct negative inotropic and chronotropic effects. Because of its cardiodepressant effects, verapamil is generally contraindicated for the treatment of increased peripheral resistance associated with heart failure.

Like all Ca^{2+}-channel blockers, diltiazem increases coronary blood flow and decreases blood pressure. Similar to verapamil, it inhibits atrioventricular nodal conduction, although to a lesser degree than verapamil. Diltiazem is effective in reducing hypertension and has fewer negative inotropic and chronotropic effects than do β-blockers.

Dihydropyridines (e.g., nifedipine) are relatively selective arteriolar dilators. These drugs reduce peripheral resistance, arterial pressure, and afterload on the heart. These effects are larger in hypertensive than in normotensive individuals. However, if the drug has a relatively sudden onset of action, the decrease in blood pressure can produce reflex sympathoexcitation, tachycardia, and augmented cardiac contractility. These effects may be counteracted by the cardiodepressant action of some Ca^{2+}-channel blockers, such as verapamil, but usually not by dihydropyridines at doses typically used for treatment of hypertension. Nevertheless, because of the potential to exacerbate cardiac disease, slow-release, sustained action formulations of dihydropyridine-type drugs are preferred for chronic therapeutic applications, such as the treatment of hypertension.

In contrast to verapamil and diltiazem, dihydropyridines have no significant effect on AV nodal conduction in vivo. The efficacy of dihydropyridines for treatment of mild to moderate hypertension is similar to the β-blockers and diuretics. Although dihydropyridines are effective antihypertensive drugs when used alone, their use in combination with low doses of β-blockers can be particularly effective in some hypertensive patients because reflex increases in heart rate and plasma renin activity can be attenuated by the β-blocker. However, β-blockers should not be used in combination with Ca^{2+} channel blockers, such as verapamil or high doses of dihydropyridines, in patients with limited cardiac reserve because of the potential to produce deleterious cardiac depression.

Nicardipine, isradipine, and felodipine are dihydropyridine Ca^{2+} channel blockers similar to nifedipine. At lower doses, they increase coronary blood flow in patients with coronary artery disease without causing myocardial depression. They also decrease systemic vascular resistance and have a potent antihypertensive effect. At higher doses, they can produce negative inotropy and exacerbate heart failure in patients with left ventricular dysfunction. They have little or no effect on cardiac conduction and have been approved for treatment of hypertension alone or in combination with thiazide diuretics or β-blockers.

Felodipine, unlike some other Ca^{2+} channel blockers, has minimal effect on cardiac function. It has a relatively long duration of action and in an extended-release formulation is appropriate for treatment of hypertension with a once-daily dose. A reflex increase in heart rate frequently occurs during the first week of therapy with many Ca^{2+} channel blockers, but this effect subsides over time and can be inhibited by β-blockers. Amlodipine has a long plasma half-life and is an effective antihypertensive drug with once-daily dosing.

Orally active direct vasodilators

The orally active direct vasodilators, hydralazine and minoxidil, lower blood pressure by directly and preferentially relaxing arterial smooth muscle. Their selectivity for arterioles is greater than that of the Ca^{2+}-channel blockers. The mechanism by which hydralazine reduces blood pressure is not known. The vasodilators minoxidil, pinacidil, and diazoxide bind to ATP-sensitive

Box 12-3 Conditions requiring rapid blood pressure reduction

Malignant hypertension
Pheochromocytoma
Hypertensive encephalopathy
Refractory hypertension of pregnancy
Acute left ventricular failure
Aortic dissection
Coronary insufficiency
Intracranial hemorrhage

K^+-channels, causing them to open. This allows K^+ to partially equilibrate along its concentration gradient, which shifts the membrane potential toward the K^+ hyperpolarizing reversal potential. The net effect is to reduce the probability of arterial smooth muscle depolarization and resultant contraction.

Drugs for hypertensive emergencies

Under some clinical circumstances, blood pressure must be reduced rapidly for a relatively short period of time (Box 12-3). Several of the antihypertensive agents already discussed can be given parenterally for this purpose. Other drugs are used exclusively to rapidly reduce blood pressure, including the directly acting vasodilators nitroprusside and diazoxide, and the short-acting ganglionic blocker trimethaphan.

Nitroprusside rapidly decomposes to release nitric oxide gas that activates guanylate cyclase, which increases intracellular cGMP concentrations, particularly in veins (see Chapter 16). Diazoxide, a preferential arteriolar dilator, is a K^+ channel opener that is used only for short-term treatment of severe hypertension because of its hyperglycemic properties. Trimethaphan is a ganglionic nicotinic receptor antagonist that blocks neurotransmission through all autonomic ganglia.

Side effects, clinical problems, and toxicity

Diuretics

Lower doses of diuretics are used to treat hypertension than to treat edema. Larger doses do not produce greater blood pressure reduction, but they significantly increase the incidence and severity of side effects, particularly decreased plasma K^+ and increased uric acid concentrations. There is some concern that diuretic-produced hypokalemia may increase the incidence of sudden cardiac death. Diuretics may also impair glucose tolerance and increase serum lipid concentrations. Monitoring of serum K^+, employing relatively low doses of thiazide diuretics and including a K^+-sparing diuretic or K^+ supplements in the drug regimen, should all be considered when thiazide and/or loop diuretics are used. In addition, K^+ depletion can be reduced when ACE inhibitors or angiotensin receptor antagonists are used in combination with diuretics. Additional details on the side effects of diuretics are given in Chapter 13.

Angiotensin inhibitors

African-American patients often have normal or subnormal plasma renin activity and thus respond less predictably or require higher doses of ACE inhibitors than do Caucasians. However, combining ACE inhibitors and diuretics lowers blood pressure in most patients and also reduces the incidence of diuretic-induced hypokalemia. ACE inhibitors have a low incidence of side effects and are generally well tolerated. The most common side effect is a persistent dry cough, which occurs in 10% to 30% of patients. A much less common side effect is angioedema, or swelling of some mucous membranes, which can be life threatening if it occurs in the airways. ACE is an alternative nomenclature for the enzyme kininase II, which degrades the irritant and proinflammatory peptides bradykinin and substance P. Inhibition of kininase II, and consequent accumulation of these peptides, is most likely the mechanism by which the ACE inhibitors precipitate cough and angioedema. Because angiotensin receptor antagonists do not inhibit ACE, they have much less potential to produce these side effects.

Both ACE inhibitors and angiotensin receptor antagonists can produce hyperkalemia, particularly in patients with impaired renal function, or if used with K^+-sparing diuretics or nonsteroidal antiinflammatory drugs. Glomerular filtration in some patients with renal artery stenosis may be dependent on angiotensin-mediated constriction of the efferent glomerular arterioles. Inhibition of angiotensin function in these patients may precipitate renal failure. In addition, angiotensin may play a role in some tissue growth and differentiation during development. Drugs that interfere with angiotensin's actions are contraindicated for use during pregnancy or in women who are breast-feeding.

Drugs affecting the sympathetic nervous system

Side effects of β-blocker therapy are discussed in Chapter 10. It is preferable to use selective β_1-antagonists in patients with asthma or diabetes, but any β-blocker should be used with some caution. Because β_1-receptor blockade impairs sympathetic stimulation of the heart, β-blockers can impair exercise tolerance. Abrupt cessation of β-blockers has been

CLINICAL PROBLEMS

Thiazide diuretics

K^+ and Mg^{2+} loss
Increase in cholesterol concentrations
Dysrhythmias

Angiotensin inhibitors

Hyperkalemia
Dry cough
Angioedema
Teratogenesis

β-Blockers

Use with caution in patients with bronchial asthma
Abrupt withdrawal may precipitate cardiac problems

α-Methyldopa

Positive direct Coombs' test result (usually but not always false)
Accumulates in patients with impaired renal function

Clonidine

Sudden withdrawal of drug produces rebound hypertension
CNS side effects

Guanadrel

Interacts with tricyclic antidepressants

Calcium channel blockers

Cardiodepression
Hypotension
Headache
Peripheral edema

Direct vasodilators

Headache
Palpitations
Tachycardia
Fluid retention

Hydralazine

Lupus-like syndrome

associated with tachycardia, angina pectoris, and (rarely) myocardial infarction (see Chapter 10).

Centrally acting sympatholytics are notable for causing less orthostatic hypotension than do many other antihypertensives. They also do not impair renal function and thus are suitable for patients with renal insufficiency. α-Methyldopa is the preferred drug for treatment of hypertension during pregnancy. The side effects of these drugs are discussed in Chapter 10. A special problem associated with clonidine and other centrally acting α_2-agonists is a dramatic sympathetic hypertensive response that occurs in some patients after abrupt withdrawal of therapy. For this reason, termination of these drugs should be done gradually, and clonidine-like drugs should be used cautiously, or not at all, in potentially noncompliant patients.

Drugs that deplete peripheral sympathetic nerve terminals of norepinephrine are not used as commonly as other classes, due primarily to side effects related to widespread sympathetic impairment. These include orthostatic hypotension, sexual dysfunction, and gastrointestinal disturbance. Reserpine, although once widely used, may precipitate clinical depression in susceptible patients because of its CNS actions. However, some of these drugs may be useful for therapy of catecholamine-secreting tumors or excessive sympathoexcitation. Of the peripherally acting drugs, doxazosin, prazosin, or other α_1-adrenergic receptor antagonists have been used to treat mild to moderate hypertension, usually in conjunction with a diuretic. These drugs are discussed further in Chapter 10. However, compared to thiazide diuretics, antihypertensive therapy with α_1-blockers increases the risk of adverse cardiovascular events in individuals older than 55 years of age (ALLHAT) and are not the preferred drugs for use in this patient population.

Ca^{2+} channel blockers

Most side effects of Ca^{2+} channel blockers result from excessive vasodilation, cardiodepression, or excessive reflex sympathoexcitation. Short-acting formulations of Ca^{2+} channel blockers may increase mortality risk in patients with heart disease. Extended release formulations, or drugs with long half-lives, are preferred for treatment of hypertension in all patients. Generally, side effects, such as dizziness, headache, and flushing, diminish or disappear with time or when the drug dose is decreased. Although true withdrawal symptoms are not observed with these drugs, sudden withdrawal of large doses of Ca^{2+} channel blockers can produce peripheral and coronary vasoconstriction and precipitate angina.

Direct vasodilators

Because of the marked lowering of blood pressure produced by these drugs, fluid retention and reflex tachycardia are common. These compensatory reactions may be so pronounced that they mask part of the antihypertensive action of the direct vasodilators. For this reason, a diuretic and a β-blocker are usually given with a vasodilator to offset these compensatory responses.

Other side effects of the vasodilator drugs are discussed in Chapter 16.

The side effects of drugs used for hypertensive emergencies can be significant. The usual side effects of diazoxide are fluid retention, tachycardia, and hyperglycemia. Nitroprusside reacts with blood and tissue to release cyanide ions, which are converted to thiocyanate by the liver. Other side effects of nitroprusside are discussed in Chapter 16. Side effects of trimethaphan are those expected of ganglionic blockade, and include mydriasis, cycloplegia, constipation, and urinary retention (see Chapter 9). Tachyphylaxis occurs a day or two after the hypotensive action of trimethaphan develops.

Other considerations

Although the goal of antihypertensive therapy is to reduce end-organ damage associated with chronically elevated blood pressure, the effects of therapy on other cardiovascular risk factors must also be considered. End-organ damage is not related exclusively to blood pressure. If an antihypertensive drug effectively lowers blood pressure but increases the influence of other risk factors for cardiovascular disease, the benefit of therapy may be reduced. In some studies, thiazide diuretics did not decrease the incidence of coronary artery disease, despite their ability to significantly reduce blood pressure. This may be related to the modest elevation of low-density lipoprotein and total triglycerides produced by K^+-losing diuretics, although the causative link or potential clinical significance of this finding has not been established. Other risk factors that can be affected by antihypertensive drugs include alterations in plasma glucose, K^+, and uric acid concentrations. In particular, insulin resistance is now recognized to be prevalent in patients with hypertension. Elevated insulin is a risk factor for coronary artery disease. Thus, it is noteworthy that thiazide diuretics and β-blockers increase, ACE inhibitors and prazosin decrease, and Ca^{2+}-channel blockers have no effect on insulin resistance. However, because of wide interpatient variability in risk factors and disease, therapeutic generalizations are difficult, and antihypertensive drug therapy must be tailored to each patient individually.

New horizons

Several new approaches to the pharmacological therapy of hypertension may be available in the United States in the near future. Many that combine two distinct pharmacological activities into one chemical moiety are being evaluated. These include β-blockers with additional properties, such as ACE inhibition, or direct vasodilation. Other drugs that increase the open time of K^+ channels in vascular smooth muscle are being developed. Another approach is to decrease the metabolism of endogenous vasodilator substances, such as atrial natriuretic peptide. Endothelial cells exert tonic control over vascular smooth muscle contraction by releasing mediators, such as nitric oxide, eicosanoids, and endothelin. Newer therapies may focus on enhancing or interfering with the actions of these mediators. Finally, discovery of drugs, such as rilmenidine and moxonidine, which decrease sympathetic nervous system activity, presumably by activating imidazoline receptors in the brainstem may have fewer side effects than currently available centrally acting sympatholytics.

TRADE NAMES

In addition to generic and fixed-combination preparations, the following are some of the trade-named materials available in the United States. (See also Chapter 10 for β-blockers and sympatholytics, Chapter 13 for diuretics, Chapter 15 for angiotensin receptor blockers and aldosterone antagonists, and Chapter 16 for vasodilators).

Angiotensin-converting enzyme inhibitors

Benazepril (Lotensin)
Captopril (Capoten)
Enalapril (Vasotec)
Fosinopril (Monopril)
Lisinopril (Prinivil, Zestril)
Quinapril (Accupril)
Ramipril (Altace)

Calcium channel blockers

Amlodipine (Norvasc)
Diltiazem (Cardizem)
Nicardipine (Cardene)
Nifedipine (Procardia, Adalat)
Verapamil (Calan, Isoptin)

Emergency agents

Diazoxide (Hyperstat)
Trimethaphan (Arfonad)

FURTHER READING

ALLHAT Collaborative Research Group. Major outcomes in high-risk hypertensive patients randomized to angiotensin-converting enzyme inhibitor or calcium channel blocker vs diuretic. The antihypertensive and lipid-lowering treatment to prevent heart attack trial (ALLHAT). *JAMA* 2002; 288:2981-2997.

Chobanian AV, Bakris GL, Black HR, et al. Seventh report of the Joint National Committee on prevention, detection, evaluation, and treatment of high blood pressure. *Hypertension* 2003; 42:1206-1252.

Kaplan NM. Kaplan's Clinical Hypertension. 8th ed. New York, Lippincott Williams & Wilkins, 2002.

Self-assessment questions

1. Which of the following statements about thiazide diuretics is *false*?

a. They produce natriuresis and kaliuresis.
b. They decrease total peripheral resistance.
c. They reduce the activity of the sympathetic nervous system.
d. They are not effective in anephric patients.
e. They are often used in combination with other drugs.

2. Which of the following statements about minoxidil is *false*?

a. It hyperpolarizes vascular smooth muscle cells by opening ATP-sensitive K^+ channels.
b. Its most common use is for the initial treatment of mild hypertension.
c. Fluid retention can mask its full antihypertensive action.
d. It is often used in combination with β-blocking drugs.
e. It dilates arteries more than veins.

3. Which type of antihypertensive drug, when given alone, often produces marked reflex tachycardia and renin release?

a. β-Adrenergic receptor blockers
b. Directly-acting vasodilators
c. Drugs that deplete sympathetic nerve terminals of norepinephrine
d. Centrally acting sympatholytics

4. Which of the following statements about dihydropyridine-type drugs is *false*?

a. They block α_1-adrenergic receptors on blood vessels.
b. They reduce total peripheral resistance.
c. They reduce the entry of Ca^{2+} into vascular smooth muscle cells.
d. They have little effect on atrioventricular conduction at therapeutic concentrations.

5. Sedation is a side effect of which of the following drugs used for the treatment of hypertension?

a. Nifedipine
b. Clonidine
c. Hydralazine
d. Losartan
e. Prazosin

6. Which of the following statements about ACE inhibitors is *false*?

a. They can lower blood pressure in individuals who do not have elevated plasma renin activity.
b. They reduce secretion of aldosterone.
c. They can produce hyperkalemia when used in combination with a potassium-sparing diuretic.
d. They can produce reflex bradycardia.
e. They are teratogenic.

CHAPTER 13

Diuretics: Drugs that increase the excretion of water and electrolytes

Kambiz Kalantarinia
Mark D. Okusa

Major Drugs	
Osmotic diuretics	Loop diuretics, types I and II
Carbonic anhydrase inhibitors	Potassium-sparing agents
Thiazides and related agents	

Therapeutic overview

The term **diuretic** classically refers to an agent that increases the rate of urine flow. However, on the basis of this definition, water is a diuretic because its ingestion is followed by an enhanced rate of urine production. Nevertheless, the diuresis induced by water is not accompanied by a substantial increase in the excretion of electrolytes, which distinguishes it from the effects of the agents described in this chapter. The primary effect of diuretics is an increase in solute excretion, mainly Na^+ salts. The increase in urine flow is secondary to this and is a response to the osmotic force of the additional solute within the tubule lumen. Drugs that increase the net urinary excretion of Na^+ salts are called **natriuretics.**

Despite variations in dietary salt intake, the kidneys adjust the excretion of Na^+ and water to maintain the extracellular fluid (ECF) volume within narrow limits. In pathophysiological states a deleterious expansion of the ECF leads to edema, and this is characteristic of congestive heart failure, cirrhosis of the liver, nephrotic syndrome, and renal failure. Dietary Na^+ restriction is the mainstay of treatment; however, frequently, ECF expansion persists and diuretic drugs are needed. The prevalence of edema-forming states in clinical medicine has led to the widespread use of diuretics to enhance excretion of salts (mainly NaCl) and water.

In addition to treatment of edema, diuretics are also efficacious in other disorders. They are used in treatment of hypertension, nephrogenic diabetes insipidus, hyponatremia, nephrolithiasis, hypercalcemia, and glaucoma. The major classes of drugs are listed in the Major Drugs box, and their therapeutic applications are given in the Therapeutic Overview box. Although all diuretics generally enhance salt and water excretion to reduce ECF volume, their mechanisms of action differ. Most diuretics (loop diuretics, thiazides, amiloride, and triamterene) have well-described effects on specific transport proteins on the luminal (or apical) plasma membrane, adjacent to the tubular fluid, of renal epithelial cells. Others inhibit carbonic anhydrase (acetazolamide), exert osmotic effects (mannitol), or block cytoplasmic receptors (spironolactone). In addition, the major effect of each class of drugs is limited to specific nephron segments (Fig. 13-1), thus they have different functional characteristics. All diuretics promote natriuresis and diuresis, but knowledge of their specific sites of action is important in selecting an appropriate drug

Abbreviations	
ATP	adenosine triphosphate
ECF	extracellular fluid
ENaC	epithelial Na^+ channels
GFR	glomerular filtration rate
GI	gastrointestinal

THERAPEUTIC OVERVIEW

Goal

To increase excretion of salt and water

Thiazide diuretics

Hypertension
Congestive heart failure (mild)
Renal calculi
Nephrogenic diabetes insipidus
Chronic renal failure (as an adjunct to loop diuretic)
Osteoporosis

Loop diuretics

Hypertension, in patients with impaired renal function
Congestive heart failure (moderate to severe)
Acute pulmonary edema
Chronic or acute renal failure
Nephrotic syndrome
Hyperkalemia
Chemical intoxication (to increase urine flow)

Potassium-sparing diuretics

Chronic liver failure
Congestive heart failure, when hypokalemia is a problem

Carbonic anhydrase inhibitors

Cystinuria (to alkalinize tubular urine)
Glaucoma (to decrease intraocular pressure)
Periodic paralysis that affects muscle membrane function
Acute mountain sickness (to counteract respiratory alkalosis)
Metabolic alkalosis

Osmotic diuretics

Acute or incipient renal failure
Reduce intraocular or intracranial pressure (preoperatively)

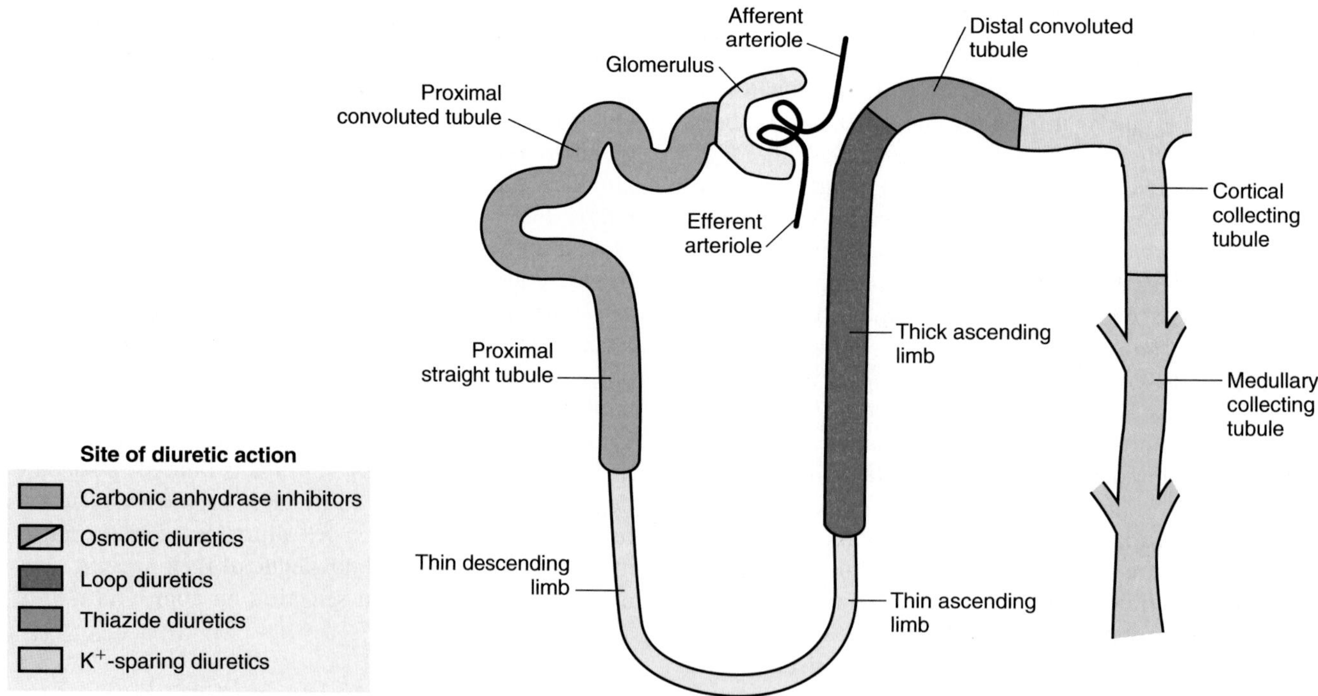

Figure 13-1 Nephron segments and sites of diuretic action. Sites of action of diuretics are color coded.

and anticipating and preventing complications. Also, because each class of drugs exerts effects at specific targets, a combination of two or more drugs will often result in additive or synergistic effects.

Diuretics are used in treatment of edema to normalize the volume of the ECF compartment without distorting electrolyte concentrations. The size of the ECF compartment is largely determined by the total body content of Na^+, which, in turn, is determined by the balance between dietary intake and excretion. When Na^+ accumulates faster than it is excreted, ECF volume expands. Conversely, when Na^+ is lost faster than it is ingested, ECF volume will be depleted. Diuretics produce a transient natriuresis and reduce total body content of Na^+ and the volume of the ECF. The effect is moderated, however, after 1 to 2 days, when a new equilibrium is attained. At this time, a balance between intake and excretion is achieved and body weight stabilizes. This "braking" phenomenon, in which there is a refractoriness to effects of the diuretic, is not a true tolerance but results from activation of compensatory salt-retaining mechanisms. Specifically, contraction of the ECF volume activates the sympathetic nervous system (see Chapter 10), with a resultant increase in release of angiotensin II, aldosterone, and antidiuretic hormone that may lead to a compensatory increase in Na^+ reabsorption. Moreover, continued delivery of Na^+ to more distal nephron segments induced by loop diuretics, and its compensatory reabsorption, may lead to structural hypertrophy of these cells, thereby enhancing Na^+ reabsorption.

Mechanisms of action

Because of the specific effects of different diuretics on particular nephron segments, it is important to review the normal physiology of each segment.

Renal epithelial transport

The normal human glomerular filtration rate (GFR) is approximately 180 L/day. Thus, assuming that the plasma Na^+ concentration is 140 mM/L, 25,200 mmol of Na^+ is filtered each day. To maintain Na^+ balance, the kidney must reabsorb more than 99% (24,950 mmol) of the filtered load of Na^+. This staggering amount of solute and water reabsorption is achieved by the combined effects of the million nephrons in each human kidney. Renal epithelial cells transport solute and water from the apical cell membrane to the basolateral cell membrane. The polarization of structures that differentiate the apical membrane from the basolateral membrane allows the vectorial transport of solute and water (Fig. 13-2). The basolateral cell membrane consists of a

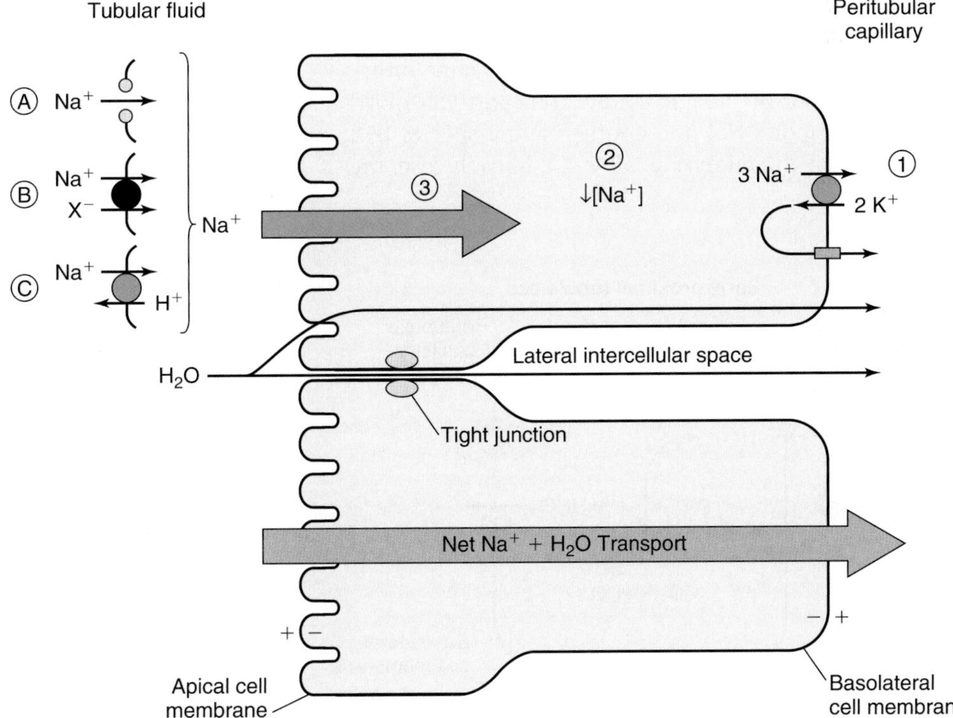

Figure 13-2 Polarized renal epithelial cells. Distinct transporters are present in apical cell and basolateral cell membranes to mediate the net transepithelial transport of Na^+ and water. Operation of the basolateral cell membrane Na^+, K^+-ATPase *(1)* initiates the movement of Na^+ and water by decreasing the intracellular Na^+ concentration *(2)* and maintaining a negative interior potential in the cell. Na^+ enters the cell from the lumen *(3)* down an electrochemical gradient via three types of transport mechanisms: channel **(A)**, symport **(B)**, and antiport **(C)**. *X*, Glucose, amino acids, and phosphate.

lateral membrane adjacent to the lateral intercellular space and a basal membrane adjacent to the interstitial fluid. The basolateral membrane expresses the ubiquitous Na^+, K^+-ATPase (the Na^+ pump). The apical cell membrane adjacent to the tubular fluid expresses three types of specialized Na^+ transporters. The essential elements of transcellular Na^+ movement are shown in Figure 13-2. Two steps are involved: an efflux of Na^+, mediated primarily by the Na^+, K^+-ATPase across the basolateral cell membrane, and an influx of Na^+ across the luminal membrane.

Three Na^+ ions are extruded from the cell into the interstitial space; simultaneously, two K^+ ions enter the cell (Fig. 13-2). The decreased intracellular Na^+, due to its active efflux, provides a chemical gradient for Na^+ entry through the apical membrane. These events result in an electronegative cell interior (a potential difference of approximately 60 mV), which attracts positively charged Na^+ from the lumen. The concentration gradient then favors passive efflux to the intercellular space of the K^+ that entered the cell. Because the ECF concentration of K^+ is low relative to Na^+, a recycling of K^+ between the cell and interstitial fluid is necessary for the Na^+ pump to function.

As mentioned earlier, specialized transport proteins are present in the apical cell membrane and are responsible for mediating Na^+ entry. Some Na^+ entry is mediated by proteins that form a pore or channel that permits Na^+ to enter by passive diffusion (Fig. 13-2, *A*). In other cells, Na^+ entry is facilitated by two types of carrier-mediated transport (Fig. 13-2). A cotransport (symport) pathway transports Na^+ and another solute species (such as Cl^- or amino acids) in the same direction (Fig. 13-2, *B*), and a countertransport (antiport) pathway transports Na^+ and another solute species (H^+) in the opposite direction (Fig. 13-2, *C*). In each case, the low intracellular Na^+ concentration caused by the active Na^+, K^+-ATPase pump provides the electrochemical gradient for Na^+ entry.

This transepithelial transport causes the osmolality of the lateral intercellular spaces to increase as a result of the accumulation of solute. This produces an osmotic gradient that permits water to flow by two routes (Fig. 13-2):

- Transcellular water flow in segments that are permeable to water
- Paracellular water flow (between cells, through tight junctions); bulk flow through the paracellular pathway carries with it solute as a result of solvent drag

Tubular reabsorption: Transport by the proximal tubule The GFR of healthy adults ranges from 1.7 to 1.8 ml/min/kg. Approximately two-thirds of the water and NaCl filtered at the glomerulus is reabsorbed by the proximal tubule segment. HCO_3^-, glucose, amino acids, and other organic solutes are also reabsorbed. In the primary pathway of water flow, water moves from lumen to cell to interstitial fluid to capillary, as a direct result of the transepithelial osmotic gradient. When GFR increases, salt and water excretion also increases, but fractional reabsorption in the proximal tubule does not change. This is called **glomerulotubular balance.** It moderates but does not entirely eliminate the effects of alterations in the GFR of salt and water excretion.

The transport of Na^+, HCO_3^-, and Cl^- are important to the proximal tubule actions of diuretics. Na^+ is reabsorbed primarily with HCO_3^- in the early proximal tubule segment, whereas Na^+ is reabsorbed primarily with Cl^- in the late proximal tubule (Fig. 13-3). In the apical cell membrane of the early proximal tubule, Na^+

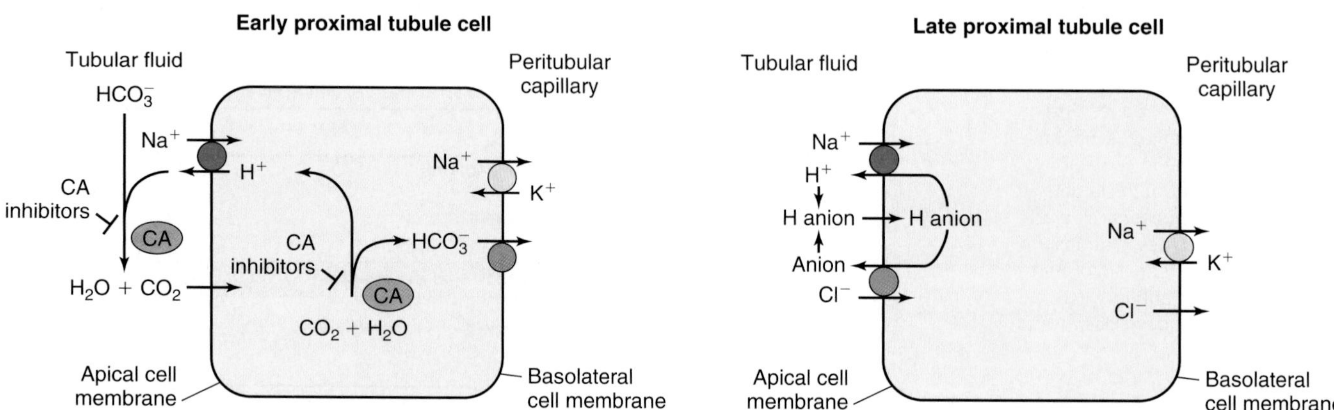

Figure 13-3 Transport by proximal tubule cells. Models for Na^+ transport in early and late proximal tubules are depicted. *CA*, Carbonic anhydrase.

entry is coupled to H^+ transport into the lumen by a Na^+-H^+ antiporter. H^+ extruded from the cell across the apical membrane into the tubular fluid combines with HCO_3^- to form H_2CO_3. In the presence of carbonic anhydrase, H_2CO_3 is split rapidly to CO_2 and water. CO_2 rapidly enters the cell, via simple diffusion, and is rehydrated to again form carbonic acid. Because the concentration of cellular H^+ is low, the reaction proceeds as follows: $CO_2 + H_2O \rightarrow H_2CO_3 \rightarrow H^+ + HCO_3^-$.

Thus a constant supply of H^+ is furnished for countertransport with Na^+. HCO_3^- that accumulates is cotransported with Na^+ across the basolateral cell membrane into the interstitial fluid and, subsequently, into the blood. The cytoplasmic hydration reaction does occur spontaneously but at a rate inadequate to allow reabsorption of the HCO_3^- load filtered (approximately 4000 mEq/day). Because of the presence of carbonic anhydrase, however, little or none of the filtered HCO_3^- is excreted. The net effect of coupling of the Na^+-H^+ antiporter to the carbonic anhydrase–mediated hydration and rehydration of CO_2 is preservation of HCO_3^-. The final step is its transfer from the interstitial fluid into peritubular capillaries.

In the late proximal tubule, Na^+ is reabsorbed primarily with Cl^-. The manner in which net Na^+ and Cl^- is reabsorbed is secondary to activation of two parallel countertransport pathways. The first is a Na^+, H^+ antiporter, in which inward Na^+ transport is coupled to outward transport of H^+. In addition, a Cl^--base (formate) exchanger is present that transports Cl^- from lumen to cell in exchange for a base. The parallel operation of both exchangers results in net Na^+ and Cl^- absorption by the late proximal tubule. Passive transport of Na^+ and Cl^- also occurs between cells through the paracellular pathway.

Reabsorptive transport systems of the proximal tubule deliver large amounts of fluid and solutes to the interstitial space. This raises pressure in the interstitium, which must be lowered for reabsorption to continue. The permeable peritubular capillary can easily carry away reabsorbed fluids and solutes. Pushed by interstitial pressure and pulled by the oncotic pressure of intracapillary proteins (higher in postglomerular than in preglomerular capillaries), filtered fluid and solutes return to the blood.

The transport protein mediating Na^+, H^+–antiport activity in the kidney has been the object of intense interest. The first eukaryotic Na^+, H^+–antiporter cloned was called NHE1 and encoded a protein predicted to have 10 to 12 transmembrane-spanning domains and a hydrophilic C-terminal domain. Since then, other isoforms (NHE2-5) with homologous structures have been identified. Virtually all measured Na^+, H^+ activity and Na^+ transport in the proximal tubule is mediated by NHE3. NHE3 is subject to regulation by a variety of factors, including angiotensin II, which increases its activity.

In summary, the convoluted and straight portions of the proximal tubule reabsorb approximately 70% of filtered water and Na^+, 69% of Cl^-, 85% of HCO_3^-, and 50% of K^+ filtered through the glomerular membranes (Table 13-1). These percentages are relatively constant, even when filtered quantities increase or decrease. As a result, minor fluctuations in GFR do not influence fluid and electrolyte excretion very much. The driving force for reabsorption of water and electrolytes is the Na^+, K^+-ATPase. Passive movements of other ions and water are initiated and sustained by active transport of Na^+ across basolateral cell membranes. Osmotic equilibrium with plasma is maintained to the end of the proximal tubule. Most of the filtered HCO_3^- is not actually reabsorbed directly from the lumen; instead it is converted to CO_2 and water in the vicinity of the brush border membranes, within which large concentrations of the catalyst carbonic anhydrase are found. The direction of this reaction is $H_2CO_3 \rightarrow CO_2 + H_2O$ (established by the high concentration of carbonic acid in luminal fluid resulting from the secretion of H^+). A carbonic anhydrase in the cytoplasm catalyzes formation of carbonic acid. Cellular H^+ is then exchanged for luminal Na^+, and HCO_3^- is reabsorbed across the basolateral cell membranes. In this indirect way, filtered HCO_3^- is reabsorbed.

Tubular reabsorption: Transport by the loop of Henle

Diuretics have no discernible actions in the descending limb of the loop of Henle. These cells do not contain specialized transport systems and are relatively impermeable to Na^+ and Cl^-. They do permit water to diffuse from the lumen to the medullary interstitium, where higher osmotic pressures are encountered.

The transport functions of the thick ascending limb are an important site of action of the loop (also called high-ceiling) diuretics (Fig. 13-4). Approximately 25% to 35% of filtered Na^+ and Cl^- is reabsorbed by the loop

Table 13-1 Summary of reabsorption in the proximal tubule*

	mEq/day		
Component	Filtered	Reabsorbed	Entering Loop
Na^+	25,200	17,640	7,560
Cl^-	19,440	13,414	6,026
K^+	810	405	405
HCO_3^-	4,320	3,825	648
H_2O	180 liters	126 liters	54 liters

*Representative values for a 70-kg human.

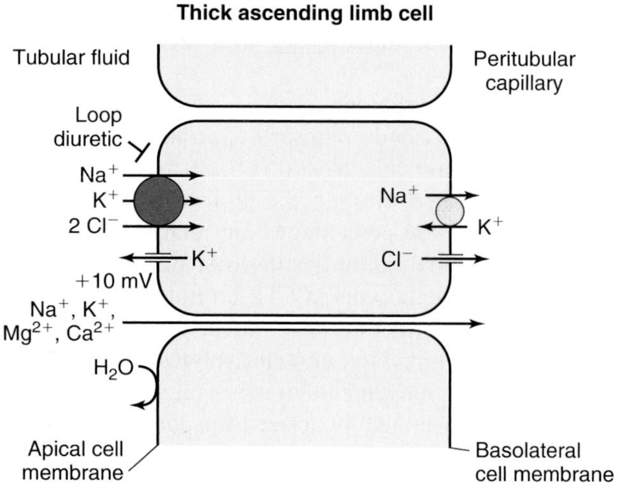

Figure 13-4 Transport by thick ascending limb cells. Model for ion transport by thick ascending limb. This segment, also referred to as the *diluting segment,* is impermeable to water, and thus the tubular lumen concentration of ions decreases.

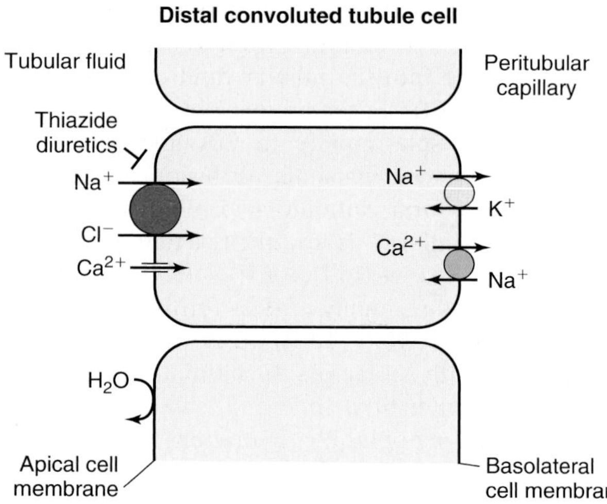

Figure 13-5 Transport by distal convoluted tubule cells. Model for a distal convoluted tubule cell. As in the case for the thick ascending limb, this segment is relatively impermeable to water.

of Henle. The Na^+, K^+-ATPase in the basolateral membrane provides the gradient for Na^+ and Cl^- absorption. Na^+ entry across the apical membrane is mediated by an electroneutral transport protein that binds one Na^+, one K^+, and two Cl^- ions and is referred to as the Na^+-K^+-$2Cl^-$ cotransporter. Although the ascending limb of the loop is highly permeable to Na^+, K^+, and Cl^-, it is impermeable to water. Thus, the continuous reabsorption of these ions without reabsorption of water dilutes the luminal fluid, thus the name, diluting segment. Na^+ entry down an electrochemical gradient drives the uphill transport of K^+ and Cl^-. This system depends on the simultaneous presence of these three ions in the luminal fluid. Once inside the cell, K^+ passively reenters the lumen (K^+ recycling) via conductive K^+ channels in the apical membrane. Cl^-, on the other hand, exits the cell via conductive Cl^- channels in the basolateral membrane. Depolarization of the basolateral membrane occurs as a consequence of Cl^- efflux, creating a lumen-positive (relative to the interstitial fluid) transcellular potential difference of approximately 10 mV. This drives paracellular cation transport, including Na^+, Ca^{2+}, and Mg^{2+}. Inhibition of the Na^+-K^+-$2Cl^-$ cotransporter not only results in excretion of Na^+ and Cl^- but also in excretion of divalent cations, such as Ca^{2+} and Mg^{2+}.

Based on its molecular structure, the Na^+-K^+-$2Cl^-$ cotransporter belongs to a family referred to as electroneutral Na^+-Cl^- cotransporters. It also includes the Na^+-Cl^- cotransporter, sensitive to thiazide diuretics. These proteins have a similar structure to the transporter described previously and appear to be upregulated by reduction of intracellular Cl^- activity and cell shrinkage. Bartter's syndrome (a renal tubular disorder) type I kindreds apparently have mutations in the gene encoding the Na^+-K^+-$2Cl^-$ transporter. Types II and III of this syndrome result from mutations in channels.

The well-recognized countercurrent mechanism in the renal medulla depends on the activity of this cotransport system, and drugs that inhibit this pathway diminish the ability of the kidney to excrete urine that is either more concentrated or more dilute than plasma.

In summary, fluid is reabsorbed from the lumen of the descending limb of the loop as it progresses deeper into the medullary areas of higher osmotic pressure. Electrolyte concentrations increase to a maximum at the bend and then gradually decrease as the Na^+-K^+-$2Cl^-$ cotransport mechanism and Na^+ pump, working in tandem, achieve reabsorption of Na^+, K^+, and Cl^-. The thick ascending limb reabsorbs 25% of filtered NaCl and 40% of K^+, but not water, whereas the entire loop reabsorbs 15% of the fluid.

Tubular reabsorption: Transport by the distal convoluted tubule In contrast to the proximal tubule and loop of Henle, there is less reabsorption of water and electrolytes in the distal convoluted tubule. It reabsorbs approximately 10% of the filtered load of NaCl. Similar to the thick ascending limb, this segment is impermeable to water, and the continuous reabsorption of NaCl further dilutes tubular fluid. NaCl entry across the apical membrane is mediated by an electroneutral Na^+-Cl^- cotransporter sensitive to thiazide diuretics (Fig. 13-5). Unlike the Na^+-K^+-$2Cl^-$ cotransporter of the thick ascending limb, this cotransporter does not require participation of K^+. As in other segments, the basolateral Na^+, K^+-ATPase provides the low intracellular Na^+

concentration that facilitates downhill transport of Na^+. The distal convoluted tubule does not have a pathway for K^+ recycling, and therefore the transepithelial voltage is near zero. Therefore, Ca^{2+} and Mg^{2+} reabsorption is not driven by electrochemical forces. Instead, Ca^{2+} crosses the apical membrane via a Ca^{2+} channel and exits the basolateral membrane via a Na^+-Ca^{2+} exchanger. Thus, by inhibiting Na^+-Cl^- cotransport, thiazide diuretics indirectly affect Ca^{2+} transport through changes in intracellular Na^+. Another mechanism of increased Ca^{2+} reabsorption with thiazide diuretics is an increase in the intracellular concentrations of calcium-binding proteins.

The thiazide-sensitive Na^+-Cl^- cotransporter is also composed of 12 transmembrane-spanning domains homologous to the Na^+-K^+-$2Cl^-$ transporter. Recently, inactivating mutations have been found in the human gene encoding this transporter in patients with Gitelman's syndrome, characterized by hypotension, hypokalemia, hypomagnesemia and hypocalciuria, similar to the effects of thiazides. Pseudohypoaldosteronism type II is an autosomal dominant disease characterized by hypertension, hyperkalemia, and sensitivity to thiazide diuretics. It has been suggested that an activating mutation of the Na^+-Cl^- cotransporter is responsible. Recently, two protein kinases have also been linked to the pathogenesis of this syndrome. They are found in the distal nephron and are thought to control the activity of Na^+-Cl^- cotransporters.

Tubular reabsorption: Transport by the collecting tubule The collecting tubule is the final site of Na^+ reabsorption, and approximately 3% is reabsorbed by this segment. Although the collecting tubule reabsorbs only a small percentage of the filtered load, two characteristics are important for diuretic action. First, this segment is the site of action of aldosterone, a hormone controlling Na^+ reabsorption and K^+ secretion (see Chapter 33). Second, virtually all K^+ excreted results from its secretion by the collecting tubule. Thus, it contributes to the hypokalemia seen with diuretics.

The collecting tubule is composed of two cell types with separate functions. **Principal cells** are responsible for transport of Na^+, K^+, and water, whereas **intercalated cells** are primarily responsible for secretion of H^+ or HCO_3^-. Intercalated cells are of two types, A and B. The A type is responsible for secretion of H^+ via a H^+-ATPase (primary active ion pump) in the apical cell membrane, whereas the B type secretes HCO_3^- via a Cl^-/HCO_3^- exchanger in the apical membrane. In contrast to more proximal cells, the apical membrane of principal cells does not express cotransport or countertransport systems; rather it expresses separate channels that permit selective conductive transport of Na^+ and K^+ (Fig. 13-6). Na^+ is reabsorbed through a conductive Na^+ channel. The low intracellular Na^+ as a result of the basolateral Na^+, K^+-ATPase generates a favorable electrochemical gradient for Na^+ entry through Epithelial Na^+ channels (ENaC). Because Na^+ channels are present only in the apical cell membrane of principal cells, Na^+ conductance causes depolarization, resulting in an asymmetrical voltage across the cell and a lumen-negative transepithelial potential difference. This, together with a high intracellular-to-lumen K^+ gradient, provides the driving force for K^+ secretion.

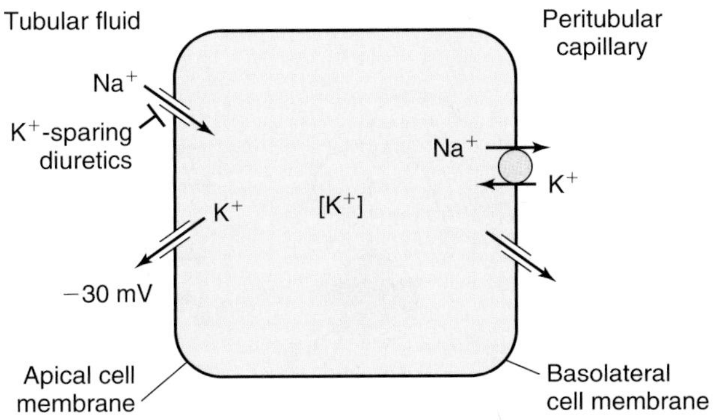

Figure 13-6 Transport by principal cells of the collecting tubule. The principal cell contains both Na^+ and K^+ channels in the apical cell membrane. The Na^+ channel in the apical cell membrane depolarizes the membrane and provides an asymmetrical transepithelial voltage profile that favors K^+ secretion.

The molecular identity of this amiloride-sensitive Na^+ channel has recently been determined with the cloning of ENaC. These channels are made of three subunits, α, β, and γ with 30% homology between them. It has been proposed that ENaC is a heterotetrameric protein, that is, $\alpha\beta\alpha\gamma$ and several factors regulate this channel, including hormones, such as vasopressin, oxytocin, and signaling elements, such as G proteins and cyclic AMP (cAMP) and intracellular ions (Na^+, H^+, and Ca^{2+}). These hormones alter Na^+ reabsorption by either increasing the number of channels expressed at the cell surface or by increasing conductance through increasing the probability of open channels and not the single channel conductance.

Mutations of ENaC could result in either gain of function as seen in Liddle's syndrome, associated with hypertension and hypokalemia, or loss of function as in pseudohypoaldosteronism, associated with hypotension and hyperkalemia. The amount of Na^+ and K^+ in the urine is tightly controlled by aldosterone, which acts on principal cells after release from the adrenal cortex. Aldosterone penetrates the basolateral membrane of principal cells and binds to a cytosolic mineralocorticoid receptor (Fig. 13-7), where its activation causes

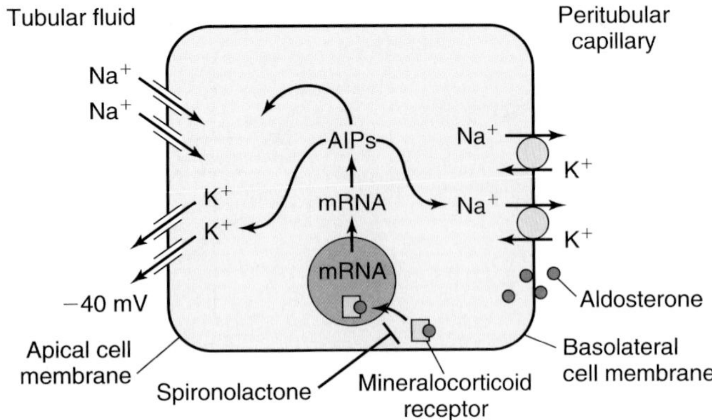

Figure 13-7 Effects of aldosterone. The principal cell is the primary target for aldosterone. Aldosterone binds to cytoplasmic receptors, which translocate into the nucleus and initiate synthesis of new proteins (aldosterone-induced proteins [AIPs]). AIPs induce newly synthesized Na^+ channels and Na^+, $-K^+$-ATPase and increase the translocation of existing transporter from the cytosol to the surface membrane.

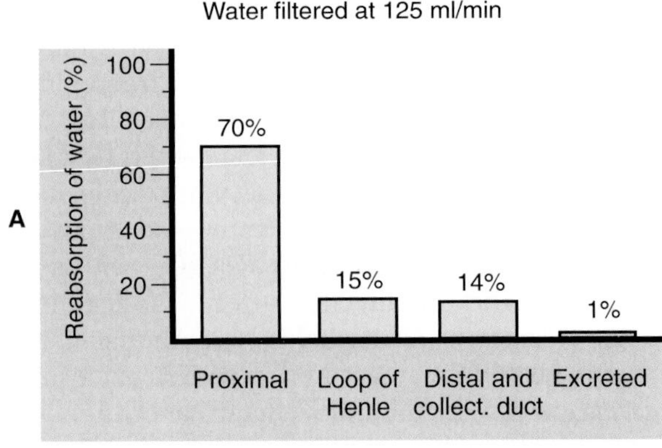

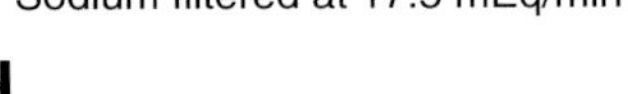

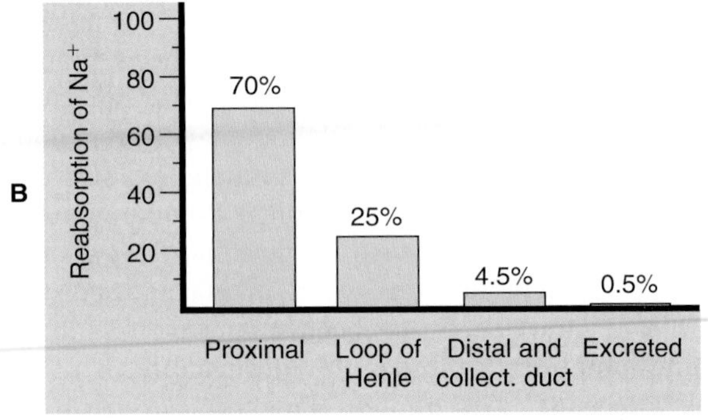

Figure 13-8 Summary of renal reabsorption of filtered water **(A)** and Na^+ **(B)** in a 70-kg human.

the receptor-aldosterone complex to translocate to the nucleus. In the nucleus, this complex induces formation of specific messenger RNAs encoding proteins that enhance Na^+ conductance in apical cell membranes and Na^+, K^+-ATPase activity in basolateral cell membranes. As a result, transepithelial Na^+ transport is increased, further depolarizing the apical membrane. An increase in the lumen-negative potential, in turn, enhances K^+ secretion through K^+ channels in the apical membrane.

The final equilibratory steps take place in medullary collecting tubules, where small amounts of NaCl and K^+ are reabsorbed. In the presence of antidiurietic hormone, water is transported out of the lumen into the interstitium. The direction of water movement is determined by the medullary tonicity established by the countercurrent mechanism. A quantitative summary of the fractional reabsorption of water and Na^+ of each tubule segment is shown in Figure 13-8. The proximal tubule reabsorbs more Na^+ than water; the entire distal tubule and medullary collecting system reabsorbs less than 5% of filtered Na^+.

Tubular secretion and bidirectional transport of organic acids and bases

Except for osmotic agents and competitive aldosterone inhibitors, all diuretics in clinical use release or accept a H^+ at the pH of body fluids and are subsequently secreted into the proximal tubular lumen. Thus, these drugs exist as both uncharged molecules and charged organic ions, and H^+ concentrations in body fluids determine the nature of drug transport and action.

Proximal tubular secretion of diuretic anions and cations into tubular fluid illustrates the influence of electrical charge on drug delivery to their sites of action and on their rapid decline in plasma. Two generic systems that transport organic ions from blood to urine reside in the proximal tubule. One handles organic acids (anions as the A^- form of acid HA), and the second transports organic bases (cations as BH^+ form) of base B (see Chapter 3). Their chief characteristics are the following:

- At least one step is active and against the concentration gradient, although energy is furnished indirectly.
- They are saturable.
- They are susceptible to competitive inhibition by other organic ions.

The lack of specific structural requirements supports the idea that these two mechanisms underlie urinary excretion of many endogenous and environmental chemicals. Many of these are solutes of low molecular weight that bind to plasma proteins and thus are not filtered through glomerular membranes. In addition to most of the diuretics, organic acids and bases that are secreted include acetylcholine and choline, bile acids, uric acid, para-amino hippuric acid, epinephrine, norepinephrine, histamine, antibiotics, and morphine.

Tubular transport of organic acids and bases is illustrated in Figure 13-9. Organic anions (OA^-) are taken up by the basolateral cell membrane through indirect coupling to Na^+ (Fig. 13-9, *A*). The Na^+, K^+-ATPase maintains a steep inward Na^+ gradient, which provides energy for entry of Na^+-coupled dicarboxylate (α-ketoglutarate). The operation of a parallel dicarboxylate/OA^- exchange drives the uphill movement of OA^- into the cell. The cell is now loaded with OA^-, which then enters the lumen by facilitated diffusion. The mechanism may involve anion exchange or conductive transport.

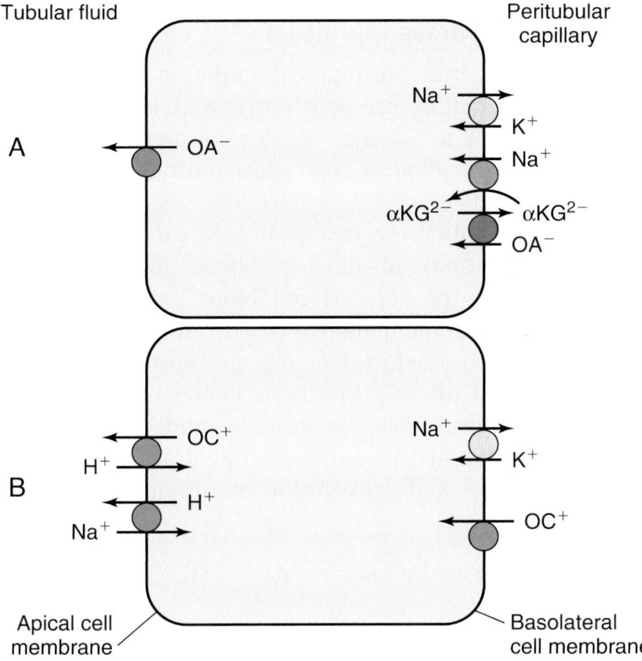

Figure 13-9 Transport of organic anions **(A)** and cations **(B)**. *OA^-*, Organic anion; *OC^+*, organic cation; αKG^{2-}, α-ketoglutarate.

Organic cations (OC^+) gain entry from interstitial fluid across basolateral cell membranes (Fig. 13-9, *B*). Their entry is aided by carrier-facilitated diffusion. Once inside the cell, OC^+ enter the lumen through countertransport with H^+. The operation of this cation exchange is dependent on the parallel operation of the Na^+-H^+ antiporter.

Diuretics

General considerations

The five major types of diuretics are listed in Table 13-2. The primary site of action is the renal tubule, with transport of Na^+, Cl^-, HCO_3^-, water, and, to some extent, K^+, H^+, and organic ions, affected. The apical membrane of each cell type expresses different transport mechanisms, which supports the following assertions:

- The pattern of excretion of electrolytes depends on the class of agent administered.
- The maximal response is limited by its site of action.
- The effect of two or more drugs from different classes is additive or synergistic, if their sites or mechanisms of action are different.

Table 13-2 Sites and mechanisms of action of diuretics

Type	Prototype	Sites of Action	Mechanism
Osmotic	Mannitol	Proximal tubule Descending loop of Henle Collecting duct	↓Na^+ resorption by osmotic action ↑In medullary blood flow Washout of medullary tonicity
Carbonic anhydrase inhibitors	Acetazolamide	Proximal tubule	Inhibits carbonic anhydrase and increases HCO_3^- excretion
Thiazides	Hydrochlorothiazide chlorthalidone	Distal convoluted tubule	Inhibits luminal cotransport (Na^+, Cl^-)
Loop diuretics			
Type I	Ethacrynic acid	Cortical and medullary TALH	Inhibits luminal cotransport (Na^+, K^+, $2Cl^-$)
Type II	Furosemide	Cortical and medullary TALH	Inhibits luminal cotransport (Na^+, K^+, $2Cl^-$)
Potassium-sparing agonists	Spironolactone Triamterene, Amiloride	Cortical collecting tubule Cortical collecting tubule	Competes for aldosterone receptor Inhibits luminal Na^+ channels

TALH, Thick ascending loop of Henle.

Osmotic diuretics

Osmotic diuretics are unique because they do not interact with receptors or directly block a renal transport mechanism. Their activity depends entirely on the osmotic pressure they exert in solution.

Mannitol, urea, glycerol, and isosorbide are the primary osmotic diuretics, with **mannitol** most widely used. A typical structure is shown in Figure 13-10. Mannitol produces a diuresis secondary to (1) an increase in osmotic pressure in the proximal tubule fluid and loop of Henle, which retards passive reabsorption of water, and (2) an increase in renal blood flow and washout of medullary tonicity. Glomerular filtration of mannitol into the tubular fluid retards passive water reabsorption primarily by the proximal tubule and thin limbs of the loop of Henle. In effect, the osmotic force of nonreabsorbable solute in the lumen opposes the osmotic force of reabsorbable Na^+. The isosmolality of urine is preserved because mannitol molecules replace reabsorbed Na^+. The reabsorbed fraction of water is reduced, increasing the amount of water entering the loop of Henle. The luminal concentration of Na^+ decreases when Na^+ is transported and water fails to follow it, resulting in a change in Na^+ concentration gradient and a backward flux of Na^+ into the lumen, with ultimately a small increase in excretion. Overzealous administration of mannitol may result in hypernatremia, hyperkalemia, and volume depletion.

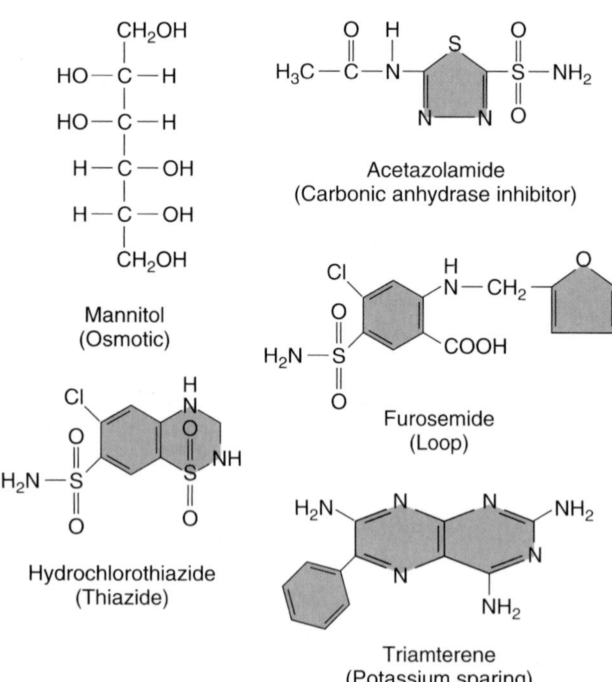

Figure 13-10 Structures of individual members of the five major classes of diuretic drugs.

Mannitol diffuses from the blood into the interstitial space, where the increased osmotic pressure draws water from the cells to increase ECF volume. This increases medullary renal blood flow, which washes out the medullary osmotic gradient created by countercurrent forces. Thus, the NaCl concentration in the thick ascending limb is reduced, indirectly diminishing the efficiency of the Na^+-K^+-$2Cl^-$ cotransport system and decreasing transport of Na^+ and water. Ascending limb cells are thus an important site of natriuretic action.

Carbonic anhydrase inhibitors

Acetazolamide, the prototypical carbonic anhydrase inhibitor, has limited use as a diuretic. It is used primarily to reduce intraocular pressure in glaucoma and to treat metabolic alkalosis, due to its ability to enhance HCO_3^- excretion.

Carbonic anhydrase is a metalloenzyme found in high concentrations in renal proximal tubule cells, ciliary processes of the eye, red blood cells, choroid plexus, intestine, and pancreas. There are five mammalian isozymes, of which two are relevant to its action in the proximal tubule. Type IV is expressed in basolateral and apical cell membranes, and type II is expressed in cytoplasm. Carbonic anhydrase catalyzes hydration of CO_2 and dehydration of carbonic acid, as follows:

$$H_2O + CO_2 \leftrightarrow H_2CO_3 \leftrightarrow HCO_3^- + H^+ \qquad (1)$$

The prevailing direction of the reaction is established by pH; normally CO_2 is hydrated, resulting in H^+ generation. The H^+ is then exchanged for Na^+, which enters the cell.

Acetazolamide inhibition of carbonic anhydrase reduces H^+ concentration in the tubule lumen and decreases availability of H^+ for Na^+/H^+ exchange. There is a resulting increase in HCO_3^- and Na^+ in the proximal portion of the lumen. Although some HCO_3^- is reabsorbed at other tubular sites, approximately 30% of the filtered load appears in the urine after carbonic anhydrase inhibition. A hyperchloremic metabolic acidosis results from HCO_3^- depletion, which renders subsequent doses of acetazolamide ineffective. The chemical structure of acetazolamide is shown in Figure 13-10.

Loop diuretics

Loop diuretics generate larger responses than those produced by thiazides. Acting on the thick ascending limb, loop diuretics can inhibit the reabsorption of as much as 25% of the glomerular filtrate (Fig. 13-11) and are often effective when thiazides do not suffice. Despite their efficacy loop diuretics are remarkably safe when used properly.

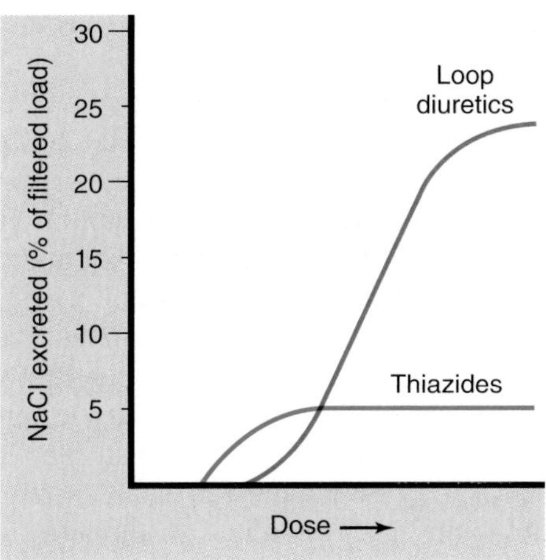

Figure 13-11 Dose-response curves comparing thiazides with loop diuretics.

Four loop diuretics are available in the United States: ethacrynic acid, furosemide, torsemide, and bumetanide. **Ethacrynic acid** and **furosemide** are prototypes of loop I and II drugs, respectively. Bumetanide is considerably more potent and differs pharmacokinetically but is otherwise similar to the older drugs. Furosemide inhibits reabsorption of Na^+ and Cl^- by the thick ascending limb (Fig. 13-1) by competing with Cl^- for a binding site on the Na^+-K^+-$2Cl^-$ cotransporter. Ethacrynic acid reacts with sulfhydryl groups, a reaction formerly considered to precede diuresis. However, this is no longer thought to be the case because several natriuretic compounds with similar structures do not react with sulfhydryl groups. Ethacrynic acid also inhibits Na^+, K^+-ATPase but only in excessive concentrations. Because the loop of Henle is responsible for accomplishing the countercurrent multiplication that generates a concentrated medullary interstitium, loop diuretics prevent formation of a concentrated urine.

In addition to their ability to enhance Na^+ and Cl^- excretion, loop diuretics also enhance Ca^{2+} and Mg^{2+} excretion. Because transepithelial Na^+ and Cl^- transport through the Na^+-K^+-$2Cl^-$ cotransporter elaborates a lumen-positive potential, furosemide inhibits this transporter and reduces the lumen-positive potential. This reduces the gradient for passive Mg^{2+} and Ca^{2+} absorption through paracellular pathways.

Under Na^+-replete conditions, loop diuretics produce an increase in GFR as well as a redistribution of blood from medulla to cortex. The increase in GFR results in part from release of vasodilatory prostaglandins. GFR is also controlled by tubuloglomerular feedback. This system relies on a unique anatomical arrangement, where a segment of nephron is juxtaposed between afferent and efferent arterioles of the glomerulus. This segment, the macula densa, lies between the cortical thick ascending limb and the distal convoluted tubule. The apical cell membrane of macula densa cells expresses a furosemide-sensitive Na^+-K^+-$2Cl^-$ cotransporter. Tubular fluid flow is somehow sensed by macula densa cells, which causes afferent arterioles to constrict and GFR to decrease. There is evidence that Na^+ and Cl^- transport by the Na^+-K^+-$2Cl^-$ cotransporter is the critical sensing step, because furosemide abolishes tubuloglomerular feedback and increases GFR. This suggests that inhibition of tubuloglomerular feedback by furosemide participates in producing an increase in GFR.

Loop diuretics reach their sites of action by first entering the tubular fluid through proximal tubular secretion. Drugs that block tubular secretion (e.g., probenecid) influence the temporal response to diuretics but do not abolish their effects.

Thiazide diuretics

Thiazide diuretics, such as **hydrochlorothiazide,** were developed in an effort to find compounds that increase excretion of Na^+ and Cl^- rather than Na^+ and HCO_3^-, as occurs with carbonic anhydrase inhibition. Their major site of action is the distal convoluted tubule (see Fig. 13-1), where they inhibit electroneutral NaCl absorption. The distal convoluted tubules also express high-affinity receptors for thiazides.

Thiazide diuretics inhibit Na^+ and Cl^- transport in distal convoluted tubules, increasing delivery to more distal portions of the nephron. There, a small fraction of excess Na^+ is reabsorbed and replaced with K^+. Because only 15% or less of the glomerular filtrate reaches the distal convoluted tubule, the magnitude of their effect is more limited than that observed with drugs acting in the thick ascending limb. The distal convoluted tubule is relatively impermeable to water absorption, which contributes to urinary dilution, therefore, urinary dilution is impaired in the presence of thiazide diuretics.

In addition to enhancing Na^+ and Cl^- excretion, thiazide diuretics contribute to urinary excretion of other ions. Because some are weak carbonic anhydrase inhibitors, HCO_3^- transport by the proximal tubule is affected. Chlorothiazide can inhibit HCO_3^- transport, but most thiazides are only weak inhibitors of carbonic anhydrase.

Thiazide diuretics decrease Ca^{2+} excretion, unlike the loop diuretics, which increase Ca^{2+} excretion. Sustained decreases in Ca^{2+} excretion resulting from the long-term administration of thiazide diuretics are accompanied by mild elevations in serum Ca^{2+}. Because of this, these agents are useful for management of nephrolithiasis and osteoporosis. The mechanisms that contribute to this include effects on Ca^{2+} transport at both proximal and distal convoluted tubules.

Thiazide diuretics enhance Mg^{2+} excretion by unknown mechanisms, and long-term use can lead to hypomagnesemia. Thiazides can cause urate excretion to be reduced, and this can lead to hyperuricemia. ECF volume contraction also plays a role.

Potassium-sparing diuretics

The K^+-sparing diuretics comprise three pharmacologically distinct groups: steroid aldosterone antagonists, pteridines, and pyrazinoylguanidines. Their site of action is the collecting tubule, where they interfere with Na^+ reabsorption and indirectly with K^+ secretion. Their diuretic activity is weak because fractional Na^+ reabsorption in the collecting tubule usually does not exceed 3% of the filtered load. For this reason, K^+-sparing drugs are ordinarily used in combination with thiazides or loop diuretics to restrict K^+ loss and sometimes augment diuretic action.

Spironolactone and eplerenone, analogs of aldosterone and its major metabolite, canrenone, bind to mineralocorticoid receptors in the kidney and elsewhere, acting as competitive inhibitors of aldosterone (see Chapter 33). Aldosterone antagonists decrease Na^+ conductance at the apical membrane of principal cells, thereby reducing the lumen-negative potential. This results in a decrease in the electrical gradient for K^+ secretion.

Triamterene (see Fig. 13-10) and amiloride are structurally different from spironolactone but have the same functional effects. Both drugs are organic bases secreted into the lumen by proximal tubular cells, and both block the apical membrane Na^+ channel of principal cells and reduce Na^+ conductance. Similar to spironolactone, they cause the lumen-negative potential and the electrical gradient for K^+ secretion to be abolished. Although they are weak diuretics and natriuretics, K^+ is conserved. Amiloride also blocks Na^+/H^+ exchange, Na^+/Ca^{2+} exchange, and Na^+,K^+-ATPase, but it only blocks the Na^+ channel at therapeutic doses. Amiloride also decreases Ca^{2+} and H^+ excretion, also as a consequence of a decrease in the lumen-negative potential.

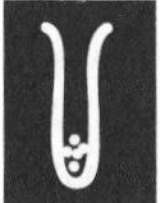

Pharmacokinetics

The pharmacokinetic parameters of the diuretic agents are summarized in Table 13-3.

Mannitol is not readily absorbed from the intestine and is administered IV. It distributes in ECF and is

Table 13-3 Pharmacokinetic parameters

Drug	Administration	Onset (hrs)	$t^1/_2$ (hrs)	Disposition
Thiazides				
Chlorothiazide	Oral	1-3	6-12	R (main) B
	IV	0.25	2	R (main) B
Hydrochlorothiazide	Oral	1	8-12	R (main) B
Chlorthalidone	Oral	2-4	24	R (main) B
Metolazone	Oral	1	12-24	R (main) B
Indapamide	Oral	1-2	18-36	R (main) B
Loop diuretics				
Furosemide	Oral	1	2	R (40%) M
	IV	5-10 min	2	R (40%) M
Ethacrynic acid	IV	0.25	3	R (main) M*
Bumetanide	Oral	0.5-1	4-6	M*
	IV	0.25	0.5-1	M*
Torsemide	Oral	1	3-4	R,M (80%)
	IV	10 min	3-4	R,M (80%)
Carbonic anhydrase inhibitors				
Acetazolamide	Oral	1	5	R
Methazolamide	Oral	2-3	14	R
Potassium-sparing diuretics				
Spironolactone	Oral	1-2 days	2-3 days	R,M,B
Eplerenone	Oral	1-2 hrs	4-6 hrs	R,M,B
Triamterene	Oral	2	12-16	R,M,B
Amiloride	Oral	2	24	R,M,B

R, Renal excretion (parent drug); *M*, metabolized; *B*, biliary excretion.
*Active metabolite.

excreted almost entirely by glomerular filtration, with approximately 90% appearing in the urine within 24 hours. Less than 10% is reabsorbed by the renal tubule, and an equal amount is metabolized in the liver.

Isosorbide and **glycerol** are administered orally to reduce intraocular pressure before ophthalmological surgical procedures. **Urea** is administered IV as an aqueous solution containing dextrose, or invert sugar, and is rarely given by mouth because it induces nausea and emesis. Urea, glycerol, and isosorbide are metabolized extensively.

Acetazolamide is well absorbed from the gastrointestinal (GI) tract. More than 90% of the drug is plasma-protein bound. Because it is relatively insoluble in lipid, it does not readily penetrate cell membranes or cross the blood-brain barrier. The highest concentrations are found in tissues that contain large amounts of carbonic anhydrase (e.g., renal cortex, red blood cells). Renal effects are noticeable within 30 minutes and are usually maximal at 2 hours. Acetazolamide is not metabolized but is excreted rapidly by glomerular filtration and proximal tubular secretion. It has a half-life of approximately 5 hours, and renal excretion is essentially complete in 24 hours. Methazolamide is absorbed more slowly, with a half-life of approximately 14 hours.

Ethacrynic acid, administered intravenously, has a rapid onset and is rapidly excreted. It is conjugated with glutathione, forming an ethacrynic acid–cysteine adduct more potent than the parent drug. Because ethacrynic acid is poorly lipid soluble, its apparent volume of distribution is small. Plasma protein binding is extensive, and the compound and its metabolites are excreted in urine by filtration and proximal tubule secretion. Elimination by the intestine is augmented through biliary transport, and this accounts for approximately one-third of the administered dose. Higher rates of ototoxicity associated with this drug, as compared to other loop diuretics, limit its use.

Absorption of administered doses of **furosemide** from the GI tract is good but could vary from 10% to 100%. Bumetanide and torsemide have better absorptions in the range of 80% to 100%, making conversion of IV to oral doses of these drugs easier. Bumetanide has the shortest elimination half-life, that is, 1 hour, and torsemide the longest, 3 to 4 hours. The half-life of furosemide is about 2 hours. Furosemide is practically insoluble in lipid and almost totally bound to plasma protein. Half of furosemide is excreted unchanged in the urine and the rest after conjugation to glucuronic acid in the kidney. A significant proportion of bumetanide and torsemide are metabolized in the liver, and, as a result, their elimination half-life is prolonged in presence of cirrhosis.

The several thiazides differ considerably with respect to their pharmacokinetics and pharmacodynamics. **Hydrochlorothiazide,** the most commonly prescribed compound in the United States, has a bioavailability of about 70%. It has a large apparent volume of distribution and a rapid onset of action. Unlike hydrochlorothiazide, GI absorption of chlorothiazide is dose-dependent.

As a group, thiazide diuretics have longer half-lives compared to loop diuretics and are mostly prescribed once a day. The longest half-life is seen with indapamide, chlorthalidone, and polythiazide. Plasma protein binding varies from 10% to 95% but does not prevent access to its site of action. Free drug enters the tubular fluid by filtration and by organic acid secretion and to its site of action via the distal convoluted tubular fluid.

The highly lipid soluble members of the thiazide family possess larger apparent volumes of distribution and lower renal clearances but have the same mechanism of action and similar maximal responses. Indapamide, bendroflumethiazide, and polythiazide are primarily metabolized in the liver. The other classes are not metabolized, and the major route of elimination is by glomerular filtration and proximal tubular secretion of unchanged drug. Biliary excretion is a less prominent route.

Spironolactone is discussed in Chapter 33. Triamterene has good bioavailability and is metabolized in the liver to an active metabolite, which is excreted in the urine. The half-life of this active metabolite increases in renal insufficiency but is unchanged in liver disease. Amiloride is not metabolized, and, because it is excreted in the urine, renal insufficiency increases its half-life.

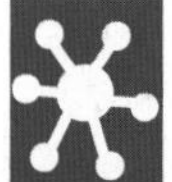

Relation of mechanisms of action to clinical response

Osmotic diuretics

Mannitol is the osmotic agent of choice because its properties best satisfy the requirements of an efficient osmotic diuretic. It is nontoxic, freely filtered through glomeruli, essentially nonreabsorbable from tubular fluid, and not readily metabolized. Urea, glycerol, and isosorbide are less efficient because they penetrate cell membranes. Consequently, as urea, glycerol or isosorbide is reabsorbed, luminal concentrations decrease, and the tendency to retain filtered fluid diminishes. Mild hyperkalemia may develop acutely in patients treated with mannitol. Mannitol may also produce a modest excretion of K^+, HCO_3^-, phosphate, Ca^{2+}, and Mg^{2+}.

Mannitol has been administered prophylactically to prevent acute renal failure associated with severe trauma, cardiovascular and other complicated surgical procedures, or therapy with cisplatin and other nephrotoxic drugs. Mannitol does not increase GFR or renal blood flow in humans.

Because osmotic drugs reduce the volume and pressure of the aqueous humor by extracting fluid from it, they are used for short-term treatment of acute glaucoma. Similarly, infusions of mannitol are used to lower the elevated intracranial pressure caused by cerebral edemas associated with tumors, neurosurgical procedures, or similar conditions. Osmotic agents redistribute body fluids, increase urine flow rate, and accelerate renal elimination of filtered solutes, which are often the goals for treatment for many clinical disorders. Mannitol is occasionally used to promote renal excretion of bromides, barbiturates, salicylates, or other drugs following overdoses.

Carbonic anhydrase inhibitors

Acetazolamide is used to treat chronic open-angle glaucoma. Because aqueous humor has a high HCO_3^- concentration, it is used to reduce aqueous humor formation. Acetazolamide is also used to prevent and/or treat acute mountain sickness, to alkalinize the urine, and treat metabolic alkalosis. Carbonic anhydrase inhibitors are occasionally used to treat epilepsy.

The popularity of carbonic anhydrase inhibitors as diuretics has waned because:

- Tolerance develops rapidly.
- Increased urinary excretion of HCO_3^- results in development of systemic acidemia.
- More effective and less toxic agents have been developed.

Nevertheless, acetazolamide is administered for short-term therapy, especially in combination with other diuretics, to patients who are resistant to other agents. As noted earlier, use of a combination of diuretics is based on their additive or synergistic effects at different sites along the nephron.

Loop diuretics

Loop agents are very efficacious at low dosages. NaCl losses are equivalent to those obtained with thiazides; at high doses, massive amounts of salt are excreted. However, two factors limit the magnitude of the response:

- The existing salt and water balance.
- Delivery of drug to its site of action.

Contraction of ECF volume lessens the response by enhancing proximal and distal tubular reabsorption of Na^+. Renal insufficiency causes less drug to reach the transporter (Na^+-K^+-$2Cl^-$) because glomeruli, proximal tubular pathways, or both, have been compromised.

The value of loop diuretics in pulmonary edema may be attributed, in part, to their stimulation of prostaglandin synthesis in kidney and lung. Furosemide and ethacrynic acid increase renal blood flow for brief intervals, promoting the urinary excretion of prostaglandin E. IV injection of furosemide also reduces pulmonary arterial pressure and peripheral venous compliance. Indomethacin, an inhibitor of prostaglandin synthesis (see Chapter 17) interferes with these actions.

Common indications for loop diuretics are listed in the Therapeutic Overview box. Often, their use overlaps those of thiazides, with some major differences. For example, the greater efficacy of loop agents often evokes a diuresis in edemas that are cardiovascular, renal, or hepatic in origin. On the other hand, it has been reported that thiazides and related drugs, especially longer-acting agents, are more efficacious than loop agents in reducing blood pressure. Loop diuretics increase Ca^{2+} excretion and therefore are used to lower serum Ca^{2+} concentrations in patients with hypercalcemia. Loop diuretics also increase K^+ excretion and are useful in treating acute and chronic hyperkalemia.

Thiazide diuretics

In general, thiazide diuretics are used in treatment of hypertension, congestive heart failure, and other conditions in which a reduction in ECF volume is beneficial. Many large clinical studies have proved the efficacy and tolerability of these agents in treatment of hypertension. As a result, this class of diuretics is recommended as monotherapy or in combination with other agents in treatment of hypertension. The blood presure reduction in patients with hypertension results in part from contraction of the ECF volume (see Chapter 12). This occurs acutely, leading to a decrease in cardiac output with a compensatory elevation in peripheral resistance. Vasoconstriction then subsides, enabling cardiac output to return to normal. Augmented synthesis of vasodilator prostaglandins has been reported and may be a crucial factor for long-term maintenance of a lower pressure, even though ECF volume tends to return toward normal.

In addition to their use in treatment of edematous disorders and hypertension, thiazide diuretics are also used in other disorders. Because they decrease renal Ca^{2+} excretion, they are used in treatment of calcium nephrolithiasis and osteoporosis. Thiazide diuretics are also used in treatment of nephrogenic diabetes insipidus, where tubules are unresponsive to vasopressin and patients undergo a water diuresis. Often the volume of dilute urine excreted is large enough to lead to intravascular volume depletion, if it is not offset by an adequate intake of fluid. Chronic administration of thiazides increases urine osmolality and reduces flow. The mechanism hinges on excretion of Na^+ and its removal from the ECF, which contracts ECF volume. The proximal tubule then avidly reabsorbs Na^+. Urine flow rate diminishes and urine osmolality increases when Na^+ transport in the distal convoluted tubule is inhibited. Drug therapy in this instance is most effective when used in combination with dietary salt restriction.

Potassium-sparing diuretics

Spironolactone and eplerenone are most effective in patients with primary hyperaldosteronism (adrenal adenoma or bilateral adrenal hyperplasia) or secondary hyperaldosteronism (congestive heart failure, cirrhosis, nephrotic syndrome). These drugs prevent binding of aldosterone to a cytosolic receptor in principal cells of the collecting tubule (see Chapter 33). They are also used to correct hypokalemia. These drugs can also be added to drug regimens, including thiazide, or loop diuretics, to further reduce ECF volume and prevent hypokalemia. They are especially appropriate for treatment of cirrhosis with ascites, a condition associated with secondary hyperaldosteronism. This class is as effective, if not more so, than loop or thiazide diuretics in this setting, because thiazide and loop diuretics are highly protein bound and enter the tubular fluid primarily by proximal tubular secretion. Tubular secretion of these agents in patients with cirrhosis and ascites decreases due to competition with toxic organic metabolites. Because thiazide and loop diuretics act at the apical cell membrane, decreased tubular secretion and lower concentrations inside the tubules reduce their effectiveness. Inhibitors of aldosterone, on the other hand, do not depend on filtration or secretion, because they gain access to their receptors from the blood side. A combination of a loop diuretic with spironolactone can be used to increase natriuresis when the diuretic effect of an aldosterone inhibitor alone is inadequate.

Although their natriuretic action is weak, these agents lower blood pressure in patients with mild or moderate hypertension and are often prescribed for this purpose. Recent trials suggest reduction in morbidity and mortality associated with addition of spironolactone to standard treatment of heart failure.

Triamterene or amiloride is generally used in combination with K^+-wasting diuretics, especially when it is clinically important to maintain normal serum K^+ (e.g., patients with dysrhythmias, receiving a cardiac glycoside, or with low serum K^+). Fixed-combination preparations are generally not appropriate for initial therapy but may be more expedient once the dosage is demonstrated to be correct. Because the site and mechanism of action of these drugs differ from those of thiazides and loop agents, they are sometimes administered together to increase the response in patients who are refractory to a single drug.

Diuretic resistance

During therapy with a loop diuretic, a patient may no longer respond to a previously effective dose. Chronic use of loop diuretics is associated with an adaptive response by nephron segments distal to their site of action. Distal tubule cells following chronic loop diuretic administration are characterized by cellular hypertrophy, hyperplasia, increased activity, and expression of Na^+-Cl^--cotransporter and increased Na^+-K^+-ATPase activity. This adaptation is thought to be due to higher rates of solute delivery to distal nephron segments, as well as an increase in aldosterone. The net result is a reduction of natriuresis normally expected from loop diuretic administration, due to a compensatory increase in Na^+ reabsorption by distal tubule cells. Combined use of a loop and a thiazide diuretic counteracts the adaptive response following chronic diuretic use.

Additional factors may contribute to resistance, including a high NaCl intake, progressive renal failure, concomitant use of a nonsteroidal antiinflammatory agent, reduced GI absorption stemming from edema of the bowel, or hypoalbuminemia and albuminuria. Solutions include combined use of a loop and another diuretic, especially a thiazide.

Side effects, clinical problems, and toxicity

Repeated use of diuretics is frequently associated with shifts in **acid-base balance** and changes in serum electrolytes. Shifts frequently encountered in patients on continuous diuretic therapy include K^+ depletion and hyperuricemia. Patients at risk include the elderly, those with severe disease, those taking cardiac glycosides, and the malnourished. Such changes are difficult to avoid in most patients unless counteractive measures are taken. Supplemental intake of K^+ (dietary or oral KCl) or concomitant use of K^+-sparing with thiazide or loop diuretics is often used to circumvent this problem.

Paradoxical diuretic-induced edema may occur in patients with hypertension, if diuretics are abruptly withdrawn after long-term use. This occurs because long-term use results in a persistently elevated plasma renin activity and a secondary aldosteronism. If it is necessary to discontinue diuretic therapy, a stepwise reduction over a few weeks combined with a reduction in Na^+ intake is recommended. The main problems are summarized in the Clinical Problems box.

CLINICAL PROBLEMS

Thiazides

Depletion phenomena (hypokalemia, dilutional hyponatremia, hypochloremic alkalosis, hypomagnesemia), retention phenomena (hyperuricemia, hypercalcemia), metabolic changes (hyperglycemia, hyperlipidemia, insulin resistance), hypersensitivity (fever, rash, purpura, anaphylaxis), and azotemia in patients with poor renal function.

Loop diuretics

Hypokalemia; hyperuricemia; metabolic alkalosis; hyponatremia; hearing deficits, particularly with ethacrynic acid; watery diarrhea with ethacrynic acid

Carbonic anhydrase inhibitors

Metabolic acidosis, drowsiness, fatigue, CNS depression, paresthesia

Potassium-sparing diuretics

Aldosterone inhibitors: hyperkalemia, gynecomastia, hirsutism, menstrual irregularities

Triamterene: hyperkalemia, megaloblastic anemia in patients with cirrhosis

Amiloride: hyperkalemia, increase in blood urea nitrogen, glucose intolerance in diabetes mellitus

Osmotic diuretics

Acute increase in ECF volume and serum potassium concentration, nausea and vomiting, headache

Osmotic diuretics

Acute expansion of ECF volume engendered by osmotic diuretics increases the workload of the heart. Patients in **cardiac failure** are especially susceptible, and pulmonary edema may develop. Therefore, they should not be treated with these drugs. Underlying heart disease in the absence of frank congestive heart failure, though not an absolute contraindication, is a serious risk factor. Mannitol is sometimes given to restore urine flow in patients in oliguric or anuric states induced by extrarenal factors (e.g., hypovolemia, hypotension). In these cases, the response to a test dose should be evaluated before therapeutic quantities are administered.

Severe volume depletion and hypernatremia may result from prolonged administration of mannitol unless Na^+ and water losses are replaced. Mild hyperkalemia is often observed, but intolerable K^+ elevations are not likely, except in patients with diabetes, adrenal insufficiency, or severely impaired renal function.

Carbonic anhydrase inhibitors

Among the side effects of carbonic anhydrase inhibitors are metabolic acidosis, drowsiness, fatigue, CNS depression, and paresthesia. Hypersensitivity reactions are rare.

Thiazide diuretics

Thiazides (and loop diuretics), whose action is exerted proximal to the K^+ secretory sites, increase the excretion of K^+. The fraction of patients in whom hypokalemia develops or who show evidence of K^+ depletion while undergoing long-term treatment is variable. Some younger people with hypertension may have no effect or become only slightly hypokalemic. A clinical trial showed no difference in mortalities and cardiac-related events between hypertensive patients taking thiazides and patients treated with β-adrenergic receptor blocking drugs. Mild hypokalemia should be avoided in cirrhotic patients, those taking cardiac glycosides, diabetics, and the elderly. Disturbances in insulin and glucose metabolism can often be prevented, if K^+ depletion is avoided.

Although Mg^{2+} is primarily reabsorbed in the proximal tubule, thiazides and loop diuretics can accelerate its excretion. Mg^{2+} depletion in patients on long-term diuretic therapy is occasionally reported and is considered by some to be a risk factor for ventricular dysrhythmias. Addition of K^+-sparing diuretics reportedly prevents Mg^{2+}-loss.

Thiazides increase the serum concentration of urate by increasing proximal tubular reabsorption and reducing tubular secretion. Hyperuricemia develops in more than 50% of patients on long-term thiazide therapy. In most, the elevation is modest and does not precipitate gout, unless the patient has primary disease or a gouty diathesis. Currently, there is no reason to believe that the risk of hyperuricemia outweighs the benefits of thiazide therapy in most patients.

Thiazide diuretics produce clinically significant reductions in plasma Na^+ (hyponatremia) in some patients. Although the magnitude of the hyponatremia is variable, values of less than 100 mEq/L have been reported, which can be life threatening.

Long-term treatment with thiazide diuretics could result in small increases in serum lipid and lipoprotein concentrations. Low-density lipoprotein-cholesterol and triglyceride concentrations may increase during short-term therapy, but total cholesterol and triglyceride concentrations are usually found to return to baseline values in studies of more than 1 year. This action may be linked to glucose intolerance and may be a consequence of K^+ depletion.

Because most complications of thiazide therapy are direct manifestations of their pharmacological effects, adverse events are usually predictable. The list in the Clinical Problems box includes adventitious hazards that have no apparent relationship to the known pharmacology of the drugs. Although relatively uncommon, these hazards are usually more serious. Thiazides also reduce the clearance of lithium, and, as a rule, should not be administered concomitantly with it. Although not absolutely contraindicated, their use in pregnant women is not recommended unless the anticipated benefit justifies the risk. Thiazides cross the placenta and appear in breast milk. Anuria and a known hypersensitivity to sulfonamides are absolute contraindications.

Loop diuretics

Loop diuretics also increase excretion of K^+, Ca^{2+}, Mg^{2+}, and H^+, and their use is associated with all the electrolyte depletion phenomena associated with thiazide use. Similarly, carbohydrate intolerance and hyperlipidemia have also been observed.

Vertigo and deafness sometimes develop in patients receiving large IV doses of loop diuretics. Coadministration of an aminoglycoside antibiotic is known to produce additive effects. Additional drug interactions occur with indomethacin (decreased activity), warfarin (displacement from plasma protein), and lithium (decreased clearance and increased risk of toxicity). All diuretics are contraindicated in anuric patients.

Potassium-sparing diuretics

The most serious adverse effect of spironolactone therapy is hyperkalemia. Serum K^+ should be monitored periodically even when the drug is administered with a K^+-wasting diuretic. Gynecomastia may occur in men, possibly as a consequence of the binding of canrenone to androgen receptors. Decreased libido and impotence have been reported. Menstrual irregularities, hirsutism, or swelling and breast tenderness may develop in women. Triamterene and amiloride may cause hyperkalemia, even when a K^+-wasting diuretic is part of the therapy. The risk is highest in patients with limited renal function. Additional complications include elevated serum blood urea nitrogen and uric acid, glucose intolerance, and GI tract disturbances. Triamterene may contribute to, or initiate, formation of renal stones, and hypersensitivity reactions may occur in patients receiving it. Some drug-drug interactions involving diuretics are given in Table 13-4.

Table 13-4 Potential drug interactions

Drug Class or Agent	Diuretic	Problem
β-Adrenergic blockers	Thiazides	Increase in blood glucose, urates, and lipids
Digitalis glycosides	Thiazides, loop diuretics	Hypokalemia resulting in increased digitalis binding and toxicity
Angiotensin-converting enzyme inhibitors	Potassium-sparing diuretics	Hyperkalemia, cardiac effects
Aminoglycosides	Loop diuretics	Ototoxicity, nephrotoxicity
Adrenal steroids	Thiazides, loop diuretics	Enhanced hypokalemia
Chlorpropamide	Thiazides	Hyponatremia

New horizons

Novel diuretics that can antagonize water transport are currently in development or are in clinical trials. There are two ways to block water transport:

- Antagonize the action of vasopressin with selective V_2-vasopressin receptor antagonists.
- Antagonize renal epithelial water channels.

The use of a vasopressin V_2 receptor antagonist has been shown to be effective in inducing water diuresis in animals. Such an effect in humans could be advantageous in treatment of disorders in which water excretion is low, as a result of high vasopressin concentrations. Congestive heart failure, cirrhosis, and nephrotic syndrome are conditions characterized by

ECF volume expansion resulting from NaCl and water retention. A decrease in cardiac output (congestive heart failure) or in effective arterial volume (cirrhosis, nephrotic syndrome) stimulate vasopressin release and reduce water excretion. The effect of the excess vasopressin on collecting tubule cells leads to hyponatremia. Antagonism of V_2 receptors in such circumstances could facilitate water excretion. Also, treatment of patients with chronic hyponatremia secondary to inappropriate antidiuretic hormone secretion could be facilitated with a selective V_2 receptor antagonist.

Alternatively, water excretion could be enhanced through use of agents that inhibit water channels. Our understanding of membrane water transport has advanced significantly with the molecular characterization of a new family of water transport proteins, referred to as aquaporins. The first water channel identified was aquaporin-1. This channel, which is constitutively active, was cloned after its purification from red blood cell membranes. Of the 10 aquaporins identified, at least 7 are expressed in kidney. Aquaporin-1 is expressed at high levels in the proximal tubule and descending limb, and its high expression level correlates with the high water permeability in these nephron segments. Aquaporin-2 is abundantly expressed in the principal cells of the collecting duct and regulates water reabsorption in response to vasopressin. Recent studies indicate that it is involved in several inherited and acquired disorders of water balance, such as inherited and acquired forms of nephrogenic diabetes insipidus. Aquaporins-3 and -4 are expressed on the basolateral membranes of collecting duct cells and allow water to exit the cells following its absorption from the apical membrane. Although expressed in kidneys, less is known about other aquaporins. The development of drugs that selectively antagonize aquaporins-1 or -2, which would, in turn, lead to selective inhibition of water transport in proximal or distal tubules, could lead to therapeutic intervention in disorders of water balance.

Recent clinical studies have targeted the natriuretic peptide family in mediating natriuresis in disorders of heart failure (see Chapter 15). The renal hemodynamic effects of A and B natriuretic peptides include increased GFR, afferent arteriolar dilation, and efferent arteriolar constriction. Additionally, they have direct effects to block Na^+ transport in the inner medullary collecting duct as well as block aldosterone release. Nesiritide, a recombinant human B natriuretic peptide, is currently used for the treatment of fluid retention in congestive heart failure.

TRADE NAMES

In addition to generic and fixed-combination preparations, the following trade-named materials are some of the important compounds available in the United States.

Acetazolamide (Diamox)
Amiloride hydrochloride (Midamor)
Bendroflumethiazide (Naturetin)
Benzthiazide (Aquatag, Proaqua, Exna)
Bumetanide (Bumex)
Chlorothiazide (Diuril)
Chlorthalidone (Hygroton)
Cyclothiazide (Anhydron)
Eplerenone (Inspra)
Ethacrynic acid (Edecrin)
Furosemide (Lasix)
Hydrochlorothiazide (Esidrix, Hydrodiuril)
Hydroflumethiazide (Diucardin, Saluron)
Indapamide (Lozol)
Methazolamide (Neptazane)
Methyclothiazide (Enduron)
Metolazone (Diulo, Zaroxolyn)
Nesiritide (Natrecor)
Polythiazide (Renese)
Quinethazone (Hydromox)
Spironolactone (Aldactone)
Torsemide (Demadex)
Triamterene (Dyrenium)
Trichlormethiazide (Metahydrin, Naqua)

FURTHER READING

Ellison DH. Diuretic resistance: physiology and therapeutics. *Semin Nephrol* 1999; 19(6):581-597.

Nielsen S, Frøkiær J, Marples D, et al. Aquaporins in the kidney: from molecules to medicine, *Physiol Rev* 2002; 82:205-244.

Okusa MD, Ellison DH. Diuretics: physiology and pathophysiology. In Seldin DW, Giebisch G (eds): *The Kidney*, 3rd ed, Philadelphia, Lippincott Williams & Wilkins, 2000, pp 2877-2922.

Self-assessment questions

1. The loop diuretics have their principal diuretic effect on the:

a. Ascending limb of loop of Henle.
b. Distal convoluted tubule.
c. Proximal convoluted tubule.
d. Distal pars recta.
e. Collecting duct.

2. Quantitative reabsorption of water and electrolytes:

a. Is greatest in the loop of Henle.
b. Particularly NaCl is against an electrochemical gradient.
c. Is driven by the Na^+ pump.
d. Is characterized by *b* and *c* only.
e. Is characterized by all of the above.

3. Spironolactone:

a. Competes for aldosterone receptors.
b. Inhibits the excretion of K^+.
c. Acts at the late distal tubule.
d. Is characterized by *b* and *c*.
e. Is characterized by all of the above.

4. Potential side effects of the thiazide diuretics include:

a. Hypokalemia, hyperglycemia, hyperlipidemia.
b. Hypokalemia, ototoxicity, hyperuricemia.
c. Hypokalemia, alkalosis, nausea/vomiting.
d. Increase in blood urea nitrogen, hyperkalemia, metabolic acidosis.
e. Hypermagnesemia, hypercalcemia, fever.

CHAPTER 14

Antiarrhythmic drugs

Peter S. Fischbach

Major Drugs

Drugs that block myocardial Na^+ channels

β-Adrenergic receptor blockers

Drugs that block myocardial K^+ channels

Drugs that block myocardial Ca^{2+} channels

Therapeutic overview

The heart is a four-chambered pump that circulates blood to the body. During normal function, blood is circulated in quantities sufficient to provide adequate oxygen and nutrients to maintain aerobic metabolism. To function efficiently, the heart needs to contract sequentially (atria and then ventricles) and in a synchronized manner. It also needs adequate time between contractions for chamber filling (diastole). This need for relaxation distinguishes cardiac from smooth and skeletal muscle, which can contract tetanically. The heart has an electrical system that allows rapid and organized spread of activation, which can then convert the electrical signal into mechanical energy.

Electrical activation originates in specialized pacemaker cells of the sinoatrial (SA) node, located in the high right atrium near the junction with the superior vena cava. After exiting the SA node, the electrical signal spreads rapidly throughout the atrium leading to contraction. However, the atria are electrically isolated from the ventricles by the fibrous atrioventricular (AV)-ring, with electrical propagation between atrium and ventricles occurring solely through the AV node and His-Purkinje system. The AV node delays the electrical impulse as it passes from atrium to ventricles, providing additional filling time prior to ejection. The signal then rapidly spreads throughout the ventricles using the Purkinje system, allowing a synchronized contraction.

When orderly propagation of the electrical signal is perturbed, the function of the heart may be adversely affected. Slowed electrical conduction through some cardiac regions, as occurs with first degree heart block or bundle branch block in the ventricles, is generally well tolerated. Other abnormalities may lead to clinical symptoms, and in its most extreme form, cardiovascular collapse. Abnormalities in heart rhythm are called **arrhythmias** and may result in abnormally fast or slow heart rates. Options for clinical management of arrhythmias have been rapidly expanding and include drugs, mechanical devices, such as pacemakers and defibrillators, as well as transcatheter therapies, such as radiofrequency ablation.

Antiarrhythmic Drugs

As discussed in the Therapeutic Overview box, currently available antiarrhythmic drugs work by one of two mechanisms. They either directly alter the function of ion channels that participate in a normal heart beat, or they interfere with neuronal control. Although antiarrhythmic drugs are intended to restore normal sinus rhythm and/or suppress initiation of abnormal rhythms, their use is hampered by the omnipresent risk of proarrhythmias. In the most famous example, the Cardiac Arrhythmia Suppression Trial showed that, even though

Abbreviations

AV	atrioventricular
CNS	central nervous system
GI	gastrointestinal
IV	intravenous
NAPA	*N*-acetylprocainamide
SA	sinoatrial

ventricular arrhythmias predictive of sudden death could be suppressed by Na^+-channel-blocking drugs, their use was associated with an increased incidence of sudden death. Likewise, even though intravenous (IV) lidocaine reduces ventricular arrhythmias in patients with acute myocardial infarction, it does not decrease but may actually increase mortality.

THERAPEUTIC OVERVIEW

Goal	To treat abnormal cardial impulse formation or conduction
Effects	Modify ion fluxes, block Na^+, K^+, or Ca^{2+} channels, modify β-adrenergic receptor-activated processes
Drug action	**Uses**
Na^+ channel blockade	Paroxysmal supraventricular tachycardia, atrial fibrillation or flutter, ventricular tachycardia
	Ventricular tachycardia, digoxin-induced arrhythmias
	Ventricular tachycardia, atrial fibrillation
β-Adrenergic receptor blockade	Paroxysmal supraventricular tachycardia, atrial or ventricular premature beats, atrial fibrillation or flutter
Prolong repolarization	(Na^+, K^+ blockade) Ventricular tachycardia, atrial fibrillation or flutter*
Ca^{2+} channel blockade	Paroxysmal supraventricular tachycardia, atrial fibrillation or flutter
Other	
Adenosine	Paroxysmal supraventricular tachycardia
Digitalis glycosides	Atrial fibrillation or flutter with increased ventricular rate

*Only amiodarone.

Antiarrhythmic drugs are used for all forms of tachycardia. However, they are not effective for long-term therapy of symptomatic bradycardia. Antiarrhythmic drugs may be administered IV acutely or orally for long-term prophylaxis. Recently, mechanical therapies have become preferred for many patients. However, drugs continue to be used as adjunctive therapy, and their complex interactions with these mechanical devices must be appreciated.

Much is now known about the currents and channels that regulate cardiac function, although the precise actions of many antiarrhythmic drugs are still incompletely understood. The activity of individual cardiac myocytes depends on the ion channels in the sarcolemmal membrane, which vary in different regions of the heart. There is also significant variability within particular cardiac regions. For example, the endocardium, mid-myocardium, and epicardium of the ventricles have very different properties. Electrical activity may also be modified by changes in extracellular pH and ions, as during myocardial ischemia. Electrical activity is due to differences in ion concentrations across cell membranes caused by energy-dependent processes. Membrane potential is modulated by channels that open or close in a voltage- and time-dependent manner, allowing specific ions to enter or exit down their electrochemical gradients. As in other excitable tissues, action potentials are propagated throughout the myocardium. Arrhythmias result from disorders in impulse formation, conduction, or both.

Mechanisms of action

Cardiac electrophysiology

An understanding of the mechanisms by which antiarrhythmic drugs act requires an understanding of normal cardiac electrophysiology, because many channels, pumps, and exchangers are targets for these drugs.

Resting potential Cardiac myocytes, like other excitable cells, maintain a transmembrane electrical gradient, with the interior of the cell negative with respect to the exterior. This transmembrane potential is generated by an unequal distribution of charged ions between intracellular and extracellular compartments (Box 14-1). Ions can only traverse the sarcolemmal membrane through selective channels or via pumps and exchangers. The resting potential is an active, energy-dependent process, relying on these channels, pumps and exchangers, and large intracellular immobile anionic proteins. Critical components include the

Box 14-1 Typical ion concentrations

Ion	Extracellular	Intracellular	Approximate Equilibrium Potential (mV)*
Na^+	145 mM	10 mM	+50
K^+	4 mM	140 mM	−90
Ca^{2+}	2 mM	10^{-7} M	+140

*Calculated from Nernst equation.

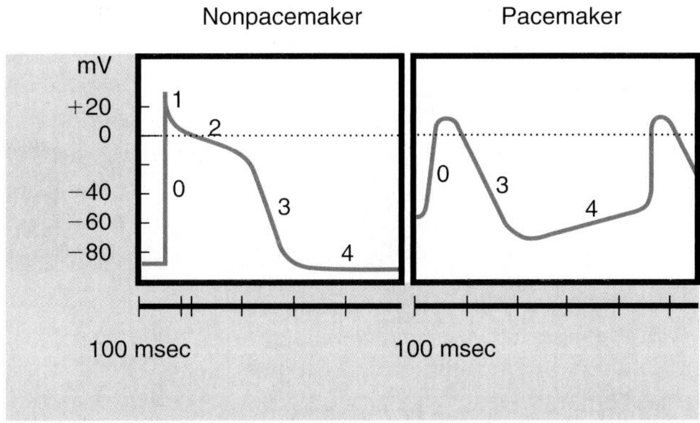

Figure 14-1 Phase of action potential (with respect to potential on extracellular side of cell membrane) in a nonpacemaker cell *(left)* and in a pacemaker cell *(right)*. Numbers refer to phases. **Nonpacemaker cell:** 0, rapid depolarization: 1, initial repolarization; 2, action potential plateau; 3, repolarization; 4, resting potential. **Pacemaker cell:** 0, rapid depolarization; 3, plateau and repolarization; 4, slow diastolic depolarization (pacemaker potential).

Na^+/K^+-ATPase and the inwardly rectifying K^+ channel (I_K). The Na^+/K^+-ATPase exchanges 3 Na^+ ions from the inside of the cell for 2 K^+ ions from the outside, resulting in a net outward flow of positive charge.

Their unequal distribution across the membrane leads to both electrical and chemical forces causing charged ions to move into or out of the cell. If a membrane is permeable to only a single ion, then for that ion, there is an "equilibrium potential" at which there is no net driving force. This can be calculated using the Nernst equation;

$$E_x = RT/F \ln[X]_0/[X]_i \quad (1)$$

where R = the gas constant; T = absolute temperature; F = the Faraday constant; and X is the ion in question. Because the usual intracellular and extracellular concentrations of K^+ are 4 and 140 mM, respectively, its equilibrium potential is −94 mV. At rest, the sarcolemmal membrane is nearly impermeable to Na^+ and Ca^{2+} but highly permeable to K^+. Therefore, the resting potential of most cardiac myocytes approaches the equilibrium potential for K^+ (−80 to −90 mV). However, the sarcolemmal membrane is dynamic, with a constantly changing permeability to various ions and resultant changes in membrane potential. The membrane potential at any given moment can be calculated based on knowledge of ion concentrations and permeabilities but is beyond the scope of this text.

Action potentials As illustrated in Figure 14-1, the cardiac action potential is divided into five phases.

Injection of current into a cardiac myocyte, or local current flow from an adjoining cell, can cause the membrane potential to depolarize (become less negative). If the resting potential exceeds a certain **threshold,** voltage-gated Na^+ channels open (Fig. 14-2). Electrical and chemical gradients drive Na^+ into the cell, making the membrane potential less negative. During **phase 0—rapid depolarization** of the action potential, Na^+ influx is the dominant conductance, and the membrane potential approaches its equilibrium potential (+50 mV). However, Na^+ channels are open for only a very short time and close quickly. They also cycle through an **inactivated** state in which they are unable to open and participate in another action potential. Therefore, if a significant percentage of Na^+ channels are in the inactivated state, the cell is refractory to further stimulation. The maximal rate of depolarization defines how fast electrical impulses can be passed from cell to cell, determining conduction velocity within a tissue. Slowing of conduction due to inhibition of Na^+ channels is the basis for the actions of Class I antiarrhythmic drugs. Action potentials in nonpacemaker cells are referred to as **fast responses** because their rate of depolarization is extremely rapid.

In pacemaker cells, like those in the SA and AV nodes, the resting membrane potential is less negative, and Na^+ channels are inactivated and do not participate in initiation of the action potential. In these cells, phase 0 is mediated almost entirely by increased conductance of Ca^{2+} through opening of voltage-gated Ca^{2+} channels (see Fig. 14-1). These "**slow**" action potentials exhibit much slower depolarization.

The voltage and time dependence of currents through individual ion channels are unique. Na^+ channels open at more negative voltages than Ca^{2+} channels, and current kinetics are quite different. Physical structures, known as activation and inactivation gates, help regulate the flow of ions. Because of these gates, Na^+ channels are believed to exist in at least three distinct states during the cardiac action potential, as shown in Figure 14-2. At the resting potential, most Na^+ channels are in a **resting** state, available for activation. Upon depolarization, most channels become **activated,**

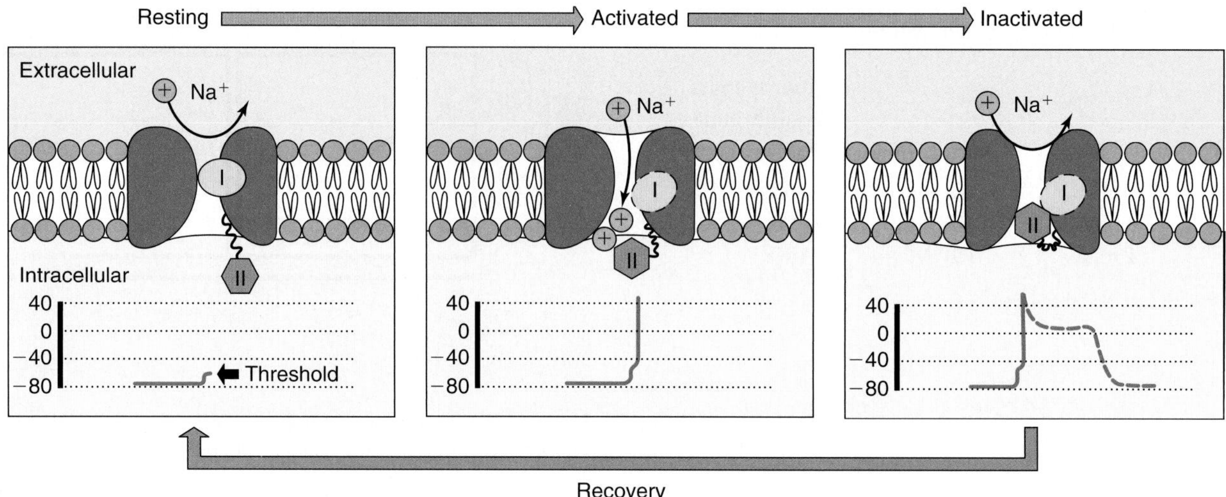

Figure 14-2 Postulated conformational arrangements of cardiac Na^+ channels compatible with concept of resting, activated, and inactivated states. Transitions between resting, activated, and inactivated states are dependent on membrane potential and time. Activation gate is shown as I and inactivation gate as II. Potentials typical for each state are shown under each channel schema as a function of time.

allowing Na^+ to flow into the cell and cause a rapid depolarization. Na^+ channels quickly become **inactivated,** limiting the time for Na^+ entry to a few milliseconds or less.

Near the end of phase 0, an overshoot of the action potential occurs. This is the most positive potential achieved and represents an abrupt transition between the end of depolarization and the onset of repolarization, known as **phase 1—initial rapid repolarization.** This phase of initial repolarization is caused by two factors: inactivation of the inward Na^+ current (described previously) and activation of a transient outward current. The transient outward current is composed of both a K^+ and Cl^- component.

Phase 2—plateau phase of the cardiac action potential is one of its most distinguishing features. In contrast to action potentials in nerves and other cells (see Chapter 30), the cardiac action potential has a relatively long duration of 200 to 500 msec, depending on the cell (see Fig. 14-1). The plateau results from a voltage-dependent decrease in K^+ conductance (the inward rectifier) and is maintained by influx of Ca^{2+} through Ca^{2+} channels that inactivate only slowly at positive membrane potentials. During this phase, another outward K^+ current, the delayed rectifier, is slowly activated, which nearly balances the maintained influx of Ca^{2+}. As a result, there is only a small change in potential during the plateau because net current flow is small.

As the plateau phase transitions to repolarization, the voltage activated Ca^{2+} channels close, leaving the outward hyperpolarizing K^+ current unopposed, known as **phase 3—repolarization.** The hyperpolarizing current during phase 3 is carried through three distinct K^+ channels, the slowly activating delayed rectifier (I_{Ks}), the rapidly activating delayed rectifier (I_{Kr}), and the ultra rapidly activating delayed rectifier (I_{Kur}). The importance to ventricular repolarization of these currents is highlighted by the clinical significance of abnormalities of these channels. The potentially lethal "long QT syndrome" results from abnormalities in the ion channels responsible for repolarization, causing a delay in repolarization and producing an arrhythmic substrate in the ventricles.

In a nonpacemaker cell, **phase 4—resting potential,** is characterized by a return of the membrane to its resting potential. Atrial and ventricular myocytes maintain a constant resting potential awaiting the next depolarizing stimulus, established by a voltage activated K^+ channel, I_{K1}. The resting potential remains slightly depolarized relative to the equilibrium potential of K^+, due to an inward depolarizing leak current likely carried by Na^+. During the terminal portions of phase 3, and all of phase 4, voltage-gated Na^+ channels are recovering from the inactivated into the resting state and preparing to participate in another action potential. In a pacemaker cell, however, there is a **slow depolarization** during diastole. This brings the membrane potential near threshold for activation of a regenerative inward current, which initiates a new action potential (see Fig. 14-1). This is called phase 4 depolarization. In a pacemaker cell in the SA node, phase 4 depolarization brings the membrane potential to a level near the threshold for activation of the inward Ca^{2+} current.

Mechanisms underlying cardiac arrhythmias

Arrhythmias result from disorders of impulse formation, conduction, or both. Several factors may contribute, such as ischemia with resulting pH and electrolyte abnormalities, excessive myocardial fiber stretch, excessive discharge of or sensitivity to autonomic transmitters, and/or exposure to chemicals or toxic substances. Disorders of impulse formation can involve no change in the pacemaker site (e.g., sinus bradycardia or tachycardia) or development of an ectopic pacemaker. Ectopic activity may arise because of emergence of a latent pacemaker, because many cells of the conduction system are capable of rhythmic spontaneous activity. Normally these latent pacemakers are prevented from spontaneously discharging because of the dominance of the rapidly firing SA nodal pacemaker cells. Under some conditions, however, they may become dominant because of abnormal slowing of SA firing rate or abnormal acceleration of latent pacemaker firing rate. Such ectopic activity may result from injury due to ischemia or hypoxia, causing depolarization. Two areas of cells with different membrane potentials may result in current flow between adjacent regions (injury current), which can depolarize normally quiescent tissue to a point where ectopic activity is initiated. Finally, development of oscillatory afterdepolarizations can initiate spontaneous activity in normally quiescent tissue. These afterdepolarizations can occur at the end of phase 3 (Fig. 14-3) and, if large enough in amplitude, reach threshold and initiate a burst of spontaneous activity. Toxic concentrations of digitalis or norepinephrine can initiate such effects. This mechanism has also been proposed to explain ventricular arrhythmias in patients with the long QT syndrome.

Disorders of impulse conduction can result in either bradycardia, as occurs with AV block, or in tachycardia, as when a reentrant circuit develops. Figure 14-4 shows an example of a hypothetical **reentrant circuit.** In order for a reentrant circuit to develop, a region of unidirectional block must exist, and the conduction time around the alternative pathway must exceed the refractory period of the tissue adjacent to the block. Before development of unidirectional block (Fig. 14-4, *A*), impulse propagation initially branches as a result of the anatomical properties of the circuit. Some of these impulses collide and extinguish on the other side of the branch point. If an area of unidirectional block develops, impulses around the branch do not collide and become extinguished but may reexcite tissue proximal to the site of block, establishing a circular pathway for continuous reentry (Fig. 14-4, *B*). Clinical examples include AV reentrant tachycardia (Wolff-Parkinson-White syndrome), AV nodal tachycardia, atrial flutter, and incisional/scar (atrial or ventricular) tachycardia. A long reentry pathway, slow conduction, and a short effective refractory period all favor reentrant circuits.

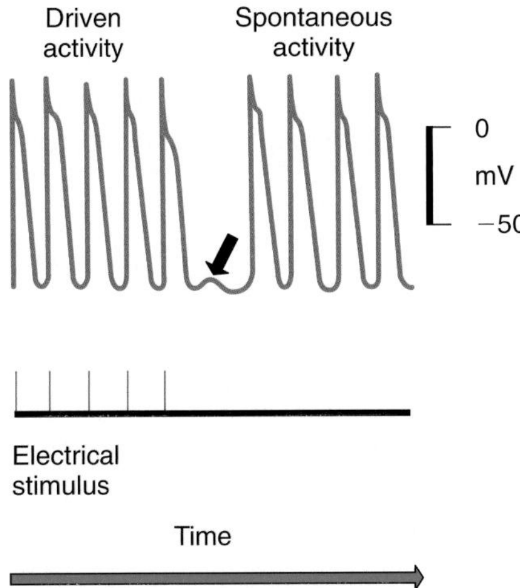

Figure 14-3 Development of oscillatory delayed afterdepolarization *(arrow)* that leads to spontaneous activity, as observed with cardiac glycosides. First five action potentials were elicited by electrical stimuli *(bottom trace)*, followed by an afterdepolarization, which was subthreshold initially but attained threshold subsequently, leading to spontaneous discharges.

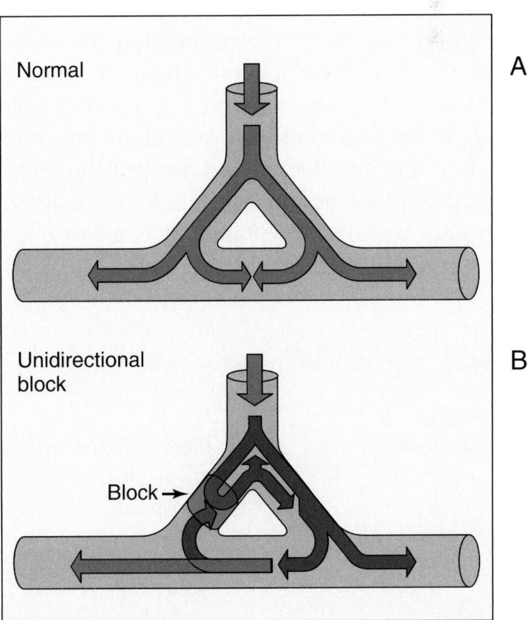

Figure 14-4 Hypothetical reentrant circuit. **A,** Normally electrical excitation branches around the circuit and becomes extinguished because of collision. **B,** An area of unidirectional block develops in one of the branches, allowing excitation of the blocked area by an impulse traveling from the opposite direction. This can lead to reexcitation and reentry.

Antiarrhythmic drugs

Antiarrhythmic drugs affect normal cardiac function and, therefore, have the potential for many serious adverse effects. In the most dramatic example, antiarrhythmic drugs have the potential to actually be proarrhythmic. Therefore, treatment of a tachycardia, which is clinically a nuisance but not life threatening, may initiate a life-threatening ventricular arrhythmia—truly a case of the cure being worse than the disease. Such potentially serious side effects requires vigilance to ensure proper dosing, proper serum levels, a thorough knowledge of drug-drug interactions, and close follow-up.

There is no universally accepted classification scheme for antiarrhythmic agents. The most commonly used scheme, the Vaughan-Williams classification, is based on the presumed primary mechanism of action of individual drugs (Table 14-1). This scheme classifies agents that block voltage-gated Na^+ channels in Class I, those with sympathetic blocking actions in Class II, those that prolong action potential duration and refractoriness in Class III, and those with Ca^{2+}-channel blocking properties in Class IV. However, classification is complicated by the fact that many drugs have multiple actions. As shown in Table 14-2, these drugs often have multiple effects on various targets. Although this scheme is useful in learning the properties of antiarrhythmic agents, all classifications are of limited use for treatment of arrhythmias because of their complex pathophysiology. New classification schemes have emerged, including the "Sicilian Gambit" in 1993. These authors proposed that because all classification systems are fraught with limitations, all clinically relevant actions should be considered and not just the presumed mechanism of drug action. Although this system has failed to gain popular acceptance, it is as an excellent resource for study of these drugs.

Class I antiarrhythmics

Class I agents are subdivided into three groups based on their effects (Table 14-3). Class IA agents slow the rate of rise of phase 0 of the action potential (and slow conduction velocity) and prolong the ventricular refractory period, although not altering resting potential. They directly decrease the slope of phase 4 depolarization in pacemaker cells, especially those arising outside the SA node. Class IB drugs slow conduction and shorten the action potential in nondiseased tissue. The IB agents preferentially act on depolarized myocardium, binding to Na^+ channels in the inactivated state. Drugs in Class IC markedly depress the rate of rise of phase 0 of the action potential. They shorten the refractory period in Purkinje fibers, although not altering the refractory period in adjacent myocardium.

Class IA **Quinidine** was one of the first antiarrhythmic agents used clinically. It has a wide spectrum of activity and has been used to treat both atrial and ventricular arrhythmias. However, its use has significantly diminished due to its high incidence of proarrhythmias and availability of other agents. Quinidine shares most properties with quinine (see Chapter 52). In addition to blocking voltage-gated Na^+ channels, quinidine inhibits the delayed rectifier K^+ channel and has both anticholinergic and antiadrenergic effects. The effect of quinidine on the heart depends on its level of parasympathetic input and the dose. A slight increase in heart rate is seen at low doses due to cholinergic blockade, whereas higher concentrations depress spontaneous diastolic depolarization in pacemaker cells, overwhelming its anticholinergic actions and slowing heart rate.

Quinidine administration results in a dose-dependent depression of responsiveness in atrial and ventricular muscle fibers. The maximum rate of phase 0 depolarization and its amplitude are depressed equally

Table 14-1 Classification of antiarrhythmic agents

Class I (blockers of fast Na^+ channels)	Class II (β-blockers)	Class III (blockers of K^+ channels)	Class IV (blockers of Ca^{2+} channels)
IA	Propranolol	Bretylium	Verapamil
Quinidine	Metoprolol	Amiodarone	Diltiazem
Procainamide	Nadolol	Sotalol	
Disopyramide	Atenolol	Dofetilide	
IB	Acebutolol	Ibutilide	
Lidocaine	Pindolol		
Phenytoin	Sotalol		
Tocainide	Timolol		
Mexiletine	Esmolol		
IC			
Flecainide			
Propafenone			

Table 14-2 Antiarrhythmic drug actions*

	Channels					Receptors				Pumps
	Na^+									Na^+, K^+
Drug	**Fast**	**Medium**	**Slow**	**Ca^{2+}**	**K^+**	**α**	**β**	**M_2**	**P**	**ATPase**
Lidocaine	○									
Mexiletine	○									
Tocainide	○									
Moricizine	●									
Procainamide		○			•					
Disopyramide		•			•			○		
Quinidine		•			●	○		○		
Propafenone		●					●			
Flecainide		●			•					
Encainide			●							
Bepridil	○			●	•					
Verapamil	○			●		•				
Diltiazem				•						
Bretylium					●	▲	▲			
Sotalol					●		●			
Amiodarone	○			○	●	•	•	•		
Ibutilide	△				●					
Propranolol	○						●			
Atropine								●		
Adenosine									△	
Digoxin								△		●
Dofetilide					●					

Antagonist; relative potency—○, low; •, moderate; ●, high; △, agonist; ▲, agonist/antagonist; M_2, cardiac muscarinic receptors; P, purinergic receptors.

*Drug targets are arranged in columns. Drugs are listed in order of their predominant actions, so that symbols form a diagonal. Other actions appear as deviations from the diagonal. Relative potency is designated by the size of the symbol. Na^+ channel blockers are listed in order of decreasing potency and rate of association (fast, medium, slow).

Table 14-3 Differences among class I antiarrhythmic drugs

Class	Phase O Depression	Repolarization	Action Potential Duration
IA	Moderate	Prolonged	Increased
IB	Weak	Shortened	Decreased
IC	Strong	No effect	No effect

at all membrane potentials. Quinidine also decreases excitability; actions that are often referred to as "local anesthetic" properties.

Quinidine also prolongs repolarization in Purkinje fibers and ventricular muscle, resulting in an increase in action potential duration. An increased refractoriness known as "postrepolarization refractoriness" has been observed. The indirect anticholinergic properties of quinidine are not a factor in its actions on ventricular muscle and Purkinje fibers.

Procainamide, like quinidine, increases the effective refractory period and decreases conduction velocity in the atria, His-Purkinje system, and ventricles. Although having weaker anticholinergic actions than quinidine, it also has variable effects on the AV node. Procainamide increases the threshold for excitation in atrium and ventricle, as well as slowing phase 4 depolarization–a combination that decreases abnormal automaticity. Procainamide is used in treatment of atrial arrhythmias, such as premature atrial contractions, paroxysmal atrial tachycardia, and atrial fibrillation of recent onset, in addition to being effective for most ventricular arrhythmias. Due to proarrhythmia risks, treatment should be limited to hemodynamically significant arrhythmias. Long-term therapy is complicated by the need for frequent dosing and side effects (see later).

Disopyramide suppresses atrial and ventricular arrhythmias and has a longer duration of action than other drugs in its class. Although effective in treating atrial arrhythmias, disopyramide is only approved to treat ventricular arrhythmias in the United States. Despite prominent anticholinergic effects, disopyramide has a pronounced negative inotropic effect, which is so prominent it has been used in therapy of hypertrophic cardiomyopathy. The electrophysiological effects of disopyramide are nearly identical to those of quinidine and procainamide. However, its anticholinergic effects are far more prominent and limit its utility. Disopyramide blocks voltage-gated Na^+ channels, thereby depressing action potentials. Disopyramide also reduces conduction velocity and increases the refractory period in atria. Postrepolarization refractoriness does not occur. Interestingly, abnormal atrial automaticity may be abolished at disopyramide concentrations that fail to alter conduction velocity or refractoriness. Conduction velocity slows and the refractory period increases in the AV node via a direct action, which is offset to a variable degree by its anticholinergic actions. Action potential duration is prolonged, which results in an increase in refractory period of the His-Purkinje and ventricular muscle tissue. Slowed conduction in accessory pathways has been demonstrated. Like quinidine, the effect of disopyramide on conduction velocity depends on extracellular K^+ concentrations. Hypokalemic patients may respond poorly to its antiarrhythmic action, whereas hyperkalemia may accentuate its actions.

Class IB **Lidocaine** is a local anesthetic (see Chapter 30) that has long been used to treat arrhythmias. Unlike quinidine, lidocaine blocks both activated and inactivated Na^+ channels and does so rapidly. Lidocaine's block of Na^+ channels in the inactivated state leads to greater effects on myocytes with long action potentials, such as Purkinje and ventricular cells, compared with atrial cells. The rapid kinetics of lidocaine at normal resting potentials result in recovery from block between action potentials, with no effect on conduction velocity. In partially depolarized cells (such as those injured by ischemia) lidocaine significantly depresses membrane responsiveness, leading to conduction delay and block. Lidocaine also elevates the ventricular fibrillation threshold.

Mexiletine is a derivative of lidocaine that is orally active. Its actions and side effects are similar to those of lidocaine. As with other members of class IB, mexiletine slows the maximal rate of depolarization of the cardiac action potential, and exerts a negligible effect on repolarization. Mexiletine also blocks the Na^+ channel with rapid kinetics, making it more effective in control of rapid, as opposed to slow, ventricular tachyarrhythmias and ineffective in treating atrial arrhythmias.

Phenytoin is an anticonvulsive agent (see Chapter 27) that has been used as an antiarrhythmic agent for decades. Its actions are similar to those of lidocaine. It depresses membrane responsiveness in the ventricular myocardium and His-Purkinje system to a greater extent than in the atrium.

Class IC **Flecainide** was initially developed as a local anesthetic and, subsequently, found to have antiarrhythmic effects. Flecainide blocks Na^+ channels, causing slowing of conduction in all parts of the heart, most notably in the His-Purkinje system and ventricles. There are minor effects on repolarization. Flecainide also inhibits abnormal automaticity.

Propafenone also results in conduction slowing due to Na^+ channel blockade. Propafenone is also a weak β-adrenergic receptor antagonist with a much lower potency than propranolol, as well as an L-type Ca^{2+} channel blocker.

Class II antiarrhythmics: β-adrenergic blockers

The antiarrhythmic properties of β-adrenergic receptor antagonists result from two major actions: (1) blockade of myocardial β_1-adrenergic receptors, and (2) direct membrane-stabilizing effects at higher concentrations related to blockade of Na^+ channels. A more complete discussion of these drugs is provided in Chapter 10.

Propranolol is the prototypical β-adrenergic receptor blocker, and, in addition to blocking β_1-receptors in the heart, also has direct membrane-stabilizing effects in atrium, ventricle, and His-Purkinje system. It causes a slowing of SA nodal and ectopic pacemaker automaticity and decreases AV nodal conduction velocity by virtue of its ability to block intrinsic sympathetic activity. There is little change in action potential duration and refractoriness in atrium, ventricle, or AV node. Currently used β-blockers (see Table 14-1) may be differentiated by their pharmacokinetics, selectivity for β_1-receptors, lipophilicity, and intrinsic sympathomimetic effects (see Chapter 10).

Class III antiarrhythmics

In the late 1980s, the Cardiac Arrhythmia Suppression Trial was undertaken using Na^+ channel blockers (encainide and flecainide) in patients following myocardial infarction to suppress arrhythmias. The study was terminated because of an increased mortality in patients treated with Na^+ channel blockers. Subsequently, attention has been focused on delaying repolarization and prolonging the refractory period.

Amiodarone is classified as a Class III agent due to its action potential prolonging effects, however, it has an extremely complex and incompletely understood spectrum of actions. In addition to prolonging action potentials as a result of blockade of several types of K^+ channels, amiodarone also blocks both Na^+ and Ca^{2+} channels (Class I and IV effects) as well as being a noncompetitive β-receptor blocker (Class II effect). The acute effects of amiodarone administration also differ from chronic effects, which may, in part, be explained by its complex pharmacokinetics (see later).

Sotalol prolongs the action potential by inhibiting the delayed rectifier K^+ channel. Sotalol is available as either the isolated *d*-isomer or as the racemic *d,l*-mixture. In addition to its action potential prolonging effects, *d,l*-sotalol is a nonselective β-adrenergic blocking agent (Class II effect) without membrane stabilizing effects and a low lipid solubility. β-blocking effects are most evident at low doses, with action potential prolonging effects predominating at high doses. The *d*-isomer, which is a pure Class III agent and devoid of β-blocking action, was found in clinical trials to increase mortality in post-infarcted patients. *d*-Sotalol and several other agents were thought to selectively block myocardial K^+ channels involved in initiating action potential repolarization. However, development of *d*-sotalol was halted when it was found to be associated with increased mortality.

Ibutilide is structurally related to sotalol. Like other Class III agents, it leads to action potential prolongation. Its unique property is that, in addition to blocking the delayed rectifier K^+ channel, it also activates a slow inward Na^+ channel, both of which delay repolarization.

Bretylium is a unique Class III agent first introduced for treatment of essential hypertension but, subsequently, shown to suppress ventricular fibrillation associated with acute myocardial infarction. Bretylium selectively accumulates in sympathetic ganglia and postganglionic adrenergic neurons and inhibits norepinephrine release. Bretylium has been demonstrated experimentally to increase action potential duration and effective refractory period without changing heart rate.

Dofetilide is a "pure" Class III agent that selectively blocks the rapid component of the delayed rectifier K^+ current (I_{Kr}). At clinically relevant concentrations, dofetilide has no effect on any other K^+, Na^+ or Ca^{2+} channels, and no adrenergic receptor blockade. The increase in effective refractory period is observed in both atria and ventricles. Dofetilide has been approved for use in atrial arrhythmias. Its effects are dependent on the concentration of extracellular K^+ and are exaggerated by hypokalemia, which is important in patients receiving diuretics. Conversely, hyperkalemia decreases its effects, which may limit its efficacy in conditions such as myocardial ischemia.

Class IV antiarrhythmics

Ca^{2+}-channel-blocking drugs are discussed in Chapter 12. Ca^{2+} channel blockers are used to slow the rate of AV-conduction in patients with atrial fibrillation or to slow ectopic atrial pacemakers. Ca^{2+} channel blockers have also been used for treating idiopathic left ventricular tachycardia arising from the posterior fascicle.

Nonclassified antiarrhythmics

Adenosine is an endogenous nucleoside produced from metabolism of adenosine triphosphate. Adenosine activates the same G-protein coupled outward K^+ current as acetylcholine (see Chapter 9). Adenosine receptors are located on atrial myocytes, and myocytes in the SA and AV nodes, and stimulation leads to hyperpolarization of the resting potential. Effects include a decrease in slope of phase 4 spontaneous depolarizations and shortening of action potential durations. Effects are most dramatic in the AV node and results in transient conduction block. This effect terminates tachycardias, which utilize the AV node as a limb of a reentrant circuit. There is no effect on ventricular myocardium, because this K^+ channel does not occur in ventricle.

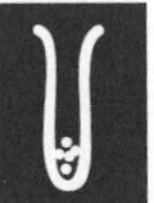

Pharmacokinetics

Pharmacokinetic parameters of selected antiarrhythmic drugs are summarized in Table 14-4. Pharmacokinetics of β-adrenergic blockers are discussed in Chapter 10 and Ca^{2+}-channel blocking drugs in Chapter 12.

Quinidine is readily absorbed from the gastrointestinal (GI) tract. It is metabolized in liver and excreted by the kidneys. Therefore, both hepatic and renal functions must be assessed in patients to prevent the accumulation of toxic concentrations in plasma. **Procainamide** is metabolized in liver by acetylation to N-acetylprocainamide (NAPA), which has Class III actions and a longer serum half life than procainamide. In the United States, approximately half of the population (90% of Asians) is homozygous for the N-acetyl transferase gene and are termed rapid acetylators (see Chapter 3). These individuals have a higher concentration of plasma NAPA than of procainamide at steady state. When its concentration exceeds 5 ng/ml, NAPA can contribute to the antiarrhythmic actions of procainamide because of its Class III actions that prolong repolarization. Concentrations greater than 20 ng/ml have been associated with adverse effects, including *torsades de pointes*.

Lidocaine is inactive when administered orally because of a high first-pass metabolism. It is therefore usually given IV for acute treatment of cardiac arrhythmias. Because most drug is metabolized, liver function is important. The main route of metabolism is N-dealkylation, which produces metabolites with only mild antiarrhythmic activity but potent central nervous system (CNS) toxicity.

Mexiletine does not have a large first-pass effect, with a bioavailability in the range of 90% to 100%. However, its half-life is about 35% less in smokers than nonsmokers, probably due to induction of hepatic enzymes. Other inducers, such as barbiturates, phenytoin,

Table 14-4 Selected pharmacokinetic parameters

Drug	% Plasma Protein Bound	Half-Life (hrs unless noted)	Disposition	Therapeutic Serum Concentration (μg/ml)
Class IA				
Quinidine (O, IV)	80	5-7	M/R (50%)	2-5
Procainamide (O, IV)	15	2.5-5	M (20%)/R (50%)	4-10
Disopyramide (O)	35-65	4.5	M (30%)/R (50%)	2-5
Class IB				
Lidocaine (IV)	60	1-2	M (90%)/R (10%)	10-20
Mexiletine (O)	50-60	9-11	M/R (20%)*	0.5-2
Phenytoin (O, IV)	70-95	22	M (90%)/R	10-20
Class IC				
Flecainide (O)	40	13	M (60%)/R (30%)*	0.2-1
Propafenone (O)	—	2-10	M*	0.2-1.5
Class III				
Amiodarone (O, IV)	96	20-100 days	M/bile	1-2.5
Sotalol (O)	0	10-15	R	1-4
Ibutilide (IV)	40	3-4	M/R	—
Dofetilide	60-70	7-10	M (minimal)/R	—
Bretylium	0	8-13	R	—
Nontyped				
Adenosine	—	<10 seconds	RBC	—

O, Oral; *IV*, intravenous; *M*, hepatic metabolism; *R*, renal elimination as unchanged drug (% by this pathway if known); *RBCs*, metabolized by red blood cells; *, polymorphic metabolism. Class II and Class IV drugs are covered in Chapters 10 and 12, respectively.

and rifampin, also increase metabolism of mexiletine. Antacids, cimetidine, and narcotic analgesics slow its absorption from the GI tract.

The long plasma half-life of **phenytoin** shows considerable interpatient variation. Drugs that influence liver microsomal drug metabolism can significantly alter its half-life. Considerable interpatient diversity is also observed for **flecainide**; metabolism and renal elimination are the major pathways of inactivation.

Therapy with several antiarrhythmic drugs is complicated by the fact that they are predominantly metabolized by a specific cytochrome P450 that is genetically polymorphically distributed, with a bimodal pattern of distribution in Caucasians. Seven percent of Caucasians (1% of Asians and African-Americans) are homozygous for mutations that result in low levels of, or no, active enzyme. These people, usually termed **poor metabolizers**, show a very slow elimination of many drugs, including several antiarrhythmics (e.g., flecainide, mexiletine, propafenone, disopyramide, metoprolol, timolol). They also show greater β-blockade when given usual doses of β-blockers and have higher plasma concentrations of flecainide or mexiletine and exhibit greater Na^+ channel blockade when given usual doses. Because they cannot be routinely identified before initiation of therapy, all patients must be started at low doses.

Amiodarone's pharmacokinetics are extremely complex. It is metabolized by *N*-deethylation by cytochrome P-450s (CYP3A4) to *N*-desethylamiodarone. Serum concentrations of this potentially active metabolite are highly variable and may relate to the large interindividual variability in CYP3A4 activity. Amiodarone is eliminated by biliary excretion with negligible excretion in urine. Amiodarone and its metabolite cross the placenta and appear in breast milk.

Ibutilide's pharmacokinetics are highly variable. Eight metabolites are generated by progressive oxidation, with renal excretion. Only one possesses any antiarrhythmic effects and its concentrations are low. Due to extensive first-pass metabolism, ibutilide must be given IV.

Adenosine is taken up by erythrocytes and vascular endothelial cells and metabolized to inosine and adenosine monophosphate. Hepatic and renal dysfunction do not effect its metabolism. Its effects are potentiated by nucleoside transport blockers, such as dipyridamole, and antagonized by methylxanthines, like caffeine and theophylline.

Relation of mechanisms of action to clinical response

Quinidine has potent anticholinergic properties. These properties cause opposite effects to those due to its direct effects in parasympathetically innervated regions of the heart. After initial administration, there may be a small SA nodal tachycardia and an increase in AV nodal conduction velocity (decrease in PR interval) as a result of its indirect anticholinergic effects. These are usually followed by direct effects, including a decrease in heart rate and a slowing of AV nodal conduction velocity (increase in PR interval). At therapeutic concentrations, the QRS complex often shows slight widening as a result of a decrease in ventricular conduction velocity. The QT interval is lengthened because of the prolonged action potential in the ventricular myocardium.

Procainamide and **disopyramide** depress automaticity in SA nodal cells as well as ectopic pacemakers. Procainamide has much less anticholinergic effect than quinidine. Therefore, its effects on heart rate and AV nodal conduction velocity are more direct and usually involve a decrease in heart rate and a slight prolongation of the PR interval. Disopyramide, however, has similar, if not more, potent anticholinergic properties than quinidine. Therefore, it has the same indirect and direct effects on heart rate and AV conduction velocity as quinidine. When disopyramide is given for treatment of atrial flutter or fibrillation, a digitalis glycoside will often be coadministered to minimize its anticholinergic properties. Procainamide and disopyramide block Na^+ channels and slightly prolong the QRS complex. However, the major metabolite of procainamide, NAPA, is a potent Class III agent and prolongs the QT interval during oral therapy. Therefore, a widening of the QRS complex and a lengthening of the QT interval are also observed after administration of these agents. Both compounds are broad-spectrum antiarrhythmics used to treat supraventricular and ventricular arrhythmias.

Lidocaine has little effect on automaticity within the SA node over a relatively large concentration range, and hence heart rate remains relatively normal. Conversely, lidocaine suppresses automaticity in ectopic ventricular pacemakers and Purkinje fibers. Shortening of the action potential and effective refractory period is possible and is more prominent in Purkinje fibers than in ventricular myocardium. Lidocaine has little effect on AV nodal conduction and at therapeutic concentrations has minimal effect on the resting electrocardiogram. Lidocaine is used exclusively for ventricular arrhythmias, especially those associated with acute myocardial infarction. It has no efficacy in treatment of supraventricular arrhythmia, such as atrial flutter or fibrillation. Lidocaine is used for the treatment of digitalis-induced arrhythmias.

Phenytoin depresses the automaticity of both SA nodal cells and ectopic pacemakers. Though devoid of anticholinergic properties it increases AV nodal conduction velocity by an unknown mechanism. Phenytoin results in a small decrease in the PR and QT intervals on electrocardiogram. Its use is limited to management of postoperative arrhythmias and digitalis toxicity in pediatric patients.

Flecainide and **propafenone** depress SA nodal automaticity and slow AV nodal conduction. They may produce conduction block in patients with preexisting AV nodal conduction disturbances. At therapeutic concentrations, prolongation of the PR and QRS intervals are seen. Both drugs also cause conduction slowing in accessory pathways contributing to their effectiveness in treating AV reentrant tachycardia. Drugs in Class IC should be used with extreme caution in patients with structural heart disease and anyone with concerns for myocardial ischemia.

β-Adrenergic receptor blockers at therapeutic doses prolong the PR interval with occasional shortening of the QT interval. These drugs are reasonably efficacious in suppressing ventricular ectopic pacemakers and are first-line therapy for most supraventricular and ventricular arrhythmias. They have been demonstrated to be effective in decreasing overall mortality rate following a myocardial infarction. β-Adrenergic receptor antagonists, such as metoprolol and acebutolol (but not propranolol) have a greater selectivity for β_1-receptors than for β_2-receptors (see Chapter 10). There are also differences between these compounds with regard to their effects on cardiac channels and their intrinsic sympathomimetic activities. Esmolol, a short acting agent, may be used for acute conversion or ventricular rate control.

Bretylium is used in emergency treatment of ventricular fibrillation.

Amiodarone is considered a Class III agent because of its prolongation of the action potential and refractory period. It profoundly depresses SA nodal automaticity and that of ectopic pacemakers. Effects on the electrocardiogram include prolongation of the PR, QRS, and QT intervals. It has become perhaps the most widely used agent due to its effectiveness in suppressing ventricular and supraventricular arrhythmias refractory to other drugs, however, its systemic toxicity and highly variable half-life make it necessary to use extreme caution during therapy.

Sotalol is marketed as the racemic mixture for treatment of life-threatening ventricular arrhythmias. At low doses, its predominant antiarrhythmic effect results from β-adrenergic blockade. At higher doses, its effects on K^+ channels predominate, thereby increasing atrial and ventricular refractoriness. Sotalol prolongs repolarization and increases the QT interval. The risk for a drug-induced, potentially life-threatening ventricular arrhythmia *(torsades des pointes)*, is 3% to 5% and necessitates initiation of therapy in an inpatient setting. Like amiodarone, sotalol has a profound effect on SA node activity and can magnify SA node dysfunction. It is used in treatment of supraventricular arrhythmias and ventricular arrhythmias but should be reserved for use in life-threatening arrhythmias, due to its high risk of ventricular proarrhythmias.

Ibutilide is used for conversion of atrial fibrillation or flutter. It is an alternative to electrical cardioversion and is effective in 60% to 80% of patients. Like other QT prolonging drugs, its use is associated with a relatively high incidence of *torsades des pointes.*

Ca^{2+}-channel blockers are most effective in treating supraventricular arrhythmias, which involve reentry and may also be effective in treating arrhythmias resulting from enhanced automaticity. Their ability to slow AV nodal conduction velocity and refractoriness makes them useful for controlling ventricular rate. Ca^{2+}-channel blockers are rarely used to treat ventricular arrhythmias, although they may be effective for treating a form of idiopathic fascicular ventricular tachycardia.

Digitalis glycosides slow conduction velocity and increase the refractory period in the AV node. They may be useful in treatment of supraventricular tachycardias, such as atrial flutter and fibrillation, by slowing conduction through the AV node and helping to control ventricular rate.

Adenosine is useful for terminating reentrant supraventricular tachycardias that involve the AV node, where it causes conduction block. Adenosine has a serum half-life of approximately 5 seconds, limiting its clinical usefulness to bolus IV therapy.

Side effects, clinical problems, and toxicity

Major problems are summarized in the Clinical Problems box, although information about β-blockers and Ca^{2+}-channel blockers are given in Chapters 10 and 12.

CLINICAL PROBLEMS

Drug	Problems
Quinidine	Diarrhea, precipitates arrhythmias; *torsades de pointes,* elevates digoxin concentrations, vagolytic effects
Procainamide	Arrhythmias, granulocytopenia, fever, rash, lupus-like syndrome
Disopyramide	Precipitates congestive heart failure, anticholinergic effects
Lidocaine	CNS effects (dizziness, seizures), first-pass metabolism
Phenytoin	CNS effects, allergy
Mexiletine	CNS and GI effects
Flecainide	Negative inotropic effect, proarrhythmogenic, CNS side effects
Propafenone	CNS effects, proarrhythmogenic
β-Blockers	Negative inotropic and chronotropic effects; precipitates congestive heart failure, AV conduction block
Bretylium	Hypotension, nausea
Amiodarone	Hypotension, pneumonitis, bradycardia; precipitates congestive heart failure, photosensitivity, thyroid abnormalities
Sotalol	Modest negative inotropic and chronotropic effects, *torsades des pointes*
Verapamil	Hypotension, negative inotropic and chronotropic effects
Dofetilide	*Torsades de pointes*
Ibutilide	*Torsades de pointes*
Adenosine	Atrial fibrillation, bronchospasm, prolonged AV block, flushing

Quinidine's use is limited by adverse side effects that are generally dose related and reversible. Common effects include diarrhea, upper-GI distress, and lightheadedness. The most worrisome side effects are related to its cardiac toxicity and include AV and intraventricular conduction block, ventricular tachyarrhythmias, and depression of myocardial contractility. "Quinidine syncope," which is a loss of consciousness resulting from ventricular tachycardia, may be fatal. This devastating side effect is more common in women and may occur at therapeutic or subtherapeutic concentrations. Quinidine is a potent inhibitor of CYP2D6 and CYP3A4 and interacts with many other drugs.

Procainamide administration may result in hypotension, AV block, intraventricular block, ventricular tachyarrhythmias, and complete heart block. Decreased dosing or discontinuation of drug is necessary, if severe depression of conduction (severe prolongation of the QRS interval) or repolarization (severe prolongation of the QT interval) occurs. Long-term treatment is problematic due to induction of a lupus-like syndrome. Increased antinuclear antibody titers are present in over 80% of patients treated for over 6 months; whereas 30% of patients develop a clinical lupus-like syndrome. Symptoms may disappear within a few days of cessation of therapy, although clinical tests remain positive for several months. Prolonged administration should be accompanied by hematological studies because agranulocytosis may occur. Procainamide has little potential to produce CNS toxicity.

Disopyramide's negative inotropic effects may precipitate heart failure in patients with or without preexisting depression of left ventricular function. Parasympatholytic effects, including urinary retention, dry mouth, blurred vision, constipation, and worsening of preexisting glaucoma (see Chapter 9), may require discontinuation of therapy. Disopyramide should not be used in patients with uncompensated congestive heart failure, glaucoma, hypotension, urinary retention, and baseline prolonged QT interval.

Lidocaine does not have negative hemodynamic effects at therapeutic concentrations and is well tolerated, even in significant ventricular dysfunction, however, excessively rapid injection or high doses may cause asystole. Most toxic side effects are caused by its local anesthetic effects on the CNS, and include drowsiness, tremor, nausea, hearing disturbances, slurred speech paresthesias, disorientation, and at high doses, psychosis, respiratory depression, and convulsions.

Mexiletine and **tocainamide** have similar actions and side effects as lidocaine, but pharmacokinetic differences allow their oral use. At higher concentrations, mexiletine may produce reversible nausea and vomiting, and CNS effects (dizziness/light-headedness, tremor, nervousness, coordination difficulties, changes in sleep habits, paresthesias/numbness, weakness, fatigue, tinnitus and confusion/clouded sensorium). Most are manageable with downward dose titration. Mexiletine can inhibit ventricular escape rhythms and is contraindicated in the presence of preexisting second- or third-degree AV block, unless the patient has an indwelling pacemaker.

Phenytoin at high levels is associated with adverse CNS effects, including vertigo, nystagmus, ataxia, tremors, slurring of speech, and sedation. Because of its long half-life and the nonlinear relationship between dose and clearance, considerable variations in response to an oral dose are typical. Rapid IV administration may produce transient hypotension from peripheral vasodilation and direct negative inotropic effects.

Flecainide's side effects include dizziness, blurred vision, headache, and nausea. Data from the Cardiac Arrhythmia Suppression Trial suggest that all Class IC drugs are thought to carry an added proarrhythmic risk, and their use has been reserved for life-threatening arrhythmias, particularly in structural heart disease. Flecainide may also slow conduction in a reentrant circuit without terminating it. This may lead to accelerating the ventricular rate during atrial flutter because fewer atrial beats are blocked due to the slower cycle length, and it may also lead to converting a rapid but self-limited AV-reentrant (accessory pathway mediated) tachycardia into a slower but persistent arrhythmia.

Propafenone may cause new or worsened arrhythmias. Similar to flecainide, most proarrhythmic events occurred during the first week of therapy, although late events were observed, suggesting that an increased risk is present throughout treatment. Agranulocytosis has been reported in patients receiving propafenone, generally within the first 2 months of therapy and resolving upon discontinuation. Liver metabolism necessitates careful administration to patients with hepatic dysfunction. Also, a small segment of the population has a genetic abnormality of CYP2D6, which is responsible for propafenone's metabolism.

β-Adrenergic receptor antagonists should be used with caution when combined with other drugs that also slow AV nodal conduction velocity because their effects may be synergistic. β-Adrenergic receptor antagonists are generally contraindicated in patients with existing AV nodal conduction disturbances, congestive heart failure, or bronchial asthma. Their toxicity and side effects are described in Chapter 10.

Amiodarone therapy is fraught with multiple complications, both cardiac and systemic. Major side effects of IV administration are hypotension, heart block, and bradycardia. Oral therapy is frequently complicated by toxic effects, some lethal. The most feared noncardiac complication is pulmonary fibrosis. Pulmonary fibrosis has an insidious onset and may occur as early as 7 weeks or as late as years after starting treatment. It is more frequent in patients receiving doses exceeding 400 mg but was seen in a patient taking 200 mg per day. Close monitoring of pulmonary status is required during chronic amiodarone therapy, because this is a potentially fatal condition that may not resolve with discontinuation. Other serious side effects include hypothyroidism, hyperthyroidism, photosensitivity, rash, slate-blue skin discoloration, severe nausea, and chemical hepatitis. In terms of cardiac toxicity, although amiodarone prolongs the QTc dramatically, the risk of *torsade des pointes* is relatively low compared with other Class III agents. Amiodarone magnifies any sinus node dysfunction and may require pacemaker placement, if ongoing therapy is necessary.

Sotalol has fewer systemic side effects than amiodarone but a higher incidence of ventricular proarrhythmias. In patients with a history of ventricular tachycardia, the use of sotalol was associated with an incidence of *torsade des pointes* of 4%. In patients with no history of ventricular arrhythmias, the risk was approximately 1%. Because of this risk, initiation of therapy should be performed as an inpatient. The β-receptor blocking effects of sotalol make it contraindicated in patients with asthma. Sotalol exacerbates sinus node dysfunction and may aggravate second- and third-degree AV block with suppression of ectopic ventricular pacemakers. Therefore, its use for patients with such conditions should be restricted unless a functioning pacemaker is present. Other contraindications include congenital or acquired long QT syndromes, cardiogenic shock, and uncontrolled congestive heart failure.

Dofetilide prolongs repolarization and the QTc, which increases the risk of *torsade des pointes*. A clinical trial that evaluated the use of dofetilide in patients following myocardial infarction demonstrated no increased mortality, which is different than results from trials with sotalol or flecainide and encainide. The risks of *torsade des pointes* in patients treated for atrial fibrillation is 0.8%. Dofetilide should not be used in patients with a prolonged QTc at baseline.

Bretylium is not considered a first-choice antiarrhythmic agent because of its toxicity and side effects. It is primarily used to stabilize cardiac rhythm in patients with ventricular fibrillation or recurrent tachycardia resistant to other treatments. Its most severe side effect is persistent hypotension, caused by peripheral vasodilation due to adrenergic nerve blockade. Also, catecholamine release can transiently enhance ectopic pacemaker activity and cause increases in myocardial oxygen consumption in patients with ischemic heart disease. Nausea and vomiting are also common side effects.

Adenosine leads to transient AV-block, which is generally well tolerated. Prolonged AV-block may be observed in patients with AV-node disease, and profound sinus bradycardia may be observed in patients with sick sinus syndrome. Patients following heart transplantation have also been documented to have a prolonged effect from adenosine. Adenosine shortens the refractory period of atrial myocytes, which may lead to initiation of atrial fibrillation. In patients with Wolff-Parkinson-White syndrome, this may result in rapid conduction across the accessory pathway, which is not blocked by adenosine and ventricular fibrillation. Adenosine may also trigger bronchospasm in patients with asthma. Although the half life of adenosine is less than 10 seconds, the bronchospasm may persist for up to 30 minutes. The mechanism is unknown.

New horizons

Antiarrhythmic therapy is rapidly changing. Increasingly, mechanical therapy via transcatheter methods, such as radiofrequency ablation or implanted devices, such as pacemakers and defibrillators, are being used to control abnormal heart rhythms. Antiarrhythmic drug therapy is being used in conjunction with these therapies, and an appreciation of the interactions between drugs and devices is important. Antiarrhythmic drugs can dramatically affect the performance of implanted devices. Certain compounds may increase the amount of energy devices need to either pace or defibrillate the heart. Amiodarone, flecainide, lidocaine, propafenone, and mexiletine all lead to increased defibrillation thresholds, whereas sotalol and dofetilide cause them to decrease.

All antiarrhythmic drugs interact with ion channels that participate in the normal action potential, and therefore interfere with the normal function of the heart. Identification of ion channels that may participate in pathological states only would make ideal drug targets. One possibility is the ATP-gated K^+ channel. This large conductance K^+ channel is found in many tissues, including heart, pancreas, and vasculature. It is normally tonically inhibited by physiological intracellular concentrations of ATP. When intracellular ATP falls and the ATP/ADP ratio is altered, the channel opens, leading to rapid repolarization and a shortened refractory period. This predisposes the tissue to reentrant arrhythmias. The ability to block this channel, which does not participate in the normal action potential, is an attractive target.

Similarly, targeting ion channels specific to a heart chamber of interest presents an interesting possibility. For example, the ultra-rapidly activating component of the inward rectifier potassium channel (I_{Kur}) has been identified in humans in atrium only and not ventricles. If it were possible to target channels in the atrium, the risk of ventricular proarrhythmia would be abolished and make drug therapy much safer.

New uses for old drugs are also being investigated. Examples include the use of Na^+ channel blockers, such as mexiletine for long QT syndrome type 3 and the use of quinidine for the short QT syndrome. Both of these are potentially lethal abnormalities of cardiac repolarization with no current effective medical therapy.

TRADE NAMES

In addition to generic and fixed-combination preparations, the following trade-named materials are some of the important compounds available in the United States. See Chapters 10 and 12 for trade names of β-adrenergic receptor blocking drugs and Ca^{2+}-blocking drugs, respectively.

Amiodarone (Cordarone)
Bretylium (Bretylol)
Disopyramide (Norpace)
Dofetilide (Tikosyn)
Flecainide (Tambocor)
Ibutilide (Corvert)
Lidocaine (Xylocaine)
Mexiletine (Mexitil)
Phenytoin (Dilantin)
Procainamide (Procan SR, Pronestyl)
Propafenone (Rythmol)
Quinidine (Quinidex, Extentabs, Quinaglute, Quinora)
Tocainide (Tonocard)

FURTHER READING

Roden DM. Drug-induced prolongation of the QT interval. *N Engl J Med* 2004; 350(10):1013-1022.

Varro A, Biliczki P, Iost N, et al. Theoretical possibilities for the development of novel antiarrhythmic drugs. *Curr Med Chem* 2004; 11(1):1-11.

Wijffels MC, Crijns HJ. Recent advances in drug therapy for atrial fibrillation. *J Cardiovasc Electrophysiol* 2003; 14(9 suppl):S40-S47.

Self-assessment questions

1. Which electrophysiological actions does amiodarone possess?
   a. Class I
   b. Class II
   c. Class III
   d. Class IV
   e. All of the above

2. The plateau (phase 2) of a nonpacemaker cardiac cell is caused by:
   a. An increased conductance to all ions and a delayed efflux of Ca^{2+}, which balances a slowly decreasing efflux of K^{+}.
   b. A reduced conductance to all ions and a delayed influx of Ca^{2+}, which balances a slowly decreasing efflux of K^{+}.
   c. A reduced conductance to all ions and a delayed influx of Ca^{2+}, which balances a slowly increasing efflux of K^{+}.
   d. A reduced conductance to all ions and a delayed influx of Ca^{2+}, which balances a slowly increasing influx of K^{+}.
   e. None of the above.

3. Which of the following agents is not orally active?
   a. Propranolol
   b. Quinidine
   c. Lidocaine
   d. Verapamil
   e. Phenytoin

4. The use of propranolol as an antiarrhythmic agent is contraindicated in patients with:
   a. Severe AV node block.
   b. Uncompensated heart failure.
   c. Bronchial asthma.
   d. None of the above.
   e. *a, b,* and *c.*

5. All of the following are associated with chronic amiodarone use *except:*
   a. Hyperthyroidism.
   b. Chemical hepatitis.
   c. Depression.
   d. Hypothyroidism.
   e. Photosensitivity.

6. Which of the following are associated with a risk of inducing *torsades de pointes?*
   a. Sotalol
   b. Procainamide
   c. Verapamil
   d. Ibutilide
   e. Amiodarone

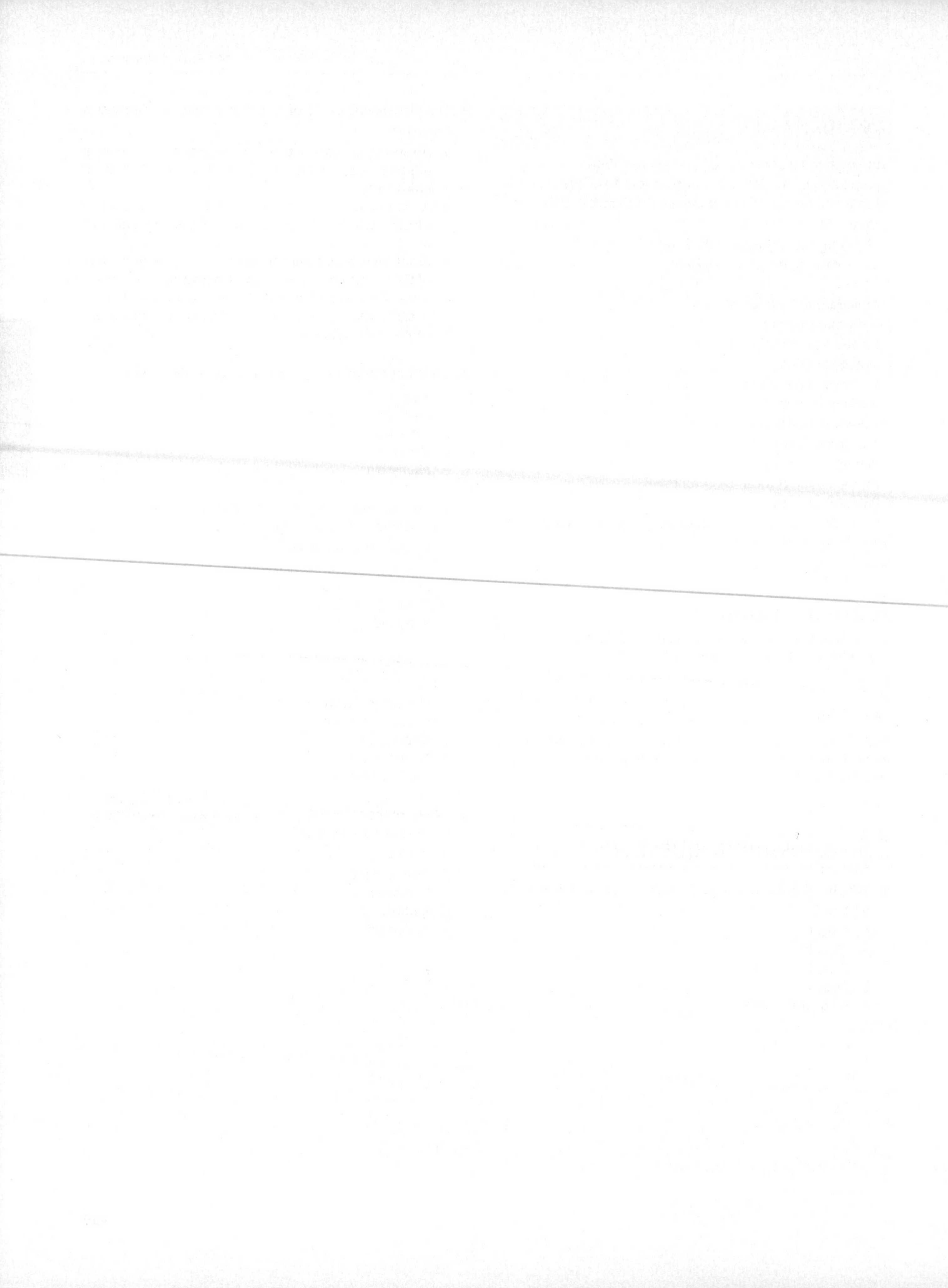

CHAPTER 15

Drugs to treat heart failure

Benedict R. Lucchesi

Major Drugs

Angiotensin-converting enzyme inhibitors	Diuretics
β-Adrenergic receptor blockers	Cardiac glycosides
Angiotensin receptor blockers	Sympathomimetic inotropic agents
Aldosterone antagonists	Phosphodiesterase inhibitors
	Intravenous vasodilators

Therapeutic overview

Heart failure is a state in which the heart is unable to provide adequate perfusion of peripheral organs to meet their metabolic requirements. A heterogeneous group of disorders (Box 15-1) can lead to a **reduction in cardiac output** and progressing to congestive heart failure (CHF) accompanied by **peripheral and pulmonary edema.**

Although there have been major advances in recent years in management of patients with CHF, it continues to be common and is often fatal. Therapeutic advances have enhanced survival, however, morbidity and mortality continue to be major public health concerns.

In the year 2000, it was estimated that 4.7 million people in the United States had heart failure. Epidemiological data suggest that **ischemic heart disease** and **hypertension** with or without diabetes mellitus are primary risk factors. The median survival after initial diagnosis is 1.7 years for men and 3.2 years for women. The incidence continues to increase as effective management of patients with myocardial infarction allows them to return home, albeit with a potential for continued progression to a state of cardiac decompensation. **Sudden cardiac death** is common in patients with heart failure, contributing to 50% of all 287,000 deaths in the United States last year, whereas progressive pump failure accounts for most of the remainder. Heart failure is a **progressive** disorder, which may initially be asymptomatic. Patients are classified as:

- Class I (asymptomatic)
- Class II (mild)
- Class III (moderate)
- Class IV (severe)

In a patient with **acute heart failure,** the short-term aim is stabilization by providing symptomatic treatment through intravenous interventions. Management of **chronic heart failure** is multifaceted, with the long-term aims of relieving symptoms and improving hemodynamics to improve quality of life and decrease mortality.

Neurohormonal responses to the failing heart

The major underlying cause of heart failure is an impairment of myocardial contractile function. The associated decrease in **stroke volume** and **cardiac output** initiates a multifaceted sequence of neurohormonal and vascular events that affect **preload, afterload,** and **heart rate.** For many years, heart failure was

Abbreviations

ACE	angiotensin-converting enzyme
ARB	angiotensin receptor blocker
AV	atrioventricular
BNP	B-natriuretic peptide
cAMP	cyclic adenosine monophosphate
CHF	congestive heart failure
RAAS	renin–angiotensin–aldosterone system
SA	sinoatrial
SNS	sympathetic nervous system

Box 15-1 Factors contributing to heart failure

Ischemic heart disease—leading cause of congestive heart failure
Hypertensive heart disease—antecedent history of hypertension
Cardiomyopathies—Dilated, hypertrophic, restrictive, alcoholic, postpartum, postinflammatory
Valvular heart disease
Cardiomyopathy of overload (high output failure)—Arteriovenous fistula, severe anemia, Paget's disease
Other factors
- Direct toxicity, including Adriamycin, external radiation, chest wall trauma, illicit drug use
- Endocrine and metabolic diseases
- Infectious agents—Bacterial, viral (including HIV), fungal, Lyme disease
- Infiltrative disease
  - Cardiac amyloidosis, hemochromatosis

attributed to left ventricular dysfunction, which was corrected by use of positive inotropic agents, such as digoxin. It is now clear that heart failure represents a highly complex series of events that include **neuroendocrine activation.** This has resulted in reevaluation of the approach to management. Whereas the hemodynamic model may still apply to patients with **acute failure,** the new model focuses on prevention of progression in the outpatient setting by preventing or delaying development of left ventricular remodeling.

Left ventricular remodeling

Remodeling of the heart occurs through complex structural changes in one or more cardiac chambers, especially the ventricles. These result in an increase in **end-diastolic** and **end-systolic volume** along with changes in cardiac shape and left ventricular mass. Impaired contractility was previously thought to be responsible for heart failure, although a specific biochemical abnormality could not be identified. This idea has given way to the concept that heart failure involves endogenous neurohormones and cytokines in response to an initial **"index event,"** usually an acute injury to the heart or genetic mutation. **Coronary artery disease** and **hypertension** account for most cases, with **myocardial infarction** being a major contributor. Any insult, whether acute myocardial infarction, essential hypertension, aortic stenosis, or volume overload due to aortic insufficiency, idiopathic cardiomyopathy, or inflammatory disease, leads to activation of specific mediators involved in the remodeling process.

Neurohormonal systems defend against changes in intravascular volume and act to maintain regional blood flow and regulate systemic blood pressure. Initially, they compensate for the decline in ventricular function and mask the underlying deficiency. Chronic activation of multiple compensatory mechanisms perpetuates progression to irreversible myocyte injury and worsening of cardiac function. Initiating factors include: stretch of the ventricular myocardium, increased cytokine and growth factor production, nitric oxide production, tumor necrosis factor, natriuretic peptides, free radical meditated oxidative stress, ischemia, activation of myocardial metalloproteinases, proapoptotic factors, and/or chronic inflammation. Heart failure is usually accompanied by an increase in **sympathetic nervous system** (SNS) activation along with chronic up-regulation of the **renin-angiotensin-aldosterone system** (RAAS) and effects of **aldosterone** on heart, vessels, and kidneys. CHF should be viewed as a complex, interrelated sequence of events involving hemodynamic, nonhemodynamic, genetic, energetic, and neurohormonal events.

Sympathetic nervous system

In the failing heart, the loss of contractile function leads to a decline in cardiac output and a decrease in arterial blood pressure. The baroreceptors sense the hemodynamic changes and initiate countermeasures to maintain support of the circulatory system. Activation of the SNS serves as a compensatory mechanism in response to a decline in left ventricular stroke volume. This helps maintain adequate cardiac output by increasing myocardial contractility and heart rate (β_1-adrenergic receptors) as well as increasing vasomotor tone (α_1-adrenergic receptors) to maintain systemic blood pressure (see Chapters 10 and 11). Over the long term, this **hyperadrenergic state** leads to irreversible myocyte damage, cell death, and fibrosis. In addition, the augmentation in peripheral vasomotor tone increases left ventricular afterload, placing an added stress upon the left ventricle and an increase in myocardial oxygen demand, factors involved in ventricular remodeling. The frequency and severity of cardiac arrhythmias are enhanced in the failing heart, in part, due to the increased adrenergic tone.

Systolic heart failure

The most frequent cause for chronic systolic dysfunction is **ischemic cardiomyopathy,** characterized by a reduction in the ventricular ejection fraction and enlargement of the left ventricle, due to a failure of the left ventricle to empty as a result of impaired myocardial contractility or pressure overload. This results from destruction of myocytes, impaired myocyte function, or fibrosis. Chronic pressure overload, secondary to untreated long-standing hypertension or aortic stenosis, decreases the left ventricular ejection fraction by increasing resistance to forward flow. Initially, the increase in the left ventricular end-diastolic pressure (volume) results in a compensatory enhancement in stroke volume due to the pressure-induced lengthening of the sarcomeres that invokes the **Frank-Starling mechanism** (Fig. 15-1), thereby partially compensating for the failing ventricle. The marked diastolic derangement in filling and the decreased ventricular distensibility do not permit adequate stretch of the myocytes because it occurs under conditions that require an increase in cardiac output. Therefore, in the presence of systolic heart failure, the Frank-Starling mechanism fails to adequately increase stroke volume in response to exercise.

The compensatory increase in sympathetic tone plus the activation of the RAAS system maintains arterial blood pressure. However, homeostatic mechanisms also increase total peripheral resistance (left ventricular afterload). Circulating blood volume is also increased, further contributing to maintenance of arterial pressure. Over the long term, this places an additional burden on the failing heart. Moreover, because increases in peripheral resistance decrease tissue perfusion for a given blood pressure and tissue perfusion is more important than blood pressure, these mechanisms may not be advantageous in the long term.

Energy efficiency is reduced in chronic heart failure because a greater wall tension is required to develop the necessary intraventricular pressure, and peripheral resistance is increased. Energetic efficiency decreases further when relaxation is inhibited in the hypertrophied heart and when the heart rate is increased by activation of the SNS, resulting in a reduced stroke volume.

Chronic pressure overload, as in uncontrolled hypertension, contributes to hypertrophy. Stretching of the sarcolemma and the ensuing influx of Na^+, and increased angiotensin II concentrations in plasma are possible causes. The number of myocardial cells does not increase in adults, but each cell enlarges. Remodeling may occur in association with such hypertrophy. Remodeling involves a shift of isoforms of functional proteins, such as myosin, creatine kinase, and Na^+, K^+-ATPase. These are adaptive events but may ultimately contribute to ventricular remodeling. Furthermore, the hypertrophied heart loses compliance (i.e., the ability to relax).

Diastolic heart failure

Diastolic dysfunction may result from impaired early diastolic relaxation, increased stiffness of the ventricular wall, or both. Hypertension, valvular disease, or congenital abnormalities lead to development of diastolic dysfunction, with hypertrophied or poorly compliant ventricular walls impeding filling of the left ventricle. **Diastolic relaxation** is an energy dependent process, which is impaired by myocardial ischemia and a temporary loss of energy production. In this case, ventricular filling can be achieved only at a greater than normal filling pressure due to reduced left ventricular wall compliance. Abnormalities may be attributable, in part, to an increase in interstitial connective tissue. Hypertrophic myocytes exhibit abnormal Ca^{2+} cycles characterized by prolonged Ca^{2+} transients and impaired

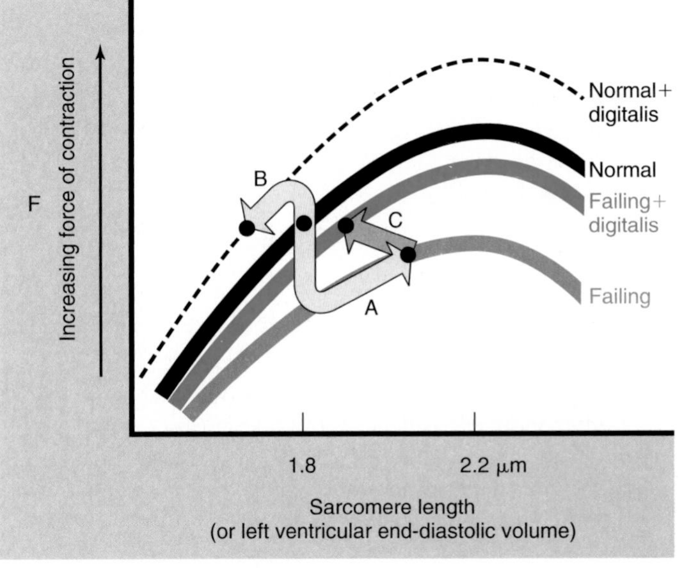

Figure 15-1 Frank-Starling ventricular function curve. Force of contraction, expressed as left ventricular dP/dt (rate of pressure development during early systolic phase) is a function of (1) left ventricular volume before the onset of contraction or (2) sarcomere length. The length of the sarcomere, the unit between two Z lines of a myofibril, in the normal heart is 1.7 to 1.8 μm at the endocardial and epicardial layers and 2.0 μm in the middle layer. The reduced force of contraction in a failing heart is partly compensated for by an increase in the end-diastolic volume, which increases the length of the sarcomere, thereby increasing the force of contraction or the stroke volume (**A,** *arrow*). Positive inotropic interventions in the normal heart are canceled by shortening of the muscle (**B,** *arrow*). Digitalis glycosides shift the ventricular function curve and reduce the end-diastolic volume required for the muscle to develop the necessary force of contraction (**C,** *arrow*).

relaxation. Current evidence implicates the local activity of angiotensin II and elevated circulating levels of aldosterone, both of which are implicated in the development of **myocardial fibrosis.** They lead to deposition of excessive amounts of collagen and a decrease in ventricular compliance, increased chamber stiffness, or a decrease in distensibility. Patients with diastolic dysfunction may have a normal cardiac output, suggesting that pharmacological management will differ from patients with systolic heart failure.

Approaches to treatment of heart failure are summarized in the Therapeutic Overview box. In the patient with **acute failure,** the short-term aim is to stabilize the patient by achieving an optimal hemodynamic status and providing symptomatic treatment through use of intravenous interventions. Management of **chronic heart failure** most often involves a combination of interventions. Most patients should be administered a regimen consisting of digoxin and diuretics along with an ACE inhibitor and β-blocker. Several new agents (such as aldosterone antagonists) may provide further benefit.

THERAPEUTIC OVERVIEW

Problem

Reduced force of contraction
Decreased cardiac output
Increased total peripheral resistance
Inadequate organ perfusion
Development of edema
Decreased exercise tolerance
Ischemic heart disease
Sudden death
Ventricular remodeling and decreased function

Goals

Alleviation of symptoms, improve quality of life
Arrest ventricular remodeling
Prevent sudden death

Nondrug therapy

Reduce cardiac work; rest, weight loss, low Na^+ diet

Drug therapy

Chronic heart failure
- ACE inhibitors, β-adrenergic receptor blockers, angiotensin II receptor blockers, aldosterone antagonists, digoxin, diuretics

Acute heart failure
- Intravenous diuretics, inotropic agents, phosphodiesterase inhibitors, vasodilators

Mechanisms of action

Angiotensin-converting enzyme inhibitors

Baroreceptor mediated activation of the SNS leads to an increase in renin release and formation of angiotensin II (see Chapter 11), which causes intense vasoconstriction and stimulates aldosterone production (Fig. 15-2). This is decreased by the ACE inhibitors, which inhibit formation of angiotensin II from angiotensin I, as discussed in Chapter 12.

Angiotensin II acts through AT_1 and AT_2 receptors, although most of its actions occur through AT_1 receptor activation. Although the AT_2 receptor is distributed widely in fetal tissues, its distribution is limited in adults. Angiotensin II mediates cell growth, vasoconstriction, Na^+ and fluid retention, and sympathetic activation (Table 15-1). The central role of the RAAS in the development and progression of cardiovascular disease

Table 15-1 Effects of angiotensin II

Site of Action	Response
Vascular smooth muscle	Vasoconstriction—increased renal and peripheral resistance, increased left ventricular afterload, vessel wall hyperplasia, hypertrophy initiated by AT_1 receptors
Heart	Positive inotropic effect by opening voltage gated Ca^{2+} channels, myocardial hypertrophy, activation of matrix metalloproteinases, myocardial fibrosis initiated by AT_1 receptors, increase in release of norepinephrine
Adrenal cortex	Increased aldosterone synthesis and release, release of catecholamines from adrenal medulla
Kidney	Reduction in renal blood flow and excretory functions, increase in Na^+ channels in the apical membrane of renal tubules, increased number of Na^+,K^+-ATPase in the basal lateral membrane, increased renal tubular reabsorption of Na^+, increased K^+ excretion
Sympathetic nervous system	Increased norepinephrine release and inhibition of reuptake (increase in peripheral resistance, stimulation of renin release)
Central nervous system	Release of vasopressin, increased fluid retention, activation of the sympathetic nervous system

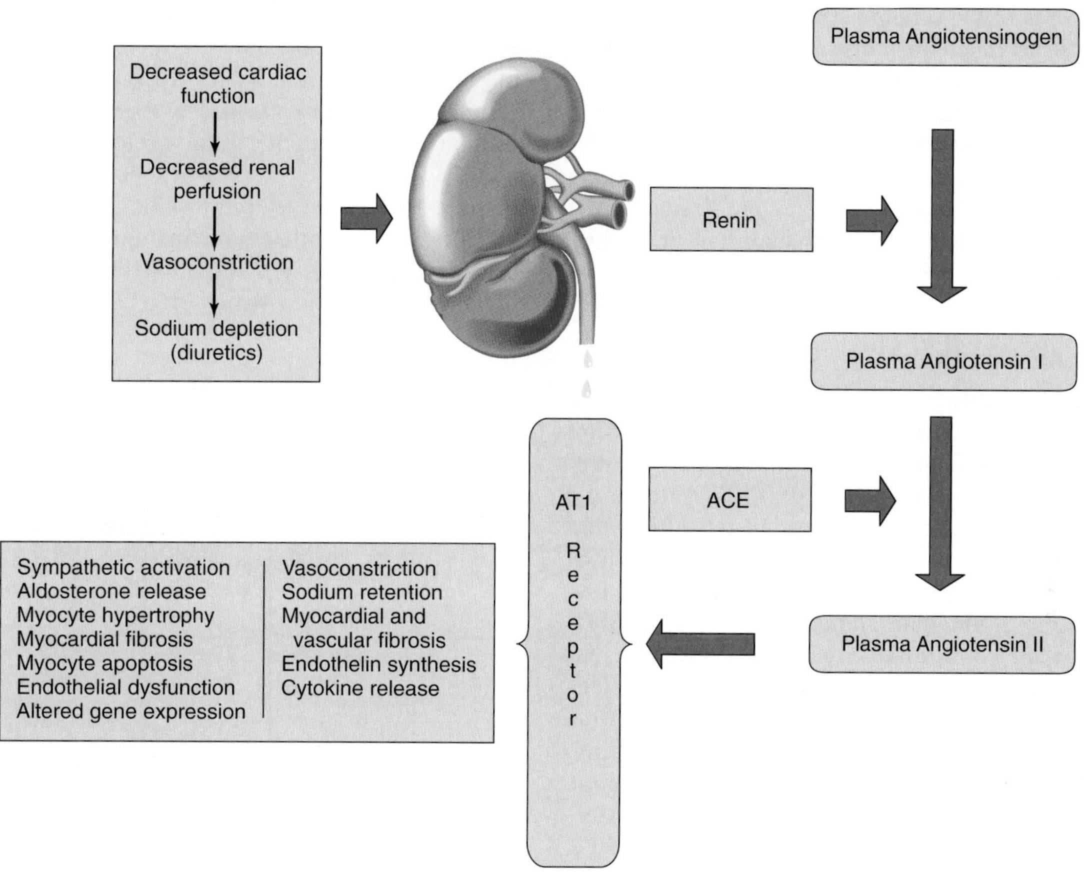

Figure 15-2 Renal release of renin leading to the formation of angiotensin II and subsequent activation of AT1 receptor–mediated events.

and, in particular, CHF is well established. In addition to regulation of blood pressure and maintenance of fluid and electrolyte balance, short-term activation of the RAAS in heart failure improves cardiac output through fluid and Na^+ retention (increased preload), whereas long-term activation results in vasoconstriction, increased afterload, and decreased cardiac output. These mechanisms, together with SNS activation, induce a vicious cycle of increased preload, afterload, and cardiac workload, leading to increased myocardial oxygen consumption, loss of myocytes through apoptosis, and progressive worsening heart failure.

β-Adrenergic receptor blocking drugs

There is overwhelming evidence to support the use of β-blockers in CHF, however, the mechanism(s) involved remain unclear. Part of their beneficial effects may derive from slowing of heart rate, which would improve coronary blood flow and decrease myocardial oxygen consumption. This would lessen the frequency of ischemic events and potential for development of a lethal arrhythmia. Activation of the SNS can provoke arrhythmias by increasing cardiac automaticity, increasing triggered activity leading to ventricular arrhythmias, which may account for the ability of β-blockers to reduce the incidence of sudden cardiac death in patients with ischemic heart disease and heart failure.

β-Blockers inhibit the adverse effects of the SNS in patients with heart failure. Whereas cardiac adrenergic drive initially serves as a compensatory mechanism to support the failing heart, long-term activation leads to a down-regulation of β_1-adrenergic receptors and an uncoupling from adenylyl cyclase (see Chapter 2), thereby reducing myocardial contractility. β-Blockers may be beneficial through resensitization of the down-regulated receptor, improving myocardial contractility.

Angiotensin II receptor blockers

Another approach is to block AT_1 receptors with the use of **angiotensin receptor blockers** (ARBs). The currently available drugs selectively block AT_1 receptors and replicate many of the actions of ACE inhibitors, although they do not block AT_2 receptors. Activation of AT_2 receptors may cause vasodilation, preventing hypertrophy of vascular smooth muscle and cardiomyocytes, production of bradykinin, and release of nitric oxide. There is also overexpression of AT_2 receptors in the failing heart. There may also be non-ACE dependent formation of angiotensin II by enzymes, such as chymase, cathepsin G, trypsin, and tissue plasminogen activator. An ARB might block the deleterious actions mediated by AT_1 receptors while preserving the desirable effects of AT_2 receptor activation. Although the hemodynamic and clinical effects may appear similar, ACE inhibitors and ARBs should not be regarded as being identical.

Aldosterone antagonists

The elevated circulating angiotensin II levels in the patient with CHF lead to greatly increased production of aldosterone (see Chapter 33), an important mediator in the progressive development of CHF. Aldosterone binds to mineralocorticoid receptors in renal epithelial cells and promotes Na^+ retention, Mg^{2+} and K^+ loss, sympathetic activation, parasympathetic inhibition, myocardial and vascular fibrosis, baroreceptor dysfunction, impaired arterial compliance, and vascular damage. Aldosterone antagonists include **spironolactone** and **eplerenone,** which may reduce norepinephrine release from cardiac sympathetic nerves and increase plasma K^+. The elevated concentrations of aldosterone in CHF led to the concept that inhibition of aldosterone receptors could be beneficial, and competitive aldosterone antagonists are now part of the therapeutic armamentarium.

Cardiac glycosides

The **cardiac glycosides** increase the force of myocardial contraction, alter electrophysiological properties in specialized regions, and have extracardiac actions associated with toxicity. Cardiac glycosides influence the heart through a direct inhibition of membrane **Na^+,K^+-ATPase** as well as an indirect increase in vagal tone (Table 15-2). Their cardiotoxic effects are an overextension of the same mechanisms responsible for their positive inotropic actions.

Cardiac glycosides increase contractile force, however, unlike catecholamines, they do not increase the rate of relaxation. By decreasing the activity of the Na^+,K^+-ATPase, they cause a progressive gain in intracellular Na^+ with each cardiac cycle. This increase promotes Ca^{2+} influx by Na^+/Ca^{2+} exchange (Fig. 15-3). The net result is to increase intracellular Ca^{2+}, enhancing the Ca^{2+} transient resulting from an augmented Ca^{2+} loading of the sarcoplasmic reticulum. In the presence of a digitalis glycoside a new steady state is achieved where an

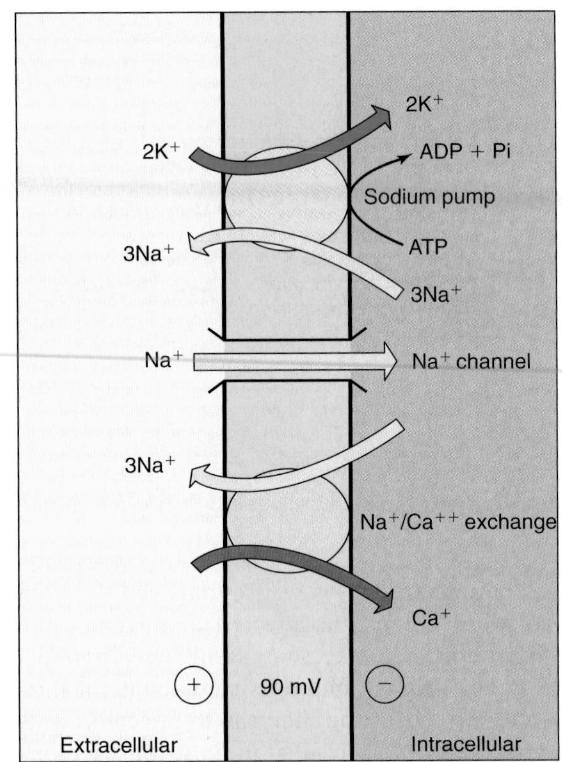

Figure 15-3 Membrane ion flux of Na^+ and Ca^{2+} in heart. Glycoside-induced inhibition of Na^+,K^+-ATPase secondarily promotes Na^+/Ca^{2+} exchange.

Table 15-2 Effects of cardiac glycosides on electrophysiological properties of the heart

	Direct	Indirect (increased vagal tone)
SA Node	No effect at therapeutic dose	No effect at therapeutic dose
Atrial muscle	High dose increases rate of spontaneous depolarization	High dose decreases rate of spontaneous depolarization
AV node	Increased refractory period Decreased conduction velocity	Decreased conduction velocity Increased refractory period
His-Purkinje system	Increased refractory period Decreased conduction velocity High dose increases triggered activity Toxic doses enhance pacemaker	Increased refractory period Decreased conduction velocity None

increased amount of Ca^{2+} is released following depolarization, increasing force development (stroke volume).

Electrophysiological effects of cardiac glycosides vary among different regions of the heart. They decrease **automaticity** within the SA and AV nodes due to an increase in parasympathetic tone along with a concomitant decrease in sympathetic tone. The increase in parasympathetic tone on the AV node leads to a decrease in conduction velocity and an increase in effective refractory period. Thus, digitalis glycosides *indirectly* decrease heart rate and impair impulse transmission across the AV node.

The major *direct* effects are in the atrial muscle, AV node, and ventricles (Table 15-2). In atria, they prolong the effective refractory period and decrease conduction velocity, effects opposite to those elicited by their *indirect* actions. However, the *direct* effects in the AV node summate with the *indirect* actions to further impair conduction velocity and increase the refractory period.

There are also significant **extracardiac effects** of digitalis glycosides. Most cells express membrane Na^+,K^+-ATPases, but those in excitable tissues have a higher affinity for cardiac glycosides. Whether or not a cell is affected depends on factors, such as the Na^+ pump reserve, the presence or absence of Na^+/Ca^{2+} exchangers, and the role of Na^+ or Ca^{2+} in its function.

Neurons of the autonomic nervous system are particularly sensitive to glycoside-induced Na^+ pump inhibition, probably due to an increased baroreceptor sensitivity. Cardiac glycosides increase parasympathetic discharge, as discussed previously. Stimulation of the chemoreceptor trigger zone is responsible for nausea and vomiting. At sympathetic nerve terminals, Na^+ pump inhibition facilitates neurotransmitter release, which is responsible for the transient vasoconstriction observed after rapid intravenous administration.

Digoxin also causes vasoconstriction by increasing intracellular Ca^{2+} in vascular smooth muscle. In CHF, the hemodynamic response is characterized by a decreased heart rate (due to augmented baroreceptor responsiveness), increased forearm blood flow and cardiac index, and a decreased sympathetic tone to skeletal muscle. These beneficial changes may be secondary to a reduction in neurohumoral activation, which may distinguish the cardiac glycosides from other positive inotropic agents.

Diuretics

Diuretics are widely used in treatment of congestive heart failure to reduce extracellular fluid volume (see Chapter 13). Their primary parenteral use is in patients with **acute** heart failure for correction of volume overload. In the most severe cases, intravenous infusions of a loop diuretic (e.g., furosemide) can initiate a rapid, predictable, and sustained diuresis (see Chapter 13). The diuretic is titrated according to an estimated "dry" weight, based on optimal filling pressures and symptoms, without exacerbating symptomatic hypotension.

Sympathomimetics

Epinephrine and **norepinephrine** are β-adrenergic receptor agonists that produce a marked positive inotropic response and have α_1-agonist activity that elicits peripheral vasoconstriction (see Chapter 10). Both agents have limited utility in patients with severe heart failure but can offer significant inotropic support for short-term intervention (minutes to hours) in life-threatening situations while more definitive measures are initiated.

Dopamine acts on prejunctional D_2 receptors to inhibit release of norepinephrine (see Chapter 11), resulting in vasodilation. Dopamine also acts on cardiac β_1-receptors to elicit a positive inotropic action, and on vascular smooth muscle to cause vasodilation, improving blood flow to renal, mesenteric, coronary, and cerebral vascular beds.

Dobutamine is a racemic mixture that activates several adrenergic receptors. It cannot interact with dopaminergic receptors but releases norepinephrine from sympathetic nerves. The resulting hemodynamic effects are dose dependent, with a positive inotropic action at low doses as a result of β_1-receptor activity. The α_1-adrenergic mediated vasoconstriction is attributed to the (–) enantiomer, which is countered by the receptor blocking actions of the (+) enantiomer.

Phosphodiesterase inhibitors

Inamrinone and **milrinone** exert their positive inotropic actions by inhibiting cyclic adenosine monophosphate (cAMP) phosphodiesterase, the enzyme that hydrolyzes and inactivates cAMP. The effects of these drugs differ from other phosphodiesterase inhibitors, such as caffeine or theophylline, in that they are selective for a particular isozyme, phosphodiesterase III. They increase cardiac cAMP, but not cyclic guanosine monophosphate, concentrations. This promotes cAMP-dependent protein kinase phosphorylation of the Ca^{2+} channel in heart, enhancing Ca^{2+} influx and resulting in a positive inotropic action similar to that caused by catecholamines.

Vasodilators

Nitroprusside was among the earliest vasodilators to show improvement in cardiac output in patients with decompensated heart failure. Nitroprusside and other nitrovasodilators are discussed in Chapter 16. Nitroprusside reduces ventricular filling pressures by directly increasing venous compliance, resulting in a redistribution of blood from central to peripheral veins. In addition, the action of nitroprusside on the arterial side of the circulation makes it one of the most effective agents for reducing left ventricular afterload. Nitroprusside dilates the pulmonary arterioles, thereby decreasing right ventricular afterload. Reducing both preload and afterload improves myocardial energetics due to a reduction in wall stress. In contrast, nitroglycerin shows specificity for venodilation, thereby increasing venous capacitance and pooling of blood in the more dependent regions of the body.

Brain (B-type) natriuretic peptide (BNP) is secreted constitutively by ventricular myocytes in response to stretch and increased wall stress and is increased in patients with CHF. Its action is counterregulatory to many of the actions of the RAAS and SNS in heart failure. BNP binds to receptors in the vasculature, kidney, and other organs, producing potent vasodilation with rapid onset and offset of action by increasing levels of cyclic guanosine monophosphate. **Nesiritide** is recombinant human BNP approved for treatment of acute decompensated CHF. Its acute hemodynamic effects include a reduction of right atrial, pulmonary artery, and pulmonary capillary wedge pressures, as well as systemic and pulmonary vascular resistances, causing an indirect increase in cardiac output and diuresis. Nesiritide may potentially provide symptomatic relief without the increases in mortality shown with other inotropic agents, because it does not increase cAMP and Ca^{2+} in cardiomyocytes.

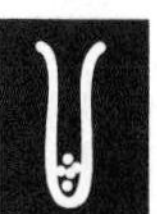

Pharmacokinetics

The pharmacokinetics of the ACE inhibitors and ARBs are discussed in Chapter 12, of the β-adrenergic receptor blockers and sympathomimetics in Chapter 10, and of the nitrovasodilators in Chapter 16.

Cardiac glycosides

Pharmacokinetic parameters of cardiac glycosides are presented in Table 15-3. Digitoxin is rarely used in the United States, although it continues to be used in Europe. Absorption of digoxin given orally varies from 45% to 85%, and because of such wide variations, patients should be maintained on a specific brand. However, bioavailability of digitoxin is consistently high.

Digoxin is excreted mainly by the kidneys, whereas digitoxin is metabolized in the liver. Digitoxin is excreted into bile and undergoes enterohepatic cycling. The reabsorbed metabolites are cardioactive and contribute to its extended half-life. There are large interpatient variations in digitoxin metabolism, partly because intestinal flora exert a significant role.

Variations may be minimized by maintenance of predetermined concentrations in plasma. However, a given plasma concentration may be therapeutic in some patients and toxic in others, due to differences in sensitivity caused by various factors (Box 15-2). Because monitoring the positive inotropic effect is impractical, clinical evaluation often involves the electrocardiogram. A slight (approximately 10%) increase in PR interval is not alarming; however, a greater delay in AV nodal conduction time and conduction block, or development of ventricular bigeminy or trigeminy, is a harbinger of serious toxicity.

Because digitoxin has a long half-life, steady state is not achieved until 20 days after starting therapy without a loading dose, so a loading dose is usually given. Digoxin, with its shorter half-life, may be administered without a loading dose; steady-state concentration is reached in 5 to 7 days when administered orally daily. Switching from maintenance doses of digoxin to digitoxin results in a temporary loss of effect, because digoxin is excreted from the body rapidly while digitoxin accumulates slowly. Conversely, switching from maintenance doses of digitoxin to digoxin causes a transient overdose. Recent studies suggest that "ideal" or therapeutic digoxin serum concentrations are 1.1

Table 15-3 Pharmacokinetic parameters for cardiac glycosides, phosphodiesterase inhibitors, and nesiritide.

Agent	Administration	Bioavailability	Peak Effect (hrs)	Protein Binding	(%) Disposition	Half-Life
Digoxin	Oral, IV	45-85	6	25	R (40%-90%)	36 hr
Digitoxin	Oral, IV	>90	12	90	M	6-7 days
Inamrinone	IV	—	0.5-2	40	M	2-3 hr
Milrinone	IV	—	0.5-1	—	R	0.5
Nesiritide	IV	—	1	—	M, R	18 min

IV, Intravenous; *R*, renal; *M*, metabolism.

Box 15-2 Factors leading to altered sensitivity to digoxin

Influence	Effects
Physiological influences	Increased vagal and sympathetic tone, age
Pathophysiological influences	Chronic pulmonary disease, renal dysfunction, myocardial ischemia or infarction, rheumatic or viral myocarditis, hyperthyroidism, or hypothyroidism
Abnormal plasma electrolytes	Hypokalemia or hyperkalemia, hypomagnesemia, hypercalcemia or hypocalcemia
Drug-drug interactions	Increased or decreased therapeutic effects or toxicity

to 1.2 ng/ml, whereas others favor a range of 0.5 to 1.5 ng/ml.

Phosphodiesterase inhibitors

Inamrinone and milrinone are administered parenterally. Inamrinone is usually administered as an initial loading dose followed by careful titration. Milrinone is approximately 10 times more potent and is often preferred for short-term parenteral inotropic support in patients with severe cardiac decompensation. The elimination half-lives of inamrinone and milrinone are 2.5 hours and 30 to 60 minutes, respectively, and are about doubled in CHF patients.

Nesiritide

When administered intravenously to patients with CHF, as an infusion or bolus injection, nesiritide exhibits a biphasic pattern of disposition. The mean terminal elimination half-life is approximately 18 minutes. Nesiritide is cleared by three mechanisms:

- Binding to cell surface clearance receptors with subsequent internalization and lysosomal proteolysis
- Proteolytic cleavage by endopeptidases on the vascular luminal surface
- Renal filtration

Neither titration of the infusion rate is commonly required nor is invasive hemodynamic monitoring. Therefore, patients treated with nesiritide may not require as close monitoring as may be necessary with nitrovasodilators, perhaps negating the need for intensive care unit stays.

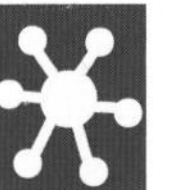

Relation of mechanisms of action to clinical response

An obvious feature of dilated cardiomyopathy is diminished systolic ventricular function, suggesting that inotropic support would be beneficial. β-Adrenergic receptor agonists, although useful for management of acute cardiac decompensation, are relatively ineffective in chronic heart failure. This is probably because long-term exposure results in receptor down-regulation. Therefore, phosphodiesterase inhibitors are used to directly increase cAMP levels and enhance Ca^{2+} cycling. Despite compelling experimental data and mechanistic rationale, most outpatient trials have demonstrated adverse outcomes, typically increased mortality with long-term use of phosphodiesterase inhibitors. The adverse events associated with positive inotropic agents for long-term management of CHF are in marked contrast to the survival benefit derived from negative inotropic therapies, such as β-adrenergic receptor blockade.

Angiotensin-converting enzyme inhibitors

ACE inhibitors now have the primary role in contemporary therapy of CHF and should be used at all costs. They must be administered in high doses, while avoiding excess hypotension. The initial dose of an ACE inhibitor must be chosen cautiously, especially in patients on diuretic therapy (most likely with intense RAAS activation); the diuretic dose must be discontinued to allow for volume expansion so as not to precipitate excessive hypotension. If the patient cannot tolerate the ACE inhibitor because of severe coughing unrelated to CHF, changing to an ARB would be the next choice.

Several clinical trials have reported significant reductions in mortality in patients receiving ACE inhibitors, even when added to the standard regimen of diuretics and digoxin. The central role of the RAAS in development and progression of cardiovascular disease, and, in particular, CHF, is well established. Short-term activation in heart failure improves cardiac output through fluid and Na^{+} retention (increased preload), whereas long-term activation results in vasoconstriction, increased afterload, and decreased cardiac output.

ACE inhibitors reduce the progression of left ventricular dysfunction in chronic heart failure and in patients recovering from an acute myocardial infarction. ACE inhibitors may also reduce the risk of acute coronary ischemic attacks. Long-term studies indicate that ACE inhibitors increase survival. An advantage in the relief of the symptoms of CHF is that they conserve K^+ by lowering aldosterone secretion, ruling out the need for K^+ supplementation.

It is currently unclear whether the beneficial effects of ACE inhibitors are solely the result of their hemodynamic actions, whether a reduction in the concentration of angiotensin II increases the concentrations of bradykinin or nitric oxide, or whether an inhibition of the SNS plays a significant role.

β-Adrenergic receptor blockers

β-Blockers that have been shown to be effective in treatment of heart failure include those that selectively block β_1-receptors, such as metoprolol, and those that block both α_1, β_1, and β_2-receptors, such as carvedilol. Their properties are discussed in Chapter 10.

In practice, β-blockers are almost always used together with ACE inhibitors (and usually with digoxin). Patients need not be taking high doses of ACE inhibitors before being considered for treatment with β-Blockers. In patients taking low doses of an ACE inhibitor, addition of a β-blocker produces a greater improvement in symptoms and reduces the risk of death. β-Blockers should not be prescribed without diuretics in patients with a history of fluid retention, because diuretics are needed to maintain Na^+ balance and prevent development of fluid retention that can accompany β-blocker therapy. Doses should be increased gradually, until side effects associated with lower doses have disappeared. Clinical trials show that 85% of patients could tolerate short- and long-term treatment with β-blockers.

β-Blockers should be prescribed to all patients with stable heart failure due to left ventricular systolic dysfunction, unless they have a contraindication to their use or cannot tolerate treatment with these drugs. Initial doses are typically much lower than those required for hypertension and are gradually increased over time for maximal therapeutic effectiveness. Because of favorable effects on survival, treatment with β-blockers should not be delayed until the patient is found to be resistant to treatment with other drugs. Although it is commonly believed (incorrectly) that patients with mild symptoms or who appear clinically stable do not require additional treatment, such patients are at high risk for morbidity and mortality and are likely to deteriorate over the next year even if treated with digoxin, diuretics, and ACE inhibitors. Therefore, patients with mild symptoms should also receive β-blockers to reduce further risk.

In summary, β-blockers are indicated in stable patients with chronic systolic heart failure and mild to moderate symptoms in combination with ACE inhibitors, diuretics, and digoxin. Therapy should be initiated slowly over several weeks with close follow-up.

Angiotensin receptor blockers

Administered with or without an ACE inhibitor, ARBs have been shown to increase left ventricular ejection fraction and reduce end-systolic and end-diastolic volumes at peak exercise in patients with heart failure. Clinical trials have shown that ARBs reduce morbidity and mortality in patients with heart failure. By acting at the receptor level, ARBs provide more complete blockade of the RAAS than ACE inhibitors, because angiotensin II may be formed by alternative enzymes, as discussed previously. These alternative pathways appear to be important, because plasma levels of angiotensin II return to pretreatment levels in some patients who receive long-term treatment with an ACE inhibitor and increase after exercise in healthy volunteers despite effective ACE inhibition. Unlike ACE inhibitors, ARBs do not activate the SNS. Potential favorable effects of ARB therapy may also be due to continued activation of AT_2 receptors, which may mediate desirable effects of vasodilation, antiproliferative effects, cell differentiation, and tissue repair. Some evidence suggests that combining an ARB with an ACE inhibitor may result in greater effects than higher doses of either drug alone.

Aldosterone antagonists

Aldosterone concentrations are elevated as much as 20-fold in patients with heart failure. It promotes Na^+ retention, Mg^{2+} and K^+ loss, sympathetic activation, parasympathetic inhibition, myocardial and vascular fibrosis, baroreceptor dysfunction, impaired arterial compliance, and vascular damage. Both spironolactone and eplerenone are reported to reduce mortality in patients with moderate or severe heart failure who are otherwise optimally treated. Current guidelines recommend using them in patients with severe symptoms, preserved renal function, and normal K^+ levels. Plasma K^+ must be monitored carefully, and caution should be exercised in patients taking K^+ supplements or using K^+ sparing diuretics due to the risk of hyperkalemia.

Clinical trials of spironolactone in patients with moderate or severe heart failure receiving an ACE inhibitor and a loop diuretic were discontinued after 24 months because of the significant benefits of spironolactone, including reductions in mortality (30%) and in hospitalization for worsening heart failure (35%), and improvement in symptoms. The benefit was not primarily diuretic but probably related to interference with aldosterone mediated myocardial fibrosis and improved endothelial function.

Cardiac glycosides

Inhibition of the Na^+,K^+-ATPase of the myocardial sarcolemma is responsible for both the positive inotropic and toxic effects of cardiac glycosides. A moderate (20% to 40%) inhibition causes a therapeutic effect, whereas greater inhibition is toxic. Thus, their therapeutic index is narrow, because a significant positive inotropic effect requires a dose that is 50% to 60% of its toxic dose.

Cardiac glycosides are the only orally effective inotropic agents approved for use in the United States. Compared to other inotropic agents, they are unique in that they exert a direct positive inotropic response in combination with an indirectly mediated bradycardia. Therefore, despite their narrow therapeutic index, they remain important inotropic agents.

Cardiac glycosides increase the force of cardiac contraction in either normal or failing hearts. Although originally thought to be effective only in patients with heart failure, they also increase force of contraction and reduce end-diastolic volume in normal hearts, which in turn decreases the force of contraction, canceling their positive inotropic effects (see Fig. 15-1, *B, arrow*). In the failing dilated heart, the increased force of contraction and decrease in end-diastolic volume make the heart's operation more nearly normal (see Fig. 15-1, *C, arrow*). Therefore, despite direct positive inotropic effects on both failing and nonfailing hearts, hemodynamic improvements are obtained only in the failing heart.

Because of autoregulatory mechanisms, a reduced force of cardiac contraction that lowers blood pressure triggers activation of the SNS and RAAS. The volume of circulating blood also may increase, which may result in decreased perfusion of certain organs. The primary beneficial effect of cardiac glycosides is a reversal of these changes and improvement in tissue perfusion.

Digoxin is especially useful in CHF patients with atrial fibrillation because it slows ventricular rate, allowing for improved filling and increasing ejection fraction or stroke volume. The net result is a reduced need for heightened sympathetic tone. This unique property makes digoxin useful in CHF patients in sinus rhythm. An additional benefit is a reduction in ventricular size in the failing heart, reducing ventricular wall tension, an important determinant of oxygen consumption. This is beneficial in patients with CHF secondary to ischemic heart disease. In patients with chronic CHF and abnormal systolic function, digoxin in combination with diuretics and ACE inhibitors reduces the frequency of hospitalizations and overall mortality.

Cardiac glycosides are useful in management of patients with chronic atrial fibrillation with a rapid ventricular response. The goal is to reduce the number of impulses from gaining access to the ventricular conducting system, thus allowing for control of ventricular rate. Other drugs (e.g., adenosine, Ca^{2+} channel blockers, β-blockers) would be additive in increasing AV nodal refractory period. Since the *indirect* effects of cardiac glycosides on atria lead to a decrease in effective refractory period and an increase in conduction velocity, use of digoxin is contraindicated in patients with Wolff-Parkinson-White syndrome (preexcitation) and atrial fibrillation. In such cases, it would increase the number of impulses traversing the bypass tract and lead to increased ventricular rate, with the potential for ventricular fibrillation.

Although digitalis glycosides have been used for over 200 years, their narrow margins of safety and limited ability to increase ventricular function in certain clinical settings are problematic. Moreover, they cannot arrest the progression of pathological changes causing heart failure, and do not prolong life in patients with CHF. However, sufficient data indicate that CHF patients maintained on digoxin experience a deterioration in cardiac function when digoxin is withdrawn, and benefit when treatment is resumed.

Diuretics

The diuretic drugs are discussed in Chapter 13. Prospective clinical trial data do not exist for evaluating their overall efficacy on mortality in patients with heart failure. However, there is little doubt that they are useful and necessary adjuncts for relief of CHF symptoms resulting from Na^+ and water retention in patients with acute and/or chronic cardiac decompensation.

Parenteral administration of diuretics is useful in treating **acute** heart failure because they reduce circulatory congestion and pulmonary and peripheral edemas. A reduction in atrial and ventricular diastolic pressure relieves stress on the ventricular wall and promotes subendocardial perfusion. Loop diuretics and thiazides are most commonly used in patients with CHF.

The renal response to parenteral loop diuretics depends upon the peak serum concentration achieved in the renal glomeruli. A low cardiac output and an increased volume of distribution can adversely alter the anticipated response by limiting the concentration at its target site. Thus, failure to achieve a response (diuretic resistance) may be due to poor renal perfusion and inadequate drug delivery. The latter may be corrected by concomitant administration of low doses of dopamine to improve renal blood flow. Although parenteral administration of loop diuretics does not directly increase myocardial contractility, there is a beneficial hemodynamic response secondary to venous dilation or increase in venous capacitance, which reduces left ventricular preload. Excessive diuresis and an excessive reduction in preload should be avoided because the decompensated heart relies upon an expanded end-diastolic volume, which serves as a compensatory mechanism for increasing stroke volume. The dosing regimen must balance the optimal relief of edema and excess loss of fluid volume, while avoiding disturbances in serum electrolytes and induction of prerenal azothermia.

Unfortunately, in more advanced CHF, the use of a single diuretic may have limited efficacy, and combination therapy may be required. With "diuretic resistance," it is common to employ a combination of a loop and a distal tubular diuretic (see Chapter 13).

Sympathomimetics

Despite the fact that **norepinephrine** and **epinephrine** increase cardiac contractility and systemic blood pressure, the major drawbacks to their use in **acute** heart failure is the intense increase in peripheral vascular constriction and increase in left ventricular afterload, thus further impairing cardiac output in an already failing heart. The peripheral vasoconstrictor effects lead to impaired tissue perfusion especially to heart, kidney, and splanchnic regions. Furthermore, activation of cardiac β_1-adrenergic receptors may result in an increased oxygen demand, leading to development of relative myocardial ischemia and potentially lethal cardiac arrhythmias.

Dopamine's combination of selective vasodilator effects and β_1-adrenergic receptor activation make it attractive for situations in which blood pressure is low and renal perfusion is poor, as in cardiogenic, traumatic, or hypovolemic shock. As discussed earlier, its renal vasodilator action is additive to the effects of furosemide, making their combined use an important adjunctive intervention in patients with **acute** cardiac decompensation and volume overload, or in "diuretic resistant" patients. Dopamine is given intravenously due to its short half-life and rapid metabolism.

Dobutamine is useful in patients with low cardiac output and an increased left ventricular end-diastolic pressure who are not hypotensive. Under such circumstances, the positive inotropic action (β_1-mediated) and the ability to reduce left ventricular afterload (β_2-mediated vasodilation) would augment stroke volume and improve organ perfusion with little increase in heart rate. However, long-term use of dobutamine is limited by the development of tolerance. In patients with **acute** decompensated heart failure who are in need of short-term inotropic support, dobutamine is preferred over dopamine. At higher doses, dobutamine will increase systemic arterial pressure and increase ventricular afterload.

Heart rate may increase during dobutamine administration. This is of particular concern in patients with atrial fibrillation, where β-adrenergic receptor activation at the AV node will increase atrial impulses to the ventricular conducting system. The short half-life of dobutamine is advantageous when unexpected hypotension, tachycardia, or tachyarrhythmia result. As with all β-agonists, dobutamine will be ineffective in patients being treated with β-blockers.

Phosphodiesterase inhibitors

Inamrinone and milrinone were introduced as oral agents for management of patients with chronic CHF, although they are now used primarily parenterally for management of **acute** heart failure. They have direct positive inotropic effects and increase the rate of myocardial relaxation. They also cause a balanced arterial and venous vasodilation, leading to decreased arterial and pulmonary vascular resistance. The result is an increased cardiac output due to an increased myocardial contractility and a decreased ventricular afterload.

Both inamrinone and milrinone are effective in patients receiving β-blockers. They may therefore serve as a "bridge to β-blockade" for long-term management of patients with severe refractory heart failure who are unable to tolerate β-blockers in the absence of added inotropic support. The increase in stroke volume and cardiac output observed with inamrinone and milrinone are due mainly to peripheral vasodilation and a decrease in left ventricular afterload. There is significant variability in the degree to which cardiac output increases and systemic vascular resistance decreases. Clinically significant hypotension has occurred with milrinone.

Vasodilators

Vasodilators used for acute or chronic treatment of heart failure should be given in doses that reduce peripheral resistance but do not cause a sharp decrease in blood pressure, that is, in doses at which most blood pressure effects are compensated for by homeostatic mechanisms. These drugs relax venous and arterial smooth muscle, thereby reducing resistance to ventricular ejection as well as increasing the capacity of the venous reservoir. This causes relief of symptoms and an increase in exercise tolerance in patients with a dilated ventricle. These changes can be achieved acutely by intravenous nitroprusside, nitroglycerin, nesiritide;

or by chronic administration of hydralazine together with isosorbide dinitrate or an ACE inhibitor (see Chapter 16).

The major hemodynamic effect of nitroglycerin is a reduction in preload and decrease in left ventricular end-diastolic pressure. However, in the presence of increased peripheral vascular resistance and with relatively high doses administered intravenously, nitroglycerin also elicits a vasodilator effect on the arterial circulation. Nitroglycerin infusion is used for patients with acute ischemic syndromes or in patients with acute decompensated heart failure secondary to ischemic heart disease. Tolerance occurs and is clinically important with prolonged administration.

Although the renal effects of BNP on the kidney and its ability to unload the heart are well documented, some data suggest that it also has direct actions on cardiac fibroblasts. BNP is found in cardiac fibroblasts and inhibits de novo collagen synthesis and increases expression of specific matrix metalloproteinases. It may therefore be beneficial in controlling synthesis and degradation of collagen deposition after myocardial injury. Also, chronic administration of BNP suppresses aldosterone secretion, despite a natriuretic response. Thus, BNP works through both renal mechanisms and suppression of the profibrotic action of aldosterone.

Intravenous infusion of nesiritide (recombinant BNP) in patients with CHF results in beneficial hemodynamic actions, including arterial and venous dilation, enhanced Na^+ excretion, and suppression of the RAAS and SNS. Nesiritide alleviates the symptoms of acute decompensated heart failure and is useful in augmenting the effects of loop diuretics in patients who fail to respond with an adequate diuresis.

CLINICAL PROBLEMS

ACE inhibitors

Dry cough, hyperkalemia, hypotension

β-Adrenergic receptor blockers

Fluid retention, fatigue, bradycardia, hypotension, worsening heart failure, hypoglycemia

Angiotensin receptor blockers

Postural dizziness

Aldosterone antagonists

Hyperkalemia, hepatotoxicity, renal failure

Cardiac glycosides

CNS: Malaise, confusion, depression, vertigo, vision
GI: Anorexia, nausea, intestinal cramping, diarrhea
Cardiovascular: Palpitations, syncope, arrhythmias, bradycardia, AV node block, tachycardia, hyperkalemia

Parenteral compounds

Must be used in hospital setting; varies with agent

Side effects, clinical problems, and toxicity

Cardiac glycosides

Digoxin toxicity remains an important clinical problem, which demands vigilance for the early recognition of disturbances of cardiac impulse formation and conduction abnormalities, along with more subtle signs related to the central nervous and gastrointestinal systems (see Clinical Problems box). Toxic effects of digoxin may occur at any serum concentration due to factors that affect sensitivity (Box 15-2) because of its low therapeutic index.

Several factors affect the sensitivity of the heart to cardiac glycosides. Binding to the Na^+, K^+-ATPase is slow and enhanced by high intracellular Na^+ and low extracellular K^+. Thus, its pharmacological and toxic effects are greater in hypokalemic patients. K^+-depleting diuretics are a major contributing factor to digoxin toxicity. Ca^{2+}, if administered rapidly intravenously, may produce serious arrhythmias in patients treated with cardiac glycosides. Tachycardia, which increases Na^+ influx, also enhances their actions. Larger doses are used in newborn and young infants than in adults because of the low sensitivity of infant heart muscle to glycosides.

When cardiac muscle is exposed to toxic concentrations of a glycoside, Na^+ pump inhibition and cellular Ca^{2+} loading become excessive. The cytoplasmic membrane becomes unstable for a short time immediately after each membrane repolarization. In normal ventricular muscle cells, membrane depolarization is followed by repolarization, in that the membrane potential reaches approximately −90 mV and remains there until the next wave of depolarization (Fig. 15-4, *A*). In digoxin toxicity, however, the membrane becomes more permeable to Na^+, Ca^{2+}, and K^+ immediately after repolarization. Movements of Na^+ and Ca^{2+} are particularly prominent because these ions are driven by both chemical and electrical gradients.

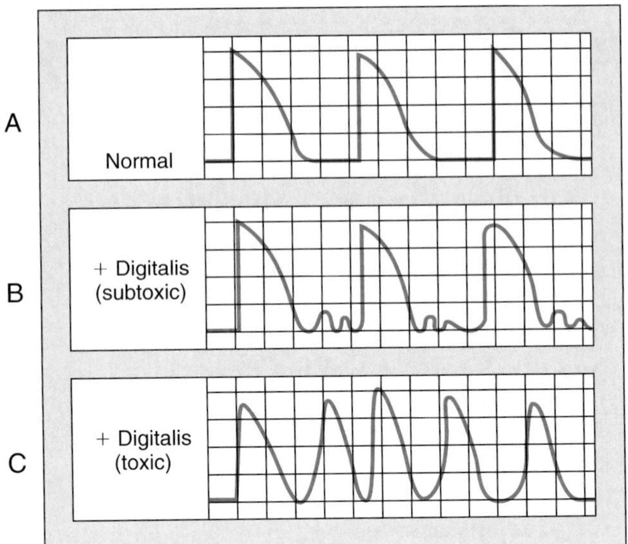

Figure 15-4 Changes in cardiac action potentials caused by subtoxic and toxic doses of cardiac glycosides. **A,** Typical action potential recordings from cardiac Purkinje fiber cells. Toxic doses produce oscillatory after depolarizations **(B)** and ventricular tachycardia **(C).**

In "mild" toxicity, the transient inward current subsides, causing the transmembrane potential to return to its resting level. This may be repeated several times, causing oscillatory **delayed afterpotentials** (Fig. 15-4, *B*). These small oscillatory delayed afterpotentials are most readily observed in cardiac Purkinje fibers and do not propagate beyond the individual cell. When their magnitude increases in advanced digoxin toxicity, the threshold potential is reached, causing the cell to be depolarized (i.e., to trigger action potentials; Fig. 15-4, *C*). Such **triggered action potentials** propagate from Purkinje fiber cells to ventricular muscle, causing the muscle to contract repetitively and no longer be under the control of the SA node. This may lead to life-threatening ventricular tachycardia and/or fibrillation.

Thyroid administration to a digitalized, hypothyroid patient may increase its dose requirement. Simultaneous use of digoxin and sympathomimetics increases the risk of cardiac arrhythmias by enhancing the formation of delayed after-depolarizations. Administration of succinylcholine results in sudden release of K^+ from skeletal muscle and may cause an increase in AV block in digitalized patients. Although β-blockers or Ca^{2+} channel blockers and digoxin may be useful in combination to control atrial fibrillation, their additive effects on AV node conduction can result in advanced or complete heart block. The reduction in plasma K^+ after administration of insulin may be associated with development of cardiac arrhythmias in patients receiving a cardiac glycoside. Caution should be exercised when combining digoxin with any drug that may cause a significant deterioration in renal function, because a decline in glomerular filtration or tubular secretion may impair its excretion.

Pharmacokinetic interactions involving digoxin are considerable. Quinidine should not be used to treat digoxin-induced arrhythmias because it increases plasma digoxin concentration, apparent volume of distribution, and renal clearance. Other drugs also interact with digoxin. Significant increases in plasma digoxin may occur with verapamil, nifedipine, amiodarone, or quinine, but only at high doses.

Ethacrynic acid, furosemide, and thiazide diuretics increase the therapeutic and toxic effects of digoxin and reduce its therapeutic index by causing K^+ depletion. Propranolol may augment bradycardia, whereas barbiturates, phenytoin, and phenylbutazone can enhance metabolism. Cholestyramine combines with digitoxin in the intestine and enhances its elimination.

Primary signs of digoxin toxicity include arrhythmias caused by suppression of AV nodal conduction. The first action taken upon suspecting digitalis toxicity is to **discontinue administration** until the adverse reaction resolves or is determined to be unrelated to the drug. Ventricular premature contractions triggered by oscillatory afterpotentials that originate in Purkinje fibers may also be superimposed. These arrhythmias may be converted to normal sinus rhythm by K^+ when the plasma K^+ concentration is low or within the normal range. K^+ is often effective against glycoside-induced arrhythmias because it:

- Stimulates Na^+ pump activity.
- Reduces glycoside binding.
- Probably alters membrane conductance to cations.

When the plasma K^+ concentration is high, antiarrhythmic drugs, such as lidocaine, procainamide, or propranolol, can be used. Although phenytoin is reported to be useful in treating arrhythmias, there have been several instances of sudden death in patients when phenytoin is administered to treat glycoside overdose. The most dramatic treatment for digoxin toxicity is a specific antibody raised against digoxin, which is administered intravenously and binds serum digoxin. The complex is excreted rapidly by the kidney.

In the more severe situation where the patient exhibits a disturbance in cardiac rhythm, additional therapy may be required. In the presence of symptomatic bradyarrhythmia or heart block, consideration should be given to the reversal of toxicity with a digoxin antibody, the use of atropine, or placement of a temporary cardiac pacemaker. However, asymptomatic bradycardia or heart block related to digoxin may require only temporary withdrawal of the drug and cardiac monitoring of the patient.

In the presence of a more severe and potentially life-threatening arrhythmia, such as bidirectional ventricular tachycardia, consideration should be given to the correction of electrolyte disorders, particularly if **hypokalemia or hypomagnesemia** are present. The antidigoxin antibody may be used to reverse potentially life-threatening ventricular arrhythmias.

Other drugs for congestive heart failure

The side effects of β-blockers are discussed in detail in Chapter 10. They are generally an extension of their therapeutic actions and include cardiac decompensation, bradycardia, hypoglycemia, and cold extremities. Initiation of treatment with a β-blocker has produced four types of adverse reactions that require careful attention and management:

- Fluid retention and worsening heart failure
- Fatigue
- Bradycardia and heart block
- Hypotension

Side effects of ACE inhibitors and ARBs are discussed in more detail in Chapter 12. ACE inhibitors often cause cough and, less commonly, development of angioneurotic edema. Both ACE inhibitors and ARBs should be discontinued before the second trimester of pregnancy due to their potential for teratogenic effects. Hypotension, oliguria, progressive azothermia, and hyperkalemia are not uncommon.

Contraindications for use of ACE inhibitors include bilateral renal artery stenosis and known allergies. High serum creatinine is a contraindication for use of ACE inhibitors or ARBs, as is the presence of hyperkalemia that will worsen on drug therapy.

Adverse effects associated with aldosterone antagonists include hyperkalemia, agranulocytosis, anaphylaxis, hepatotoxicity, and renal failure (see Chapter 33). Spironolactone has the added features of inducing gynecomastia, sexual dysfunction, and menstrual irregularities. Severe adverse effects associated with eplerenone include severe arrhythmias, life-threatening myocardial infarction, and myocardial ischemia (angina).

The sympathomimetics epinephrine and norepinephrine may cause restlessness, headache, tremor, and cardiac palpitations (see Chapter 10), as well as cerebral hemorrhage and cardiac arrhythmias. They should be used with caution in patients receiving nonselective β-blockers, because their unopposed actions on vascular α_1-adrenergic receptors can cause an acute hypertensive crisis and possible cerebral hemorrhage. The adverse effects of dopamine and dobutamine are similar and attributable to excessive sympathomimetic activity related to overdose (see Chapter 10).

Serious adverse effects attributable to the phosphodiesterase inhibitor inamrinone include ventricular arrhythmias, hypotension, and the potential for development of thrombocytopenia (10%) on prolonged administration. Long-term clinical trials of milrinone and inamrinone were associated with significant adverse effects and increased mortality in patients with heart failure. Currently, intravenous formulations of inamrinone and milrinone are approved for short-term support in patients with acute cardiac decompensation who are unresponsive to other drugs, such as diuretics or digoxin.

Adverse effects of nitrovasodilators, most commonly hypotension, are discussed in Chapter 16. Aggressive treatment with nitroprusside may result in a precipitous fall in left ventricular end-diastolic pressure, marked hypotension, and myocardial ischemia. The accompanying pulmonary vasodilation may lead to an increased ventilation-perfusion mismatch and hypoxia. Nitroprusside is contraindicated in patients with severe obstructive valvular heart disease (aortic, mitral, or pulmonic stenosis, or obstructive cardiomyopathy).

Hypotension, occasionally accompanied by bradycardia, is the major side effect associated with the administration of nesiritide, which is usually well tolerated in the supine position. The potential for hypotension is increased with concomitant administration of other drugs capable of lowering blood pressure.

New horizons

The last decade has transformed our understanding of the pathophysiology of CHF. This has led the way for development of new drugs that have demonstrated efficacy to increase survival, reduce hospitalization, and improve the quality of life for patients with CHF. Despite these advances, the prognosis for patients with established heart failure remains less than ideal, and morbidity and mortality remain unacceptably high.

The recognition that the activation of the SNS has an important role in the pathophysiology of heart failure encouraged a reexamination of the potential usefulness of β-blockers in treatment. For many years, β-blockers were contraindicated in treatment of severe left ventricular dysfunction. However, several clinical trials of β-blockers in patients following myocardial infarction showed that significant reductions in mortality were observed in patients with mild to moderate heart failure. Clinical experience with β-blockers in treatment of ventricular arrhythmias has also strengthened the case for their use in heart failure. Clinical trials with carvedilol, a β-blocker with α-blocking activity and antioxidant properties, showed a reduction in both disease progression and mortality.

Atrial and brain natriuretic peptides are known to increase Na^+ and water excretion, suppress renin and aldosterone secretion, and cause venous and arterial dilatation. Recent findings suggest that they may have favorable effects on autonomic function and antimitotic effects in the heart and blood vessels. The plasma concentration of BNP serves as a marker for the severity of CHF and may help assess the efficacy of pharmacological interventions. Small molecules that mimic the actions of BNP and are orally active are under investigation.

Nonpharmacological approaches for management of patients with heart failure are also under development or in clinical use. The most exciting, and perhaps the most controversial, has been generated by the emergence of expensive devices that significantly modify the natural history of left ventricular dysfunction and heart failure. Dyssynchrony between right and left ventricular contraction and relaxation has been identified as an independent predictor of cardiac mortality in patients with heart failure. Biventricular pacemakers synchronized to the patient's intrinsic sinus rate have been developed. One pacemaker is programmed to stimulate the right ventricle, whereas the other stimulates the left ventricle. Clinical trials show that this approach, in combination with an implantable cardioverter defibrillator, improves the quality of life and exercise duration in patients with moderate-to-severe heart failure.

Despite recent approaches to delay the progression of heart failure and prolong life, the important issue of prevention remains. Ischemic heart disease is an important contributor to development of chronic heart failure. Life-style changes discussed in Chapter 18, and the introduction of new antiatherogenic interventions, will reduce the number of patients who develop chronic heart failure. Because the mode of death in patients with CHF is sudden, there is the need for novel antiarrhythmic agents (see Chapter 14) that function during the normal cardiac cycle. Pharmacological inhibition of membrane currents activated during an ischemic event (IK_{ATP}) that heralds the onset of the lethal arrhythmic episode could provide a major benefit. Further understanding of the role of inflammation in progression of heart failure is indicated. The introduction of the neurohumoral hypothesis has brought about major changes in the management of chronic heart failure.

TRADE NAMES

In addition to generic and fixed-combination preparations, the following trade-named materials are some of the important compounds available in the United States. β-Adrenergic receptor blockers and sympathomimetics are in Chapter 10, ACE inhibitors in Chapter 12, diuretics in Chapter 13, and nitrovasodilators in Chapter 16.

Angiotensin II receptor blockers

Candesartan (Atacand)
Eprosartan (Teveten)
Irbesartan (Avapro)
Losartan (Cozaar)
Olmesartan (Benicar)
Telmisartan (Micardis)
Valsartan (Diovan)

Aldosterone antagonists

Spironolactone (Aldactone)
Eplerenone (Inspra)

Positive inotropic agents—for chronic heart failure

Digoxin (Lanoxin)

Phosphodiesterase III inhibitors

Milrinone (Primacor)
Inamrinone (Inocor IV)

B-natriuretic peptide

Nesiritide (Natrecor)

FURTHER READING

DiBianco R. Update on therapy for heart failure. *Am J Med* 2003; 115:480-488.

Braunwald E, Bristow MR. Congestive heart failure: Fifty years of progress. *Circulation* 2000; 102(suppl IV):IV-14-IV23.

Weber KT. Aldosterone in congestive heart failure. *N Engl J Med* 2001; 345:1689-1697.

Patterson JH. Angiotensin II receptor blockers in heart failure. *Pharmacotherapy* 2003; 23:173-182.

Self-assessment questions

1. The site responsible for the pharmacological and toxic actions of digitalis glycosides is:

a. β-Adrenergic receptor.
b. Na^+,K^+-ATPase.
c. protein kinase C.
d. cAMP-dependent protein kinase.
e. Ca^{2+} pump.

2. In a patient with congestive heart failure, which of the following will result in a reduction in preload?

a. Nitroprusside
b. A loop diuretic (e.g., furosemide)
c. Nitroglycerin
d. All of the above
e. *b* and *c* only

3. In a patient with congestive heart failure, which of the following would be most likely to result in afterload reduction?

a. Dobutamine
b. Captopril
c. Digoxin
d. Furosemide
e. Metoprolol

4. Which of the agents listed, *when administered in a therapeutic dose,* would produce a positive inotropic effect in the presence of β-adrenergic receptor blockade with metoprolol?

a. Digoxin
b. Milrinone
c. Dobutamine
d. Isoproterenol
e. All of the above
f. *a* and *b* only

5. Which of the following inhibits phosphodiesterase III?

a. Digoxin
b. Dobutamine
c. Milrinone
d. Propranolol

6. Eplerenone was introduced recently for the management of patients with congestive heart failure. Which of the following best describes its mode of action?

a. Inhibition of angiotensin II on the AT_1 receptor
b. Inhibition of aldosterone on its mineralocorticoid receptor
c. Inhibition of angiotensin-converting enzyme
d. Inhibition of angiotensin II on the AT_2 receptor

CHAPTER 16

Vasodilators and nitric oxide synthase

David Westfall
William T. Gerthoffer
R. Clinton Webb

Major Drugs	
Nitroglycerin (Nitrol) and nitrates	Minoxidil (Lotinen)
Angiotensin-converting enzyme inhibitors	Prazosin (Minipress)
Hydralazine (Apresoline)	Sodium nitroprusside (Nitropress)
	Sildenafil (Viagra)

Therapeutic overview

Ischemic heart disease is characterized by **angina pectoris,** chest pain that arises generally midsternally but also may radiate along the inner portion of one or both arms, or to the back. Vasodilators, specifically the **nitrates,** are mainstays in management. There are several different types of angina, depending on whether the disease is of atherosclerotic origin, the result of coronary artery spasm, or both. Angina may also be classified according to whether the pain is exertional or occurs more frequently at rest. However, irrespective of its type, the purpose of drug intervention is to bring about vasodilation of the coronary arteries, redistribution of blood flow in the heart, and/or a reduction in cardiac oxygen demand. Vasodilators, such as nitrates, provide no permanent beneficial effect on the underlying pathological condition but afford temporary symptomatic relief.

Vasodilators have important uses in management of coronary artery disease, hypertension, and congestive heart failure (CHF). Some modest success in preventing vasospasm or peripheral vascular disease has also been achieved. These drugs also play a minor role in lowering blood pressure to reduce bleeding in a surgical field. They are also increasingly popular for treatment of male impotence.

Recent studies indicate that vasodilator therapy is extremely effective in treatment of CHF. Drugs used more frequently for treating CHF are those that increase the force of cardiac contraction (see Chapter 15) or minimize Na^+ and water retention (see Chapter 13). Cardiac glycosides affect only two of several determinants of cardiac function (e.g., contractility and rate). Vasodilators can be useful in treatment of CHF by reducing preload, afterload, or both. Whether preload or afterload is affected depends on specific actions on arteriolar and venous vessels. Patients who are refractory to cardiac glycosides frequently do well if treated with vasodilators. Among the directly acting vasodilators used to treat CHF are the nitrates, hydralazine, minoxidil, and sodium nitroprusside. Angiotensin-converting enzyme (ACE) inhibitors are also of proven effectiveness in treatment of CHF.

Vasodilators are also used to treat certain peripheral vascular disorders. Direct-acting vasodilators, α_1-adrenergic receptor blockers, Ca^{2+}-channel blocking

Abbreviations	
ACE	angiotensin-converting enzyme
cAMP	cyclic adenosine monophosphate
cGMP	cyclic guanosine monophosphate
CHF	congestive heart failure
NO	nitric oxide
PDE	phosphodiesterase

drugs, and ACE inhibitors are used to treat Raynaud's phenomenon. Vasodilators are not effective in increasing blood flow when organic obstruction is significant. In some instances, vasodilator therapy may actually be harmful when blood is shunted away from diseased areas (see later).

A major goal of vasodilator therapy is to counterbalance vasoconstriction. A new direction is the development of agents that interact with endothelial cells. Endothelial cells line all vessels of the body and release factors that affect both the contractile state and growth of smooth muscle cells in the media. One of the important vasodilator factors released from the endothelium is **nitric oxide** (NO). NO, a short-lived radical, is formed from L-arginine by a class of enzymes known as NO synthases. Many drugs and endogenous substances, including acetylcholine and bradykinin, exert their vasodilator activity by stimulating synthesis of endothelial NO. Basal NO release also plays an important role in regulating vasoconstrictor tone. Endothelium-derived NO causes vasodilation in much the same way as nitrovasodilators, which owe their activity to donation of NO or a closely related molecule after their administration. Since the endothelium lies at the interface between blood and vascular smooth muscle, it has the potential of being an important target for vasodilator therapy.

A new and evolving use of direct vasodilators is in treatment of **erectile dysfunction** in men. Sildenafil, tadalafil, and vardenafil are selective inhibitors of cGMP-specific phosphodiesterase (PDE) type 5, which is responsible for degradation of cGMP in the corpus cavernosum of the penis. NO release during sexual stimulation activates guanylate cyclase, resulting in increased levels of cGMP. cGMP causes smooth muscle relaxation in the corpus cavernosum, allowing inflow of blood, and this effect is potentiated by selective PDE5 inhibitors. Sildenafil and related drugs have no direct relaxant effect on isolated human corpus cavernosum and, at recommended doses, have no effect in the absence of sexual stimulation. These drugs are highly selective for PDE5, and thus have few side effects.

Although vasodilators have useful therapeutic actions, they are not without problems. One major problem is the "steal" phenomenon. Some data indicate that use of vasodilator drugs to promote blood flow to ischemic or diseased tissue is limited. It appears that the small blood vessels around the ischemic area are already significantly dilated, therefore vasodilators may do little to enhance flow in this region. However, in normal nonischemic areas, where small vessels are not dilated, there is increased blood flow. By shunting blood to these areas, vasodilators may actually be reducing flow to the ischemic region.

Another concern is that, by decreasing peripheral vascular resistance, vasodilators cause reflex activation of the sympathetic nervous system (see Chapter 10). Enhanced sympathetic activity can lead to unwanted cardiac effects. The release of renin from juxtaglomerular cells is also enhanced by reflex sympathetic nerve stimulation caused by vasodilators. To counteract this action, β-adrenergic receptor antagonists are frequently administered in conjunction with directly acting vasodilators.

Another problem is the potential of these drugs to cause dilation of other, nonvascular, smooth muscles. Although uncommon, there are circumstances in which this is clinically significant, as in treatment of hypertension associated with the toxemia of pregnancy. In this case, vasodilators might interrupt labor by relaxing uterine smooth muscle.

A summary of the uses of these compounds is provided in the Therapeutic Overview box.

THERAPEUTIC OVERVIEW

Clinical problem	Goal of drug intervention
Hypertension	Decrease blood pressure
Congestive heart failure	Increase cardiac output and decrease oxygen consumption
Coronary artery insufficiency	Increase effective flow through coronary arteries and decrease oxygen consumption by the heart
Peripheral vascular disease	Increase blood flow to the ischemic area
Hemostasis	Slow bleeding into surgical field
Impotence	Increased erectile function

Mechanisms of action

Vasodilators act at different sites in the cascade of events that couple excitation of vascular smooth muscle to contraction (Table 16-1). Smooth muscle contraction is ultimately regulated by intracellular Ca^{2+} concentrations. Excitation-contraction coupling occurs by several mechanisms. Depolarization of vascular smooth muscle cell membranes allows Ca^{2+} entry through voltage-gated

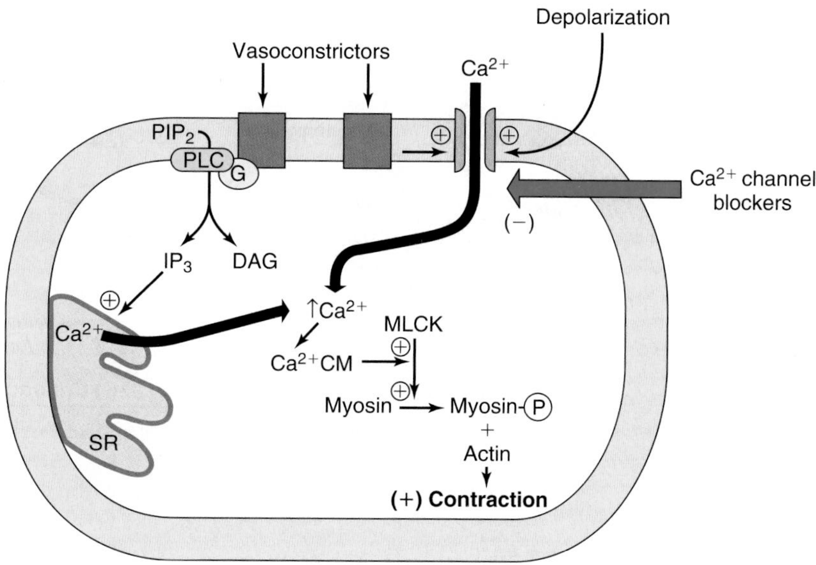

Figure 16-1 Mechanisms of contraction of vascular smooth muscle cells and its inhibition by Ca^{2+}-channel blockers. Increases in intracellular Ca^{2+} can occur by Ca^{2+} entry through channels opened by a change in membrane potential, by receptor activation, or by Ca^{2+} release from sarcoplasmic reticulum *(SR)*, an event triggered by inositol 1,4,5 trisphosphate *(IP_3)*. IP_3 is formed by hydrolysis of phosphatidylinositol 4,5-bisphosphate *(PIP_2)* by phospholipase C *(PLC)*. Ca^{2+} interacts with calmodulin (CM), which activates myosin light-chain kinase *(MLCK)*. The latter phosphorylates myosin, which interacts with actin, resulting in contraction. Ca^{2+}-channel blockers act by limiting Ca^{2+} entry through membrane channels.

Table 16-1 Mechanisms, sites of action, and uses of selected vasodilator drugs

Drug	Mechanism	Vessels Affected	Uses
Nitroglycerin and nitrates	Direct effect, conversion to NO, increase in cGMP	Venous	Angina pectoris (coronary artery disease), CHF, Raynaud's disease
Hydralazine	Direct effect, partially EDRF-dependent formation of NO,* increase in cGMP; possible K^+-channel agonist	Arteriolar	Hypertension, CHF (with nitrate)
Sodium nitroprusside	Direct effect, conversion to NO,* increase in cGMP	Arteriolar and venous	Hypertensive emergencies, acute CHF
Captopril, enalapril, and lisinopril	Inhibition of ACE	Arteriolar and venous	Hypertension, CHF
Minoxidil	Direct effect, K^+-channel agonist	Arteriolar	Refractory hypertension
Prazosin	Blockade of α_1-adrenergic receptors	Arteriolar and venous	Hypertension, Raynaud's disease
Sildenafil	Blockade of PDE type 5	Arteriolar and venous	Male impotence

See Chapter 12 for Ca^{2+}-channel blockers.
*May be NO or a chemically related unstable nitroso compound.

channels. When these channels open, Ca^{2+} flows into the cell down to its concentration gradient (Fig. 16-1). Activation of receptors for certain vasoconstrictor substances can also open Ca^{2+} channels. In addition to elevating intracellular Ca^{2+} by opening channels, receptor activation can also increase intracellular Ca^{2+} by activation of phospholipase C, which hydrolyzes phosphatidylinositol 4,5-bisphosphate to diacylglycerol and inositol 1,4,5-trisphosphate, both of which contribute to contraction (see Chapters 2 and 8). Inositol trisphosphate releases Ca^{2+} from intracellular stores, whereas diacylglycerol activates protein kinase C, an enzyme that phosphorylates several substrates involved in the contractile response. When Ca^{2+} enters the smooth muscle cell it combines with calmodulin. The Ca^{2+}-calmodulin complex activates myosin light-chain

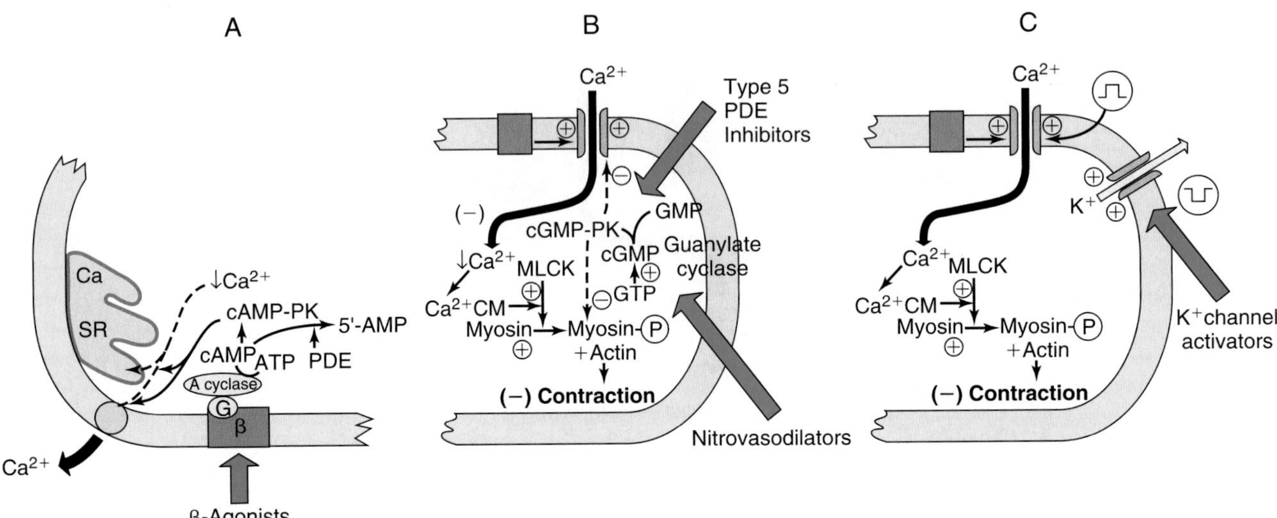

Figure 16-2 Mechanisms for relaxation of vascular smooth muscle cells. **A,** β-Adrenergic receptor agonists cause relaxation by stimulating formation of cAMP, which activates protein kinase *(PK)* and decreases intracellular Ca^{2+}. This occurs by activating Ca^{2+} pumps in the sarcoplasmic reticulum membrane or cell membrane to either sequester Ca^{2+} or pump it from the cell. **B,** Nitrovasodilators activate soluble guanylate cyclase by releasing NO or related compounds, leading to an increase in cGMP and activation of cGMP-dependent protein kinase. This substance may influence contractility by limiting Ca^{2+} entry through channels or by directly decreasing the sensitivity of contractile proteins to Ca^{2+}. Type 5 PDE Inhibitors, such as sildenafil, inhibit cGMP breakdown in cells where they are expressed (such as penile corpus cavernosum), and potentiate its vasodilatory actions. **C,** K^+-channel activators, such as minoxidil, increase K^+ conductance, which hyperpolarizes the cell, causing relaxation.

kinase, which in turn phosphorylates the myosin light chain. It is this phosphorylation that promotes interaction of myosin and actin and cross-bridge formation, leading to contraction (Fig. 16-1).

Ca^{2+} channel antagonists block or limit the entry of Ca^{2+} through voltage-gated channels, therefore reducing its availability to interact with contractile proteins (see Fig. 16-1). Thus, these drugs dilate blood vessels that have some endogenous degree of vasoconstrictor tone, or limit vasoconstriction caused by endogenous or exogenous vasoactive stimulants (see Chapter 12).

Increases in cyclic adenosine monophosphate (cAMP) are also associated with smooth muscle relaxation. When cAMP is elevated, cAMP-dependent protein kinase is activated. Vasodilation produced by this pathway includes decreased intracellular Ca^{2+} secondary to reduced influx, enhanced Ca^{2+} uptake into the sarcoplasmic reticulum, and/or enhanced Ca^{2+} extrusion through the cell membrane (Fig. 16-2, *A*). cAMP-dependent protein kinase may also phosphorylate and inhibit myosin light-chain kinase, thus inhibiting contraction. Relaxation of smooth muscle produced by β-adrenergic receptor agonists, such as isoproterenol, depends on formation of cAMP. Stimulation of β-adrenergic receptors activates adenylate cyclase, which generates cAMP from adenosine triphosphate. Drugs that inhibit PDEs, which metabolize cAMP and cGMP, can promote smooth muscle relaxation by elevating their concentrations. Drugs, such as papaverine, may act by this mechanism. PDEs exist in several isoforms, and there is considerable interest in developing agents with specificity for these isoforms (see later).

Nitrovasodilators activate a soluble guanylate cyclase in vascular smooth muscle, causing an increase in intracellular cyclic guanosine monophosphate (cGMP). cGMP in turn activates a cGMP-dependent protein kinase (Fig. 16-2, *B*). The mechanism by which cGMP-dependent protein kinase leads to smooth muscle relaxation is not entirely clear but may include decreased entry of Ca^{2+} through membrane channels. Other actions include inhibition of phosphatidylinositol hydrolysis, or stimulation of Ca^{2+} pumps, resulting in extrusion or sequestration of Ca^{2+}. cGMP-dependent protein kinase may also decrease the sensitivity of contractile proteins to Ca^{2+}. Regardless, it is clear that increases in cGMP are associated with vascular smooth muscle relaxation.

The action of nitrovasodilators appears to be quite similar to that of endothelium-derived relaxing factor. This compound is formed in, and released from, endothelial cells of blood vessels. Probably the most important stimulus controlling its release is shear forces placed on the endothelium by blood flow. Endothelial derived relaxing factor is now known to be NO. As discussed previously, NO is synthesized by enzymes known as NO synthases. Two isoforms of this enzyme are particularly important with respect to vascular biology. The "constitutive" form is present in endothelium under normal physiological conditions, and its activity is dependent upon the concentration of Ca^{2+}-calmodulin. There is also an "inducible" form of NO synthase expressed in smooth muscle in response to trauma or pathological stimuli, such as invading bacteria. The activity of this isoform does not depend on intracellular Ca^{2+}-calmodulin concentration and is not easily regulated. In severe septicemia, NO generated by this enzyme can cause harmful hypotension due to vasodilation. In all cases, NO-induced vasodilation is associated with elevated levels of cGMP.

NO may be the final common mediator for several vascular smooth muscle relaxants. In addition to nitrovasodilators, which may form NO or a related molecule, some endogenous agents that cause vasodilation do so in whole or in part by releasing NO from endothelial cells. Included among these are bradykinin, histamine, adenosine triphosphate, adenosine diphosphate, substance P, and acetylcholine (Fig. 16-3). Because the endothelium is an important structure for communicating between the blood and the vascular media, it has the potential to be an important target for vasodilator therapy.

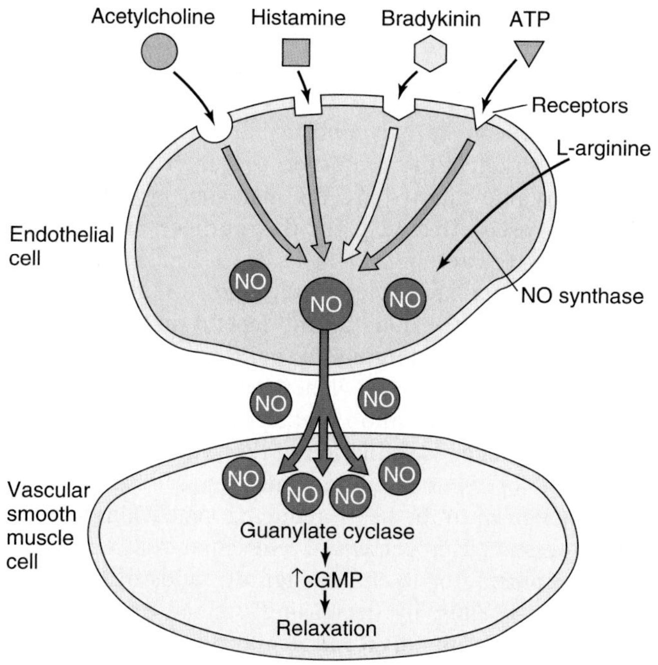

Figure 16-3 Endothelium-dependent relaxation produced by vasodilators. These substances act on endothelial cells at their respective receptors to release nitric oxide *(NO)*. The latter diffuses into the vascular smooth muscle cell, increases soluble guanylate cyclase activity and cGMP concentration, and promotes relaxation. L-Arginine is converted to NO by NO synthases.

Specific inhibitors of PDE5, which is found in high concentrations in the penile corpus cavernosum, have been found to specifically dilate blood vessels in this tissue. These drugs include sildenafil, tadalafil, and vardenafil, and appear to enhance the actions of cGMP formed in response to NO by blocking cGMP breakdown and prolonging its actions (see Fig. 16-2B). They therefore cause specific vasodilation in the presence of appropriate sexual stimulation and have become increasingly popular for treating erectile dysfunction in men.

Agents, such as minoxidil, cause vasodilation by activating K^+ channels in vascular smooth muscle. The increased K^+ conductance results in hyperpolarization of the cell membrane, and relaxation (see Fig. 16-2, *C*). The hyperpolarizing effect also counteracts stimulants that act by depolarization and promoting Ca^{2+} entry.

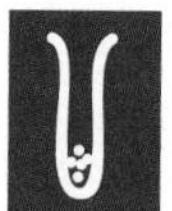

Pharmacokinetics

Selected pharmacokinetic parameter values for vasodilators are summarized in Table 16-2. Organic nitrates are almost completely absorbed from the gastrointestinal tract and fairly completely absorbed from the buccal mucosa. After sublingual administration, peak plasma concentrations are achieved in 1 to 2 minutes. Absorption is much slower with topical ointments and transdermal patches, and plasma concentrations attained with transdermal preparations are lower and more variable than those obtained with ointments. The nitrates are metabolized in liver by glutathione nitrate reductase (e.g., nitroglycerin is rapidly converted to inorganic nitrite and to denitrated metabolites). Isosorbide dinitrate is also metabolized by hepatic glutathione reductase and converted to inactive products, as well as to an active metabolite, 5-isosorbide mononitrate. This may account for its longer duration of antianginal activity. Isosorbide dinitrate is also used in therapy of intractable chronic CHF, frequently in combination with other vasodilators that cause relaxation of resistance vessels. Sublingual nitroglycerin is the mainstay of therapy in anginal attacks and is also used prophylactically. It is rapid in onset and inexpensive. Sublingual isosorbide dinitrate is also available and has a longer duration of action than nitroglycerin. The nitroglycerin aerosol spray appears to be as effective as the sublingual tablets. Transdermal patches are not as effective as

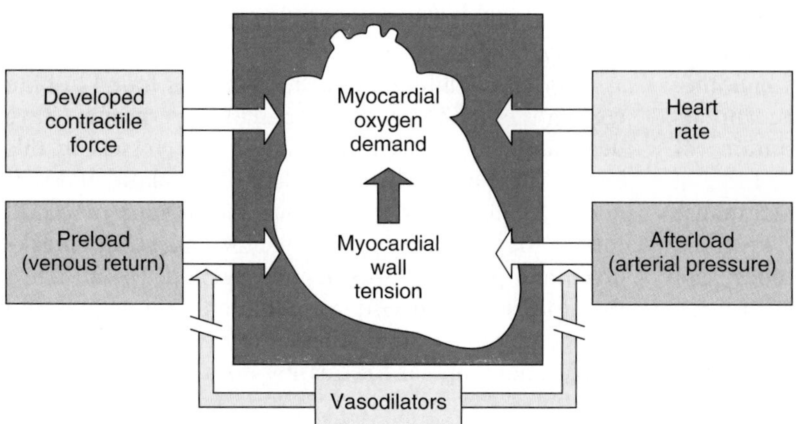

Figure 16-4 Mechanism of vasodilator action in the therapy of CHF. The four main determinants of cardiac function act to determine the myocardial oxygen demand. Nitrates decrease preload and afterload but do not affect contractile force, thereby decreasing oxygen demand. Heart rate may increase slightly as a result of the baroreceptor reflex.

Table 16-2 Pharmacokinetic parameters of vasodilators

Drug	Route of Administration	Remarks
Nitroglycerin	Sublingual	Onset 2-4 min, duration 30-60 min depending on patient activity, minimal first-pass effect, all organic nitrates metabolized by liver
	Oral	Onset 10-20 min, duration 2-3 hr, significant first-pass effect
	IV	Immediate onset, used to maintain stable blood concentration
	Transdermal	Discs or patches: slower onset, 10-18 hr variable duration; ointment less variable, duration 20-24 hr, for nocturnal angina
	Aerosol	Rapid onset, difficult to control
Isosorbide dinitrate*	Sublingual	Similar in onset to nitroglycerin, longer duration (2-4 hr)
	Oral	Onset 10-20 min, duration 4-8 hr
Erythrityl tetranitrate	Sublingual	Onset 3-5 min, duration 1-2 hr
Pentaerythritol tetranitrate	Oral	Onset 15-30 min, duration 4-8 hr
Sildenafil	Oral	Onset 30-60 min, duration 2-4 hr

*Active metabolite; oral preparations: onset varies with dose, and duration depends on extent of first-pass metabolism.

the oral, timed-release preparations, largely because of variable absorption through the skin. As a result of tolerance, transdermal patches left in place for 24 hours are ultimately ineffective for treatment of angina, even if the dose is increased. However, patches that deliver 10 mg or more nitroglycerin can be effective, if the patches are removed for a 10- to 12-hour period daily.

Type 5 PDE inhibitors are given orally, have an onset of action within about 30 minutes, and durations of action from 4 to 48 hours. They are metabolized in the liver by the cytochrome P450 system to inactive metabolites.

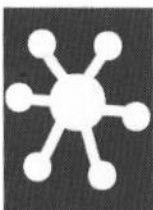

Relation of mechanisms of action to clinical response

Angina

The goal of therapy in coronary artery disease is to reduce pain and increase the patient's exercise tolerance. This can be accomplished by administration of organic nitrates, the prototype of which is **nitroglycerin.** Organic nitrates are the mainstay of antianginal therapy, used effectively for this purpose for approximately 100 years.

The pharmacological properties of the organic nitrates that make them useful depend on the underlying cause of the angina. If pain is associated with atherosclerosis, the chief benefit arises from actions on the peripheral circulation and not on coronary vessels. Nitrates produce vasodilation of the venous vasculature. Dilation of venous capacitance vessels diminishes venous return to the heart, reducing ventricular volume and pressure. This decreases ventricular wall tension, a major contributor to the oxygen demands of the heart (Fig. 16-4). Thus, by decreasing preload on the heart, oxygen needs diminish and demand is consistent with supply.

Other consequences of nitroglycerin administration also contribute to its beneficial effect in angina. For example, nitrates cause relaxation of resistance vessels of the arterial circulation. This decreases afterload placed on the heart or the impedance against which the heart must pump. Reducing afterload decreases oxygen demands of the heart, just as reducing preload does. The nitrate effect on resistance vessels generally requires somewhat higher concentrations than those needed for venodilation.

Another beneficial feature of organic nitrate actions in angina pectoris is redistribution of blood flow to the subendocardial regions of the heart, which are especially vulnerable to ischemia. Perfusion of the subendocardial region occurs most prominently during early diastole. Later in diastole, as the ventricle fills, subendocardial arteries are constricted because of pressure in the ventricles, with the subsequent decrease in perfusion of these arteries. By decreasing preload, nitrates reduce ventricular filling pressure and increase the time available for endocardial perfusion.

In management of angina pectoris caused by coronary artery spasm, the organic nitrates, in addition to effects described previously, are useful because they can dilate constricted coronary vessels. Nitrates are available in many dosage forms, including sublingual, transdermal, and longer-acting oral preparations (Table 16-2). The choice of nitrate preparation depends on the necessity for a rapid onset or a longer duration of action. Other drugs used in treatment of angina pectoris are β-adrenergic receptor antagonists and Ca^{2+} channel blocking drugs (see Chapter 12). The beneficial effect of β-blockers in angina is their ability to decrease oxygen demands of the heart. Beta-blockers decrease heart rate and ventricular contractile force (see Chapter 10). Heart rate and contractile force, together with ventricular wall tension, are major determinants of myocardial oxygen demand (see Fig. 16-4). In addition, chronic therapy with β-blockers reduces blood pressure. Thus, these drugs also decrease afterload. Unlike organic nitrates, β-blockers are not used to terminate an acute attack of angina pectoris but rather to increase exercise tolerance of the patient and to reduce the frequency of anginal attacks.

Congestive heart failure

Vasodilator therapy is now widely used for treatment of chronic congestive heart failure (CHF), particularly when the patient has not responded adequately to drugs that increase the force of cardiac contraction (see Chapter 15) or to diuretics (see Chapter 13). Increased survival of patients under a vasodilator regimen has been demonstrated. As previously described, the determinants of cardiac function are preload, afterload, contractility, and heart rate (see Fig. 16-4). Among the major mechanisms by which vasodilators increase cardiac performance are afterload reduction, preload reduction, and the resulting increased left ventricular diastolic compliance. Afterload reduction, by use of other vasodilators and high concentrations of nitrates, is accomplished by dilating arterioles and thereby decreasing systemic vascular resistance. This increases cardiac output and tissue perfusion. Venodilators, including low doses of nitrates, predominantly decrease preload, reducing systemic and pulmonary venous pressures. Ventricular volume is also affected by the decreasing preload. The venodilators do not increase the force of contraction, and the heart rate is generally unchanged, so that the work of the heart remains the same. The overall effect, therefore, is a reduction in myocardial oxygen consumption and demand on the heart. The vasodilator drugs may also improve left ventricular diastolic performance by shifting the diastolic pressure-volume curve to the left (i.e., to pump the same volume at a lower pressure). This shift also moves the ventricular function curve to the left, demonstrating an improvement in left ventricular performance.

Vasodilators used to treat CHF influence preload, afterload, or both. Among the agents used are the direct-acting agents (nitrates, hydralazine, and nitroprusside), the α_1-adrenergic receptor blocker prazosin, and the ACE inhibitors captopril, enalapril, and lisinopril (see Chapter 15). Long-term treatment with hydralazine alone is only minimally effective in treatment of CHF, but the combination of hydralazine with a nitrate, isosorbide dinitrate, effectively decreases mortality. Minoxidil is also generally not very effective when used alone.

Peripheral vascular disease

Peripheral vascular diseases are either vasospastic or occlusive. In Raynaud's disease, a vasospastic disorder, blood flow to the extremities is reduced as a result of a reversible vasoconstriction. Therefore, vasodilators may be helpful to these patients by dilating the blood vessels of the skin. Vasodilators are of limited usefulness in occlusive disease with a physical obstruction, however, and they do not generally improve flow to either skeletal muscle or skin. A wide variety of drug classes has been used in treatment of peripheral vascular diseases, including α_1-adrenergic blockers, Ca^{2+} channel blockers, prostaglandins, β-adrenergic agonists, and direct-acting vasodilators. Nitroglycerin ointment may be helpful as an adjunctive agent in Raynaud's disease. Other nonspecific vasodilators, such as cyclandelate, papaverine, ethaverine, and nicotinyl tartrate have been used, but are of questionable efficacy.

Hemostasis

Vasodilators may be used as aids during surgical procedures. They can be used to provide a more satisfactory surgical field, to minimize large blood volume losses, and to improve cardiac performance by reducing preload or afterload.

Impotence

The use of type 5 PDE inhibitors, such as sildenafil, has dramatically altered the therapeutic treatment of male erectile dysfunction. Parasympathetic nerves innervating blood vessels of penile corpus cavernosum release NO when activated during sexual activity. Sildenafil and related drugs potentiate the action of NO on cGMP by blocking cGMP breakdown, resulting in prolonged dilation of cavernosal blood vessels, thereby enhancing erection. Tadalafil and vardenafil are similar compounds with increased selectivity for PDE5 and longer durations of action.

Side effects, clinical problems, and toxicity

Major side effects of vasodilators are summarized in the Clinical Problems box. As with all vasodilators, orthostatic hypotension and tachycardia are adverse effects of nitrate therapy. Vascular headache is quite common but rapidly disappears on continued use. Tolerance to the vascular effects of nitrates does occur; however, this is not of great clinical significance, except possibly in treatment of chronic CHF. Cross-tolerance exists between nitroglycerin and other nitrate esters, but this and other nitrate tolerance can be reduced by only a short period of nitrate abstention. Orthostatic hypotension can be minimized by careful adjustment of dose and by having the patient avoid the upright position when taking rapid-acting preparations. Physical dependence has been observed in munitions workers exposed continuously to very high concentrations of nitrates. In these individuals, withdrawal from the industrial environment may result in angina. This phenomenon is not observed in patients normally taking therapeutic doses of nitrates but can occur in individuals who have been taking large doses for a long time.

Nitrates can be reduced to nitrites, which in turn can oxidize the ferrous iron of hemoglobin, converting it to methemoglobin. The latter reduces oxygen delivery to tissues. Methemoglobinemia is not a problem with normal nitrate therapy but may be observed in accidental poisoning or overdose.

Type 5 PDE inhibitors can cause abnormalities in color vision, although this is most common with sildenafil. Inhibition of PDE5 in other tissues, such as esophageal smooth muscle and brain, can result in a reduced tone of the esophageal sphincter and increased gastroesophageal reflux, as well as dyspepsia. They have also been reported to result in emotional, neurological, and psychological side effects, and have the potential to cause hypotension.

Problems associated with nitroprusside, prazosin, hydralazine, the ACE inhibitors, and minoxidil are discussed in Chapter 12.

CLINICAL PROBLEMS

Vasodilators in general
Orthostatic hypotension
Tachycardia

Nitrate vasodilators
Headache
Tolerance

Hydralazine
Lupus-like effect

Sodium nitroprusside
Thiocyanate accumulation

Minoxidil
Sodium retention
Hypertrichosis

Sildenafil
Hypotension and reflex stimulation of the heart
Problems with color vision

New horizons

Development of new vasodilators with greater specificity remains an important goal. One area with particular promise is the pharmacology of the vascular endothelium. The endothelium has a crucial function in regulation of both the contractile state and growth of vascular smooth muscle cells. It also has antithrombotic properties that inhibit adhesion and aggregation of blood cells. The important outcome of these effects is that the microvasculature is perfused without obstruction, whereas blood flow is regulated locally.

The most important approach has been to develop drugs that interact with the NO signaling cascade of the endothelium. Potential targets include:

- Drugs that activate NO synthase.
- Gene therapy to influence expression of NO synthase or other protein mediators.
- Drugs that prolong the vasodilator properties of NO.

Several other products of endothelial cells, called endothelins, have been isolated. The most prominent and well studied is a 21-amino acid peptide, endothelin-1. This compound is released in response to physiological challenges, such as hypoxia or stress, or by endogenous hormones, such as angiotensin. Endothelin-1 initially dilates smooth muscle but subsequently produces an intense, long-lasting vasoconstriction. Two types of endothelin receptors have been characterized (ET_A and ET_B). Current evidence indicates that endothelin does not act as a circulating hormone but rather as an autocrine or paracrine substance. Abnormally high levels may play a pathogenic role in some forms of vasospasm. Antagonists of endothelin receptors have been developed, and their therapeutic potential is being investigated.

Finally, recent studies have demonstrated that NO is balanced by superoxide anion generated in the vascular wall. Superoxide anion is the product of several reactions, but the principal ones in the vasculature are NADPH oxidase, xanthine oxidase, uncoupled NO synthase, and cyclooxygenase. In several vascular diseases (atherosclerosis, hypertension, etc.), the production of superoxide in blood vessel walls is increased. The reaction between NO and superoxide is so fast that it effectively removes the vasodilator action of NO. Drugs that block production of superoxide anion may be useful in vasodilator therapy that focuses on NO.

TRADE NAMES

In addition to generic and fixed-combination preparations and the drugs listed in the Major Drugs box, the following trade-named materials are some of the important compounds available in the United States.

Erythrityl tetranitrate (Cardilate)
Isosorbide dinitrate (Isordil, Sorbitrate, Dilatrate)
Nitroglycerin sublingual (Nitro-Bid, Nitrospan, Nitrolingual)
Nitroglycerin ointment (Nitrol)
Nitroglycerin transdermal (Nitrodisc, Transderm-Nitro, Nitro-Dur)
Pentaerythritol tetranitrate (Peritrate, Pentitrol)
Tadalafil (Cialis)
Vardenafil (Levitra)

FURTHER READING

Toda N, Okamura T. The pharmacology of nitric oxide in the peripheral nervous system of blood vessels. *Pharmacol Rev* 2003; 55:271-324.

Vanhoutte PM. Endothelial control of vasomotor function: From health to coronary disease. *Circ J* 2003; 67:572-575.

Webb RC. Smooth muscle contraction and relaxation. *Adv Physiol Educ* 2003; 27:201-206.

Self-assessment questions

1. All of the following are side effects of nitrovasodilators *except:*

a. Hypotension.
b. Reflex tachycardia.
c. Headache.
d. Lupus-like syndrome.
e. Tolerance.

2. Which of the following is a mixed (venous and arteriolar) dilator?

a. Hydralazine
b. Minoxidil
c. Nitrates
d. Prazosin
e. Captopril

3. In the vascular smooth muscle cell:

a. Depolarization of the membrane allows calcium entry via voltage-operated channels.
b. Inositol trisphosphate, a product of phospholipase C activation, increases intracellular Ca^{2+} by stimulating receptor-operated membrane channels.
c. Ca^{2+} combines with calmodulin to activate myosin light-chain kinase.
d. *a* and *c* are correct.
e. All are correct.

4. All of the following actions of nitrovasodilators are correct *except* that:

a. They inhibit phosphodiesterase.
b. They generate nitric oxide.
c. They increase cGMP.
d. They are similar to endothelial derived relaxing factor.
e. All are correct.

5. All of the following can be used to treat chronic congestive heart failure *except:*

a. Nitrovasodilators.
b. ACE inhibitors.
c. Minoxidil.
d. Hydralazine.
e. Prazosin.

6. Which of the following is not a property of nitric oxide synthesized by the endothelium?

a. The most important stimulus for NO synthesis is blood flow producing shear stress on the endothelium.
b. NO activates guanylate cyclase in smooth muscle leading to elevated cGMP and vasodilatation.
c. NO synthesis in the endothelium is due to activation of an inducible enzyme isoform, which is not dependent on calcium-calmodulin complex.
d. NO is a free radical and has a very short half-life in plasma (5-10 minutes).

CHAPTER 17

Prostaglandins and related autacoids

Barrie Ashby

Major Drugs

Alprostadil (PGE_1)	Misoprostol (Cytotec)
Corticosteroids	Montelukast (Singulair)
Dinoprostone (PGE_2, Cervidil)	Nonsteroidal antiinflammatory drugs
Epoprostenol (PGI_2, Flolan)	Zafirlukast (Accolate)
Latanoprost (Xalatan)	Zileuton (Zyflo)

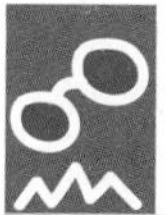

Therapeutic overview

Eicosanoids include a large family of endogenous compounds containing oxygenated unsaturated 20-carbon fatty acids. The eicosanoids include prostaglandins (PGs), thromboxanes (Txs), and leukotrienes (LTs), and exert profound effects on practically all cells and tissues, providing many potential targets for intervention in treatment of disease.

PGs may be used as drugs themselves to mimic effects they would produce if formed endogenously. Alternatively, other drugs, such as **nonsteroidal anti-inflammatory drugs** (NSAIDs, see Chapter 31) and **corticosteroids** (see Chapter 33), produce their effects by inhibiting their formation. New drugs are also being introduced to block the effects of PG or LT receptors (see Chapter 34).

A schematic overview of eicosanoid synthesis is provided in Figure 17-1. Most pathways originate with the parent compound **arachidonic acid**, a major component of membrane phospholipids. Catalysis by **cytochrome P450 monooxygenases** produces **epoxides**, whereas **cyclooxygenases** (COXs) produce PGs and Txs, and **5-lipoxygenases** produce LTs. Because of the large number of physiological actions attributed to the eicosanoids, they have diverse therapeutic applications (see Therapeutic Overview box).

Mechanisms of action

Synthesis The structures and biosynthesis of PGs are shown in Figure 17-2. PGs are derived from essential fatty acids, usually arachidonic acid (C20:4) but also eicosatrienoic acid (C20:3, present in seminal vesicles) and eicosapentaenoic acid (C20:5, derived from cold water fish). The numbering designation of arachidonic acid, 20:4, indicates 20 carbon atoms and 4 double bonds. The compounds that retain 2 double bonds in their alkyl side-chains are denoted by the subscript 2 and those that retain 3 double bonds by the subscript 3. Arachidonic acid and other fatty acids are cleaved from membrane phospholipids by the action of phospholipase A_2 and metabolized by three different types

Abbreviations

COX	cyclooxygenase
GI	gastrointestinal
LTs	leukotrienes
NSAID	nonsteroidal antiinflammatory drug
PGs	prostaglandins
Txs	thromboxanes

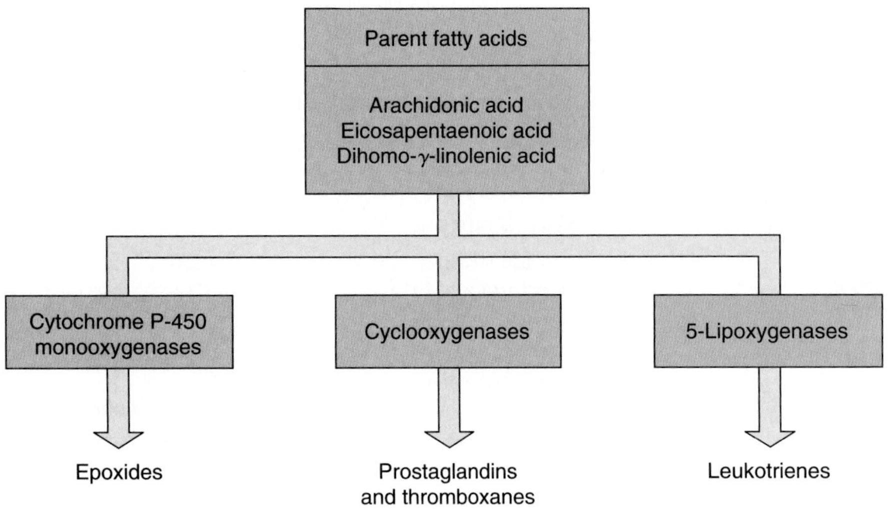

Figure 17-1 Classification of the major eicosanoids of pharmacological interest.

THERAPEUTIC OVERVIEW

Drug	Effect	Use
Corticosteroids	Block eicosanoid production	Inflammation
Prostaglandins	Increased blood flow and oxygenation by vessel relaxation	Neonatal defects Penile erection
	Increased uterine contraction	Induction of labor, abortifacient
	Reduced platelet aggregation	Peripheral vascular disease
	Reduce intraocular pressure	Glaucoma
	Suppress gastric acid secretion	Gastric ulcers
Leukotriene antagonists	Block leukotriene receptor-mediated bronchoconstriction	Asthma
Leukotriene synthesis inhibitors	Inhibit lipoxygenase	Asthma
Nonsteroidal antiinflammatory drugs	Block prostaglandin synthesis	Pain, inflammation

of enzymes: COXs, lipoxygenases, and cytochrome P-450 monooxygenases.

COXs convert arachidonic acid into the PG endoperoxides PGG_2 and PGH_2. COXs are inhibited by NSAIDS, such as aspirin and ibuprofen (see Chapter 31), leading to inhibition of PG and Tx formation. Two distinct COXs have been described designated **COX-1** and **COX-2**. COX-1 is constitutively expressed, whereas COX-2 is inducible and expressed in response to inflammatory mediators, such as cytokines and lipopolysaccharides. Corticosteroids suppress induction of COX-2 (see Chapter 33), suggesting that control of PG synthesis is involved in their antiinflammatory actions. In addition, selective COX-2 inhibitors, such as celecoxib (see Chapter 31) are useful in treating chronic inflammation because they may cause less gastric disturbance than NSAIDS by allowing formation of cytoprotective PGE_2 through COX-1.

Like the PGs, the LTs are acidic lipids derived from essential fatty acids by lipoxygenases (Fig. 17-3), which are not inhibited by NSAIDs. Three major lipoxygenases have been discovered, which catalyze incorporation of a molecule of oxygen into the 5-, 12-, or 15-position of arachidonic acid, and formation of the corresponding 5-, 12-, or 15-hydroxyperoxyeicosatetraenoic (HPETE) acids. The 5- and 15-lipoxygenases give rise to the LTs. 5-lipoxygenase is activated by a protein called 5-lipoxygenase activating protein, which is a potential target for drug intervention. LTB_4 has potent chemotactic properties for polymorphonuclear leukocytes, promoting adhesion and aggregation. LTC_4 and LTD_4 are potent constrictors of peripheral lung airways and other vessels, including coronary arteries.

Metabolism and concentration PGs are not stored but are synthesized and secreted in response to diverse

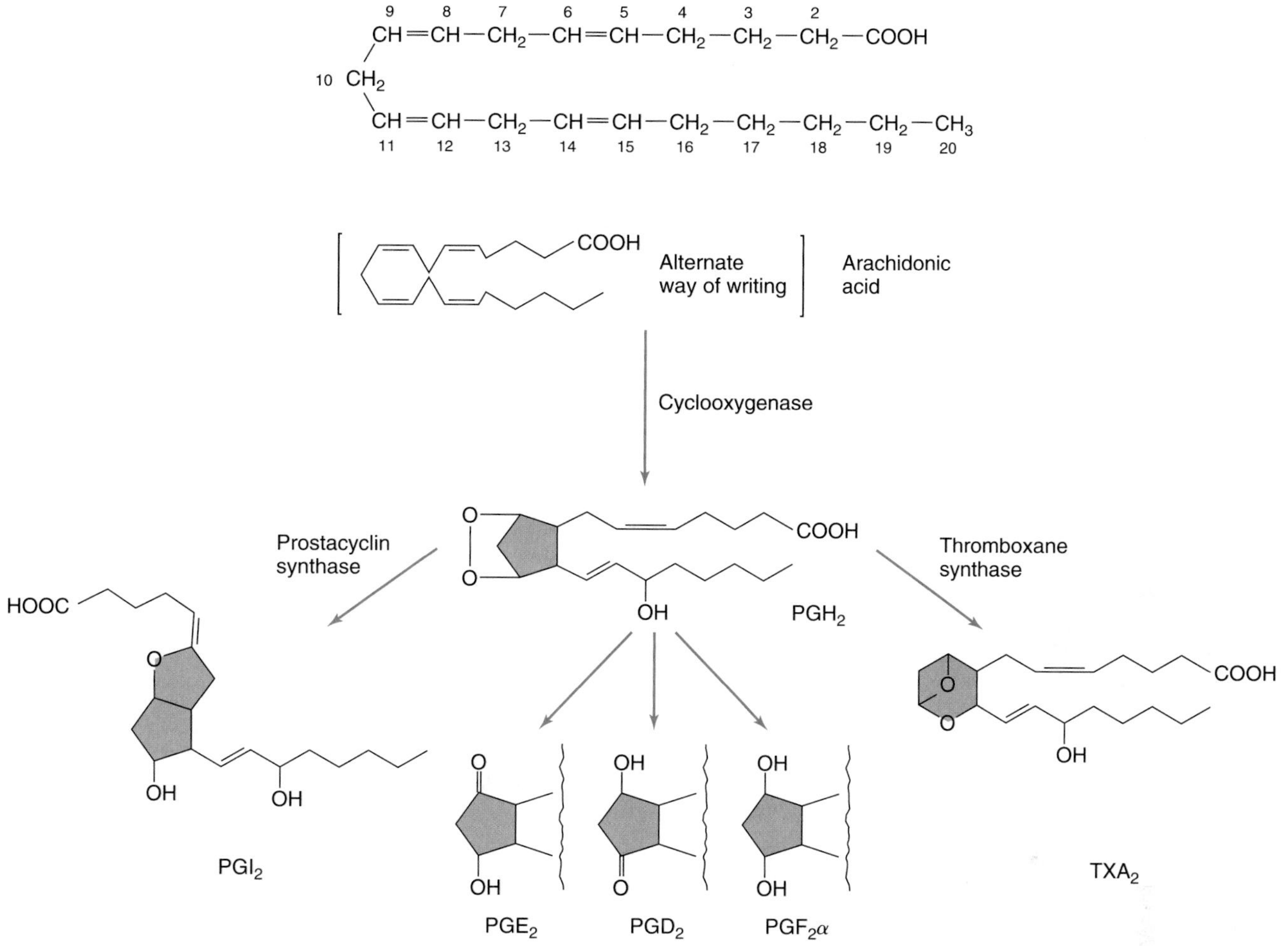

Figure 17-2 Chemical structures and biosynthesis of principal prostaglandins. *PG*, Prostaglandin; *Tx*, thromboxane; *PGI₂*, prostacyclin. (PGE_2, PGD_2, and $PGF_{2\alpha}$ differ from endoperoxide PGH_2, as indicated.)

stimuli. PGs and TxA_2 act primarily as local hormones (autocoids), with their biological activities usually restricted to the cell, tissue, or structure where they are synthesized. Concentrations of PGE_2 and $PGF_{2\alpha}$ in arterial blood are very low because of pulmonary degradation, which normally removes more than 90% of these PGs from the venous blood as it passes through the lungs. Not all cells synthesize PGs; for example, there are segments of the nephron that lack COXs or show negligible capacity to transform added arachidonic acid to PGs. In contrast, COX is abundant within the vasculature, although the principal products vary longitudinally along the vasculature and cross-sectionally within the blood vessel wall (e.g., endothelium versus vascular smooth muscle). Within the coronary circulation the larger blood vessels synthesize principally PGI_2, whereas PGE_2 predominates in microvessels.

PG receptors PGs exert their effects by binding to specific cell surface receptors, which have been pharmacologically subdivided with respect to agonist potency and the signal transduction system to which they are coupled. All PG receptors are G-protein coupled–receptors (see Chapter 2), which stimulate G-proteins to initiate transmembrane signaling. PGD_2 activates DP receptors, PGE_2 activates EP receptors, $PGF_{2\alpha}$ activates FP receptors, PGI_2 activates IP receptors, whereas TxA_2 activates TP receptors. PG receptors may stimulate (DP, EP_2, EP_4, IP) or inhibit (EP_3) adenylyl cyclase, or stimulate phospholipase C (EP_1, TP) leading to formation of diacylglycerol and inositol trisphosphate and Ca^{2+} mobilization. Many cell types possess several PG receptor subtypes and respond in a variety of ways to PGs. For example, renal tubules possess multiple PG receptors, based on the observation that low concentra-

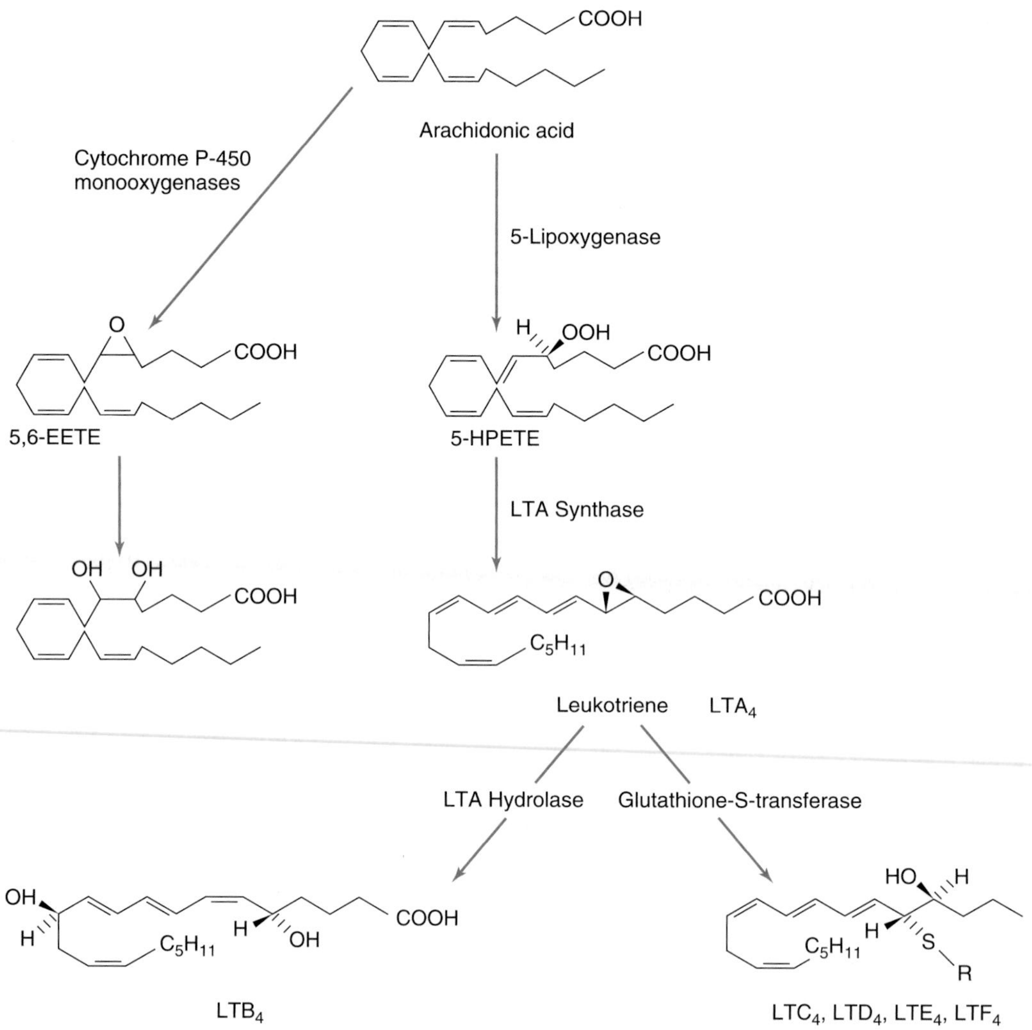

Arachidonic acid

Cytochrome P-450 monooxygenases

5-Lipoxygenase

5,6-EETE

5-HPETE

LTA Synthase

Leukotriene LTA$_4$

LTA Hydrolase

Glutathione-S-transferase

LTB$_4$

LTC$_4$, LTD$_4$, LTE$_4$, LTF$_4$

Figure 17-3 Lipoxygenase and cytochrome P450 pathways. Chemical structures and nomenclature for principal leukotrienes. LTC$_4$, LTD$_4$, LTE$_4$, and LTF$_4$ differ from LTA$_4$ in the R groups. Cytochrome P450 monooxygenases oxidize arachidonic acid to several epoxides (EETE [epoxy-eicosatetraenoic acids]) and diols. *5-HPETE,* Unstable hydroxyperoxyeicosatetraenoic acid.

tions of PGE$_1$ inhibit arginine-vasopressin induced water reabsorption through G$_i$-mediated inhibition of adenylyl cyclase, whereas higher concentrations of PGE$_1$ cause water reabsorption. The tissue specific functional changes induced by PGE$_2$ acting through four receptor subtypes include vasodilation, bronchodilation, promotion of salt and water excretion, and inhibition of lipolysis, glycogenolysis, and fatty acid oxidation. PGI$_2$ produces effects through IP receptors with wide distribution. IP receptors are highly expressed in the vasculature, reflected in the high vasodilator activity of PGI$_2$.

After being released, PGs are usually denied entrance into cells, presumably because they cannot permeate the lipid bilayer. In the lung, renal proximal tubules, thyroid plexus, and ciliary body of the eye, an active transport system is responsible for rapid uptake of PGs from extracellular fluids. PGs differ in their affinity for this transport system. PGE$_2$ and PGF$_{2\alpha}$ have a high affinity, thus accounting for removal and subsequent metabolism within the lung. In contrast, PGI$_2$ passes intact through the pulmonary circulation. It is possible to inhibit this transport system, which resembles the organic acid secretory system of the renal proximal tubules, with probenecid. The diuretic drug, furosemide, and other organic acids also inhibit this uptake in the lung, kidney, and possibly in the brain and eye. One effect of this drug class is to increase PG concentrations in blood, urine, and perhaps CSF.

A practical application of suppressing the effects of PGE$_2$ can be demonstrated in Bartter's syndrome, a disease in which there is excessive renal PG production, leading to diuresis, kaliuresis, natriuresis, and hyperreninemia. Inhibition of COX activity with NSAIDs results in improvement in patients by allowing expression of salt- and water-retaining hormonal influences, chiefly angiotensin II and arginine-vasopressin.

Tx Receptors TxA_2 (TP) receptors have been identified on the plasma membranes of platelets, blood vessels, bronchial smooth muscle, and mesangial cells of glomeruli. The platelet TxA_2 receptor activates Gq and phospholipase C. The PG endoperoxides, PGG_2 and PGH_2, also bind to Tx receptors.

There are no potent, selective antagonists of the PG or TX receptors in clinical use, although some compounds are effective *in vitro*.

LT receptors The LTs also act through specific G-protein–coupled receptors. LTB_4 binds to and activates BLT receptors, which consist of two subtypes, BLT_1 and BLT_2, both of which bind LTB_4. The cysteinyl LTs bind to and activate two CysLT receptors designated $CysLT_1$, which binds LTD_4 and LTE_4, and $CysLT_2$, which binds LTC_4. Clinically useful CysLT receptor antagonists include montelukast and zafirlukast. In addition, LT formation can be inhibited by the lipoxygenase inhibitor zileuton. All three of these agents are useful in treatment of asthma (see Chapter 34).

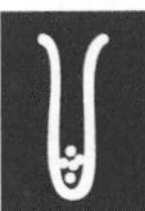

Pharmacokinetics

The pharmacokinetics of PGs, LT antagonists, NSAIDs, corticosteroids, and related drugs are discussed in Chapters 19, 31, 33, 34, and 55.

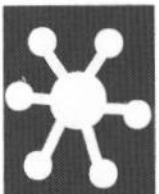

Relation of mechanisms of action to clinical response

Blood flow regulation PGE_1, PGE_2, and PGI_2 are potent vasodilators, and endogenously produced PGE_2 and PGI_2 may be local regulators in many vascular beds. Patients with peripheral vascular disease benefit from PGI_2 infusions into the femoral artery, although there are several side effects. TxA_2 is a potent constrictor of cerebral and coronary arteries, and $PGF_{2\alpha}$ constricts superficial veins in the hands. Prinzmetal's (vasospastic or variant) angina is associated with coronary artery vasoconstriction, which may be caused, in part, to TxA_2 released from activated platelets. LTC_4 and LTD_4 also constrict coronary arteries.

Platelet aggregation The dynamic interplay at the platelet-endothelium interface between proaggregatory vasoconstrictor and antiaggregatory vasodilator mediators influences the outcome of arterial insufficiency, thrombosis, and ischemia (see Chapter 19). Key components are the proaggregatory TxA_2 and the antiaggregatory PGI_2, with interventions that favor PGI_2 production and lowering TxA_2 formation having the most benefit. Aspirin irreversibly inhibits COXs by covalent acetylation. Therapeutic strategies strive to maximize the effect of aspirin on platelet COXs, while sparing as much as possible the effect of COXs on endothelial cells. Unlike the endothelium, platelets lack nuclei and cannot synthesize new COXs to replace that inactivated by aspirin. The effects of aspirin therefore continue for the life of the platelet or more than 10 days. Thus, a deficient production of Tx by platelets cannot be corrected until new platelets form. In contrast, after being inhibited, vascular COX can be replaced by resynthesis in endothelial cells. The resulting low dose aspirin strategy limits the opportunity for aspirin to enter the systemic circulation to inhibit vascular COX but still allows it to act on platelet COX in the portal circulation (from the site of absorption of aspirin to its metabolism by the liver).

Ductus arteriosus The ductus arteriosus generally closes spontaneously at birth, but, in some cases, especially infants born prematurely, it remains patent (open) so that 90% of the cardiac output is shunted away from the lungs. The patency is probably maintained as a result of high production of PGs after delivery. Indomethacin inhibits PG production and closes the ductus arteriosus. On the other hand, neonates with certain congenital heart defects depend on an open ductus arteriosus for survival until corrective surgery can be performed. These defects include interruption of the aortic arch, transposition of the great vessels, and pulmonary atresia or stenosis. PGE_1 (alprostadil) is administered by continuous intravenous infusion or by catheter through the umbilical vein to dilate the ductus.

Gastrointestinal tract PGE_1 and PGE_2 inhibit basal and stimulated gastric acid secretion and are used for treatment of ulcers, as discussed in Chapter 55. The propensity of NSAIDs to cause GI ulcers is a consequence of eliminating the PG contribution to maintenance of mucosal integrity. Because PGs and their analogs have protective actions on the gut mucosa distinct from their ability to inhibit secretory activity, they are considered cytoprotective (see Chapter 55). COX-2 inhibitors may have the advantage over NSAIDs in long-term therapy because they do not suppress the cytoprotective effects of PGs and may therefore be less likely to cause ulcers.

Inflammatory and immune responses PGs and LTs released in response to infection, and to mechanical, thermal, chemical and other injuries, participate in inflammatory responses. LTs affect vascular permeability and LTB_4 is a chemoattractant for polymorphonuclear leukocytes. PGE_2 and PGI_2 enhance edema by increasing blood flow and enhance the action of bradykinin in producing pain. Consequently, COX inhibitors are effective as analgesics and antiinflammatory agents (see Chapter 31).

Reproductive system Elevated concentrations of PGs have been measured in the circulating blood of women during labor or spontaneous abortion, suggesting that initiation and maintenance of uterine contractions may be caused by increased synthesis. In fact, labor can be induced by PGE_2 given orally; if labor does not occur within 12 hours, oxytocin is substituted. Use of PGE_2 to induce labor is accompanied by uterine hypertonus and fetal bradycardia, so its main use in gynecological practice has been as an abortifacient. In contrast to oxytocin, PGs will induce uterine contractions at all stages of pregnancy. Therefore, PGE_2 (dinoprostone) and $PGF_{2\alpha}$ (dinoprost) are used as abortifacients.

PGs are also useful in treating impotence, although they have largely been replaced for this purpose by specific phosphodiesterase inhibitors, such as sildenafil. Smooth muscle relaxing PGs, such as PGE_1 (alprostadil), enhance penile erections. Self-injection creates an erection by relaxing the smooth muscle and dilating the major artery in the penis, enhancing blood flow.

Bronchoconstriction The lungs produce many PGs and LTs. Mast cells lining the respiratory passages are the likely source of LTs. Overproduction of these substances leads to bronchoconstriction, and they are potential mediators of asthma. $PGF_{2\alpha}$ and TxA_2 are also potent bronchoconstrictors, whereas PGE_1, PGE_2, and PGI_2 are potent vasodilators. However, inhaled PGs irritate the airways and are not suitable as antiasthmatic drugs. However, LT receptor antagonists, including montelukast and zafirlukast, are useful in treating asthma (see Chapter 34).

Eye PGs of the E and F series reduce intraocular pressure by enhancing uveoscleral outflow. Topical application of latanoprost, a stable $PGF_{2\alpha}$ derivative, is useful in treating glaucoma.

Side effects, clinical problems, and toxicity

Attempts to use authentic PGI_2 or its stable analogs to forestall or ameliorate myocardial infarction, cerebral ischemia, and other manifestations of arterial insufficiency are restricted by the hypotension, headache, and flushing that attend the IV infusion of these agents.

An unwanted side effect of PGE (and $PGF_{2\alpha}$) analogs is GI hypermotility and associated diarrhea, consequences of the contractile effects of E series PGs on GI smooth muscle. However, in appropriate dosage misoprostol is usually devoid of major side effects.

Under unusual circumstances, PGs may achieve relatively high concentrations in circulating blood. For example, PGD_2 is elevated in human mastocytosis, PGE_2 in some solid tumors with metastases to bone, and PGI_2 in pregnancy. In a small group of patients with solid tumors that metastasize to bone, the associated hypercalcemia, related to elevated PGE_2 concentrations, responds to treatment with aspirin-like drugs. In late pregnancy, the gravid uterus may serve as a reservoir of PGI_2, which is released into the systemic circulation. In addition, diseases of the lung associated with the shunting of blood to the systemic circulation, thereby bypassing the lungs, can result in elevated PG concentrations in arterial blood.

CLINICAL PROBLEMS

PGE_2	GI hypermotility, vomiting, diarrhea; uterine hypertonus and fetal bradycardia in labor
PGI_2	Hypotension, headache, flushing

New horizons

New molecular techniques have greatly advanced knowledge of PG synthesis and function. All of the PG receptors have been cloned, and the functions of some have been resolved by knockout studies in mice. For example, gene knockout shows that the EP_3 receptor, localized to the preoptic hypothalamic region, is involved in fever. Gene knockout of the EP_4 receptor shows that it is involved in closure of the ductus arteriosus. Knowledge of involvement of individual eicosanoid receptor subtypes in specific cellular functions highlights the need for subtype selective antagonists. Several such agents have been synthesized but are not yet clinically available.

TRADE NAMES

All of the important compounds available in the United States are listed in the Major Drugs box.

FURTHER READING

Brink C, Dahlen SE, Drazen J, et al. International Union of Pharmacology XXXVII. Nomenclature for leukotriene and lipoxin receptors. *Pharmacol Rev* 2003; 55:195.

McAdam BF, Catella-Lawson F, Mardini IA, et al. Systemic biosynthesis of prostacyclin by cyclooxygenase (COX)-2: The human pharmacology of a selective inhibitor of COX-2. *Proc Natl Acad Sci USA* 1999; 96:272.

Whittle BJ. Gastrointestinal effects of nonsteroidal anti-inflammatory drugs. *Fundam Clin Pharmacol* 2003; 17:301.

Self-assessment questions

1. Which one of the following statements about eicosanoids is *not* true?

a. Eicosanoids are unsaturated fatty acids.
b. Eicosanoids all contain a pentane ring.
c. Eicosanoids originate primarily from arachidonic acid.
d. Eicosanoids may act through several second messengers.
e. Eicosanoid synthesis results from activation of phospholipase A_2.

2. Which one of the following statements about prostaglandins is *not* true?

a. Prostaglandin synthesis is inhibited by aspirin.
b. Prostaglandins play an important role in inflammation.
c. Prostaglandins are products of cyclooxygenase activity.
d. Prostaglandins act exclusively to stimulate adenylyl cyclase.
e. Either PGE_2 or oxytocin can be used to induce labor.

3. All of the following possess vasoconstrictor activity *except:*

a. TXA_2.
b. PGI_2.
c. $PGF_{2\alpha}$.
d. LTD_4.
e. LTC_4.

4. Which one of the following statements is *not* true?

a. Leukotrienes are products of lipoxygenases.
b. Prostaglandins act through G-protein–coupled receptors.
c. TXA_2 is a stable metabolite of arachidonic acid.
d. Prostaglandin synthesis can be inhibited by corticosteroids.
e. Prostaglandins act primarily as local hormones (autocoids).

5. Clinical indications for eicosanoids or their inhibitors include all of the following *except:*

a. Transposition of the great arteries.
b. Hypertension.
c. Patent ductus arteriosus.
d. Abortion.
e. Peptic ulcers.

6. A patient presents with wheezing and difficulty breathing. Examination reveals bronchoconstriction and inflammatory cell infiltration of the bronchi. Select the most appropriate drug to treat the condition.

a. COX-1 inhibitor
b. COX-2 inhibitor
c. Leukotriene receptor antagonist
d. PGI_2
e. LTD_4

CHAPTER 18

Lipid-lowering drugs and atherosclerosis

Melvyn Rubenfire

Major Drugs

HMG-CoA reductase inhibitors (statins)
Lovastatin (Mevacor)
Pravastatin (Pravachol)
Simvastatin (Zocor)
Fluvastatin (Lescol)
Atorvastatin (Lipitor)
Rosuvastatin (Crestor)

Niacin
Crystalline niacin (nicotinic acid)
Sustained release niacin (Niaspan, Slo-Niacin, Nicobid)

Fibric acid derivatives
Gemfibrozil (Lopid)
Fenofibrate (Tricor)
Clofibrate (Atromid-S)

Bile acid ion-exchange resins
Cholestyramine (Questran)
Colestipol (Colestid)
Colesevelam (WelChol)

Cholesterol absorption inhibitor
Ezetimibe (Zetia)

Therapeutic overview

Cardiovascular disease (CVD) is the principal cause of death and disability in middle aged and elderly men and women in the industrialized world. There were nearly 1 million deaths from CVD in the United States in 1999, representing about 40% of all deaths. An estimated 33% were premature, most of which were preventable. The prevalence of CVD is summarized in Box 18-1.

Of deaths resulting from CVD, the vast majority can be attributed to atherosclerosis and its complications. Each of the major complications of CVD, including acute coronary syndromes (myocardial infarction and unstable angina), sudden deaths, angina pectoris, stroke, claudication (exercise induced leg pain), and congestive heart failure can be reduced by appropriate lifestyle and drug treatment interventions.

The major risk factors for atherosclerosis and its complications are known and are targets for treatment (Box 18-2). Lowering low density lipoprotein (LDL) cholesterol (C) with HMG-Co A reductase inhibitors, collectively known as the **statins**, is associated with decreased rate of death, acute coronary syndromes, strokes, and need for coronary artery revascularization by bypass surgery or angioplasty in patients at risk and with established congestive heart disease. Smoking cessation, diet and exercise, controlling blood pressure, daily low dose aspirin, and increasing levels of high density lipoprotein (HDL)-C also reduce the risk for atherosclerosis-related events (Fig. 18-1). Lipid altering strategies shown to be effective include statins, niacin, fibric acid derivatives, bile acid–binding resins, intestinal bypass, and removal of LDL by plasma apheresis. In general, for every 1% lowering of cholesterol, there is a 2% reduced risk of coronary artery disease.

Pathobiology of atherosclerosis and therapeutic targets

Atherosclerosis is a systemic disease of the aorta, coronary, carotid, and peripheral arteries in response to endothelial injury by one or more risk factors (e.g.,

Abbreviations

Acetyl CoA	acetyl coenzyme A
Apo	apolipoproteins
C	cholesterol
CVD	cardiovascular disease
HDL	high-density lipoprotein
HMG-CoA	hydroxy-3-methyl-glutaryl coenzyme A
IDL	intermediate-density lipoprotein
LDL	low-density lipoprotein
Lp(a)	lipoprotein (a)
PPAR-α	peroxisome proliferator-activated receptor alpha
VLDL	very low-density lipoprotein

hypertension, oxidized LDL, tobacco, homocysteine, infection). The earliest lesions, fatty streaks, can be found in children and young men and women who die of noncardiac causes. Diffuse nonocclusive coronary plaque has been found in 25% to 50% of young adult men at post mortem. The amount of fatty streak and plaque correlates with the prevalence of classic coronary risk factors even in children. The duration of exposure to risk factors (age) and genetics (family history of premature disease) are major determinants of how and when clinical manifestations may occur.

Atherosclerosis is primarily an **inflammatory response** to injury. At least six major processes occur in development of atherosclerotic plaques (atheroma). Each is a potential therapeutic target that can be influenced by drugs, particularly the statin family of lipid lowering drugs:

- Injury of the endothelial lining facilitating entry of monocytes and adherence of platelets
- Active and passive transport of lipid particles into the subendothelial space followed by oxidation
- Conversion of monocytes to macrophages that ingest oxidized LDL and transform to foam cells that coalesce into fatty streaks
- Inflammatory T lymphocyte responses
- Smooth muscle cells and fibroblasts provide a matrix skeleton of collagen, fibrin, and calcification
- Spontaneous death or digestion of foam cells with release of cholesterol and other lipids to form a lipid pool

Histological evidence suggests plaque growth may be gradual over years, with bursts of growth from periodic intraplaque hemorrhage and repair. Gradual

Box 18-1 Prevalence of cardiovascular disease in the United States*

Hypertension	50
Coronary heart disease	12.6 (6.4 females)
Myocardial infarction	7.5
Angina pectoris	6.4
Stroke	4.6
Congestive heart failure	4.8

*Millions of persons.

Box 18-2 Known and putative coronary risk factors

Major

Age/male gender
Smoking
Hypertension
Cholesterol/LDL-C
Low HDL-C
Diabetes
Family history of premature coronary heart disease, peripheral vascular disease, or stroke

Minor

Sedentary lifestyle
Obesity
Dietary saturated fats
Triglycerides
VLDL and IDL remnants

Contributory

Chronic renal failure
Radiation therapy
Systemic lupus erythematosus

Putative

Homocysteine
Lp(a)
Small LDL particles
C-reactive protein
Chronic infection

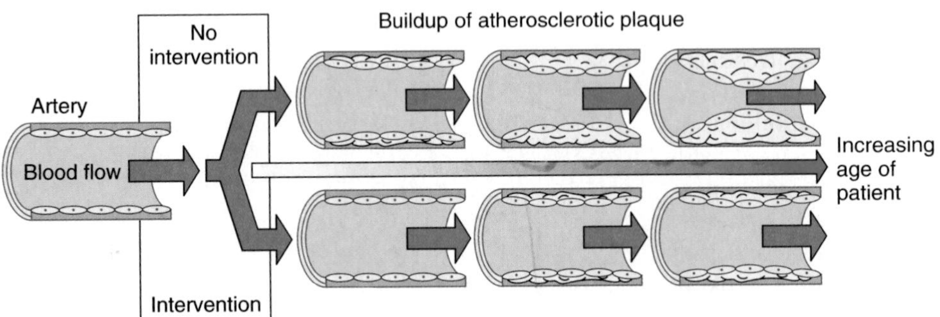

Figure 18-1 Atherosclerosis prevention. Intervention (treatment) involves (1) diet to decrease cholesterol and fats, (2) cessation of smoking, (3) drugs to reduce plasma cholesterol concentration, (4) control of blood pressure, (5) control of diabetes, and (6) regular moderate exercise.

buildup of plaque over decades can lead to coronary and other conduit arteries (carotid, femoral, popliteal) gradually narrowing, and, alternatively, can rupture leading to sudden occlusion resulting in an acute ischemic syndrome (unstable angina, myocardial infarction, stroke, death, critical limb ischemia). Fibrous plaques are prevalent in the 4th and 5th decades, and symptoms (angina, claudication) from occlusive plaques peak in the 7th decade. Ruptures and fissures of plaques, which can lead to sudden occlusion with a superimposed thrombus resulting in acute ischemic events, occur predominantly in nonocclusive lesions. The prevalence of acute coronary syndromes in healthy men and women increases with age, from very rare in the 30s to over 1% in men over 60 years and women over 70 years of age.

The type of plaque is a major determinant for risk of acute coronary events. Angina pectoris and claudication are usually caused by flow limiting partially occlusive coronary or peripheral artery stenosis (>50%-70%). The latter are composed of fibrocalcific plaques abundant in smooth muscle and fibrous tissue with or without a lipid core. The majority of persons with hemodynamically significant stenosis remain asymptomatic until an acute event occurs. Most **acute coronary events** are the result of an occluding or partially occluding thrombus at the site of rupture of the fibrous cap in a nonocclusive (20% to 75%) coronary segment or intraplaque hemorrhage.

The majority of heart attacks and sudden cardiac deaths occur in persons without a history of angina or previous symptoms. Intraplaque hemorrhage from weakening of the walls of the vasa vasorum (small adventitial arteries supplying arteries with oxygen and nutrients) can lead to plaque progression as well as sudden occlusion. Characteristics of vulnerable plaques include:

- A thin fibrous cap
- Increased inflammatory cells (macrophages and T lymphocytes capable of secreting matrix metalloproteinases that digest collagen)
- Few smooth muscle cells and collagen fibers
- A large lipid core

The **endothelium**, or luminal layer of cells of the arterial wall, provides a protective barrier and produces a wide variety of substances involved in regulating vascular tone, thrombosis, and cellular adhesion, migration, and growth. Coronary risk factors, including age, elevated LDL-C, low HDL-C, smoking, hypertension, and diabetes are associated with impaired endothelial function. Nitric oxide and prostacyclin are released in response to shear stress and autonomic tone. Each is a vasodilator with antithrombotic, antiplatelet, and antioxidant functions. Formation and release of prostacyclin and nitric oxide by the endothelium is impaired after a high fat diet and in all stages of atherosclerosis in coronary and conduit vessels with or without plaque.

Lipid-lowering therapy can improve endothelial function, reduce coronary events and strokes, relieve symptoms, prevent new plaque formation, reduce rate of progression, and even induce regression of focal narrowing. Raising HDL-C enhances endothelial function and results in removal of cholesterol from cells and lipid pools, known as **reverse cholesterol transport.** In established coronary heart disease, other atherosclerosis, and primary prevention, serum lipids are one of many interactive risk factors requiring lifestyle changes and drug therapy (see Fig. 18-1). Aspirin and other platelet antagonists (see Chapter 19) reduce risks of acute coronary syndrome and strokes by reducing thrombosis. Antihypertensive strategies (see Chapter 12) reduce wall stress and plaque rupture by various mechanisms.

Therapeutic uses of lipid-lowering drugs are summarized in the Therapeutic Overview box.

THERAPEUTIC OVERVIEW

Reduce formation and rate of progression in coronary and peripheral atherosclerosis from childhood to old age

Prevention of coronary events and strokes in apparently healthy persons at risk, particularly middle-aged and elderly

Prevention of heart attacks, strokes, need for revascularization in persons with established atherosclerosis

Prevention and treatment of pancreatitis in hypertriglyceridemia

Mechanisms of action

Cholesterol balance

The dynamics of cholesterol ingestion, synthesis, and elimination are depicted in Figure 18-2. The sole sources of exogenous cholesterol are animal based food substances, including meats and dairy products, and reabsorption of biliary cholesterol. Dietary intake can vary from 0 to 1000 mg/day; usually 30% to 75% of the total is absorbed. The normal rate of endogenous cholesterol synthesis varies from 600 to 1000 mg/day, with about 750 to 1250 mg secreted in bile daily. One-half to

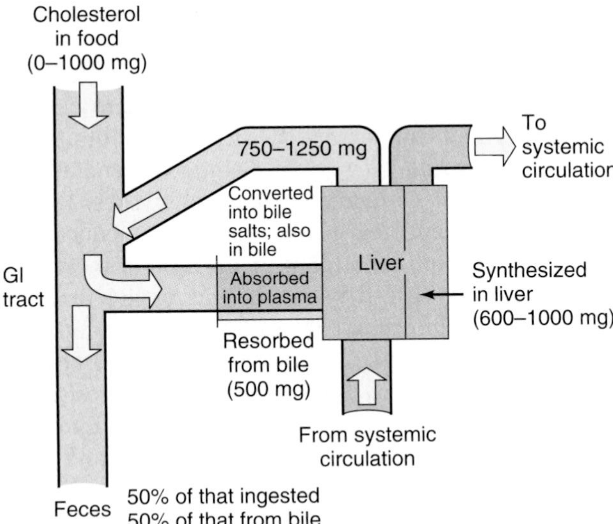

Figure 18-2 Total body balance of cholesterol, showing input by ingestion and liver synthesis, output by nonabsorption into feces, conversion into bile salts, delivery in bile salts to small intestine, partial reabsorption from bile, and delivery as lipoproteins into systemic circulation. Quantities shown are approximate daily amounts.

two-thirds of biliary cholesterol is reabsorbed, and the remainder is excreted in the stool. Total body cholesterol is estimated to be in excess of 125 g, of which greater than 90% is in cell membranes.

De novo synthesis is the major source of cholesterol. Although cholesterol can be synthesized in most cells, its main sources are the adrenals and liver. Because of the greater liver mass, hepatic synthesis is responsible for a considerable proportion.

Synthesis of cholesterol originates with acetyl CoA, a key intermediate for glycolysis, the citric acid cycle, and fatty acid degradation. The first step, an irreversible conversion of HMG-CoA to mevalonic acid, is rate limiting (Fig. 18-3). The rate of synthesis is influenced by several factors, including time of day (predominantly at night), diet composition, excessive food intake, or obesity. Diets rich in saturated fats increase serum cholesterol primarily by down-regulating hepatic clearance, whereas a diet of predominantly unsaturated fats or carbohydrates is generally associated with lower concentrations. In addition, many other factors affect the rate of cholesterol synthesis, including a dynamic equilibrium with certain lipoproteins, discussed later.

The liver is the primary organ for cholesterol uptake and degradation. Most is converted to bile acids, which in turn are secreted into the intestine to emulsify ingested fats. Bile acids are then reabsorbed and recycled. The total bile pool mass is estimated to be 2 to 3 g and is recycled about six times per day. About half the cholesterol secreted in bile is reabsorbed, and the remainder is excreted. Rapid recycling normally limits the need for rapid synthesis of bile acids. Cholesterol is also secreted in bile as free cholesterol. Because it is fairly insoluble, large amounts of bile are required. The enhanced synthesis and increased excretion of cholesterol in bile is a probable cause of cholesterol-containing gallstones in obese patients.

Lipoproteins and lipids

Cholesterol, triglycerides, and phospholipids are transported in plasma and other fluids in lipoprotein particles, which have a lipid core encased in a protein coat. Triglycerides are assembled in the liver from fatty acids and glycerol.

The largest lipoprotein particle is the **chylomicron**, composed of approximately 85% to 95% triglyceride and 3% to 6% cholesterol. The shell is composed of phospholipid, cholesterol, and several apolipoproteins (Apo). They are only present after eating but may be present in fasting persons with inadequate chylomicron metabolism. The chylomicron is formed in the gut wall, and its principal role is to transport dietary fats to adipose tissue, muscle, and liver. As it leaves the gut, it acquires apo C-II, which acts with insulin to activate lipoprotein lipase in the capillary wall. Released triglycerides are cleaved into free fatty acids and glycerol. The chylomicron remnants, containing apo A, B, and E, but having lost apo C-II and C-III, continue to circulate and are eventually removed by specific hepatic receptors. This is the principal route by which dietary fat is transported and is referred to as the **exogenous pathway.** Fasting chylomicronemia resulting from inherited or acquired deficiency of lipoprotein lipase is usually associated with triglyceride levels greater than 2000 mg/dl, which may result in life-threatening pancreatitis.

Endogenous formation and transport of triglycerides is accomplished by very low density lipoprotein **(VLDL)** particles. Synthesized principally by the liver and to a lesser extent by the gut, these particles are much smaller than chylomicrons. In contrast to chylomicrons, triglycerides in VLDL are obtained from fatty acids synthesized by the liver or released by adipose tissue and circulate to the liver. In addition to cholesterol and phospholipid, the wall of VLDL particles contains apo B-100, C-II, C-III, and E. The internal composition is 50% to 60% triglyceride and 20% to 30% cholesterol. The ratio of triglyceride to cholesterol is approximately 5:1. Apo C-II on the VLDL surface results in lipoprotein lipase activation, release of triglycerides to muscle and adipose tissues, and the remaining particles are smaller VLDL remnants. The surface apo E

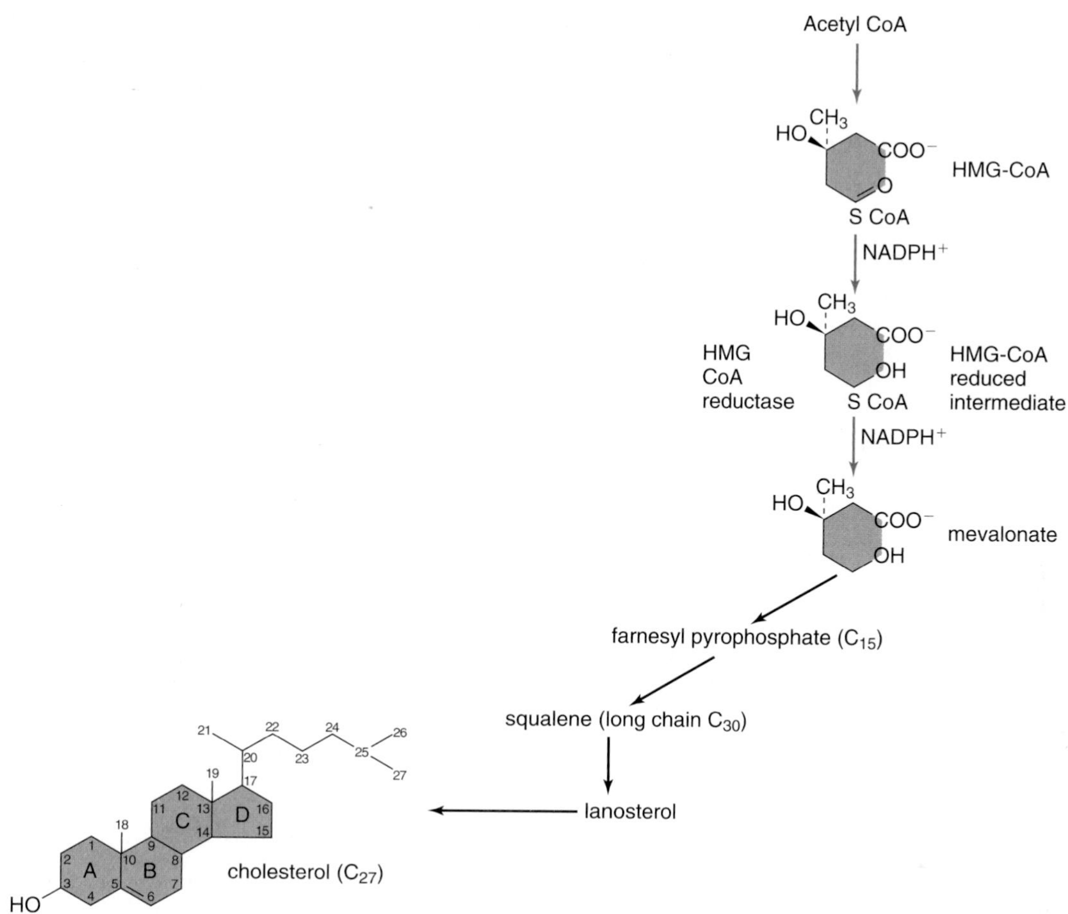

Figure 18-3 Sequence for in vivo synthesis of cholesterol from acetyl CoA.

on VLDL remnants results in clearance of some particles via the same hepatic receptors that bind chylomicron remnants (Fig. 18-4).

As VLDL particles are reduced in size with loss of triglycerides, a substantial portion are transformed to smaller and increasingly dense IDL particles. Significant amounts of these particles are cleared by the hepatic remnant receptor. The remaining apo E is lost as the particles lose further triglycerides via a hepatic endothelial lipase. The resultant contracted particles are known as **LDL**, which are approximately 2% the size of VLDL particles and 0.02% the volume of a chylomicron. LDL particles contain 50% to 60% cholesterol and less than 10% triglyceride and have one molecule of apo B-100 on their surface. LDL particles vary in density and size. The small, dense particles are usually found in association with higher levels of serum triglycerides, are highly atherogenic due to more readily crossing the endothelial barrier, are more easily oxidized, and more readily taken up by scavenger receptors. **Atherogenicity** is related to both LDL particle number and size. Every 1% increase in LDL-C increases the rate of coronary events by about 2%. Additionally, both VLDL remnants and IDL particles have been found in atheroma. Lipoprotein (a) (Lp[a]) is a small particle formed in the liver, the size of LDL particles, containing apo(a) linked to apo B. Apo(a) has a homology with plasminogen, resulting in competition for plasminogen receptors and decreasing thrombolysis.

The **LDL surface protein** apo B-100 is recognized by LDL receptors located in pits on walls of hepatocytes and other cells. When LDL particles bind, they and their receptors are endocytosed, the LDL particle is incorporated into lysosomes and separated from its receptor which is recycled. The coating of the particle is removed, and esterified cholesterol is hydrolyzed and released. The released cholesterol has three major effects on its own metabolism:

- Intracellular cholesterol affects cellular content of HMG-CoA reductase. Thus, as cholesterol concentrations increase, internal synthesis decreases.

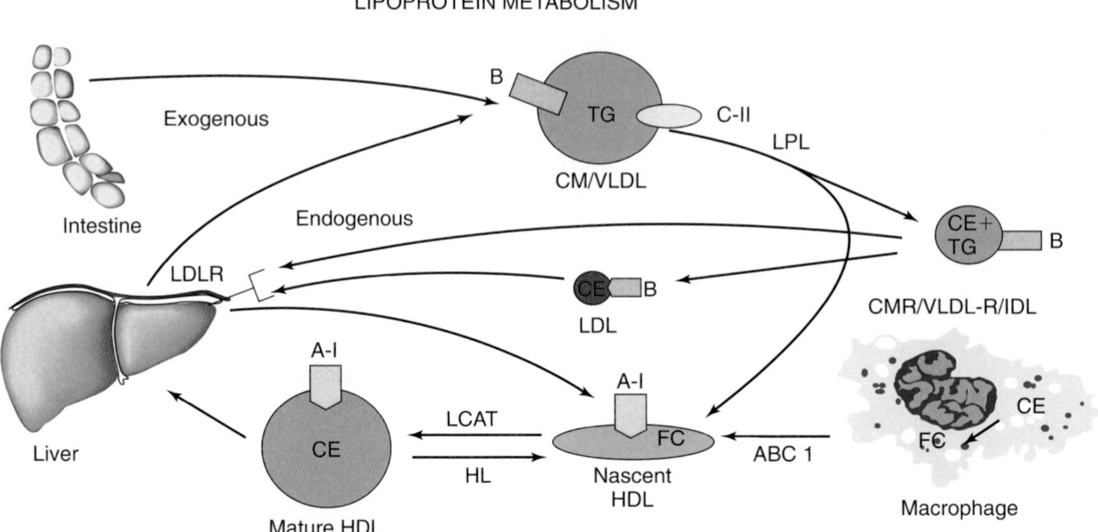

Figure 18-4 The exogenous pathway of chylomicrons *(CM)* containing triglycerides *(TG)* and the endogenous pathway beginning with VLDL are converted by lipoprotein lipase *(LPL)* to form remnants that are cleared via a hepatic remnant *(R)* receptor, or form IDL, which is acted upon by hepatic lipase to form LDL particles that are cleared by LDL receptors. The separate VLDL remnant and LDL receptors are both represented by LDLRs. Nascent HDL is formed in the circulation, receives free cholesterol from cells, and forms mature HDL. HDL particles can be removed by the liver, one mechanism of removing cholesterol, and the other HDL cholesterol is transferred to VLDL remnant particles in exchange for TGs, and cholesterol is removed by the LDL receptor. Apolipoproteins (A-I, B, C-II) are indicated by yellow, orange, and pink symbols. CE, cholesterol ester; ABC1, ATP binding cassette 1 transporter.

- Increasing concentrations of cholesterol activate intracellular acyl CoA, cholesterol acyl transferase.
- Increasing concentrations of cholesterol lower transcription of LDL receptors, whereas decreasing concentrations increase transcription. This enables cells to adjust cholesterol concentrations to their need.

The **HDL lipoprotein particle** is relatively small and dense and has a volume approximately 0.12% of the VLDL particle. The predominant apoproteins on the surface of HDL are apo A-I, A-II, C-II, and E. Nascent HDL is synthesized in the liver, intestine, and circulation as a "spin-off" fragment during lipolysis of chylomicrons or VLDL fragments (Fig. 18-4). HDL is the major vehicle for transport of cholesterol from peripheral tissues (including macrophages and endothelial cells) to the liver for use or excretion. Increased numbers of circulating HDL particles are associated with less coronary and carotid atherosclerosis and decreasing coronary events, strokes, and death rate. For every 1 mg/dl increase in HDL-C there is about a 2% to 3% decrease in risk of coronary artery disease. HDL particles improve endothelial function, reduce oxidation of LDL particles, reduce cellular damage by oxidized LDL, have anti-inflammatory properties, enhance production and prolong the half-life of prostacyclin, and inhibit platelet aggregation.

Mechanisms include removal of excess cholesterol by active transport via a cell membrane binding protein and in a passive process facilitated by interaction of HDL particles with a scavenger receptor. VLDL and IDL particles also exchange triglycerides for cholesterol with HDL particles, which is facilitated by cholesterol ester transfer protein. The clearance of these particles via remnant and LDL receptors facilitates hepatic clearance of cholesterol. Each of these mechanisms contributes to the antiatherosclerotic process known as reverse cholesterol transport. Treatment strategies designed to raise HDL levels alone or in association with decreasing triglycerides have been associated with less atherosclerosis progression, disease regression, as well as decreased coronary event rates in persons with atherosclerosis. Low levels of HDL-C (<45 mg/dl in men and 50 mg/dl in women) are associated with increasing risk for coronary disease and strokes at normal and low levels of LDL-C. Figure 18-5 demonstrates how HDL particles impact vascular endothelial function and tone. Total and HDL cholesterol are measured in the nonfasting state to assess the risk of coronary heart disease in adults.

A low total cholesterol (<200 mg/dl) and a normal or high HDL-C (>45 mg/dl in men and 55 mg/dl in women) in the absence of other risk factors or a family history of atherosclerosis generally infers a low risk. In

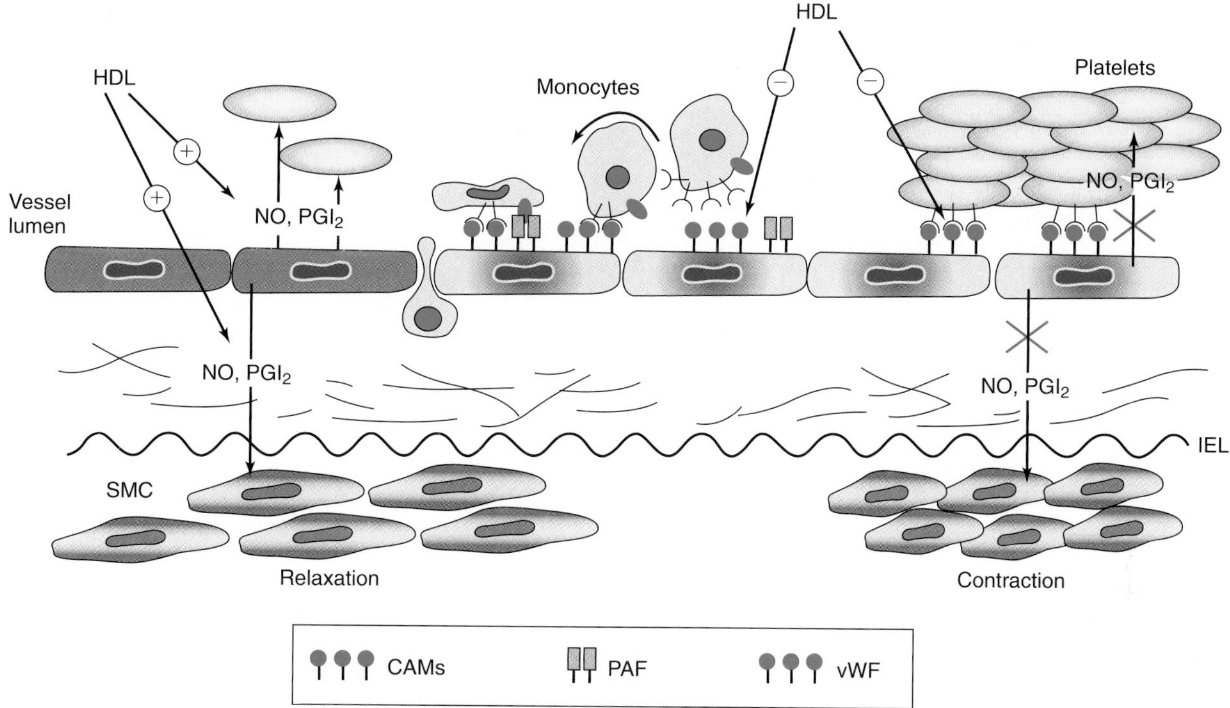

Figure 18-5 Multiple biological actions of HDL on vascular endothelium. Functional endothelial cells are in dark blue, dysfunctional endothelial cells are in light blue. *NO,* Nitric oxide; *PGI₂,* prostacyclin, *SMC,* smooth muscle cells; *CAMs,* cell adhesion molecules; *PAF,* platelet activating factor; *vWF,* von Willebrand's factor.

persons with other risk factors and an increase in total cholesterol and less than average HDL-C, lipids and lipoproteins are measured in the fasting state (about 12 hours), so as to eliminate the postprandial increase in triglycerides. Total cholesterol, triglycerides, and HDL-C are measured, and the LDL-C is calculated by the Fredrickson equation:

$$\text{LDL-C} = \text{total cholesterol} - \text{HDL-C} - \text{VLDL-C}$$

VLDL-C is calculated as triglycerides divided by 5, based on the 1:5 ratio of cholesterol to triglycerides in VLDL particles. The formula is inaccurate when the triglycerides are greater than 350 to 400 mg/dl, an indication for direct measurement of LDL-C.

Although ideal total cholesterol is less than 150 mg/dl and LDL-C is less than 100 mg/dl, the average person in the United States has cholesterol of 205 mg/dl and an LDL-C of 135 mg/dl, and those with and without coronary heart disease have similar levels. The major cause of elevated cholesterol in the United States and industrialized world is an increased intake of saturated fats. Approximately 5% of persons have primary hypercholesterolemia, which can be divided into polygenic hypercholesterolemia (3.8%), familial combined hyperlipidemia (1.5%), and familial hypercholesterolemia (0.2%). A decrease in number or activity of LDL receptors is the basis for familial hypercholesterolemia. The heterozygous form appears in about 0.2% of people, whereas the homozygous form is rare (0.000001%). Heterozygotes have serum cholesterol concentrations about twice normal and LDL-C levels greater than 240 mg/dl. Homozygotes have cholesterol concentrations six times normal and may show evidence of coronary heart disease in childhood and adolescence. Many homozygotes die before 10 to 12 years of age, and almost all experience a myocardial infarction by 20 years of age. Much more common are polygenic hypercholesterolemia and familial combined or mixed hyperlipidemia (increased cholesterol and triglycerides) in which there may be increased absorption of dietary fats and overproduction as well as decrease in clearance of lipoprotein particles. A deficiency in lipoprotein lipase activity, either inherited or acquired with obesity, excess dietary carbohydrates, and diabetes, results in high levels of fasting triglycerides (200-10,000 mg/dl) and chylomicronemia. The lipoproteins that promote atherosclerosis and the vasculoprotective effect of HDL particles are depicted in Figure 18-6.

A classic inheritable **atherogenic lipoprotein phenotype** is present in 5% to 10% of the population, nearly all diabetics, the metabolic syndrome associated with insulin resistance (hypertension, truncal obesity, elevated insulin), and nearly 50% of persons with

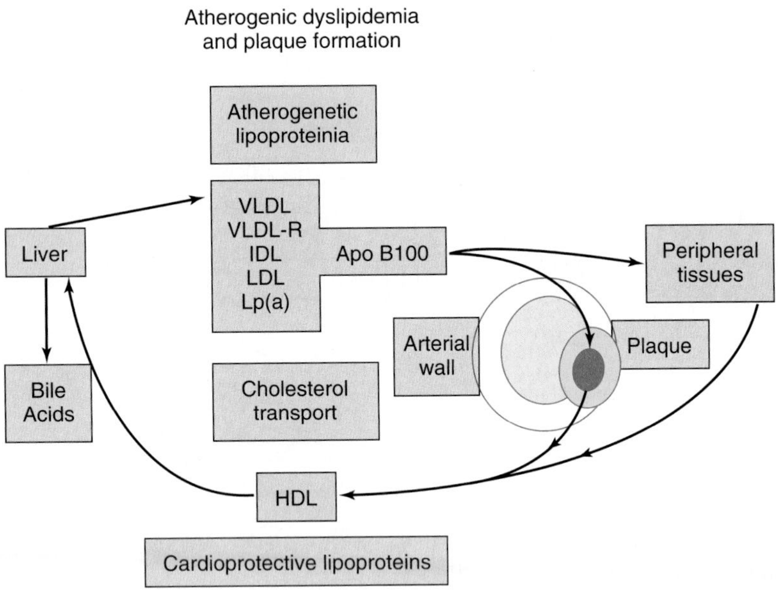

Figure 18-6 Factors contributing to atherogenesis and plaque formation. Abbreviations are as in text.

premature coronary artery disease. It consists of an increase in small dense LDL particles, a decrease in HDL particles with less of the larger buoyant type, and a moderate increase in VLDL remnant particles rich in triglycerides and cholesterol. Elevated triglyceride levels increase the risk in men and, particularly, women with elevated cholesterol. This is likely due to the association with small LDL particles and low HDL-C, and the atherogenicity of VLDL remnant particles. Elevated Lp(a) is the most common abnormal lipid in patients with a family history of premature coronary heart disease. In addition to increasing thrombosis and decreasing thrombolysis, Lp(a) is a small LDL-like particle that is easily oxidized and atherogenic. Low HDL-C and increased triglycerides and isolated low HDL-C are common causes of premature coronary artery disease. Ironically, hypercholesterolemia accounts for less than 10% of premature coronary artery disease.

Table 18-1 Selected pharmacokinetic parameters

Drug	Administration	Half-Life (hrs)	Disposition
Statins			
Rosuvastatin	Oral	20	F, R
Lovastatin	Oral	3-4	F, R
Pravastatin	Oral	1.8	F, R
Simvastatin	Oral	3	F, R
Fibric acid derivatives			
Gemfibrozil	Oral	1.5	M
Fenofibrate	Oral	20	M
Bile acid sequestrants			
Cholestyramine	Oral	NA	F
Colestipol	Oral	NA	F
Others			
Niacin*	Oral	1	M
Ezetimibe	Oral	22	M

F, Fecal excretion; *R,* renal excretion; *M,* metabolized; *NA,* not absorbed.
*Extended release preparations are available with substantially different pharmacokinetics.

Pharmacokinetics

Selected pharmacokinetic parameters of individual drugs are listed in Table 18-1.

Atorvastatin and rosuvastatin, the two most potent **statins,** have a half-life of 14 to 20 hours, compared to 2 to 4 hours for the other statins. Because of their long half-life, atorvastatin and rosuvastatin can be taken once in the morning. The statins differ in their bioavailability and in the effect of food on their absorption. Lovastatin absorption is enhanced by food, while fluvastatin and pravastatin absorption is reduced by food, so these are given at bedtime. Simvastatin, rosuvastatin, and atorvastatin absorption is unaffected by food. All statins are subject to high extraction (approximately 60%) by the liver on the first circulation. Their varying hydrophilic or lipophilic natures do not appear to correlate with lipid-lowering effects, side effects, or toxicity.

Fibrates are metabolized by the liver and excreted by the kidneys and should be discontinued in acute renal failure and used with caution in chronic renal failure. Because immunosuppressive drugs may impair

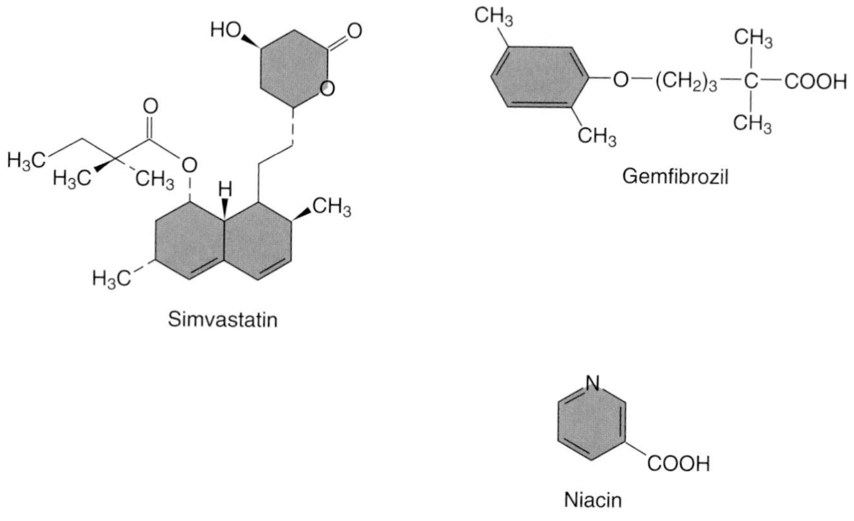

Simvastatin

Gemfibrozil

Niacin

Figure 18-7 Structures of selected lipid-lowering agents.

renal function, fibrates should be used with caution in transplant patients.

Both crystalline and slow release **niacin** are available over the counter. The minimal effective dose is about 1 g/day. The plasma half-life of crystalline niacin is approximately 1 hour. When given by mouth, peak concentrations are achieved within 1 hour.

After oral administration, **ezetimibe** is absorbed and extensively conjugated to a pharmacologically active phenolic glucuronide. After a single dose in fasting adults, mean ezetimibe peak plasma concentrations are attained within 4 to 12 hours. Food administration (high fat or nonfat meals) has no effect on its absorption. Ezetimibe and ezetimibe-glucuronide are highly bound to plasma proteins and metabolized in the small intestine and liver via glucuronide conjugation, with subsequent biliary and renal excretion.

Relation of mechanisms of action to clinical response

The effect of each drug class on lipid parameters depends, to a large extent, on the fasting levels of lipids. For example, at a triglyceride level of 1000 mg/dl **gemfibrozil** can lower triglycerides by 50%, whereas at 250 mg/dl it may be only 20%. The magnitude of effect also depends upon diet, absorption, metabolism, and other genetic factors.

HMG-CoA reductase inhibitors

The **statins** inhibit the enzyme HMG-CoA reductase, the initial rate-limiting step in cholesterol synthesis (see Fig. 18-3). Inhibition of cholesterol synthesis, particularly in hepatocytes, decreases intracellular pools, which triggers an increase in LDL receptor number and activity. This induces an increased clearance of LDL particles. Plasma concentrations of LDL-C and the number of LDL particles decrease, and less LDL is available to react with cells in blood and vessel walls. Statins also lower plasma lipids, including LDL-C and triglycerides, by inhibition of hepatic VLDL synthesis, resulting in decreased numbers of VLDL, IDL, and LDL particles. The structure of **simvastatin,** a typical HMG-CoA reductase inhibitor, is shown in Figure 18-7.

Lovastatin, pravastatin, and simvastatin are derivatives of fungal products. Fluvastatin, atorvastatin, and rosuvastatin are synthetic. Lovastatin and simvastatin are both prodrugs requiring hydrolysis in the liver to become active. Rosuvastatin and pravastatin are active drugs, and fluvastatin has active metabolites that do not reach the systemic circulation. Although atorvastatin is active, its metabolites also contribute significantly to lowering cholesterol. Statins act as **competitive inhibitors** for the active site on the reductase enzyme, with a higher affinity than HMG-CoA.

The statins vary in their abilities to alter LDL-receptors. The LDL-C lowering effect of comparable doses of each of the statins is summarized in Table 18-2, although all doses are not necessarily available commercially. Note that a **doubling of dose** results in only a **5% to 6% further reduction in LDL-C.** Statin effects on apo B, VLDL-C, IDL-C and triglycerides appear to be proportionate to the decrease in LDL-C. With cessation of therapy, lipids return to pretreatment levels within 4 weeks.

The **antiatherosclerotic** effects of statins are not explained solely by their effects on lipids. They also cause many other important effects, which are different for each drug. These include platelet inhibition and

Table 18-2 Comparative LDL-C lowering of statins within available doses

	Dose				
Statin	**5 mg**	**10 mg**	**20 mg**	**40 mg**	**80 mg**
Atorvastatin	31%	37%	43%	49%	55%
Fluvastatin	10%	15%	21%	27%	33%
Lovastatin	—	21%	29%	37%	45%
Pravastatin	15%	20%	24%	29%	33%
Rosuvastatin	38%	43%	48%	53%	58%
Simvastatin	23%	27%	32%	37%	42%

Numbers are based upon a meta-analysis of published data.

antithrombosis; enhanced fibrinolysis and effects on clotting factors; effects on tissue factors, blood viscosity and flow; reduced leukocyte adhesiveness; enhanced endothelial function; inhibition of LDL-C oxidation; reduction of circulating inflammatory markers; and atherosclerotic plaque stabilization by decreasing lipid content, reducing numbers of macrocytes and T lymphocytes, and reducing vascular smooth muscle cell growth.

In healthy middle-aged and elderly men and women with increased risk factors, there is evidence that statins can provide a 20% to 30% reduction in total and CVD mortality, coronary events, strokes, and need for coronary revascularization. The benefits are more pronounced in men and women with established vascular disease of any type (coronary heart disease, peripheral vascular disease, stroke), including the elderly, diabetics, and those with congestive heart failure. There is evidence of benefit of statins in men and women with atherosclerosis of all ages and regardless of baseline cholesterol, if above 135 mg/dl. Clinical studies show that men and women with coronary or other vascular disease, diabetes, and older men with hypertension show similar benefits regardless of levels of LDL-C; an approximate 25% reduction in total mortality, cardiovascular mortality, and recurrent fatal and nonfatal myocardial infarctions.

Statins are the lipid altering drugs of choice and should be given to all persons with atherosclerosis of any type. They are also indicated in diabetes in men and women with multiple risk factors and a 20% or greater 10-year risk of a coronary event. A reasonable approach would be to choose a dose that reduces LDL-C by 35% or greater.

Fibric acid derivatives

Phenoxyisobutyric acid, or fibric acid, is the parent compound for several drugs that lower plasma cholesterol and triglyceride concentrations, known collectively as the **fibrates** or fibric acid derivatives. Gemfibrozil, fenofibrate, and clofibrate are approved in the United States.

Fibrates have a broad spectrum of lipid modulating and pleiotropic effects related to their capacity to mimic the structure and biological functions of free fatty acids. Their mechanisms of action are only partially understood but appear to activate transcription factors belonging to the nuclear hormone receptor superfamily, the peroxisome proliferator-activated receptors (PPARs). **PPAR-α** mediates fibrate action on HDL-C levels via transcriptional induction of synthesis of major HDL apos (apoA-I and apoA-II) as well as increased synthesis of lipoprotein lipase. Fibrates decrease hepatic apo C-III transcription, reducing inhibition of lipoprotein lipase and enhancing clearance of triglyceride-rich lipoproteins. Other functions altered by PPAR-α actions of fibrates result in increased fatty acid uptake, decreased fibrinogen and high sensitivity C-reactive protein, and increased cholesterol efflux. The effect of fibrates on raising HDL and reducing triglyceride rich chylomicron and VLDL particles and lipid content is mediated by decreasing production of hepatic VLDL containing less apo C-III, and induction of hepatic and systemic expression of lipoprotein lipase. Increasing the activity of endothelial lipoprotein lipase enhances release of VLDL surface fragments to form nascent HDL, as well as by increasing production of apo A-1. Decreasing triglyceride content and number of VLDL remnants reduces the cholesterol ester transfer protein transfer of triglycerides to HDL particles in exchange for cholesterol.

The fibrates are particularly effective in modulating the atherogenic lipoprotein profile. Specifically, they reduce fasting and postprandial triglycerides by reducing VLDL, VLDL remnants, and IDL; increase LDL particle size; and increase HDL particle number and cholesterol content. The effects depend on fasting lipid parameters. **Fenofibrate** can lower LDL-C by up to 25% in patients with isolated hypercholesterolemia and has a moderate LDL-C lowering effect (15% to 25%) in hypertriglyceridemia and mixed lipid disorders. **Gemfibrozil** is neutral or can increase LDL-C by up to 10%, particularly in patients with isolated hypertriglyceridemia (see Fig. 18-7). A major antiatherosclerotic effect of fibrates results from lowering triglycerides and a resultant shift in LDL mass to the larger and buoyant particles (up to 50% change), which are less easily oxidized and less capable of entering the subendothelial space.

The fibrates also reduce the magnitude of both fasting and postprandial hyperlipidemia. Although epidemiological evidence implicating lipids in atherosclerosis is predominantly in fasting states, there is

Table 18-3 Antiatherothrombotic lipid and pleiotropic effects of niacin

Lipoprotein	Vascular	Thrombosis	Other
Increases HDL ↑ HDL-C ↑ apo A-1 ↓ apo A-2 ↑ large HDL_2	Stabilizes plaque and new lesion formation ↓ lipid core by reverse cholesterol transport	Inhibits thrombosis ↑ fibrinolysis ↓ coagulation factors	Limits ischemia and reperfusion injury, possibly by preservation of glycolysis
Reduces LDL ↓ LDL-C ↓ small LDL ↓ LDL oxidation	↓ vascular inflammation	↓ platelet adhesion and aggregation ↓ fibrinogen ↓ blood viscosity	
VLDL ↓ VLDL-C ↓ VLDL-trigs Reduces Lp(a)	Improves endothelial function ↑ nitric oxide synthase activity ↑ vasodilation		

considerable evidence that postprandial increases in triglycerides and VLDL receptors and IDL particles help explain the increase in coronary artery disease risk in diabetes and the metabolic syndrome. Impaired postprandial triglyceride metabolism is associated with endothelial dysfunction possibly related to cytotoxicity of triglycerides.

Gemfibrozil is approved in the United States for treatment of adults with very high elevations of serum triglycerides, who present a risk of pancreatitis, and who do not respond adequately to dietary changes. Gemfibrozil should also be considered in less severe hypertriglyceridemia in patients with a history of pancreatitis or recurrent abdominal pain typical of pancreatitis.

Gemfibrozil is also approved for reducing the risk of developing coronary heart disease in patients with elevation of triglycerides and LDL-C and low HDL-C without a history of or symptoms of existing coronary heart disease, who have had an inadequate response to weight loss, dietary therapy, exercise, and other drugs, such as the statins and niacin. Although there is some disagreement, clinical trials generally support the efficacy of fibrate therapy for treatment of atherosclerotic vascular disease. However, considering the safety and efficacy of statin therapy in all forms of atherosclerosis, these drugs remain the first choice when cholesterol levels are above 135 mg/dl. Fibrate therapy should be considered in patients with vascular disease or diabetes who are intolerant to statins. Additionally, fibrates can be used cautiously in combination with statins to further decrease non–HDL-C and increase HDL-C.

Niacin

Niacin was found in the mid-1950s to lower serum triglycerides and cholesterol (see Fig. 18-7). It was the first drug with lipid modulating effects shown to reduce recurrent coronary events and mortality in men who had recovered from a myocardial infarction. Following absorption, niacin is enzymatically converted to nicotinamide adenine dinucleotide. However, nicotinamide does not have hypolipidemic activity.

Niacin reduces release of fatty acids from fat stores, reduces hepatic uptake of released free fatty acids, and synthesis of VLDL triglyceride rich particles. It also increases hepatic clearance of HDL-C but inhibits uptake of apo A-1, resulting in its increased availability for development of HDL particles. The decrease in anabolism of VLDL triglyceride rich particles, which are metabolized to IDL and LDL, results in decreased LDL-C and LDL particle numbers, and an increase in the less atherogenic, larger more buoyant LDL particles.

The major antiatherosclerotic effect of niacin appears to be its ability to raise HDL-C, which is considerable and greater than that of the fibrates. In contrast to the fibrates, niacin is very effective in isolated low HDL-C. Like the statins, nonlipid pleiotropic effects of niacin are also important for preventing coronary events and progression of atherosclerosis. Table 18-3 summarizes the effects of niacin. Clinical trials have shown that niacin reduces nonfatal and recurrent myocardial infarctions and is associated with relatively less new lesion formation and more coronary plaque regression.

The effect of niacin is also highly dependent on fasting lipids. In patients with elevated triglycerides and low HDL-C, niacin would usually reduce triglycerides by 15% to 25%, increase HDL-C by 20% to 30%, and reduce LDL-C minimally. Average reduction in LDL-C by 2 g of niacin is about 15%. A slow release product that reduces the side effect of flushing, without a loss of efficacy, is available. The cholesterol-lowering effect of niacin can be enhanced by coadministration with statins and resins.

Approved indications for niacin include as an adjunct to diet for reduction of LDL-C and triglycerides, an increase in HDL-C in patients with hypercholesterolemia and mixed lipid disorders, and a history of myocardial infarction or coronary heart disease to slow progression or promote regression of atherosclerotic disease. Although it is not approved for use in isolated low HDL-C in coronary heart disease, many consider it effective. Niacin is of particular value in combination with statins. The combination results in a marked reduction of atherogenic lipoproteins (number of small dense LDL particles, Lp(a), VLDL remnants), increases HDL-C, and increases the nonlipid antiatherothrombotic effects. High doses of statins plus niacin have been shown to induce coronary artery lesion regression and reduction in event rates beyond that of statins alone. Vitamin E, which is often taken as an antioxidant supplement, interferes with the benefits of niacin, probably by inhibiting the increase in the protective HDL-2b fraction.

Bile acid sequestrants

Cholestyramine, colestipol, and **colesevelam** are bile acid absorbants approved for use in treatment of hypercholesterolemia. They are large copolymers that act by exchanging Cl^- for negatively charged bile salt anions. They are poorly absorbed and pass out of the gut with the stool. Bile resins are particularly of value in patients intolerant to statins and in combination with statins and niacin when additional lowering of LDL-C is the goal.

Prior to the statins they were the most often prescribed cholesterol lowering drug. Clinical trials demonstrated that lowering LDL-C with bile resins can reduce coronary event rates in men with hypercholesterolemia, and improve coronary endothelial function. In contrast to the statins, niacin, and fibrates, which have antiatherothrombotic properties, the resins are effective in primary and secondary prevention of coronary heart disease because of the decrease in LDL-C and apo B, having effects similar to a very low fat diet.

As previously described, the usual bile acid pool is 2 to 3 g but is recycled up to six times per day. When bile acids are removed from the enterohepatic recirculation, their synthesis is increased. The resultant increase in cholesterol synthesis also results in an increase in LDL receptors and greater hepatic uptake of LDL. Concentrations of LDL-C are reduced by 10% to 25% in response to bile acid sequestrants, in a dose dependent fashion. VLDL and plasma triglyceride concentrations may increase as much as 20%. Usually this effect disappears within 2 to 3 months, but changes are not predictable. The bile absorbants should be avoided when triglyceride levels are greater than 250 to 300 mg/dl. They have no consistent effect on HDL levels.

Cholesterol absorption inhibitor

Ezetimibe reduces blood cholesterol by inhibiting absorption of cholesterol by the small intestine. Ezetimibe does not inhibit cholesterol synthesis or increase bile acid excretion. Instead, it appears to act at the brush border of the small intestine to inhibit absorption of cholesterol, leading to a decreased delivery to the liver. This reduces hepatic cholesterol and increases LDL receptor clearance of cholesterol from the blood. This distinct mechanism is complementary to that of HMG-CoA reductase inhibitors.

Ezetimibe reduces total-C, LDL-C, apo B, and has minimal effects on triglycerides and HDL-C in hypercholesterolemia. Administration with an HMG-CoA reductase inhibitor is effective in improving serum total-C, LDL-C, apo B, triglycerides, and HDL-C beyond either treatment alone. The effects of ezetimibe given either alone or in addition to an HMG-CoA reductase inhibitor on cardiovascular morbidity and mortality have not been established. It is indicated for cholesterol and LDL lowering in patients who are intolerant of statins or in whom abnormal liver function or side effects benefit from a reduction in the statin dose.

Combination therapies

Combination therapies are often required in mixed lipid disorders, statin intolerant patients, treatment of non–HDL-C, and when targeting a low HDL-C along with elevated LDL-C.

In patients with statin induced abnormal liver function testing (2-3 times normal), combining a lower dose of a statin with ezetimibe or a bile resin can safely provide an additional 15% to 20% reduction of LDL-C. Similarly, in statin-intolerant patients, a combination of high dose niacin and bile resins or ezetimibe can reduce LDL-C by up to 40% to 50%. The strategy of combining low dose statins with ezetimibe to reduce toxicity should be used only when necessary, because some pleiotropic effects of statins may be lost.

The combination of a statin with niacin is very effective in decreasing LDL-C, apo B, triglycerides, and LDL particle numbers, while increasing HDL-C and LDL particle size. Although relatively safe, liver function should be monitored. Lovastatin plus niacin is available as a single tablet given at bedtime, which increases compliance significantly.

Generally, statins should not be used with gemfibrozil, a warning that is less of a concern with fenofibrate. In patients with hypertriglyceridemia or elevated non–HDL cholesterol, the drug of choice is a statin targeting LDL-C to less than 100 mg/dl and non–HDL-C to less than 130 mg/dl. If this is not achieved, in diabetics and patients with established atherosclerosis, careful combination of gemfibrozil with pravastatin, fluvastatin, simvastatin, and atorvastatin might be considered. Patients must be warned of the possibility of muscle weakness and pain and the potential for rhabdomyolysis. At the onset of symptoms, both drugs should be stopped and serum creatine kinase determined. Rhabdomyolysis can occur as early as a few weeks or any time thereafter and result in irreversible renal failure.

Side effects, clinical problems, and toxicity

Adverse effects of the various drug classes are listed in the Clinical Problems box.

CLINICAL PROBLEMS

Drug class	Side effects
HMG-CoA reductase inhibitors (statins)	Muscle pain and weakness, myositis, increased liver enzymes, rosuvastatin increased microalbuminuria
Bile acid sequestrants	Gastrointestinal distress, constipation, flatus, but colesevelam better tolerated
	Decrease absorption of fat soluble vitamins and some drugs
Niacin	Flushing, increase uric acid and gout, dyspepsia, dry skin, hepatotoxicity
Cholesterol absorption inhibitor	Mild gastrointestinal distress
Fibric acids	Dyspepsia, gallstones, myopathy, increase in violent deaths

HMG-CoA reductase inhibitors

The statins are very safe, except for possible drug interactions. Mild elevation in creatine kinase activity and mild elevation of hepatic alanine aminotransferase are not uncommon, and are usually, but not always, clinically insignificant. Statins should be avoided in active liver disease and avoided or given with great caution in chronic liver disease. However, there have been no confirmed cases of fatal liver disease associated with statins.

Severe rhabdomyolysis, while very rare, can occur with each statin. Muscle aches or weakness should trigger discontinuation and measurement of creatine kinase. In cardiac transplant patients receiving immunosuppressive drugs, myositis develops in 30% within 1 year of initiating lovastatin therapy. In a few patients, it progresses to severe rhabdomyolysis and acute renal failure. In the general population, the incidence of myositis is less than 1% but increases to 5% in patients on lovastatin and gemfibrozil or immunosuppressive drugs. Discontinuation of drug is recommended in patients with risk factors that may lead to renal failure secondary to rhabdomyolysis (i.e., severe infection, hypotension, major surgery, trauma, or uncontrolled seizures).

Up to 10% of patients have gastrointestinal symptoms, including diarrhea, constipation, nausea, dyspepsia, excess flatus, and abdominal pain or cramps. Other rare effects, which are difficult to confirm, include thrombocytopenia, visual blurring, alopecia, proteinuria (especially rosuvastatin), depression, insomnia, and sensory and motor neuropathy. Statins have been reported to cause erectile dysfunction, but improved endothelial function could enhance erectile function. Because these drugs inhibit cholesterol synthesis, the potential exists for inhibition of synthesis of adrenal and gonadal steroid hormones and of bile acids. However, there is substantial evidence indicating that this does not occur. The levels of other end products of mevalonic metabolism, such as dolichol, required for glycoprotein synthesis, and ubiquinone, the potent antioxidant used for mitochondrial electron transport, are not significantly affected by statins.

Statins have been used safely in children over 8 years and do not interfere with sexual maturation, menarche, or growth and development. Because their effect on fetal development and fertility is unknown, they should be avoided during pregnancy and breastfeeding.

Fibric acid derivatives

Clofibrate use has diminished because of the increased incidence of cholelithiasis and a possible increased incidence of carcinoma. Both clofibrate and gemfibrozil have been associated with increasing suicidal and accidental deaths.

Gemfibrozil and fenofibrate enhance the anticoagulant effect of warfarin and associated compounds. Doses of warfarin must often be reduced as much as 50% in patients taking these compounds. Other side effects are principally gastrointestinal and consist of abdominal pain and, less frequently, nausea, vomiting, and diarrhea. The increased ratio of cholesterol to bile in patients treated with gemfibrozil and fenofibrate makes them more susceptible to gallbladder disease.

Fibric acid derivatives should not be used in pregnancy unless the potential benefit is very high, such as in pancreatitis or severe hypertriglyceridemia (>2000 mg/dl). The contraindication of combining gemfibrozil with lovastatin and rosuvastatin has been emphasized.

Bile acid sequestrants

The bile resins are insoluble, have the consistency of course sand, and must be mixed with fluids to be ingested. They tend to cause gastrointestinal bloating, excess flatus, and constipation with nausea and indigestion. A diet high in fluids and fiber is necessary to minimize these effects.

Because of the exchange of chloride ions for bile acids, excess chloride absorption may result in a hyperchloremic metabolic acidosis. Transient rises in alkaline phosphatase, and transaminase activities have been reported.

Binding of bile acids decreases their emulsifying action, and excess fat may appear in stool. Since they may interfere with absorption of fat-soluble vitamins, supplementation is indicated. They may also interfere with intestinal absorption of thiazide diuretics, phenobarbital, thyroxine, warfarin, and digoxin, all compounds that undergo enterohepatic circulation. It is generally advisable to not administer resins with other drugs. Bedtime is a convenient and safe time for thyroid supplements, warfarin, and digoxin. A time differential of 1 hour prior and 4 hours after is recommended when coadministration is indicated. Because they are not absorbed, the resins can be safely administered to children and during pregnancy and breastfeeding.

Ezetimibe

Ezetimibe is relatively contraindicated in liver disease and renal failure where blood levels may rise significantly. It must also be used with caution in patients on cyclosporine and other immunosuppressive drugs that may alter renal function. Gemfibrozil and fenofibrate increase blood levels of ezetimibe, but their own blood levels are not affected by ezetimibe. Rare patients complain of bloating, but clinical trials show that ezetimibe has adverse events similar to placebo.

Niacin

Side effects are generally noted within 30 minutes of niacin ingestion. Intense flushing and pruritus of the trunk, face, and arms can occur. Gradual dose titration of niacin over days to weeks results in a marked reduction in flushing and tolerance in over 70% to 80% of users. Symptoms are caused by release of prostaglandin D in the skin and can be partially inhibited by ingestion of aspirin. Bedtime use of sustained release niacin reduces flushing and increases compliance.

Side effects include nausea, diarrhea, and dyspepsia and aggravation of peptic ulcer disease. Elevations of transaminase and creatine kinase concentrations are common but not generally of concern. Serum urate concentrations may increase, with an increased incidence of gouty arthritis. An increased incidence of cardiac dysrhythmias has been reported.

Lifestyle interventions and drugs in atherosclerosis

Prevention and treatment of atherosclerosis need to be comprehensive and targeted to each of the major and contributing risk factors (see Box 18-2). Both food choices and calories consumed should be tailored for weight control, lipid management, and hypertension. Because cholesterol levels increase with dietary fat and age, a basic recommendation for reducing them is to decrease caloric intake and lower the proportion of dietary fat to less than 30% and saturated fat to less than 7% to 10%. This requires a shift to foods rich in monounsaturated fats, such as olive oil, lean meat, and certain vegetables.

Patients with abnormal lipid profiles, hypertension, diabetes, and obesity should be encouraged to consult with dietitians. Simply recommending a low fat diet often results in inappropriate increases in starches and sugars, and increased triglycerides and lowered HDL-C. Smoking cessation, weight loss, and moderate exercise, along with an increase in monounsaturated fats and decrease in saturated fats will result in an increase in HDL-C, decrease in LDL-C, and improvement in the ratio of cholesterol to HDL-C.

The effect of dietary intervention varies widely. Diets high in fiber, antioxidant containing fruits and vegetables, and cold water fish rich in omega-3 polyunsaturated fats have been shown to reduce first and recurrent coronary events independent of drugs. Patients with established atherosclerosis should be placed on drug therapy with appropriate dietary advice. The argument for dietary change as a principal component in prevention of atherosclerosis is based on the following:

- Patient is in control.
- Change should be lifelong.
- Benefits are additive to drug therapy.
- Drug doses may be able to be reduced.

- Primary prevention by diet may eliminate the need for expensive drugs.

Summary

All patients with atherosclerosis of any kind, a cholesterol greater than 135 mg/dl, and a life expectancy of at least a few years should be treated with a statin. The decision for treatment should follow the most current National Cholesterol Education Program Adult Treatment Panel guidelines, which encourage use of risk stratification. Patients at high risk (>2% annual risk of a coronary event) should be treated as a coronary risk equivalent. Those at intermediate risk (1%-2% annual risk) should be treated to a target LDL-C of less than 130 mg/dl with a statin or other agent, if necessary. Intermediate and low risk persons with a family history of premature coronary heart disease would benefit from further risk stratification with measurement of the high sensitivity C-reactive protein, which reflects the inflammatory state and supplements coronary risk prediction. In coronary heart disease, other atherosclerosis or diabetes with isolated low HDL-C with or without moderate increases in triglycerides and low levels of LDL-C (<90-100 mg/dl) from diet and or statins, niacin, or possibly gemfibrozil should be considered. Strategies to increase the HDL-C with niacin and combination with statins appear fruitful.

New horizons

Future drugs will be designed to prevent the early stages of atherosclerosis and progression, induce regression, and provide plaque stability by novel mechanisms. These may include potent intracellular antioxidants that increase HDL-C and lower LDL-C and inhibit formation of vascular endothelial adhesion molecules; synthetic HDL; inhibitors of cholesterol ester transfer protein that increases HDL levels and reduces cardiovascular event rates alone or in combination with the statins; potent antiinflammatories targeted to T-lymphocytes; and inhibition of matrix metalloproteinases responsible for plaque instability.

Physician awareness, patient education, and society's ability to pay for prevention remain problematic. Only half of patients with proven coronary artery disease and elevated total cholesterol are receiving treatment, and nearly half stop therapy after 1 to 2 years despite having insurance. Statins are cost saving in patients with coronary disease and strokes. Only 35 to 40 patients with intermediate to high risk by LDL-C and C-reactive protein need to be treated to prevent one coronary event. Resolution of compliance and cost issues will determine whether continuing advances in treatment of coronary artery disease and other forms of atherosclerosis will occur.

TRADE NAMES

All of the important compounds available in the United States are listed in the Major Drugs box.

FURTHER READING

Chapman MJ. Fibrates in 2003: Therapeutic action in atherogenic dyslipidemia and future perspectives. *Atherosclerosis* 2003; 171:1-13.

Heart Protection Study Collaborative Group. MRC/BHF Heart Protection Study of cholesterol lowering with simvastatin in 20,536 high-risk individuals: A randomized placebo-controlled trial. *Lancet* 2002; 360:7-22.

Rosenson RS. Antiatherothrombotic effects of nicotinic acid. *Atherosclerosis* 2003; 171:87-96.

Self-assessment questions

1. Which of the following statements regarding cholesterol and cholesterol metabolism is *false?*
   a. The liver is the primary organ for cholesterol clearance and degradation.
   b. LDL cholesterol is formed primarily in the liver.
   c. The transport of cholesterol is primarily accomplished within particles having a surface protein.
   d. A small percent of cholesterol is derived from dietary intake.

2. HMG-CoA reductase inhibitors have each of the following characteristics *except:*
   a. They can reduce cholesterol concentrations in patients with all forms of hypercholesterolemia, including those homozygous for LDL receptor deficiency.
   b. They have considerable antiatherosclerotic properties beyond lowering LDL-C.
   c. They can produce muscle weakness and pain.
   d. They significantly lower LDL-C, apo B, and triglycerides.

3. A variety of epidemiological studies have shown a negative correlation between the concentrations of HDL and the risk of cardiovascular disease. Agents that increase HDL concentrations include all *except:*

a. Fibric acid.
b. Statins.
c. Cholesterol absorption blockers.
d. Nicotinic acid.

4. Epidemiological studies of atherosclerosis indicate that:

a. A strong correlation exists for the atherogenic phenotype of increase in small dense LDL particles, increase in triglycerides, and decreased HDL-C.
b There is an inverse correlation between triglycerides and HDL cholesterol concentrations.
c. Lp(a), an LDL like particle produced in the liver, is prothrombotic and is an independent risk factor for myocardial infarction and strokes in many populations.
d. All of the above are correct.

CHAPTER 19

Drugs to treat blood disorders

William P. Fay

Major Drugs	
Anticoagulants	Platelet function inhibitors
Fibrinolytics	Antianemia drugs

Therapeutic overview

Normally, **hemostasis** functions to prevent excessive bleeding and formation of unwanted thrombi. However, modifying pathways involved in coagulation, fibrinolysis, or platelet aggregation is useful in many patients undergoing surgery or with cardiovascular disease. Events leading to arterial thrombosis (usually a platelet thrombus) or venous thrombosis (usually a fibrin clot) or that cause clot lysis are activated and inhibited by many endogenous blood and tissue components, as well as exogenous materials. The main reasons for intervention are:

- To inhibit blood **coagulation**
- To stimulate **lysis** of an already formed but unwanted thrombus
- To inhibit **platelet** function

Certain procedures such as hip joint replacement and cardiopulmonary bypass, in which blood comes into contact with foreign materials, initiate coagulation and thrombus formation. In these settings, prophylactic administration of anticoagulants diminishes unwanted thrombus formation. Rapid activation of the fibrinolytic system to lyse the thrombus, and initiation of anticoagulation therapy to minimize further clot formation, are effective in situations where a thrombus has already formed, such as deep vein thrombosis, acute myocardial infarction, and pulmonary embolism. Clinical evidence also supports the use of drugs inhibiting platelet function in cardiovascular disease and stroke.

Anemia is a deficiency of oxygen-carrying red blood cells. Adult bone marrow is primarily responsible for maintaining hematopoiesis and requires ample supply of **iron, vitamin B_{12},** and **folate,** as well as the presence of several growth factors, particularly **erythropoietin.** A wide variety of anemias occur clinically, however, the most common involves a time-dependent iron deficiency. Most anemias are corrected by dietary correction of the imbalance of these cofactors, or more recently, by parenteral use of recombinant hematopoietic growth factors, particularly in chronic renal failure.

Therapeutic uses of drugs for treating blood disorders are summarized in the Therapeutic Overview box.

Abbreviations	
APTT	activated partial thromboplastin time
INR	international normalized ratio
PT	prothrombin time
t-PA	tissue plasminogen activator
TXA_2	thromboxane A_2
u-PA	urokinase plasminogen activator
vWF	von Willebrand factor

THERAPEUTIC OVERVIEW

Anticoagulation

Heparin and heparin derivatives, coumarins, directly acting thrombin inhibitors	Arterial thrombosis, atrial fibrillation, cardiomyopathy, cerebral emboli, hip surgery, vascular prostheses, heart valve disease, venous thromboembolism

Fibrinolysis

Streptokinase, urokinase, tissue plasminogen activator and its derivatives	Acute myocardial infarction, deep venous thrombosis Pulmonary embolism

Platelet aggregation inhibition

Aspirin	Cerebrovascular accident, stroke, after coronary artery bypass surgery, coronary angioplasty/stenting or thrombolysis, myocardial infarction, transient ischemic attack
Clopidogrel	Coronary artery disease, cerebrovascular accident, stroke, peripheral arterial disease
Glycoprotein IIb/IIIa inhibitors	Acute coronary syndromes, after coronary artery stenting

Antianemia drugs	Increase blood cell production and oxygen and carrying capacity

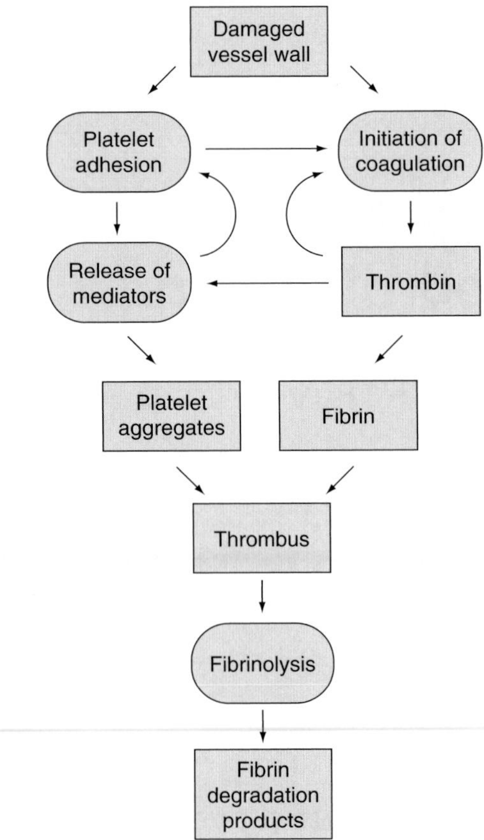

Figure 19-1 Involvement of thrombin and platelets and their interaction in thrombosis.

Mechanisms of action

The interactions of the coagulation, fibrinolytic, and platelet systems are summarized in Figure 19-1. Endothelial cells in the blood vessel lumen normally present a nonthrombogenic surface. If the endothelium is damaged, blood comes into contact with thrombogenic substances within the subendothelium, such as collagen, which activates platelets, and tissue factor, which initiates blood coagulation. Foreign surfaces, such as prosthetic vascular grafts or mechanical cardiac valves, can also trigger clotting. Removal of thrombi by the fibrinolytic system depends on generation of plasmin from plasminogen by plasminogen activators.

Coagulation

Blood coagulation occurs by sequential conversion of a series of inactive proteins into catalytically active proteases (Fig. 19-2). When the endothelium is damaged, blood comes into contact with cells that express tissue factor, a membrane-bound glycoprotein. A catalytically active complex of tissue factor and plasma factor VII is produced, which converts factor X to its enzymatically active form (X_a). In turn, factor X_a, in the presence of factor V_a and a phospholipid surface (usually that of activated platelets), converts prothrombin to thrombin. Thrombin removes small peptides from fibrinogen, converting it to fibrin monomer, which spontaneously polymerizes to form a clot. Fibrin is stabilized by factor XIII_a (transglutaminase), which introduces covalent bonds between fibrin molecules (Fig. 19-3).

In addition to clotting fibrinogen, thrombin activates platelets and converts factors V and VIII to their active forms (V_a and VIII_a). Factor VIII_a participates with activated platelets in generation of factor X_a by an

Figure 19-2 A simplified model of thrombin generation. Reactions fall into four phases, which occur preferentially on surfaces. Activated platelets provide the surface for two phases; the vascular subendothelium or nonvascular tissue provides the surface for the extrinsic phase, and foreign surfaces, such as glass and collagen, activate the contact phase. In each, a multicomponent complex is assembled, comprising an enzyme, its substrate (a proenzyme), and a cofactor. This complex affects conversion of proenzyme to its active form at a rate thousands of times faster than that of the enzyme alone.

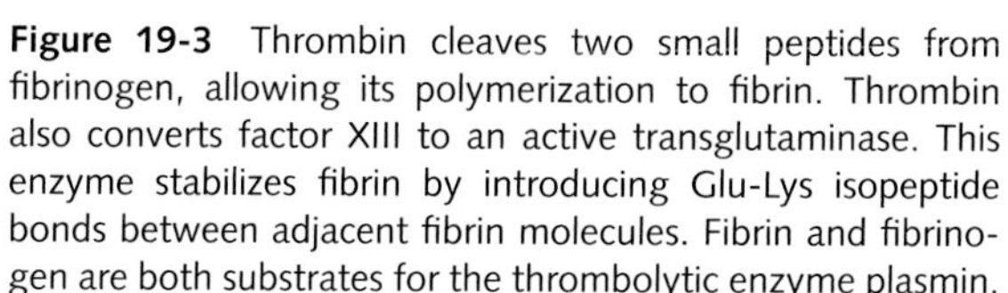

Figure 19-3 Thrombin cleaves two small peptides from fibrinogen, allowing its polymerization to fibrin. Thrombin also converts factor XIII to an active transglutaminase. This enzyme stabilizes fibrin by introducing Glu-Lys isopeptide bonds between adjacent fibrin molecules. Fibrin and fibrinogen are both substrates for the thrombolytic enzyme plasmin.

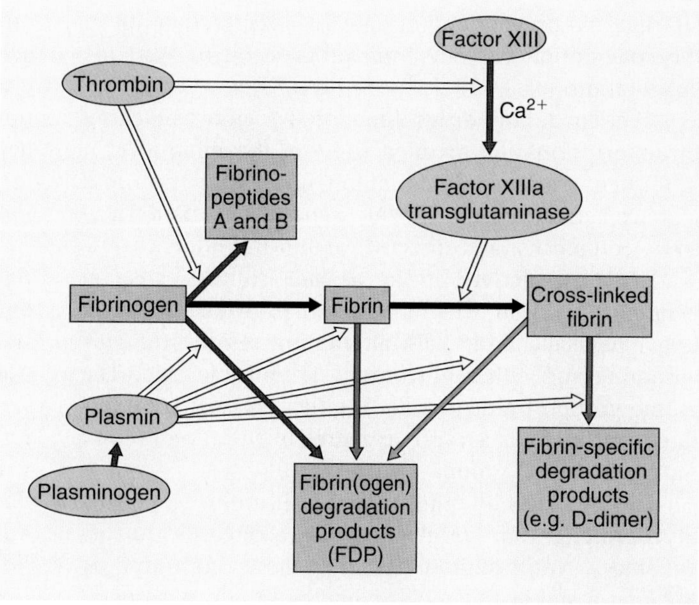

Box 19-1 Plasma protease inhibitors that regulate blood coagulation and fibrinolysis

Name	Principal target
α_1-Protease inhibitor	Elastase
α_1-Antichymotrypsin	Cathepsin C_1
Antithrombin	Thrombin, X_a, IX_a, VII_a
α_2-Macroglobulin	Plasmin, kallikrein, and other proteases
C1 inhibitor	Complement, XII_a
α_2-antiplasmin	Plasmin
Heparin cofactor II	Thrombin, X_a
Plasminogen activator inhibitor-1 (PAI-1)	t-PA, u-PA

alternative route (the intrinsic pathway). This involves factor IX, which is activated by the factor VII_a-tissue factor complex, or by factor XI_a. *In vitro,* upon contact of blood with a glass surface, the contact phase of coagulation involving factor XII, prekallikrein, and high molecular weight kininogen leads to activation of factor XI. The relevance of this pathway to initiation of coagulation *in vivo* is not clear because people with defects in these proteins seldom demonstrate excessive bleeding.

Most enzymes involved in coagulation are trypsin-like **serine proteases** with considerable homology. Plasma contains many inhibitors that regulate the coagulation cascade (Box 19-1). They prevent inappropriate clotting and prevent appropriate, localized activation of the coagulation cascade from progressing to systemic coagulation.

Anticoagulant drugs function by either blocking thrombin formation or the activity of thrombin after it is formed. Anticoagulants inhibit fibrin formation and platelet activation and include heparin and its derivatives, coumarins, and direct thrombin inhibitors.

Heparin derived from animal sources has an average molecular weight of 15 kD (5-30 kD) and is a linear polysaccharide with alternating residues of glucosamine and either glucuronic or iduronic acid. The amino group of glucosamine is either acetylated or sulfated, and there is a variable degree of sulfation ($\leq$40%) on the hydroxyl groups.

Heparin acts by binding to **antithrombin,** a plasma glycoprotein that inhibits serine protease clotting enzymes. Antithrombin inhibits these enzymes by forming a stable 1 : 1 molar complex by direct association of specific residues. Heparin binds to a lysine-rich site in antithrombin, leading to a greatly enhanced rate of inhibition, particularly of factor X_a and thrombin, but also of factors IX_a and XII_a; heparin dissociates from the complex and can then interact with another antithrombin molecule (Fig. 19-4). Although low-dose heparin acts primarily by neutralizing factor X_a, at high doses it acts by preventing thrombin-induced platelet activation, as well as factors V and VIII. Although the heparin-antithrombin complex is a very efficient inhibitor of free thrombin, clot-bound thrombin is resistant to inhibition.

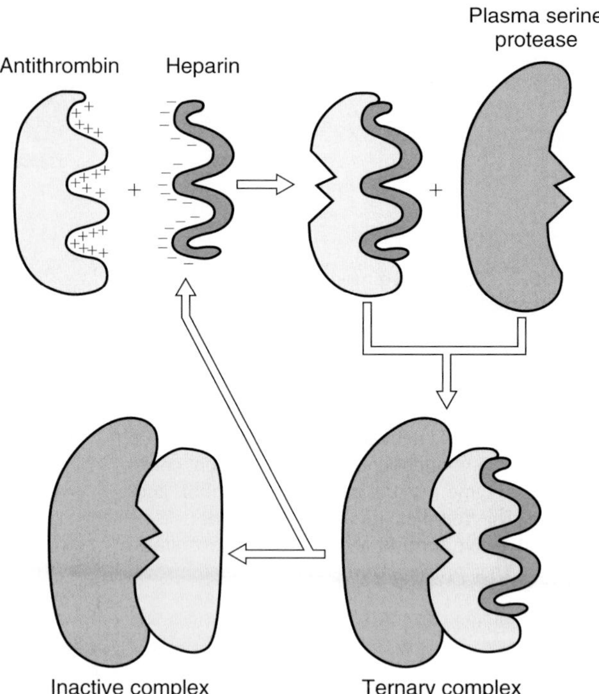

Figure 19-4 Heparin binds to a positively charged region of antithrombin and greatly increases the rate at which it interacts with plasma serine proteases. Heparin then dissociates from the ternary complex and can interact with other antithrombin molecules. This gives heparin the quality of a nonprotein enzyme. Antithrombin can inactivate thrombin and factors X_a, VII_a, and IX_a.

Heparin is heterogeneous; fractions that bind most tightly to antithrombin are responsible for most of its anticoagulant effects. Low molecular weight heparin fragments, produced hydrolytically, have a longer half-life, allowing them to be administered less frequently.

Fondaparinux is a synthetic pentasaccharide that binds to antithrombin and selectively catalyzes inactivation of factor X_a. Due to its short chain length, it does not promote thrombin inhibition, making it an antithrombin-dependent selective factor X_a inhibitor. Fondaparinux is used to prevent and treat deep venous thrombosis and does not affect platelet function.

A subset of blood coagulation proteases undergo γ-carboxylation of several glutamic acid residues. The γ-carboxyglutamic acid (GLA) residues mediate their Ca^{2+}-dependent binding to phospholipid surfaces, which

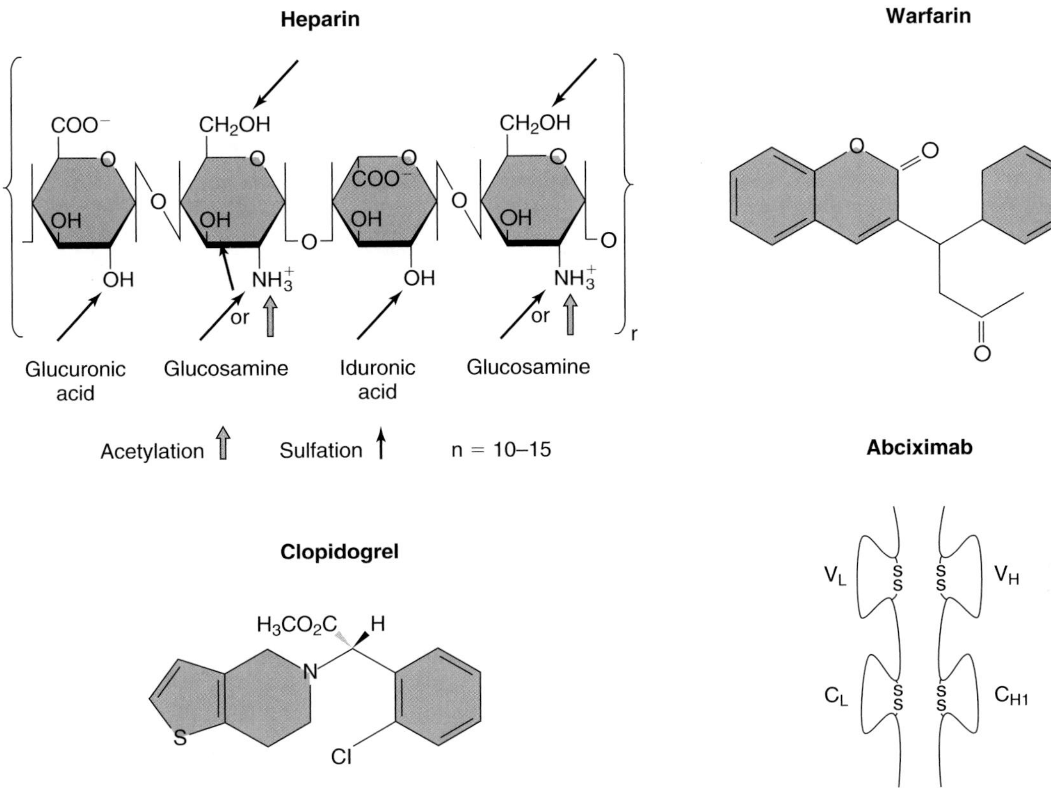

Figure 19-5 Structures of selected anticoagulants. *Top left:* Structure of a repeating unit in heparin. There is considerable variation in the extent of sulfation of different hydroxyl groups. *Lower right:* Abciximab is a Fab fragment of a chimeric human-murine monoclonal antibody. The variable *(V)* and constant *(C)* regions of the light *(L)* and heavy *(H1)* chains are shown.

is critical for proper assembly of complexes necessary to generate thrombin (see Fig. 19-1). γ-Carboxylation requires vitamin K as a cofactor; hence these proteases (factors II [prothrombin], VII, IX, X and proteins C and S) are referred to as vitamin K-dependent coagulation factors. **Coumarins,** typified by **warfarin,** are a very important class of anticoagulants. They inhibit vitamin K epoxide reductase, thereby blocking recycling of the oxidized form of vitamin K to the reduced form required for cofactor function. Coumarins inhibit synthesis of clotting factors but have no direct effect on previously synthesized factors. Therefore, plasma levels of preexisting vitamin K-dependent factors must decline before warfarin's anticoagulant effect becomes apparent, which requires several days. The first to decline is factor VII, followed by other factors with longer half-lives (Box 19-2). The full anticoagulant effect of warfarin is typically reached within 4 to 7 days. Due to genetic variations in metabolism, drug interactions, and differences in vitamin K intake, there are significant variations between individuals in the time required for a maximal effect, as well as maintenance doses required. Consequently, careful monitoring of prothrombin time (PT), a lab clotting assay, is necessary. Structures of selected anticoagulants are shown in Figure 19-5.

Box 19-2 Rates of disappearance (half-lives) of vitamin K-dependent proteins from blood

Protein	Time
Coagulation factors	
Factor VII	5 hours
Factor IX	15 hours
Factor X	1 day
Prothrombin	2-3 days
Anticoagulant proteins	
Protein C	6 hours
Protein S	10 hours

Proteins C and S, two other vitamin K-dependent factors, inhibit excessive coagulation. Thrombin binds to thrombomodulin, an endothelial cell surface protein, resulting in a different proteolytic specificity than free thrombin. In this state, it no longer cleaves fibrinogen or activates platelets; instead, it activates protein C.

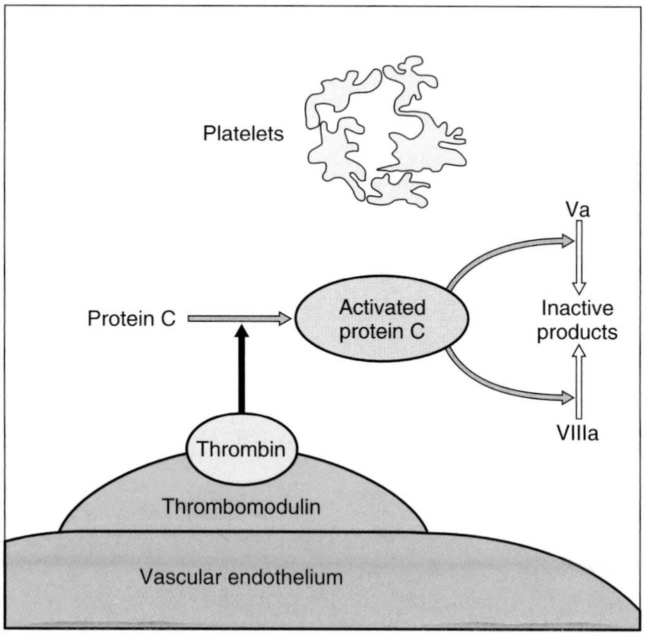

Figure 19-6 The anticoagulant protein C pathway. Thrombin bound to thrombomodulin on the surface of vascular endothelial cells has a proteolytic selectivity different from that of free thrombin. Rather than cleaving fibrinogen, it cleaves protein C to activated protein C, which then cleaves factors V_a and VIII_a to give inactive products. This process is accelerated in the presence of protein S and platelets. Both protein C and protein S are GLA-containing proteins, are vitamin K-dependent, and are affected by warfarin.

Activated protein C, in combination with protein S, proteolytically inactivates clotting cofactors V_a and VIII_a (Fig. 19-6), thereby providing a feedback inhibition to down-regulate blood clotting after vascular injury. Genetic deficiency of protein C or protein S can cause thromboembolic disease.

If a patient has an acute thrombus or is at high risk of forming one within the next few days, heparin is used, because its antithrombotic effect is immediate, whereas that of warfarin is delayed. If long-term anticoagulation is necessary, warfarin can be started as soon as therapeutic anticoagulation with heparin is achieved. After therapeutic anticoagulation with warfarin is achieved, heparin is often continued for 1 to 2 days. This overlap is commonly employed because the antithrombotic effect of warfarin can lag behind laboratory measurements of warfarin anticoagulation, which is largely affected by a reduction in the level of factor VII, which has a short half-life (see Box 19-2). If warfarin is started for prophylaxis of thrombosis, and the short-term risk is not high (e.g., a patient with atrial fibrillation being started on warfarin to lower stroke risk), heparin may be unnecessary. Most experts recommend that loading doses of warfarin should not be used, that is, the patient be started on the anticipated maintenance dose. During the first week of warfarin therapy, the coagulation response should be checked at least twice. Depending on the rapidity and stability of this measure, the time interval between subsequent determinations is gradually increased.

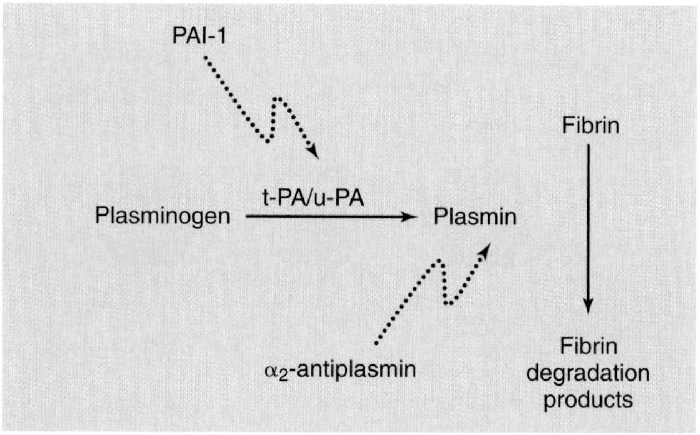

Figure 19-7 Key components of the fibrinolytic system. Dotted lines depict inhibition of t-PA and u-PA by plasminogen activator inhibitor-1 (PAI-1) and the inhibition of plasmin by α_2-antiplasmin.

There are several agents that directly inhibit thrombin. **Hirudin** is a 65-amino-acid leech salivary gland protein that directly inhibits thrombin activity. Hirudin blocks the active site of thrombin and an exosite that mediates fibrinogen binding. Recombinant hirudins, such as desirudin and lepirudin, and analogs of hirudin, such as bivalirudin, are used as anticoagulants. They must be administered intravenously and are primarily used in patients intolerant of heparin. Argatroban is a synthetic, directly acting thrombin inhibitor derived from L-arginine that reversibly binds to the thrombin active site. Argatroban and hirudin inhibit the activity of both free and clot-associated thrombin.

Fibrinolysis

Fibrin clots are lysed mainly through the proteolytic action of **plasmin,** the enzyme produced by proteolytic activation of plasminogen by plasminogen activators (Fig. 19-7). A minor aspect of clot lysis may result from release of proteolytic enzymes, such as elastase, from leukocytes. The two major classes of endogenous plasminogen activators are tissue-type plasminogen activator (t-PA) and urinary-type plasminogen activator (u-PA). Recombinant forms of these proteins are used as clot-dissolving drugs. **Streptokinase,** a protein produced by streptococci, forms a complex with plasminogen that activates free plasminogen molecules to plasmin and is also used as a thrombolytic agent. Plasmin formed by the action of PAs attacks not only fibrin but also several other proteins, including fibrinogen, factor V, and factor VIII. The recombinant forms of u-PA and t-PA may have some advantages over streptokinase because of their selectivity in binding to the fibrin clot, but streptokinase is less expensive. Streptokinase, however, is highly immunogenic and cannot be used repeatedly. Modified forms of t-PA, such as reteplase and tenecteplase, have deletions or mutations in domains responsible for clearance from the circulation. They have a prolonged half-life, which enables them to be administered as a bolus, rather than a continuous infusion to patients with acute myocardial infarction.

Platelet aggregation

Activation and subsequent aggregation of platelets is a major component of arterial thrombosis and may be involved in initiation of venous thrombosis. Interaction of platelets with vessel wall collagen appears to be a key step. Activation of platelets leads to formation and release of thromboxane A_2 (TXA_2) from arachidonic acid in platelet membranes (see Chapter 17). TXA_2 is a potent aggregating agent and vasoconstrictor. Platelet activation also causes secretion of adenosine diphosphate from storage granules. Both TXA_2 and adenosine diphosphate, which act through specific receptors, cause activation of integrin $\alpha_{IIb}\beta_{IIIa}$ receptors on the platelet surface for fibrinogen and for other adhesive proteins, including von Willebrand's factor (vWF). Fibrinogen binding to its integrin receptor mediates aggregation, whereas vWF is primarily involved in adhesion of platelets to extracellular matrices in the vessel wall. Thrombin generated locally on the surface of activated platelets greatly amplifies the response by causing further activation and mediator secretion. Although TXA_2, adenosine diphosphate, and thrombin all increase cytoplasmic Ca^{2+}, the mechanism by which thrombin activates its receptor is unique. Thrombin activates its platelet receptors (PAR1 and PAR4, respectively) by cleaving within their N-terminal domains. The newly formed N-terminus forms a "tethered ligand" that binds to the body of the receptor to induce transmembrane signaling (Fig. 19-8).

Platelet activation is inhibited by elevation of intracellular cyclic adenosine monophosphate, thus agents that increase this second messenger inhibit aggregation. The most active agent is prostacyclin, released by cells of the vessel wall (see Chapter 17). Other mediators from endothelial cells may also contribute.

The major therapeutic approach to reducing platelet aggregation is through inhibition of cyclooxygenase. **Aspirin** irreversibly inhibits platelet cyclooxygenase by acetylating a serine residue near the active site of the enzyme, thereby blocking TXA_2 formation (see Chapter 31). Aspirin also blocks synthesis of the endogenous vasodilator and platelet inhibitor prostacyclin, although at standard doses this prothrombotic effect is insignificant.

Clinical trials have shown that aspirin reduces the incidence of myocardial infarction and death from cardiac causes by 30% to 50% in patients with unstable angina. Aspirin also significantly reduces the incidence of a first myocardial infarction in men with stable angina and is effective as an antithrombotic agent after coronary angioplasty/stenting or bypass grafting. Aspirin is effective in secondary prevention of myocardial infarction. Aspirin is also recommended for use in patients with transient ischemic attacks. There are, of course, adverse effects of long-term aspirin therapy (see Chapter 31).

Clopidogrel irreversibly blocks activation of the platelet P2Y receptor by adenosine diphosphate (see Fig. 19-5). Clopidogrel is a prodrug that is metabolized by cytochrome P450 3A to an active metabolite. Clopidogrel has become a mainstay in treatment of patients with coronary artery disease, and it is also commonly administered to patients with peripheral arterial occlusive disease and cerebrovascular disease. It is routinely administered with aspirin, particularly to patients who have received coronary artery stents.

Dipyridamole acts as an antiplatelet drug by stimulating prostacyclin synthesis, enhancing its inhibitory action, inhibiting phosphodiesterase, and blocking uptake of adenosine into vascular and blood cells, leading to accumulation of this platelet-inhibitory and vasodilatory compound. At therapeutic doses, dipyridamole does not prolong bleeding time or inhibit *ex vivo* platelet aggregation. **Aggrenox** is a combination antiplatelet agent consisting of dipyridamole and aspirin, which has been found to be useful in secondary prevention of stroke.

Inhibitors of **glycoprotein IIb/IIIa** (Fig. 19-9) bind to $\alpha_{IIb}\beta_{IIIa}$, or glycoprotein IIb/IIIa, the platelet integrin receptor for fibrinogen, vWF, and other adhesive ligands. These inhibitors prevent fibrinogen cross-linking of platelets, which is the final common pathway of aggregation. These agents are administered by intravenous infusion, primarily to prevent platelet-dependent thrombosis during treatment of acute coronary artery syndromes and after implantation of intracoronary stents. **Abciximab** is the Fab fragment of a chimeric human-murine monoclonal antibody that binds to the glycoprotein IIb/IIIa receptor of human platelets (see Fig. 19-5). Abciximab also binds to the vitronectin receptor ($\alpha_V\beta_3$) present on platelets, vascular endothelial cells, and vascular smooth muscle cells. Platelet function gradually recovers after abciximab infusion is stopped. Plasma drug levels fall quickly, though platelet-bound abciximab can be detected for up

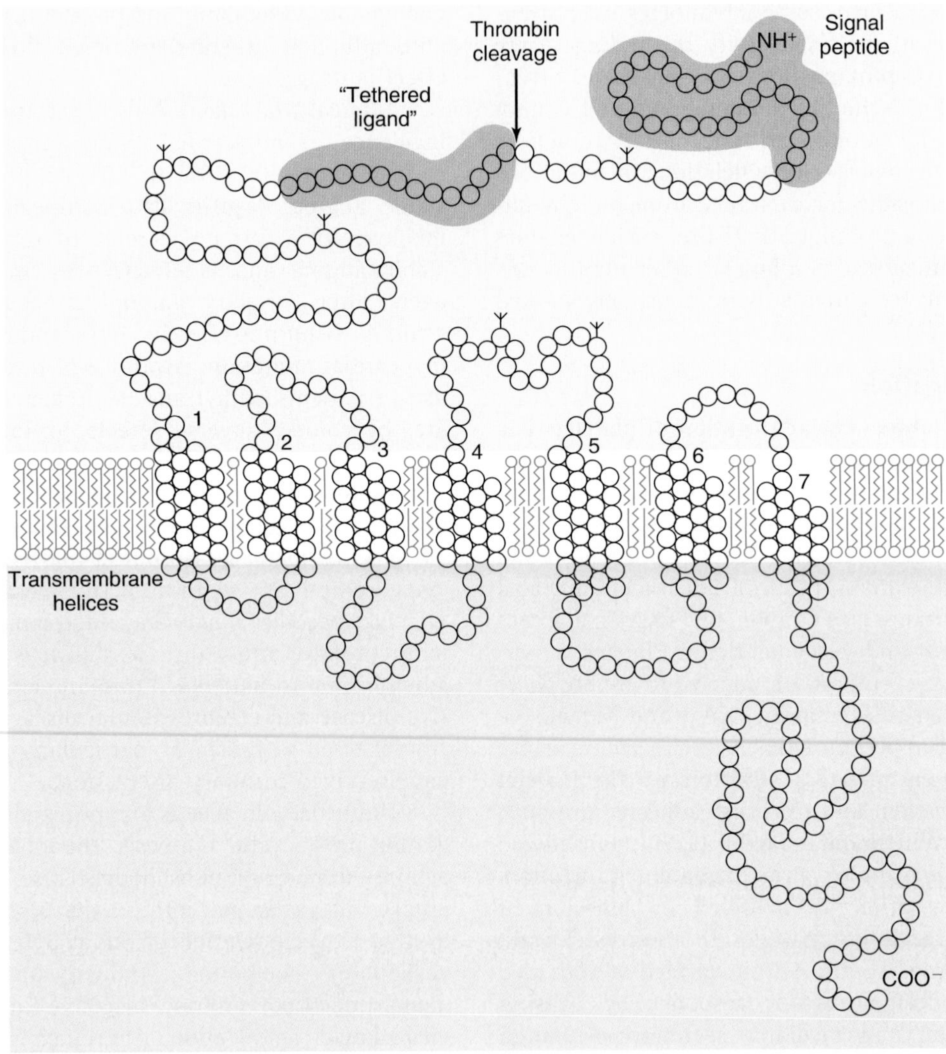

Figure 19-8 Predicted linear structure of the platelet thrombin receptor, protease activated receptor 1 *(PAR1)*. It is thought to have a characteristic seven-transmembrane domain G-protein–coupled receptor structure (see Chapter 2). However, thrombin acts by cleaving the N-terminal extracellular tail of the receptor, releasing an activation peptide and leaving a new N-terminal sequence: Ser-Phe-Lys-Lys-Arg-. This sequence acts as a "tethered ligand," which activates the receptor and is a powerful aggregating agent.

to 15 days. **Eptifibatide** is a cyclic heptapeptide containing six amino acids and one mercaptopropionyl (des-amino cysteinyl) residue. Eptifibatide inhibits platelet aggregation by blocking the binding of fibrinogen to glycoprotein IIb/IIIa. Inhibition of platelet aggregation by eptifibatide is reversible after the drug is stopped due to dissociation from the platelet surface. **Tirofiban** is a nonpeptide antagonist of the platelet glycoprotein IIb/IIIa receptor. Platelet inhibition following tirofiban is reversible after infusion is stopped.

Hematopoiesis

Production of new blood cells occurs primarily in adult bone marrow. Over 150 billion new erythrocytes, platelets, and leukocytes are produced daily in normal people, and depend importantly on availability of iron, vitamin B_{12}, folate, and a number of growth factors that regulate stem cell differentiation into particular blood cell phenotypes. Anemia caused by red blood cell deficiency is most common and is treated by iron replacement therapy until hemoglobin concentrations are normal and iron stores have been repleted. Vitamin B_{12} and folate deficiencies are also normally corrected by dietary replacement. More severe anemia, such as that occurring during renal failure, is now treated with recombinant erythropoietin or other hematopoietic growth factors (see Chapter 53). This is because erythropoietin is mainly synthesized in renal cortical cells,

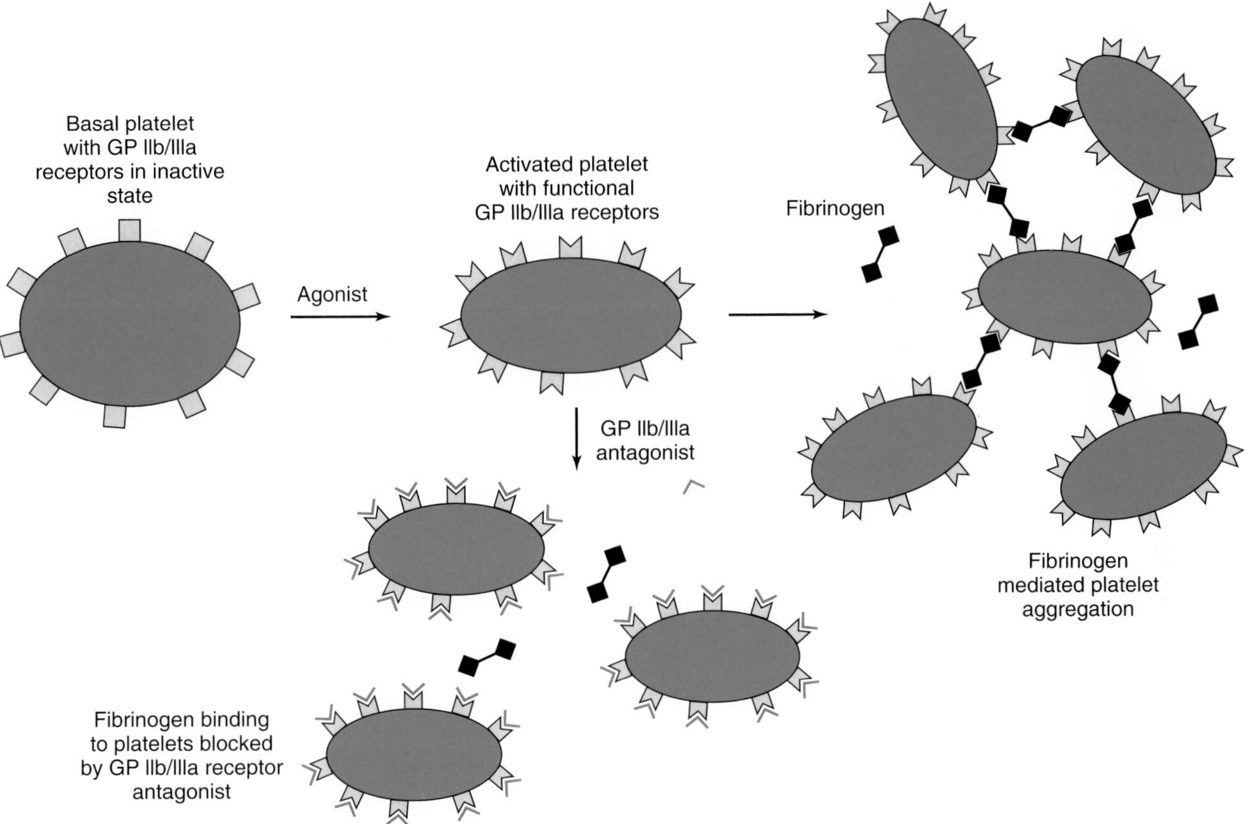

Figure 19-9 Inhibition of platelet aggregation by glycoprotein (GP) IIb/IIIa receptor antagonists. The GP IIb/IIIa receptors on unstimulated platelets exist in an inactive conformation that does not support fibrinogen binding. Activation of platelets by agonists, such as ADP, epinephrine, thrombin, and thromboxane A_2, converts the GP IIb/IIIa receptors to an active conformation capable of binding fibrinogen, which leads to the formation of platelet aggregates. Blocking of the GP IIb/IIIa receptors with antagonists, such as abciximab, eptifibatide, and tirofiban, prevents fibrinogen from cross-linking activated platelets, thereby inhibiting thrombus growth.

and the lack of its production in kidney failure can contribute significantly to loss of circulating blood cells in this condition.

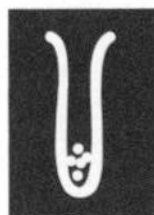

Pharmacokinetics

The principal pharmacokinetic parameters of the anticoagulants, fibrinolytic activators, and antiplatelet drugs are given in Table 19-1. Warfarin is typical of orally administered anticoagulants (see Fig. 19-5). Heparin is given by IV infusion or subcutaneously. Because of different mechanisms of action, the anticoagulant effect of heparin is immediate, whereas that of warfarin typically occurs within 3 to 7 days. Warfarin is metabolized in the liver. Warfarin is strongly bound to plasma albumin, whereas heparin is not. The half-life of low molecular weight heparins is longer than that of the naturally occurring, unfractionated compound. Thus, they are effective when administered by once or twice daily subcutaneous injection.

Aspirin is hydrolyzed in plasma to salicylic acid, with a half-life of 15 to 20 minutes, as discussed in Chapter 31. The antithrombotic effect of aspirin, however, persists for at least 2 days because circulating platelets cannot synthesize cyclooxygenase. New platelets must be produced to restore TXA_2 concentrations.

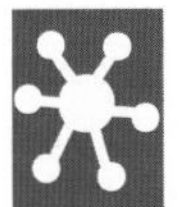

Relation of mechanisms of action to clinical response

Anticoagulants and antiplatelet compounds are commonly used to prevent thromboembolic disease. **Heparin** is effective in prevention and treatment of

Table 19-1 Selected pharmacokinetic parameters

Drug	Administration	Half-Life (hr)	Disposition	Plasma Protein Binding (%)
Unfractionated heparin	IV	1		Trace
	SC	3		
Low molecular weight heparin	IV	2	R	Trace
	SC	4		
Fondaparinux	SC	17-21	R	
Warfarin	Oral	40	M, (R)	97
Argatroban	IV	<1	M	
Lepirudin	IV	1	M, R	
Bivalirudin	IV	<1	M, R	
Aspirin	Oral	2-3	M, R	50-70
Clopidogrel	Oral	8	M, R	?
Abciximab	IV	<1 hr*		
Eptifibatide	IV	2.5	R	
Tirofiban	IV	2	R	
Streptokinase	IV	0.3	M	
Urokinase (u-PA)	IV	0.3	M	
t-PA	IV	0.2	M	

M, Metabolism; *R*, renal excretion.
*For free compound. Remains bound to platelets for up to 15 days.

venous thrombosis and pulmonary embolism and related events and can be used either for prophylaxis or treatment. For prophylaxis, it is given by once or twice daily subcutaneous injection at a dose that does not affect in vitro clotting times, such as the activated partial thromboplastin time (APTT). A higher dose is required for treatment of ongoing thrombotic processes. If unfractionated heparin is used, its anticoagulant effect must be monitored, such as by APTT. The anticoagulant response varies significantly among patients with thromboembolic disease. The risk of bleeding is increased as the dose increases. For this reason, the APTT is used to monitor the degree of anticoagulation. Due to their shorter chain lengths, **low molecular weight heparins** have a greater capacity to inhibit factor X_a than thrombin. Consequently, at standard clinical doses they produce only a mild prolonging of the APTT. Furthermore, they have a high and relatively constant bioavailability after subcutaneous injection. Consequently, self-administered low molecular weight heparins can be used to provide full anticoagulation in the outpatient setting without monitoring. Because they are cleared from the blood by the kidneys, their dosing must be adjusted in patients with renal insufficiency.

Oral **coumarin** anticoagulants are effective in primary and secondary prevention of arterial and venous thromboembolism. The one-stage prothrombin time (PT) is used to measure their anticoagulant effects. Because different clinical laboratories use different thromboplastins, a formula was developed to transform the PT to an index that allows results from different laboratories to be meaningfully compared. This index, the international normalized ratio (INR), is routinely used to report PT results. Warfarin therapy prolongs the PT and the INR.

Platelet function is assessed by measurement of bleeding time, which involves incising the forearm skin under standardized conditions and measuring the time required for bleeding to stop. Platelet aggregation in vitro can be monitored optically using an aggregometer.

Side effects, clinical problems, and toxicity

The major problem associated with antithrombotic agents is **bleeding**, even when used in therapeutic doses. Thrombocytopenia (heparin), drug interactions (warfarin), and platelet aggregation caused by other drugs also pose significant problems (see Clinical Problems box).

The anticoagulant effect of unfractionated heparin can be reversed rapidly with protamine sulfate, a positively charged molecule that binds avidly to the negatively charged heparin. Rapid reversal of the effect of

CLINICAL PROBLEMS

Heparin

Bleeding, thrombocytopenia, hypersensitivity, transient hypercoagulability when discontinued

Warfarin

Bleeding, drug interactions, some patients are resistant

Streptokinase

Bleeding, immunogenic

Urokinase and recombinant tissue plasminogen activator

Bleeding, expensive

Aspirin

Dose-dependent gastrointestinal upset, hypersensitivity, Reye's syndrome in children

Clopidogrel

Bleeding

Glycoprotein IIB/IIIA inhibitors

Bleeding, thrombocytopenia

Directly-acting thrombin inhibitors

Bleeding

Fondaparinux

Bleeding, thrombocytopenia

Iron

Gastrointestinal upset, pediatric toxicity

Erythropoietin

Hypertension

warfarin can be achieved only by transfusion of plasma containing clotting factors. If the patient is overly anticoagulated with warfarin and is not actively bleeding, anticoagulation can be restored with 24 hours in most patients by small oral doses of vitamin K.

Transient **thrombocytopenia** is a well-recognized, usually asymptomatic complication of heparin therapy. Thrombocytopenia induced by heparin is generally considered clinically significant if the platelet count falls to less than 100×10^9/L. Heparin-induced thrombocytopenia can be mediated by immune and by nonimmune mechanisms, with the immune form involving formation of complexes of heparin, platelet factor 4, and immunoglobulin. Its incidence ranges from 0.3% to 3% in patients exposed to unfractionated heparin for greater than 4 days and is less common with low molecular weight heparins than with unfractionated heparin. It is associated with arterial or venous thrombosis in a small but significant subset of patients and occasionally can be extremely serious and even fatal. Platelet counts should be monitored at regular intervals in patients receiving heparin for prolonged periods. When heparin is discontinued, platelet count usually returns to normal within 4 days.

Box 19-3 Drug interactions with warfarin

Decreased anticoagulation

Increased warfarin metabolism by cytochrome P450: barbiturates, carbamazepine, griseofulvin, rifampin
Reduced warfarin absorption: cholestyramine
Unknown mechanism: penicillins

Increased anticoagulation

Inhibition of warfarin clearance: disulfiram, amiodarone, metronidazole, sulfinpyrazone
Displacement of warfarin from plasma albumin: salicylates, chloral hydrate
Increased clearance of clotting factors: thyroid hormones
Unknown mechanism: erythromycin, anabolic steroids

Functional synergism

Inhibition of coagulation: heparin, thrombolytic agents
Inhibition of platelet function: aspirin and other nonsteroidal antiinflammatory drugs, clopidogrel, glycoprotein IIb/IIIa inhibitors

Heparin does not cross the placenta and does not produce untoward effects in the fetus. Warfarin crosses the placenta and is a teratogen. Characteristic abnormalities associated with warfarin embryopathy include nasal bridge deformities and abnormal bone formation. Fetal risk from warfarin exposure is greatest during weeks 6 to 12 of development. Any woman with the potential to become pregnant should be advised of warfarin's potential teratogenic effects, and instructed to contact her health care provider immediately, if she believes that she may be pregnant.

Because warfarin treatment often extends over months or years, the possibility of drug-drug interactions is high. This is primarily attributable to warfarin's high degree of binding to plasma albumin and its mode of elimination. Common warfarin-drug interactions are listed in Box 19-3. Hereditary resistance to warfarin is rare but has been described; those affected require 5 to 20 times the average normal dose.

New horizons

Ximelagatran is a prodrug that is converted to melagatran, a low molecular weight, direct-acting thrombin inhibitor. Ximelagatran has been studied in clinical trials of atrial fibrillation and deep venous thrombosis, the results of which suggest that it may be as safe and effective as warfarin. Potential advantages of this agent over warfarin include the fact that it can be administered at a fixed dose without anticoagulation monitoring, and that ximelagatran's anticoagulant effect is not significantly affected by diet or drug interactions. Elevations of serum levels of hepatic transaminases can occur early in the course of ximelagatran therapy, suggesting that screening for potential hepatotoxicity is necessary.

TRADE NAMES

In addition to generic and fixed-combination preparations, the following trade-named materials are available in the United States.

Anticoagulation

Heparin calcium (Calciparine)
Low molecular weight heparins
  Dalteparin (Fragmin)
  Enoxaparin (Lovenox)
  Nadroparin (Fraxiparin)
  Tinzaparin (Innohep)
Bivalirudin (Angiomax)
Fondaparinux (Arixtra)
Lepirudin (Refludan)
Vitamin K_1, phytonadione (Aquamephyton)
Warfarin sodium (Coumadin)

Fibrinolysis

Recombinant tissue plasminogen activator (Activase)
Reteplase (Retavase)
Streptokinase (Streptase, Kabikinase)
Tenecteplase (TNKase)
Urokinase (Abbokinase)

Platelet aggregation inhibition

Abciximab (ReoPro)
Clopidogrel (Plavix)
Eptifibatide (Integrilin)
Tirofiban (Aggrastat)

FURTHER READING

Esmon CT. The protein C pathway. *Chest* 2003; 124(3 suppl): 26S-32S.

Hirsh J, Fuster V, Ansell J, et al. American Heart Association/American College of Cardiology Foundation guide to warfarin therapy. *Circulation* 2003; 107:1692-1711.

Nutescu EA, Wittkowsky AK. Direct thrombin inhibitors for anticoagulation. *Ann Pharmacother* 2004; 38:99-109.

Self-assessment questions

1. Heparin:

a. Has thrombolytic activity.
b. Has most prolonged activity when given orally.
c. Acts by binding to antithrombin.
d. Inhibits the aggregation of platelets caused by TXA_2.
e. Acts by blocking hepatic vitamin K regeneration.

2. Warfarin:

a. Acts rapidly when given orally.
b. Is potentiated by barbiturates.
c. Is antagonized by protamine sulfate.
d. Affects the activity of clotting factors.
e. Is potentiated by platelet factor 4.

3. The risk of bleeding in patients receiving heparin is increased by aspirin because aspirin:

a. Inhibits heparin anticoagulant activity.
b. Inhibits platelet function.
c. Displaces heparin from plasma protein-binding sites.
d. Inhibits prothrombin formation.
e. Causes thrombocytopenia.

4. In patients taking warfarin, the antithrombotic effect is *decreased* when they are also given which of the following drugs?

a. Chloral hydrate
b. Heparin
c. Aspirin
d. Cholestyramine
e. Clopidogrel

5. Aspirin can:

a. Prevent formation of TXA_2.
b. Prolong whole blood clotting time.
c. Shorten bleeding time.
d. Inhibit fibrinolysis.
e. Inhibit the effects of warfarin.

PART IV

Drugs affecting the brain and behavior

DRUGS ACTING ON THE **central nervous system** (CNS) are among the most widely used of all drugs. Humankind has experienced the effects of mind-altering drugs throughout history, and many compounds with specific and useful effects on brain and behavior have been discovered over the last half century. Drugs used for therapeutic purposes have improved the quality of life dramatically for people with diverse illnesses, while illicit drugs have altered the lives of many others, often in detrimental ways.

Discovery of the general anesthetics was essential for the development of surgery, and continued advances in the development of anesthetics, sedatives, narcotics, and muscle relaxants have made possible the complex microsurgical procedures in use today. Discovery of the typical antipsychotics and tricyclic antidepressants in the 1950s revolutionized psychiatry and enabled many individuals afflicted with these mind-paralyzing diseases to begin to lead productive lives and contribute to society. Similarly, the introduction of l-DOPA for the treatment of Parkinson's disease in 1970 was a milestone in neurology and allowed many people who had been immobilized for years the ability to move and interact with their environment. Other advances led to the development of drugs to reduce pain or fever, relieve seizures and other movement disorders associated with neurological diseases, and alleviate the incapacitating effects associated with psychiatric disorders, including mania and anxiety.

The nonmedical use of drugs affecting the CNS has also increased dramatically. Alcohol, hallucinogens, caffeine, nicotine, and other compounds were used historically to alter mood and behavior and are still in common use. Many stimulants, depressants, and antianxiety agents intended for medical use are obtained illicitly and used for their mood-altering effects. Although the short-term effects of these drugs may be exciting or pleasurable, excessive use often leads to physical dependence or toxic effects that result in long-term alterations in the brain. This dependence is a major problem in adolescents, as the use of illicit drugs by this age group has increased significantly over the past 20 years, and very little is known about the long-term effects of these compounds on the developing brain.

Although tremendous advances have been made recently, knowledge of the brain and how it functions is still in its infancy, as is an understanding of the molecular targets through which drugs alter brain function. Much of what is known has resulted from relating observed actions on specific molecular processes to known mood-altering or behavioral actions of drugs. In addition, although many compounds have been developed with beneficial therapeutic effects for countless patients, many patients do not respond to any available medications, underscoring the need for further research and development.

This section describes drugs that affect specific neurotransmitter systems, second messengers, and the activities of neuronal circuits in the brain and are used to modify behavior, control epilepsy and movement disorders, control pain, and reduce inflammation. In addition, the use of alcohol and mind-altering, often addictive abused drugs is described. The major CNS disorders and the classes of drugs currently used for their treatment are listed in Table IV-1, along with the chapter in which they are discussed.

Table IV-1 Major CNS disorders and classes of drugs used for treatment

Disorder or Indication	Drug Group/Class	Chapter
NEURODEGENERATIVE DISORDERS		
Parkinson's disease	Dopamine-enhancing compounds	21
Alzheimer's disease	Acetylcholinesterase inhibitors	21
	NMDA receptor antagonists	
PSYCHIATRIC DISORDERS		
Psychotic disorders (schizophrenia)	Typical and atypical antipsychotics	22
Affective disorders (unipolar/bipolar depression)	Antidepressants	23
	Mood stabilizers	
Anxiety and sleep disorders	Anxiolytics	24
	Sleep-promoting drugs	
Eating disorders and obesity		26
NEUROLOGICAL DISORDERS		
Seizures	Anticonvulsants	27
Spasticity	Antispasmodic drugs	29
	Motor neuron blocking drugs	
SURGERY	General anesthetics	28
	Neuromuscular blocking drugs	29
	Local anesthetics	
PAIN	Local anesthetics	30
	Opioids	31
	Nonsteroidal antiinflammatory agents	31
	Antigout drugs	31
	Antimigraine drugs	31
DRUGS OF ABUSE		
Ethanol and related compounds	Disulfiram	25
Drug addiction and abuse	Opioids and opiates	32
	Stimulants	
	Depressants	
	Cannabinoids	
	Hallucinogens	
	Dissociative compounds	
	Inhalants	
	Anabolic steroids	
	Nicotine	

CHAPTER 20

Introduction to the central nervous system

Lynn Wecker

Understanding the actions of drugs on the central nervous system (CNS) and their rational use for the treatment of brain diseases requires an understanding of the organization and component parts of the brain. Most drugs interact with specific proteins at defined chemical synapses associated with specific neurotransmitter pathways. These interactions are responsible for the primary therapeutic actions of drugs as well as many of their unwanted side effects.

To have CNS effects, drugs must obviously be able to reach their targets in the brain. Because the brain is protected from many harmful and foreign blood-borne substances by the blood-brain barrier (BBB), the entry of many drugs is restricted. Therefore it is important to understand the characteristics of drugs that enable them to enter the CNS.

This chapter covers basic aspects of CNS function, with a focus on the cellular and molecular processes and neurotransmitters thought to underlie CNS disorders. The mechanisms through which drugs act to alleviate these disorders are emphasized.

Neurotransmission in the central nervous system

Cell types: neurons and glia

The CNS is composed of two predominant cell types, neurons and glia, each of which has many morphologically and functionally diverse subclasses. Glial cells outnumber neurons and contain many neurotransmitter receptors and transporters. They are involved in supporting neurons as well as in information transfer and integration. There are three types of glial cells: astrocytes, oligodendrocytes, and microglia (Fig. 20-1). **Astrocytes** physically separate neurons and multineuronal pathways, assist in repairing nerve injury, and modulate the metabolic and ionic microenvironment. **Oligodendrocytes** form the myelin sheath around axons, while **microglia** proliferate after injury or degeneration, move to sites of injury, and transform into large macrophages (phagocytes) to remove cellular debris.

Neurons are the major cells involved in intercellular communication because of their ability to conduct impulses and transmit information. They are structurally different from other cells, with four distinct features (Fig. 20-2):

- Dendrites
- A perikaryon (cell body or soma)
- An axon
- A nerve (or axon) terminal

Abbreviations

ACh	acetylcholine
BBB	blood-brain barrier
CNS	central nervous system
DA	dopamine
GABA	γ-aminobutyric acid

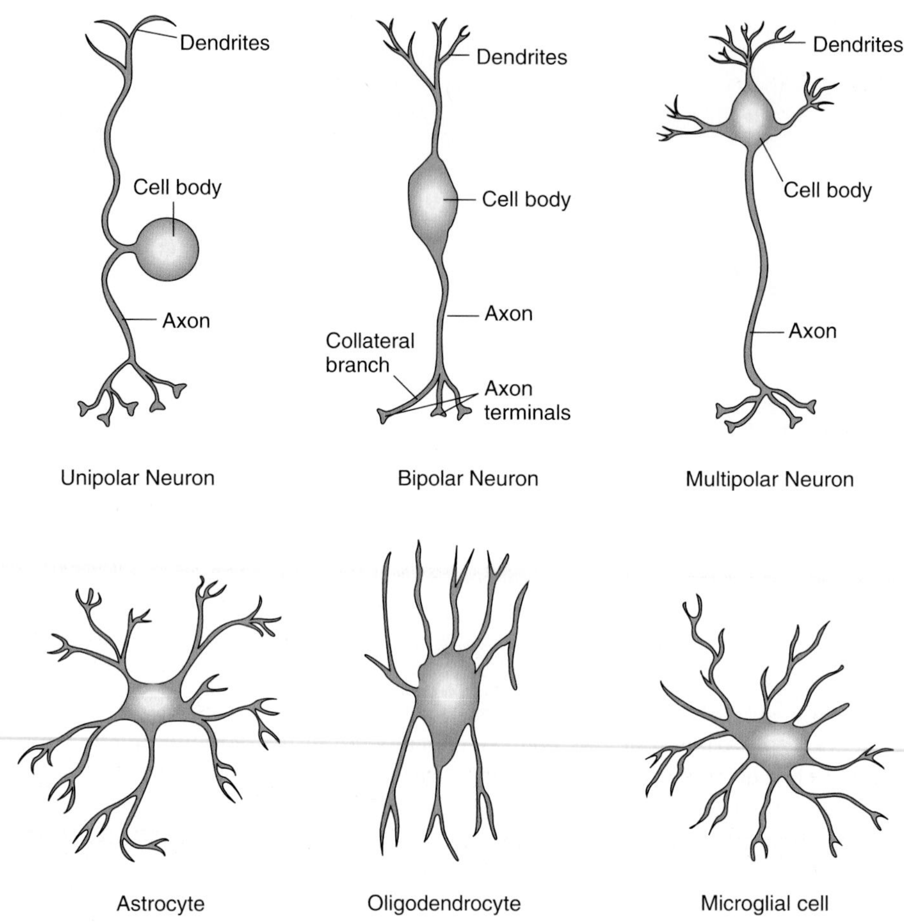

Figure 20-1 Types of cells in the CNS: Selected examples.

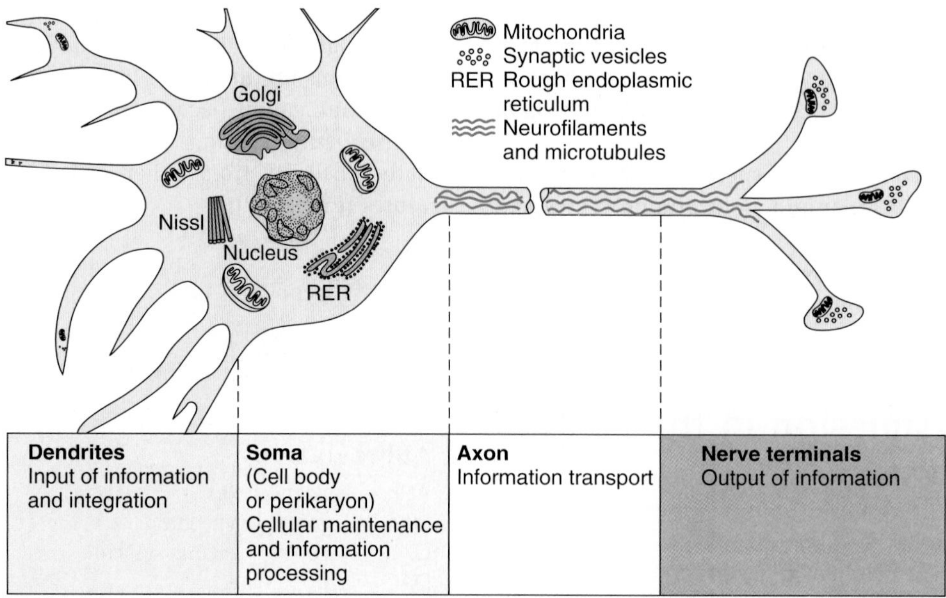

Figure 20-2 Structural components of nerve cells.

The **perikaryon** contains most of the organelles necessary for maintenance and function, including the nucleus, rough endoplasmic reticulum, ribosomes, Golgi apparatus, mitochondria, lysosomes, and cytoskeletal elements. **Dendrites** are relatively short afferent processes with similar cytoplasmic contents. The number of dendrites varies greatly between cell types, and many dendrites possess multiple spines protruding from their surface. Both dendrites and perikarya contain surface receptors to receive signals from nearby neurons. Incoming signals from the dendrites are relayed to the cell body, which transmits information to the nerve terminal via the **axon.**

The axon contains neurofilaments and microtubules, which play an important role in maintaining cell shape, growth, and intracellular transport. The movement of organelles, peptide neurotransmitters, and cytoskeletal components from their sites of synthesis in the cell body to the axon terminal (anterograde) and back to the cell body (retrograde) is called **axonal transport.** The main function of the axon is propagation of the action potential. The axon maintains ionic concentrations of Na^+ and K^+ to ensure a transmembrane potential of −65 mV. In response to an appropriate stimulus, ion channels open and allow Na^+ influx, causing depolarization toward the Na^+ equilibrium potential (+30 mV). This causes opening of neighboring channels, resulting in unidirectional propagation of the action potential. When it reaches the **nerve terminal,** depolarization causes release of chemical messengers to transmit information to nearby cells.

Nerve terminals contain all components required for synthesis, release, reuptake, and packaging of neurotransmitters into synaptic vesicles, as well as mitochondria and structural elements. They may also contain structures classically thought to be restricted to the perikaryon, such as ribosomes and machinery for protein synthesis, as well as proteolytic enzymes important in the final processing of peptide neurotransmitters.

Neurons are often shaped according to their function. Unipolar or pseudounipolar neurons have a single axon, which bifurcates close to the cell body, with one end typically extending centrally and the other peripherally (see Fig. 20-1). Unipolar neurons tend to serve sensory functions. Bipolar neurons have two extensions and are associated with the retina, vestibular cochlear system, and olfactory epithelium; they are commonly interneurons. Finally, multipolar neurons have many processes but only one axon extending from the cell body. These are the most numerous neurons and include spinal motor, pyramidal, and Purkinje neurons.

Neurons may also be classified by the neurotransmitter they release and the response they produce. For example, neurons that release γ-aminobutyric acid (GABA) generally hyperpolarize postsynaptic cells; thus GABAergic neurons are generally inhibitory. In contrast, neurons that release glutamate depolarize postsynaptic cells and are excitatory.

The synapse

Effective transfer and integration of information in the CNS requires passage of information between neurons or other target cells. The nerve terminal is usually separated from adjacent cells by a gap of 20 nm or more; therefore signals must cross this gap. This is accomplished by specialized areas of communication, referred to as **synapses.** The synapse is the junction between a nerve terminal and a postsynaptic specialization on an adjacent cell where information is received.

Most neurotransmission involves communication between nerve terminals and dendrites or perikarya on the postsynaptic cell, called **axodendritic** or **axosomatic** synapses, respectively. However, other areas of the neuron may also be involved in both sending and receiving information. Neurotransmitter receptors are often spread diffusely over the dendrites, perikarya, and nerve terminals but are also commonly found on glial cells, where they probably serve a functional role. In addition, transmitters can be stored in and released from dendrites. Thus, transmitters released from nerve terminals may interact with receptors on other axons at **axoaxonic** synapses; transmitters released from dendrites can interact with receptors on either "postsynaptic" dendrites or perikarya, referred to as **dendrodendritic** or **dendrosomatic** synapses, respectively (Fig. 20-3).

In addition, released neurotransmitters may diffuse from the synapse to act at receptors in extrasynaptic regions or on other neurons or glia distant from the site of release. This process is referred to as **volume**

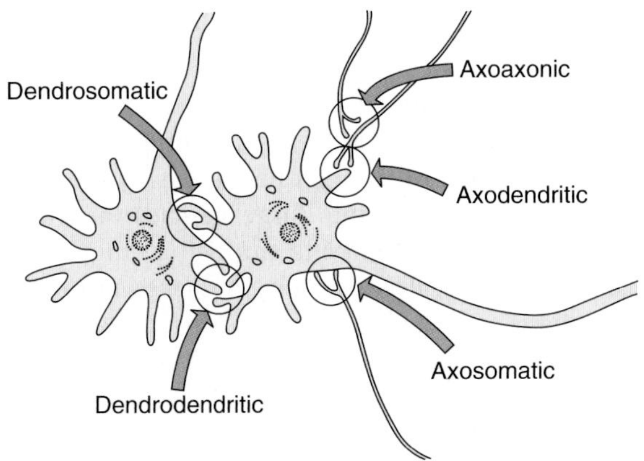

Figure 20-3 Types of synaptic connections in the CNS.

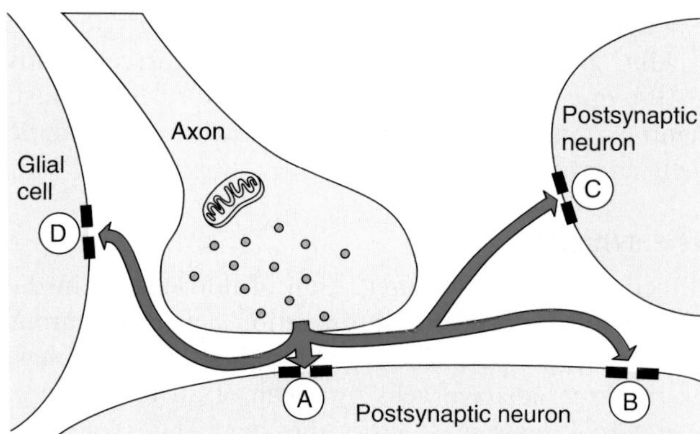

Figure 20-4 Volume transmission in the CNS. Released transmitter can activate receptors on an adjacent postsynaptic neuron at a site close to the release site **(A)** or at an extrajunctional site **(B)**, on a postsynaptic neuron distant to the release site **(C)**, or on a glial cell distant from the site of release **(D)**.

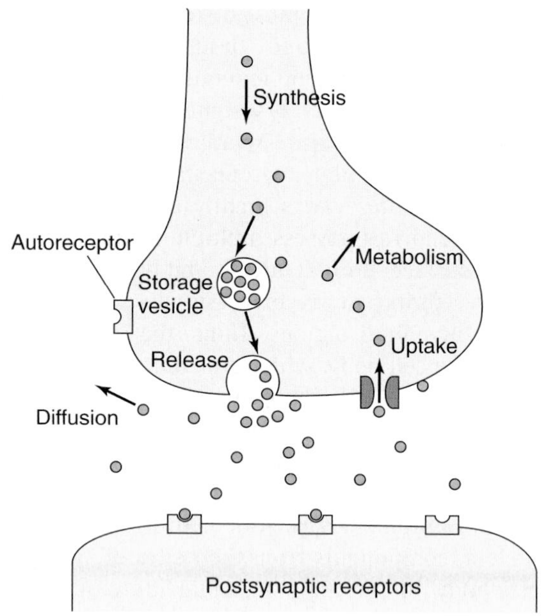

Figure 20-5 Life cycle of a neurotransmitter.

transmission (Fig. 20-4). Although its significance is not well understood, it may play an important role in the actions of neurotransmitters in brain regions where primary inactivation mechanisms are absent or dysfunctional.

The life cycle of neurotransmitters

Neurotransmitters are any chemical messengers released from neurons. They represent a highly diverse group of compounds including amines, amino acids, peptides, nucleotides, and gases (Table 20-1). Most classical neurotransmitters, first identified in peripheral neurons, play a major role in central transmission including acetylcholine (ACh), dopamine (DA), norepinephrine, epinephrine, and serotonin. Recently it has become clear that histamine is also an important neurotransmitter in the brain. The amino acid neurotransmitters include the excitatory compounds glutamate and aspartate and the inhibitory compounds GABA and glycine. All of these molecules are synthesized in nerve terminals and are generally stored in and released from small vesicles (Fig. 20-5). In addition to these small molecules, it is now clear that many peptides function as neurotransmitters. Peptide neurotransmitters are cleaved from larger precursors by proteolytic enzymes and packaged into large vesicles in neuronal perikarya. The most recent and surprising group of neurotransmitters identified include the gases nitric oxide and carbon monoxide, along with several growth factors including brain-derived neurotrophic factor and nerve growth factor. The gaseous neurotransmitters are synthesized and released upon demand, and thus are not stored in vesicles. The growth factors are stored in vesicles and released following depolarization.

Table 20-1 Representative neurotransmitters in the CNS

Category	Subcategory	Neurotransmitter
Primary amines	Quaternary amines	Acetylcholine
	Catecholamines	Dopamine
		Norepinephrine
		Epinephrine
	Indoleamines and related compounds	Serotonin
		Histamine
Amino acids	Excitatory	Glutamate
		Aspartate
	Inhibitory	GABA
		Glycine
Nucleotides and nucleosides		ATP
		Adenosine
Peptides		Cholecystokinin
		Dynorphin
		β-Endorphin
		Enkephalins
		Neuropeptide Y
		Neurotensin
		Somatostatin
		Substance P
		Vasoactive intestinal peptide
		Vasopressin
Gases		Nitric oxide
		Carbon monoxide

For many years it was assumed that a single neuron synthesized and released only *one* neurotransmitter. We know now that many classical neurotransmitters coexist with peptide neurotransmitters in neurons, and both are released in response to depolarization. ACh coexists with enkephalin, vasoactive intestinal peptide, and substance P, whereas DA coexists with cholecystokinin and enkephalin. In some cases, both substances cause physiological effects on postsynaptic cells, suggesting the possibility of multiple signals carrying independent, complementary, or mutually reinforcing messages.

Because many centrally-acting drugs act by altering the **synthesis, storage, release,** or **inactivation** of specific neurotransmitters, it is critical to understand these processes. For neurons to fire rapidly and repetitively, they must maintain sufficient supplies of neurotransmitter. Most neurons synthesize neurotransmitters locally (with the exception of peptides) and have complex mechanisms for regulating this process. Synthesis is usually controlled by either the amount and activity of synthetic enzymes or the availability of substrates and cofactors. For example, ACh synthesis is regulated primarily by substrate availability (see Chapters 8 and 9), while DA, norepinephrine, and epinephrine syntheses are regulated primarily by the activity of the synthetic enzyme tyrosine hydroxylase (see Chapters 8 and 10).

Following synthesis, neurotransmitters are concentrated in vesicles by carrier proteins through an energy-dependent process. This mechanism transports neurotransmitters into vesicles at concentrations 10 to 100 times higher than in the cytoplasm. Two families of vesicular transporters have been identified, one that transports monoamines and the other that transports amino acids. Vesicular storage protects neurotransmitters from catabolism by intracellular enzymes and maintains a ready supply of neurotransmitters for release. Although non-vesicular release of some neurotransmitters has been proposed, this appears to be rare.

The arrival of an action potential causes the nerve terminal membrane to depolarize, resulting in release of neurotransmitter into the synaptic cleft. This process is initiated by opening voltage-dependent Ca^{2+} channels in the membrane, enabling Ca^{2+} to enter the cell (see Fig. 8-3). Ca^{2+} influx leads to a complex sequence of events resulting in translocation and fusion of vesicles with the plasma membrane, releasing their contents into the synaptic cleft by exocytosis.

Following receptor activation, neurotransmitters must be inactivated to terminate their actions and allow for further information transfer. Rapid enzymatic hydrolysis of ACh terminates its action (see Chapters 8 and 9), while the actions of biogenic amines are terminated primarily by reuptake into presynaptic terminals by specific pumps (see Chapters 8 and 10). Inside the terminal, neurotransmitters can be repackaged into vesicles and re-released. The inactivation processes are important targets for drug action.

The action of any transmitter may also be terminated by simple diffusion or nonspecific (energy-independent) absorption into surrounding tissues. These processes are effective but are less important in inactivating classical small molecule neurotransmitters. They may be more important in terminating the actions of peptides and gaseous neurotransmitters.

Neurotransmitter receptors

As discussed in Chapter 2, receptors are sensors by which cells detect incoming messages. Many different types of receptors can coexist on cells, including receptors for different transmitters as well as multiple subtypes for a single transmitter. The response of a particular neuron to a neurotransmitter depends as much on the type of receptors present as on the type of transmitter released. It is important to realize that *a given neurotransmitter or drug does not always produce the same postsynaptic effect.*

Because each transmitter can activate a family of different receptors associated with distinct signal transduction mechanisms, a single transmitter may cause completely different effects on different cells (see Chapter 2). The function of the neuron is to integrate these multiple messages, from a single transmitter or from multiple transmitters, to control the impulse activity of its own axon.

Organization of the central nervous system

An understanding of the effects and side effects of drugs affecting the CNS requires a basic understanding of CNS organization. This organization can be viewed from anatomical, functional, or chemical perspectives.

Anatomical and functional organization

The gross anatomy of the brain includes the cerebrum or cerebral hemispheres; subcortical structures including the thalamus and hypothalamus (the diencephalon); the midbrain; and the hindbrain composed of the pons, medulla, and cerebellum (Fig. 20-6).

The cerebrum, or cerebral cortex, is the largest part of the human brain and is divided into apparently symmetrical left and right hemispheres. These have different functions, however, with the right hemisphere

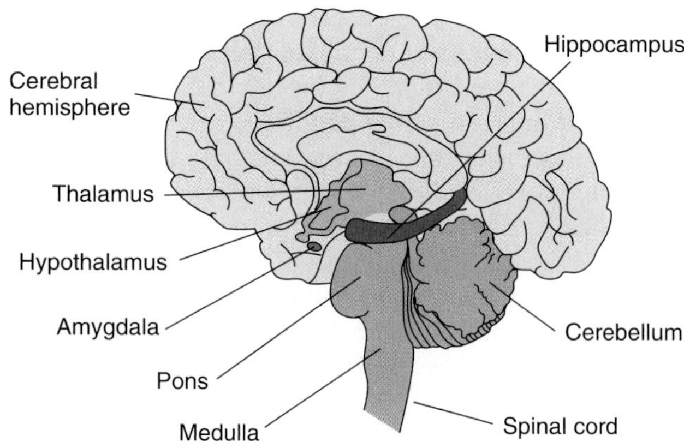

Figure 20-6 Gross anatomical structures in the brain.

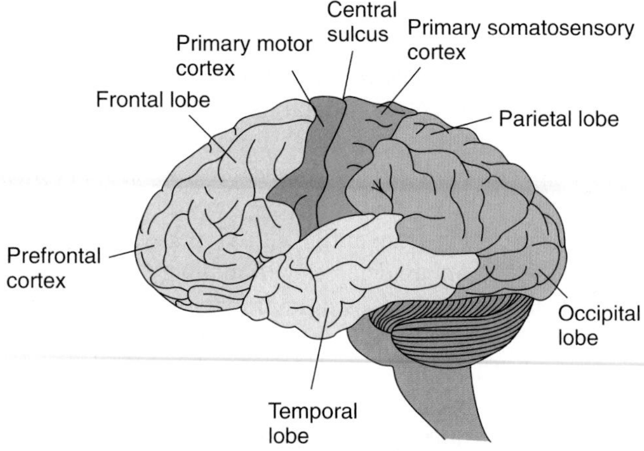

Figure 20-7 Regions of the cerebrum.

associated with creativity and the left with logic and reasoning. Most sensory, motor, and associational information is processed and many somatic and vegetative functions are integrated in the cerebral cortex.

The cerebral cortex contains four regions, the frontal, parietal, occipital, and temporal lobes (Fig. 20-7). The frontal lobe extends anterior from the central sulcus and contains the motor and prefrontal cortices. It is associated with higher cognitive functions and long-term memory storage; the posterior portion is the primary motor cortex and controls fine movements. The parietal lobe, between the occipital lobe and central sulcus, is associated with sensorimotor integration and processes information from touch, muscle stretch receptors, and joint receptors. This area contains the primary somatosensory cortex. The temporal lobe is located laterally in each hemisphere and is the primary cortical target for information originating in the ears and vestibular organs; it is involved in vision and language. The occipital lobe is located in the posterior cortex and is involved in visual processing. It is the main target for axons from thalamic nuclei that receive inputs from the visual pathways and contains the primary visual cortex.

The thalamus and hypothalamus are part of the diencephalon (see Fig. 20-6). The thalamus has both sensory and motor functions. Sensory information enters the thalamus and is transmitted to the cortex. The hypothalamus is involved in homeostasis, emotion, thirst, hunger, circadian rhythms, and control of the autonomic nervous system. It also controls the pituitary gland. The limbic system, often referred to as the "emotional brain," consists of several structures beneath the cerebral cortex that integrate emotional state with motor and visceral activities. The hippocampus is involved in learning and memory; the amygdala in memory, emotion, and fear; and the ventral tegmental area/nucleus accumbens septi in addiction.

The medulla, pons, and often midbrain are referred to as the brainstem and are involved in vision, hearing, and body movement (see Fig. 20-6). The medulla regulates vital functions such as breathing and heart rate, while the pons is involved in motor control and sensory analysis and is important in consciousness and sleep. The cerebellum is associated with the regulation and coordination of movement, posture, and balance. The cerebellum and brainstem relay information from the cerebral hemispheres and limbic system to the spinal cord for integration of essential reflexes. The spinal cord receives, sends, and integrates sensory and motor information.

Chemical organization

The effects of drugs are determined primarily by the type and activity of cells in which their molecular targets are located and the types of neural circuits in which those cells participate. Thus, an understanding of the chemical organization of the brain is particularly useful in pharmacology. CNS diseases often affect neurons containing specific neurotransmitters, and drugs often activate or inhibit synthesis, storage, release, or inactivation of these neurotransmitters. Many neurotransmitter systems arise from relatively small populations of neurons localized in discrete nuclei in the brain that project widely through the brain and spinal cord.

Dopaminergic systems Neurons synthesizing DA have their cell bodies primarily in two brain regions, the midbrain containing the substantia nigra and adjacent ventral tegmental area, and the hypothalamus (Fig. 20-8). Nigrostriatal DA neurons project to the striatum (caudate nucleus, putamen) and are involved in control of posture and movement; these neurons degenerate

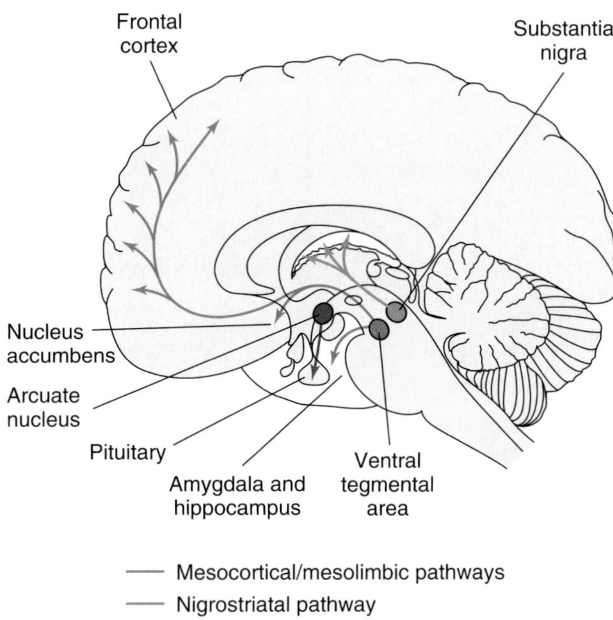

Figure 20-8 Dopaminergic pathways in the brain.

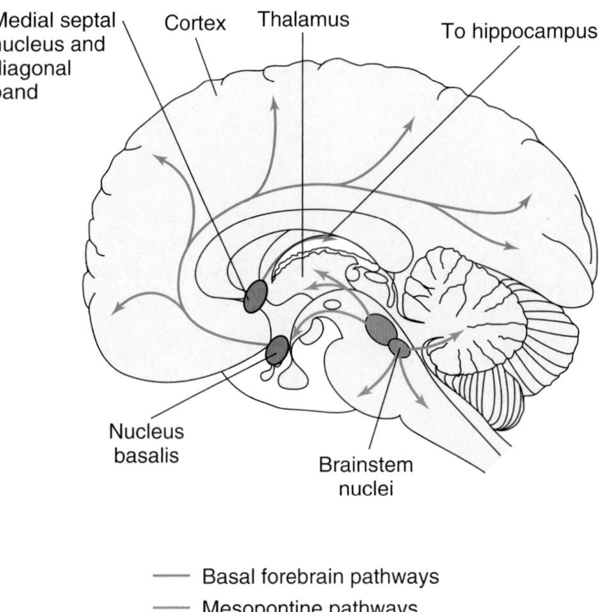

Figure 20-9 Cholinergic pathways in the brain.

in Parkinson's disease. The ventral tegmental neurons extend to the cortex and limbic system referred to as the mesocortical and mesolimbic pathways, respectively, and are important for complex target-oriented behaviors, including psychotic behaviors. Those neurons projecting from the ventral tegmental area to the nucleus accumbens septi are believed to be involved in addiction. DA is also synthesized by much shorter neurons originating in the arcuate and periventricular nuclei of the hypothalamus that extend to the intermediate lobe of the pituitary and into the median eminence, known as the tuberoinfundibular pathway. These neurons regulate pituitary function and decrease prolactin secretion. Drugs used for the treatment of Parkinson's disease (see Chapter 21) stimulate these DA systems, while drugs used for the treatment of psychotic disorders such as schizophrenia (see Chapter 22) block them.

Cholinergic systems Three primary groups of cholinergic neurons are found in the brain; those originating in ventral areas of the forebrain (nucleus basalis and nuclei of the diagonal band and medial septum), the pons, and the striatum (Fig. 20-9). Neurons from the nucleus basalis project to large areas of the cerebral cortex, while septal and diagonal band neurons project largely to the hippocampus. These pathways are important in learning and memory and degenerate in Alzheimer's disease. Thus, treatment of this disorder involves the use of acetylcholinesterase inhibitors in attempts to alleviate this cholinergic deficit (see Chapter 21). Neurons originating in the pons project to the thalamus and basal forebrain and have descending pathways to the reticular formation, cerebellum, vestibular nuclei, and cranial nerve nuclei; they are involved in arousal and REM sleep. Finally, there are small cholinergic interneurons in the striatum that are inhibited by nigrostriatal DA neurons, forming the basis for the use of muscarinic receptor antagonists in treating Parkinson's disease (see Chapter 21).

Serotonergic systems Serotonergic neurons originate primarily in the raphe nucleus and have widespread projections (Fig. 20-10). Neurons from the rostral raphe project to the limbic system, thalamus, striatum, and cerebral cortex, whereas caudal raphe neurons descend to the spinal cord. Serotonergic pathways have broad influences throughout the brain and are important for sensory processing and homeostasis. They play a role in psychotic behaviors (see Chapter 22), depression and obsessive-compulsive disorder (see Chapter 23), and eating behavior (see Chapter 26) and are major targets for drugs used to treat these diseases.

Noradrenergic systems Neurons synthesizing norepinephrine have their cell bodies primarily in the locus coeruleus in the pons and project anteriorly to large areas of the cerebral cortex, thalamus, hypothalamus, and olfactory bulb (Fig. 20-11). Other noradrenergic neurons originate in the midbrain (lateral tegmental region) and have ascending pathways to the limbic system and descending projections to the cerebellum and spinal cord, with fibers passing in the ventrolateral

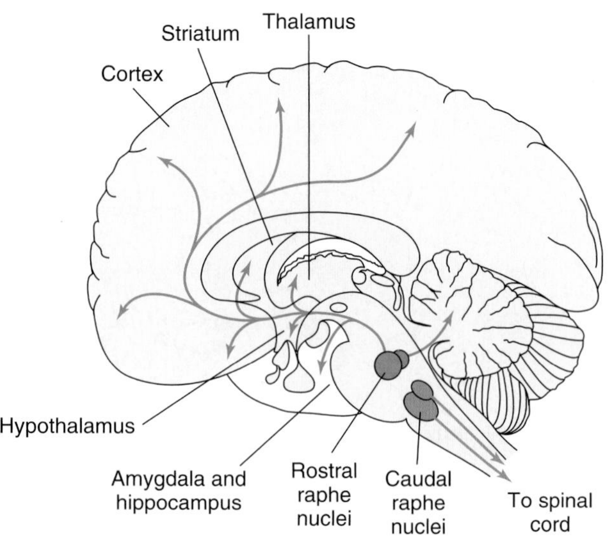

Figure 20-10 Serotonergic pathways in the brain.

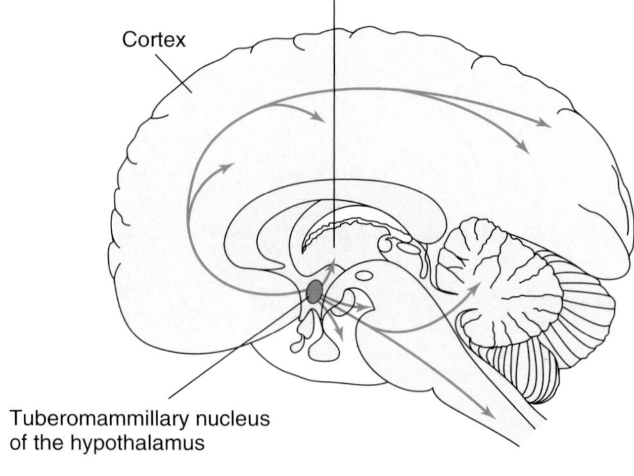

Figure 20-12 Histaminergic pathways in the brain.

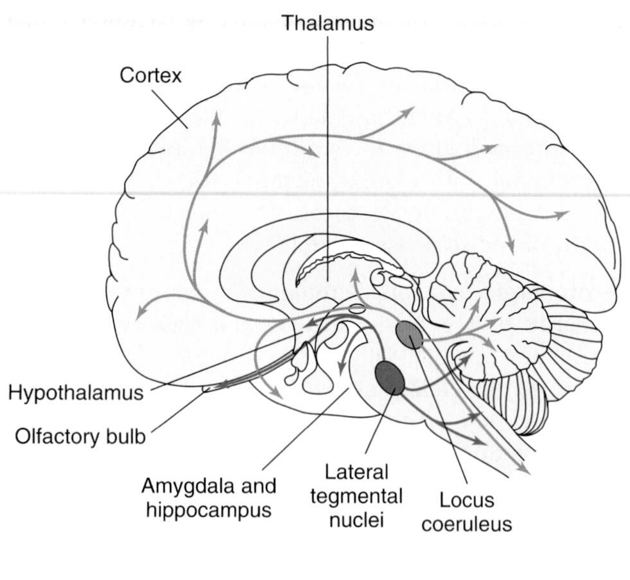

Figure 20-11 Noradrenergic pathways in the brain.

column. Noradrenergic pathways are involved in controlling responses to external sensory and motor stimuli, arousal and attention, and learning and memory and may be important in major depression (see Chapter 23). Midbrain neurons also play important roles in control of autonomic and neuroendocrine function.

Histaminergic systems All known histaminergic neurons originate in magnocellular neurons in the posterior hypothalamus, referred to as the tuberomammillary nucleus (Fig. 20-12). These neurons form long ascending connections to many telencephalic areas, including all areas of the cerebral cortex, the limbic system, caudate putamen, nucleus accumbens, and globus pallidus. Also, long descending neurons project to mesencephalic and brainstem structures including cranial nerve nuclei, the substantia nigra, locus coeruleus, mesopontine tegmentum, dorsal raphe, cerebellum, and spinal cord. Histaminergic neurons play a major role in arousal, in coupling neuronal activity with cerebral metabolism, and in neuroendocrine regulation.

Amino acid neurotransmitter systems Amino acid neurotransmitters are not restricted to specific pathways but are widespread throughout the brain and spinal cord. GABAergic neurons play a major inhibitory role in most brain regions and are important in anxiety and insomnia. Drugs for treating these disorders function to increase GABAergic activity (see Chapter 24). Glutamate is also widely distributed in the brain and functions opposite to GABA; that is, it is primarily excitatory. Recently, antagonists of specific glutamate *N*-methyl-D-aspartate receptors have been introduced for the treatment of Alzheimer's disease, although the underlying rationale is somewhat unclear (see Chapter 21).

A summary of major neurotransmitter pathways and the specific brain disorders in which they play important roles is presented in Table 20-2.

Table 20-2 Neurotransmitter pathway/disorder summary

Neurotransmitter	Associated Structures or Pathways	Functions	Associated Disorders
Dopamine	Nigrostriatal	Posture and movement	Parkinson's disease
	Mesolimbic/mesocortical	Target-oriented behaviors Addiction Reinforcement	Psychoses, drug abuse, depression
	Tuberoinfundibular	Hypothalamic and pituitary regulation Decrease prolactin secretion	Hyperprolactinemia
Acetylcholine	Intrastriatal	Motor activity	Parkinson's disease
	Basal forebrain	Learning/memory	Alzheimer's disease
	Mesopontine	Arousal and REM sleep	Narcolepsy (?)
Serotonin	Raphe	Broad homeostatic functions	Depression/suicide, psychoses, obsessive compulsive disorder, anxiety
	Telencephalic and diencephalic projections	Sensory processing	
Norepinephrine	Locus coeruleus	Learning/memory	Depression
	Midbrain reticular formation	Attention/arousal	Narcolepsy
Histamine	Tuberomammillary	Arousal Cerebral metabolism Neuroendocrine	?
GABA	Widespread	Anxiolytic	Anxiety
		Anticonvulsant	Seizures
Glutamate	Widespread	Pro-convulsant	Seizures
		Synaptic plasticity (LTP) Learning/memory	

Drug action in the central nervous system

The blood-brain barrier

As mentioned, drugs acting on the brain must be able to gain access to their targets. Because of its unique importance, the brain is "protected" by a specialized system of capillary endothelial cells known as the blood-brain barrier (BBB). Unlike peripheral capillaries that allow relatively free exchange of substances between cells, the BBB limits transport through both physical (tight junctions) and metabolic (enzymes) barriers (see Chapter 3). The primary BBB is formed by firmly connected endothelial cells with tight junctions lining cerebral capillaries. The secondary BBB surrounds the cerebral capillaries and is composed of glial cells.

There are several areas of the brain where the BBB is relatively weak, allowing substances to cross. These circumventricular organs include the pineal gland, area postrema, subfornical organ, vas-cular organ of the lamina terminalis, and median eminence.

Factors that influence the ability of drugs to cross the BBB include size, flexibility and molecular conformation, lipophilicity and charge, enzymatic stability, affinity for transport carriers, and plasma protein binding. In general, large polar molecules do not pass easily through the BBB, while small, lipid-soluble molecules such as barbiturates cross easily. Most charged molecules cross slowly if at all. It is clear that the BBB is the rate-limiting factor for drug entry into the CNS.

The BBB is not formed fully at birth, and drugs that may have restricted access in the adult may enter the newborn brain readily. Similarly, the BBB can be compromised in conditions such as hypertension, inflammation, trauma, and infection. Exposure to microwaves or radiation has also been reported to open the BBB.

While the action of many CNS-active drugs is based on their ability to cross the BBB, it may also be advantageous for a drug to be restricted from entering the brain. For example, l-DOPA, used for the treatment of Parkinson's disease, must enter the brain to be effective. When administered alone, only 1% to 3% of an administered dose reaches the brain; the rest is metabolized by plasma DOPA decarboxylase to DA, which cannot cross the BBB. Thus l-DOPA is administered in combination with carbidopa, which inhibits DOPA decarboxylase and does not itself cross the BBB, thereby increasing the amount of l-DOPA that enters the brain (see Chapter 21).

Target molecules

Most centrally-acting drugs produce their effects by modifying cellular and molecular events involved in synaptic transmission. The distribution of these targets determines which cells are affected by a particular drug and is the primary determinant of the specificity of drug action. Drugs acting on the CNS can be classified into several major groups, based on the distribution of their specific target molecules. Drugs that act on molecules expressed by all types of cells (DNA, lipids, and structural proteins) have "general" actions. Other drugs act on molecules that are expressed specifically in neurons and not other cell types. These drugs are **neuron-specific** and interact with the transporters and channels that maintain the electrical properties of neurons. Many drugs interact specifically with the macromolecules involved in the synthesis, storage, release, receptor interaction, and inactivation processes associated with particular neurotransmitters. The targets for these **transmitter-specific** drugs are expressed only by neurons synthesizing or responding to specific neurotransmitters; consequently, these drugs have more-discrete and limited actions. The targets for transmitter-specific drugs can be any of the macromolecules involved in the life cycle of specific transmitter molecules (Fig. 20-13). Last, some drugs mimic or interfere with specific signal transduction systems shared by a variety of different receptors. Such **signal-specific** drugs affect responses to activation of various receptors that use the same pathway for initiating signals. Although all of these drug groups are found in clinical practice, the transmitter-specific drugs represent the largest class. Because the distribution of their target molecules is more limited than that of the general, neuron-specific, or even signal-specific classes, administration of these compounds often results in a greater specificity of drug action and is reflected clinically by a lower incidence of unwanted side effects.

All drugs have multiple actions. No drug causes only a single effect, because few, if any, drugs bind to only a single target. At higher concentrations, most drugs can interact with a wide variety of molecules, often resulting in cellular alterations. Some drugs have potent actions on so many different processes in the CNS that it is difficult to identify their primary targets. While some drugs may cause their therapeutic effects by combinations of specific actions, others may exert their primary effects through their interaction with a single cellular target. The window of selectivity of any particular drug will dramatically influence its incidence of unwanted side effects.

Levels of neuronal activity

Drug actions on neuronal systems in the CNS are largely dependent on the level of their **tonic activity.** In the absence of synaptic input, neurons can exist in either of two states. They can be quiescent by maintaining a constant and uniform hyperpolarization of their cell membrane, or they can initiate action potentials at uniform intervals by spontaneous graded depolarizations. A system with intrinsic spontaneous activity has different characteristics than those of a quiescent system. Although both can be activated, only a spontaneously active system can be inhibited. Drugs that inhibit neuronal function (CNS depressants) may have quite different effects depending on the activity of the neuronal system involved. Systems with a tonic activity (either intrinsic or externally driven) are inhibited by CNS depressants, while the activity of a quiescent system is unaffected.

The activity of a tonically active neural network can be increased or decreased by excitatory or

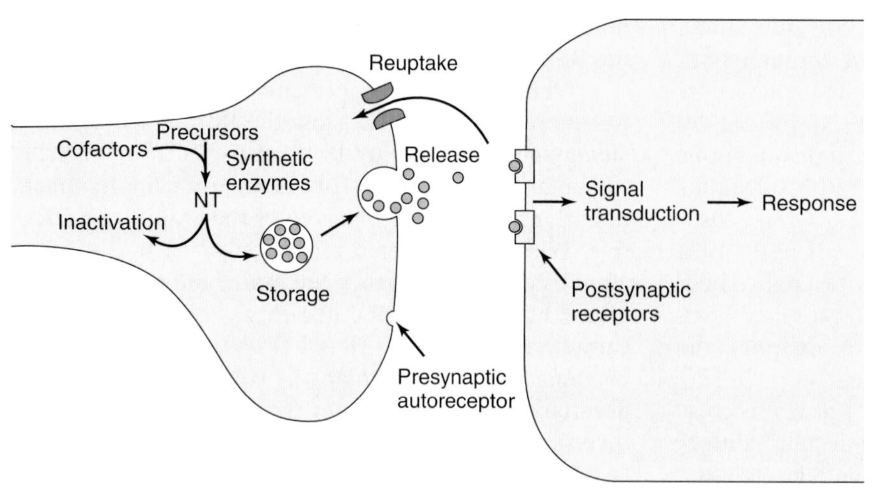

Figure 20-13 Sites of drug action in the CNS.

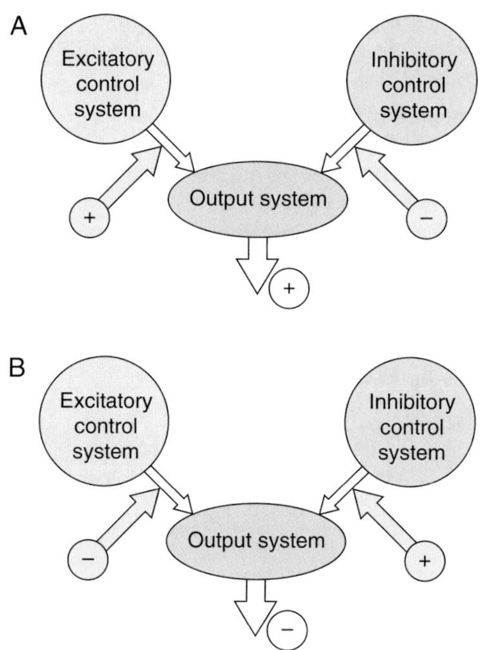

Figure 20-14 Hierarchical control systems in the CNS. **A,** Neuronal output can be increased by increasing tonic excitatory control or decreasing tonic inhibitory control. **B,** Output can be reduced by decreasing tonic excitatory control or increasing tonic inhibitory control.

inhibitory control systems, respectively. This type of bidirectional regulation implies that the effect of a drug cannot be predicted solely on the basis of its effect on isolated neurons. A drug that reduces neuronal firing can activate a neural system by reducing a tonically active inhibitory input. Conversely, a drug that increases neuronal firing can inhibit a neural system by activating an inhibitory input (Fig. 20-14). Thus, in some circumstances a "depressant" drug may cause excitation and a "stimulant" drug may cause sedation. A well-known example is the stimulant phase that is observed frequently after ingestion of ethanol (see Chapter 25), a general neuronal depressant. The initial stimulation is attributable to the depression of an inhibitory control system. This occurs only at low concentrations of ethanol; higher concentrations cause a uniform depression of nerve activity. A similar "stage of excitement" can be observed during induction of general anesthesia, which is also caused by the removal of tonically active inhibitory control systems (see Chapter 28).

Normal physiological variations in neuronal activity can also alter the effects of centrally-acting drugs. For example, anesthetics are generally less effective in hyperexcitable patients, and stimulants are less effective in more sedate patients. This is attributable to the presence of varying levels of excitatory and inhibitory control systems, which alter sensitivity to drugs. Other stimulant and depressant drugs administered concurrently also alter responses to centrally-acting drugs. Depressants are generally additive with other depressants, and stimulants are additive with stimulants. For example, ethanol potentiates the depression caused by barbiturates, and the result can be fatal. However, the interactions between stimulant and depressant drugs are more variable. Stimulant drugs usually antagonize the effects of depressant drugs, and vice-versa. Because such antagonism is caused by activation or inhibition of competing control systems and not by neutralization of the effect of the drugs on their target molecules, concurrently administered stimulants and depressants usually do not completely cancel the effects of both substances.

Adaptive responses

Adaptive mechanisms exist in all cells to control signaling. Adaptation can occur at several levels, predominantly at the receptors themselves. Two mechanisms are involved, sensitization and desensitization. As discussed in Chapter 2, sensitization is a process whereby a cell becomes more responsive to a given concentration of compound, whereas desensitization is a process whereby a cell becomes less responsive. Receptor sensitization and desensitization play a major role in the action of drugs in the CNS, in terms of both therapeutic effects and side effects induced.

Chronic activation of receptors, as occurs typically following long-term agonist administration, decreases the density of receptors in the postsynaptic cell membrane, whereas chronic decreases in synaptic activation, as a result of long-term antagonist administration, increases receptor density (see Fig. 2-18). Such changes occur slowly and are only slowly reversible, because increasing receptor density requires synthesis of new receptors, and reversing such an increase requires degrading these new receptors. Thus, changing receptor density usually represents a long-term (days to weeks) adaptive response to changes in synaptic input.

Postsynaptic cells can also regulate the efficiency with which receptor activation is coupled to changes in cell physiology. These changes usually occur at the level of the coupling of a receptor to channel opening or second-messenger production and can be extremely rapid in onset. Often, a change in coupling efficiency results from increases or decreases in covalent modifications of the receptors, G proteins, channels, or enzymes responsible for signal transduction (see Chapter 2).

Adaptive responses to long-term drug administration are thought to underlie many desired therapeutic effects as well as unwanted side effects. For example, the therapeutic effects of antidepressants take several weeks to develop, corresponding to the time it takes for adrenergic and serotonergic receptor systems to adapt to the enhanced levels of the biogenic amines (see Chapter 23). Similarly, evidence suggests that antipsychotic-induced tardive dyskinesia may result from the up-regulation of D_2 receptors caused by chronic receptor antagonism (see Chapter 22).

Overall, it is clear that determining the mechanisms by which drugs affect CNS function is challenging. Clearly the mechanisms by which psychoactive drugs exert their effects at a molecular level are only beginning to be understood. Manipulating brain chemistry and physiology with specific drugs and observing the effects on integrated behavioral parameters is one of the few approaches available currently for relating the function of brain cells with complex integrated behaviors. Such information will be useful in the future for the rational design of drugs for the treatment of various CNS diseases. It will also be satisfying to understand more about the genesis and control of human thought and emotion. Although understanding the actions of drugs on the CNS poses a great challenge, it also promises great rewards.

FURTHER READING

Cooper JR, Bloom FE, Roth RH: *The biochemical basis of neuropharmacology*, 8th edition, New York, 2003, Oxford University Press.

Self-assessment questions

1. The mechanisms of action of which of the following neurotransmitters is terminated by enzymatic degradation?

a. ACh
b. Norepinephrine
c. DA
d. Serotonin
e. Epinephrine

2. Which of the following is true concerning the synthesis and storage of biogenic amine neurotransmitters?

a. They are stored in and released from vesicles in nerve terminals.
b. They are synthesized in perikarya.
c. Their concentration in the presynaptic cytosol is greater than in the vesicles.
d. They are passively transported into vesicles.
e. They are transported down axons by anterograde transport.

3. Which of the following represents an adaptive response to the long-term use of agonists?

a. Increased synthesis of receptors
b. Decreased degradation of receptors
c. Decreased density of postsynaptic receptors
d. Increased density of postsynaptic receptors
e. None of the above

4. Which types of neurons originate primarily in the substantia nigra and hypothalamus?

a. Noradrenergic
b. Serotoninergic
c. Dopaminergic
d. GABAergic
e. Histaminergic

5. What characteristics increase the likelihood that a drug will penetrate the blood-brain barrier and enter the CNS?

a. Negative charge
b. High degree of lipophilicity
c. High molecular weight
d. Positive charge
e. High degree of binding to plasma proteins

6. Why does ethanol, a CNS depressant, cause an initial phase of excitation following ingestion?

a. It activates excitatory glutamate receptors.
b. It inhibits GABAergic inhibition.
c. It reduces activity of a tonically active inhibitory system.
d. It blocks serotonin reuptake.
e. It is metabolized to aspartate, an excitatory compound.

CHAPTER 21

Treatment of Parkinson's and Alzheimer's diseases

Lynn Wecker
Dave Morgan

Major Drugs

Parkinson's disease

Increased DA synthesis
- Entacapone (Comtan)
- Entacapone/L-DOPA/carbidopa (Stalevo)
- L-DOPA (Larodopa)
- L- DOPA/carbidopa (Atamet, Madopar, Medopar, Sinemet)

Decreased DA catabolism
- Selegiline (Eldepryl)

DA receptor agonists
- Apomorphine (Apokyn)
- Bromocriptine (Parlodel)
- Pergolide (Permax)
- Ropinirole (Requip)
- Pramipexole (Mirapex)

Others
- Amantadine (Symmetrel)
- Benztropine (Cogentin)
- Trihexyphenidyl (Artane)

Alzheimer's disease
- Donepezil (Aricept)
- Galantamine (Reminyl)
- Memantine (Namenda)
- Rivastigmine (Exelon)
- Tacrine (Cognex)

Therapeutic overview

Parkinson's disease

Parkinson's disease is a progressive neurodegenerative disorder caused by a loss of **dopamine** (DA) neurons in the **substantia nigra** and the presence of Lewy bodies (eosinophilic cytoplasmic inclusions) in surviving DA neurons. The disease is characterized by resting **tremor, bradykinesia** (slowness), **rigidity,** and **postural instability** (impaired balance), the latter appearing late in the course of the disease. Long-term disability is typically related to worsening motor fluctuations and **dyskinesias, dementia,** or imbalance, and death results from the complications of immobility, including pulmonary embolism or aspiration pneumonia.

Although evidence implicates environmental and genetic factors in Parkinson's disease, its etiology remains unknown. While the term *Parkinson's disease* refers to the idiopathic disease, **parkinsonism** refers to disorders that resemble Parkinson's disease but have a known cause and variable rates of progression and responses to drug therapy. These include encephalitis lethargica, multiple small strokes, and traumatic brain injury (pugilistic parkinsonism). In addition, parkinsonism can be induced by the long-term use of typical antipsychotic drugs and results from poisoning by manganese, carbon monoxide, or cyanide.

Parkinson's disease is one of the few neurodegenerative diseases whose symptoms can be improved with drugs. In the late 1960s it was discovered that orally ingested l-DOPA improved symptoms dramatically. Primary treatments for Parkinson's disease now include

Abbreviations

ACh	acetylcholine
AChE	acetylcholinesterase
BBB	blood-brain barrier
ChE	cholinesterase
DA	dopamine
DOPA	3,4-dihydroxyphenylalanine
MAO	monoamine oxidase
NMDA	*N*-methyl-D-aspartate

drugs that increase DA **synthesis**, decrease DA **catabolism**, and stimulate DA **receptors;** secondary compounds antagonize **muscarinic** cholinergic receptors, enhance DA **release**, and may antagonize ***N*-methyl-D-aspartate** (NMDA) glutamate receptors.

Alzheimer's disease

Alzheimer's disease is a progressive dementing disorder resulting from widespread degeneration of synapses and neurons in the cerebral cortex and hippocampus as well as some subcortical structures. Its defining pathological characteristics are the presence of extracellular senile plaques and intracellular neurofibrillary tangles. The plaques in Alzheimer's brain consist of an amyloid core surrounded by dystrophic (swollen, distorted) neurites and activated glia secreting a number of inflammatory mediators. The amyloid core consists of aggregates of a polymerized 40-42 amino acid peptide (Aβ) that is an alternate processing product of the transmembrane amyloid precursor protein and several accessory proteins. The neurofibrillary tangles are intracellular filaments composed of the microtubule associated protein tau, which is highly phosphorylated at unusual amino acid residues.

Both plaques and tangles are present in brain regions with the greatest degree of neuron and synapse loss and largely absent from regions that are spared (e.g., cerebellum). Although the best correlate of the severity of dementia is synapse loss, the amount of neurofibrillary tangles appears more closely related to neuron loss than the amount of plaque pathology. The loss of these largely glutamatergic neurons intrinsic to the cortices is responsible for most clinical manifestations of Alzheimer's disease.

While several neurotransmitter systems deteriorate in Alzheimer's disease, one of the first and most pronounced reductions occurs within the **acetylcholine (ACh)** containing projections from the nucleus basalis in the basal forebrain to the cerebral cortex. The septohippocampal cholinergic pathway is similarly affected, while the intrinsic striatal cholinergic system remains largely intact. Muscarinic cholinergic receptors in the cerebral cortex and hippocampus remain more or less intact, but nicotinic cholinergic receptors decline.

Current drug treatments for Alzheimer's disease increase cholinergic transmission by the use of **acetylcholinesterase** (AChE) **inhibitors** and blocking the excitotoxic effects of glutamate at NMDA receptors with the antagonist **memantine.**

Patients with both Parkinson's and Alzheimer's diseases may manifest neuropsychiatric disturbances secondary to their primary disease, including psychoses, depression, anxiety, and agitation. These can be treated with the atypical antipsychotics, antidepressants, and anxiolytic compounds discussed in Chapters 22 to 24. A summary of the treatment of Parkinson's and Alzheimer's diseases is provided in the Therapeutic Overview Box.

THERAPEUTIC OVERVIEW

Parkinson's disease

Pathology
- Degeneration of nigrostriatal DA neurons
- Presence of Lewy bodies in surviving neurons

Treatment
- Drugs to increase DA synthesis
- Drugs to inhibit DA catabolism
- DA receptor agonists
- Muscarinic cholinergic receptor antagonists

Alzheimer's disease

Pathology
- Degeneration of basal forebrain cholinergic neurons
- Presence of amyloid plaques and neurofibrillary tangles
- Neuron and synapse loss in cerebral cortex and hippocampus

Treatment
- AChE inhibitors to increase ACh
- NMDA glutamate receptor antagonists

Mechanisms of action

Parkinson's disease drugs

Current strategies for the treatment of Parkinson's disease are directed at increasing dopaminergic activity in the striatum to compensate for the loss of nigrostriatal DA neurons (see Fig. 20-8). The major drugs used include compounds that increase the synthesis and decrease the catabolism of DA or directly stimulate DA receptors; secondary compounds block muscarinic cholinergic receptors, enhance DA release, and perhaps antagonize NMDA receptors.

Increased DA synthesis L-DOPA was introduced for the treatment of Parkinson's disease in 1970. It is the precursor of DA and crosses the **blood-brain barrier** (BBB), whereas DA does not. L-DOPA increases DA synthesis but does not stop progression of the disease. When given alone, only 1% to 3% of an administered dose of l-DOPA reaches the brain; the rest is metabolized

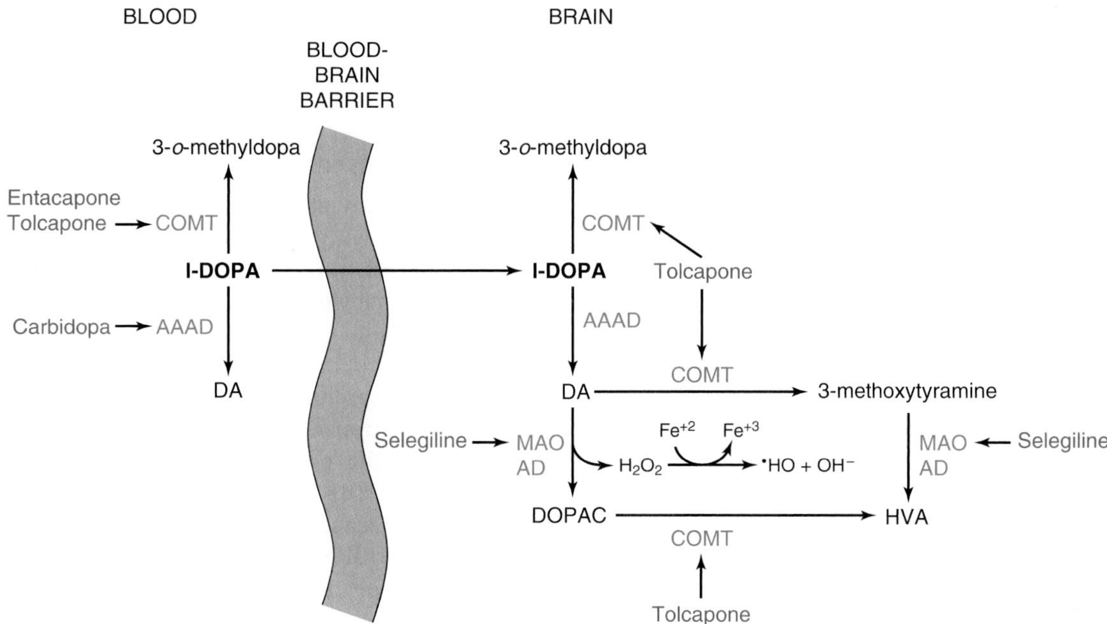

Figure 21-1 Peripheral and central metabolism of l-DOPA and DA depicting the sites of action of enzyme inhibitors. *AAAD,* Aromatic l-amino acid decarboxylase; *AD,* aldehyde dehydrogenase; *COMT,* catechol-*O*-methyltransferase; *MAO,* monoamine oxidase.

peripherally as shown in Figure 21-1. To prevent its peripheral metabolism and increase its availability to the brain, l-DOPA is administered with **carbidopa,** an **aromatic l-amino acid decarboxylase** inhibitor that does not cross the BBB. Carbidopa does not have any therapeutic benefit when used alone but increases the amount of l-DOPA available to the brain. However, as a consequence of peripheral inhibition of aromatic l-amino acid decarboxylase, more precursor is metabolized by plasma **catechol-*O*-methyltransferase** producing 3-*o*-methyldopa. To overcome this, the inhibitors **tolcapone** or **entacapone** are used in combination with l-DOPA/carbidopa. These compounds prolong the plasma half-life of l-DOPA, increasing the time the drug is available to cross the BBB. They also prevent the buildup of 3-*o*-methyldopa, which competitively inhibits l-DOPA transport across the BBB. Entacapone does not cross the BBB, and its actions are limited to the periphery. However, tolcapone does cross the BBB and also prevents the formation of 3-*o*-methyldopa in brain, as well as the catabolism of DA (Fig. 21-1).

Decreased DA catabolism Another approach to increase brain DA levels involves the use of the **monoamine oxidase** type B (MAO-B) irreversible inhibitor **selegiline** to inhibit the catabolism of DA in the brain (see Fig. 21-1). In addition, by inhibiting the catabolism of DA to DOPAC, selegiline decreases production of the byproduct hydrogen peroxide, limiting the possible formation of free radicals that form when the peroxide reacts with ferrous iron.

DA receptor agonists As their name implies, DA receptor agonists directly stimulate DA receptors. **Bromocriptine** and **pergolide** are ergot derivatives with agonist activity at D_2 receptors. Bromocriptine is also a partial agonist at D_1 receptors, while pergolide is a full agonist at D_1 receptors. **Ropinirole** and **pramipexole** are newer, non-ergot derivatives that selectively activate D_2 and D_3 receptors. The non-ergot DA agonist **apomorphine** has been approved recently as an injectable drug for use in patients with advanced disease, particularly for patients who experience episodes of immobility despite l-DOPA therapy.

Other compounds The **antimuscarinic** compounds **trihexyphenidyl** and **benztropine** act by inhibiting muscarinic cholinergic receptors in the striatum (see Fig. 20-9). Normally, nigrostriatal DA neurons inhibit ACh release from striatal interneurons. In Parkinson's disease, the loss of nigrostriatal DA neurons leads to increased firing of striatal cholinergic neurons, with a consequent overstimulation of muscarinic receptors. The muscarinic cholinergic receptor antagonists block this effect.

The antiviral drug **amantadine,** which is used for the treatment and prophylaxis of influenza, has several actions that appear beneficial in Parkinson's disease. Amantadine moderately increases DA release and has antimuscarinic activity. In addition, although the role of glutamate in Parkinson's disease is unclear, amantadine antagonizes NMDA glutamate receptors, possibly protecting neurons from the excitotoxic actions of excessive glutamate.

Alzheimer's disease drugs

Current strategies for the treatment of Alzheimer's disease are directed primarily at increasing cholinergic activity to compensate for the loss of basal forebrain cholinergic neurons (see Fig. 20-9). Most available compounds are AChE inhibitors, including **donepezil, galantamine, rivastigmine,** and **tacrine;** the latter has been largely replaced by the others because of hepatotoxicty. All of these drugs cross the BBB and are reversible AChE inhibitors. Tacrine, donepezil, and galantamine are specific for AChE, whereas **rivastigmine** inhibits both AChE and butyrylcholinesterase (ChE). As a consequence of AChE inhibition, ACh released from remaining cholinergic terminals is not rapidly hydrolyzed, leading to prolonged cholinergic receptor activation. In addition, galantamine stimulates presynaptic nicotinic cholinergic receptors in the brain through an allosteric mechanism, enhancing ACh release.

Because the AChE inhibitors indirectly enhance the effects of ACh released from nerve terminals by preventing its catabolism, their effects are more pronounced on active than on quiescent cholinergic neurons. This helps retain the spatial and temporal patterning of cholinergic activity in the brain, unlike directly-acting agonists, which would tonically activate all receptors.

Memantine is the first low-affinity NMDA receptor channel blocker approved to treat Alzheimer's disease. Memantine is a derivative of amantadine (see above) and binds to the open state of the glutamate NMDA receptor to block ion flux through this channel (see Chapter 2). NMDA receptors are critical to learning and memory and neural plasticity in the brain and serve an integrating function by remaining closed until a sufficient dendritic depolarization occurs to overcome blockade of the channel by Mg^{2+}. Once open, Na^{+} and Ca^{2+} enter the cell, with Ca^{2+} activating multiple signaling cascades. Excessive opening of the channel can be associated with excitotoxicity in neurons, involving both osmotic and apoptotic mechanisms. Although this may contribute to neurodegeneration in Alzheimer's disease, there is no evidence yet that memantine protects neurons or modifies the course of the disease. It is hypothesized that the low-affinity antagonism of the NMDA receptor prevents tonic activation while still permitting opening of the channel during periods of elevated activity critical for memory formation.

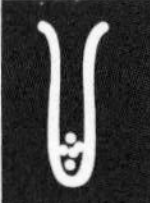

Pharmacokinetics

Parkinson's disease drugs

L-DOPA is rapidly absorbed by the gastrointestinal tract but competes with dietary protein for both intestinal absorption and transport across the BBB. The half-life of the immediate-release form of l-DOPA is only 60 to 90 minutes and thus, controlled-release formulations are available to minimize the number of daily doses required and prolong therapeutic plasma concentrations. As mentioned, carbidopa increases plasma levels and the half-life of l-DOPA and allows more l-DOPA to cross the BBB. The catechol-*O*-methyltransferase inhibitors entacapone and tolcapone also prolong the half-life of l-DOPA approximately two-fold.

Entacapone and tolcapone are rapidly absorbed, highly bound to plasma proteins, and almost completely inactivated prior to excretion. Selegiline is rapidly absorbed and metabolized to N-desmethylselegiline, amphetamine, and methamphetamine with half-lives of 2, 18, and 20 hours, respectively.

The pharmacokinetic profiles of the DA receptor agonists vary widely. It should be noted that ropinirole is metabolized by *CYP1A2,* which is stimulated by smoking and the proton pump inhibitor omeprazole. Omeprazole is used to treat gastrointestinal problems and is often used by the elderly; thus a potential for drug interactions exists.

Selected pharmacokinetic parameters for drugs used for Parkinson's disease are listed in Table 21-1.

Table 21-1 Selected pharmacokinetic parameters

Drug	Half-Life (hrs)	Plasma Protein Binding (%)	Disposition/ Excretion
PARKINSON'S DISEASE DRUGS			
Entacapone	0.4-0.7; 2.4 (biphasic)	98	B
Tolcapone	2-3	>99.9	R
Selegiline	7-9	—	R
Bromocriptine	5-7	90-96	B
Pergolide	20-27	90	R
Ropinirole	6	40	M, R
Pramepexole	8 (young) 12 (elderly)	15	R
ALZHEIMER'S DISEASE DRUGS			
Donepezil	70	96	M, R
Galantamine	7	18	M, R
Rivastigmine	1.5	40	Plasma ChE, R
Memantine	70	45	R

M, Metabolized; *R,* renal; *B,* biliary.

Alzheimer's disease drugs

All drugs used to treat Alzheimer's disease have good oral bioavailability but differ widely in their pharmacokinetic profiles (see Table 21-1). Donepezil, which has a very long half-life, is highly bound to plasma proteins and is metabolized in the liver by *CYP2D6* and *CYP3A4*. Its primary metabolite is equally effective as the parent compound in blocking AChE activity. More than 50% of a dose of donepezil is excreted unchanged, and its hepatic metabolism does not appear to lead to drug interactions or limitations in special populations. In contrast, galantamine is metabolized by *CYP2D6* and *CYP3A4*, and inhibitors of both of these metabolic pathways increase its bioavailability. In addition, poor metabolizers (7% of the population with a genetic variation with decreased *CYP2D6* activity) exhibit a significant reduction in clearance of galantamine.

Unlike the other AChE inhibitors, rivastigmine is metabolized by plasma ChE. Population pharmacokinetic analysis has shown that nicotine increases the clearance of rivastigmine by 23%.

Memantine has a long half-life, with approximately 75% of an administered dose excreted unchanged in the urine. The renal clearance of memantine involves active tubular secretion that may be altered by pH-dependent reabsorption. Thus memantine clearance can be decreased by alkalinization of urine—that is, use of carbonic anhydrase inhibitors or bicarbonate increases the concentration of memantine and elevates the risk of adverse responses.

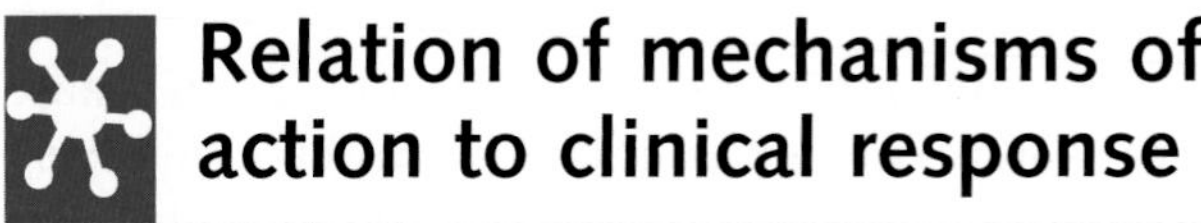

Relation of mechanisms of action to clinical response

Parkinson's disease

The combination of l-DOPA/carbidopa remains the most effective symptomatic treatment for Parkinson's disease to date, and both immediate- and controlled-release formulations are available, the latter of benefit for patients exhibiting wearing-off effects. The catechol-*O*-methyltransferase inhibitors do not provide any therapeutic benefit when used alone but may increase a patient's responses to l-DOPA, especially by reducing motor fluctuations in patients with advanced disease. However, there may be an increased incidence of dyskinesia requiring decreased doses of l-DOPA.

The DA receptor agonists are effective as monotherapy early in the disease or as an adjunct to l-DOPA in later stages. These compounds are not as efficacious as l-DOPA and have a lower propensity to cause dyskinesias or motor fluctuations. As monotherapy, these compounds are effective for 3 to 5 years, at which time l-DOPA/carbidopa must be initiated. As adjunctive therapy in advanced disease, DA receptor agonists contribute to clinical improvement and allow a reduction in the dose of l-DOPA required.

Apomorphine is effective to treat episodes of immobility ("off" times) in patients with advanced disease. However, apomorphine has strong emetic effects and an antiemetic must be administered prophylactically prior to its use.

Selegiline enhances clinical responses to l-DOPA and is approved as an adjunct in patients experiencing clinical deterioration during l-DOPA therapy. There is little evidence that it has more than modest benefit when used alone.

Antimuscarinics are useful in some patients for controlling tremor and drooling and may have additive therapeutic effects at any stage in the disease. They may be used for short-term monotherapy in tremor-predominant disease but have little value for akinesia or impaired postural reflexes. In contrast, amantadine helps alleviate mild akinesia and rigidity but does not alter tremor. Like the antimuscarinics, it may be useful for short-term monotherapy in patients with mild to moderate disease prior to initiation of l-DOPA.

It still is unclear whether any of the currently available treatments for Parkinson's disease alter disease progression.

Alzheimer's disease

The cognitive benefits of the AChE inhibitors in Alzheimer's disease, while statistically significant, are very modest and fairly controversial. Only a fraction of patients respond, and those who do typically show only a slight improvement in functional ability (daily activities), disturbed behaviors, and cognitive function (6-12 month reversal of cognitive impairments). This initial improvement is followed by subsequent decline, albeit from this elevated level of performance. Some degree of benefit has been reported to be retained for several years. Perhaps most importantly, reports claim these drugs can delay institutionalization, a considerable benefit from both a pharmacoeconomic and quality of life perspective. They may also benefit dementias resulting from other causes, such as vascular dementias.

Memantine has been used since the beginning of 2004 in the U.S. but for several years previously in Europe. Memantine improves daily activities and cognitive function scores in moderate to severe cases of Alzheimer's disease, but these effects are also modest. After a period of initial improvement, patients continue to deteriorate. Importantly, patients on donepezil benefit significantly from memantine, suggesting that these two drugs acting through different mechanisms are additive in improving cognitive function.

Side effects, clinical problems, and toxicity

Parkinson's disease

The peripheral side effects of l-DOPA include actions on the gastrointestinal and cardiovascular systems. Vomiting may be caused by stimulation of DA neurons in the area postrema, which is outside the BBB. The peripheral decarboxylation of l-DOPA to DA in plasma can activate vascular DA receptors and produce orthostatic hypotension, while the stimulation of α- and β-adrenergic receptors by DA can lead to cardiac arrhythmias, especially in patients with preexisting conditions.

Central nervous system effects include depression, anxiety, agitation, insomnia, hallucinations, and confusion, particularly in the elderly, and may be attributed to enhanced mesolimbic and mesocortical dopaminergic activity (see Fig. 20-8). The tricyclic antidepressants or selective serotonin reuptake inhibitors (see Chapter 23) may be used for depression, but the latter may cause worsening of motor symptoms. The atypical antipsychotics clozapine and quetiapine are beneficial for psychotic reactions and do not exacerbate the motor symptoms like the typical antipsychotics (see Chapter 22).

Although l-DOPA/carbidopa remains the most effective treatment for Parkinson's disease to date, for most patients it is effective for only 3 to 5 years. As the disease progresses, even with continued treatment, the duration of therapeutic activity from each dose decreases. This is known as the **"wearing off"** effect, and many patients fluctuate in their response between mobility and immobility, known as the **"on-off"** effect. In addition, after 5 years of continued drug treatment, as many as 75% of patients experience dose-related **dyskinesias**, characterized by chorea and dystonia, inadequate therapeutic responses, and toxicity at subtherapeutic doses. These effects may represent an adaptive process to alterations in plasma and brain levels of l-DOPA and involve alterations in expression of DA and NMDA receptors.

Tolcapone induced fatal hepatitis in 3/60,000 patients and has been taken off the market in Canada but not the U.S. Because of the risk of potentially fatal, acute fulminant liver failure, tolcapone should be used only in patients who have failed to respond to other drugs and who are experiencing motor fluctuations. Baseline liver function tests should be performed before starting tolcapone and should be repeated for the duration of therapy. If patients do not demonstrate a clinical response within 3 weeks, the drug should be withdrawn. Tolcapone is contraindicated in patients with compromised liver function.

DA receptor agonists cause side effects similar to those with l-DOPA, including nausea and postural hypotension. These compounds cause more central nervous system related effects than l-DOPA, including hallucinations, confusion, cognitive dysfunction, and sleepiness. Several studies have reported that patients maintained on DA receptor agonists develop increased impulsivity and exhibit pathological gambling, perhaps reflecting stimulation of the midbrain dopaminergic ventral tegmental-nucleus accumbens pathway thought to mediate addictive behaviors (see Chapter 20).

Selegiline can also cause nausea and orthostatic hypotension. At doses recommended for Parkinson's disease, which inhibit MAO-B but not MAO-A, selegiline is unlikely to induce a tyramine interaction (see Chapters 10 and 23). Selegiline may cause rare toxic interactions with fluoxetine and meperidine and can increase the adverse effects of l-DOPA, particularly dyskinesias and psychoses in the elderly.

Selegiline must be used with caution in patients taking any drug enhancing serotonergic activity, including the antidepressants, dextromethorphan, and tryptophan (see Chapter 23). Combinations of these compounds could induce "serotonin syndrome," a serious condition characterized by confusion, agitation, rigidity, shivering, autonomic instability, myoclonus, coma, nausea, diarrhea, diaphoresis, flushing, and even death (see Chapter 23).

The muscarinic receptor antagonists all cause typical anticholinergic effects as discussed extensively in Chapter 9. Because Parkinson's disease is predominantly an age-related disorder, and older people show increased vulnerability to other dysfunctions including dementia and glaucoma, anticholinergics must be used with caution in the elderly because these drugs impair memory, exacerbate glaucoma, and may cause urinary retention.

Amantadine may produce hallucinations and confusion, nausea, dizziness, dry mouth, and an erythematous rash of the lower extremities. Symptoms may worsen dramatically if it is discontinued, and amantadine should be used with caution in patients with congestive heart disease or acute angle-closure glaucoma.

Alzheimer's disease

All AChE inhibitors are relatively free of serious side effects with the exception of tacrine, which has been replaced by the other compounds because of significant hepatotoxicity. As expected, these compounds have a high incidence of peripheral cholinergic effects such as nausea, vomiting, anorexia, and diarrhea. Rivastigmine is associated with a greater incidence of these effects than the other drugs; it is uncertain if inhibition of ChE activity is responsible. Fortunately, many of these effects demonstrate tolerance, and gradual dosage escalation permits many patients to tolerate their full therapeutic doses. Adverse events with memantine were low in clinical trials, with none exceeding twice the placebo values in 5% or more of patients. High doses can produce dissociative anesthetic type effects similar to ketamine, including confusion, hallucination, hypnosis, and stupor (see Chapter 28).

Common side effects associated with drugs used for Parkinson's and Alzheimer's diseases are listed in the Clinical Problems Box.

CLINICAL PROBLEMS

Parkinson's disease

L-DOPA
- Nausea and vomiting, orthostatic hypotension, cardiac arrhythmias
- Depression, anxiety, hallucinations, sleepiness
- Limited effectiveness, fluctuations in response, and dyskinesias after 3-5 years of treatment

DA receptor agonists
- Nausea and vomiting, orthostatic hypotension, cardiac arrhythmias
- Marked depression, confusion, hallucinations, sleepiness
- Impulsivity

Alzheimer's disease

ChE inhibitors
- Nausea, vomiting, diarrhea, anorexia

Memantine
- Dizziness, headache, confusion, constipation

New horizons

The treatment of Parkinson's disease has focused largely on drugs that slow or ameliorate symptoms of this disorder. To this end, newer and more efficacious MAO-B inhibitors and DA receptor agonists are under development. These include rasagiline, which is a novel MAO-B inhibitor with efficacy as monotherapy and as an adjunct to l-DOPA, and rotigotine, which is a DA receptor agonist delivered transdermally. An additional drug in development is istradefylline, an adenosine A_{2a} receptor antagonist.

Recently studies have begun to focus on developing compounds with neuroprotective and restorative actions to slow down, and perhaps stop, the progression of disease. Along these lines, several compounds are being tested including antiinflammatory agents and neuroimmunophilin ligands that have been shown to promote regeneration in animal models.

Several new approaches have been proposed for the treatment of Alzheimer's disease. Compounds that have been suggested include vitamin E, vitamin C, and the herbal supplement ginkgo biloba. A limited number of studies have shown modest benefit from these agents, but effects are small in terms of cognitive improvement.

Epidemiological studies have indicated that women taking hormone replacement have had a reduced risk of dementia prevalence, but thus far, controlled trials have not found benefits of estrogen treatment or hormone replacement therapy in early stage dementia. Similarly, although epidemiological studies identified reduced risk of dementia for those chronically using non-steroidal antiinflammatory drugs, no benefit has been determined in controlled trials; prevention trials are in process. The cholesterol-lowering statins are also associated with reduced prevalence of Alzheimer dementia; placebo-controlled prospective trials are in progress.

Much attention is focusing on drugs designed to reduce the accumulation of the Aβ peptide in hopes of modifying disease progression. Approaches include drugs to block protease enzymes involved in formation of the Aβ peptide (the β and γ secretases), drugs to dissolve fibrillar plaques, or drugs to enhance the removal of Aβ peptide. In the latter context, preliminary data when using a vaccine against Aβ peptide indicated some stabilization of cognitive function, albeit after a fraction of the patients developed meningoencephalitic symptoms. The wide variety of mechanistically distinct approaches to treating Alzheimer's disease offers encouragement that this personally, socially, and economically devastating illness may be treated effectively in the near future.

TRADE NAMES

All the major drugs used for Parkinson's and Alzheimer's diseases in the United States are listed in the Major Drugs box.

FURTHER READING

Drugs for Parkinson's disease: treatment guidelines. *Med Lett* 2004; 2:41-46.

Reisberg B, Doody R, Stoffler A, et al. Memantine in moderate to severe Alzheimer's disease. *N Engl J Med* 2003; 348:1333-1341.

Tariot PN, Federoff HJ. Current treatment for Alzheimer's disease and future prospects. *Alzheimer Dis Assoc Disord* 2003; Suppl 4:S105-113.

Self-assessment questions

1. Which of the following activates D_2 receptors directly?

a. L-DOPA
b. Bromocriptine
c. Amantadine
d. Selegiline
e. All of the above

2. The tremor of Parkinson's disease occurs:

a. At rest and is alleviated by β-adrenergic receptor antagonists.
b. At rest and is worsened by bromocriptine.
c. Mainly with intentional movement and is increased by l-DOPA.
d. At rest and is reduced by benztropine or amantadine.

3. Carbidopa administration:

a. Reduces the decarboxylation of l-DOPA in brain.
b. Reduces the decarboxylation of l-DOPA in plasma.
c. Reduces the signs and symptoms of Parkinson's disease.
d. Slows the neurodegeneration of Parkinson's disease.
e. Reduces the half-life of l-DOPA in brain.

4. The most common adverse event associated with the use of AChE inhibitors is:

a. Gastrointestinal distress.
b. Blurring of vision.
c. Hypertension.
d. Renal insufficiency.
e. Allergic reactions.

CHAPTER 22

Treatment of psychotic disorders

Lynn Wecker
Glenn Catalano

Major Drugs	
Typical antipsychotics	**Atypical antipsychotics**
Chlorpromazine (Thorazine)	Aripiprazole (Abilify)
Fluphenazine (Permitil, Prolixin)	Clozapine (Clozaril)
Haloperidol (Haldol)	Olanzapine (Zyprexa)
Pimozide (Orap)	Quetiapine (Seroquel)
Thioridazine (Mellaril)	Risperidone (Risperdal)
Thiothixene (Navane)	Ziprasidone (Geodon)

Therapeutic overview

Psychotic behaviors are characterized by disturbances of reality and perception, impaired cognitive functioning, and disturbances of affect (mood). The most common psychotic disorder is **schizophrenia**, but others include severe mood disorders (such as bipolar disorder or major depression), anxiety disorders (such as post-traumatic stress disorder), organic disorders (such as delirium or dementia), some personality disorders, and the effects of many different psychoactive substances.

Schizophrenia affects 2.2 million Americans (1% of the population), and most cases develop between 16 and 30 years of age. Schizophrenia interferes with a person's ability to think clearly, manage emotions, make decisions, and relate to others. The symptoms of schizophrenia fall into two clusters, positive and negative. **Positive symptoms** are characterized by delusions and hallucinations and **reality distortions,** which include thought disorders and bizarre and agitated behaviors. **Negative symptoms** include a flattened affect and emotional and social withdrawal. In addition, many schizophrenics exhibit **cognitive impairments** manifest by attentional and short-term memory deficits.

Although schizophrenia is of unknown etiology, evidence supports a role for **genetic** and **environmental** factors, including **neurodevelopmental** abnormalities that may involve defects in the normal pattern of neuronal proliferation and migration, alterations in neurotransmitter receptor expression, and aberrant neuronal myelination. Evidence supporting a role for genetic factors includes findings that relatives of schizophrenics have a higher risk of illness as compared with the general population and that there is a higher concordance of schizophrenia in monozygotic (50%) as compared with dizygotic (15%) twins. In fact, a child born to two schizophrenic parents has a 40 times greater risk of developing the illness than the general population.

Structural studies have demonstrated that brains of schizophrenics have enlarged cerebral ventricles; atrophy of cerebral cortical layers; a decreased number of synaptic connections in the prefrontal cortex; and alterations in neocortical, limbic, and subcortical structures. Functional abnormalities include reduced cerebral blood flow and reduced glucose utilization in the prefrontal cortex.

Although consistent neurochemical alterations have not been found in schizophrenia, studies have implicated changes in the expression or function of several neurotransmitter receptors including those for

Abbreviations	
ACh	acetylcholine
DA	dopamine
5-HT	serotonin

dopamine (DA), serotonin (5-HT), acetylcholine (ACh), and glutamate. Other studies have suggested that schizophrenia may involve alterations in signaling pathways, particularly those involving *fos* and neuregulin, as well as a decreased expression of oligodendrocyte-associated genes, including proteolipid protein, the most abundant myelin-related protein.

Psychotic behaviors are treated pharmacologically with **antipsychotic** drugs, which have been classified into two categories, the **typical** and **atypical** compounds. The typical antipsychotics, often called first-generation or traditional compounds, include the prototypes **chlorpromazine** and **haloperidol,** which were introduced in the 1950s. The atypical antipsychotics, referred to as second-generation or novel antipsychotics, were developed recently and represent a more heterogeneous group that includes compounds such as **clozapine** and **risperidone.** The typical and atypical antipsychotics differ significantly with respect to their mechanisms of action, ability to relieve positive versus negative symptoms, and side effect profiles. Most importantly, many schizophrenic patients who fail to respond to the typical compounds show significant improvement following administration of atypical antipsychotics. It is also critical to understand that within the schizophrenic population, few patients achieve full recovery with or without medication. About 30% exhibit good responses, 30% demonstrate partial improvement, and 20% to 25% are resistant to all drugs. Thus schizophrenia likely represents a heterogeneous disorder.

Therapeutic issues related to the treatment of psychotic disorders are summarized in the Therapeutic Overview box.

THERAPEUTIC OVERVIEW

Typical antipsychotics

Alleviate positive symptoms

Bind to and block 70% to 80% of D_2 receptors at clinically effective doses

Atypical antipsychotics

Alleviate both positive and negative symptoms

May improve cognitive impairments

Bind to and block 40% to 60% of D_2 receptors at clinically effective doses

Bind to and block 70% to 90% of $5\text{-}HT_{2A}$ receptors at clinically effective doses

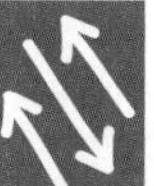

Mechanisms of action

Typical antipsychotics

The typical antipsychotics comprised the first group of compounds developed for the treatment of schizophrenia. Based on chemical structure, these compounds fall into 3 groups (Fig. 22-1):

- Phenothiazines
- Thioxanthines
- Butyrophenones

Chlorpromazine was the first antipsychotic approved for use and is the prototypical phenothiazine, characterized by a 3-ring structure. Thiothixene is representative of the thioxanthines, and haloperidol is representative of the butyrophenones.

The effects of the typical antipsychotics are due to blockade of postsynaptic DA receptors, specifically D_2 receptors. Indeed, a positive linear correlation exists between the therapeutic potency of typical antipsychotics and their ability to bind to and block D_2 receptors (Fig. 22-2). Inhibition of these receptors in mesolimbic and mesocortical regions (see Fig. 20-8) are believed to mediate the ability of these compounds to relieve some behavioral manifestations of schizophrenia. On the other hand, blockade of these receptors in the basal ganglia underlie the motor side effects of these compounds, and inhibition of these receptors in the tuberoinfundibular pathway in the hypothalamus leads to increases in prolactin secretion from the pituitary gland (see Fig. 20-8).

Acute administration of the typical antipsychotics increases the firing rate of both mesolimbic and nigrostriatal DA neurons as a compensatory response to DA receptor blockade. However, long-term administration inactivates these pathways via **depolarization blockade.** Because the therapeutic effects of the typical antipsychotics require several weeks to become apparent, it is believed that this inactivation of mesolimbic DA neurons mediates the time-dependent amelioration of psychotic symptoms. Long-term administration of antipsychotics also leads to an upregulation of DA receptors as a consequence of the depression of DA activity.

In addition to blocking DA receptors, the typical antipsychotics may also block muscarinic cholinergic receptors, α_1-adrenergic receptors, histamine receptors, and $5\text{-}HT_2$ receptors. These actions underlie many of the side effects associated with these compounds.

The typical antipsychotics are of benefit primarily in alleviating the positive symptoms of schizophrenia.

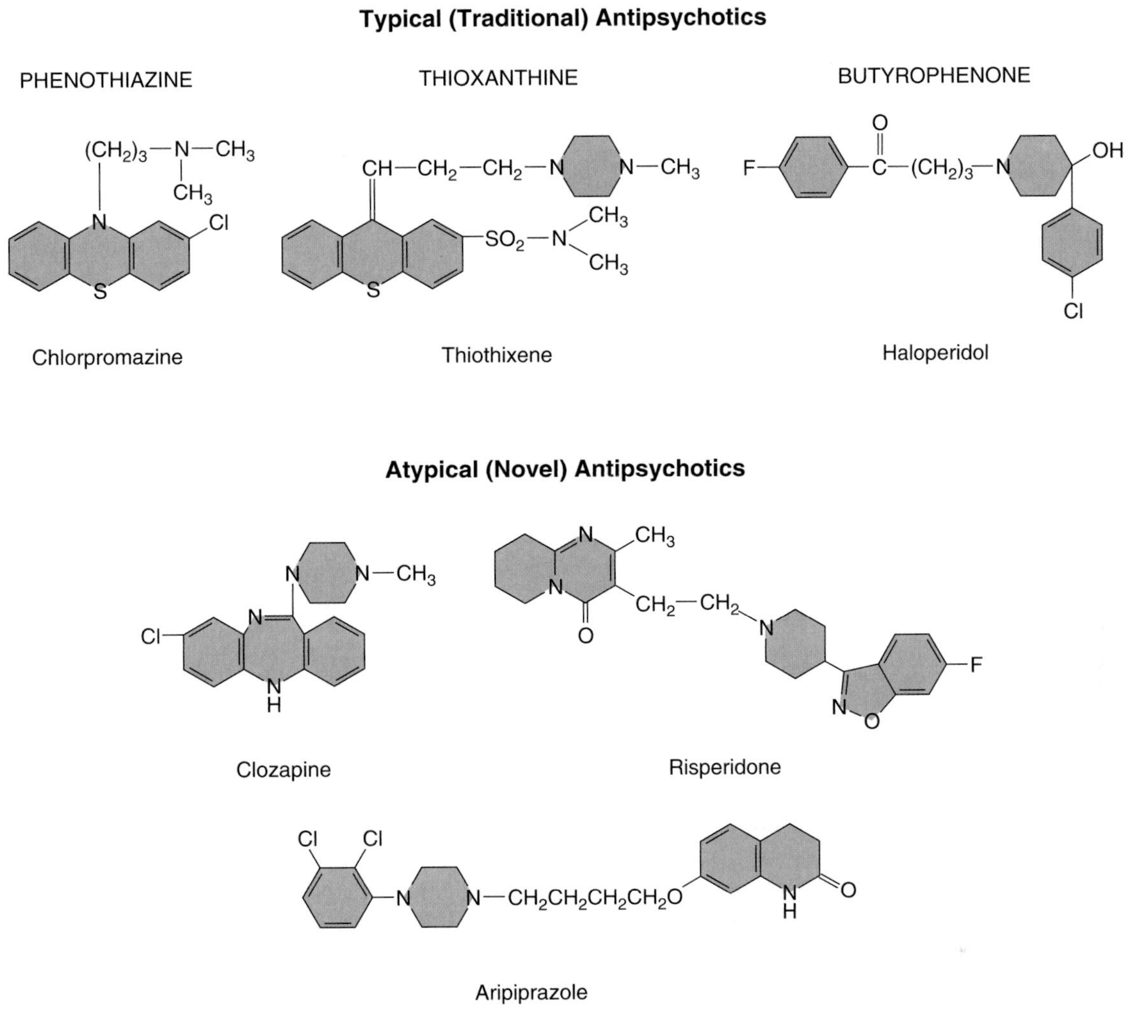

Typical (Traditional) Antipsychotics

PHENOTHIAZINE — Chlorpromazine

THIOXANTHINE — Thiothixene

BUTYROPHENONE — Haloperidol

Atypical (Novel) Antipsychotics

Clozapine

Risperidone

Aripiprazole

Figure 22-1 Structures of various antipsychotic agents.

Atypical antipsychotics

The atypical antipsychotics represent a somewhat heterogeneous group of compounds with large differences in chemical structure (Fig. 22-1), receptor antagonist activity, and therapeutic and side effect profiles. These compounds vary more in potency and range in treating specific symptoms as compared with the typical compounds. As heterogeneous as the group is, however, these compounds share several commonalities. They all occupy and block fewer D_2 receptors than the typical antipsychotics (40% to 60% as compared with >70-80%), and they all block a high number (70% to 90%) of 5-HT_{2A} receptors. Because of their lower occupancy of D_2 receptors, the atypical antipsychotics have a lower propensity than the typical compounds to induce motor side effects. In addition, they have an increased ability to alleviate the negative symptoms of schizophrenia, and the rate of relapse is lower than that following administration of typical antipsychotics.

Clozapine was the first atypical antipsychotic drug to be characterized and is effective in a significant population of schizophrenics who fail to respond to typical antipsychotic drugs. In addition to having a low affinity for D_2 receptors, clozapine was the first antipsychotic demonstrated to have selective effects on specific DA pathways—that is, it produces a depolarization blockade of mesolimbic and mesocortical, but not nigrostriatal, DA neurons. Thus, in contrast to typical antipsychotics, clozapine does not disrupt DA function in the nigrostriatal pathway. Two of the newer compounds, olanzapine and quetiapine, both demonstrate similar anatomical specificity for DA pathways.

Clozapine also exhibits a high affinity for D_4 receptors as well as for 5-HT_{2C} receptors. The contribution of these effects to the actions of clozapine remains

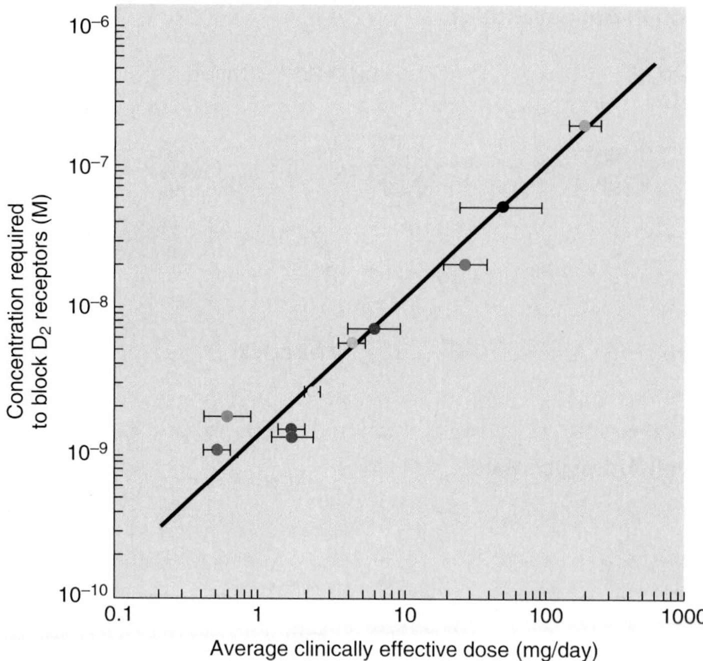

Figure 22-2 Correlation between the therapeutic dose of antipsychotics and the concentration to block D_2 receptors.

unknown. However, several other atypical antipsychotics—including olanzapine, risperidone and ziprasidone—also have a very high affinity for 5-HT_{2A}, 5-HT_{2C}, and D_4 receptors.

In addition to actions at these receptors, clozapine and olanzapine increase regional blood flow in cerebral cortex through an undefined mechanism, an action that may contribute to the beneficial effects of these compounds on cognitive functions such as working memory and attention.

The newest atypical drug, aripiprazole, is unlike others in this group, because it is a partial agonist at D_2 and 5-HT_{1A} receptors and a full antagonist at 5-HT_{2A} receptors. Thus its therapeutic and side effect profile differs somewhat from other atypical antipsychotics.

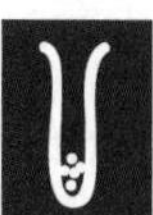

Pharmacokinetics

The antipsychotics are readily but erratically absorbed after oral administration, and most undergo significant first pass metabolism. Most of these compounds are highly lipophilic and protein bound, with variable half-lives following oral administration. In general, most antipsychotics are oxidized by hepatic microsomal enzymes to inactive metabolites and excreted as glucuronides. A major exception is thioridazine, which is metabolized to the active product mesoridazine, which is more potent than the parent compound. Depot formulations of some antipsychotics (e.g., fluphenazine decanoate, haloperidol decanoate, and risperidone) are available and can be used for maintenance therapy administered intramuscularly at 2- to 4-week intervals. For patients who have difficulty taking oral medications, risperidone and olanzapine are available as rapidly dissolving oral wafers. In addition, for management of acute psychotic episodes, antipsychotics can be administered intramuscularly, although ziprasidone and olanzapine are currently the only atypical antipsychotics available in this formulation. The risperidone-dissolving wafer provides rapid relief of symptoms as well. Haloperidol is available in an intravenous form, which is commonly used in intensive care settings. However, because intravenous haloperidol bypasses first-pass metabolism, it is effectively twice as potent as oral haloperidol dosing. In general, once an effective dose is established, a regimen of single daily oral dosing is effective for symptomatic treatment. Pharmacokinetic parameters are summarized in Table 22-1.

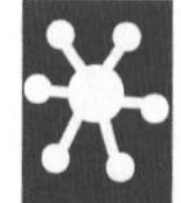

Relation of mechanisms of action to clinical response

The positive (hallucinations, delusions, paranoia, and thought disorders) and negative (depressive manifestations) symptoms and cognitive impairments characteristic of schizophrenia respond differently to currently

Table 22-1 Selected pharmacokinetic parameters for antipsychotics following oral administration

Drug	Half-Life (hrs)	Plasma-Protein Binding (%)	Disposition/ Excretion
TYPICAL ANTIPSYCHOTICS			
Chlorpromazine	8-35	>90	M, R
Fluphenazine	14-24	>90	M, R, B
Haloperidol	12-36	92	M, R, B
Pimozide	50-60	>90	M, R
Thioridazine	6-40	>90	M, R
Thiothixene	30-40	>90	M, R
ATYPICAL ANTIPSYCHOTICS			
Aripiprazole	75-94	>99	M, R, B
Clozapine	4-66	97	M, R, B
Olanzapine	21-54	93	M, R, B
Quetiapine	5-10	83	M, R, B
Risperidone	20-24	90	M, R
Ziprasidone	5-10	>99	M, R, B

M, Metabolism; *B*, biliary; *R*, renal.

available drugs. In addition, the intensity of these symptoms varies among patients as well as in particular patients over time, such that a patient may exhibit predominantly one set of symptoms at any particular time. However, in general, positive symptoms respond to both typical and atypical compounds, whereas the negative symptoms and cognitive impairments respond better to atypical than typical antipsychotics.

The DA hypothesis of psychotic behavior is based on findings that the chronic administration of amphetamine and other compounds that increase DA release lead to psychotic behaviors, the administration of compounds that enhance dopaminergic activity such as l-DOPA can induce psychotic behaviors, and a linear correlation exists between the therapeutic efficacy of the typical antipsychotics and their ability to block DA receptors (see Fig. 22-2). Similarly, a role for 5-HT in schizophrenia is based on evidence that many hallucinogens are structurally related to 5-HT. The newer atypical antipsychotics block 5-HT_2 receptors with high potency, leading to a reduction and/or resolution of the hallucinations. Thus, both DA and 5-HT clearly play a role in the manifestations of psychotic behavior.

The atypical antipsychotics block both 5-HT_2 and D_2 receptors and alleviate both positive and negative symptoms of schizophrenia, while the typical antipsychotics block only D_2 receptors at therapeutic doses and alleviate only the positive symptoms. Therefore, the idea has emerged that DA plays a major role in the manifestation of positive symptoms, whereas 5-HT plays a major role in the manifestation of negative symptoms.

It is critical to understand that DA receptor blockade occurs rapidly after initial antipsychotic treatment, whereas a maximal therapeutic response is not observed for several weeks and correlates with the induction of depolarization blockade of mesolimbic DA neurons. The long-term consequences of 5-HT blockade are less well understood.

Based on evidence that the atypical antipsychotics may improve the cognitive impairment exhibited by schizophrenics, in concert with their ability to increase blood flow and enhance ACh release in prefrontal cortex, studies have suggested a role for altered cholinergic systems in the cognitive impairment in psychotic behavior. This idea is underscored by the vast literature supporting a role for ACh in learning and memory and the role of impaired cholinergic activity in Alzheimer's disease (see Chapter 21).

The short-term goal of management of a psychotic episode is to reduce positive symptoms. The long-term goal includes the prevention of relapse, because it is believed that multiple psychotic episodes negatively affect the long-term outcome. Relapse of psychosis generally stems from noncompliance and not development of tolerance to the drug. Relapse is best prevented with continuous rather than intermittent drug therapy.

The choice of antipsychotic drug is based on the particular symptoms manifested by the patient as well as on sensitivity to undesirable side effects and prior therapeutic response to a particular agent. Although the typical antipsychotics have been first-line compounds, the use of atypicals is increasing because of their limited side effect profile, leading to better compliance. While clozapine has not been considered a first-line drug because of multiple significant side effects (including agranulocytosis, seizures, and myocarditis), it is clearly of tremendous benefit for patients who fail to respond to other antipsychotics.

In addition to their use in schizophrenia, several antipsychotics have been of therapeutic benefit in other neuropsychiatric disorders. Many of the atypical antipsychotics (including risperidone, quetiapine, and olanzapine) are effective as the primary treatment or as an augmenting agent with mood stabilizers in the treatment of bipolar disorder, regardless of whether psychotic features were present at the time. The antipsychotics are often prescribed concomitantly with antidepressants and mood stabilizers for schizoaffective disorder (see Chapter 23). Haloperidol and pimozide are used to treat behavioral syndromes accompanied by motor disturbances, specifically Gilles de la Tourette's syndrome.

Although the clinical outcome in schizophrenic patients is improved greatly with antipsychotic drug therapy, their quality of life is improved through the use of psychosocial interventions. Clinical outcomes appear to be more positive in patients who can engage in an occupation, maintain family contact, and function in a social environment.

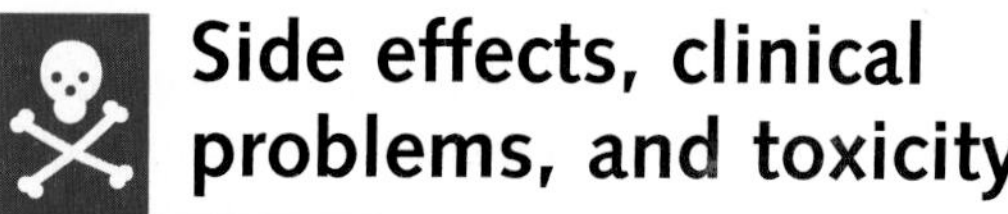

Side effects, clinical problems, and toxicity

Although most antipsychotics are relatively safe, they can elicit a variety of neurological, autonomic, neuroendocrine, and metabolic side effects. Many side effects are an extension of the general pharmacological actions of these drugs and result from the blockade of receptors for several neurotransmitters (Table 22-2), whereas other side effects are specific to particular compounds.

Typical antipsychotics

All typical antipsychotics block muscarinic cholinergic receptors, leading to dry mouth, urinary retention, and memory impairment (see Chapter 9). These effects are more common with the lower-potency agents such as chlorpromazine and thioridazine. They also block α_1-adrenergic and histamine (H_1) receptors, producing orthostatic hypotension and reflex tachycardia and sedation, respectively. Blocking DA receptors in the pituitary gland results in elevated prolactin secretion, and this hyperprolactinemia may lead to menstrual irregularities in females and breast enlargement and galactorrhea in both sexes. In addition, thioridazine has a propensity to prolong the cardiac QT interval, predisposing to a risk for ventricular arrhythmias. High-dose thioridazine therapy (>800 mg/day) has been associated with the development of retinitis pigmentosa. Thioridazine should be used with caution at all times, whether it is used as monotherapy or with other agents. As thioridazine is metabolized by *CYP2D6*, using it concurrently with a *CYP2D6* inhibitor (such as paroxetine or fluoxetine) could greatly increase serum thioridazine levels, leading to an increase in adverse events.

Blocking DA receptors in the basal ganglia leads to **acute extrapyramidal symptoms** including dystonia, parkinsonism, and akathisia. Acute dystonic reactions, characterized by spasms of the facial or neck muscles, may be evident, as well as a parkinsonian syndrome characterized by bradykinesia, rigidity, tremor, and shuffling gait. Akathisia or motor restlessness may also be apparent. These symptoms occur early (1-60 days) after initiation of drug treatment, improve if the antipsychotic is terminated, and if severe enough to cause non-compliance, may be treated with centrally active anticholinergic compounds such as those used for Parkinson's disease (see Chapter 21).

In general, the high-potency butyrophenones such as haloperidol are associated with a greater incidence of extrapyramidal side effects, whereas the low-potency phenothiazines such as chlorpromazine are associated with a greater incidence of autonomic side effects and sedation.

Following months to years of therapy, two late-onset effects may become apparent—perioral tremor, characterized by "rabbit-like" facial movements, and **tardive dyskinesia**, characterized by involuntary and

Table 22-2 Side effect profile of representative antipsychotic drugs

Drug	Anticholinergic	Antiadrenergic (α_1)	Antihistaminergic (H_1)
TYPICAL ANTIPSYCHOTICS			
Chlorpromazine	++	++++	+++
Fluphenazine	–	+++	++
Haloperidol	–	+++	–
Pimozide	–	–	–
Thioridazine	+++	++++	–
Thiothixene	–	+++	+++
ATYPICAL ANTIPSYCHOTICS			
Aripiprazole	–	++	++
Clozapine	+++	+++	+++
Olanzapine	+++	++	+++
Quetiapine	++	++	+++
Risperidone	–	+++	++
Ziprasidone	–	+++	++

The symbols represent the relative potency of each compound to produce anticholinergic (dry mouth, constipation, cycloplegia), antiadrenergic (sedation, postural hypotension) or antihistaminergic (sedation, weight gain) effects. The highest activity (++++) represents an inhibition constant (K_i) of <1 nM; +++, K_i from 1-10 nM; ++, K_i from 10-100 nM; +, K_i from 100-1,000 nM; and –, K_i > 1,000 nM.

excessive movements of the face and extremities. Severe tardive dyskinesia can be disfiguring and cause impaired feeding and breathing. There is no satisfactory treatment for tardive dyskinesia, and stopping drug treatment may unmask the symptoms, apparently exacerbating the condition. Tardive dyskinesia is thought to result from the hypersensitivity or upregulation of DA receptors that occurs following chronic DA receptor blockade induced by the antipsychotics. Together, clinician and patient must weigh the risks and benefits when considering whether to stop the antipsychotic medication or switch to another agent (i.e., from a typical to an atypical antipsychotic) once symptoms manifest themselves.

An idiosyncratic and potentially lethal effect of the typical antipsychotics is known as **neuroleptic malignant syndrome,** which occurs in 1 to 2% of patients and is fatal in almost 10% of those affected. It is most commonly seen in young males recently treated with an intramuscular injection of a typical antipsychotic agent. This syndrome is observed early in treatment and is characterized by a near-complete collapse of the autonomic nervous system, causing fever, muscle rigidity, diaphoresis, and cardiovascular instability. Immediate medical intervention with the DA receptor agonist bromocriptine (see Chapter 21) and the skeletal muscle relaxant dantrolene (see Chapter 29) is recommended to treat this condition.

Antipsychotics are not the only class of medications that can cause these types of side effects. In fact, any medication with significant D_2 receptor blockade may induce extrapyramidal symptoms, akathisia, neuroleptic malignant syndrome, and other side effects normally associated with antipsychotics. Prochlorperazine, metoclopramide, promethazine, and trimethobenzamide are agents used in gastroenterology that can have similar side effects.

Atypical antipsychotics

In general, the side effect profile of the atypical antipsychotics differs from that of typical antipsychotics. While the typical antipsychotics have a narrow therapeutic window in terms of acute extrapyramidal side effects, clozapine and the newer atypical compounds are associated with a very low incidence of these problems and most do not produce hyperprolactinemia. Risperidone has been associated with increased prolactin levels in some patients. While these compounds are not devoid totally of the ability to induce tardive dyskinesia or neuroleptic malignant syndrome, their incidence is lower than with the typical antipsychotics.

The most prominent side effects of the atypical compounds are metabolic and cardiovascular. Many of these compounds cause substantial weight gain (particularly olanzapine and clozapine) and the development of insulin resistance, leading to the onset of diabetes mellitus. While the development of diabetes mellitus is believed to be caused by all atypical antipsychotics, it has been most commonly observed with olanzapine and clozapine. The atypical antipsychotics also cause increased plasma lipids, with as much as a 10% increase in cholesterol levels. Olanzapine and, to a lesser extent, quetiapine are the atypical agents most likely to induce hyperlipidemia. Like the typical antipsychotic thioridazine, the atypical compound ziprasidone can also increase the cardiac QT interval predisposing to arrhythmias. Quetiapine is very sedating and has also been associated with significant hypotension, especially during the titration phase of treatment.

Clozapine is the only atypical compound that causes agranulocytosis, characterized by leukopenia. Because this condition can be fatal, weekly blood cell counts must be performed for the first 6 months of treatment. After that time, if counts are stable, blood counts are done every other week. The incidence of agranulocytosis with the other atypical antipsychotics is minimal and no greater than that associated with the use of typical antipsychotics.

The major problems associated with the use of the antipsychotics are listed in the Clinical Problems box.

CLINICAL PROBLEMS

Typical antipsychotics

- High propensity to produce extrapyramidal symptoms and tardive dyskinesia
- Hyperprolactinemia
- Sedation
- Moderate weight gain
- Postural hypotension
- Neuroleptic malignant syndrome
- Prolonged QT interval, risk of ventricular arrhythmias (thioridazine)

Atypical antipsychotics

- Diabetes mellitus
- Hypercholesterolemia
- Sedation
- Seizures and agranulocytosis (clozapine)
- Hyperprolactinemia (risperidone)
- Moderate to severe weight gain (clozapine, olanzapine)
- Prolonged QT interval, risk of ventricular arrhythmias (ziprasidone)

New horizons

The development of new antipsychotic drugs is a major focus for research, especially because 20 to 25% of diagnosed schizophrenics are resistant to all currently available drugs. In addition, many schizophrenics are non-compliant because of the troublesome side effects associated with the use of currently available drugs. Thus, there is a great need to develop newer compounds with efficacy for more patients and decreased side effects.

While much attention has focused on the role of DA and 5-HT in schizophrenia, as our understanding of the etiology of the disorder increases, so will the potential to develop compounds directed at newer targets. One such area of research is on glutamatergic neurotransmission. The glutamate *N*-methyl-D-aspartate receptor antagonist phencyclidine ("angel dust") mimics schizophrenia more accurately than any other compound. The behavioral effects of phencyclidine prompted investigators to postulate a glutamatergic deficiency in the etiology of schizophrenia, and recent studies have demonstrated that partial deletion of the gene encoding these receptors leads to the same behavioral abnormalities observed following phencyclidine. Thus, attempts to enhance the activity of the *N*-methyl-D-aspartate receptor in schizophrenics with glycine or serine, both of which stimulate allosteric sites on the receptor, have resulted in some symptomatic improvement.

The challenge remains to develop drugs that are effective in the schizophrenic population resistant to currently available antipsychotic agents and to improve side effect profiles to enhance patient compliance.

TRADE NAMES

In addition to generic and fixed-combination preparations and the drugs listed in the Major Drugs box, the following trade-named materials are some of the important compounds available in the United States.

Typical antipsychotics

Loxapine (Loxitane)
Molindone (Moban)
Perphenazine (Trilafon)
Trifluoperazine (Stelazine)
Prochlorperazine (Compazine)

FURTHER READING

Drugs for Psychiatric Disorders: treatment guidelines. *Med Lett* 2003; 1:69-76.

Meltzer HY. What's atypical about atypical antipsychotic drugs? *Current Opin Pharmacol* 2004; 4:53-57.

Wong AHC, Van Tol HM. Schizophrenia: from phenomenology to neurobiology, *Neurosci Biobehav Revs* 2003; 27:269-306.

Self-assessment questions

1. Which of the following side effects of antipsychotic drugs should be treated immediately?
   a. Mild slowing of gait
   b. Production of breast milk in a non-nursing woman
   c. Neuroleptic malignant syndrome
   d. Constipation
   e. All of the above

2. Which of the following statements are correct regarding typical antipsychotic drugs?
   a. Clinical potency correlates with binding to D_2 receptors.
   b. Long-term treatment increases the firing rate of dopamine neurons.
   c. Long-term treatment results in the supersensitivity of dopamine receptors.
   d. The drugs differ in efficacy, as well as potency.
   e. a and c

3. Tardive dyskinesia is thought to result from which of the following?
   a. Dopamine receptor supersensitivity
   b. Depolarization blockade of mesolimbic dopamine neurons
   c. Blockade of serotonin receptors
   d. Anticholinergic properties of the drugs
   e. None of the above

4. Which of the following is considered the most serious side effect of clozapine?
   a. Parkinsonian symptoms
   b. Hyperprolactinemia
   c. Tardive dyskinesia
   d. Agranulocytosis
   e. Akathisia

5. Which of the following actions distinguishes newer (atypical) antipsychotics from typical antipsychotics?
   a. Low incidence of extrapyramidal effects
   b. Selective effect on mesolimbic dopamine neurons
   c. Little hyperprolactinemia
   d. Lower incidence of sedation
   e. a, b, and c

CHAPTER 23

Treatment of affective disorders

Lynn Wecker
Glenn Catalano

Major Drugs

Tricylic antidepressants
Amitriptyline (Elavil)
Clomipramine (Anafranil)
Desipramine (Norpramin)
Imipramine (Tofranil)
Nortriptyline (Pamelor)

Selective serotonin reuptake inhibitors
Citalopram (Celexa)
Escitalopram (Lexapro)
Fluoxetine (Prozac, Sarafem)
Fluvoxamine (Luvox)
Paroxetine (Paxil)
Sertraline (Zoloft)

Atypicals
Bupropion (Wellbutrin, Zyban)
Mirtazapine (Remeron)
Nefazodone (Serzone)
Trazodone (Desyrel)
Venlafaxine (Effexor)

Monoamine oxidase inhibitors
Phenelzine (Nardil)
Tranylcypromine (Parnate)

Mood stabilizer
Lithium (Eskalith, Lithobid)

Therapeutic overview

Depression is a **heterogeneous** disorder that involves bodily functions and moods and thoughts and is characterized by feelings of sadness, anxiety, guilt, and worthlessness; disturbances in sleep and appetite; fatigue and loss of interest in daily activities; and difficulties in concentration. In addition, individuals with depression are often obsessed with suicidal ideations. Symptoms of depression can last for weeks, months, or years, and depression is a major cause of **morbidity** and **mortality.** In any given year, 9.5% of the population (about 18.8 million U.S. adults) suffers from a depressive illness, and depression is a factor in more than 30,000 suicides per year in the U.S., making it one of the most widespread of all **life-threatening** disorders. Although depression can affect any age, the current mean age of onset is 25 to 35 years. Of particular concern is that the rate of depression and **suicide** among children, adolescents, and the elderly is increasing at an alarming pace and often goes unrecognized.

Depression is a symptom of many different illnesses. It may arise secondary to substance abuse (alcohol, steroids, cocaine, etc.), secondary to a medical illness (pancreatic carcinoma, hypothyroidism, etc.), or secondary to a major life stress event. However, it may also arise from unknown causes.

Three of the most important psychiatric illnesses that present with depressive symptoms are major depression, dysthymia, and bipolar depression. **Major depression** (also referred to as unipolar depression) may be totally disabling (interfering with work, sleeping, and eating); episodes may occur several times during a lifetime and may progress to psychosis. **Dysthymia** is less severe and involves long-term chronic symptoms that do not disable but keep a person from functioning at their highest level. Finally, **bipolar disorder (manic-depressive disease)** is a syndrome in which there are

Abbreviations

DA	dopamine
5-HT	serotonin
MAO	monoamine oxidase
MAOI	monoamine oxidase inhibitor
NE	norepinephrine
SSRI	selective serotonin reuptake inhibitor
TCA	tricyclic antidepressant

cycling mood changes characterized by severe highs and gut-wrenching lows, which may worsen to a psychotic state. In addition, depression is often associated with co-morbid anxiety disorders.

Major depression, dysthymia, and the depression associated with anxiety disorders are treated with compounds classified as **antidepressants.** These compounds fall into 3 broad categories:

- The **amine reuptake inhibitors,** which include the **tricyclic antidepressants** (TCAs) and the **selective serotonin reuptake inhibitors** (SSRIs)
- The **monoamine oxidase inhibitors** (MAOIs)
- The **atypical** drugs, which represent a heterogeneous group of compounds.

Although their specific mechanisms of action differ, these drugs all share the ability to increase **monoaminergic neurotransmission** in the brain, primarily increasing the activities of pathways utilizing **serotonin** (5-HT) and **norepinephrine** (NE) and possibly **dopamine** (DA) as neurotransmitters.

Although the molecular and cellular etiology of depression remains unknown, it is generally accepted that depression involves impaired monoaminergic neurotransmission leading to alterations in expression of specific genes. This is supported by studies demonstrating that antidepressants increase expression of the transcription factor CREB and brain-derived neurotrophic factor, both of which are critical for maintaining normal cell structure in limbic regions of the brain that are targets for monoaminergic projections. In addition, postmortem and imaging studies have demonstrated neuronal loss and shrinkage in the prefrontal cortex and hippocampus in depressed patients, some of which could be reversed by antidepressants.

Within the past several years, as evidence of adult **neurogenesis** has become increasingly clear, the idea has emerged that depression may be due to impaired neurogenesis in adult hippocampus. Studies have demonstrated that new neurons can proliferate from progenitor cells in the hippocampus. This process is impaired by stress and stress hormones such as the glucocorticoids and is enhanced by antidepressants. Furthermore, it has been shown that neurogenesis is required for antidepressants to exert their behavioral effects in laboratory animals. Thus, impaired monoaminergic transmission in specific brain regions may lead to a decreased expression of transcription or growth factors required for maintaining neurogenesis, resulting in depression.

In contrast to unipolar depression, **bipolar disorder** is characterized by depressive cycles with manic episodes, interspersed with periods of normal mood. The characteristics of the depressive phase resemble those of unipolar depression, while the manic phase manifests as increased psychomotor activity and grandiosity, feelings of euphoria, poor judgment and recklessness, extreme irritability, and symptoms sometimes resembling psychotic behavior. Bipolar disorder affects 2 million people in the U.S., often begins in adolescence or early adulthood, and may persist for life. Evidence suggests a role for genetic factors, because the concordance rate in identical twins is 61 to 75%. However, the disorder cannot be attributed to a single major gene, suggesting multifactorial inheritance.

The treatment of bipolar disorder has changed drastically over the past decade. **Lithium** has been the mainstay of treatment for many years, particularly for control of the manic phase. However, the anticonvulsants, valproic acid and carbamazepine, have been frequently used as well, especially in cases in which the bipolar disorder was characterized by rapid cycling. Recently, the atypical antipsychotic drugs risperidone, olanzapine, and quetiapine have been approved as monotherapy for bipolar disorder (see Chapter 22). Lamotrigine is an anticonvulsant that has also recently been approved for maintenance therapy of bipolar disorder (see Chapter 27). Antidepressants may also be warranted to treat the depressive phase of the illness, and the combination of the atypical antipsychotic olanzapine and the SSRI fluoxetine was recently approved for use in bipolar disorder.

This chapter focuses on the pharmacology of the antidepressants and lithium. The anticonvulsants are discussed in Chapter 27. Therapeutic issues related to the use of these compounds are summarized in the Therapeutic Overview box.

THERAPEUTIC OVERVIEW

Major depression and dysthymia

Tricyclic antidepressants
Monoamine oxidase inhibitors
Selective serotonin reuptake inhibitors
Atypical antidepressants

Bipolar (manic-depressive) disorder

Lithium
Antidepressants
Antipsychotics
Anticonvulsants

Mechanisms of action

The antidepressants may be generally classified according to their mechanisms of action as amine reuptake inhibitors, MAOIs, and mixed-action atypical drugs–the latter representing a heterogenous group that includes compounds often referred to as second- or third-generation antidepressants.

Amine reuptake inhibitors and atypical compounds

The TCAs were the first group of antidepressants developed in the 1950s. Imipramine was the first compound demonstrated to have antidepressant efficacy and is the prototype TCA. The TCAs have a 3-ring structure with a side chain containing a tertiary or secondary amine attached to the central ring, resembling the phenothiazine antipsychotics (Fig. 23-1). The tertiary amines include imipramine, amitriptyline, trimipramine, and doxepin; the secondary amines include desipramine, nortriptyline, and protriptyline.

The TCAs block the reuptake of NE and/or 5-HT into noradrenergic and/or serotonergic nerve terminals, respectively (Fig. 23-2) by specific interactions with their plasma membrane transporters. As a consequence of this inhibition, the actions of NE and 5-HT released from these neurons are not rapidly terminated, resulting in a prolonged stimulation of NE and/or 5-HT receptors. The TCAs do not affect the reuptake of DA by

Tricyclic Antidepressants (TCAs)

Imipramine

Nortriptyline

Serotonin Selective Reuptake Inhibitors (SSRIs)

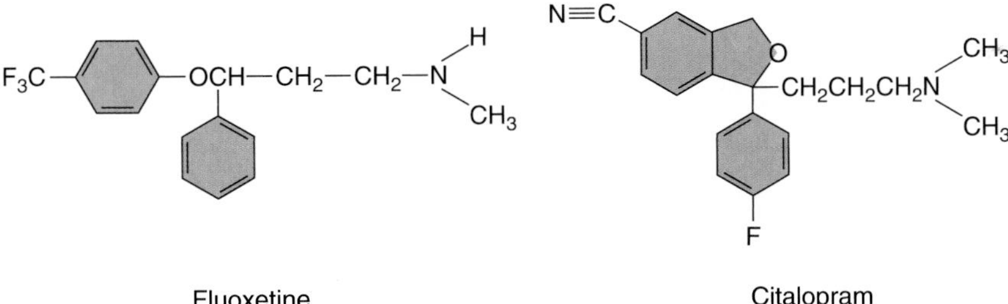

Fluoxetine

Citalopram

Atypical Compounds

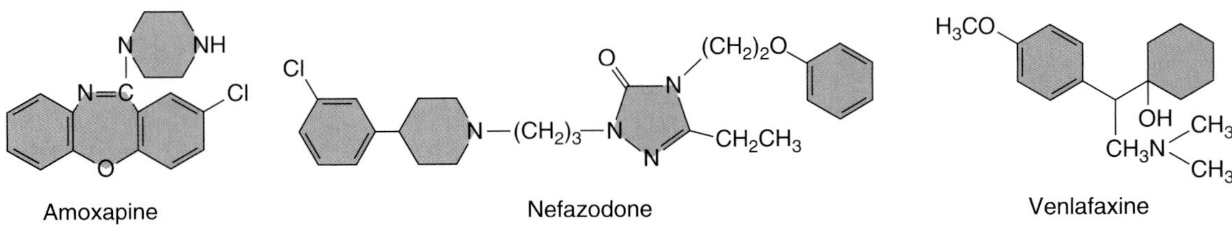

Amoxapine

Nefazodone

Venlafaxine

Monoamine Oxidase Inhibitors (MAOIs)

Phenelzine

Tranylcypromine

Figure 23-1 Structures of prototypical antidepressants.

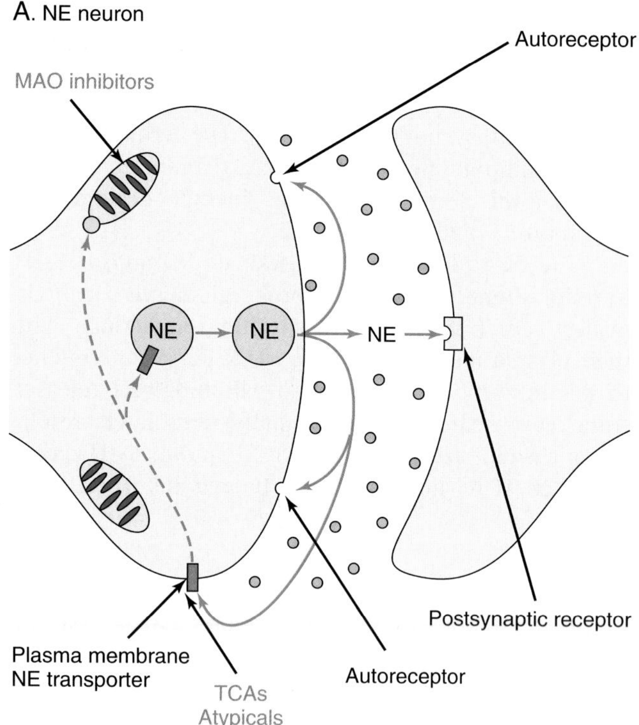

Table 23-1 Relative selectivity of antidepressants for amine reuptake

Compound	NE	5-HT	DA
TRICYCLICS			
Amitriptyline	++	+++	–
Clomipramine	+++	++	–
Desipramine	+++	–	–
Imipramine	++	+++	–
Nortriptyline	++	+++	–
SSRIs			
Citalopram	–	+++	–
Fluoxetine	+	++++	–
Fluvoxamine	–	+++	–
Paroxetine	++	++++	+
Sertraline	+	++++	++
ATYPICALs			
Bupropion	–	–	+
Mirtazapine	–	–	–
Nefazodone	++	+	+
Trazodone	–	+	–
Venlafaxine	+	+++	–

The symbols represent the relative potency of each compound to inhibit the reuptake of the amines. The highest activity (++++) represents an inhibition constant (K_i) of <1 nM; +++, K_i from 1-10 nM; ++, K_i from 10-100 nM; +, K_i from 100-1,000 nM; and –, K_i > 1,000 nM.

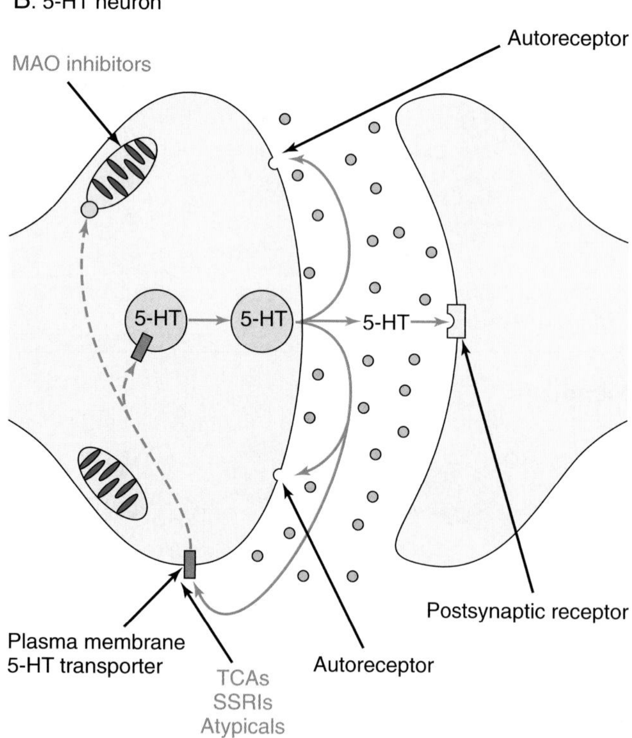

Figure 23-2 A noradrenergic and serotonergic synapse and sites at which antidepressants may exert their actions. TCAs, SSRIs, and some atypical antidepressants inhibit the reuptake transporter for NE and/or 5-HT. Monoamine oxidase, which is targeted by MAO inhibitors, is localized at the outer mitochondrial membrane.

dopaminergic nerve terminals, and their selectivity for the NE versus the 5-HT transporter differs among the different compounds (Table 23-1). Although trimipramine belongs to this group, it has not been demonstrated to have activity at any amine membrane transporter.

In addition to inhibiting NE and 5-HT reuptake, the TCAs also block muscarinic cholinergic receptors, α_1-adrenergic receptors, and histamine H_1 receptors. These actions underlie many of their side effects.

As their name implies, the SSRIs have the highest affinity for the 5-HT transporter. Several of these compounds, however, inhibit the NE and DA transporters as well, particularly sertraline and paroxetine, which inhibit NE and DA reuptake at the upper end of their dose ranges (see Table 23-1).

As mentioned, the atypical compounds are a very heterogeneous group of drugs. Among these, amoxapine, maprotiline, and nefazodone are relatively selective inhibitors of NE reuptake, whereas venlafaxine resembles the SSRIs in selectivity (see Table 23-1). Trazodone is a weak inhibitor of 5-HT reuptake, bupropion weakly inhibits DA reuptake, and mirtazapine appears devoid of activity at any reuptake transporter, similar to trimipramine.

Trazodone, nefazodone, mirtazapine, and several TCAs have also been shown to block 5-HT_{2A} receptors with a high potency, and these drugs are at least 5-fold

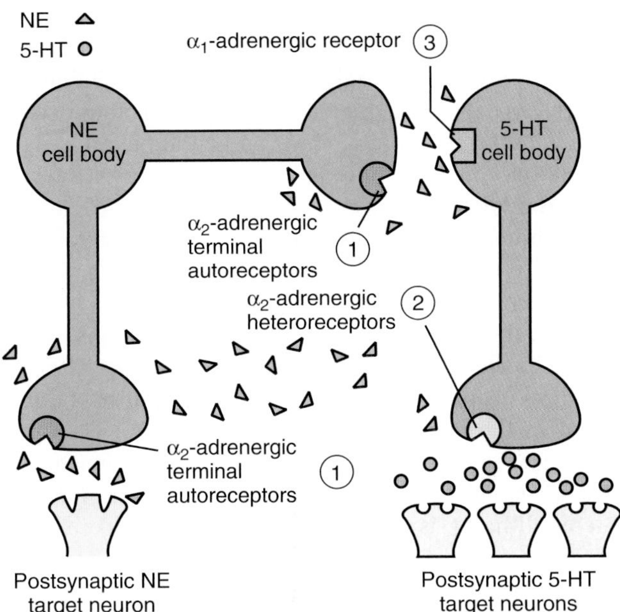

Figure 23-3 Receptor mechanisms controlling NE and 5-HT release. *1*, Stimulation of α_2-adrenergic autoreceptors on NE nerve terminals decreases NE release by a negative feedback process. *2*, Stimulation of α_2-adrenergic heteroreceptors on 5-HT nerve terminals decreases 5-HT release. *3*, Stimulation of α_1-adrenergic receptors on 5-HT dendrites and perikarya increases the firing of 5-HT neurons. Thus a drug that blocks α_2 but not α_1-adrenergic receptors, increases NE and 5-HT release.

more potent *in vitro* as antagonists of this receptor than as inhibitors of 5-HT reuptake. These receptors are widely distributed throughout the brain at regions containing 5-HT nerve terminals, and their stimulation produces depolarization. Interestingly, chronic antagonism of these receptors leads to their paradoxical down regulation, although the role of this mechanism in mediating the antidepressant actions of these compounds remains to be elucidated.

Mirtazapine also blocks α_2-adrenergic receptors on noradrenergic and serotonergic nerve terminals and on noradrenergic dendrites (Figure 23-3). Stimulation of α_2 autoreceptors on noradrenergic neurons decreases NE release, while stimulation of α_2 heteroreceptors on serotonergic neurons inhibits 5-HT release. In addition, stimulation of α_1-adrenergic receptors on serotonergic cell bodies and dendrites increases their firing rate. Thus, mirtazapine, by inhibiting α_2 autoreceptors, enhances noradrenergic cell firing and the release of NE, which activates α_1-adrenergic receptors to increase 5-HT release while concurrently blocking α_2 heteroreceptors, further facilitating the release of 5-HT.

Monoamine oxidase inhibitors

The MAOIs currently available in the U.S. for the treatment of depression are phenelzine and tranylcypromine (see Figure 23-1). These compounds are irreversible or long-lasting inhibitors of MAO and are non-selective—that is, they inhibit both MAO-A and MAO-B. These enzymes are distinct gene products with MAO-A present in human placenta, intestinal mucosa, liver, and brain—responsible for catabolism of 5-HT, NE, and tyramine; and MAO-B present in human platelets, liver, and brain—responsible predominantly for the catabolism of DA as well as tyramine. These enzymes are located in the outer membrane of mitochondria and maintain low cytoplasmic concentrations of the monoamines, facilitating inward-directed transporter activity (i.e., monoamine reuptake).

Research with selective MAOIs has shown that inhibition of MAO-A is necessary for antidepressant activity. Inhibition of MAO causes an increase in monoamine concentrations in the cytosol of the nerve terminal. All the effects of the MAOIs have been attributed to enhanced aminergic activity secondary to enzyme inhibition.

Lithium

Although lithium has been the standard prophylactic agent for bipolar disorder for decades, its cellular mechanisms of action remain unclear. Currently, three actions of lithium have been postulated to mediate its clinical efficacy. The first is interference with receptor-activated phosphoinositide turnover (see Chapter 2). Lithium blocks the hydrolysis of inositol phosphate to free inositol, thereby reducing free inositol concentrations and depleting further formation of phosphatidylinositol in the cell membrane. Hence, the effects of agonists working through this signaling system will be blunted. Lithium has also been shown to inhibit 5-HT_{1A} and 5-HT_{1B} autoreceptors on serotonergic dendrites and nerve terminals, thereby preventing feedback inhibition of 5-HT release. Last, sustained lithium exposure enhances glutamate reuptake by glutamatergic neurons, thereby decreasing the time glutamate is present at glutamatergic synapses and dampening its ability to stimulate its receptors. Clearly, additional studies are needed to elucidate the actions of lithium that underlie its unique efficacy in bipolar disorder.

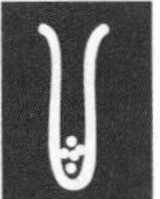

Pharmacokinetics

Pharmacokinetic parameters of representative antidepressants are presented in Table 23-2. In general, antidepressants are readily absorbed, primarily in the small intestine, and undergo significant first-pass hepatic metabolism. Peak plasma concentrations are achieved

Table 23-2 Pharmacokinetic parameters of representative antidepressant drugs

Compound	Elimination Half-Life (hrs)	Plasma Protein Binding (%)	Disposition/ Elimination
TRICYCLICS			
Amitriptyline	9-25	90-95	M, R
Clomipramine	19-37	97	M, R, B
Desipramine	14-24	90-95	M, R
Imipramine	6-18	90	M, R
Nortriptyline	18-38	90	M, R
SSRIs			
Citalopram	35	80	M, R
Escitalopram	27-32	56	M, R
Fluoxetine	1-3 days (acute) 4-6 days (chronic)	95	M, R
Fluvoxamine	15-20	80	M, R
Paroxetine	20	95	M, R, B
Sertraline	26	98	M, R, B
ATYPICALs			
Bupropion	14	85	M, R, B
Mirtazapine	20-40	85	M, R, B
Nefazodone	3-4	>99	M, R
Trazodone	4-8	90-95	M, R
Venlafaxine	3-4	30	M, R

M, Metabolism; *R*, renal; *B*, biliary.

within hours after ingestion, with steady-state concentrations achieved after 4 to 7 days at a fixed dose.

Most amine reuptake inhibitors and atypical antidepressants are extensively bound to plasma proteins, in general are oxidized by hepatic microsomal enzymes to inactive metabolites, and are excreted in the urine as glucuronides or sulfates. A small amount may be excreted in the feces via the bile. Some antidepressants, especially fluoxetine and the tertiary-amine TCAs, are metabolized to active compounds, which themselves have antidepressant efficacy. For example, desipramine and nortriptyline are major metabolites of imipramine and amitriptyline, respectively. Nefazodone and trazodone are metabolized relatively rapidly into active compounds with varying half-lives. Some have properties similar to those of the parent compounds, which may contribute to their antidepressant activity.

The MAOIs are absorbed readily following oral administration, and maximal inhibition of MAO occurs in 5 to 10 days. The binding of these compounds to MAO leads to their cleavage to active products (hydrazines), which are inactivated primarily by acetylation. Because phenelzine inhibits MAO irreversibly and tranylcypromine inhibits it persistently but non-covalently, their biological effects outlast their physical presence in the body—that is, a loss of enzyme activity persists after the drugs are metabolized and eliminated. New enzyme must be synthesized for MAO activity to return to normal, a process that takes several weeks. It is important to note that the rate of inactivation of these compounds by acetylation depends on genotype, and "slow acetylators" may exhibit an exaggerated effect when given these compounds.

Lithium is most often administered as a carbonate salt but is also administered as a citrate salt. Orally administered lithium is rapidly absorbed and is present as a soluble ion unbound to plasma proteins. Peak plasma concentrations are reached 2 to 4 hours after an oral dose. Approximately 95% of a single dose is eliminated in the urine with a half-life of 20 to 24 hours, and steady-state plasma concentrations are reached 5 to 6 days after initiation of treatment. About 80% of filtered lithium is reabsorbed by the renal proximal tubules.

Lithium has a low therapeutic index; therapeutic levels are 0.6-1.4 mEq/liter, and toxicity is manifest at 1.6-2.0 mEq/liter. Thus, the concentration of lithium in plasma must be monitored routinely to ensure adequate therapeutic levels without toxicity.

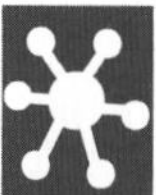

Relation of mechanisms of action to clinical response

Currently available TCAs have similar efficacies for most types of depression, significantly improving symptoms in 65% to 75% of patients. The mood-elevating properties of antidepressants are associated with a blunting or amelioration of the depressive state, such that there is an improvement in all signs and symptoms, although rates of improvement of individual symptoms may differ. A major problem, however, is that it takes several weeks for the maximal therapeutic benefit of these compounds to become apparent. This limitation is particularly disturbing given the propensity for depressed patients to commit suicide.

The temporal discrepancy between the therapeutic efficacy of the antidepressants and their ability to immediately facilitate monoaminergic transmission remains unresolved. However, repeated administration of many antidepressants has been shown to produce numerous adaptive changes in the brain, particularly at serotonergic and noradrenergic receptors. For example, studies have shown that acute administration of SSRIs stimulates both somatodendritic and terminal autoreceptors on serotonergic neurons to decrease firing and inhibit 5-HT release. However, chronic administration of

SSRIs downregulates or desensitizes these autoreceptors, producing a disinhibition, thereby promoting neuronal firing and 5-HT release. Similarly, several TCAs have been shown to reduce responses elicited by activation of central β-adrenergic receptors and cause a decrease in their density following chronic administration. Because these and other adaptive changes induced by antidepressants take weeks to develop, it has been suggested that they are crucial to the clinical efficacy of these drugs.

Because of the frequency of recurrences of depression, attention has focused on whether antidepressants can prevent recurrences and if so, how long they should be given. Eighty percent of recurrently depressed patients maintained for 3 years on the same dose of imipramine used earlier to treat their acute episode had no recurrence of a serious depressive episode. Prophylactic effects of other antidepressants have been described as well. Studies have found that 50% of patients who have a depressive episode will have a recurrence. Of patients who have two depressive episodes, 70% will have a third episode. If a patient has three depressive episodes, there is a 90% chance there will be another. Therefore, if a patient has three depressive episodes, he/she should remain on long-term antidepressant therapy. If the patient has two episodes that are severe (they reach psychotic proportions or the patient becomes suicidal), the clinician should consider maintaining the patient on long-term antidepressant therapy at that time. However, it is not yet clear when, if ever, patients can be taken off long-term maintenance treatment without the risk of recurrence of a depressive episode.

Side effects, clinical problems, and toxicity

Amine reuptake inhibitors and atypical compounds

Many of the most common side effects of the TCA and atypical drugs result from their antagonist actions at H_1 histaminergic, muscarinic cholinergic, and α_1-adrenergic receptors, leading to marked sedative effects; atropine-like effects, including dry mouth, constipation, and cycloplegia; and prazosin-like effects such as orthostatic hypotension, respectively (Table 23-3). As a group these drugs are more potent at blocking H_1 than muscarinic and α_1-adrenergic receptors. In fact, doxepin is so highly antihistaminergic that it is often used by dermatologists to treat allergic rashes. These side effects are especially bothersome in elderly patients, with postural hypotension a particularly severe problem because it

Table 23-3 Side effect profile of representative antidepressant drugs

Compound	Anticholinergic	Antiadrenergic (α_1)	Antihistaminergic (H_1)
TRICYCLICS			
Amitriptyline	++	++	+++
Desipramine	+	+	++
Imipramine	+	++	+++
Nortriptyline	+	++	+++
SSRIs			
Citalopram	–	–	+
Fluoxetine	–	–	–
Fluvoxamine	–	–	–
Paroxetine	++	–	+
Sertraline	+	+	–
ATYPICALs			
Bupropion	–	–	–
Mirtazapine	+	+	++++
Nefazodone	–	++	++
Trazodone	–	++	+
Venlafaxine	–	–	–
MAOIs			
Phenelzine	–	–	–
Tranylcypromine	–	–	–

The symbols represent the relative potency of each compound to produce anticholinergic (dry mouth, constipation, cycloplegia), antiadrenergic (sedation, postural hypotension) or antihistaminergic (sedation, weight gain) effects. The highest activity (++++) represents an inhibition constant (K_i) of <1 nM; +++, K_i from 1-10 nM; ++, K_i from 10-100 nM; +, K_i from 100-1,000 nM; and –, K_i > 1,000 nM.

can lead to falls and broken bones. Clinically, doxepin and amitriptyline have the most pronounced orthostatic hypotensive effects of the TCAs. This is not a clinically significant problem for the SSRIs, which have low affinities for α_1-adrenergic receptors.

Although the atypical compounds are somewhat less potent than TCAs in blocking muscarinic cholinergic receptors, maprotiline and mirtazapine do have anticholinergic effects (see Table 23-3). The SSRI paroxetine also inhibits muscarinic cholinergic receptors and produces anticholinergic side effects; however, it does not do so to the same extent as the TCAs, reflecting a dose-related difference. Other SSRIs and other atypical antidepressants are very weak antagonists at muscarinic cholinergic receptors and do not cause anticholinergic side effects.

Of the atypical antidepressants, amoxapine, maprotiline, mirtazapine, nefazodone, and trazodone are sedating; the latter was used as a soporific agent for many years. Venlafaxine and bupropion cause little drowsiness. Among the SSRIs, paroxetine is most likely to induce sedation. Although trazodone and nefazodone are equally potent at blocking α_1-adrenergic receptors, nefazodone causes less orthostatic hypotension than trazodone. Nefazodone is associated with hepatic failure and received a "black box" warning from the Food and Drug Administration. Amoxapine also produces orthostatic hypotension. Amoxapine is a metabolite of loxitane, which is a typical antipsychotic agent. Therefore, amoxapine can have the same side effects as any antipsychotic agent, including dystonic reactions, tardive dyskinesia, and neuroleptic malignant syndrome (see Chapter 22). The TCAs affect the heart through a combination of anticholinergic activity, inhibition of amine reuptake, and direct depressant effects. Although these effects may be manifested by a mild tachycardia, conduction disturbances and electrocardiographic changes can occur. The quinidine-like depressant effects on the myocardium can precipitate slowing of atrioventricular conduction or bundle-branch block or premature ventricular contractions. These effects are much more common in patients with preexisting cardiac problems. Abnormalities of cardiac conduction occur in <5% of patients receiving therapeutic doses of TCAs, with most being clinically insignificant. The majority of the SSRIs have virtually no effect on the heart. There have been a number of cases (some fatal) of citalopram-induced cardiac conduction delay in patients who have taken an overdose of this compound. One of citalopram's metabolites is cardiotoxic, and when patients take an overdose, this metabolite increases enough to cause changes in the electrocardiogram and clinical symptoms. Therefore, citalopram should probably not be a first-line agent in patients with pre-existing cardiac disease.

TCAs can lower seizure thresholds and are potentially epileptogenic, but this occurs in less than 0.5% of patients; the incidence is even lower in patients receiving SSRIs. Many of the other antidepressants can induce seizures, and this is a particularly pronounced problem with maprotiline and bupropion, especially in patients receiving high doses. In fact, bupropion is contraindicated for use in any patient with a history of seizures. By contrast, the incidence of seizures is very low in patients receiving trazodone, nefazodone, or mirtazapine.

TCA-induced toxicity of the central nervous system can produce delirium, especially in the elderly, which is easily recognizable. Such delirium is usually preceded by what appears to be a worsening of depression. This may lead to administration of increased doses of the TCA, with further worsening of the delirium. In most cases, the antimuscarinic activity of the TCAs is the driving force behind the delirium. If the patient is hospitalized, physostigmine can be used to reverse the delirium. The incidence of insomnia, nervousness, restlessness, and anxiety appears to be relatively high in patients taking fluoxetine. It has an activating effect that can be anxiogenic in some patients and should be started at a lower dose in those with an anxiety component to their illness and to avoid night time dosing. Venlafaxine has side effects similar to those of SSRIs. Bupropion can cause nervousness and insomnia, as well as tremors and palpitations, and has more of a stimulant than a sedative effect; therefore, it should not be administered in the evening.

An important side effect of many of the antidepressants including the MAOIs is weight gain, which reduces patient compliance. Most SSRIs have an anorectic effect and therefore do not cause any clinically significant weight gain, although paroxetine has been reported to cause weight gain over time. Bupropion also does not cause weight gain, and venlafaxine can cause weight loss. Mirtazapine can cause significant weight gain, perhaps because of its potent antihistamine activity.

Sexual dysfunction—including abnormal ejaculation, anorgasmy, impotence, and decreased libido—are receiving increasing attention in patients receiving antidepressants. These effects occur at least as frequently in patients treated with TCAs or MAOIs as in patients receiving SSRIs. There appears to be little impairment of sexual function in patients treated with bupropion or mirtazapine and perhaps nefazodone. However, care must be taken, since nefazodone has been recently associated with the development of priapism, whereas it has long been known as a potential occurrence with the structurally similar trazodone.

Most TCAs show little evidence of teratogenicity in humans. However, imipramine, nortriptyline, and amitriptyline may pose some risk for possible human teratogenicity. Although there have been a few isolated reports of possible birth defects in the offspring of mothers taking a TCA, the conclusion drawn from several extensive retrospective analyses performed is that there is no association between TCA exposure during pregnancy and the occurrence of fetal malformations or defects. However, signs and symptoms of withdrawal or TCA intoxication can occur in newborns of mothers who take a TCA late in pregnancy. The SSRIs and venlafaxine also show little evidence of teratogenicity, but with no adequate studies in humans. Bupropion is the only newer antidepressant that has no evidence that it is teratogenic or embryocidal. However, further research is warranted, given the relatively short time these agents have been in use and their increasing use as maintenance therapies.

Patient tolerability is better for all the newer antidepressants than for the TCAs. As with all drugs, though, there are side effects. The SSRIs and venlafaxine cause nausea (15%-35%), vomiting, and diarrhea to a much greater extent than do the TCAs. The incidence of nausea and vomiting in patients treated with trazodone, nefazodone, mirtazapine, or bupropion is generally less than that seen in patients treated with SSRIs or venlafaxine. Headaches commonly occur in patients on SSRIs and venlafaxine.

An important central side effect of TCAs and SSRIs is induction of mania or hypomania in depressed patients with a bipolar disorder. This manic overshoot requires urgent care since a patient can switch from deep depression to an agitated manic state overnight. Anecdotally, fluoxetine is felt to be the drug most likely to induce such an overshoot and bupropion the least likely to do so. This also occurs in patients treated with MAOIs.

Many SSRIs are potent inhibitors of several cytochrome P450 enzymes and thus can lead to potentially dangerous drug interactions. Fluoxetine and paroxetine inhibit *CYP2D6*, whereas fluvoxamine inhibits both *CYP1A2* and *CYP3A4*. Sertraline, escitalopram, citalopram, and venlafaxine have little if any effect on cytochrome P450s. The majority of the TCAs are substrates of the cytochrome P450 system, so using them concurrently with SSRIs may lead to increased serum TCA concentrations and potential toxicity. The SSRIs have the potential to lead to serious consequences if combined with other compounds that increase brain levels of 5-HT or stimulate 5-HT receptors. Among these are the MAOIs and other antidepressants, as well as meperidine and dextromethorphan, which are potent inhibitors of 5-HT reuptake, and tryptophan, which can enhance 5-HT synthesis. This interaction can lead to a condition known as **serotonin syndrome.** This syndrome is characterized by alterations in autonomic function (fever, chills, diarrhea), cognition and behavior (agitation, excitement, hypomania), and motor systems (myoclonus, tremor, motor weakness, ataxia, hyperreflexia) and may often resemble neuroleptic malignant syndrome (see Chapter 22). Currently it is believed that activation of 5-HT receptors in the brainstem and spinal cord may mediate these effects. The incidence of the disorder is not known, but as the use of SSRIs increases, it may become more prevalent. Thus, a heightened awareness is required for prevention, recognition, and prompt treatment. This involves discontinuation of the suspected drugs, administration of 5-HT antagonists such as cyproheptadine or methysergide, administration of the skeletal muscle relaxant dantrolene, and other supportive measures. The syndrome usually resolves within 24 hours but can be fatal.

Poisoning accounts for about 20% of all suicides, and TCAs are the most commonly used drugs in such cases. TCA overdose can produce coma, seizures, hypertension, and cardiac abnormalities, with death resulting primarily from cardiac arrest. A lethal dose of a TCA may be as low as 1 gram, which is roughly 4 or 5 days of medication. In general, the SSRIs and the other atypical compounds (except amoxapine and maprotiline) are much safer in overdoses than the TCAs. However, as noted earlier, there have been reports of cardiac conduction problems associated with citalopram overdose.

Monoamine oxidase inhibitors

The side effects of the MAOIs are an extension of their pharmacological effects, reflecting enhanced catecholaminergic activity. Primary side effects are central nervous system excitation (hallucinations, agitation, hyperreflexia, and convulsions), a large suppression of REM sleep that may lead to psychotic behavior, and drug interactions, the latter of which are potentially life-threatening. The MAOIs have not been associated with extensive human teratogenicity.

The interaction between the MAOIs and the other antidepressants may produce serotonin syndrome, as discussed. In addition, because MAOIs lead to increased intracellular stores of NE within adrenergic nerve terminals, these compounds can enhance the action of indirectly acting sympathomimetics that stimulate the release of NE from these sites. Of major importance is the potential for the MAOIs to induce a hypertensive reaction following the ingestion of tyramine-containing compounds, an action known as the **"cheese" effect.** Tyramine, which is an indirectly acting sympathomimetic, is normally metabolized by MAO within the gastrointestinal tract following ingestion. When MAO activity in the gastrointestinal tract is inhibited, such as occurs following the oral administration of MAOIs, tyramine is not metabolized and enters the circulation, where it can release stored NE from sympathetic nerve endings. Because the amount of NE in the adrenergic nerve ending is increased as a consequence of MAO inhibition, the result is a massive increase in NE released into the synapse, with a resultant hypertensive crisis (see Chapter 10). Therefore, patients taking MAOIs are maintained on a tyramine-restricted diet. While hypertensive crises are associated with tyramine ingestion during MAOI treatment, in all actuality, hypotension is a much more common side effect of MAOI treatment.

Lithium

Numerous side effects occur in patients treated with lithium, involving the central nervous system, thyroid, kidneys, and heart.

Subclinical hypothyroidism can develop in patients taking lithium. Although obvious hypothyroidism is rare, a benign, diffuse, nontender thyroid enlargement (goiter), indicative of compromised thyroid function, occurs in some patients. This results from the ability of lithium to interfere with the iodination of tyrosine and, consequently, the synthesis of thyroxine (see Chapter 37).

Lithium blocks the responsiveness of the renal collecting tubule epithelium to vasopressin, leading to a nephrogenic diabetes insipidus. In addition, polydipsia and polyuria are frequent problems, the latter due to uncoupling of vasopressin receptors from their G proteins. It is important to monitor patients' renal function during treatment with lithium.

Lithium can cause substantial weight gain, which may be detrimental to health but also leads to patient noncompliance. Lithium may also cause nausea and diarrhea as well as daytime drowsiness. All these effects are quite common, even in patients with therapeutic plasma concentrations. Other side effects include allergic reactions, particularly an exacerbation of acne vulgaris or psoriasis. It may also cause a fine hand tremor in some patients.

Lithium is an important human teratogen, and there is evidence of human fetal risk. It has been noted to cause Ebstein's anomaly, which is an endocardial cushion defect. It is also secreted in breast milk, so breast-feeding should be discouraged in mothers receiving lithium.

Potential changes in the plasma concentration of lithium resulting from changes in renal clearance can be dangerous because lithium exhibits a very narrow therapeutic index. The major drug class that poses a problem when administered with lithium is the class of thiazide diuretics, which block Na^+ reabsorption in renal distal tubules. The resulting Na^+ depletion promotes reabsorption of both Na^+ and lithium from proximal tubules, reducing lithium excretion and elevating its plasma concentrations. Similarly, nonsteroidal antiinflammatory agents can decrease lithium clearance and elevate plasma lithium concentrations, leading to lithium toxicity. Difficulties can arise if a patient on lithium becomes dehydrated, as that may also increase serum lithium levels to the toxic range.

Lithium toxicity is related both to its absolute plasma concentration and its rate of rise. Symptoms of mild toxicity occur at the peak of lithium absorption and include nausea, vomiting, abdominal pain, diarrhea, sedation, and fine hand tremor. Because lithium is often administered concomitantly with antipsychotics, which may exhibit anti-nausea effects, it is critical to be aware of the potential of these compounds to mask the initial signs of lithium toxicity. More serious toxicity, which occurs at higher plasma concentrations, produces central effects, including confusion, hyperreflexia, gross tremor, cranial nerve and focal neurological signs, and even convulsions and coma. Cardiac dysrhythmias may also occur, and death can result from severe lithium toxicity. The problems associated with the use of the antidepressants are summarized in the Clinical Problems box.

CLINICAL PROBLEMS

Amine reuptake inhibitors and atypicals

Anticholinergic, antihistaminergic and antiadrenergic effects
Sexual dysfunction
Seizures
Myocardial depression leading to ventricular arrhythmias

Selective serotonin reuptake inhibitors

Nervousness, agitation, sweating and fatigue, sexual dysfunction
"Serotonin syndrome"

Monoamine oxidase inhibitors

CNS excitation, suppression of REM sleep, hepatotoxicity
"Serotonin syndrome"
"Cheese effect"

Lithium

CNS—tremors, mental confusion, decreased seizure threshold
Thyroid—decreased function
Renal—polydipsia, polyuria, induced diabetes insipidus
Cardiac—dysrhythmias

New horizons

Although the introduction of the SSRIs and atypical antidepressants represent major advances in the treatment of depression, these compounds still have limitations related to efficacy, tolerability, and rapidity of action. Unfortunately, only about 50% of patients treated with standard doses of currently available antidepressants exhibit favorable responses after 6 to 8 weeks of treatment, while others exhibit suboptimal improvement and some individuals do not respond at all. Some lack of response may be attributed to patient compliance, as many individuals cannot tolerate the side effects of these compounds. While the side effects of the newer compounds are clearly less severe than those seen with the TCAs, they are not without their own problems, especially causing sexual dysfunction and weight gain. Last, slow response time is a major issue because many depressed individuals are prone to suicidal ideations.

Clearly, new approaches to the pharmacological treatment of depression are needed. One approach involves increasing the safety profile of currently available agents that may be better tolerated by patients. Indeed, the first transdermal MAOI that avoids the potential for the cheese effect has recently been approved.

Additional approaches include developing compounds aimed at new targets, including drugs that promote neurogenesis and agents that normalize the hypothalamic-pituitary-adrenal axis, which is hyperactive in many depressed patients. The challenge remains to develop therapeutic agents that are effective in the population of depressive patients that are resistant to currently available antidepressant medications and to decrease side effects to enhance patient compliance.

TRADE NAMES

In addition to generic and fixed-combination preparations and the drugs listed in the Major Drugs box, the following trade-named materials are some of the important compounds available in the United States.

Amoxapine (Asendin)
Doxepin (Adapin, Sinequan)
Maprotiline (Ludiomil)
Protriptyline (Vivactil)
Trimipramine (Surmontil)

FURTHER READING

Drugs for Psychiatric Disorders: Treatment Guidelines. *Med Lett* 2003; 1:69-76.

Nemeroff CB, Owens MJ. Treatment of mood disorders. *Nature Neurosci* Supp 2002; 5:1068-1070.

Schloss P, Henn FA. New insights into the mechanisms of antidepressant therapy. *Pharmacol Therap* 2004; 102:47-60.

Self-assessment questions

1. Which of the following adverse side effects caused by the tricyclic antidepressant drugs is *not* the consequence of blockade of H_1 receptors, muscarinic cholinergic receptors, or α_1-adrenergic receptors?
   a. Orthostatic hypotension
   b. sedation
   c. blurred vision
   d. urinary retention
   e. increase in intraventricular conduction time

2. The neurotransmitter most likely to be involved in the beneficial antidepressant effects of fluoxetine is:
   a. Norepinephrine.
   b. Serotonin.
   c. Dopamine.
   d. GABA.
   e. Acetylcholine.

3. Fluoxetine is comparable to a tricyclic antidepressant, such as imipramine, in causing:
   a. Orthostatic hypotension.
   b. Dry mouth and blurred vision.
   c. Nausea and vomiting.
   d. Urinary retention.
   e. Alleviation of the symptoms of depression.

4. A 47-year-old man with bipolar depressive illness also has a history of glomerulonephritis. He is actively manic and needs treatment. Which one of the following drugs would be *most* appropriate for the treatment of his mania?
   a. Imipramine
   b. Carbamazepine
   c. Lithium carbonate
   d. Diazepam
   e. Buspirone

5. Which drug can enhance both noradrenergic and serotonergic neurotransmission in the brain by blocking α_2-adrenoceptors?
   a. Imipramine
   b. Mirtazapine
   c. Phenelzine
   d. Fluoxetine
   e. Bupropion

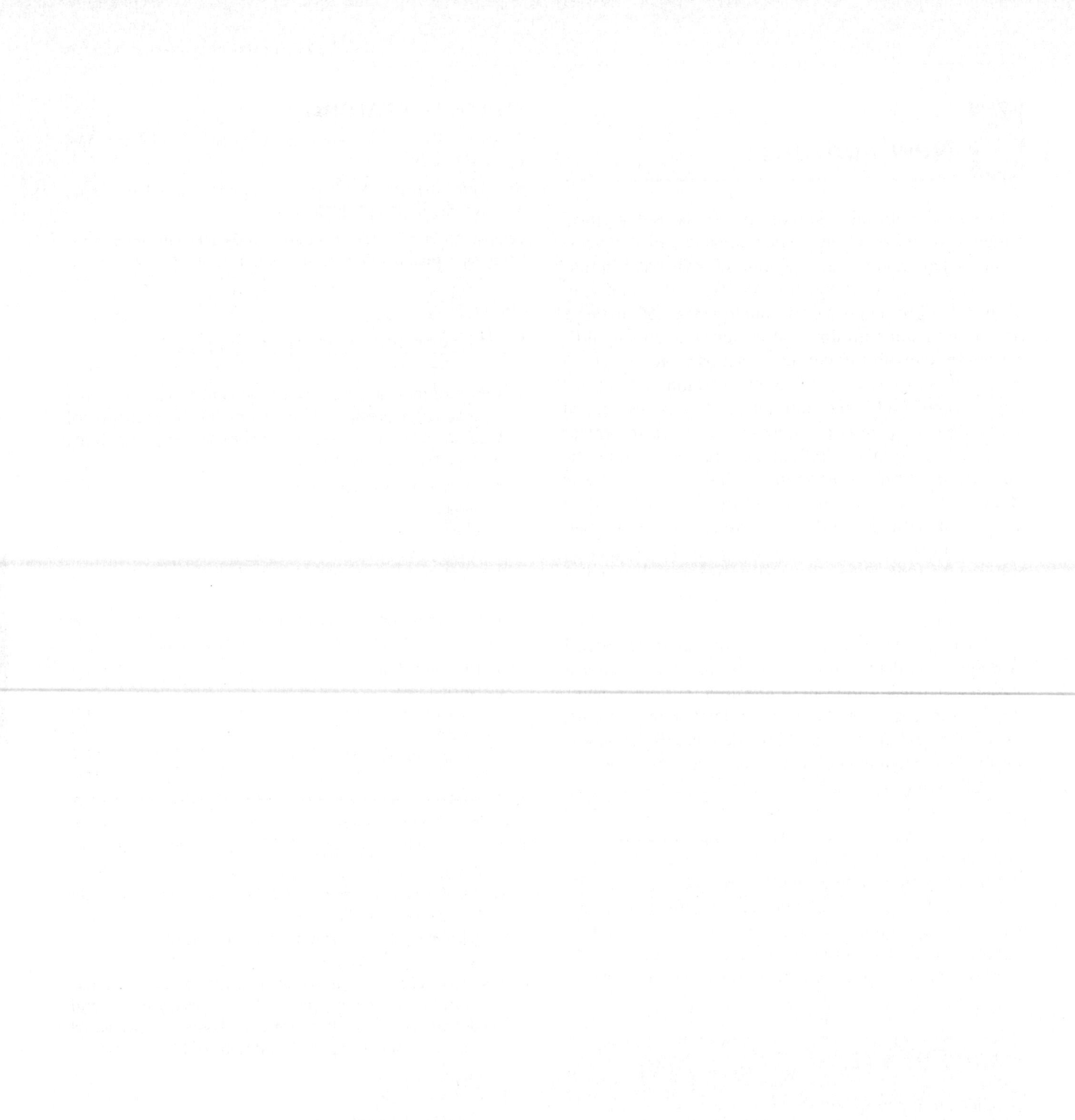

CHAPTER 24

Treatment of anxiety and sleep disorders

Lynn Wecker
Glenn Catalano

Major Drugs	
Anxiolytics	**Insomnia**
Alprazolam (Xanax)	Flurazepam (Dalmane)
Buspirone (BuSpar)	Temazepam (Restoril)
Chlordiazepoxide (Librium)	Triazolam (Halcion)
Clonazepam (Klonopin)	Zaleplon (Sonata)
Diazepam (Valium)	Zolpidem (Ambien)
Lorazepam (Ativan)	**Antagonist**
Oxazepam (Serax)	Flumazenil (Mazicon, Romazicon)
Propranolol (Inderal)	

Therapeutic overview

The term **anxiety** refers to a pervasive feeling of apprehension, and specific **anxiety disorders** affect 19 million U.S. adults. Anxiety is characterized by diffuse symptoms such as feelings of helplessness, difficulties in concentrating, irritability and insomnia, as well as somatic symptoms including gastrointestinal disturbances, muscle tension, excessive perspiration, tachypnea, tachycardia, nausea, palpitations, and dry mouth.

Anxiety disorders are **chronic** and relentless and can progress if not treated. The anxiety disorders include:

- **Panic disorder**
- **Obsessive-compulsive disorder**
- **Posttraumatic stress disorder**
- **Social phobia**
- **Social anxiety disorder**
- **Generalized anxiety disorder**
- **Specific phobias**

Each disorder has its own distinct features, but they are all bound together by the common theme of excessive, irrational fear of impending doom, loss of control, nervousness, and dread. Depression often accompanies anxiety disorders, and when it does, it should be treated (see Chapter 23).

In many cases, anxiety symptoms may be mild and require little or no treatment. However, at other times symptoms may be severe enough to cause considerable distress. When patients exhibit anxiety so debilitating that lifestyle, work, and interpersonal relationships are severely impaired, they may require drug treatment. Although these compounds may be of great benefit, concurrent psychological support and counseling are absolute necessities for the treatment of anxiety and cannot be overemphasized.

Three classes of drugs, referred to as the **anxiolytics**, are used to treat anxiety disorders and include:

- **Benzodiazepines** and **buspirone**
- **Antidepressants**
- **β-Adrenergic blocking agents**

The benzodiazepines are the most commonly prescribed anxiolytics in the United States. Prior to the introduction of these compounds in the 1960s, the major drugs used to treat anxiety were primarily sedatives and hypnotics and included meprobamate, glutethimide, barbi-

Abbreviations	
CNS	central nervous system
GABA	γ-aminobutyric acid
5-HT	serotonin

turates, and alcohols. Unfortunately, these compounds have a high abuse potential and potent respiratory depressant effects and led to a high incidence of drug dependence, overdose, and death. Although the benzodiazepines are not devoid of side effects or abuse potential, they have a wide margin of safety, with anxiolytic activity achieved at doses that do not induce clinically significant respiratory depression.

In addition to their use as anxiolytics, the benzodiazepines have also become drugs of choice for the treatment of **insomnia,** which often accompanies anxiety and depression. It has been estimated that 30% of all adults in the U.S. have insomnia, characterized by difficulty initiating and maintaining sleep. The benzodiazepines and subtype-selective benzodiazepine agonists **zaleplon** and **zolpidem,** in addition to several over-the-counter antihistamine preparations, are useful for insomnia.

Just as central nervous system (CNS) **depressants** such as the benzodiazepines and related compounds are useful for insomnia, CNS **stimulants** are used to treat the **hypersomnias,** which are characterized by excessive sleep or sleepiness and include narcolepsy, cataplexy, and related disorders. Such drugs include modafinil, amphetamines, and methylphenidate. The pharmacology of these compounds is discussed in Chapters 10 and 32.

This chapter focuses on the pharmacology of the benzodiazepines, buspirone, and related compounds. The pharmacology of the antidepressants is discussed in Chapter 23 and that of β-adrenergic receptor blockers in Chapter 10.

Therapeutic issues related to both anxiety and insomnia are summarized in the Therapeutic Overview box.

THERAPEUTIC OVERVIEW

Anxiety disorders

Benzodiazepines
Buspirone
Antidepressants
β-Adrenergic receptor blockers

Insomnia

Benzodiazepines
Subtype-selective benzodiazepine agonists
Antihistamines
Antidepressants

Hypersomnia

CNS Stimulants

Mechanisms of action

Compounds affecting the $GABA_A$ receptor

The **benzodiazepines** exert their effects through allosteric interactions at the γ-aminobutyric acid type A ($GABA_A$) receptor. $GABA_A$ receptors are pentameric ligand-gated ion channels, and stimulation of these receptors by GABA leads to the influx of chloride and a resultant hyperpolarization of the postsynaptic cell (see Chapter 2). This hyperpolarization renders the cell less likely to fire in response to an incoming excitatory stimulus, thus mediating the inhibitory effects of GABA throughout the CNS.

$GABA_A$ receptors contain a primary agonist binding site for GABA as well as multiple allosteric sites that can be occupied by numerous pharmacological compounds, as depicted in Figure 24-1. Benzodiazepines bind to one of these modulatory sites, often referred to as the benzodiazepine binding site or benzodiazepine receptor, whereas compounds such as the barbiturates and the poison picrotoxin bind to other sites on the receptor. When benzodiazepines bind to the benzodiazepine binding site, they induce a conformational change in the receptor, resulting in an increased frequency of chloride ion channel opening upon stimulation of the receptor by GABA. They are referred to as **positive allosteric modulators** in that they increase the effect of the natural agonist but have no effect in the absence of agonist.

Benzodiazepines are not the only group of compounds that bind to this allosteric site. The **β-carbolines** such as harmine and harmaline also interact with this site. However, when these compounds bind, they

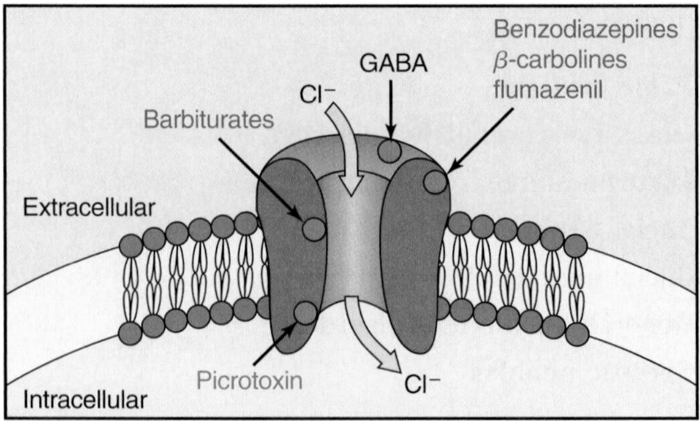

Figure 24-1 The $GABA_A$ receptor depicting the membrane-associated protein composed of 5 subunits, the chloride channel, and relative location of binding sites for GABA, benzodiazepines, barbiturates, and picrotoxin.

allosterically reduce chloride conductance by decreasing the affinity of GABA for its binding site. Because the β-carbolines increase CNS excitability and may produce anxiety and precipitate panic attacks, effects opposite to those of the benzodiazepines, they are called **inverse agonists** (see Chapter 2). The inverse agonists block the effects of the benzodiazepines but have no therapeutic use. However, they are found in nature and are thought to be responsible for the psychedelic properties of some plant species.

A third group of compounds that bind to the benzodiazepine site on the $GABA_A$ receptor are competitive antagonists such as **flumazenil.** As a competitive antagonist, flumazenil occupies the benzodiazepine site with high affinity but does not have any ability to activate it and does not affect GABA-mediated chloride ion influx. Rather, flumazenil competitively antagonizes the actions of the benzodiazepines and is used therapeutically to treat benzodiazepine overdose. Flumazenil also competitively antagonizes the effects of the inverse agonists, because they also bind at the same allosteric site.

The last group of compounds that bind to the benzodiazepine site on the $GABA_A$ receptor include **zaleplon** and **zolpidem,** agents used to treat insomnia. These compounds are chemically unrelated to the benzodiazepines but are sometimes termed benzodiazepine agonists because they bind to the same site as the benzodiazepines on the $GABA_A$ receptor. However, these compounds have a different pharmacological profile than the benzodiazepines because they bind only to a subset of $GABA_A$ receptor subtypes containing a specific subunit composition, whereas the benzodiazepines bind to all these receptors irrespective of their subunit composition (see Relation of Mechanisms of Action to Clinical Response). A summary of the mechanisms of action of compounds affecting the $GABA_A$ receptor is presented in Table 24-1.

Buspirone

Buspirone is a member of a new series of anti-anxiety drugs unrelated chemically to the benzodiazepines or the barbiturates. Buspirone is as effective as the benzodiazepines as an anxiolytic but does not have anticonvulsant, muscle relaxant, or sedative effects. Buspirone is a partial agonist at serotonin $5\text{-}HT_{1A}$ receptors, and it is currently thought that this action mediates its anxiolytic effects. Buspirone has no affinity for either GABA or benzodiazepine binding sites on $GABA_A$ receptors but has moderate affinity for dopamine D_2 receptors. This is why buspirone was initially investigated as a possible treatment for schizophrenia. While it was not effective for psychosis, it decreased symptoms of anxiety. For that reason it has been used in the treatment of anxiety, even though the role of D_2 receptors in anxiety is unclear.

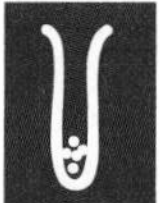

Pharmacokinetics

In general, the benzodiazepines are well absorbed after oral administration and reach peak blood and brain concentrations within 1 to 2 hours. Clorazepate is an exception, because it is the only benzodiazepine that is rapidly converted in the stomach to the active product N-desmethyldiazepam. The rate of conversion of clorazepate is inversely proportional to gastric pH.

The duration of action of the benzodiazepines varies considerably, and the formation of active metabolites plays a major role in their effects (Table 24-2). Diazepam, chlordiazepoxide, and lorazepam are available for injection. Lorazepam is well absorbed following intramuscular injection, but absorption of diazepam and chlordiazepoxide is poor and erratic

Table 24-1 Agents affecting the $GABA_A$ receptor

Site of Action	Compound	Mechanism	Action
GABA binding site	GABA	Agonist	Promotes chloride influx Hyperpolarization
	Muscimol	Agonist	Promotes chloride influx Hyperpolarization
	Bicuculline	Competitive antagonist	Blocks effects of GABA
Benzodiazepine binding site	Benzodiazepines	Allosteric agonist	Potentiates effects of GABA
	β-Carboline	Allosteric inverse agonist	Inhibits effects of GABA Inhibits effects of benzodiazepines
	Flumazenil	Competitive antagonist	Blocks effects of benzodiazepines
	Zolpidem Zaleplon	Subtype-selective benzodiazepine agonists	Potentiates effects of GABA at specific receptor subtypes
Barbiturate binding site	Barbiturate	Allosteric agonist	Potentiates effects of GABA
Chloride Channel	Picrotoxin	Noncompetitive antagonist	Blocks chloride influx

following intramuscular injection and should be avoided. When administered intravenously as an anticonvulsant or for induction of anesthesia, diazepam enters the brain rapidly and is redistributed into peripheral tissues, providing CNS depression for less than 2 hours. In contrast, lorazepam is less lipid soluble and depresses brain function for as long as 8 hours after intravenous injection.

The benzodiazepines and their active metabolites are highly bound to plasma proteins, being greatest for diazepam (99%) and lowest for alprazolam (70%). The distribution of diazepam and other benzodiazepines is complicated somewhat by a considerable degree of biliary excretion, which occurs early in their distribution. This enterohepatic recirculation occurs with metabolites as well as parent compounds and may be important clinically for compounds with a long elimination half-life. The presence of food in the upper bowel delays reabsorption and contributes to the late resurgence of plasma drug levels and activity.

Table 24-2 Pharmacokinetic parameters for representative benzodiazepines following oral administration

Drug	Onset of Action*	Half-Life†
Alprazolam	Intermediate	Intermediate
Chlordiazepoxide	Intermediate	Long
Clorazepate	Rapid	Long
Diazepam‡	Rapid	Long
Flurazepam	Rapid	Long
Halazepam	Intermediate	Long
Lorazepam‡	Intermediate	Intermediate
Oxazepam	Slow	Short
Prazepam	Slow	Long
Temazepam	Slow	Intermediate
Triazolam	Rapid	Short

*Rapid = 15-30 min; Intermediate = 30-45 min; Slow = 45-90 min.
†Short, <10 hours; Intermediate, 10-36 hours; Long >48 hours.
‡Also administered by injection.

The benzodiazepines are metabolized extensively by the hepatic cytochrome P450 system (Fig. 24-2). The major biotransformation reactions are N-dealkylation and aliphatic hydroxylation, followed by conjugation to inactive glucuronides that are excreted in the urine. The long-acting benzodiazepines clorazepate, diazepam, chlordiazepoxide, prazepam, and halazepam are dealkylated to the active compound N-desmethyldiazepam (nordiazepam). This compound has an elimination half-life of 30 to 200 hours and is responsible for the long duration of action of these compounds. N-desmethyldiazepam is hydroxylated to oxazepam, which forms a glucuronide conjugate. Alprazolam undergoes hydroxylation followed by glucuronidation, and lorazepam is directly glucuronidated.

Flurazepam is a long-acting drug that is converted to desalkylflurazepam, a long-acting active metabolite. Relatively little flurazepam and desalkylflurazepam are excreted unchanged in urine, as they are biotransformed in the liver. Hence their elimination half-lives in young adults is long and is even longer in older patients and those with liver disease.

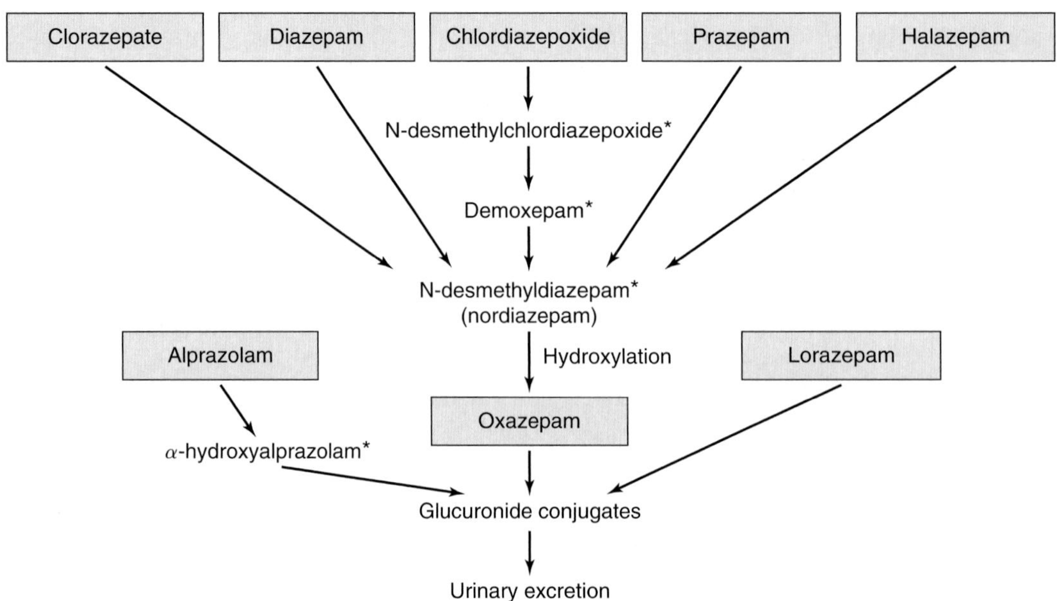

Figure 24-2 Major metabolic interrelationships among the benzodiazepines. *Active metabolite.

The subtype-selective benzodiazepine receptor agonists zolpidem and zaleplon have short elimination half-lives of 2.5 and 1 hour, respectively. They are metabolized extensively, and the inactive metabolites are excreted as glucuronides.

Buspirone is rapidly absorbed and undergoes extensive first-pass metabolism. It is highly bound to plasma proteins and oxidized to an active metabolite. The elimination half-life is about 2 to 3 hours, and less than 50% of the drug is excreted in the urine unchanged.

Flumazenil is administered intravenously and has a very short duration of action. It is metabolized by the liver and excreted in the urine with a half-life of approximately 1 hour. Its antagonist activity is manifest within 1 to 2 minutes, a peak effect is seen in 6 to10 minutes, and its duration of action is about 1 hour.

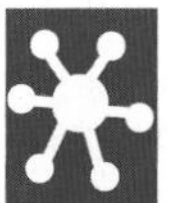

Relation of mechanisms of action to clinical response

All the effects of the benzodiazepines are a consequence of their actions in the CNS to enhance GABAergic neurotransmission and thereby cause CNS depression.

Anxiety is managed effectively with the benzodiazepines—particularly alprazolam, lorazepam, and clonazepam. Their intermittent use for acute attacks or limited long-term use (4-8 weeks) for recurring symptoms is often beneficial. However, all benzodiazepines should be used cautiously in patients with a history of addiction or more-chronic and severe emotional disturbances. Panic attacks respond favorably to alprazolam, which has been shown to possess antidepressant activity similar to the tricyclic antidepressants, which are also used for treatment of panic attacks (see Chapter 23). A debilitating anxiety secondary to another illness can be controlled by short-term treatment with anxiolytic drugs while treatment for the primary condition is implemented.

Buspirone offers an attractive alternative to benzodiazepines for the long-term therapy of less-severe and longer-term forms of anxiety such as generalized anxiety disorder. It produces little sedation and does not produce physical or psychological dependence. This makes buspirone especially useful in patients with a history of substance abuse or dependence. However, the onset of its anxiolytic activity is delayed, making it less suitable for control of an acute anxiety attack. Buspirone is indicated for the management of generalized anxiety disorder and may be more effective than benzodiazepines for chronic states of anxiety in which irritability and hostility are manifest. However, patient compliance is often poor, especially in individuals who have been treated previously with benzodiazepines.

In addition to the benzodiazepines, buspirone, and the antidepressants, β-adrenergic receptor blockers such as propranolol (see Chapter 10) are useful for treatment of performance anxiety or "stage fright." These compounds are effective in suppressing the somatic and autonomic symptoms of anxiety but do not alter emotional symptoms. The α_2-adrenergic receptor agonist, clonidine, has also been reported to have anxiolytic properties.

Sedation is the most common effect of the benzodiazepines, and its intensity and duration depend on the dose and concentration of drug in plasma and brain. Although flurazepam, temazepam, and triazolam are used for treatment of insomnia, they may lead to daytime sedation because of their long duration of action. Oxazepam has a shorter duration of action and would be less likely to cause this problem. The benzodiazepines decrease the latency of sleep onset (time to go to sleep), increase the amount of time spent in stage 2 sleep, and increase total sleep time. However, REM sleep, as well as stage 4 (slow wave) sleep are depressed. If the benzodiazepines are discontinued, a rebound increased REM sleep occurs, characterized by "bizarre" dreams. Tolerance occurs to the sedative but not the anxiolytic effect of the benzodiazepines.

The subtype-selective benzodiazepine agonists zaleplon and zolpidem, which are chemically unrelated to the benzodiazepines, produce sedation without anxiolytic, anticonvulsant, or muscle relaxant effects. They have been shown to be highly efficacious for the treatment of transient and chronic insomnia. These compounds decrease sleep latency and increase total sleep time without affecting REM sleep. In patients who often need to ambulate in the night, zaleplon is often preferred because of its shorter duration of action; it causes less confusion and less somnolence on awakening. Other compounds used for insomnia include the antihistamines hydroxyzine and diphenhydramine (see Chapter 54). The antihistamines do not exhibit cross-tolerance with the benzodiazepines and do not produce physical or psychological dependence.

Owing to their ability to produce sedation and anterograde amnesia and reduce the anxiety, stress, and tension associated with surgical or diagnostic procedures, benzodiazepines are used both as preanesthetic medications and for induction and maintenance of anesthesia (see Chapter 28). For procedures that do not require anesthesia—such as endoscopy, cardioversion, cardiac catheterization, specific radiodiagnostic procedures, and reduction of minor fractures—benzodiazepines may be administered orally, intramuscularly, or intravenously.

The benzodiazepines produce skeletal muscle relaxation by inhibiting polysynaptic reflexes. However, most evidence suggests that, with the exception of diazepam, skeletal muscle relaxation occurs only with doses of the benzodiazepines that have significant CNS depressant effects. Diazepam has a direct depressant effect on monosynaptic reflex pathways in the spinal cord and thus produces skeletal muscle relaxation at doses that do not induce sedation. This effect renders diazepam of benefit for relief of skeletal muscle spasms, spasticity, and athetosis.

In addition to these major indications, the benzodiazepines have also been found to be of use for treatment of alcohol withdrawal. Because the benzodiazepines exhibit cross-tolerance with alcohol, have anticonvulsant activity, and do not have major respiratory depressant effects, they have become the drugs of choice for treatment of acute alcohol withdrawal symptoms. In particular, chlordiazepoxide, lorazepam, diazepam, and oxazepam have now replaced other sedatives for this purpose. Choosing between these medications for alcohol withdrawal is often based on metabolic considerations. If a patient has hepatic impairment, lorazepam or oxazepam are often preferred to treat the symptoms of alcohol withdrawal, as they are metabolized in both liver and kidney. If hepatic dysfunction is not an issue, the use of drugs primarily metabolized by the liver (such as chlordiazepoxide and diazepam) would be appropriate.

Although all benzodiazepines act at benzodiazepine binding sites on $GABA_A$ receptors, they differ in their pharmacological profiles. For example, some anxiolytic benzodiazepines are non-sedating, while other benzodiazepines are used selectively for their sedative properties. Similarly, the incidence of muscle relaxation differs among compounds, and not all benzodiazepines have anticonvulsant activity. Such differences may be attributed to two primary factors, the type of $GABA_A$ receptor involved and the nature of the interaction of the benzodiazepine with its binding site.

Current evidence indicates that multiple $GABA_A$ receptors exist in the brain. These receptors have different subunit compositions as well as different anatomical distributions. Studies have shown that receptors containing α_2 subunits may mediate anxiolytic effects of the benzodiazepines, whereas other effects (sedation, skeletal muscle relaxation) may be mediated by receptors containing α_1 subunits. This may explain why zolpidem and zaleplon, which have full agonist activity at receptors containing α_1 subunits, are sedating but not anxiolytic.

In addition to receptor subtype selectivity, the divergent pharmacological and behavioral profiles of the benzodiazepines may be explained on the basis of differences in intrinsic efficacy. The benzodiazepines exhibit a broad range of intrinsic efficacies, and studies have shown that partial agonists with anxiolytic and anticonvulsant activities are non-sedating and do not cause muscle relaxation. Thus, as we learn more about benzodiazepine receptor subtypes and the nature of the interactions between these receptors and drugs, therapeutic compounds with selective and specific pharmacological and behavioral profiles may be developed.

As mentioned, flumazenil is a competitive antagonist at benzodiazepine receptors and is approved for use to reverse the sedative effects of the benzodiazepines following overdose, anesthesia, or sedation for brief surgical or diagnostic procedures. Flumazenil does not have any activity on its own and does not antagonize the effects of the opioids, non-benzodiazepine sedatives, or anesthetic agents. In addition, although flumazenil can antagonize the sedative effects of the benzodiazepines, it may not be effective in reversing respiratory depression. Flumazenil is of great benefit in cases of overdose, and it has been reported that in unconscious adults, flumazenil causes regaining of consciousness sufficient such that gastric lavage, bladder catheterization, electroencephalography, and other procedures could be avoided.

Side effects, clinical problems, and toxicity

Systemic effects

The adverse reactions most frequently encountered with benzodiazepine use are an extension of their CNS depressant effects and include sedation, lightheadedness, ataxia, and lethargy. The mild sedative actions of these drugs vary quantitatively. For example, lorazepam has a prolonged sedative action compared with the other benzodiazepines, even though it clears the body rapidly. Occasional reactions observed with hypnotic doses of the benzodiazepines include impaired mental and psychomotor function, confusion, euphoria, delayed reaction time, uncoordinated motor function, dysarthria, headache, and xerostomia. Rare reactions may include syncope, hypotension, blurred vision, altered libido, skin rashes, nausea, menstrual irregularities, agranulocytosis, lupus-like syndrome, edema, and constipation.

Anterograde memory disturbances have been observed in patients taking diazepam, chlordiazepoxide, and lorazepam. Thus, patients cannot recall information acquired after drug administration. This effect has been attributed to interference with the memory consolidation process and may be beneficial when the benzodiazepines are administered parenterally for presurgical or diagnostic procedures such as endoscopy. In this situation, patients should be warned of this effect, especially if they are being treated on an outpatient basis. When administered orally, most benzodiazepines do not cause this effect.

Adverse reactions associated with the intravenous use of benzodiazepines include pain during injection, thrombophlebitis, hypothermia, restlessness, cardiac arrhythmias, coughing, apnea, vomiting, and a mild anticholinergic effect. Deaths from overdose rarely occur. Patients have taken as much as 50 times the therapeutic doses of benzodiazepines without causing mortality. This particular property of these drugs is another example of how they differ from the potent respiratory depressant sedatives and hypnotics. Unlike the barbiturates, the benzodiazepines have only a mild effect on respiration when given orally, even with toxic doses. However, when they are administered parenterally or are taken in conjunction with other depressants such as alcohol, all benzodiazepines have the potential of causing significant respiratory depression and death.

Adverse reactions of buspirone include dizziness, drowsiness, dry mouth, headaches, nervousness, fatigue, insomnia, weakness, lightheadedness, and muscle spasms.

The most frequent side effects associated with the use of both zolpidem and zaleplon are headache and dizziness. In addition, zaleplon may cause back and chest pain, migraines, anticholinergic gastrointestinal effects, nervousness, and difficulty concentrating. Zolpidem appears devoid of these effects, but its use may lead to confusion and ataxia. There have also been reports of zolpidem inducing delirium, psychotic reactions, and nightmares.

Drug withdrawal and dependence

The benzodiazepines are well known to produce physical dependence, and withdrawal reactions ensue upon abrupt discontinuation. However, the dependence associated with the benzodiazepines is not the same as that observed with alcohol, narcotics, or the barbiturates. Although physical dependence is more likely to occur with high drug doses and long-term treatment, it has also been reported after usual therapeutic regimens. The onset of withdrawal symptoms is related to the elimination half-life and is more rapid in onset and more severe after discontinuation of the shorter-acting benzodiazepines such as oxazepam, lorazepam, and alprazolam. With the longer-acting benzodiazepines, the onset of withdrawal is much slower because of their longer half-lives and slower disappearance from the plasma. Therefore, doses of the benzodiazepines with short half-lives should be decreased more gradually. In addition, alprazolam, estazolam, and triazolam, which have a chemical structure (triazolo ring) that differs from the other benzodiazepines and are referred to as triazolobenzodiazepines, cause more serious withdrawal reactions than the other compounds.

The withdrawal symptoms accompanying abrupt discontinuation from the benzodiazepines are generally autonomic and include tremor, sweating, insomnia, abdominal discomfort, tachycardia, systolic hypertension, muscle twitching, and sensitivity to light and sound. In rare instances, severe withdrawal reactions may develop, characterized by convulsions. These reactions are usually manifest in individuals maintained on high doses of the benzodiazepines for prolonged (more than 4 months) periods of time. In addition to these autonomic manifestations, abrupt withdrawal of benzodiazepines can often cause patients to "rebound," exhibiting symptoms of anxiety and insomnia sometimes worse than before drug treatment was initiated.

The benzodiazepines have been reported to have a high abuse potential. However, evidence suggests that psychological dependence occurs mainly in people with a history of drug abuse; appropriate therapeutic use by persons not predisposed to drug abuse should not lead to abuse of the benzodiazepines.

The abuse liability of zaleplon and zolpidem is less than that of the benzodiazepines when used at the doses recommended. However, when used at higher doses, zolpidem may lead to some physical dependence, and abrupt discontinuation may lead to withdrawal, although less severe than that observed with the benzodiazepines.

When administered chronically, buspirone causes less tolerance and potential for abuse than the other compounds and does not produce a rebound effect after discontinuation.

Adverse reactions to flumazenil include nausea, dizziness, headache, blurred vision, increased sweating, and anxiety. In addition, panic attacks have been reported to occur in some patients. Flumazenil can precipitate convulsions in individuals physically dependent on benzodiazepines as well as in patients maintained on benzodiazepines for seizure disorders. Flumazenil must be used with caution in patients taking benzodiazepines and tricyclic antidepressants, because it may antagonize the anticonvulsant effect of the benzodiazepines and unmask the epileptogenic effect of the tricyclic antidepressant. Cardiac arrhythmias have been reported in some instances.

Drug interactions

The benzodiazepines and the subtype-selective benzodiazepine agonists are powerful CNS depressants, and additive effects are apparent when they are administered with other CNS depressants. These include ethanol, antihistamines, other sedative/hypnotic agents, antipsychotics, antidepressants, and narcotic analgesics. Because ethanol is readily available and widely used, the CNS depressant interaction between the benzodiazepines and subtype-selective benzodiazepine agonists and ethanol is common. Individuals may experience episodes of mild to severe ataxia and "drunkenness" that severely retards performance levels. No single compound is considered safer than another in combination with ethanol. Therefore it is imperative that physicians caution their patients not to drink alcoholic beverages while taking these compounds. This is especially important for patients not exposed previously to the benzodiazepines. Individuals who have been drinking alcohol and taking benzodiazepines for long periods of time experience this interaction, but to a milder degree.

Another drug interaction is a consequence of the biotransformation of the benzodiazepines. Because many of the benzodiazepines are metabolized by the hepatic P450 system, therapeutic agents that inhibit P450s decrease the biotransformation of the long-acting compounds. The histamine (H_2) receptor antagonist cimetidine, as well as oral contraceptives, prolong the elimination half-life of the benzodiazepines by inhibiting their metabolism. Cisapride is a potent inhibitor of *CYP3A4* and can cause significant increases in blood levels of many medications, including alprazolam, midazolam, and triazolam. Conversely, compounds that induce this enzyme, such as the barbiturates and carbamazepine, increase their rate of metabolism. Of course, the biotransformation of benzodiazepines that proceed by a route other than hepatic oxidation is unaltered. Although the benzodiazepines are biotransformed via P450s, they do not significantly induce P450 activity and do not accelerate the metabolism of other agents biotransformed via this system.

Contraindications and precautions

As with any drug or class of drugs, the benzodiazepines should be avoided in patients with a known hypersensitivity to these agents. Alprazolam, clorazepate, diazepam, halazepam, lorazepam, and prazepam are contraindicated in individuals with acute narrow-angle glaucoma because of their anticholinergic side effects. In addition, because of the considerable lipid solubility of most benzodiazepines, they cross the placenta and are secreted in mother's milk. It should be noted that the benzodiazepines may be teratogenic and should be avoided in pregnant and nursing women.

Again, because of the hepatic biotransformation of these compounds, special care must be taken when prescribing benzodiazepines for individuals with hepatic dysfunction and for the elderly and debilitated population. These patients generally have a diminished liver detoxifying capacity and often show cumulative toxicity in response to the usual adult dosage, especially of agents metabolized to active metabolites with long half-lives (diazepam, chlordiazepoxide). The elderly are also more prone to acute depression of attention, alertness, motor dexterity, and sensory acuity as well as memory disturbance and confusion. For this reason, doses in the elderly should be started at 25% of the usual adult dose and administered less frequently.

As with other psychoactive medications, precautions should be given with respect to administration of the drug and the amount of the prescription for severely depressed patients or for those in whom there is reason to expect concealed suicidal ideation or plans.

Clinical problems associated with the use of these compounds are summarized in the Clinical Problems box.

CLINICAL PROBLEMS

Benzodiazepines and subtype-selective agonists

Sedation, lightheadedness, ataxia, lethargy
Anterograde amnesia
Addiction liability, physical dependence
Potentiates alcohol intoxication
Rebound anxiety

Buspirone

Dizziness, drowsiness, dry mouth, headaches
Delay in anxiolytic effect

New horizons

It is obvious that there is a need for newer, better-tolerated, and more efficacious treatments for anxiety and insomnia, especially drugs without abuse potential.

To this end, our understanding of the role of different $GABA_A$ receptor subtypes in the brain is of paramount importance. If each of the pharmacological actions of the benzodiazepines could be ascribed to a specific receptor subtype, then it may be possible to develop compounds with selective actions on these receptors.

Additional approaches to the development of newer compounds depend on our understanding the molecular and cellular events mediating the pathophysiology of stress and stress-related disorders. During the past several years, studies have suggested that the ability to cope with stress involves corticotrophin-releasing factor signaling pathways and that these peptides and their receptors play a major role in generating stress responses. This may represent a new target for development of anxiolytic compounds.

Similarly, as more is learned about the cellular and molecular events regulating specific functional pathways in the brain, research should provide better agents to treat sleep disorders. Sleep-promoting fatty acid amides, neurosteroids, prostaglandins, and peptides are of special interest. New sleep-promoting treatments promise to be more selective in producing natural sleep without disturbing the normal sleep cycle.

TRADE NAMES

In addition to generic and fixed-combination preparations and the drugs listed in the Major Drugs box, the following trade-named materials are some of the important compounds available in the United States.

Clorazepate (Tranxene)
Estazolam (ProSom)
Halazepam (Paxipam)
Prazepam (Centrax)
Quazepam (Doral)

FURTHER READING

Argyropoulos SV, Sandford JJ, Nutt DJ. The psychobiology of anxiolytic drugs. Part 2: pharmacological treatments of anxiety. *Pharmacol Therap* 2000; 88:213-227.

Drugs for Psychiatric Disorders: treatment guidelines. *Med Lett* 2003; 1:69-76.

Littner M, Johnson SF, McCall WV, et al. Practice parameters for the treatment of narcolepsy: an update for 2000. *Sleep* 2001; 24:451-66.

Self-assessment questions

1. The proposed mechanism of CNS depression by benzodiazepines is:

a. A decreased release of norepinephrine from brain locus coeruleus neurons.
b. A decreased Na^+ ion influx at channels located in neuronal postsynaptic membranes.
c. A facilitated $GABA_A$-receptor activity to open chloride ion channels.
d. An antagonist activity at excitatory glutamate receptors.
e. None of the above.

2. Which of the following is least sedative, will NOT potentiate the effects of alcohol, and has no appreciable dependence liability?

a. Chlordiazepoxide
b. Amobarbital
c. Alprazolam
d. Meprobamate
e. Buspirone

3. The mechanism of anxiolytic activity of buspirone is proposed to relate to:

a. A direct action on chloride channels to enhance hyperpolarizing effects at brain inhibitory synapses.
b. A decrease in muscarinic cholinergic function in the brain "punishment" regions.
c. A partial agonist activity at brain $5\text{-}HT_{1A}$ receptors.
d. An agonist activity at brain adrenergic receptors.
e. An antagonist activity at brain dopaminergic receptors.

4. Diazepam resembles other general CNS-depressant drugs in:

a. Promoting psychological dependence.
b. Leading to the development of seizures on sudden withdrawal after long-term treatment with large doses.
c. Demonstrating a cross-dependence pattern to alcohol.
d. All of the above are correct.
e. a and c are correct.

5. Tolerance develops fairly rapidly to most effects of the benzodiazepines, *except* for:

a. Anxiety.
b. Anticonvulsant activity.
c. Sedation.
d. Motor relaxation.
e. None of the above.

CHAPTER 25

Ethanol and related compounds

Richard A. Deitrich
John D. Palmer

Major Drugs	
Disulfiram (Antabuse)	Naltrexone (ReVia)

Therapeutic overview

Ethanol belongs to a class of compounds known as the central nervous system (CNS) depressants that includes the barbiturate and nonbarbiturate sedative/hypnotics, as well as the benzodiazepines. Although these latter compounds are used for their sedative and anxiolytic properties, ethanol is not prescribed for these purposes. Rather, ethanol is used primarily as a social drug, with only limited application as a therapeutic agent. It has been used by injection to produce irreversible nerve block or tumor destruction and is effective for treatment of **methanol** and **ethylene glycol** poisonings, because it can inhibit competitively the metabolism of these alcohols to toxic intermediates.

In cultures in which ethanol use is accepted, the substance is misused and abused by a fraction of the population and is associated with social, medical, and economic problems, including life-threatening damage to most major organ systems and **psychological** and **physical dependence** in people who use it excessively. It is estimated that in the U.S., 65% to 70% of the population uses ethanol and more than 10 million individuals are alcohol-dependent. An additional 10 million are subject to negative consequences of alcohol abuse such as arrests, automobile accidents, violence, occupational injuries, and deleterious effects on job performance and health. About 50% of all traffic deaths are estimated to involve alcohol, and the annual cost of alcohol-related problems in the United States is over $180 billion. In the primary care setting, about 15% of patients exhibit an "at risk" pattern of alcohol use or an alcohol-related health problem. A medical history designed to elicit information on alcohol use is an essential feature of a modern medical work-up. Clearly, alcohol abuse is a significant public health problem.

This chapter covers the behavioral and toxicological problems associated with the use of ethanol and reviews the deleterious effects of other alcohols. The pharmacology of the benzodiazepines is presented in Chapter 24 and that of the barbiturates in Chapters 27 and 28. General issues related to abuse of CNS depressants are in Chapter 32.

Abbreviations	
ADH	alcohol dehydrogenase
ALDH	aldehyde dehydrogenase
BAC	blood alcohol concentration
CNS	central nervous system
GABA	γ-aminobutyric acid
GI	gastrointestinal
5-HT	serotonin
NAD	nicotinamide adenine dinucleotide
NADH	nicotinamide adenine dinucleotide, reduced
NADPH	nicotinamide adenine dinucleotide phosphate, reduced

The uses of ethanol and treatment of ethanol abuse are summarized in the Therapeutic Overview box.

THERAPEUTIC OVERVIEW

Ethanol is used:
- Topically to reduce body temperature and as an antiseptic
- By injection to produce irreversible nerve block by protein denaturation
- By inhalation to reduce foaming in pulmonary edema
- In treatment of methanol and ethylene glycol poisoning

Ethanol abuse may be treated with:
- Psychotherapy
- Disulfiram
- Naltrexone

Mechanisms of action of ethanol

For many years alcohol and the general anesthetic agents were assumed to share a common mechanism of action, requiring millimolar concentrations for either to produce effects and an excellent correlation between their oil:water partition coefficients and their ability to depress the CNS (Chapter 28). Before the advent of ether, ethanol was used as an "anesthetic" agent for surgical procedures. Pharmacological and genetic evidence also indicated that ethanol, like general anesthetics, "fluidizes" or "disorders" the physical structure of cell membranes, particularly those low in cholesterol. This idea was supported by studies indicating that neuronal cell membranes from mice tolerant or genetically resistant to the effects of ethanol are not readily disordered by ethanol, whereas those from mice sensitive to ethanol are more easily fluidized.

Ethanol may interfere with the packing of molecules in the phospholipid bilayer of the cell membrane, increasing membrane fluidity. However, this bulk fluidizing effect is small and probably not responsible primarily for its CNS depressant effects. Nevertheless, it may play a role in disrupting membranes surrounding neurotransmitter receptors or ion channels. Ethanol has been shown to affect most ion channels and receptors, and recent evidence indicates that ethanol binds directly to lipophilic areas either near or in receptor proteins.

Table 25-1 Ion channels functionally affected by ethanol

Channel	Effects	Ethanol Concentration (mM)
Sodium (voltage-gated)	Inhibited	100 and higher*
Potassium (voltage-gated)	Facilitated	50-100
Calcium (voltage-gated)	Inhibited	50 and higher
Calcium (glutamate-activated)	Inhibited	20-50
Chloride (GABA-gated)	Facilitated	10-50
Chloride (glycine-gated)	Facilitated	10-50
Sodium-potassium ($5HT_3$-gated)	Facilitated	10-50

*100 mM ethanol is 460 mg/dl.

The ion channels influenced by ethanol are listed in Table 25-1. Ethanol may have either inhibitory or facilitatory effects, depending on the channel, but its resultant action is CNS depression. Because the barbiturates and benzodiazepines exhibit cross-tolerance to ethanol, and their CNS depressant effects are additive with those of ethanol, they may share a common mechanism, perhaps through the γ-aminobutyric acid (GABA) $GABA_A$-benzodiazepine-chloride channel complex (Chapter 24). Ethanol may also exert some of its effects by inhibition of NMDA glutamate receptors or activation of serotonin (5-HT) $5\text{-}HT_3$ receptors.

Animal studies have shown that low concentrations of ethanol promote activation of G_s, enhancing adenylyl cyclase activity (Chapter 2). Whether this plays an important role in the CNS effects of ethanol is not known, but it has been suggested that this may provide a biochemical marker of a genetic predisposition to alcoholism.

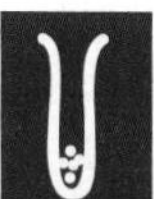

Pharmacokinetics

Ethanol

Alcohol taken orally is absorbed throughout the gastrointestinal (GI) tract. Absorption depends on passive diffusion and is governed by the concentration gradient and the mucosal surface area. Food in the stomach will dilute the alcohol and delay gastric emptying time, thereby retarding absorption from the small intestine (where absorption is favored because of the large surface area). High ethanol concentrations in the GI tract cause a greater concentration gradient and therefore hasten absorption. Absorption continues until the alcohol concentration in the blood and GI tract are at

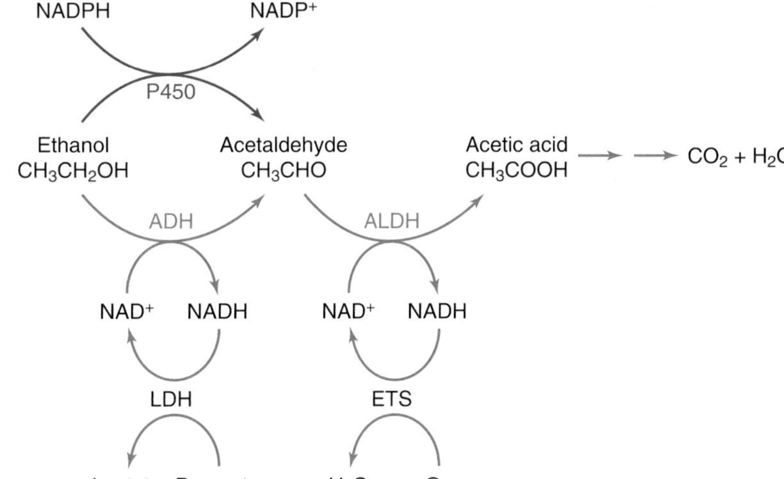

Figure 25-1 Metabolism of ethanol by ADH, ALDH and cytochrome P450. *ETS,* Electron transport system; *LDH,* lactate dehydrogenase.

equilibrium. Because ethanol is rapidly metabolized and removed from the blood, eventually all the alcohol is absorbed.

Once ethanol reaches the systemic circulation, it is distributed to all body compartments at a rate proportional to blood flow to that area; its distribution approximates that of total body water. Because the brain receives a high blood flow, high concentrations of ethanol occur rapidly in the brain.

Ethanol undergoes significant first-pass metabolism. Most (>90%) of the ethanol ingested is metabolized in the liver, with the remainder excreted through the lungs and in urine. **Alcohol dehydrogenase** (ADH) oxidizes ethanol to acetaldehyde, which is oxidized further by **aldehyde dehydrogenase** (ALDH) to acetate (Fig. 25-1). Acetate is oxidized primarily in peripheral tissues to CO_2 and H_2O. Both ADH and ALDH require the reduction of nicotinamide adenine dinucleotide (NAD^+), with 1 mole of ethanol producing 2 moles of reduced NAD^+ (NADH). The NADH is reoxidized to NAD^+ by conversion of pyruvate to lactate by lactate dehydrogenase and the mitochondrial electron transport system. During ethanol oxidation, the concentration of NADH can rise substantially, and NADH product inhibition can become rate-limiting. Similarly, with large amounts of ethanol, NAD^+ may become depleted, limiting further oxidation through this pathway. At typical blood alcohol concentrations (BACs), the metabolism of ethanol exhibits zero-order kinetics—that is, it is independent of concentration and occurs at a relatively constant rate (Fig. 25-2). Fasting decreases liver ADH activity, decreasing ethanol metabolism.

Ethanol may also be metabolized to acetaldehyde in the liver by cytochrome P450, a reaction that requires 1 molecule of reduced nicotinamide adenine dinucleotide phosphate (NADPH) for every ethanol molecule (see Fig. 25-1). Although P450-mediated oxidation does not normally play a significant role, it is important with high concentrations of ethanol (≥100 mg/dl), which saturate ADH and deplete NAD^+. Because this enzyme system also metabolizes other compounds, ethanol may alter their metabolism. In addition, this system may be inhibited or induced (Chapter 3), and induction by ethanol may contribute to the oxidative stress of chronic alcohol consumption by releasing reactive oxygen species during metabolism.

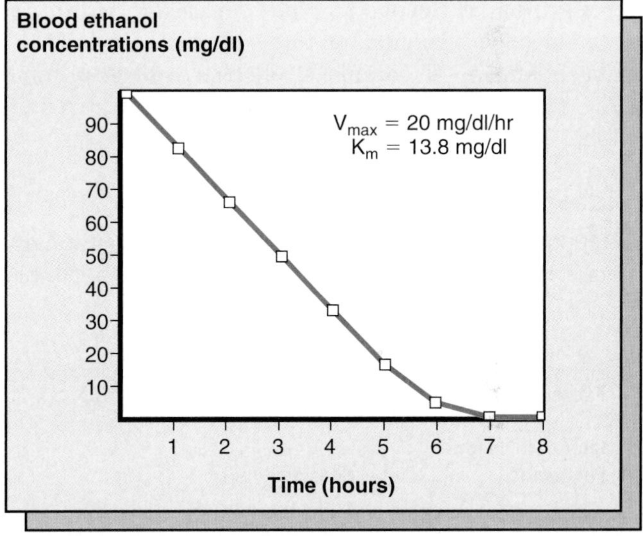

Figure 25-2 Disappearance of ethanol after oral ingestion follows zero-order kinetics.

A third system capable of metabolizing ethanol is a peroxidative reaction mediated by catalase, a system limited by the amount of hydrogen peroxide available, which is normally low. Small amounts of ethanol are also metabolized by formation of phosphatidylethanol and ethyl esters of fatty acids. The significance of these pathways is unknown.

Significant genetic differences exist for both ADH and ALDH that affect the rate of ethanol metabolism. Several forms of ADH exist in human liver with differing affinities for ethanol. Caucasians, Asians, and African-Americans express different relative percentages of the genes and their respective alleles that encode subunits of ADH, contributing to racial differences in the rate of ethanol metabolism. Similarly, there are genetic differences in ALDH. About 50% of Asians have an inactive ALDH, caused by a single base change in the gene that renders them incapable of oxidizing acetaldehyde efficiently, especially if they are homozygous. When they consume ethanol, high concentrations of acetaldehyde are achieved, leading to flushing and other unpleasant effects. People with this condition rarely become alcoholic. The unpleasant effects of acetaldehyde accumulation forms the basis for the aversive treatment of chronic alcoholism with disulfiram. The pharmacokinetics of ethanol are summarized in Table 25-2.

Other alcohols

Methanol, which may be accidentally or intentionally ingested, is metabolized by ADH and ALDH in a manner similar to ethanol, but at a much slower rate, forming formaldehyde and formic acid. Because ethanol can compete with methanol for ADH and saturate the enzyme, ethanol can be used successfully for methanol intoxication.

The dihydric alcohol ethylene glycol, found in antifreeze products, and isopropyl or rubbing alcohol, are also metabolized by ADH; thus, ethanol can be used as a competitive antagonist for these compounds.

Table 25-2 Pharmacokinetic considerations of ethanol

Pharmacokinetic Parameter	Considerations
Route of administration	Topically, orally, inhalation, by injection into nerve trunks, or intravenously for poison management
Absorption	Slight topically Complete from stomach and intestine by passive diffusion Rapid via lungs
Distribution	Total body water; volume of distribution is 68% of body weight in men and 55% in women; varies widely
Metabolism	>90% to CO_2 and H_2O by liver and other tissues Follows zero-order kinetics Rate is about 100 mg/kg/hr of total body burden; higher or lower with hepatic enzyme induction or disease
Elimination	Excreted in expired air, urine, milk, sweat

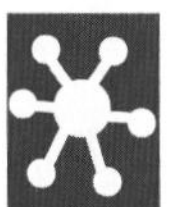

Relation of mechanisms of action to clinical response

Behavior

Like general anesthetics and most CNS depressants, ethanol decreases the function of inhibitory centers in the brain. This releases normal mechanisms controlling social functioning and behavior, leading to an initial excitation. Thus ethanol is described as a **disinhibitor** or **euphoriant.** The higher integrative areas are affected first, with thought processes, fine discrimination, judgment, and motor function impaired sequentially. These effects may be observed with BACs of 0.05% or lower. Specific behavioral changes are difficult to predict and depend to a large extent on the environment and the personality of the individual. As BACs increase to 100 mg/dl, errors in judgment are frequent, motor systems are impaired, and responses to complex auditory and visual stimuli are altered. Patterns of involuntary motor action are also affected. Ataxia is noticeable, with walking becoming difficult and staggering common as the BAC approaches 0.15% to 0.2%. Reaction times are increased and the person may become extremely loud, incoherent, and emotionally unstable. Violent behavior may occur. These effects are the result of depression of excitatory areas of the brain. At BACs of 0.2% to 0.3%, intoxicated people may experience periods of amnesia or "blackout" and fail to recall events occurring at that time.

Anesthesia occurs when BAC increases to 0.25% to 0.30%. Ethanol shares many properties with general anesthetics but is less safe because of its low therapeutic index (see Chapter 2). It is also a poor analgesic. Coma in humans occurs with BAC above 0.3%, and the lethal range for ethanol, in the absence of other CNS depressants, is 0.4% to 0.5%, though people with much higher concentrations have survived. Death from acute ethanol overdose is relatively rare compared with the frequency of death resulting from combinations of

Table 25-3 Physiological and behavioral states as a function of blood ethanol concentrations

Blood Ethanol Concentrations (mg/dl)	%	Reactions
0-50	0-0.05	Loss of inhibitions, excitement, incoordination, impaired judgment, slurred speech, body sway
50-100	0.05-0.1	Impaired reaction time, further impaired judgment, impaired driving ability, ataxia
100-200	0.1-0.2	Staggering gait, inability to operate a motor vehicle
200-300	0.2-0.3	Respiratory depression, danger of death in presence of other CNS depressants, blackouts
>300	>0.3	Unconsciousness, severe respiratory and cardiovascular depression, death
>1200	>1.2	Highest known blood concentration with survival in a chronic alcoholic

alcohol with other CNS depressants, such as barbiturates and benzodiazepines. Death is due to a depressant effect on the medulla, resulting in respiratory failure.

Physiological and behavioral changes as a function of BAC are summarized in Table 25-3.

Blood alcohol concentration

Measures of blood alcohol concentration (BAC) are important for providing adequate medical care to intoxicated individuals. BAC is calculated based on the amount of ethanol ingested, the percentage of alcohol in the beverage (usually volume/volume, with 100 proof equivalent to 50% ethanol by volume), and the density of 0.8 g for each milliliter of ethanol. BACs are expressed in a variety of ways. The legal limit for operating a motor vehicle in most states is 80 mg/dl or 0.08%. An example of a typical calculation for a 70 kg person ingesting 1 oz, or 30 ml, of 80 proof distilled spirits is as follows:

$$(80\text{ proof}/2 = 40\%)(30\text{ ml}) = 12\text{ ml } 100\% \text{ ethanol (by volume)}$$

$$(12\text{ ml})(0.8\text{ g/ml}) = 9.6\text{ g ethanol (by weight)}$$

If absorbed immediately and distributed in total body water (assuming blood is 80% water and body water content averages 55% of body weight in women and 68% in men):

$$\underset{(\text{male})}{\text{BAC}} = \frac{9.6\text{ g}}{(70\text{ kg})(0.68)} \times 0.8 = 0.16\text{ g/L}, 16\text{ mg/dl}, 0.016\%$$

$$\underset{(\text{female})}{\text{BAC}} = \frac{9.6\text{ g}}{(70\text{ kg})(0.55)} \times 0.8 = 0.2\text{ g/L}, 20\text{ mg/dl}, 0.02\%$$

The average rate at which ethanol is metabolized in non-tolerant individuals is 100 mg/kg body weight/hr, or 7 g/hr in a 70 kg person. Chronic alcoholics metabolize ethanol faster because of induction of P450s. In the calculation above, a male with a body burden of 9.6 g of ethanol would metabolize the alcohol totally in less than 2 hours.

Drinks in one hour

Body weight (pounds)	1	2	3	4	5
100	30	60	90	120	150
120	25	50	75	100	125
140	22	44	66	88	110
160	19	39	58	78	97
180	17	34	52	69	86
200	16	31	47	62	78

Blood alcohol concentration (BAC) mg/dl

Figure 25-3 Approximate percentages of ethanol in blood *(BAC)* in male subjects of different body weights, calculated as percentage, weight/volume (w/v), after indicated number of drinks. One drink is 12 oz of beer, 5 oz of wine, or 1 oz of 80 proof distilled spirits. People with BACs of 0.08% (80 mg/dl) or higher are considered intoxicated in most states; those with BACs of 0.05 to 0.079% (50-79 mg/dl) are considered impaired. *Light pink area,* impaired; *dark pink area,* legally intoxicated. BAC can be 20% to 30% higher in female subjects. Notice the small number of drinks that can result in a state of intoxication.

Figure 25-3 shows approximate maximum BACs in men of various body weights ingesting one to five drinks in one hour. Rapid absorption is assumed. This figure emphasizes how little consumption is required to impair motor skills and render a person unable to drive safely.

The BAC varies with hematocrit; that is, people living at higher altitudes have a higher hematocrit and a lower water content in blood. It is therefore essential to know whether the BAC was determined by using whole blood, serum, or plasma. Urine, cerebrospinal fluid, and vitreous concentrations of ethanol have also been used in estimating BAC.

Because expired air contains ethanol in proportion to its vapor pressure at body temperature, the ratio of ethanol concentrations between exhaled air and blood alcohol (1/2100) forms the basis for the breathalyzer test, in which BAC is extrapolated from the alcohol content of the expired air.

BACs can also be calculated from the weight and sex of the person if the amount of ethanol consumed orally is known. However, this estimate is somewhat higher than actual concentrations because of rapid first-pass metabolism following oral administration. BACs are higher in women than in men after consumption of comparable amounts of ethanol, even after correcting for differences in body weight. This can be attributed to both the volume of distribution and first-pass metabolism of ethanol in women. Women have a smaller volume of distribution than men because, on average, they have a greater percentage of adipose tissue that does not contain as much water as do other tissues. In addition, the first-pass metabolism of ethanol, which occurs primarily in gastric tissue, is less in women than men because ADH activity in the female gastric mucosa is less than that in the male. Thus, with low doses of ethanol, first-pass metabolism is lower in women, leading to higher BACs; at higher doses, the percentage of ethanol that undergoes first-pass metabolism is relatively small. Women are also more susceptible to alcoholic liver disease for this reason as well as a consequence of interactions with estrogen. This applies to both nonalcoholic and alcoholic women and partially explains the increased vulnerability of women to the deleterious effects of acute and chronic alcoholism. It was once assumed that higher BACs in women were entirely the result of differences in apparent volumes of distribution between men and women; however, they do not account entirely for this difference.

Side effects, clinical problems, and toxicity

Tissue-specific effects of ethanol

Ethanol has detrimental effects on many organs and tissues, and knowledge of these actions is important for understanding its hazards. Deleterious effects of ethanol on the liver and other organs resulting from chronic alcoholism are listed in the Clinical Problems box.

CLINICAL PROBLEMS

Effects of ethanol on the liver

Increased: $NADH/NAD^+$ ratio, acetaldehyde concentration, lipid content, protein accumulation, collagen deposition, cytochrome P450 content, oxygen uptake, production of free radicals and lipoperoxidation products

Decreased: protein export, production of coagulation factors, gluconeogenesis

Centrilobular hypoxia, proliferation of endoplasmic reticulum

Altered drug metabolism

Hepatitis, scarring, cirrhosis with portal hypertension, hepatocellular death

Effects of ethanol on other organs

Gastritis and GI tract bleeding

Peptic ulcer disease

Pancreatitis

Cardiomyopathy and cardiac dysrhythmias

Myopathy and peripheral neuropathy

Cancers of upper GI tract

Fetal alcohol syndrome

Wernicke-Korsakoff syndrome

The gastrointestinal tract The oral mucosa, esophagus, stomach, and small intestine are exposed to higher concentrations of ethanol than other tissues of the body and are susceptible to direct toxic effects. Acute gastritis resulting in nausea and vomiting results from ethanol abuse, and bleeding, ulcers, and cancer of the upper GI tract are possible consequences.

The liver Ethanol metabolism by the liver causes a large increase in the $NADH/NAD^+$ ratio, which disrupts liver metabolism. The cell attempts to maintain NAD^+ concentrations in the cytosol by reducing pyruvate to lactate, leading to increased lactic acid in liver and blood. Lactate is excreted by the kidney and competes with urate for elimination, which can increase blood urate concentrations. Excretion of lactate also apparently leads to a deficiency of zinc and magnesium. A more direct effect of increased NADH concentrations in the liver is increased fatty acid synthesis, because NADH is a necessary cofactor. Since NADH participates in the citric acid cycle, the oxidation of lipids is depressed, further contributing to fat accumulation in liver cells.

The increase in $NADH/NAD^+$ ratio and the inability to regenerate NAD^+ may cause hypoglycemia and ketoacidosis. The former occurs in the non-eating user of alcohol when hepatic glycogen stores are exhausted

(72 hours) and gluconeogenesis is inhibited as a result of the increased NADH/NAD$^+$ ratio. The metabolic acidosis observed in nondiabetic alcoholics is an anion gap acidosis, with an increase in the plasma concentration of β-hydroxybutyrate and lactate.

Acetaldehyde may also play a prominent role in liver damage. If there is an initial insult to the liver, the concentration of ALDH decreases and acetaldehyde is not removed efficiently and can react with many cell constituents. For example, acetaldehyde blocks transcriptional activation by peroxisome proliferator-activated receptor α. Normally, fatty acids activate this receptor, and this action of acetaldehyde may contribute to fatty acid accumulation in liver. Acetaldehyde also increases collagen in the liver.

During ethanol ingestion, the intestine releases increased amounts of lipopolysaccharide (endotoxin), which is taken up from the portal blood by the Kupffer cells of the liver. In response to this, these cells release tumor necrosis factor-alpha (TNF-α) as well as a host of other proinflammatory cytokines. In the face of depleted glutathione and S-adenosylmethionine, liver cells die. This process of secondary liver injury occurs over and above the primary liver injury caused directly by ethanol. In spite of this, there are many heavy drinkers who never develop severe liver damage, indicating a substantial genetic effect in producing alcoholic hepatic damage.

The use of acetaminophen by alcoholics may result in hepatic necrosis. This reaction can occur with acetaminophen doses that are less than the maximum recommended (4 g per 24 hours). Ethanol has this effect because it induces the cytochrome P450 responsible for formation of a hepatotoxic acetaminophen metabolite, which cannot be detoxified when glutathione stores are depleted by ethanol or starvation. This condition is characterized by greatly elevated serum aminotransferase concentrations. *N*-Acetylcysteine is given orally to provide the required glutathione substrate in such patients.

The pancreas Ethanol use is a known cause of acute pancreatitis, and repeated use can lead to chronic pancreatitis, with decreased enzyme secretion and diabetes mellitus as possible consequences.

The endocrine system Large amounts of ethanol decrease testosterone concentrations in males and cause a loss of secondary sex characteristics and feminization. Ovarian function may be disrupted in premenopausal females who abuse alcohol, and this may be manifest as oligomenorrhea, hypomenorrhea, or amenorrhea. Ethanol also stimulates release of adrenocortical hormones by increasing secretion of adrenocorticotropic hormone.

The cardiovascular system Alcoholic cardiomyopathy is a consequence of chronic ethanol consumption. Other cardiovascular effects include mild increases in blood pressure and heart rate, and cardiac dysrhythmias. Cardiovascular complications also result from hepatic cirrhosis and accompanying changes in the venous circulation that predispose to upper GI bleeding. Coagulopathy, secondary to hepatic dysfunction and bone marrow depression, increase the risk of bleeding.

Epidemiological studies have demonstrated an association between alcohol use and a reduced risk of cardiovascular disease, including nonfatal myocardial infarction and fatal coronary heart disease. Alcohol increases the levels of high-density lipoprotein cholesterol. However, the biological foundations of the observed cardioprotective effects of alcohol have not been established. It is not likely that there will be primary prevention trials.

Ethanol relaxes blood vessels, and in severe intoxication, hypothermia resulting from heat loss as a consequence of vasodilatation may occur.

The kidney Ethanol has a diuretic effect unrelated to fluid intake that results from inhibition of antidiuretic hormone secretion, which decreases renal reabsorption of water.

The immune system Alcoholics are frequently immunologically compromised and are subject to infectious diseases. The mortality resulting from cancers of the upper GI tract and liver is also excessively high in alcoholics. Although the mechanism of this latter effect is unknown, alcohol consumption is a known risk factor for cancer, and this may be related to vitamin A metabolism.

The nervous system There are several well-documented neurological conditions resulting from excessive ethanol intake and concomitant nutritional deficiencies. These include Wernicke-Korsakoff syndrome, cerebellar atrophy, central pontine myelinosis and demyelinization of the corpus callosum, and mamillary body destruction.

Tissue specific effects of other alcohols

Methanol has a toxicological profile quite different from that of ethanol. The metabolic products of methanol, formaldehyde and formic acid, are responsible for causing optic nerve damage which can lead to blindness and severe acidosis. Maintenance of the airways and ventilation are required with methanol intoxication. Management also includes attempts to remove residual methanol, treatment of the acidosis, and administration of intravenous ethanol to reduce formation of toxic metabolic products and provide the time necessary to remove methanol by dialysis, which is the treatment of choice.

Ingestion of ethylene glycol may cause severe CNS depression and renal damage. In addition, the glycolic acid produced from metabolism by ADH can cause metabolic acidosis, whereas the oxalate formed is responsible for renal toxicity. Management of intoxication in this context is similar to that for methanol.

Isopropanol is a CNS depressant that is more toxic to the CNS than ethanol. Signs and symptoms of intoxication are similar to those of ethanol intoxication, but toxicity is limited because isopropanol produces severe gastritis with accompanying pain, nausea, and vomiting. In severe intoxication, hemodialysis is used to remove isopropanol from the body.

Fetal alcohol syndrome

Although fetal alcohol syndrome has been recognized from early times, it was rediscovered in the 1970s, and the general public is well aware of the deleterious effects of drinking on the health of the fetus. Consequences of maternal ingestion of alcohol can include miscarriage, stillbirth, low birth weight, slow postnatal growth, microcephaly, mental retardation, and many other organic and structural abnormalities. The incidence of fetal alcohol syndrome in some parts of the U.S. is estimated to be as high as 1 in 300 births. It is the most common cause of birth defects that is entirely preventable.

Tolerance and dependence

Both acute and chronic tolerance occur in response to ethanol use. Acute tolerance can occur in a matter of minutes and rapidly dissipates when ethanol is applied directly to nerve cells. Chronic tolerance occurs in people who ingest alcohol daily for weeks to months, with very high tolerances developing in some individuals. BACs must be approximately double to produce effects in tolerant as opposed to nontolerant people. This is much less, however, than that observed in those who use opiate drugs, in whom a tolerance of 10- to 30-fold can be demonstrated. The development of tolerance to alcohol has greater implications than that to other agents, because organ systems are exposed to much higher concentrations of ethanol, with deleterious consequences particularly to the liver. Because the liver becomes injured as a function of the dose and duration of ethanol exposure, metabolism of ethanol may be impaired in late-stage alcoholism with serious liver damage.

Both psychological and physical dependence are characteristic of chronic alcohol use. The clinical manifestations of ethanol withdrawal are divided into early and late stages. Early symptoms occur between a few hours and up to 48 hours after relative or absolute abstinence. Peak effects occur around 24 to 36 hours. Tremor, agitation, anxiety, anorexia, confusion, and signs of autonomic hyperactivity occur individually or in combinations. Seizures occurring in the early phase of withdrawal may reflect altered neurotransmission at $GABA_A$ (reduced) and NMDA (enhanced) receptors. Late withdrawal symptoms (delirium tremens) occur one to five days following abstinence and while relatively rare, can be life-threatening if untreated. Signs of sympathetic hyperactivity, agitation, and tremulousness characterize the onset of the syndrome. There are sensory disturbances including auditory or visual hallucinations, confusion, and delirium. Death may occur, even in treated patients. Complicating factors in alcohol withdrawal include trauma from falls or accidents, bacterial infections, and concomitant medical problems such as heart and liver failure. The alcohol withdrawal syndrome is more likely to be life-threatening than that associated with opioids.

Management of withdrawal is directed toward protecting and calming the person while identifying and treating underlying medical problems. Clinical data have demonstrated that the longer-acting benzodiazepines (chlordiazepoxide, diazepam or lorazepam) have a favorable effect on clinically important outcomes, including the severity of the withdrawal syndrome, risk of delirium and seizures, and incidence of adverse responses to the drugs used. The benzodiazepines are the treatment of choice. The phenothiazine antipsychotics and haloperidol are less effective in preventing seizures or delirium. Phenobarbital is problematic because its long half-life makes dose adjustment difficult, and in high doses, it may cause respiratory depression. β-Adrenergic receptor blockers and centrally acting α_2-adrenergic receptor agonists are useful as adjuvants to limit autonomic manifestations. Neither class of drugs reduces the risk of seizures or delirium tremens.

Treatment of acute intoxication

Emergency treatment of acute alcohol intoxication includes maintenance of an adequate airway and support of ventilation and blood pressure. In addition to depressant actions on the CNS, other organs, including the heart, may be affected. It is also important to assess the level of consciousness relative to the BAC, because other drugs may influence the apparent degree of intoxication. Acetaminophen concentration should also be determined. A short-acting opioid receptor antagonist is generally administered as a precaution. Glucose may need to be administered in the event of hypoglycemia, ketoacidosis, or dehydration. Loss of body fluids may necessitate intravenous infusion of fluids containing K^+, Mg^{2+}, and PO_4^-. Thiamine and other vitamins, such as folate and pyridoxine, are usually administered with intravenous glucose to prevent neurological deficits. Extreme caution is needed when one is modifying Na^+ concentrations in such patients, however, because overcorrection has been associated with central pontine myelinolysis.

Alcoholism

Diagnosis and genetic factors

It is difficult to diagnose chronic alcoholism. Success depends on obtaining a reliable history from the patient or from a member of the patient's family. Even if a diagnosis can be made, it is frequently difficult to manage the problem because treatment is often initiated when the disorder is already well advanced.

Over the past 10 to 15 years, the role of genetic factors in the development of chronic alcoholism has been identified with the hope that early intervention may be more successful. Results of studies involving family members of alcoholics and twins support a predisposition and an increased risk among close relatives. This conclusion that primary alcoholism is genetically influenced is based on several interesting findings.

Studies indicate a threefold to fourfold higher risk of alcoholism primarily in sons but also in some daughters of alcoholic parents. Comparisons in identical twins versus fraternal twins should reveal whether alcoholism is related to childhood environment. Because both types of twins have similar backgrounds, if alcoholism is related to childhood environment, its incidence should be the same in identical and fraternal twins. Most studies show that there is a twofold higher concordance for alcoholism in identical twins than in fraternal twins. In another study, alcoholic risk was assessed in male children of alcoholics raised by adoptive parents who were nonalcoholic. A threefold to fourfold higher risk of alcoholism was found in these males. Being raised by alcoholic adoptive parents did not increase the risk for alcoholism. In some studies, in fact, there was a protective effect.

Other studies have categorized alcoholics into several subgroups. One is the alcoholism most frequently seen in males and is associated with criminality; the second is a subtype observed in both sexes and influenced by the environment. Genetic predisposition, however, is merely one of several factors leading to alcoholism. Studies are attempting to reveal biological markers with which to identify potential alcoholics (e.g., differences in blood proteins, enzymes involved in ethanol degradation, and enzymes concerned with brain neurotransmitters and signaling components, including G proteins) to encourage such people to seek assistance sooner.

Treatment

Effective management of chronic alcoholism includes social and environmental as well as medical approaches and involves the family of the person undergoing treatment. Several types of treatment are available, including group psychotherapy (e.g., Alcoholics Anonymous) that may be rendered in private and public clinics outside of a hospital setting. Hypnotherapy, psychoanalysis, and aversive therapy with **disulfiram** also have been used.

Disulfiram inhibits ALDH, and in the presence of ethanol, causes a rise in blood acetaldehyde concentrations, producing flushing, headache, nausea and vomiting, sweating, and hypotension. Disulfiram also inhibits dopamine β-hydroxylase, the enzyme that converts dopamine to norepinephrine in sympathetic neurons (see Chapter 8). Thus, in an alcoholic taking disulfiram, there is an altered ability to synthesize norepinephrine, possibly contributing to the hypotension when alcohol is taken in conjunction with disulfiram. Recently, naltrexone, a pure opioid receptor antagonist, was approved as an adjunct for treatment of alcoholics. Short-term, double-blind, placebo-controlled trials showed that naltrexone decreased craving, the number of drinking days, the number of drinks per occasion, and the relapse rate. The mechanism is not known, nor is it known whether there will be long-term benefits.

While the only proven cure for advanced liver damage is transplantation, other drugs are being tried. These include prednisolone, vitamin E, S-adenosylmethionine, precursors of glutathione, propylthiouracil, polyunsaturated lecithin and colchicine. In general, management regimens have had variable success rates, with many being effective over the long term in no more than 10% to 15% of participants.

New horizons

New drugs have been proposed for treatment of alcohol craving and prevention of relapse. Data from animal studies and limited clinical trials have suggested 5-HT reuptake blockers as being possible useful agents. Studies also implicate dopamine in the reward pathway as a target for a variety of drugs of abuse (Chapter 32), which might lead to the development of useful drugs that act on dopamine receptors. Perhaps the combination of naltrexone with 5-HT reuptake blockers will yield improved results. A newer drug, calcium *N*-acetylhomotaurine (acamprosate), an analog of GABA, is used currently in Europe and is undergoing clinical trials in the U.S. as a single treatment and in combination with other drugs. Studies suggest that acamprosate may help maintain abstinence from ethanol in alcoholic patients who have withdrawn from alcohol and want to maintain their abstinence.

Much effort is being expended in finding genes associated with a risk for alcoholism, as well as a predisposition to liver and other organ damage. Data from both human and animal studies are revealing new avenues for development of tools for early detection of risk.

TRADE NAMES

All of the drugs approved for use in the United States are listed in the Major Drugs box.

FURTHER READING

Menon KUN, Cores GJ, Shah VH. Pathogenesis, diagnosis and treatment of alcoholic liver disease. *Mayo Clinic Proc* 2001; 76:1021-1029.

Mukamal KJ, Conigrave KM, Mittleman MA, et al. Roles of drinking pattern and type of alcohol consumed in coronary heart disease in men. *N Engl J Med* 2003; 348:109-118.

Sokol RJ, Delaney-Black V, Nordstrom B. Fetal alcohol spectrum disorder. *JAMA* 2003; 290:2996-2999.

Self-assessment questions

1. An adequate medical history from a patient should include information concerning alcohol usage because alcohol may be implicated in:
   a. Cardiovascular disease.
   b. Liver malfunction.
   c. Cancer of the larynx and pharynx.
   d. Mental retardation of children.
   e. All of the above.

2. Ascites resulting from chronic excessive alcohol intake is most likely caused by:
   a. Obstructed hepatic venous return.
   b. Increased osmolality of the blood.
   c. Increased blood uric acid concentrations.
   d. Increased magnesium excretion.
   e. Increased blood lactate concentrations.

3. Current evidence indicates that genetic risk for developing alcoholism is:
   a. Mediated by a single gene.
   b. Greater in men than women.
   c. Caused by inheritance of altered genes encoding liver ADH.
   d. Caused by high concentrations of acetaldehyde.
   e. Caused by inheritance of genes coding for increased dopamine concentrations in the reward pathways of the brain.

4. Women's risk for alcohol-induced disorders is greater than that in men in which organ?
   a. Pancreas
   b. Stomach
   c. Larynx
   d. Liver
   e. Heart

5. Flushing reactions in response to ethanol in Asians resemble the response to ethanol in people who have taken:
   a. Benzodiazepines.
   b. Barbiturates.
   c. Antihistamines.
   d. Disulfiram.
   e. Chloral hydrate.

6. Which of the following may occur as a consequence of the metabolism of ethanol by the cytochrome P450 system and also its induction by ethanol?
   a. Increased rate of metabolism of other drugs.
   b. When ethanol is present, a decreased rate of metabolism of some drugs.
   c. Increased production of carcinogenic compounds from procarcinogens.
   d. Increased clearance of ethanol.
   e. All of the above.

CHAPTER 26

Treatment of eating disorders and obesity

Lynn M. Crespo
Lynn Wecker

Major Drugs

Phentermine (Adipex-P, Fastin, Ionamin, Obenix, Phentercot, Phentride, Teramine, Zantryl)
Diethylpropion (Tenuate, Tepanil)
Mazindol (Mazanor, Sanorex)
Sibutramine (Meridia)
Orlistat (Xenical)

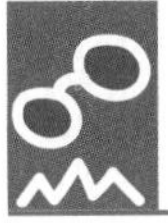

Therapeutic overview

Anorexia nervosa and **bulimia nervosa** are two commonly recognized eating disorders that affect women primarily in which there is an exaggerated concern about body weight and shape. Anorexia is the more disabling and lethal, characterized by the obsessive pursuit of thinness that results in serious, even **life-threatening** weight loss. Bulimia differs from anorexia because many individuals are of normal body weight. Bulimic patients indulge in binge eating, followed by excessive inappropriate behavior to lose weight, such as vomiting, the use of laxatives, or compulsive exercising. Anorexic and bulimic patients have common characteristics, and although the physiological disturbances from the latter are less severe than the former, both are associated with serious medical complications. Treatment involves the management of these complications and restoring and maintaining normal body weight through psychotherapy and pharmacotherapy with **antidepressants.**

Anorexia/cachexia is not primarily an eating disorder but is manifest by cancer patients. It is often very debilitating and is associated with weakness, fatigue, and significantly, decreased survival time and responses to cytotoxic therapeutic compounds. The **progestational agents** and **corticosteroids** stimulate appetite and cause weight gain in these patients.

Obesity is increasing at an alarming rate in the United States, with approximately 50% of adults classified as overweight and 25% as obese. Childhood obesity is also reaching epidemic proportions. Obesity is a significant risk factor for many common conditions, including type 2 diabetes mellitus; hypertension; dyslipidemia; coronary artery disease; congestive heart failure; stroke; hepatic steatosis; sleep apnea; osteoarthritis; and endometrial, breast, prostate, and colon cancers. Additionally, mortality rates from all causes increase with obesity. Weight reduction lowers the risk of morbidity and mortality from all diseases and is currently accepted as one of the most preventable health risk factors. Drugs available currently for treatment of obesity include the centrally active agents **diethylpropion, mazindol, phentermine,** and **sibutramine** and the peripherally active gastrointestinal (GI) lipase inhibitor **orlistat.**

Binge-eating disorder is characterized by binge eating, similar to bulimia, but these individuals do not exhibit any subsequent counteracting or weight-reduction behaviors. Although this disorder has been

Abbreviations

CNS	central nervous system
DA	dopamine
GI	gastrointestinal
5-HT	serotonin
NE	norepinephrine

classified with anorexia and bulimia, binge-eating disorder is manifest by about one third of obese patients enrolled in weight loss clinics; thus, its relationship to obesity is beginning to be recognized.

The etiology of eating disorders and the involvement of developmental, social, and biological factors are beyond the scope of this chapter. Pharmacological treatment of eating disorders is presented in the Therapeutic Overview box.

THERAPEUTIC OVERVIEW

Anorexia and bulimia

Baseline medical and psychological assessment
Psychotherapy is cornerstone of treatment
Antidepressants may be of benefit

Anorexia/cachexia

Associated with advanced cancers
Corticosteroids and progestational agents stimulate appetite and weight gain

Obesity

Significant risk factors should be present before initiating drug therapy
Patients with concurrent diseases such as diabetes and hypertension require close monitoring
Exercise and a supervised dietary plan are essential
Centrally active drugs that enhance DA and NE may be of benefit
Peripherally active drugs that decrease fat absorption (orlistat) may be of benefit

Mechanisms of action

Drugs that promote eating

Based on evidence that individuals with anorexia and bulimia are prone to mood disturbances, the pharmacological treatment of these disorders has focused on use of antidepressants. Evidence supports the efficacy of these compounds for treatment of bulimia. Antidepressants in all classes including the **tricyclic antidepressants, monoamine oxidase inhibitors,** and **selective serotonin reuptake inhibitors** have been shown to be equally efficacious. However, because of side effects associated with the use of tricyclic antidepressants and monoamine oxidase inhibitors (Chapter 23), selective serotonin reuptake inhibitors may be considered first-line agents. Antidepressants reduce binge eating, vomiting, depression, and improve eating habits in bulimia but do not affect poor body image. Imipramine, desipramine, phenelzine, amitriptyline, and trazodone have all been used with some success, but currently, **fluoxetine** is the only approved antidepressant for treatment of bulimia. It is unclear whether the effectiveness of these compounds is due primarily to their antidepressant action or whether they are directly orexigenic (appetite stimulating). These compounds are ineffective for binge-eating disorder and have limited benefit for anorexia. Their mechanisms of action are discussed in Chapter 23.

Similar to the goal for therapy with anorectic and bulimic patients is the need to stimulate appetite in individuals with anorexia/cachexia. In concert with nutritional counseling, **progestational agents** such as **megestrol** acetate, as well as **corticosteroids** such as **dexamethasone,** have been shown to stimulate appetite and cause weight gain in these patients. The mechanisms of action of these compounds are discussed in Chapters 33 and 35.

Anti-obesity drugs

Drugs approved for the treatment of obesity include the centrally active agents and the GI lipase inhibitor orlistat.

All centrally active compounds, with one exception (mazindol), are β-phenethylamine derivatives and resemble the neurotransmitters dopamine (DA) and norepinephrine (NE), as well as the sympathomimetic amphetamine (Fig. 26-1). The **amphetamines,** which stimulate release of DA and NE, are well recognized for their ability to suppress appetite and were used for this purpose. However, their pronounced sympathomimetic effects (Chapter 10), as well as potential for abuse (Chapter 32), led to their discontinuation for this indication. Similarly, the sympathomimetic **phenylpropanolamine,** which was the only weight loss drug available over the counter and was also present in several nasal decongestants, has recently been withdrawn from the market in the United States because of a reported risk of hemorrhagic stroke (Chapter 10).

The four centrally active drugs currently approved for treatment of obesity include **diethylpropion, mazindol, phentermine,** and **sibutramine.** All of these compounds increase synaptic concentrations of NE or DA, although notable differences exist among them.

Phentermine is structurally similar to amphetamine (see Fig. 26-1) but produces less central nervous system (CNS) stimulation and therefore has a lower abuse potential. Phentermine increases release of both NE and DA and decreases food consumption through an inhibitory effect on the appetite control center in the

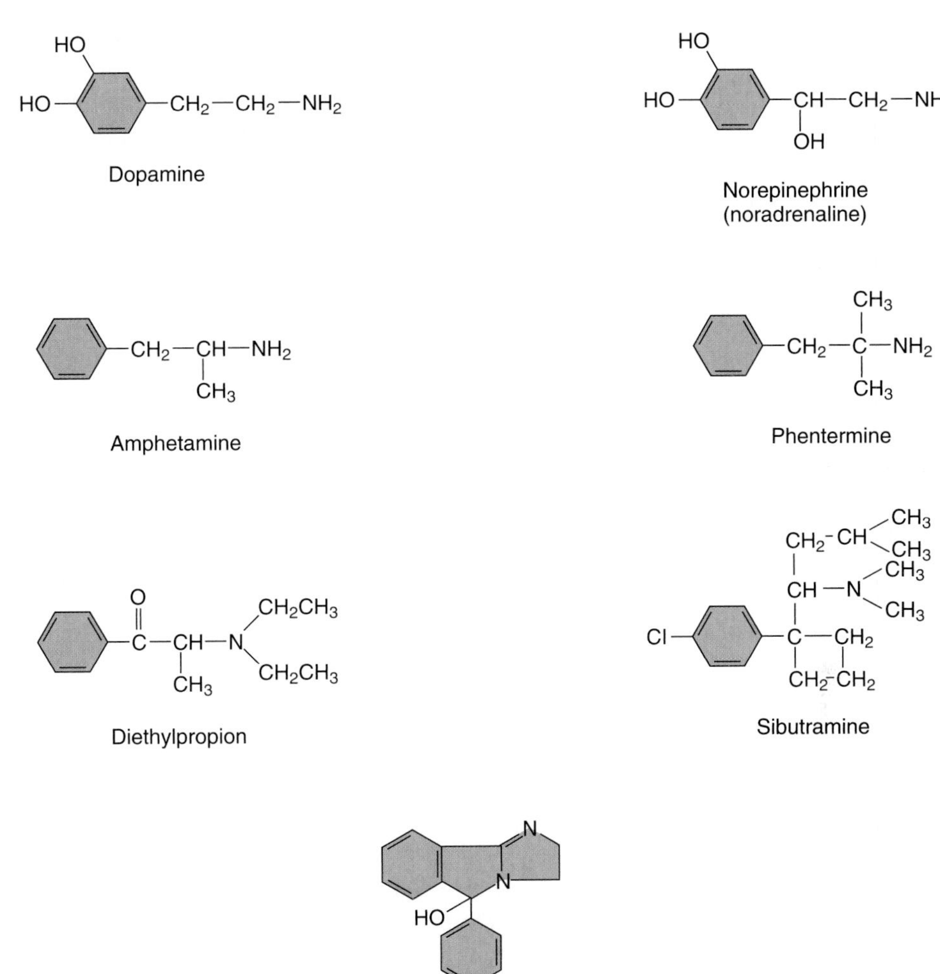

Figure 26-1 Structures of the centrally active drugs to treat anorexia compared with the endogenous neurotransmitters NE and DA and amphetamine.

lateral hypothalamus; its effect on metabolic rate is equivocal.

Mazindol exerts its effects through inhibition of NE reuptake and direct stimulation of hypothalamic activity. It also has a thermogenic action to stimulate oxygen consumption and enhance NE stimulation in brown fat. Mazindol has fewer CNS stimulant effects than amphetamine and is also considered to have a low abuse potential.

Diethylpropion stimulates NE release and causes even less CNS stimulation than mazindol; it is considered to have the lowest potential for abuse.

Sibutramine is first in a new class of drugs that works by inhibiting amine reuptake. Sibutramine and its two active metabolites inhibit the reuptake of NE, DA, and serotonin (5-HT) with the potency order of NE > 5-HT > DA. Sibutramine has no direct receptor agonist activity and induces weight loss by both suppressing appetite and increasing thermogenesis. Involvement of the CNS versus actions of this compound on peripheral systems is unknown.

The drugs used today primarily enhance noradrenergic and not serotonergic activity. Although 5-HT plays a role in the regulation of eating behavior via an inhibitory effect on the appetite control center in the lateral hypothalamus, no serotonergic agents are currently approved for treatment of obesity. Fenfluramine and dexfenfluramine, both of which release 5-HT, were used for this indication but were taken off the market because of an increased risk of valvular heart disease. Similarly, both fluoxetine and sertraline may be useful but are not currently approved.

Orlistat is the only prescription weight-loss drug that does not suppress appetite. Rather, orlistat inhibits GI lipase activity, thereby decreasing production of free fatty acids from triglycerides. Orlistat is a synthetic derivative of lipstatin, a naturally occurring lipase inhibitor produced by *Streptomyces toxytricini*. Normal

GI lipases are essential for the dietary absorption of long chain triglycerides and facilitate gastric emptying and secretion of pancreatic and biliary substances. Because the body has limited ability to synthesize fat from carbohydrates and proteins, most accumulated body fat in humans comes from dietary intake. Orlistat reduces fat absorption up to 30% in individuals whose diets contain a significant fat component. Reduced fat absorption translates into significant calorie reduction and weight loss in obese individuals. In addition, the lower luminal free fatty acid concentrations also reduce cholesterol absorption.

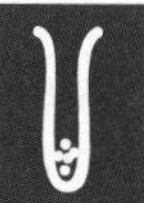

Pharmacokinetics

The pharmacokinetics of the antidepressants are discussed in Chapter 23; those of the corticosteroids are discussed in Chapter 33, and those of the progestational agents are discussed in Chapter 35.

All centrally acting anorectic drugs are well absorbed from the GI tract and reach peak plasma levels within two hours. However, they differ somewhat in their pharmacokinetic profiles (Table 26-1).

Diethylpropion is rapidly absorbed and is subject to extensive first-pass hepatic metabolism via N-dealkylation and reduction, producing active metabolites with half-lives of approximately 4 to 8 hours that are excreted mainly by the kidneys.

Mazindol is available for once-daily dosing; however, some physicians prescribe it in multiple, smaller doses throughout the day. Mazindol undergoes extensive hepatic metabolism, and 50% is excreted in the urine as conjugated metabolites.

Phentermine is available in both immediate- and sustained-release formulations, but use of the latter is questionable, as its half-life is 12 to 24 hours.

Sibutramine is inactive and undergoes extensive first-pass hepatic metabolism to its active mono- and di-desmethyl metabolites, which are further metabolized and excreted by the kidneys. The active metabolites have elimination half-lives of 14 to 18 hours. The cytochrome P450 enzyme responsible for the metabolism of sibutramine is **CYP3A4**, which also metabolizes other compounds (see Chapter 3). Thus, changes in plasma levels of sibutramine, as well as its metabolites, have been noted when it is co-administered with ketoconazole, erythromycin, and cimetidine, and the use of these drugs can decrease its effectiveness.

Orlistat must be administered with meals containing fat to exert its effects. Timing of drug ingestion, before or after the meal, and the fat/fiber ratio of the meal do not affect its ability to inhibit fat absorption. In spite of its effects on fat absorption and GI motility, orlistat does not change the pharmacodynamic or pharmacokinetic profiles of most drugs, except for the fat-soluble vitamins, for which malabsorption has been documented. Orlistat is 99% bound to plasma proteins, primarily lipoproteins and albumin. It has a half-life of about 1 to 2 hours and is metabolized within the GI tract to inactive compounds. The metabolites undergo some biliary excretion, and the unabsorbed drug is eliminated in the feces.

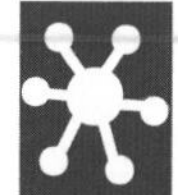

Relation of mechanisms of action to clinical response

Anorexia nervosa, bulimia nervosa, and binge-eating disorder have multifactorial etiologies, and as such, drug therapy alone is likely to be ineffective. Studies indicate that antidepressants do not lead to the remission of bulimia, although a single course of drug is better than placebo. In addition, with continued treatment, patients have a high rate of relapse. Thus, although antidepressants have been shown to be efficacious for bulimia, their long-term utility remains to be determined.

All centrally active anti-obesity drugs increase synaptic concentrations of biogenic amines in the CNS, leading to their anorectic effect. In addition, increases

Table 26-1 Selected pharmacokinetic parameters

Drug	Half-Life (hrs)	Metabolism and Elimination
Diethylpropion	4-8 for metabolites	>70% first-pass hepatic metabolism >75% renal excretion
Mazindol	<24	Hepatic metabolism 50% renal excretion of unchanged drug
Phentermine	12-24	Renal excretion
Sibutramine	14-18 for metabolites	Hepatic metabolism required to activate compound >75% renal excretion

in peripheral amine levels may promote thermogenesis contributing to weight loss. Although clinical studies have demonstrated that use of these drugs produces more weight loss than placebo when used as an adjunct to a supervised diet and exercise routine, their effects were maximal during the first 6 months of use, and continued treatment did not lead to further weight loss; as a matter of fact, weight regain usually occurs within 6 months after discontinuation. Unfortunately, it is unclear whether chronic use of these drugs continues to decrease mechanisms controlling appetite or whether tolerance develops. Further studies are needed to understand the loss of effectiveness after chronic use.

Orlistat has no effect on appetite-regulating pathways in the CNS and as such, there is no potential for CNS tolerance or abuse. Continued treatment with orlistat increases the intake of low fat-containing foods and decreases high fat intake by patients, perhaps reflecting the desire to decrease the GI side effects that accompany its use. In addition to decreasing fat absorption, orlistat decreases cholesterol absorption and reduces plasma LDL cholesterol beyond that produced by weight loss alone in obese individuals, an added benefit of this drug.

Side effects, clinical problems, and toxicity

The centrally active anorexigenics have similar side-effect profiles, related to their ability to increase central and peripheral aminergic activity. Use is contraindicated in patients with a history of stroke, coronary artery disease, congestive heart failure, or arrhythmias. Sibutramine can increase both systolic and diastolic blood pressure, and baseline blood pressure should be obtained prior to initiating therapy; regular monitoring is required thereafter.

In addition to their effects on the cardiovascular system, these drugs also cause insomnia and tremors and induce anxiety through their CNS actions.

These drugs should be used as monotherapy and are contraindicated in patients receiving sympathomimetic amines, tricyclic antidepressants, selective serotonin reuptake inhibitors, or monoamine oxidase inhibitors, because documented cases of hypertensive crises exist. In addition, for compounds such as sibutramine that affect serotonin, a serotonin syndrome can be precipitated (see Chapter 23). A minimum drug-free period of 14 days is required for anyone using MAO inhibitors before therapy is initiated with these agents.

Because of their CNS stimulation, these drugs carry a potential for abuse. Although they have less abuse potential than amphetamine, they are contraindicated in abusers of cocaine, phencyclidine, and methamphetamine.

Glaucoma can be exacerbated as a result of the mydriasis produced by these agents and is also a contraindication to their use.

Increased insulin sensitivity has been reported in type 2 diabetics receiving mazindol and diethylpropion, and thus careful monitoring of serum glucose, insulin, and oral hypoglycemic agents is required in these patients; sibutramine leads to better metabolic control in type 2 diabetics.

As a consequence of significant hepatic metabolism of these agents, a potential for drug interactions exists.

Orlistat is unique for treatment of obesity as it does not carry a risk of cardiovascular side effects. Since its actions involve the GI system, its adverse effects are limited to this area. The most commonly reported GI complaints, which occur in as many as 80% of individuals, are most pronounced in the first 1 to 2 months and decline with continued use. Malabsorption of fat-soluble vitamins (A, D, E, and K) as well as β-carotene occur, but no notable changes in the pharmacokinetic profiles of other drugs have been reported. Long-term use of orlistat has not resulted in any documented cases of serious reactions.

Side effects associated with use of the anti-obesity drugs are listed in the Clinical Problems box.

CLINICAL PROBLEMS

Diethylpropion, Mazindol, Phentermine
- Dry mouth, headaches, nervousness, insomnia

Sibutramine
- Constipation, insomnia, headache, dry mouth
- Tachycardia and hypertension

Orlistat
- Decreased absorption of fat-soluble vitamins
- Soft and oily stools and anal leakage
- Cramping, diarrhea, flatulence

New horizons

The potential to develop new drugs to affect eating behaviors is increasing as our understanding of the basic pathways and neurotransmitters involved expands.

Currently, most research is focused on treatment of obesity rather than anorexia and bulimia. Obesity has become a national epidemic and is linked with a high rate of morbidity and mortality from other causes. Anorexia and bulimia are less well understood, and psychotherapy remains the cornerstone of therapy. However, as the role of specific neurotransmitters becomes more clearly defined, new treatment options may become available. Preliminary studies suggest that the 5-HT antagonist cyproheptadine may lead to weight gain in non-bulimic anorexic patients.

Orexigenic signals appear to be redundant in the body and involve numerous peptides, hormones, and neurotransmitters. When body fat stores decrease, serum concentrations of leptin (secreted by adipocytes) and insulin (secreted by the pancreas) decrease. Concurrently, endocrine cells within the stomach secrete ghrelin. Alterations in these hormones are sensed in the arcuate nucleus of the hypothalamus and stimulate production of orexigenic signals involving agouti-related protein, neuropeptide Y, galanin, and melanin-concentrating hormone. These are potential targets for drug development. NPY and galanin stimulate food consumption, each with different effects on intake of energy sources such as protein, fat, and carbohydrates.

Leptin has been extensively studied, and obese individuals have been shown to be leptin resistant. Axokine is an injectable weight loss drug in clinical trials. It is an analog of ciliary neurotrophic factor that signals the satiety center in the brain to decrease food intake by activating the central leptin pathway distal to the leptin receptor. Inhibitors of tyrosine phosphatase-IB, an enzyme involved in leptin resistance, has shown promise in preclinical trials to increase leptin receptor sensitivity, similar to effects of sulfonylureas on insulin receptors.

Other approaches include ghrelin receptor antagonists to block central stimulation of appetite. However, preliminary results with ghrelin and ghrelin antagonists have been disappointing.

In addition to ongoing drug development for central or peripheral inhibition of appetite, research is also targeting thermogenesis. Specific β_3-adrenergic receptor agonists would stimulate breakdown of fat for energy metabolism by directly activating adipocytes yet avoiding sympathetic stimulation and cardiovascular effects.

As obesity has rapidly become a major health and economic issue, development of better drugs to combat this epidemic may become a dominant strategy in treatment and prevention of many diseases associated with obesity.

TRADE NAMES

All of the drugs approved for use in the United States are listed in the Major Drugs box.

FURTHER READING

Halpern A, Mancini MC. Treatment of obesity: an update on anti-obesity medications. *Obesity Revs* 2003; 4:25-42.

Korner J, Aronne LJ. The emerging science of body weight regulation and its impact on obesity treatment. *J Clin Invest* 2003; 111:565-570.

Zhu AF, Walsh BT. Pharmacologic treatment of eating disorders. *Can J Psychiatry* 2002; 47:227-234.

Self-assessment questions

1. A 47-year-old obese man requires pharmacological intervention for weight loss. He has a history of hypertension and angina. Which of the following drugs would be *best* for this patient?

a. Diethylpropion
b. Fluoxetine
c. Orlistat
d. Phentermine
e. Sibutramine

2. A 23-year-old anorexic patient requires drug therapy to assist her with weight maintenance. Which of the following drugs would have the *least* risk of cardiovascular complications?

a. Fluoxetine
b. Amitriptyline
c. Desipramine
d. Imipramine
e. Phenelzine

MATCHING

Match the following drugs to the statement that BEST describes it. Each answer may be used once, more than once, or not at all.

3. Inhibits intestinal lipase activity.

4. Has two active metabolites that are more potent than the parent compound at inhibiting reuptake of serotonin, norepinephrine, and dopamine.

a. Amitriptyline
b. Fluoxetine
c. Mazindol
d. Orlistat
e. Sibutramine

CHAPTER 27

Treatment of seizure disorders

Janet L. Stringer

Major Drugs

Carbamazepine (Tegretol)
Diazepam (Valium)
Ethosuximide (Zarontin)
Lamotrigine (Lamictal)
Lorazepam (Ativan)
Phenytoin (Dilantin)
Valproate (Depakene, Depakote)

Therapeutic overview

Epilepsy is a chronic disorder characterized by recurrent, self-limited **seizures.** Seizures occur when there is abnormal, excessive firing of neurons synchronized throughout a localized or generalized population of neurons. About 0.5% of the population suffers from epilepsy, with most patients having their first seizure before 18 years of age. Recurrent seizures, if frequent, interfere with a patient's ability to carry out day-to-day activities. However, judicious use of antiepileptic medications allows about 75% of patients to remain seizure-free.

The goal of antiepileptic drug therapy is to prevent seizures while minimizing side effects, by using the simplest drug regimen. If seizures continue after drug therapy begins and dose increases are inadvisable because of side effects, one should try at least one and sometimes another drug as monotherapy before considering the use of two drugs simultaneously. Discontinuation of antiepileptic medication after several seizure-free years depends on the diagnosis (type of seizure and epileptic syndrome), cause, and response to therapy. Antiepileptic drugs may be discontinued in patients with certain epileptic syndromes but should be continued for life in patients with others such as recurrent seizures secondary to a structural lesion.

Antiepileptic medication is selected according to seizure type. This chapter covers the classification and purported underlying pathophysiology of seizure types and the actions of drugs used for specific types of seizures. The principal therapeutic uses of drugs covered in this chapter are listed in the Therapeutic Overview box.

THERAPEUTIC OVERVIEW

Partial (focal) seizures

Carbamazepine
Lamotrigine
Phenytoin

Generalized tonic-clonic (grand mal) seizures

Carbamazepine
Phenytoin
Valproate

Absence (petit mal) seizures

Ethosuximide
Valproate

Status epilepticus

Diazepam or lorazepam
Phenytoin

Abbreviations

EEG	electroencephalogram
GABA	γ-aminobutyric acid
NMDA	*N*-methyl-D-aspartate

Mechanisms of action

The current classification of seizure types (Table 27-1) recognizes two broad categories: those that arise in part of one cerebral hemisphere and are accompanied by focal electroencephalographic (EEG) abnormalities **(partial** or **focal seizures),** and those with clinical and EEG features that indicate the initial simultaneous involvement of all, or large parts, of both cerebral hemispheres **(generalized seizures).**

Partial seizures arise when pathophysiological changes in one region of the brain initiate a seizure. The seizures are termed **simple** if consciousness is unaltered and **complex** if consciousness is impaired or lost. In partial complex seizures, motor activity often appears as a complicated and seemingly purposeful movement. If the seizure focus synchronizes and activates neurons in surrounding areas, the partial seizure can **secondarily generalize** to involve the entire brain. These mechanisms are depicted in Figure 27-1.

In generalized seizures, large areas of the brain are involved at the onset. Generalized seizures are subclassified by the presence or absence of specific patterns of motor convulsions and include **generalized tonic-clonic seizures** in which widespread convulsions occur; **absence seizures,** characterized by impaired consciousness only; and other types (see Table 27-1). Little is understood about the onset of generalized tonic-clonic seizures, although there are some clues about the cellular mechanisms underlying absence seizures, which are characterized by the sudden appearance of spike-wave discharges synchronized throughout the brain. The EEGs recorded during an absence seizure compared with a generalized tonic-clonic seizure are shown in Figure 27-2. Thalamocortical circuits are thought to play a major role in the pathogenesis of absence seizures. These neurons generate depolarizations, based on Ca^{2+} currents, that generate normal and possibly abnormal thalamocortical rhythms, including spike-wave discharges.

All people are capable of experiencing seizures. Brain insults such as fever, hypoglycemia, hyponatremia, and extreme acidosis or alkalosis can trigger a

Table 27-1 Classification of seizures, frequency, and clinical manifestations

Seizure Type	Frequency (%)	Clinical Manifestations
PARTIAL (FOCAL) SEIZURES		
Simple partial	10	No impairment of consciousness; focal motor, sensory, autonomic or psychic disturbance
Complex partial (temporal lobe)	35	Impaired consciousness; dreamy dysaffective state, with or without automatisms
Partial seizures, secondarily generalized	10	
GENERALIZED SEIZURES		
Tonic-clonic (grand mal)	30	Loss of consciousness, falling Rigid extension of trunk and limbs (tonic phase) Rhythmic contraction of arms and legs (clonic phase)
Absence (petit mal)	10	Impaired consciousness with staring spells, with or without eye blinks
Others, including myoclonic, atonic (atypical), clonic, tonic	4	Variable depending on seizure type
UNCLASSIFIED EPILEPTIC SEIZURES	1-8	Includes all other seizures

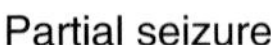

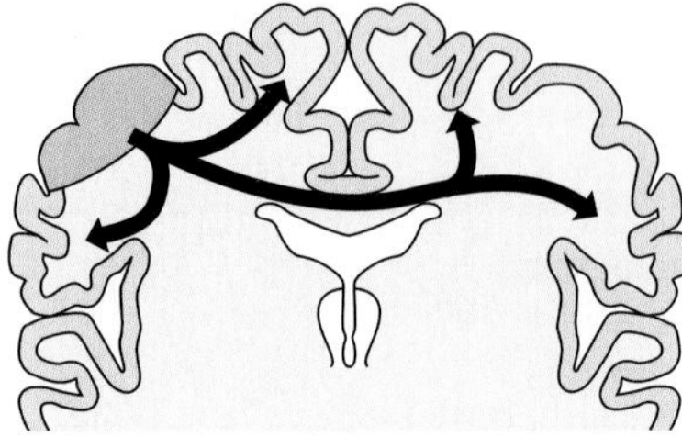

Partial seizure
secondarily generalized

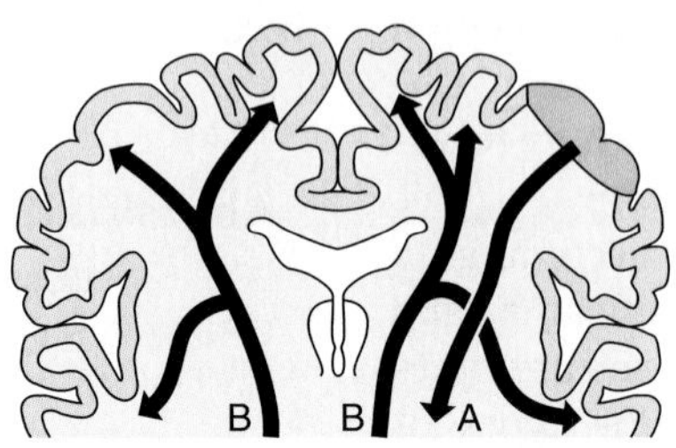

Figure 27-1 Seizure spread. In the partial (focal) seizure, activity begins in a localized area and spreads to adjacent and contralateral cortical regions. In the partial seizure, secondarily generalized, the locally-generated seizure activates subcortical regions *(A)*, which leads to activation of additional neurons *(B)*, resulting in seizure spread throughout the entire cortex.

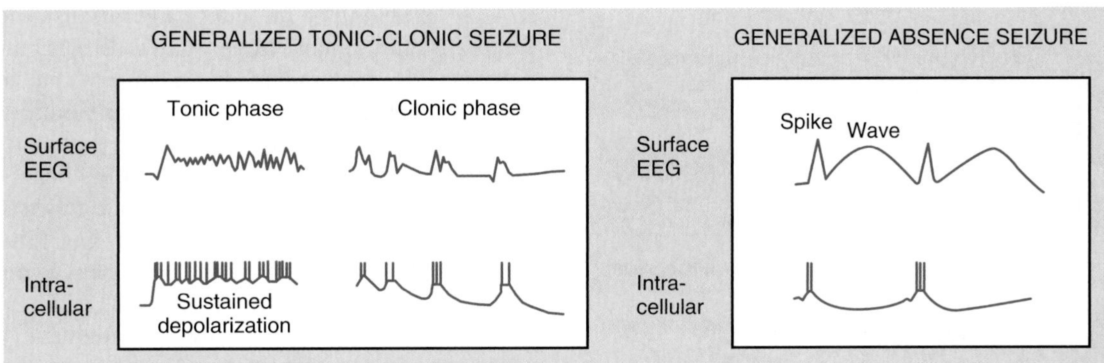

Figure 27-2 Comparison of electrical changes during a tonic-clonic and an absence seizure. A generalized tonic-clonic seizure begins with a tonic phase of rhythmic high-frequency discharges (recorded by surface EEG) with cortical neurons undergoing sustained depolarization, and the generation of protracted trains of action potentials (recorded intracellularly). Subsequently, the seizure converts to a clonic phase, characterized by groups of spikes on the EEG and periodic neuronal depolarizations with clusters of action potentials. During absence seizures, a spike-and-wave discharge is recorded on the surface EEG; during the spike phase, neurons generate short-duration depolarizations and a burst of action potentials but neither exhibit sustained depolarization or produce sustained repetitive firing of action potentials, unlike during tonic-clonic seizures. This difference may explain why drugs that are effective against sustained firing *in vitro* are effective against tonic-clonic seizures, but not absence seizures, in humans.

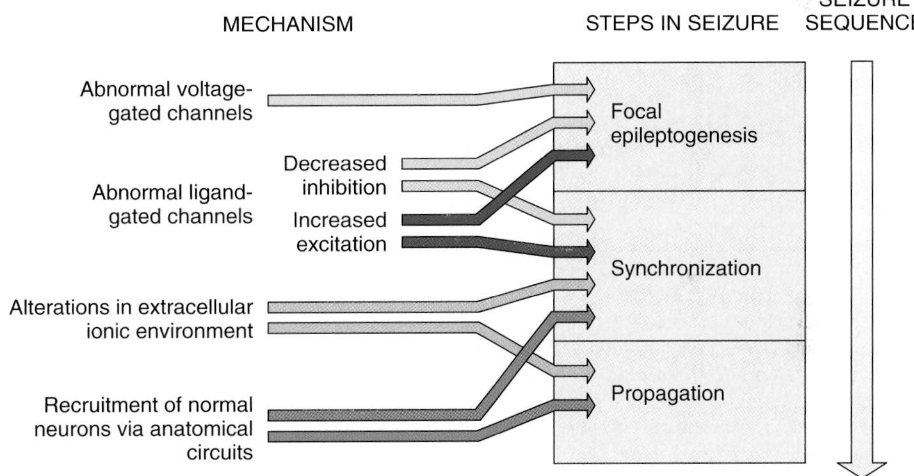

Figure 27-3 Cellular and synaptic mechanisms generating epileptic seizures. A seizure can be divided into three phases: *(1)* focal epileptogenesis (initiation); *(2)* synchronization of the surrounding neurons; and *(3)* propagation of the seizure discharge to other areas of the brain. Arrows indicate where each of the mechanisms on the left participates in these phases.

seizure, but if the condition is corrected, seizures do not recur. The causes of isolated seizures and **epilepsy** (recurrent seizures) are summarized in Box 27-1.

Status epilepticus exists when seizures recur within a short time period, such that baseline consciousness is not regained between seizures. A patient is considered to be in status epilepticus if seizures last at least 30 minutes. Status epilepticus can lead to systemic hypoxia, acidemia, hyperpyrexia, cardiovascular collapse, and renal shutdown and is a medical emergency.

Several mechanisms are involved in the genesis and spread of epileptic discharges (Fig. 27-3). The first includes alterations in neuronal membrane function as a consequence of changes in voltage-regulated ion channels. Examples of drugs useful in this

Box 27-1 Causes of seizures

- Birth and perinatal injuries
- Vascular insults
- Head trauma
- Congenital malformations
- Metabolic disturbances (e.g., serum Na^+, glucose, Ca^{2+}, urea)
- Drugs or alcohol, including withdrawal from barbiturates and other CNS depressants
- Neoplasia
- Infection
- Genetic
- Idiopathic
- Hyperthermia in children

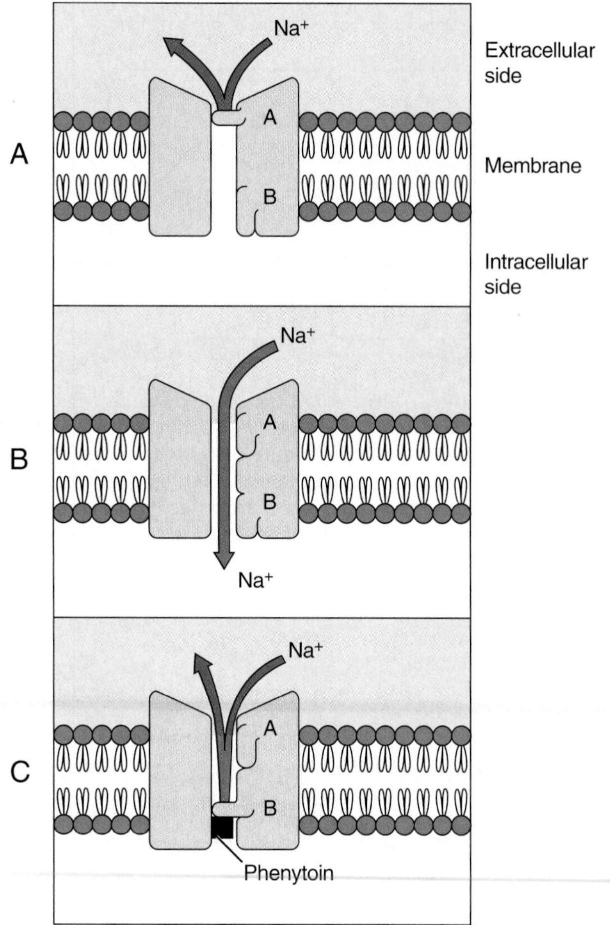

Figure 27-4 Action of phenytoin on Na^+ channel. **A,** Resting state in which Na^+ channel activation gate *(A)* is closed. **B,** Arrival of an action potential causes depolarization and opening of activation gate *(A)*, and Na^+ flows into the cell. **C,** When depolarization continues, an inactivation gate *(B)* moves into the channel. Phenytoin prolongs the inactivated state of the Na^+ channel, presumably by preventing reopening of the inactivation gate *(B)*.

setting are **carbamazepine, phenytoin, lamotrigine,** and **topiramate,** which reduce repetitive firing of neurons by producing a use-dependent blockade of Na^+ channels (Fig. 27-4). By prolonging the inactivated state of the Na^+ channel and thus the relative refractory period, these drugs do not alter the first action potential but rather reduce the likelihood of repetitive action potentials. Neurons retain their ability to generate action potentials at the lower frequencies common during normal brain function. Because these drugs block repetitive firing, they are better at controlling tonic-clonic seizures than absence seizures (see Fig. 27-2).

The second broad mechanism of seizure onset that can be influenced by drugs involves changes in ligand-gated ion channels. Excessive neuronal firing may occur as a consequence of either decreased inhibition or increased excitation of neurons. γ-Aminobutyric acid (GABA) is the major inhibitory neurotransmitter in the forebrain and opens ligand-gated Cl^- channels (see Chapter 24), hyperpolarizing neurons and rendering epileptic firing less likely. In experimental animals, increased GABA-mediated inhibition has antiepileptic activity, whereas decreased inhibition can lead to seizures. $GABA_A$ receptors contain binding sites for both the benzodiazepines and barbiturates (see Chapter 24). Binding of a benzodiazepine (diazepam, clonazepam, lorazepam) enhances the effectiveness of GABA-mediated inhibition by increasing the frequency of Cl^--channel opening when GABA combines with its receptor. Barbiturates interact with the receptor at a binding site adjacent to the Cl^- channel but separate from the benzodiazepine site. Some barbiturates have **GABA-mimetic** (direct action on Cl^- channels) and **GABA-potentiating** effects (prolonging the opening of Cl^- channels achieved by a given amount of GABA). Barbiturates that are effective antiepileptic compounds (suppressing seizures with minimal sedation) have strong GABA-potentiating actions but little or no GABA-mimetic actions. Some barbiturates suppress seizures but are not useful clinically because they have strong sedative effects. GABA activity may also be enhanced by either decreasing its reuptake or inhibiting its catabolism. **Tiagabine** blocks reuptake of GABA from the synapse, thus prolonging its action. Similarly, **vigabatrin,** which is not yet marketed in the United States, is an irreversible inhibitor of GABA transaminase, the enzyme mediating the catabolism of GABA. Another antiepileptic drug, **gabapentin,** was designed as a lipophilic GABA analog (hence its name) but does not stimulate $GABA_A$ receptors. Although its mechanism of action is currently unknown, gabapentin may alter GABA metabolism, reuptake, or release.

The excessive neuronal firing that occurs following decreased inhibition releases **adenosine,** which has been postulated to be an endogenous antiepileptic agent. Adenosine is a neuromodulator that interacts with its receptors to inhibit neuronal firing. **Carbamazepine** appears to interact directly with the adenosine system, leading to enhanced neuronal inhibition. This, in turn, makes it harder for a seizure to begin, synchronize, and spread.

Another mechanism of seizure onset and spread of epileptic discharges that can be influenced by drugs involves changes in ligand-gated ion channels that promote neuronal firing directly. Excitatory neurotransmission is mediated predominantly by **glutamate** or related excitatory neurotransmitters. Both **NMDA** and the **AMPA** glutamate receptors may play a role in seizure onset. Antagonists of both of these receptor types have anticonvulsant effects in experimental models of seizures, but side effects have limited their use in humans. Studies have suggested, however, that part of the mechanism of action of both **lamotrigine** and **topiramate,** and perhaps **phenobarbital,** may involve inhibition of glutamate receptors.

A fourth mechanism by which drugs may interrupt the origin and spread of epileptic discharges is through alterations in the extracellular concentrations of K^+ and Ca^{2+}. During seizures, the extracellular concentrations of K^+ increase and those of Ca^{2+} decrease. Both changes cause greater excitability of neurons and may promote seizure initiation and spread. The ability of **phenytoin** to produce frequency-dependent blockade of action potentials is augmented when the extracellular K^+ concentration is elevated to that found during seizure activity. This renders phenytoin more effective in epileptic tissue than in normally functioning brain areas.

The mechanisms of action of **valproic acid** and **ethosuximide,** drugs used for treatment of absence seizures, remain uncertain. Studies suggest that valproic acid may act by increasing concentrations of GABA in the brain, while some evidence indicates that **ethosuximide** may block absence seizures by reducing Ca^{2+} currents in thalamic neurons.

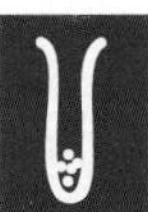

Pharmacokinetics

The pharmacokinetic parameters of the primary antiepileptic agents are summarized in Table 27-2. Because antiepileptic drugs are used to treat a chronic medical condition, they must be absorbed orally and cross the blood-brain barrier. Most antiepileptic drugs are metabolized by the hepatic cytochrome P450 system with the metabolites excreted by the kidney; several antiepileptic drugs have active metabolites.

Many antiepileptic drugs are highly bound to plasma proteins, which is clinically important because the usual determinations of blood concentrations indicate total drug (bound plus free) in serum, even though it is only free drug that is active. The half-life of antiepileptic agents varies with the age of the patient and exposure to other drugs.

The metabolism of **phenytoin** is characterized by saturation, or zero-order kinetics (Chapter 3). At low doses, there is a linear relationship between the dose and the serum concentration of the drug. At higher doses, however, there is a much greater rise in serum concentration for a given increase in dose (nonlinear) because, when serum concentrations rise above a certain value, the liver enzymes that catalyze phenytoin metabolism become saturated. The dose at which this transition occurs varies from patient to patient but is usually between 400 and 600 mg/day (Fig. 27-5). Because of this kinetic pattern, doses of phenytoin must be individualized.

Carbamazepine is metabolized in the liver to produce an epoxide, which is relatively stable and accumulates in the blood. This metabolite has antiepileptic properties, and some believe that it contributes to the neurotoxicity that can develop in patients taking carbamazepine. Carbamazepine also induces its own metabolism, with the rate of metabolism increasing during the first four to six weeks. After this time, larger doses become necessary to maintain constant serum concentrations.

Ethosuximide has a long half-life, which allows for once-a-day dosing. However, the gastrointestinal side effects are frequently intolerable with once-a-day

Table 27-2 Pharmacokinetic parameters

Drug	Half-Life (hrs)*	Disposition	Bound to Plasma Proteins (%)
Carbamazepine	10-15†	M (60%),‡ R (40%)	75
Ethosuximide	30-60	M (80%), R (20%)	<10
Lamotrigine	7-70	M (80%), R (20%)	55
Phenytoin	12-36	M (95%), R (5%)	90
Valproic acid	8-17	M (>95%)	90

M, Metabolized (in liver); *R*, eliminated unchanged by renal mechanisms.
*Age dependent.
†After repeated doses.
‡Produces an active metabolite.

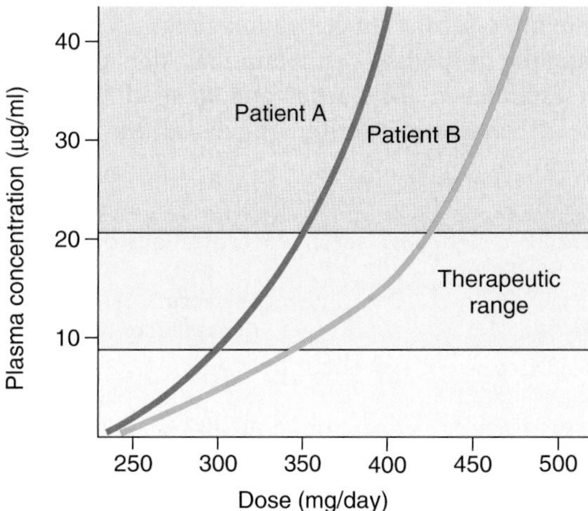

Figure 27-5 Relationship between the dose and steady-state plasma concentration of phenytoin illustrated for 2 patients. In both patients there is a linear relationship between the dose and plasma concentration at low doses. As the dose increases, there is a transition to a non-linear relationship. This transition occurs at different doses in each patient.

dosing and are significantly reduced with divided dosing. Divided dosing reduces the peak plasma concentration and thereby reduces the incidence of side effects.

Lamotrigine exhibits negligible first-pass metabolism and is inactivated and excreted as a glucuronic acid.

Valproic acid is metabolized approximately equally by hepatic microsomes and mitochondria and is excreted as a glucuronide conjugate.

Phenobarbital induces liver microsomal enzyme systems and accelerates its own metabolism and that of other drugs taken concurrently. **Primidone** is metabolized in the liver to phenobarbital and to phenylethylmalonamide, which also has some antiepileptic action.

Many antiepileptic drugs are available as brand name and generic products, and differences in formulation result in a wide range of bioavailability among different preparations of a given drug. This can lead to problems in seizure control when formulations are changed and should be considered when prescribing antiepileptic drugs.

Relation of mechanisms of action to clinical response

As mentioned, antiepileptic medication is selected according to seizure type, and the goal of therapy is to prevent seizures and minimize side effects. To this end, relative serum concentration ranges for producing therapeutic responses with minimal side effects have been established for partial and generalized seizures. These "therapeutic" serum concentration ranges are listed in Table 27-3 and have been determined empirically from general clinical experience in diverse and heterogeneous populations of epileptic patients. Thus, one should not take these values as absolute recommendations for individual patients, but they may be used as a guide.

The general strategy for treating **status epilepticus** involves support of cardiovascular and respiratory systems and treatment of seizure activity. Initially, a rapid-acting antiepileptic such as diazepam (10 mg at a rate of 1-2 mg/min) or lorazepam (4 mg at a rate of 1 mg/min) should be administered intravenously to stop the seizures; the doses should be repeated after 5 minutes if a response is not obtained. Because the effects of these compounds wear off rapidly, therapy with phenytoin or fosphenytoin (20 mg/kg administered intravenously at a rate of 30-50 mg/min) should also be instituted. Because phenytoin can produce hypotension or cardiac dysrhythmias if administered too rapidly, the patient must be monitored closely.

Side effects, clinical problems, and toxicity

Antiepileptic drugs cross the blood-brain barrier and have potential to cause systemic and neurological toxicity. The problems encountered are listed in the Clinical Problems box. Side effects of antiepileptic drugs occur in 30% to 50% of patients. However, these are frequently tolerable and require monitoring only. In other cases, side effects can be reduced or eliminated by changing the dose or administration schedule. In 5% to 15% of patients, another antiepileptic drug must be prescribed because of toxicity. Serious idiosyncratic effects, such as allergic reactions, are rare but can be life-threatening. They usually occur within several

Table 27-3 Effective serum concentrations of antiepileptic drugs required for specific seizure types

Drug	Therapeutic Serum Concentration (μg/ml)	Indication
Carbamazepine	4-12	Partial, including secondarily generalized Generalized tonic-clonic (grand mal)
Ethosuximide	40-100	Absence (petit mal)
Lamotrigine	2-20	Partial, including secondarily generalized Atypical absence, myoclonic, atonic
Phenytoin	5-25	Generalized tonic-clonic (grand mal)
	10-20	Partial, including secondarily generalized
Valproate*	50-150	Generalized tonic-clonic (grand mal) with absence seizure Absence (petit mal)
	50-100	Atypical absence, myoclonic, atonic

*First choice for absence if primary generalized tonic-clonic seizure is also present.

CLINICAL PROBLEMS

Carbamazepine

Autoinduction of metabolism
Nausea and visual disturbances (dose-related)
Granulocyte suppression
Aplastic anemia (idiosyncratic)

Ethosuximide

Stomach aches and vomiting
Hiccups

Lamotrigine

Rash

Phenytoin

Ataxia and nystagmus (dose-related)
Cognitive impairment
Hirsutism, coarsening of facial features, gingival hyperplasia
Saturation metabolism kinetics

Valproic acid

Tremor
Nausea and vomiting
Elevated liver enzymes
Weight gain

weeks or months of starting a new drug and tend to be dose-independent. Felbamate-related aplastic anemia occurs in approximately 1 in 5,000 patients. Most antiepileptic drugs should be introduced slowly to minimize side effects.

Patients often experience nausea and visual disturbances during initiation of carbamazepine therapy, and these can be minimized by slow introduction of the drug. Carbamazepine may have hematological effects, particularly leukopenia or sometimes thrombocytopenia, which may disappear with continued use. The most problematic hematological effect is depression of granulocytes in the blood. If good seizure control is achieved and other serious side effects are absent, an absolute granulocyte count of 1000/mm^3 or more is acceptable. An aplastic anemia syndrome is associated with carbamazepine but is very infrequent (less than 1 in 50,000). An infrequent dose-related side effect of carbamazepine is inappropriate antidiuretic hormone secretion leading to hyponatremia. Measurement of serum concentrations of carbamazepine to assess toxicity can be problematic because the epoxide metabolite may also cause toxicity.

Dose-related side effects of ethosuximide include gastrointestinal problems (stomach aches and vomiting) and hiccups. Tolerance to these effects develops. Ethosuximide may also lead to bone marrow suppression, but this is rare.

Dose-related side effects of lamotrigine include dizziness, headache, diplopia, nausea, and sleepiness. A rash can occur as either a dose-related or idiosyncratic reaction but seems to be most closely related to the rate of increase in the dose. Ataxia can sometimes occur.

In general, phenytoin is quite safe. Dose-related side effects include ataxia and nystagmus, commonly detected when total serum concentrations exceed 20 µg/ml. Other side effects of long-term phenytoin therapy are hirsutism, coarsening of facial features, gingival hyperplasia, and osteomalacia. These should be considered when prescribing phenytoin for children. Less-common reactions are hepatitis, a lupus-like connective tissue disease, lymphadenopathy, and pseudolymphoma.

Valproic acid may produce nausea, vomiting, and lethargy, particularly early in therapy. The availability of enteric-coated tablets of valproic acid has led to a significant decrease in the gastrointestinal side effects. Elevation of liver enzymes and blood ammonia levels in patients receiving valproic acid is common. Fatal hepatitis may occur in patients taking valproic acid, but overall the risk is small (approximately 1 in 40,000). The risk of fatal hepatitis is increased considerably in patients less than 2 years of age treated with multiple antiepileptic drugs. Two uncommon dose-related side effects of valproic acid are thrombocytopenia and changes in coagulation parameters, secondary to depletion of fibrinogen. However, these changes usually are not serious. Other side effects of valproic acid are weight gain, alopecia, and tremor.

Phenobarbital frequently produces depression of central nervous system function, resulting in sedation and depression. Side effects of phenobarbital in children include motor hyperactivity, irritability, decreased attention, and mental slowing.

Antiepileptic drugs during pregnancy

Because antiepileptic agents are taken for many years or a lifetime, the issue of taking these drugs during pregnancy is important. During pregnancy, seizures increase in frequency in 25% of epileptic women, do not change in frequency in 50%, and decrease in frequency in 25%. The possibility of seizures puts both the mother and child at risk. The teratogenic properties of antiepileptic drugs are also a concern. Fetal exposure to phenytoin, carbamazepine, valproate, and phenobarbital has been associated with congenital anomalies, including cardiac, urinary tract, and neural tube defects and cleft palate, but most pregnant patients exposed to antiepileptic drugs deliver normal infants. Children of mothers who have epilepsy are at increased risk for malformations even if antiepileptic drugs are not used during pregnancy. Whenever possible, the woman should be counseled before she becomes pregnant. If discontinuation of antiepileptic medication is not an option, single-drug therapy and the smallest dose of the antiepileptic agent should be used.

A deficiency of vitamin K–dependent clotting factors may develop in newborn infants of mothers who have received phenobarbital, primidone, or phenytoin during pregnancy, and this can result in serious hemorrhage during the first 24 hours of life. This can be prevented by administering vitamin K to the newborn shortly after birth.

Drug interactions

Antiepileptic drugs can induce or inhibit certain isozymes of cytochrome P450, resulting in drug interactions, not only with other antiepileptic drugs but also with a wide range of therapeutic agents. In general, enzyme inducers decrease serum concentrations of other drugs, while enzyme inhibitors increase concentrations. In addition, many antiepileptic drugs are highly bound to plasma proteins, which can also lead to significant drug interactions. For example, valproic acid may increase the toxicity of phenytoin by displacing phenytoin from plasma binding sites. It is important to be aware of the possibility of drug interactions as a consequence of the pharmacokinetic characteristics of the antiepileptic drugs.

New horizons

Over the past 70 years, compounds have been discovered to have antiepileptic properties, either accidentally or through screening with animal models of seizures. More recently the focus has been on countering putative epileptogenic mechanisms. For example, augmentation of inhibition in the brain should have an antiepileptogenic effect. In fact, two of the newer antiepileptic drugs act to augment inhibition in the brain. Tiagabine acts by slowing reuptake of GABA from the synaptic cleft, while vigabatrin inhibits irreversibly GABA transaminase, the main enzyme that catabolizes GABA. Both drugs produce an increase in brain GABA levels. A number of generalized epilepsies have Mendelian inheritance and are associated with single gene mutations. Almost all of these mutations have been found in genes that encode ion channels. While it is not yet known how these genetic polymorphisms result in an epilepsy phenotype, understanding the underlying mechanisms and being able to treat patients with these inherited epilepsies is an area of intense research.

Another area of considerable interest is the role of cortical malformations in development of epilepsy. Many cortical malformations are associated with seizures that are impossible to control with currently available drugs. High-resolution magnetic resonance imaging scanning has detected very small malformations in patients who were previously classified as having cryptogenic epilepsy. Understanding how these malformations lead to seizures could provide the basis for developing appropriate therapy for these patients.

In addition to pharmacological therapy, some patients with seizures benefit from surgery. One goal of surgical therapy is to remove identifiable lesions such as arteriovenous malformations, brain tumors, abscesses, and hematomas. The overall results have been gratifying. Another goal of surgery has been to treat patients who are refractory to drug therapy. Seizures in such patients must originate in a well-circumscribed region of the brain that can be removed without risk of producing a major neurological handicap. Epilepsy surgery is usually undertaken at a specialized comprehensive epilepsy center.

TRADE NAMES

In addition to generic and fixed-combination preparations and the drugs listed in the Major Drugs box, the following trade-named materials are some of the important compounds available in the United States.

Secondary antiepileptic drugs, including adjuncts

Acetazolamide (Diamox)
Clonazepam (Klonopin)
Felbamate (Felbatol)
Gabapentin (Neurontin)
Levetiracetam (Keppra)
Methsuximide (Celontin)
Oxcarbazepine (Trileptal)
Phenobarbital (Luminal and others)
Primidone (Mysoline)
Tiagabine (Gabitril)
Topiramate (Topamax)
Zonisamide (Zonegran)

FURTHER READING

Browne TR, Holmes GL. Primary care: epilepsy. *N Engl J Med* 2001; 344:1145-1151.

Chang BS, Lowenstein DH. Mechanisms of disease: epilepsy. *N Engl J Med* 2003; 349:1257-1266.

Drugs for epilepsy: treatment guidelines. *Med Lett* 2003; 1:57-64.

Self-assessment questions

1. A 6-year-old girl and her mother come to see you because the girl's teacher has observed episodes of staring and inability to communicate. These episodes last 3 to 5 seconds and occur 10 to 20 times during the school day. An EEG shows synchronized 3-per-second spike-wave discharges generalized over the entire cortex. Which antiepileptic medication would you try first in this young girl?
   a. Phenytoin
   b. Clonazepam
   c. Primidone
   d. Carbamazepine
   e. Ethosuximide

2. A young patient's seizures have been well controlled with phenytoin for many years. He recently has had two seizures, and you determine that the phenytoin concentration in his blood is low because of his recent growth. You increase the phenytoin dose, calculating the increased dose based on his weight gain (same mg/kg as before). Several weeks later the patient calls up and tells you that he has not had any seizures but he is having trouble walking and is dizzy. Which of the following statements best describes what has happened?
   a. The patient did not follow your instructions and has been taking too many pills.
   b. After the dose increase, phenytoin was eliminated by zero-order kinetics and serum concentrations were in the toxic range.
   c. His metabolism of phenytoin has increased as a result of induction of liver microsomal enzymes.
   d. His phenytoin concentrations are too low.
   e. An inner ear infection has developed.

3. What is the best initial treatment for a 3-year-old girl experiencing generalized tonic-clonic seizures daily?
   a. Brain surgery to remove the focus of her seizures
   b. Monotherapy with primidone
   c. Treatment with carbamazepine
   d. Treatment with phenytoin
   e. No drug therapy at this time

4. Generalized tonic-clonic seizures are characterized by a sustained depolarization of cortical neurons with action potentials. Which of the following characteristics of a new drug for the treatment of generalized tonic-clonic seizures would you like to see?
   a. Adenosine agonist
   b. Block GABA receptors
   c. Block of repetitive neuronal firing
   d. Block synchronization of inhibitory neurons
   e. NMDA antagonist

5. A 45-year-old woman with new-onset seizures is started on an antiepileptic drug. She initially does well, but she has 2 seizures about 4 weeks after the start of treatment. She has taken the same number of pills each day, but her plasma concentration of the drug has decreased. Which antiepileptic drug is she taking?
   a. Ethosuximide
   b. Primidone
   c. Phenytoin
   d. Carbamazepine
   e. Valproic acid

6. Seizures can be caused by all of the following, *except*
   a. Hyponatremia
   b. Alkalosis
   c. Brain tumor
   d. Mental retardation
   e. Drug withdrawal

CHAPTER 28

General anesthetics

Yung-Fong Sung
Stephen G. Holtzman

Major Drugs

Inhalational anesthetics
Desflurane (Suprane)
Enflurane (Ethrane)
Halothane (Fluothane)
Isoflurane (Forane)
Nitrous oxide
Sevoflurane (Ultane)

Antagonist drugs
Flumazenil (Mazicon, Romazicon)
Naloxone (Narcan)

Intravenous anesthetics
Etomidate (Amidate)
Fentanyl (Sublimaze)
Ketamine (Ketalar)
Midazolam (Versed)
Propofol (Diprivan)
Remifentanil (Ultiva)
Thiopental (Pentothal)

Therapeutic overview

Modern surgical procedures would not be possible without anesthetics to block the traumatic emotional and physical pain that would otherwise be experienced by the patient. Such agents have been available since the 1840s, when diethyl ether was first used successfully to anesthetize patients undergoing surgery.

General anesthesia can be viewed as a controlled, reversible state of **loss of sensation** and consciousness. The ideal general anesthetic state comprises **analgesia; amnesia;** loss of consciousness (absence of awareness); relaxation of skeletal muscles; suppression of somatic, autonomic, and endocrine reflexes; and hemodynamic stability. Although most objectives of general anesthesia can be achieved with diethyl ether, this inhalational agent has become obsolete because of its flammability and explosiveness. Other general anesthetic agents are available and are classified based on their route of administration—by inhalation or intravenous (IV) injection.

The induction of anesthesia produced by the IV administration of an anesthetic agent is more rapid, smoother, and more pleasant for the patient than that produced by an inhalational anesthetic agent, with its slower onset, vapors that may be unpleasant, and face-mask delivery system. In addition to their use for the induction of anesthesia, hypnotic and opioid drugs are often administered intravenously for anesthesia management. In **balanced anesthesia,** a combination of various anesthetic agents is used, each in small doses, to reduce the chance of significant side effects. This is now common practice.

The safe and effective use of general anesthetics is a dynamic process that must be individualized for each patient and surgical situation. Further, the needs of both the surgical team and the patient may change during a procedure, altering anesthetic requirements. For example, there may be a need to blunt the tachycardia and hypertension that result from an intense sympathetic nervous system stimulus, produce greater relaxation of skeletal muscle, or provide additional analgesia. All interventions must be reversible and tissue hypoxia must be prevented.

The primary therapeutic considerations are summarized in the Therapeutic Overview box.

Abbreviations

CNS	central nervous system
ED_{50}	median effective dose
GABA	γ-aminobutyric acid
IV	intravenous
MAC	minimum alveolar concentration
NMDA	*N*-methyl-D-aspartate
PCO_2	carbon dioxide tension (partial pressure)

THERAPEUTIC OVERVIEW

Requirements of anesthetic drugs

Inhalational
- Chemical stability
- Minimal irritation upon inhaling
- Speed of onset (time to loss of consciousness)
- Ability to produce analgesia, amnesia, and muscle relaxation
- Minimal side effects, especially cardiovascular and respiratory depression and toxicity to the liver
- Speed and safety of emergence
- Minimal metabolism

Intravenous
- Chemical stability
- No pain at injection site
- Speed of onset
- Minimal side effects
- Ability to produce analgesia, amnesia, and muscle relaxation
- Speed and safety of emergence
- Rapid metabolism or redistribution

Mechanisms of action

Inhalational anesthetics

The molecular basis for the anesthetic action of inhalational agents is poorly understood. Although most inhalational anesthetics contain an ether (-O-) link and a halogen, no obvious structure-activity relationships have been defined, suggesting that they do not exert their effects through specific cell-surface receptors, unlike most other therapeutic agents acting on the central nervous system (CNS) (Fig. 28-1).

The potency of an inhalational anesthetic is expressed in terms of the minimum alveolar concentration (MAC), which is a concentration that prevents 50% of patients from responding to a painful stimulus, such as a skin incision. MAC is analogous to the median effective dose (ED_{50}) and is used to express the relative potency of gaseous drugs. Meyer and Overton observed that the potencies of anesthetic agents correlate highly with their lipid solubilities, as measured by the oil:gas partition coefficient (Table 28-1; Fig. 28-2). Indeed, this relationship holds not only for agents in clinical use but also for inert gases that are not used clinically, such as xenon and argon. This correlation has given rise to several theories of anesthetic action, none of which has been substantiated.

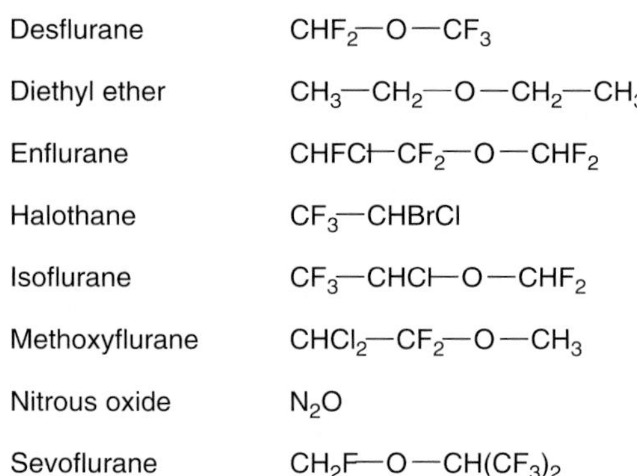

Desflurane	$CHF_2—O—CF_3$
Diethyl ether	$CH_3—CH_2—O—CH_2—CH_3$
Enflurane	$CHFCl—CF_2—O—CHF_2$
Halothane	$CF_3—CHBrCl$
Isoflurane	$CF_3—CHCl—O—CHF_2$
Methoxyflurane	$CHCl_2—CF_2—O—CH_3$
Nitrous oxide	N_2O
Sevoflurane	$CH_2F—O—CH(CF_3)_2$

Figure 28-1 Chemical structure of inhalational anesthetic agents.

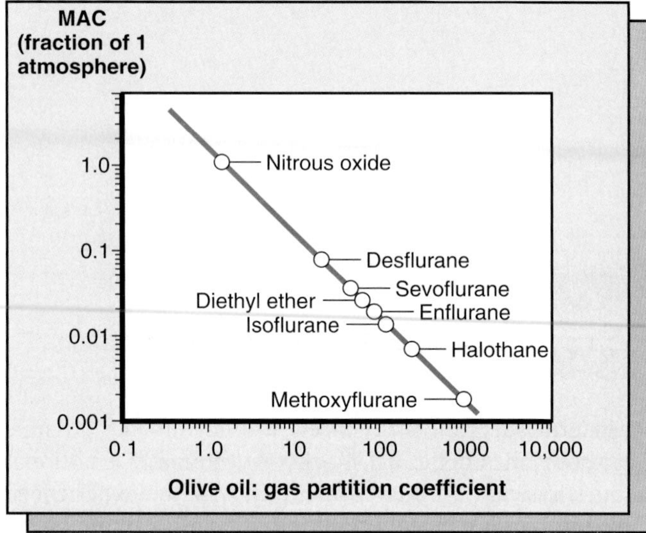

Figure 28-2 The potency of an inhalational anesthetic agent is determined by its lipid solubility, as measured by its oil:gas partition coefficient.

According to the volume expansion theory, molecules of an anesthetic dissolve in the phospholipid bilayer of the neuronal membrane, causing it to expand and impede opening of ion channels necessary for generation and propagation of action potentials. Another hypothesis suggests that anesthetic molecules bind to specific hydrophobic regions of lipoproteins in the neuronal membrane that are part of, or close to, an ion channel. The resulting conformational change in the protein prevents effective operation of the channel. Anesthetics also have been considered to alter the fluidity of membrane lipids, which could also prevent or limit increases in ion conductance.

Alternatively, "nonspecific" effects of anesthetics may occur at specific cell-surface receptors for neurotransmitters or neuromodulators. For example, clinically relevant concentrations of halogenated inhalational

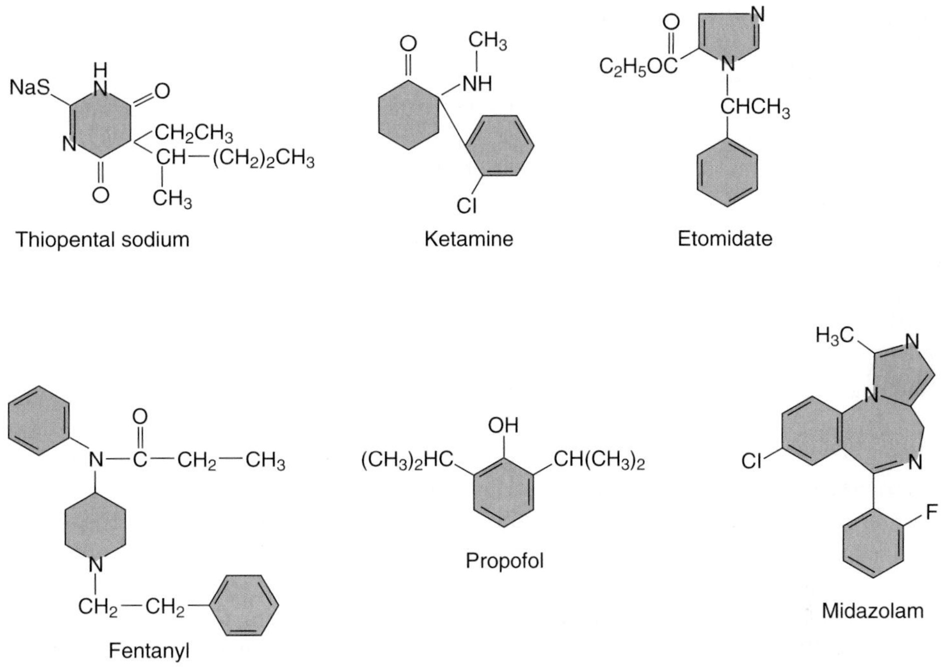

Thiopental sodium

Ketamine

Etomidate

Fentanyl

Propofol

Midazolam

Figure 28-3 Structures of representative IV general anesthetic drugs.

Table 28-1 Characteristics of inhalational anesthetic agents

Anesthetic Agent	Blood:Gas Partition Coefficient	Oil:Gas Partition Coefficient	MAC (% of 1 atmosphere)	Approximate Percentage of Anesthetic Dose Metabolized
Desflurane	0.42	19	7.0	0.5
Diethyl ether*	12	65	1.9	—
Enflurane	1.9	98	1.7	3
Halothane	2.3	225	0.75	15
Isoflurane	1.4	98	1.2	0.5
Methoxyflurane*	13	825	0.16	60
Nitrous oxide	0.47	1.4	105.0	Nil
Sevoflurane	0.63	53	2.0	3

*No longer used clinically.

anesthetics increase Cl^- conductance induced by γ-aminobutyric acid (GABA) in *in vitro* neuronal preparations. Because GABA is the principal inhibitory neurotransmitter in the brain, activation or enhancement of GABA-mediated Cl^- conductance would inhibit CNS neuronal activity. Similarly, nitrous oxide decreases cation conductance in the ion channel controlled by the *N*-methyl-D-aspartate (NMDA) glutamate receptor, thereby blocking the actions of the principal excitatory neurotransmitter in the brain, and all inhalational anesthetics inhibit the activity of neuronal nicotinic acetylcholine receptors. Thus, through mechanisms as yet undefined, inhalational anesthetics disrupt the function of ligand-gated ion channels, increasing inhibitory and decreasing excitatory synaptic transmission.

Intravenous anesthetics

Most IV anesthetic agents contain ring structures (Fig. 28-3) and have well-documented effects at specific cell-surface receptors. For example, the barbiturates and benzodiazepines act at two distinct recognition sites on the $GABA_A$ receptor-Cl^- channel complex to potentiate GABA-mediated Cl^- conductance and neuronal inhibition (see Chapter 24). The depressant effects of morphine-like opioids on neuronal activity are mediated by the μ-opioid receptor and those of agonist-antagonist opioids by the μ- and κ-opioid receptors (see Chapter 31). Ketamine appears to act by blocking neuronal excitation; it binds to the phencyclidine receptor, a site within the cation channel gated by the NMDA glutamate receptor, and inhibits cation conductance through the channel. The mechanisms of action of etomidate and propofol remain obscure, although a facilitatory effect on the $GABA_A$ receptor-Cl^- ionophore complex may be involved. In clinically relevant concentrations *in vitro,* both drugs block specific high-affinity neuronal uptake of GABA without affecting its release. Propofol also has inhibitory effects on NMDA glutamate receptors.

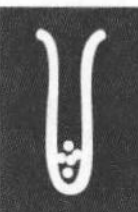

Pharmacokinetics

Inhalational anesthetics

The depth of anesthesia is determined by the concentration of an anesthetic in the brain. Therefore, to produce concentrations adequate for surgery, it is necessary to deliver an appropriate amount of drug to the brain. Unlike most drugs, inhalational anesthetics are administered as gases or vapors. Therefore, a specific set of physical principles applies to the delivery of these agents.

In a mixture of gases, the **partial pressure** of an anesthetic agent is directly proportional to its fractional concentration in the mixture (Dalton's Law). Thus, as depicted in Figure 28-4, in a mixture of 5% halothane, 70% nitrous oxide, and 25% oxygen—which might be used during mask induction of anesthesia—the partial pressures of the component gases are 38, 532, and 190 mm Hg, respectively, at 1 atmosphere (760 mm Hg) of pressure.

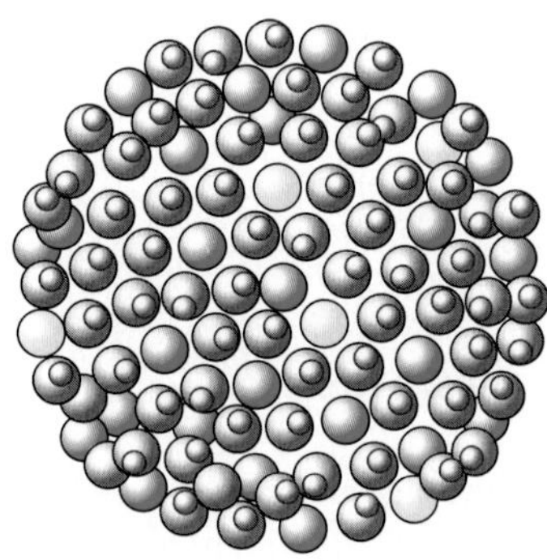

	Concentration %		Partial pressure (mm Hg)
Nitrous oxide	70	(x 760 =)	532
Oxygen	25	(x 760 =)	190
Halothane	5	(x 760 =)	38
	100%	(=)	760 mm Hg (1 atmosphere)

Figure 28-4 The partial pressure of a gas in a mixture of gases is directly proportional to its concentration.

When a gas is dissolved in the blood or other body tissues, *its partial pressure is directly proportional to its concentration but inversely proportional to its solubility in that tissue.* The concept of partial pressure is of central importance, because the partial pressure of a gas is the driving force that moves the gas from the anesthetic machine to the lungs, from the lungs to the blood, and from the blood to the brain. At theoretical equilibrium, the partial pressures are equal in all body tissues, alveoli, and the inspired gas mixture. Because solubility varies from tissue to tissue as a consequence of differences in tissue lipophilicity, the concentration of anesthetic must also vary from tissue to tissue if partial pressures are equal throughout the body. The partial pressure (or concentration) of the anesthetic in the inspired gas mixture is the factor controlled most easily by the anesthesiologist. This is accomplished by adjusting the anesthetic machine to optimize partial pressures during induction and/or maintenance.

The rate of induction of anesthesia by inhalational agents is affected by numerous factors, including those that reduce **alveolar ventilation,** which represents the product of the rate of respiration and tidal volume less the pulmonary dead space (Table 28-2). Thus, if a patient is administered respiratory depressants such as barbiturates or opioid analgesics preoperatively, the rate of respiration or tidal volume decreases, thereby reducing alveolar ventilation in the absence of assisted ventilation. Alveolar dead space is substantial in patients with pulmonary diseases such as emphysema and atelectasis, which result in decreased alveolar ventilation and rate of anesthesia induction.

The path followed by an inhalational anesthetic during induction of, and emergence from, anesthesia is diagrammed in Figure 28-5. Induction is facilitated by factors that maintain a high partial pressure of the anesthetic in the inspired gas mixture, alveolar space, and arterial blood to deliver as much of the gas to the brain as quickly as possible. The alveolar membrane poses no

Table 28-2 Factors affecting the rate of induction with an inhalational anesthetic

Condition	Rate of Induction
↑Concentration of anesthetic in inspired gas mixture	↑
↑Alveolar ventilation	↑
↑Solubility of anesthetic in blood (blood:gas partition coefficient)	↓
↑Cardiac output	↓

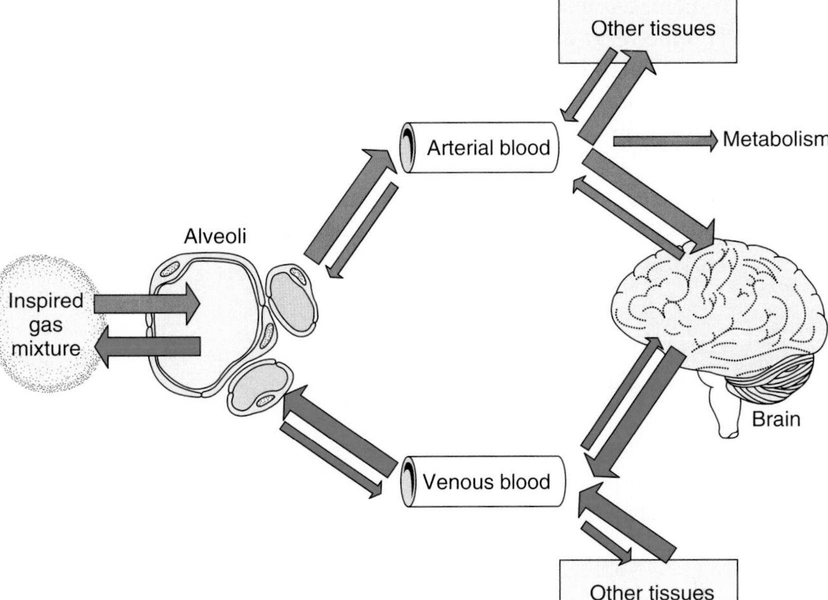

Figure 28-5 Pathway of an inhalational anesthetic agent during induction of *(red arrows)* and emergence from *(blue arrows)* anesthesia. The large arrows indicate the direction of net movement.

barrier to gases, permitting unhindered diffusion in both directions. Therefore, once the anesthetic gas reaches the alveolar space, it obeys the law of mass action and moves down its partial-pressure gradient into arterial blood. At the initiation of anesthetic administration, the partial pressure of the anesthetic in the alveolar space is much higher than that in blood. Thus, the partial-pressure gradient between the alveolar space and the arteriolar blood is high, and initially the gas moves rapidly into blood. As the partial pressure of the anesthetic agent in blood increases, the gradient between the alveolar space and blood decreases and uptake slows (Fig. 28-6).

Another important factor in the rate of rise of the arterial partial pressure of an anesthetic gas is its solubility in blood. This relationship is expressed as the **blood : gas partition coefficient.** The higher the solubility of an anesthetic gas in blood, the more must be dissolved to produce a change in partial pressure (because partial pressure is inversely proportional to solubility). This relationship is illustrated for nitrous oxide and halothane in Figure 28-7.

Nitrous oxide has a blood : gas partition coefficient of 0.47, so relatively little must be dissolved in blood for its partial pressure in blood to rise. This also is true for **desflurane** and **sevoflurane.** In contrast, blood serves as a large reservoir for **halothane,** retaining at equilibrium 2.3 parts for every 1 part in the alveolar space. Induction therefore depends *not* on dissolving the anesthetic in blood but on raising arterial partial pressure to drive the gas from blood to brain. Therefore, the rate of rise of arterial partial pressure and speed of induction are fastest for gases that are least soluble in blood (see Fig. 28-6). The blood : gas partition coefficients of inhalational anesthetics are listed in Table 28-1.

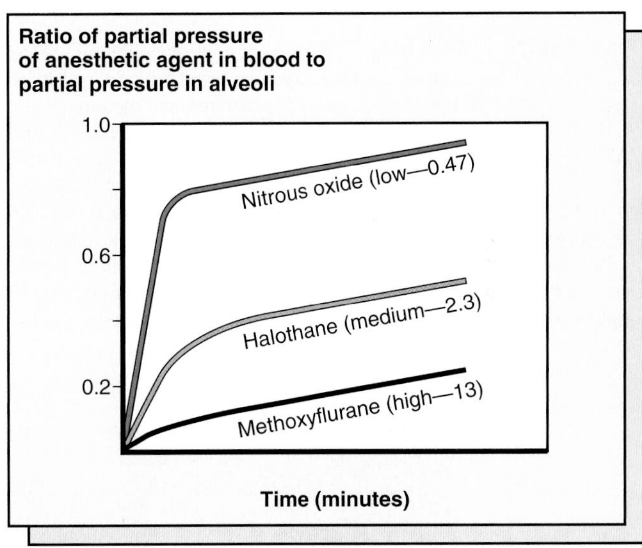

Figure 28-6 Rate of rise of partial pressure of an inhalational anesthetic agent in arterial blood is determined by its solubility in blood (blood : gas partition coefficient).

Because **cardiac output** is the primary determinant of the rate of pulmonary blood flow, it would seem that an increase in cardiac output, and thus an increase in pulmonary blood flow, would accelerate induction of anesthesia. However, the opposite is true. The rate of anesthetic induction decreases with increasing cardiac output. An increased pulmonary blood flow means that the same volume of gas from the alveoli diffuses into a larger volume of blood per unit of time. The initial consequence is a reduced concentration of anesthetic (and partial pressure) in blood. In addition, increases in cardiac output typically increase perfusion of tissues other than brain, such as muscle, thereby increasing the apparent volume of distribution of the anesthetic. In a patient with heart failure, blood loss, or other conditions resulting in decreased cardiac output, the volume of distribution of an anesthetic is reduced and the rate of induction is increased.

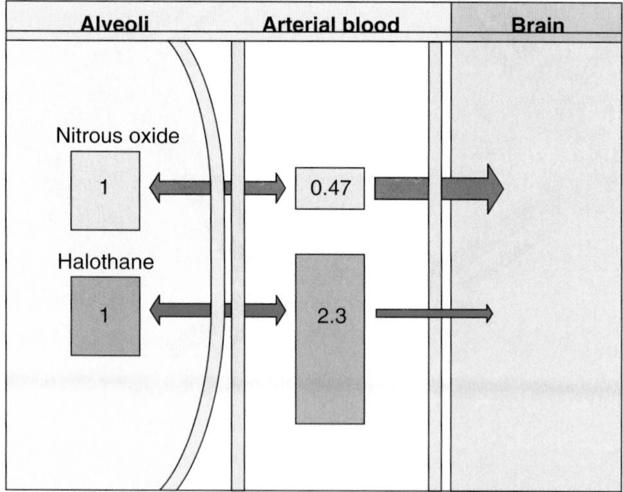

Figure 28-7 The solubility of an inhalational anesthetic in blood determines how rapidly its partial pressure rises in blood and brain with a change in partial pressure in the inspired gas mixture. If the alveolar space and blood were a closed system and nitrous oxide and halothane were allowed to equilibrate between the two, there would be 0.47 parts of nitrous oxide in blood for every 1 part in alveoli, and 2.3 parts of halothane in blood for every 1 part in alveoli. An increase in the partial pressure of nitrous oxide in the inspired gas mixture results in almost a fivefold larger increase in its partial pressure in blood than would a similar increase in the partial pressure of halothane in the inspired gas mixture, driving nitrous oxide into the brain more rapidly.

The transfer of an anesthetic from arterial blood to brain depends on factors analogous to those involved in movement of gas from alveoli to arterial blood. These include the partial pressure gradient between blood and brain, the solubility of the anesthetic in brain, and cerebral blood flow. The brain is part of the **vessel-rich group** of tissues that compose 9% of body mass but receive 75% of cardiac output. The anesthetic uptake curve levels off (see Fig. 28-6), reflecting attainment of equilibrium by the vessel-rich group of tissues. In contrast, the muscle group constitutes 50% of body mass but receives only 18% of cardiac output. Fat represents 19% of body mass and receives 5% of cardiac output, whereas the **vessel-poor group,** bone and tendon, accounts for 22% of body mass yet receives less than 2% of cardiac output. Thus, about 41% of total body mass receives a mere 7% of cardiac output. As a consequence, in most surgical procedures, poorly perfused tissues do not contribute meaningfully to the apparent volume of distribution of the inhalational anesthetic, and true total equilibration does not occur. The importance of tissue perfusion as a factor determining the uptake of an anesthetic is illustrated for halothane in Figure 28-8.

When administration of an anesthetic is terminated, the anesthetic gas flows from the venous blood

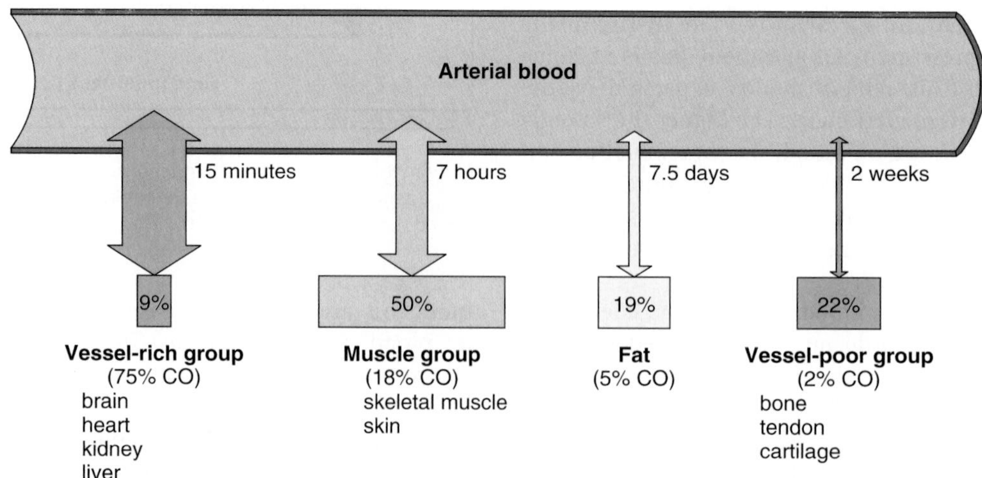

Figure 28-8 The rate at which an inhalational anesthetic agent is taken up by a tissue depends on the fraction of the cardiac output (CO) that the tissue receives. The approximate time for halothane to equilibrate between blood and tissues is indicated next to the arrows; the percentage of body mass that the tissue represents is shown in the boxes. The numbers in parentheses represent the relative percentage of CO received by each tissue group.

to the alveolar space (see Fig. 28-5). Factors that affect the rate of elimination of an inhalational anesthetic are analogous to those that determine its rate of uptake. Therefore, the rate of loss of an anesthetic gas during emergence from anesthesia is directly proportional to its rate of uptake, and emergence is a mirror image of induction.

Although inhaled anesthetics are cleared from the body largely via the lung, most undergo some degree of hepatic metabolism, and several metabolites have been implicated in organ toxicity. The extensive metabolism of **methoxyflurane**, 50% to 60% of an administered dose, results in the release of fluoride ions, which can reach nephrotoxic concentrations during long surgical procedures; therefore, methoxyflurane is no longer used. The extent of biotransformation of other inhalational anesthetics ranges from approximately 15% for halothane to negligible amounts for nitrous oxide (see Table 28-1). Inhalational anesthetics that are not appreciably metabolized generally exhibit less-toxic sequelae.

Intravenous anesthetics

When IV anesthetics are administered, movement of drug from blood to brain determines its onset of action. A good IV anesthetic drug should be effective within one "arm-to-brain blood circulation." The short-acting barbiturates, propofol and etomidate, are the fastest to induce anesthesia; that is, 30 to 50 seconds from injection to loss of the eyelash reflex, or one arm-to-brain circulation. On the other hand, a benzodiazepine requires several minutes to induce a similar response. Because blood flow to the brain is also important, the onset of action may be delayed in a patient with extremely low cardiac output and therefore a relatively low blood flow to the brain.

The duration of effect of a single induction dose of an IV anesthetic is determined by its rate of redistribution or metabolism. Redistribution from the brain into less-well-perfused tissues (i.e., abdominal viscera, skeletal muscle) is the predominant mechanism responsible for termination of action. Redistribution can occur within minutes of induction of anesthesia with a single dose of anesthetic, resulting in recovery of reflex activity and consciousness. The IV induction agents have varying speeds of onset, durations of action, and rates of redistribution. The pharmacokinetic and physicochemical characteristics of the ideal IV anesthetic are listed in Box 28-1.

Box 28-1 Characteristics of an Ideal Intravenous Anesthetic Drug

Physicochemical

- Water soluble
- Stable on shelf and to light exposure
- Lipophilic
- Small injection volume

Pharmacokinetic

- Rapid onset of action
- Short duration of action
- Nontoxic metabolites

Pharmacodynamic

- Wide margin of safety
- No interpatient variability in effects
- Nonallergenic
- Nontoxic to tissues

Thiopental has been used widely for IV induction because of its rapid and smooth onset and its short duration of action. It is highly lipid soluble, rapidly crosses the blood-brain barrier, and is rapidly redistributed from brain to other body tissues. These pharmacokinetic characteristics preclude its use as a maintenance agent for lengthy procedures. However, because of its long terminal elimination half-life, thiopental accumulates in the body, and its duration of action increases with repeated administration, causing some patients to remain unconscious after surgery is completed (Table 28-3). Thiopental is metabolized primarily in the liver to water-soluble metabolites that are excreted in the urine. The pharmacokinetic properties of other barbiturates used as IV anesthetics, such as **methohexital**, are generally similar to those of thiopental.

Induction of anesthesia with **diazepam** is relatively slow, often taking several minutes. It has a long redistribution half-life (30-60 minutes), a long duration of action, and a long terminal elimination half-life (see Table 28-3). It is metabolized by the microsomal enzyme system in liver, and most of its metabolites are pharmacologically active and have long half-lives. **Midazolam** is a water-soluble benzodiazepine twice as potent as diazepam. It takes midazolam 2 to 3 minutes to induce anesthesia, which is faster than diazepam but slower than thiopental.

Propofol is twice as potent as thiopental. Loss of consciousness occurs within one arm-to-brain circulation time. The induction dose is much lower in the elderly and slightly higher in younger children. Propofol can be used for both induction and maintenance of anesthesia. The duration of sleep after administration of a single dose is 5 to 10 minutes. To achieve a more sustained effect after induction, the patient should be given another bolus dose within 5 minutes or receive a continuous infusion; the latter is preferred to ensure smooth maintenance and constant plasma concentrations. The redistribution half-life of propofol is 5 to 10 minutes, and a long terminal-elimination half-life suggests that propofol may accumulate in tissues after prolonged use.

Table 28-3 Comparison of intravenous anesthetic induction agents in healthy adults

	Water Soluble	Solution Characteristics	Dose (mg/kg)	Elimination Half-Life (hrs)	Active Metabolites
HYPNOTICS					
Diazepam	No	Clear, yellow, propylene glycol-alcohol-benzoate	0.3-0.5	30-60	Three
Etomidate	No	Acidic propylene glycol	0.3-0.4, 0.1-0.25*	1-1.5	None
Methohexital	Yes	Clear, pale yellow	1.5-2.5, 1.0*	3-6	None
Midazolam	Yes	Clear	0.2-0.4, 0.1-0.2*†	2-6	One
Propofol	No	Milky emulsion	2.0-4.0, 1.0-2.0*	3-12	None
Thiopental	Yes	Clear, pale yellow; alkaline	3.0-6.0, 4.0-7.0,† 2.0-3.0*	3-8	One
OPIOIDS					
Alfentanil	Yes	Clear	0.02-0.075	1.5-2.0	None
Fentanyl	Yes	Clear	0.002-0.015	3-4	None
Meperidine	Yes	Clear	0.5-2	3-5	None
Morphine	Yes	Clear	0.1-0.15‡	1.5-2.5	One
Remifentanil	Yes	Clear	0.0005-0.001	0.16-0.33	None
Sufentanil	Yes	Clear	0.001-0.008	2.5-3.0	None
OTHER					
Ketamine	Yes	Clear	1.0-3.0, 2.0-4.0†	2-3	None

*Elderly/geriatric.
†Children.
‡Contraindicated in children <1 month old.

Ketamine, which is used for anesthesia induction, sedation, and analgesia, has a duration of action of 11 to 16 minutes.

Morphine, the prototypical opioid analgesic, is given subcutaneously or intramuscularly in doses of 8 to 15 mg to allay anxiety and ease pain before, during, and after surgery. It is administered IV in substantially higher doses in combination with an inhalational or IV anesthetic for the induction and maintenance of anesthesia, especially for cardiac or other major surgery. Morphine is being replaced gradually in this role by fentanyl and newer analogs of fentanyl such as sufentanil and remifentanil. Because of its low lipophilicity, morphine crosses the blood-brain barrier slowly, and plasma concentrations may not accurately reflect those in brain. Morphine is metabolized in the liver, primarily to morphine-6-glucuronide, which retains considerable morphine-like activity but has limited access to the CNS (see Chapter 31). Other opioids commonly used in anesthesia differ from morphine in their potency, rate of onset, and duration of action but are generally similar in their pharmacological activity (see Table 28-3 and Chapter 31).

The physicochemical properties of some IV anesthetic drugs render them insoluble in water at physiological pH, necessitating use of solvents or adjusting the pH of the injectate (see Table 28-3), either of which can lead to problems. The alkaline pH of a 2.5% solution of thiopental makes it unsuitable for mixing with acidic drugs, especially opioids and muscle relaxants. Thiopental solutions also cause tissue damage if injected intraarterially or extravascularly. Acidic **etomidate** solutions can cause pain and thrombophlebitis after intravascular injection. All alcohol-based solvents and buffers are venous irritants, causing pain when injected intravenously. Thus, a diazepam solution is sometimes mixed with a solution of the local anesthetic lidocaine to make the injection less painful. Midazolam, in contrast, is water soluble and poses no special problems for IV administration. Propofol emulsion causes pain on injection, a problem that may be resolved by newer formulations.

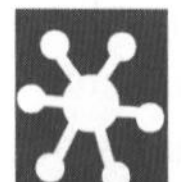

Relation of mechanisms of action to clinical response

Inhalational anesthetics

As indicated, the MAC is used to express the relative potency of gaseous drugs and is the concentration that prevents 50% of patients from responding to a painful stimulus. Clearly, one should administer an inhalational anesthetic at a concentration higher than 1.0 MAC to achieve an acceptable level of surgical anesthesia in which there is no movement in 100% of patients. Thus, although 1.0 MAC defines the ED_{50}, a level of anesthesia satisfactory for most surgical procedures is achieved at an alveolar gas concentration of 1.3 MAC, which is equal to or greater than the ED_{99}, the concentration that prevents greater than 99% of patients from responding to a painful stimulus.

Because doses of inhalational anesthetics are additive, a 0.5 MAC of compound "A" can be combined with a 0.5 MAC of compound "B" to give an inspired-gas mixture that has a MAC of 1.0. For example, 1.0 MAC of halothane is 0.75% (5.7 mm Hg, or 5.7 torr at 1.0 atmosphere of pressure) and 1.0 MAC of isoflurane is 1.15% (8.7 torr). Therefore, an inspired gas mixture containing 0.375% halothane and 0.575% isoflurane has a MAC of 1.0.

Except for nitrous oxide, all inhalational anesthetics in clinical use are sufficiently potent to produce surgical anesthesia when administered in a mixture containing at least 25% oxygen. Although MAC is not a prime factor in determining the inhalational anesthetic selected, it does provide a convenient point of reference for comparing their properties. For example, it can be useful to compare the extent of hypotension or relaxation of skeletal muscle produced by two different anesthetic agents administered at a MAC of 1.0.

The MAC is independent of the duration of the surgical procedure, remaining unchanged with time, and is unaffected by the sex of the patient. It also is relatively independent of the type of noxious stimulus applied (e.g., pressure versus heat). Indeed, increasing the intensity of the noxious stimulus, within limits, has little effect on MAC, although higher anesthetic concentrations are required for some traumatic surgical manipulations. MAC is also relatively unaffected by the acid-base status of the patient and is independent of the patient's body mass. However, at a fixed alveolar concentration, it takes longer to anesthetize a larger patient because of differences in the apparent volume of distribution. Although the MAC of an anesthetic is relatively independent of many patient and surgical variables, it is affected by age. The anesthetic requirement is higher in infants and lower in geriatric patients.

The general health of the patient also affects the anesthetic requirement. Not surprisingly, it is lower in debilitated patients than in otherwise healthy ones. Another consideration is the presence of other drugs. In general, the MAC of an inhalational anesthetic is reduced in patients receiving other CNS depressants. In surgical patients, these drugs are commonly opioid analgesics, antianxiety agents, sedatives, or IV anesthetics used for induction. Indeed, CNS depressants are frequently administered preoperatively or intraoperatively to lower the MAC for an inhalational anesthetic.

Nitrous oxide, which cannot be used safely by itself to produce surgical levels of anesthesia, is a common component of anesthetic-gas mixtures. A concentration of 70% nitrous oxide in an inspired gas mixture lowers the MAC of the halogenated agent by one half to two thirds. Alcoholic patients who have acquired a tolerance to the CNS depressant effects of ethanol often have an increased anesthetic requirement, as do patients who are tolerant to barbiturates and benzodiazepines. CNS stimulants also cause the anesthetic requirement to be increased. Although a stimulant is unlikely to be administered to a hospitalized patient, the widespread abuse of stimulants increases the probability of encountering patients undergoing emergency surgery with appreciable tissue concentrations of cocaine or amphetamine.

Intravenous anesthetics

The onset of induction of anesthesia with IV agents is determined by administering a single dose and monitoring for a loss of reflex, for example, the lash or cough reflex. Factors that alter the apparent volume of distribution, including protein binding, alter the amount of drug required to obtund body reflexes. An insufficient dose of a single IV agent may lead to transient excitation, which varies for different agents. Excitation may be manifest as hiccups with methohexital, myoclonic twitches with etomidate, and non-purposeful movements with propofol and thiopental. Thiopental may cause laryngeal spasm in an asthmatic patient, especially if the dose is insufficient or the patient is inadequately premedicated.

Most IV anesthetics do not have muscle relaxant effects, and those classified as hypnotics have no analgesic properties; thiopental has anti-analgesic effects, as noted previously. Ketamine may produce hypnotic (dissociative), amnestic, and analgesic effects. Because it does not reduce cardiac output or blood pressure, ketamine is a useful induction agent in hypovolemic patients. However, ketamine often causes "bad dreams," especially in adults, unless it is combined with a small dose of a benzodiazepine.

Side effects, clinical problems, and toxicity

Inhalational anesthetics

All inhalational anesthetics reduce spontaneous respiration in a concentration-dependent manner by depressing medullary centers in the brainstem. They decrease the responsiveness of chemoreceptors in respiratory centers to elevations in carbon dioxide tension (P_{CO_2}) in blood and cerebrospinal fluid, which normally

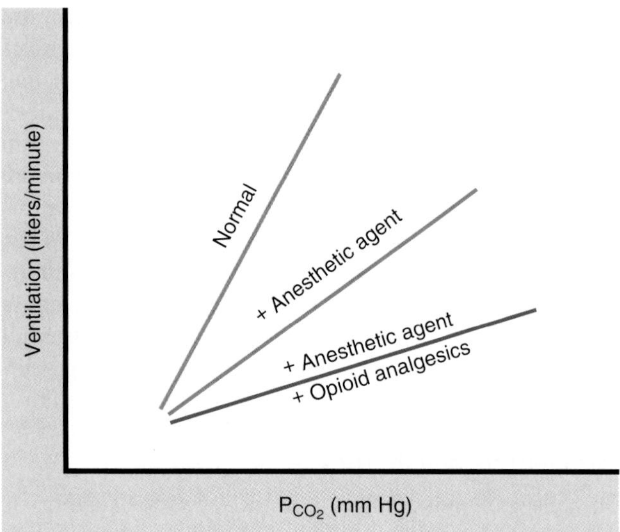

Figure 28-9 Anesthetic agents reduce the ventilatory response to increases in the arterial carbon dioxide tension (P_{CO_2}) in blood and cerebrospinal fluid. This effect is exacerbated by opioid analgesics.

serve as a potent stimulus for increasing minute ventilation. The result is a shift to the right and flattening of the P_{CO_2} ventilation-response curve (Fig. 28-9). Thus, the ventilatory response to hypercapnia is attenuated. Opioids also reduce the responsiveness of brainstem chemoreceptors to elevations in P_{CO_2} and shift the P_{CO_2} ventilation-response curve in a similar manner. When an opioid is given concurrently with an inhalational anesthetic, the effects of the two on respiration are additive and often synergistic, as shown in Figure 28-9. Carbon dioxide exerts a local effect on the cerebral vasculature by dilating small vessels. The resultant increase in intracranial pressure is a cause for concern in patients with head trauma.

All inhalational anesthetics depress the force of myocardial contraction in a concentration-dependent manner in isolated heart preparations. In patients, the effects on myocardial function varies depending on the agent, the concentration needed for surgical anesthesia, and the drug's effects on the sympathetic nervous system. Nitrous oxide has minimal effects on cardiovascular function, whereas halothane significantly depresses most cardiovascular variables. The cardiovascular effects of other anesthetics fall between those of nitrous oxide and halothane. In addition to directly depressing myocardial contractility and reducing cardiac output, halothane depresses the central outflow of the sympathetic nervous system, depresses the baroreceptor reflex, and relaxes peripheral vascular smooth muscle, the latter attributable to a direct action and to the elevated blood concentrations of carbon dioxide resulting from depression of brainstem respiratory centers. The overall effect is hypotension and decreased organ perfusion. Halothane also sensitizes the myocardium to dysrhythmias induced by catecholamines, an action shared to a lesser extent with enflurane. Therefore, caution must be exercised when one is administering pressor drugs to counteract the hypotension induced by these anesthetics.

The liver and kidney are the most prominent targets of undesirable effects of anesthetics. Generally, metabolites of the anesthetics are implicated in organ toxicity, but it is often difficult to determine which toxic effects are attributable to the anesthetic itself or to its metabolites. Some adverse effects are secondary to the anesthetic-induced decrease in cardiac output and blood flow to the liver or may result from blood transfusions administered during surgery. **"Halothane hepatitis"** occurs in 1/10,000 to 1/20,000 patients, with fatal hepatic necrosis occurring in about half. A metabolite of halothane is postulated to form a hapten that triggers an immune response. Liver function tests commonly show abnormalities for 1 or more days after administration of inhalational anesthetics. Although halothane has been administered safely countless times, it is now used less frequently, particularly in the U.S., in favor of newer halogenated agents, because of the specter of hepatic toxicity.

Renal blood flow and glomerular filtration rate are decreased during general anesthesia, resulting in decreased urine formation. Enflurane and sevoflurane undergo some metabolism in the liver and release free fluoride ions, which can be nephrotoxic in sufficiently high concentrations during lengthy surgical procedures. Although fluoride ions released from enflurane and sevoflurane do not reach concentrations toxic to the kidney, it is best not to use either agent in patients with impaired renal function. Halothane, though metabolized to an appreciable extent (see Table 28-1), does not release significant amounts of free fluoride.

Halogenated inhalational anesthetics, and halothane in particular, can precipitate **malignant hyperthermia** in genetically susceptible patients. Depolarizing neuromuscular blocking agents, notably succinylcholine (see Chapter 29), can also trigger this reaction, which is manifest as a sustained contraction of the musculature with a dramatic increase in oxygen consumption and an increased body temperature. The syndrome results from a failure of the sarcoplasmic reticulum to re-sequester Ca^{2+}, preventing the dissociation of actin and myosin filaments of muscle. The resultant hyperthermia is an emergency requiring prompt treatment, including rapid cooling and administration of the skeletal muscle relaxant dantrolene (see Chapter 29). Overall, malignant hyperthermia occurs in 1/15,000 to 1/50,000 cases. The combined use of halothane and succinylcholine is associated with the highest incidence, and the combined use of a halogenated anesthetic other than halothane and a non-depolarizing muscle relaxant is associated with the lowest incidence.

As indicated, nitrous oxide lacks sufficient potency to produce surgical levels of anesthesia safely by itself and does not relax skeletal muscles. It can produce analgesia comparable to that produced by a therapeutic dose of morphine at concentrations of 20% and cause amnesia at concentrations of 60%. At a concentration of 40%, nitrous oxide can induce a state of behavioral disinhibition and raucousness in patients not receiving other drugs. It is this action of nitrous oxide that has given the agent the name "laughing gas." Most often, nitrous oxide is administered in combination with a halogenated anesthetic to lower the anesthetic requirement for the latter, as well as to promote rapid induction (see Fig. 28-6). The minimal effect of nitrous oxide on cardiovascular function is another advantage of its use.

Nitrous oxide diffuses into enclosed air-filled cavities in the body, where it exchanges with nitrogen. Because of a difference in their blood : gas partition coefficients, blood can carry much more nitrous oxide than nitrogen. Nitrous oxide diffuses out of blood and into air-filled cavities about 35 times faster than nitrogen leaves those cavities and enters the blood. This results in an increase in pressure and distention of enclosed air-filled, nitrogen-containing spaces. This situation might be encountered in patients with an occlusion of the middle ear, pneumothorax, obstructed intestine, or air emboli in the bloodstream, or after a pneumoencephalogram. These conditions, if not absolute contraindications to the use of nitrous oxide, are at least signals for caution.

Nitrous oxide also oxidizes components of vitamin B_{12}, which decreases the availability of this vitamin and inhibits the activity of methionine synthetase, a vitamin B_{12}-dependent enzyme. This results in a decrease in protein and nucleic acid synthesis, megaloblastic anemia, and other signs of vitamin B_{12} deficiency. Inhalation of nitrous oxide for as little as 2 hours can result in a detectable decrease in methionine synthetase activity, and megaloblastic anemia has been observed in severely ill patients several days after exposure. Generally, clinical problems do not occur unless exposure is lengthened from hours to days. However, long-term exposure to low concentrations of nitrous oxide has been linked to neuropathies stemming from vitamin B_{12} deficiency. There is also some evidence that ongoing occupational exposure to nitrous oxide reduces fertility in women.

The cardiovascular effects of enflurane are similar to those of halothane, although cardiac dysrhythmias occur less frequently. Analgesia and skeletal muscle relaxation following administration of enflurane are superior to halothane. Concentrations of enflurane above its MAC, especially during hypocapnia, can cause a characteristic seizure activity on an electroencephalogram, coupled with increased motor activity in the non-medicated patient. This excitatory effect of enflurane has minimal or no adverse consequences to the patient. Nevertheless, it may be a consideration in patients with known seizure disorders. Isoflurane, a structural isomer of enflurane, does not evoke seizures. In fact, it suppresses electrical activity of the brain and can, in combination with thiopental, provide some protection against hypoxic injury.

Desflurane and sevoflurane are successors to isoflurane, and their effects on respiration and cardiovascular function appear to be similar to those of isoflurane. Sevoflurane has the advantages of rapid onset during induction and rapid washout during emergence. Because sevoflurane does not cause respiratory irritation, it can be used for mask induction in adults and especially in children. However, the disadvantages of releasing fluoride ions during metabolism and of interacting with the soda lime in the rebreathing circuit of anesthesia systems hindered its clinical development for almost 20 years. In the 1990s, sevoflurane became the most popular anesthetic agent in Japan. Its record of safety in 2 million patients led to acceptance in the United States.

Desflurane, like sevoflurane, has the advantages of rapid uptake and wash out. Its extremely low blood : gas partition coefficient allows the depth of anesthesia to be adjusted rapidly. However, respiratory irritation prevents its use for mask induction, and special vaporizers must be used because of its high vapor pressure. In spite of some undesirable characteristics, both sevoflurane and desflurane are now widely used in the United States, especially in ambulatory or day surgery settings.

Intravenous anesthetics

Like all barbiturates, thiopental is contraindicated in patients who may be allergic to barbiturates or with a familial history of acute intermittent porphyria. Because it depresses respiration, thiopental should not be used when instrumentation for supporting respiration is not available. Thiopental is contraindicated in patients with cardiovascular instability, such as in shock, because it decreases myocardial contractile force and dilates peripheral vessels. Because thiopental decreases pain threshold, thereby exerting an anti-analgesic effect, it must be combined with an analgesic drug before surgery. Thiopental causes postoperative nausea and vomiting less frequently than inhalational anesthetics but more frequently than propofol.

Because diazepam is a respiratory depressant, its use as a sole induction agent is contraindicated in ultra short procedures, in patients with chronic obstructive airway disease, or where no facilities exist for airway and respiratory management. When equivalent doses for induction are compared, midazolam depresses cardiovascular function to the same extent as thiopental. However, a smaller dose of midazolam given incrementally does not cause myocardial depression, and because of its prominent amnestic effect, can produce a pleasant induction in patients with severe hypovolemia.

Flumazenil acts competitively at the benzodiazepine recognition site of the $GABA_A$ receptor complex to reverse the residual sedative effects of benzodiazepine agonists (see Chapter 24). Because of its receptor selectivity, flumazenil does not antagonize the depressant effects of drugs other than benzodiazepines. Flumazenil may not reverse the respiratory-depressant effects of benzodiazepines completely. Therefore flumazenil cannot replace equipment for airway management and resuscitation. Although flumazenil acts rapidly, within one arm-to-brain circulation time, its duration is short. Therefore, re-sedation may occur after reversal (so-called residual sedation), especially in patients receiving a large dose of a long-acting benzodiazepine, requiring additional doses of flumazenil. Flumazenil can precipitate a withdrawal syndrome in patients who are physically dependent on a benzodiazepine.

Etomidate is not suitable for IV infusion for maintenance of anesthesia because it causes pain on injection, myoclonus, and thrombophlebitis at the injection site. Its propensity to cause nausea and vomiting postoperatively limits its use in an outpatient setting. Although the effects of etomidate on the cardiovascular and respiratory systems are relatively benign, small increases in heart rate and dysrhythmias have been reported. Etomidate has also been shown to suppress the synthesis and release of corticosteroids.

The use of propofol is contraindicated in any person with hypersensitivity to the drug. Respiratory and cardiovascular support systems must be available during propofol use because it is a respiratory and cardiovascular depressant. Its use in obstetrical procedures should be avoided until there is adequate data on the safety of propofol to the fetus.

Ketamine is related structurally to phencyclidine, and both drugs have many pharmacological actions in common. Although ketamine produces analgesia and amnesia, skeletal muscle tone is maintained. At appropriate doses, the patient may appear to be awake but is unresponsive to or dissociated from the environment (hence the term *dissociative anesthesia*). Although ketamine is indicated for use as a general anesthetic, its practical usefulness for maintenance of anesthesia is limited by its cardiovascular stimulant actions and in particular by the high incidence of unpleasant dreams and other dysphoric episodes occurring in patients during emergence from anesthesia. For these reasons, ketamine is used primarily as an induction agent in patients in hypovolemic shock and for brief painful procedures, such as changing burn dressings, where its analgesic and amnestic effects are advantageous. A benzodiazepine is often co-administered to minimize postoperative psychotomimetic reactions.

Because opioids are potent respiratory depressants, they should be used only where equipment is available to provide assisted ventilation. Postoperative nausea and vomiting are common side effects. The rapid IV administration of morphine can evoke histamine release from mast cells, which in turn causes arterial and venous dilatation and hypotension. This effect can be prevented by pretreatment with H_1 and H_2 receptor blockers, such as diphenhydramine and cimetidine, respectively (see Chapter 54). All μ-agonist opioid drugs, especially fentanyl and its derivatives, cause rigidity of respiratory muscles, often necessitating use of muscle relaxants so that assisted ventilation can be provided. Remifentanil, the newest potent and ultrashort acting μ-opioid receptor agonist, has an onset of action as rapid as that of alfentanil. It is metabolized rapidly by plasma and tissue esterases and has a terminal elimination half-life of 10 to 15 minutes. It is often one of the components in "balanced-anesthesia," where it is given as a continuous infusion, titrating to the desired effect. Because remifentanil is so short-acting, patients should be given a longer-acting opioid or other analgesic 10 to 15 minutes prior to emergence from anesthesia.

The specific opioid antagonist naloxone can be administered postoperatively to reverse any respiratory depression produced by opioid analgesics and to arouse a patient. However, because it reverses all effects of opioids, including analgesia, it should not be used routinely. The duration of action of naloxone is short, necessitating repeated administration. Because of its exquisite selectivity, naloxone will not reverse depressant effects of drugs other than opioids.

CLINICAL PROBLEMS

Inhalational agents

Depressed respiratory drive because of lower response to CO_2 or to hypoxia
Depressed cardiovascular drive
Enlarged gaseous space (nitrous oxide)
Malignant hyperthermia

Intravenous agents

Depressed respiratory drive because of lower response to CO_2 or to hypoxia
Depressed cardiovascular drive
Muscular rigidity (opioids, ketamine)
Hallucinations and emergence delirium (ketamine)
Inhibited steroidogenesis (etomidate)
Reduced pain threshold (thiopental)

New horizons

Efforts to reduce the rising cost of health care in the U.S. may result in 70% to 75% of all surgical procedures being performed in ambulatory surgical facilities. Surgery in hospitals will be reserved for patients requiring the most intensive medical care. This trend has important implications in terms of drug development. Because most surgical patients are discharged within hours of their surgery, the effects of anesthetic drugs have to be dissipated rapidly and completely, enabling the patient to have a clear sensorium and no residual postoperative nausea or impairment of motor function, judgment, or memory. This requires inhalational anesthetic agents that have a faster onset and offset of action than those available currently. It is uncertain if such agents can be developed. Therefore, IV drugs that are inactivated rapidly by simple mechanisms (such as plasma esterase activity) will be relied on more heavily for general anesthesia because their effects disappear within moments of terminating drug administration. Newer drugs should possess the characteristics of the ideal agent listed in Box 28-1.

Inhalational agents will still be used widely. They should have good potency and low solubility in blood for rapid onset and offset of effects, and they should undergo minimal biotransformation, because the metabolites of inhalational anesthetics are responsible for some undesirable side effects.

TRADE NAMES

In addition to generic and fixed-combination preparations and the drugs listed in the Major Drugs box, the following trade-named materials are some of the important compounds available in the United States.

Intravenous anesthetics and adjuvants

Alfentanil (Alfenta)
Diazepam (Valium)
Droperidol (Inapsine)
Meperidine (Demerol)
Methohexital (Brevital)
Sufentanil (Sufenta)

FURTHER READING

Antognini JF, Carstens E. *In vivo* characterization of clinical anaesthesia and its components. *Br J Anaesth* 2002; 89:156-166.

Campagna JA, Miller KW, Forman A. Mechanisms of actions of inhaled anesthetics. *N Engl J Med* 2003; 348:2110-2124.

Self-assessment questions

1. Cardiac output and blood pressure are reduced *most* by:
   a. Nitrous oxide.
   b. Halothane.
   c. Ketamine.
   d. Isoflurane.
   e. Fentanyl.

2. The ventilatory response to carbon dioxide is blunted during anesthesia with:
   a. Halothane.
   b. Morphine.
   c. Enflurane.
   d. Isoflurane.
   e. All of the above.

3. The MAC of an inhalational anesthetic is higher:
   a. In an obese patient than in a patient of average body weight.
   b. During a long surgical procedure than during a short surgical procedure.
   c. In an infant than in an elderly patient.
   d. In a patient pretreated with morphine than in an otherwise drug-free patient.
   e. In males than in females.

4. A competitive receptor antagonist is available for reversing the undesirable postoperative effects of:

a. Thiopental.
b. Halothane.
c. Propofol.
d. Midazolam.
e. Isoflurane.

5. Potential advantages of fentanyl over morphine for the induction or maintenance of anesthesia include:

a. Superior relaxation of skeletal muscles.
b. Absence of postoperative nausea and vomiting.
c. Lack of depressant effect on spontaneous respiration.
d. All of the above.
e. None of the above.

6. Nitrous oxide does all of the following *except:*

a. Relax skeletal muscles.
b. Produce analgesia.
c. Produce amnesia.
d. Increase the pressure in enclosed air-filled cavities in the body.
e. Reduce the anesthetic requirement for a concurrently administered halogenated inhalational agent.

CHAPTER 29

Skeletal muscle relaxants

Lynn Wecker
Kenneth P. Minneman

Major Drugs

Neuromuscular blockers	Antispasmodic agents
Atracurium (Tracrium)	Baclofen (Lioresal)
Gallamine (Flaxedil)	Cyclobenzaprine (Flexeril)
Pancuronium (Pavulon)	Dantrolene (Dantrium)
Rocuronium (Zemuron)	Metaxalone (Skelaxin)
Succinylcholine (Anectine, Quelicin)	Methocarbamol (Robaxin)
Tubocurarine (Intocostrin)	Tizanidine (Zanaflex)
Vecuronium (Norcuron)	**Motor nerve blocker**
	Botulinum Toxin (BoTox)

Therapeutic overview

Drugs that relax skeletal muscle are classified according to their use and mechanisms of action and include the **neuromuscular blocking agents** that produce muscle paralysis required for surgical procedures and the **antispasmodic drugs** that alleviate skeletal muscle spasms associated with specific disorders such as multiple sclerosis, cerebral palsy, stroke, or spinal injury.

The introduction of the neuromuscular blockers in the early 1940s marked a new era in anesthetic and surgical practice. Today, many surgical procedures are performed more safely and rapidly with the aid of drugs that produce skeletal muscle paralysis. These drugs interrupt transmission at the skeletal neuromuscular junction and are classified according to their action as either **depolarizing** or **nondepolarizing.**

The antispasmodic drugs include compounds that relax skeletal muscle either through actions on the **central nervous system** (CNS) and **spinal reflexes,** such as baclofen, or through a direct action on skeletal muscle; the latter are often referred to as **directly-acting skeletal muscle relaxants** and include compounds such as **dantrolene.** The antispasmodic compounds are used to alleviate skeletal muscle cramping and tightness caused by specific neurological disorders. Although these drugs are not curative, their ability to relieve symptoms enables patients to successfully pursue other treatments, such as physical therapy.

Recently, another class of compounds has emerged for producing local paralysis of skeletal muscle. The only compound currently in this class is **botulinum toxin,** approved initially for treatment of muscle disorders of the eye (blepharospasm and strabismus). Botulinum toxin is now approved for elective cosmetic purposes and produces muscle paralysis by blocking release of **acetylcholine** (ACh) from motor nerves.

Clinical uses of these compounds are listed in the Therapeutic Overview box.

Abbreviations

ACh	acetylcholine
AChE	acetylcholinesterase
CNS	central nervous system
GABA	γ-aminobutyric acid

THERAPEUTIC OVERVIEW

Neuromuscular blocking drugs

Endotracheal intubation
Reduce muscle contractility and depth of anesthesia required for surgery
In the intensive care unit to prevent high airway pressures, decrease oxygen consumption, and abolish muscle rigidity in patients on mechanical ventilation
Prevent bone fractures during electroconvulsive therapy

Antispasmodic drugs

Reduce muscle spasms in neurological disorders

Motor nerve blockers

Blepharospasm and strabismus
Elective cosmetic purposes

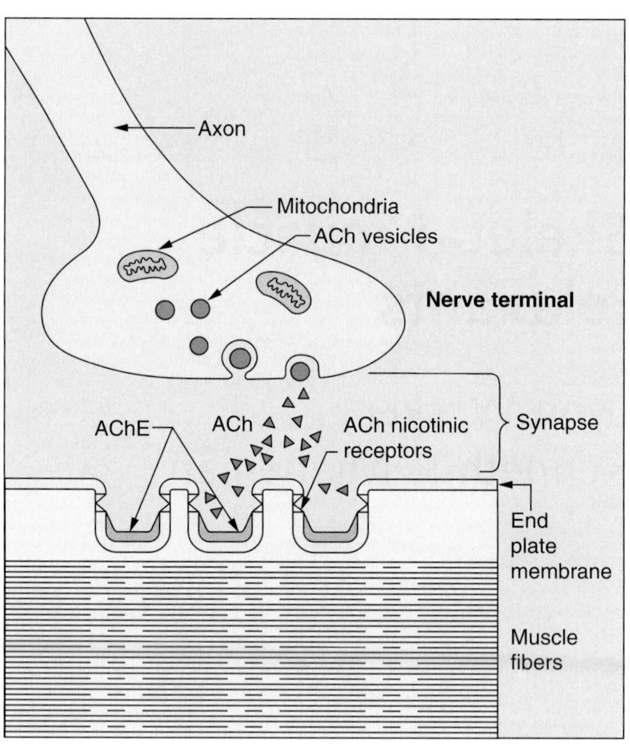

Figure 29-1 Acetylcholine *(ACh)* release, diffusion across the synaptic cleft, binding to nicotinic receptors, and hydrolysis by acetylcholinesterase *(AChE)* in the absence of blocking drugs.

Mechanisms of action

Neuromuscular blocking drugs

Skeletal muscles are innervated by somatic motor nerves that originate in the spinal cord, terminate at muscle cells, and release ACh as their neurotransmitter (see Chapters 8 and 9). Upon arrival of an action potential, ACh is released from synaptic vesicles by exocytosis, crosses the synapse, and interacts with skeletal muscle nicotinic cholinergic receptors to depolarize the postsynaptic membrane (see Chapter 2). When the membrane reaches threshold, a muscle action potential is generated and propagates along the fiber to initiate excitation-contraction coupling. The action of ACh is terminated very rapidly by hydrolysis by **acetylcholinesterase** (AChE) located in the synaptic junction. Neuromuscular transmission is depicted in Figure 29-1.

Neuromuscular blocking agents interfere with neurotransmission by either (1) occupying and activating the nicotinic receptor for a prolonged period of time, as with the **depolarizing** agents; or (2) competitively antagonizing the actions of ACh on nicotinic receptors, as with the **nondepolarizing** agents. Not surprisingly, the structures of the depolarizing agents resemble that of ACh, whereas the nondepolarizing agents are bulky, rigid molecules. A comparison of the structure of ACh with prototypical depolarizing (succinylcholine) and nondepolarizing (tubocurarine, atracurium, and pancuronium) neuromuscular blockers is shown in Figure 29-2.

As mentioned, the **nondepolarizing blockers** are competitive antagonists at nicotinic receptors. They have no agonist activity but competitively occupy the receptor binding site. The first compound, *d*-tubocurarine, was extracted from plants by native South Americans to coat their darts and rapidly paralyze their prey. This led to the development of synthetic compounds including the benzylisoquinolines (atracurium) and the aminosteroids (pancuronium).

Nondepolarizing neuromuscular blocking drugs decrease the ability of ACh to open the ligand-gated cation channels in skeletal muscle, producing flaccid paralysis. Muscle contraction is partially impaired when 75% to 80% of receptors are occupied and inhibited totally when 90% to 95% are occupied. Required concentrations vary with the drug, the muscle and its location, and the patient.

Because nondepolarizing blockers compete with ACh, the blockade can be reversed by increasing the concentration of ACh. This is done by inhibiting AChE, which hydrolyzes ACh (Chapters 8 and 9). Neostigmine, pyridostigmine, and edrophonium are all AChE inhibitors used clinically to reverse neuromuscular

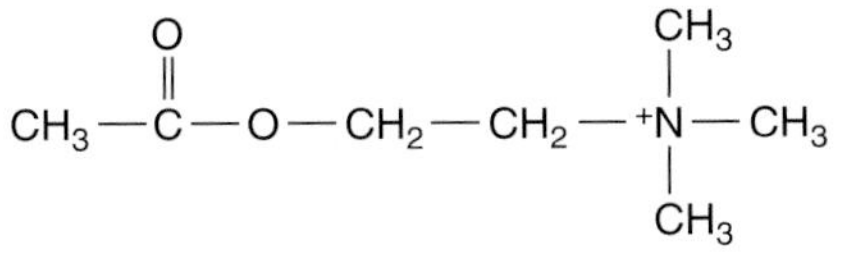

Acetylcholine

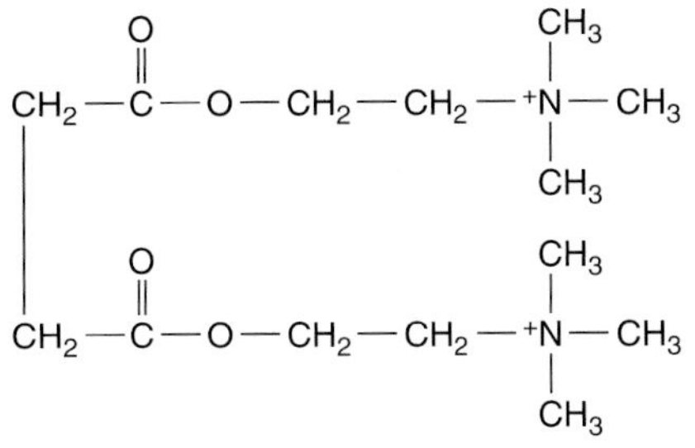

Succinylcholine

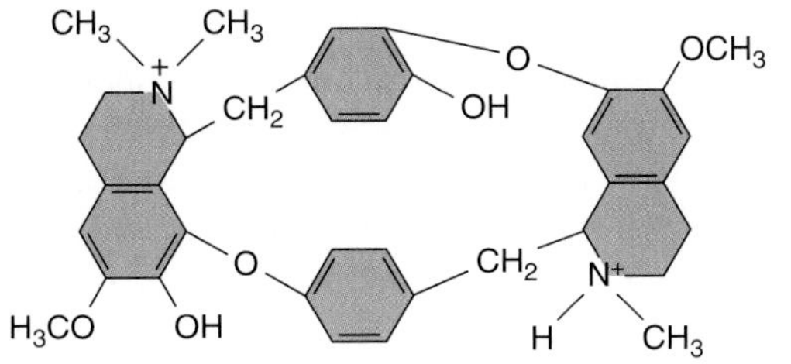

d-(+) Tubocurarine

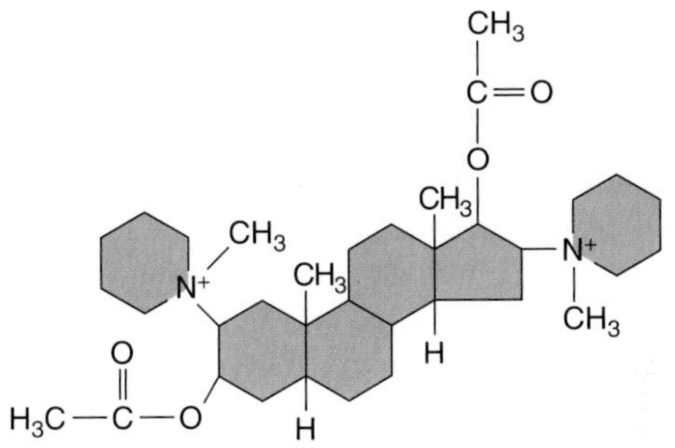

Pancuronium

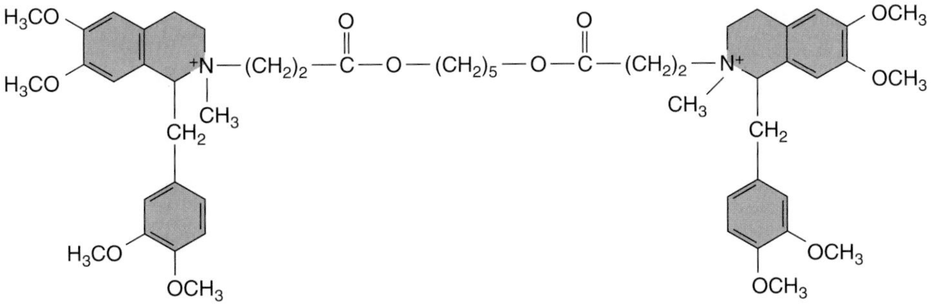

Atracurium

Figure 29-2 Competitive nondepolarizing blocking agents.

block caused by nondepolarizing blockers. However, if the concentration of the competitive blocking agent is greater than that needed for blockade of 95% of the receptors, AChE inhibitors will be unable to increase ACh sufficiently to reverse the block.

There is only one **depolarizing agent** in clinical use, succinylcholine (see Fig. 29-2). This compound binds to and activates muscle nicotinic receptors in the same manner as ACh. However, succinylcholine is not metabolized by AChE, resulting in receptor occupation for a prolonged period. Succinylcholine is hydrolyzed primarily by pseudocholinesterase, which is not present in high concentrations at the neuromuscular junction, resulting in prolonged muscle depolarization. The neuromuscular block resulting from succinylcholine is characterized by two phases. The first, termed *phase I* block, is a consequence of prolonged depolarization, rendering the membrane unresponsive to further stimuli. It is characterized by initial muscle fasciculations followed by a flaccid paralysis that is not reversed, but augmented, by administration of AChE inhibitors.

With continued exposure to succinylcholine, *phase II* block occurs during which the membrane repolarizes but is still unresponsive, reflecting a desensitized state of the nicotinic cholinergic receptor. This phase progresses to a state in which the block appears similar to that produced by nondepolarizing agents—that is, it becomes responsive to high concentrations of ACh and can be reversed by AChE inhibitors.

Antispasmodic agents

The antispasmodic or spasmolytic agents act on either the brain and spinal reflexes to affect descending pathways that control α-motor neuron excitability or on the muscle itself to interfere with excitation-contraction coupling.

Cyclobenzaprine, methocarbamol, and metaxalone all relax skeletal muscle by unknown mechanisms. They depress the CNS and do not have direct actions on the neuromuscular junction or skeletal muscle.

Baclofen is a structural analog of γ-aminobutyric acid (GABA) that decreases spasticity by interacting with $GABA_B$ receptors on pre- and post-synaptic terminals of spinal interneurons. Presynaptic interaction allows hyperpolarization of the membrane, which restricts Ca^{2+} influx and decreases release of excitatory neurotransmitters. Postsynaptic interactions with sensory afferent terminals cause membrane hyperpolarization and increases in K^+ conductance, enhancing presynaptic inhibition. Baclofen may also inhibit γ-motor neuron activity and reduce muscle spindle sensitivity, leading to inhibition of mono- and polysynaptic spinal reflexes.

Benzodiazepines such as diazepam act on $GABA_A$ receptors to increase their affinity for GABA (see Chapter 24). Diazepam also increases presynaptic inhibition in the spinal cord by reducing mono- and polysynaptic reflexes.

Tizanidine is a clonidine derivative with short-acting α_2-adrenergic receptor agonist actions. Tizanidine inhibits release of excitatory amino acids such as glutamate and aspartate and facilitates the action of glycine, an inhibitory neurotransmitter, on presynaptic terminals of the spinal cord.

Dantrolene has direct effects on skeletal muscle. It inhibits Ca^{2+} release from the sarcoplasmic reticulum, thereby uncoupling motor nerve excitation and muscle contraction.

Motor nerve blockers

Botulinum neurotoxins are produced by the anaerobic bacterium *Clostridium botulinum*. There are seven serotypes (A-G), all of which block ACh release. Botulinum toxin interferes with proteins involved in the exocytotic release of synaptic vesicles containing ACh; therefore, it produces flaccid paralysis. Botulinum toxin also affects muscle-spindle afferent pathways, which suggests a direct effect on γ-motor nerve endings.

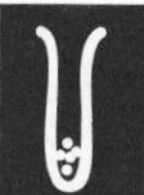

Pharmacokinetics

Neuromuscular blocking drugs

Neuromuscular blocking drugs have different pharmacokinetic properties (Table 29-1) that influence the choice of drug for particular patients in particular situations. Because these drugs are positively charged, they cross membranes poorly and are generally limited in distribution to the extracellular space. However, small amounts of pancuronium, vecuronium, and pipecuronium cross membranes. Pancuronium also crosses the placenta but not in sufficient amounts to cause problems in the fetus when used during a cesarean section.

The use of pancuronium, metocurine, tubocurarine, or gallamine is discouraged in patients with impaired renal function because appreciable fractions of these drugs are cleared by renal filtration. Atracurium is inactivated almost entirely by metabolism, two-thirds enzymatic and one-third by spontaneous non-enzymatic breakdown. Vecuronium and pancuronium undergo significant hepatic metabolism, and their 3-hydroxy metabolites have much less neuromuscular blocking activity than do the parent drugs. Succinylcholine and mivacurium are metabolized by plasma pseudocholinesterase, with minimal hydrolysis by AChE.

Antispasmodic agents

Baclofen is rapidly absorbed after oral administration. It has a therapeutic half-life of 3.5 hours and is excreted primarily unchanged by the kidney; 15% is metabolized in the liver. Baclofen crosses the blood-brain barrier readily.

Dantrolene is metabolized primarily in the liver and eliminated in urine and bile. After oral administration, its half-life is 15 hours. Benefits may not be apparent for a week or more.

The pharmacokinetics of diazepam are discussed in Chapter 24.

The oral bioavailability of tizanidine is low because of extensive first-pass metabolism. Its half-life is approximately 3 hours, and less than 3% is excreted unchanged in urine.

Table 29-1 Selected pharmacokinetic parameters

Compound	Onset (min)	Duration of Action (min)*	Metabolism	Elimination	Protein Binding (%)
Alcuronium	3-6	Intermediate	Unchanged	R 80%-90% B 15%-20%	75
Atracurium	3-6	Intermediate	Carboxylesterase and nonenzymatic	R 6%-10%	80
Cisatracurium	5-7	Intermediate	Carboxylesterase and nonenzymatic	R < 10% B < 10%	nd
Doxacurium	4-6	Long	Plasma ChE (75%)	R 25%-50%	30-35
Gallamine	4-6	Intermediate	Unchanged	R 95% B < 1%	15
Mivacurium	2-4	Short	Plasma ChE (100%)	R < 10%	nd
Pancuronium	4-6	Long	Hepatic (35%)	R 40%-60% B 10%-20%	85
Pipecuronium	3-6	Long	Hepatic (20%)	R 40%-60% B 10%-20%	nd
Rocuronium	2-4	Intermediate	Hepatic (35%)	R 20%-30% B 50%-60%	nd
Succinylcholine	1-2	Ultrashort	Plasma ChE (100%)	R < 10%	nd
Tubocurarine	4-6	Long	Hepatic (50%)	R 45%-60% B 10%-40%	35-55†
Vecuronium	2-4	Intermediate	Hepatic (35%)	R 20%-30% B 50%-60%	70

*Duration: Ultrashort = <10 min; Short = 10-30; Intermediate = 30-90 min; Long = >90 min.

†Additional drug; binds to cartilage and connective tissue.

R, Renal; *B*, biliary; *nd*, not determined due to rapid metabolism in plasma.

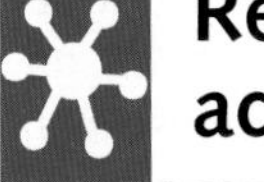

Relation of mechanisms of action to clinical response

Neuromuscular blocking drugs

The choice of neuromuscular blocking agent is based primarily on the speed of onset, the duration of neuromuscular block required, and the importance of side effects. The duration of blockade required is, in turn, influenced by the anatomical location of the surgery and the condition of the patient. Relative potency is not a principal consideration, despite a 100-fold variation in the doses of different drugs needed to attain 95% blockade.

Several factors—such as patient age, weight, and renal function—can influence the choice of a particular compound used; also, the electrolyte content of body fluids can influence the degree of blockade achieved with a given dose of a particular muscle relaxant. The actions of tubocurarine and atracurium, for example, are potentiated in neonates as compared with children and adults, but succinylcholine is less potent in neonates. Such pharmacokinetic considerations can explain some differences in effectiveness between patients of different ages.

The actions of nondepolarizing blocking agents are often potentiated by inhalational anesthetics (see Chapter 28) and also by low concentrations of extracellular K^+ or Ca^{2+}, as may occur after use of diuretics or in renal dysfunction. Elevated K^+ or Ca^{2+} and reduced Mg^{2+} concentrations, however, may counteract drug actions through changes in ACh release in response to depolarization or changes in membrane potential at the muscle endplate.

In most surgical procedures in which neuromuscular blocking agents are used, the drugs enter the systemic circulation and are distributed widely. Spontaneous respiration is usually inhibited, and ventilatory support must be available. The rate of neuromuscular block and recovery varies with different muscles. Muscles of respiration are usually among the last to be paralyzed and the first to recover. It is not practical, however, to attempt selective blockade of one anatomical area for prolonged periods because of the widespread distribution of these drugs.

In patients with burns, denervated muscles, spinal cord injury, or other trauma, sensitivity to neuromuscular blocking drugs may vary. In some burn patients, for example, doses of atracurium or metocurine may need to be 2 to 3 times greater than normal.

Because of its rapid onset and short duration of action, succinylcholine is used primarily for facilitation of endotracheal intubation and for relaxation during extremely short surgical procedures.

Antispasmodic agents

Spasticity is a common neurological problem present in patients with damage of central motor pathways. It is characterized by hyperexcitability of α-motoneurons in the spinal cord, because of an imbalance of excitatory and inhibitory neurotransmitters. Antispasmodic drugs alter the function of neurotransmitters in the CNS and at peripheral neuromuscular sites.

Cyclobenzaprine, methocarbamol, and metaxalone are approved for use as adjunctive treatment with physical therapy and rest for certain types of muscle spasticity. Methocarbamol is also recommended for treatment of muscle spasticity associated with tetanus poisoning.

Dantrolene is the drug of choice for treatment of malignant hyperthermia. Malignant hyperthermia is a rare and potentially lethal disorder characterized by hypermetabolism, tachycardia, hypertension, premature ventricular contractions, rigidity, cyanosis, and rapid temperature increase. The hyperthermic response is not ameliorated by typical antipyretic drugs such as aspirin or acetaminophen. Malignant hyperthermia may develop in susceptible patients exposed to halogenated anesthetic gases with or without succinylcholine (see Chapter 28).

Motor nerve blockers

Botulinum toxin A is approved for treatment of muscle disorders of the eye, including blepharospasm and strabismus, characterized by excessive neuromuscular contractility, and for elective cosmetic purposes. Botulinum toxin is also injected into muscles suffering from "repetitive use" disorders such as "tennis elbow" and "violinist wrist" and a recent use is to treat chronic spasticity of skeletal muscle in cerebral palsy. The objective is to permit the contralateral muscle to grow while the normally spastic muscle is relaxed.

When botulinum toxin is injected intramuscularly, it induces partial chemical denervation and diminishes involuntary contracture without causing complete paralysis. The onset of weakness varies from a few days to 2 weeks, depending on the time the toxin takes to reach the inside of the nerve terminal and begin its block. Effects last for about 3 months, by which time function begins to recover by sprouting of nerve terminals and formation of new synaptic contacts. Patients will then need additional injections to sustain the effects. Some patients may develop tolerance by formation of neutralizing antibodies to the toxin.

Because botulinum toxin inhibits ACh release from all parasympathetic and cholinergic postganglionic sympathetic neurons, it may be useful for treating patients with conditions such as hyperhidrosis and detrusor sphincter dyssynergia.

Side effects, clinical problems, and toxicity

Neuromuscular blocking agents

The major side effects of the neuromuscular blocking drugs are **cardiovascular effects** and **histamine release.** Their significance varies, with the older compounds exhibiting greater effects and the newer drugs having fewer effects.

Although nondepolarizing neuromuscular blocking drugs are generally selective for nicotinic cholinergic receptors in skeletal muscle, cholinergically innervated parasympathetic and sympathetic ganglia and cardiac parasympathetic neuroeffector junctions can all be affected if drug concentrations are sufficiently high. Tubocurarine produces a significant degree of ganglionic blockade, metocurine less, and other agents essentially none at normal doses. Because of its similarity in structure to ACh, succinylcholine binds to ganglionic nicotinic and cardiac muscarinic receptors and stimulates cholinergic transmission. Pancuronium and alcuronium exert a direct blocking effect on muscarinic (M_2) receptors at doses used for neuromuscular blockade, but tubocurarine, metocurine, and atracurium produce muscarinic blockade only at much higher concentrations. Pancuronium, succinylcholine, and gallamine also produce direct muscarinic effects that result in cardiac dysrhythmias. Pancuronium also causes tachycardia and hypertension by blocking norepinephrine reuptake.

The reduced cardiac effects of the newer agents greatly increase their safety margins. For instance, vecuronium is essentially free of cardiac and histamine effects.

Histamine release is a major problem with tubocurarine and to a lesser extent with succinylcholine, metocurine, and mivacurium. Because of its marked histamine release and ganglionic blockade leading to hypotension and reflex tachycardia, tubocurarine is now seldom used, except as a pre-curarizing agent prior to administration of succinylcholine.

The main disadvantage of atracurium is histamine release, which occurs in about 30% of patients. Histamine release also occurs with cisatracurium but does not result in clinical signs or cardiovascular effects. Mivacurium may cause histamine release at high doses, but at clinical doses it has no cardiovascular effects. Doxacurium does not release histamine, and even at high doses, it does not produce cardiovascular effects. Alcuronium may cause blood pressure to fall under certain conditions during anesthesia induced or maintained with halothane, although this effect is less than with other nondepolarizing drugs. Alcuronium produces mild histamine release. Pancuronium produces no histamine release or ganglionic blockade but causes moderate increases in heart rate, blood pressure, and cardiac output because of sympathomimetic and anticholinergic effects. Rocuronium does not produce histamine release or cardiovascular effects.

Long-term use of several neuromuscular blockers in the intensive care unit to maintain controlled ventilation has resulted in prolonged periods of paralysis. Indications for **reversal** of neuromuscular block are postoperative residual curarization—that is, the inability of the patient to breathe adequately following discontinuation of anesthesia, or when it is impossible to artificially ventilate the patient after administration of a muscle relaxant. Although many criteria, such as the ability of the patient to sustain voluntary activities (adequate swallowing, coughing, eye opening, and head lifting) are used to evaluate the return of muscle function immediately after use of muscle relaxants, monitoring the response to electrical stimulation is one of the most accurate methods to detect residual neuromuscular blockade. Other methods include electromyography, mechanomyography, and accelerography.

The K^+ efflux elicited by succinylcholine is dangerous in patients with **neurological diseases** such as hemiplegia, paraplegia, intracranial lesion, peripheral neuropathy, and in patients with extensive soft-tissue damage such as burns. Plasma K^+ concentrations ≥13 mM produce cardiac arrhythmias and arrest. In these patients, a marked resistance to nondepolarizing neuromuscular agents called "extrajunctional chemosensitivity" is present, probably because of an increased number of extrajunctional receptors. In addition, a combination of succinylcholine and halothane may potentiate a malignant hyperthermia syndrome in patients predisposed to this condition.

Neuromuscular blocking agents must be used with caution in patients with underlying neuromuscular, hepatic, or renal disease or electrolyte imbalance. Patients with neuromuscular disorders such as myasthenia gravis may be resistant to succinylcholine because of a decrease in the number of ACh receptors; the dose of muscle relaxants must be reduced by 50 to 75% in such patients. Myasthenic patients are also more likely than normal patients to develop a phase II block in response to succinylcholine, particularly when repeated doses have been administered. Use of long-acting muscle relaxants such as pancuronium, pipecuronium, and doxacurium must be avoided. Intermediate- and short-acting nondepolarizing drugs can be administered with close monitoring of neuromuscular transmission. Lambert-Eaton Myasthenic Syndrome, an autoimmune presynaptic neuromuscular disorder in which the stimulated release of ACh is reduced at the neuromuscular junction, is another disease in which patients are very sensitive to muscle relaxants.

Special consideration is required for use of neuromuscular blockers in patients with renal or hepatic disease. Prolonged neuromuscular block has been reported in these patients with gallamine, metocurine, alcuronium, pancuronium, vecuronium, rocuronium, and tubocurarine. These drugs are all water-soluble compounds that depend on glomerular filtration, tubular excretion, and tubular reabsorption for clearance. The larger volume of distribution in the edematous renal patient, a reduced renal clearance, and decreased plasma protein binding can cause prolonged elimination. The drug of choice in patients with renal disease is atracurium, because of its unique degradation that is unaffected by renal or hepatic dysfunction.

Hepatic disease also prolongs the duration of neuromuscular blockade. The liver is especially important in metabolism of steroid-type relaxants such as vecuronium and rocuronium. In patients with cholestasis or cirrhosis, uptake of drug into the liver is decreased; thus, plasma clearance is also decreased, leading to a prolonged effect. Because pseudocholinesterase is produced in the liver, in patients with hepatic disease, a decrease in its production may prolong the effect of succinylcholine. Again, since the liver is not involved in elimination of atracurium, it is the drug of choice in patients with hepatic failure.

Drug interactions occur between neuromuscular blockers, anesthetics, Ca^{2+}-channel blockers, and some antibiotics. Many volatile anesthetic agents enhance the action of the nondepolarizing neuromuscular blockers by decreasing the open time of the ACh receptor, which increases ACh binding affinity. Enflurane has the strongest effect, followed by halothane. The local anesthetic bupivacaine potentiates blockade by nondepolarizing and depolarizing agents, and lidocaine and procaine prolong the duration of action of succinylcholine by inhibiting pseudocholinesterase.

Ca^{2+}-channel blockers, and to a lesser extent β-adrenergic blockers, potentiate neuromuscular blocking drugs. Antibiotics that interact with neuromuscular blocking agents are aminoglycosides, tetracyclines, polymyxin, and clindamycin. Aminoglycosides decrease ACh release and lower postjuctional sensitivity to ACh. Tetracyclines chelate Ca^{2+} and reduce ACh release.

CLINICAL PROBLEMS

Fasciculations and postoperative myalgias, particularly in the neck, shoulders, and chest
Masseter muscle spasm
Increased intraocular pressure
Increased intraabdominal and intracranial pressure
Bradycardia and cardiac arrest
Malignant hyperthermia
Histamine release
Tachycardia and hypertension

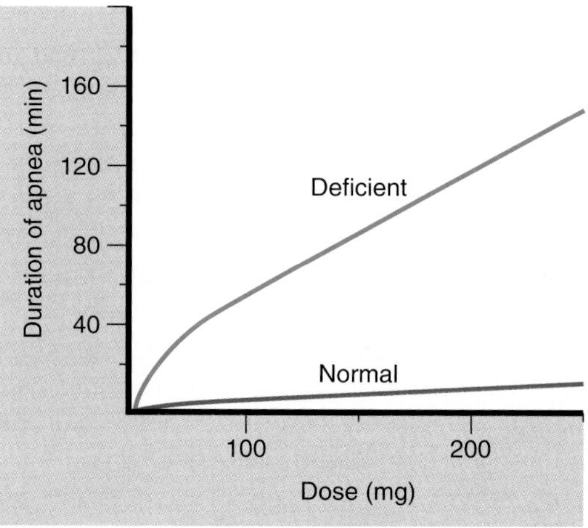

Figure 29-3 Length of time patients display apnea after IV dose of succinylcholine. Normal and deficient refer to the plasma pseudocholinesterase activity in each patient group.

Lincomycin and clindamycin block nicotinic receptors and depress muscle contractility, enhancing neuromuscular blockade. The duration of action of vecuronium, pancuronium, doxacurium, and pipecuronium is also reduced in patients taking phenytoin or carbamazepine. These anticonvulsants decrease the affinity of nicotinic receptors for neuromuscular blockers and increase the number of receptors on muscle fibers. The duration of action of vecuronium is also prolonged in patients treated with cimetidine. Mg^{2+} sulfate, used to treat preeclampsia, prolongs the effect of nondepolarizing relaxants and inhibits the effect of succinylcholine.

Genetic variations in pseudocholinesterase activity result in either lower concentrations of normal enzyme or an abnormal enzyme. A dose of 1 to 2 mg/kg succinylcholine in normal patients produces neuromuscular blockade lasting <15 min; in an enzyme-deficient patient, the same dose may last much longer. This is illustrated in Figure 29-3, with block defined as the duration of apnea. Trauma, alcoholism, pregnancy, use of oral contraceptives, and other conditions in which pseudocholinesterase activity is changed can alter the duration of neuromuscular block produced by succinylcholine.

Primary problems in the use of neuromuscular blocking agents are summarized in the Clinical Problems box.

Antispasmodic agents

CNS depression including drowsiness occurs to a variable extent with the centrally acting agents. Side effects of baclofen include hypotension, dizziness, drowsiness, weakness, fatigue, and depression. Baclofen may interfere with attention and memory in elderly or brain-injured patients.

Adverse effects of dantrolene are muscle weakness, drowsiness, dizziness, diarrhea, and seizures; chronic use may result in hepatotoxicity.

Side effects of botulinum toxin vary with the site of injection. For example, in patients injected in the neck for treating cervical dystonia, dysphagia may develop. Other side effects include influenza-like illness, brachial plexopathy, and gallbladder dysfunction.

New horizons

Neuromuscular blocking drugs are now commonly used in anesthesia during surgical procedures and on a long-term basis to allow controlled ventilation in patients in intensive care units. However, this practice is not without problems, including prolonged muscle paralysis after termination of treatment. In recent years, the search for new neuromuscular relaxants has concentrated on finding a drug with a rapid onset and shorter and more predictable duration of action with minimal side effects. Nonetheless, the withdrawal of rapacuronium from the market in 2001 has delayed the search for a new succinylcholine alternative. New nondepolarizing neuromuscular blockers such as G-1-64, GW280430A, and SZ1677 represent important advances on the way to finding an "ideal" muscle relaxant.

At present, clinically used reversal agents are inhibitors of AChE such as neostigmine, pyridostigmine, and edrophonium; however, because of the widespread distribution of AChE, they cause many side effects including bradycardia, hypotension, and bronchoconstriction. The cyclodextrin derivate (Org25969) is a new reversal agent that reverses rocuronium-induced block faster than standard treatment with neostigmine and atropine yet has few significant hemodynamic changes. However, more research must be done before it can be introduced into clinical practice.

Other agents used for reversal of neuromuscular blockade, such as 2,4-diaminopyridine, are also being used to treat neuromuscular disorders such as the Lambert-Eaton Myasthenic syndrome.

TRADE NAMES

In addition to generic and fixed-combination preparations and the drugs listed in the Major Drugs box, the following trade-named materials are some of the important compounds available in the United States.

Neuromuscular blockers

Alcuronium (Alloferin)
Cisatracurium (Nimbex)
Doxacurium (Nuromax)
Metocurine (Metubine)
Mivacurium (Mivacron)
Pipecuronium (Arduan)

FURTHER READING

Lee C. Conformation, action, and mechanism of action of neuromuscular blocking muscle relaxants. *Pharmacol Ther* 2003; 98:143-169.

Raj PP. Botulinum toxin therapy in pain management. *Anesthesiol Clin N Am* 2003; 21:715-731.

Sparr HJ. Choice of the muscle relaxant for rapid-sequence induction. *Eur J Anaesthesiol* 2001; 18(suppl 23):71-76.

Self-assessment questions

1. Which of the following neuromuscular blocking drugs cause histamine release?

a. Vecuronium
b. Metocurine
c. Tubocurarine
d. *b* and *c*
e. All of the above

2. At therapeutic concentrations the primary action of doxacurium is to:

a. Block acetylcholine release.
b. Inhibit acetylcholinesterase.
c. Block muscarinic receptors.
d. Block ion channels opened by activation of nicotinic receptors.
e. Block nicotinic receptors at motor end plates.

3. Which of the following neuromuscular blocking agents has the shortest duration of action?

a. Doxacurium
b. Mivacurium
c. Succinylcholine
d. Atracurium

4. Metabolism is the main route of elimination for all of the following agents *except*:

a. Gallamine.
b. Succinylcholine.
c. Mivacurium.
d. Atracurium.
e. Pancuronium.

5. Potential therapeutic uses of neuromuscular blockers include:

a. Diagnosis of myasthenia gravis.
b. Control of ventilation during surgery.
c. Endotracheal intubation.
d. *b* and *c*.
e. All of the above.

CHAPTER 30

Local anesthetics

Gary R. Strichartz

Major Drugs	
Bupivacaine* (Marcaine, Sensorcaine)	Mepivacaine (Carbocaine, Isocaine, Polocaine)
Chloroprocaine (Nesacaine)	Procaine (Novocain)
Etidocaine (Duranest)	Ropivacaine (Naropin)
Levobupivacaine (Chirocaine)	Tetracaine‡ (Pontocaine)
Lidocaine† (Dilocaine, Lidoject, Octocaine, Xylocaine)	

*In Japan the drug name is bupivacaine.
†In the UK the drug name is lignocaine.
‡In the UK the drug name is amethocaine.

Therapeutic overview

Local anesthetics reversibly block the generation and conduction of action potentials in all excitable cells. By rendering painful stimuli imperceptible in a specific part of the body, these drugs have many uses in medicine ranging from dental to obstetric procedures. These anesthetics may be applied locally by subcutaneous infiltration for the removal of a superficial skin lesion or may be applied to the spinal cord as a regional anesthetic for a hip replacement procedure or for the management of postoperative pain. Thus the selection of a local anesthetic depends on the pharmacokinetic profile required for each specific use as well as the side effect profile of the compound, factors summarized in the Therapeutic Overview box.

THERAPEUTIC OVERVIEW

Factors in drug selection

Speed of onset
Duration of effect
Side effects
Seizures
Cardiovascular depression

Mechanisms of action

Local anesthetics act directly on nerve cells to block their ability to transmit impulses down their axons. By blocking action potential propagation in nociceptive neurons, local anesthetics eliminate sensations of pain. Local anesthetics are not specific to any nerve cell type but act on all sensory, motor, and autonomic neurons and all neurons in the central nervous system (CNS). Thus the actions of these compounds can be restricted by administering them locally. Certain practical pharmacokinetic properties make these agents particularly useful in temporarily blocking the sensory transmission of pain impulses. The greatest advantage of local anesthetics is their reversibility—that is, once the drug is eliminated by metabolism or excretion or removed from its site of action by vascular resorption, its action is terminated and the nerve resumes normal function. There are generally no long-term consequences from the use

Abbreviations

CNS	central nervous system
IV	intravenous
VGSC	voltage-gated sodium channels

of local anesthetics. Thus, these drugs are highly effective in providing regional or localized reversible pain relief.

The molecular targets for local anesthetics are the **voltage-gated sodium channels (VGSCs),** which exist in all neurons. These channels are responsible for producing the regenerative action potentials that occur along axons and carry messages from cell bodies to nerve terminals. VGSCs are usually closed at normal resting membrane potentials, which prevents the high concentration of sodium in the extracellular fluid from entering the cell. When membranes are depolarized, these channels open and allow sodium to flow into the cell down its concentration gradient. This influx of positively charged ions leads to further depolarization, causing more channels to open and leading to a self-regenerating action potential. Sustained depolarization causes:

- Spontaneous inactivation of VGSC, which shuts off sodium influx
- Concurrent opening of voltage-gated potassium channels

The resultant potassium efflux through these and non-voltage-gated potassium channels returns the membrane potential to its normal resting value. This mechanism is depicted in Figure 30-1.

The cellular physiological mechanism by which local anesthetics block the conduction of nerve impulses is well understood. These drugs bind selectively to VGSC at the intracellular surface near the pore's vestibule and thereby block the pathway for Na^+ and prevent the channels from opening (Fig. 30-2). By blocking sodium influx, these drugs prevent the depolarization necessary for action potential propagation and, at sufficient concentrations, block impulse conduction. Because local anesthetics dissociate from the VGSC in seconds, once drug administration is stopped, the drug diffuses away from the nerve and/or is absorbed by the local circulation, and impulse activity is restored.

The ability of local anesthetics to block VGSC is highly dependent on the conformation (or state) of the channel. Sodium channels exist in three major states (Fig. 30-3). In the *resting* closed state the channels do not allow sodium influx and are highly sensitive to depolarization-induced opening. In the *open* state, the channels allow sodium influx, whereas in the *inactivated* closed state, they do not allow sodium influx and are not opened by depolarization. Local anesthetics have different potencies for binding to these different states. They are much more likely to bind when the channels are open or inactivated and are less likely to bind to the resting state. This modulation of affinity is called state dependence and has great practical importance. Because local anesthetics preferentially block nerves in which sodium channels are open or inactivated, they are more potent in rapidly firing nerves than in nerves in which action potentials occur less frequently. Because sensory neurons fire at greater frequencies in response to more intense noxious stimuli, the effectiveness of impulse blockade is greater under these conditions.

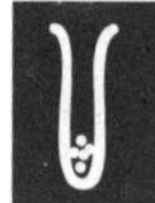

Pharmacokinetics

The structures of the local anesthetics have a direct bearing on their therapeutic actions (Fig. 30-4). All

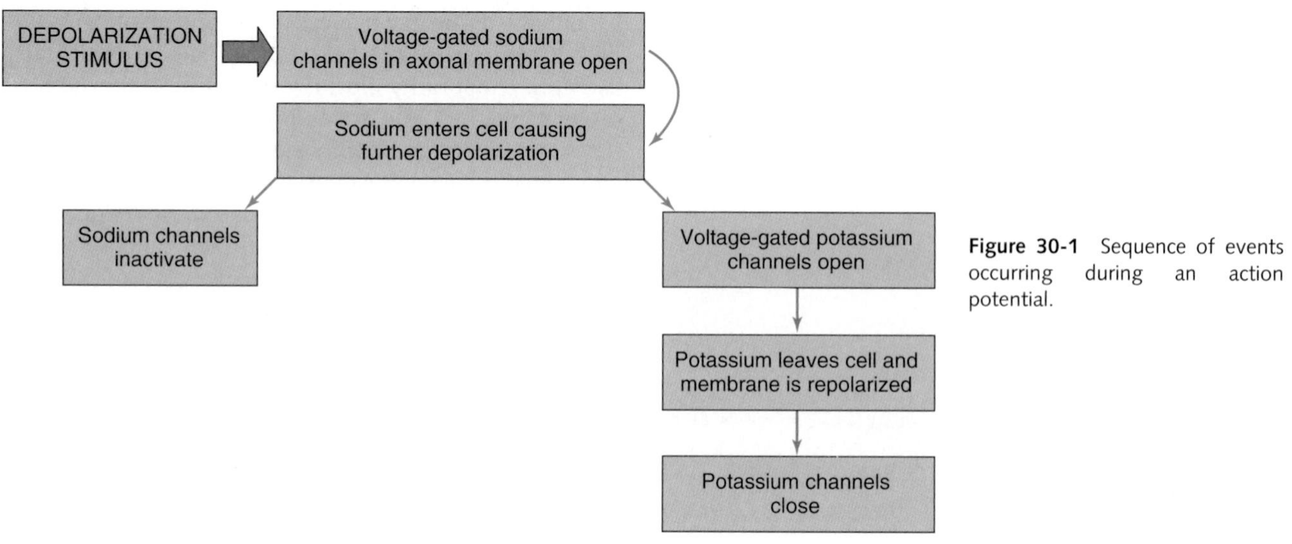

Figure 30-1 Sequence of events occurring during an action potential.

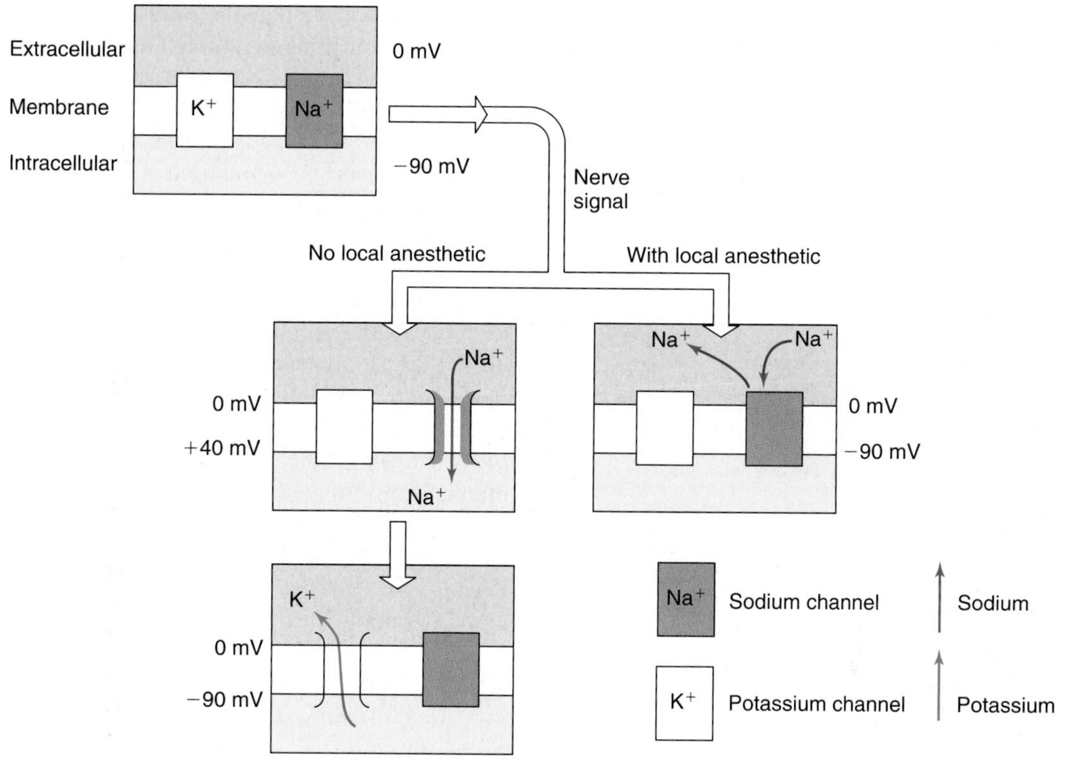

Figure 30-2 Transmission of nerve impulses under normal conditions and its prevention in the presence of a local anesthetic agent (producing nerve block).

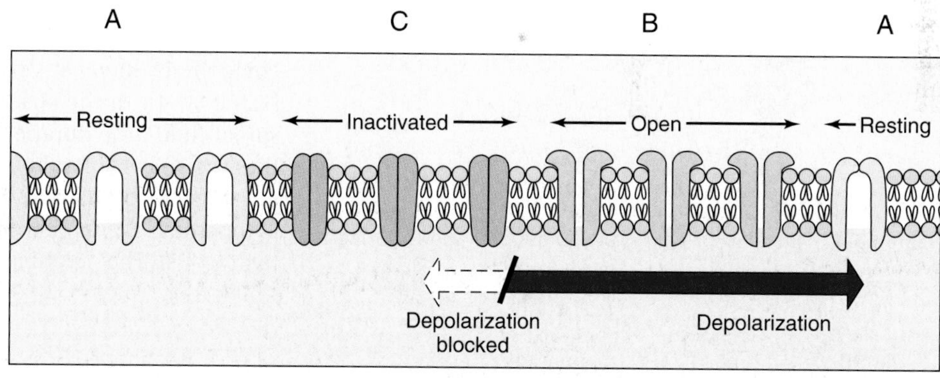

Figure 30-3 Unidirectional nature of axonal impulse conduction. Sodium channels are depicted in the resting **(A)**, open **(B)**, or inactivated **(C)** state. The inactivated channels prevent the depolarization from proceeding in more than one direction.

contain a hydrophobic group (generally an aromatic moiety) linked by either an ester or an amide bond to a relatively hydrophilic group (usually a tertiary amine, which can be protonated) through an alkyl chain of intermediate length. The hydrophilic group renders water solubility and enables the drug to diffuse to the nerves to be blocked. Similarly, the hydrophobic group renders lipid solubility and enables the drug to penetrate the sheathing, perineural tissue, and neuronal cell membrane to reach its binding site on the hydrophilic inner surface of the VGSC. In addition, more hydrophobic local anesthetics bind more tightly to their active site in the channel. Thus both the charged tertiary amine and the linking ester or amide facilitate diffusion of the agent to the target tissue, and the hydrophobic property aids the drug in its passage through the membranes to ultimately reach its site of action.

Because local anesthetics must cross the neuronal cell membrane to reach their binding site on the VGSC, sufficient amounts of the drugs must be in their nonionized form to gain entry to the cell. However, the charged form of the compound is thought to be most active. Thus, an important aspect of the chemistry of these agents is their pK_a. Local anesthetics are weak bases, with pK_a values of 8 to 9. At physiological pH (~7.4), most (80-90%) of the drug is in the charged cationic form (see Chapter 3). However, sufficient amounts of drug exist in the uncharged state to cross the nerve cell membrane, and once inside the cell, it is the predominant cationic species that binds to the channel proteins.

Determinants of the rate of onset of clinical local anesthesia include the drug concentration and potency, binding to local tissues, the rate of metabolic local biotransformation (for ester-linked agents), and the degree of vascularity at the site of drug injection. The last factor is of primary importance because any diffusion of the agent into blood reduces drug concentration at the nerve fibers. Vasoconstrictors, such as epinephrine, are frequently injected with local anesthetics to diminish local blood flow and reduce systemic absorption. Although such vasoconstrictors extend the duration of action of local anesthetics, they are more effective in prolonging the actions of the less lipid-soluble agents (lidocaine, chloroprocaine, and mepivacaine) than those of the more lipid-soluble agents (etidocaine and bupivacaine). Some combinations of local anesthetics with fixed concentrations of vasoconstrictor drugs are commercially formulated.

Local anesthetics vary considerably in the rates at which they are converted to inactive metabolites. Because all of these compounds diffuse into the systemic circulation to some extent, metabolism becomes a prominent factor in the potential ability of these agents to produce undesirable side effects or overt toxicity. In addition to drug biotransformation, the binding to plasma proteins (α_1-acid glycoprotein and serum albumin) also causes the concentration of free drug in the circulation to be reduced.

The ester local anesthetics including procaine and tetracaine (see Fig. 30-4) are rapidly hydrolyzed to inactive products by plasma cholinesterase (butyrylcholinesterase) and liver esterases. Thus these compounds have a very short half-life in the body (Table 30-1). In the absence of esterase activity (e.g., in spinal fluid), the duration of "spinal" (intrathecal) anesthesia is considerably extended. The amide local anesthetics, by contrast, are metabolized by hepatic cytochrome P450s through N-dealkylation, followed by hydrolysis. The relative rates of biotransformation of

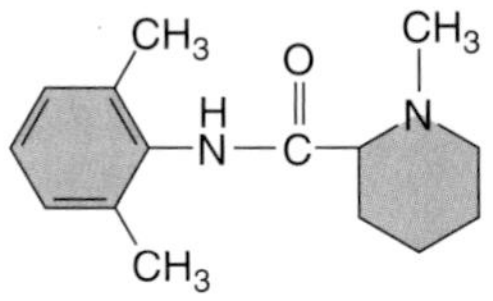

Mepivacaine

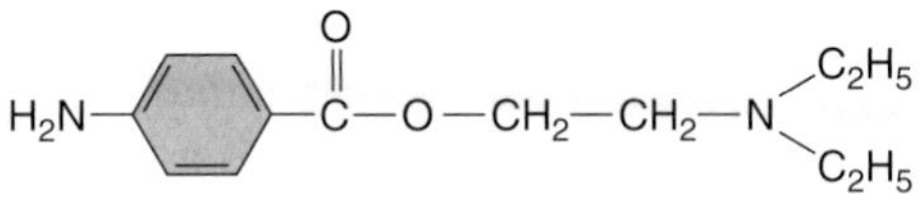

Procaine

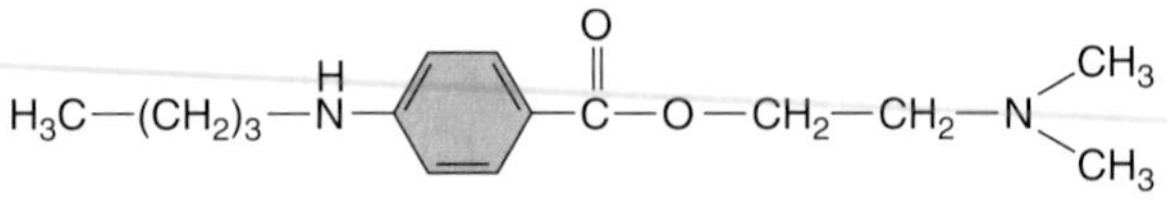

Tetracaine

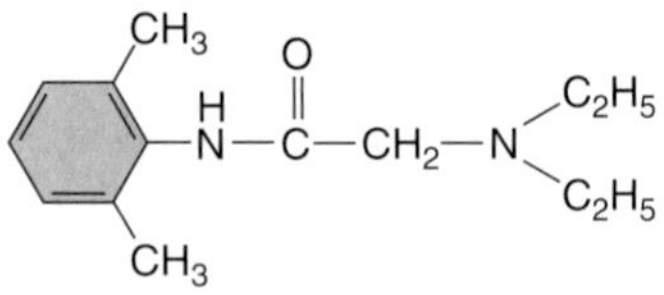

Lidocaine

Figure 30-4 Structures of typical local anesthetics shown in their free base form.

Table 30-1 Pharmacokinetic parameters

Drug	Route of Administration	Elimination Half-Life (hrs)	Disposition	Plasma Protein Bound (%)‡	Onset Time (min)
Mepivacaine	PN	1.9-3.2 (adults) 2.7-9.0 (neonates)	R, M (main)	75	3-20
Bupivacaine	PN	2.7 (adults) 8.1 (neonates)	R, M-	95	10-20
Lidocaine	PN, IV†	1.5-2.0	M* (95%), R	70	3-15
Procaine	PN, IV†	<3 min	M	10	5-20
Etidocaine	PN	2.5	M, R	95	3-5

M, Metabolism; *PN*, perineural; *R*, renal.

*Large first-pass effect; significant pulmonary biotransformation.

†Intravenous lidocaine and procaine used at very low concentrations to relieve neuropathic pain may have effects lasting weeks to months.

‡Binding of local anesthetics to plasma proteins is rapidly reversible, such that a substantial fraction of the drug bound at equilibrium becomes free during hepatic extraction, making it a substrate for biotransformation.

these local anesthetics vary depending on their specific chemical structure (see Table 30-1). Some metabolic products (e.g., *N*-demethylation products of lidocaine) also possess weak local anesthetic activity.

Bupivacaine and etidocaine are bound to plasma proteins extensively, with nonspecific tissue binding also occurring near the injection site. These agents are more likely to cause toxicity in patients with preexisting liver disease as a result of the reduced drug biotransformation and lower plasma protein concentration in these patients (plasma proteins are synthesized in the liver).

Relation of mechanisms of action to clinical response

Anatomical, physiological, and chemical factors all play an important role in determining the susceptibility of nerve fibers to blockade by local anesthetics during clinical procedures. Because the sodium channels present in different types of neurons have similar affinities for local anesthetics, these drugs block impulse conduction in all nerve cells, including sensory, motor, autonomic, and CNS neurons. Sodium channels also play an important role in other electrically excitable cells. Thus, local anesthetics can also have prominent effects on skeletal and cardiac muscle. Their effects on cardiac sodium channels form the basis for their therapeutic use in the treatment of certain cardiac dysrhythmias (see Chapter 14). Their effects on smooth and cardiac muscle also contribute to their toxicity (see later discussion). However, local anesthetics are not equally potent and effective in all cells where sodium channels are present, and they exhibit some selectivity for different neuronal and muscle cell types. This selectivity is determined by the rate of drug penetration, firing rate, and axonal size and location within the nerve bundle and importantly, by the "margin of safety" for nerve impulse transmission. This last factor, a measure of how well transmission can overcome deficits in excitability, differs among different fiber types and also at different zones in a neuron. It is likely to be highest in the trunk region of an axon, lower at distal and central branch regions, and lower also at the impulse generating sites such as the distal terminals of sensory fibers.

It also takes longer and a higher dose of drug to block nerves in a highly vascularized region, a requirement that can be reduced by the co-injection of vasoconstrictors. For peripheral nerve blocks in general, less than 10% of the injected dose actually reaches the nerve to provide impulse blockade. Correspondingly, clinical solutions of local anesthetics (e.g., 1% lidocaine HCl, equal to about 40 mM) are far more concentrated than the solutions (about 1 mM) that achieve impulse blockade on bare axons.

Neurons differ substantially in terms of their diameter, degree of myelination, and frequency of firing, and all of these factors influence the ability of local anesthetics to produce blockade. The three major types of nerve fibers are classified as A, B, or C (Fig. 30-5). A fibers are myelinated and have the fastest conduction

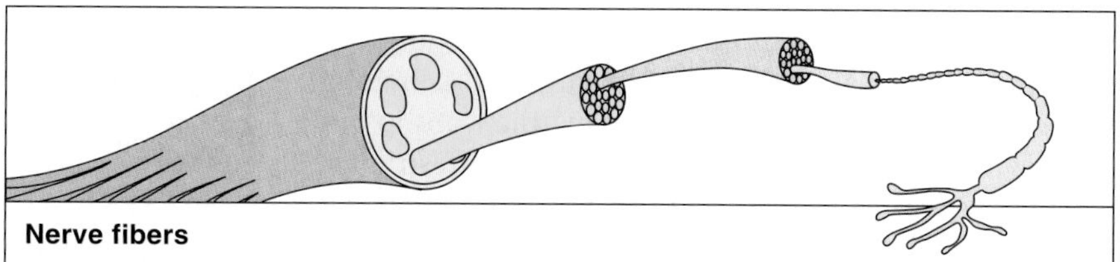

Nerve fibers			
Fiber type	A	B	C*
Diameter μm	2–20	<3	<1.5
Conduction velocity (m/sec)	5–100	3–15	0.1–2.5
Myelinated	Yes	Yes	No
		Preganglionic, autonomic, vascular smooth muscle	Pain, temperature, postganglionic, autonomic

Subtypes of A fibers	Aα	Aβ	Aγ	Aδ*
	Efferent, motor, somatic, reflex activity	Afferent, innervate muscle, touch sensation, pressure sensation	Efferent, muscle spindle tone	Afferent, pain, cold, temperature, tissue damage indication*

* Pain transmission fibers.

Figure 30-5 Nerve fibers according to anatomical type.

velocity, B fibers are myelinated with a slower conduction velocity, and C fibers are unmyelinated and have the slowest conduction velocity. Most pain impulses in humans are carried by the Aδ and C fibers. The Aδ fibers, which are distributed primarily in skin and mucous membranes, are the smallest subtype of A fibers (2-5 μm diameter) and are associated with a sharp, pricking pain termed "fast pain." C fibers, which are more widely distributed, are smaller than Aδ fibers (<1.5 μm diameter) and are associated with a duller, long-lasting, burning pain termed "slow pain."

Local anesthetics block the smaller diameter, myelinated fibers first, and rapidly firing neurons are generally blocked at lower drug concentrations than the more slowly firing neurons (state dependency as discussed earlier). Thus, B and Aδ fibers are blocked first, followed by blockade of C fibers. Aγ fibers, which set the length of muscle spindles, are similar in diameter and conduction velocity to Aδ fibers and thus will be blocked along with the Aδ fibers. Blockade of impulses in Aγ fibers produces a flaccid paralysis and probably accounts for the early signs of motor weakness and paralysis. Hence, fast pain fibers (Aδ) are inhibited prior to a loss of touch or pressure sensations (Aβ fibers), slow pain (C fibers), or motor function (Aα fibers).

The anatomical location of different nerve types also influences the ability of local anesthetics to produce nerve block. For example, peripheral nerves are never affected uniformly by a local anesthetic because a concentration gradient of the drug from the mantle to the core of the nerve is established during the onset of the block; a steady-state distribution of drug in the nerve is rarely achieved. Thus, a dynamic block results from both the rapid influx of the drug into the nerve and a slower efflux from the nerve after injection of a concentrated bolus. Axons in the mantle are generally exposed to higher drug concentrations than are axons in the core, where drug diffusion is more restricted. Although these principles help explain the differential sensitivity of nerve fibers to local anesthetics, it is difficult to predict what will happen in every given situation. Sensory modalities are lost in the following general order: cold, warmth, pain, touch, and deep pressure. As indicated above, motor functions appear to be more resistant to blockade by local anesthetics, but this may result from the relatively complex motor tasks that are tested in the clinical setting, wherein the patient can recruit several different groups of muscles to accomplish a similar movement. Indeed, when simple muscle movements—for example, extensor postural thrust—are isolated in experimental animals during peripheral nerve block, their deficiencies are greater and longer in duration than the loss of pain sensitivity.

Local anesthetics are generally less effective in inflamed tissues than in normal tissues because inflammation usually results in a local metabolic acidosis, which decreases the pH in surrounding tissues. At an acidic pH, the proportion of drug in its non-protonated form is reduced markedly resulting in insufficient amounts of the unionized form to penetrate cell membranes (see Chapter 3). Thus, the ability of the drug to reach its site of action can be greatly reduced.

Local anesthetic drugs are used widely to provide temporary pain relief in localized regions of the body. By varying the drug, its concentration and dose, and the method of administration, one can obtain a wide range of effects. A localized, intensely numb area of skin can be achieved for a short time by infiltrating the area with a short-acting drug. On the other hand, a sensory block can be achieved by administering a dilute solution of a long-acting local anesthetic through an indwelling catheter to the epidural space, providing complete anesthesia while preserving most motor function, including uterine motility. Anesthetics are used to simultaneously provide analgesia and muscle relaxation through spinal or epidural administration. In addition, dilute solutions of local anesthetics mixed with opioids are being used increasingly for postoperative pain relief (see Chapter 31). These combinations provide effective analgesia and have the advantage of using a lower total dose of the narcotic drug than normally would be required for conventional therapies. Finally, local anesthetics are used as both diagnostic and therapeutic tools in the management of more complicated acute and chronic pain states.

Side effects, clinical problems, and toxicity

Because termination of local anesthetic action ultimately depends on the movement of the drug into the systemic circulation, side effects and toxicity can result from properly conducted nerve blocks as well as from accidental intravenous (IV) injection. CNS effects may manifest as depression or stimulation, or both, depending on the neural pathways affected. Depression of cortical inhibitory neurons, without the balancing depression of excitatory nerves, may result in tremor and restlessness and culminate in overt clonic convulsions, coma, and respiratory failure (see Clinical Problems box). However, a variety of signs and symptoms, including general depression and drowsiness, are common clinical consequences. Seizures can be treated

CLINICAL PROBLEMS

CNS seizures and convulsions at high concentrations of agent
Blockade of cardiac sodium channels (also used therapeutically for antiarrhythmic effects; see Chapter 14)

or prevented by the IV injection of diazepam along with oxygen administration to protect against hypoxemia in the convulsing patient. An overdose of local anesthetic can result in the reduced transmission of impulses at the neuromuscular junction and at ganglionic synapses, producing weakness or muscle paralysis. Support of respiration is an important component of treatment. Smooth muscle is only minimally affected by local anesthetics.

Local anesthetics have potentially deleterious effects on cardiac pacemaker activity, electrical excitability, conduction times, and contractile force. Dysrhythmias are possible when high blood concentrations of anesthetic agents are attained. For example, cocaine, a potent local anesthetic that was widely used clinically several decades ago and is now a prominent drug of abuse, has side effects on the heart and the CNS (see Chapter 32). Among the local anesthetics in current use, bupivacaine is considered to be the most cardiotoxic. On the other hand, lidocaine is used therapeutically to depress abnormal pacemaker-derived and ectopic activity in certain arrhythmogenic states (see Chapter 14).

Local hypersensitivity reactions can result from the use of some ester-type local anesthetics, particularly procaine and related compounds. These can be ameliorated by the systemic administration of antihistamines.

New horizons

Although the local anesthetics are important therapeutic compounds for pain management, their usefulness is somewhat limited by their potential side effects. The therapeutic profile of these agents would be improved significantly if one were able to:

- Control and predict the duration of block.
- Enhance selectivity for pain suppression relative to motor and autonomic blockade.
- Improve safety, especially cardiotoxicity.

To this end, studies have focused on identifying different types of VGSC in various tissues. The idea is that selectivity for pain suppression may be possible by designing drugs that selectively target channels expressed uniquely in peripheral pain fibers. Although several VGSCs have been identified, their local anesthetic binding sites are often quite similar. While more highly selective local anesthetics have not yet been identified, further studies will ultimately determine the utility of this approach.

TRADE NAMES

All of the important compounds available in the United States are listed in the Major Drugs box.

FURTHER READING

Lai J, Hunter JC, Porreca F. The role of voltage-gated sodium channels in neuropathic pain. *Current Opin Neurobiol* 2003; 3:291-297.

Mao J, Chen LL. Systemic lidocaine for neuropathic pain relief. *Pain* 2000; 87:7-17.

Wang GK, Strichartz, GR. Therapeutic Na^+ channel blockers beneficial for pain syndromes. Drug development research. *Research Overview* 2002; 54:154-158.

Self-assessment questions

1. Which of the following is true of local anesthetics?
   a. Their molecular sites of action are voltage-dependent sodium channels.
   b. They bind selectively to the intracellular surface and block the entry of sodium into the cell.
   c. The binding of local anesthetics to sodium channels is completely reversible.
   d. The ability to block the sodium channel depends on the conformational state of the channel.
   e. All of the above.

2. Which of the following is true about local anesthetics?
   a. They are weak acids.
   b. They are largely in the charged cationic form at normal body pH.
   c. The charged form of the drug readily penetrates the cell membrane because of the presence of a hydrophilic group.
   d. The protonated form of the drug blocks the sodium channel.
   e. *b* and *d*.

3. All of the following are correct *except:*

a. Local anesthetics form salts by combining with acids.
b. Local anesthetics possess both hydrophilic and hydrophobic groups.
c. Anesthetics with amide linkages have longer durations of actions than those with ester linkages.
d. The effectiveness of the local anesthetic is reduced by vascular reabsorption/uptake.
e. All of the above are correct.

4. Toxic effects of local anesthetics include all of the following *except:*

a. Cardiac dysrhythmias.
b. Seizures.
c. Hypersensitivity.
d. CNS depression.
e. All of the above.

CHAPTER 31

Drugs to control pain

Stephen G. Holtzman
Yung-Fong Sung

Major Drugs

Opioid analgesics	Acetaminophen (Tylenol)
Nonsteroidal antiinflammatory drugs	Antigout drugs
	Antimigraine drugs

Therapeutic overview

In *Paradise Lost,* John Milton wrote that "Pain is perfect misery, the worst of evils, and excessive, overturns all patience." **Pain** is a subjective symptom, an unpleasant sensory or emotional experience that is associated typically with actual or potential tissue damage and is the most common reason for seeking medical care. **Analgesia** is a state in which no pain is felt despite the presence of normally painful stimuli. Drugs that alleviate pain without major impairment of other sensory modalities are termed **analgesics** and fall into three major categories: the opioid analgesics, the non-opioid analgesics, and analgesics used to treat specific pain syndromes.

The **opioid analgesics** include compounds that relieve moderate-to-severe pain through actions mediated by a specific family of cell-surface receptors. Morphine is the prototypical opioid and is one of two analgesics (codeine is the other) found in opium, the milky exudate of the poppy plant *(Papaver somniferum).* It was the first alkaloid to be isolated in 1806 by Sertürner, who named the substance after the Greek god of dreams, *Morpheus.*

Narcotic is a term still used to refer to opioids, and has its origins in Federal legislation (1914 Harrison Narcotic Act). Medically, a narcotic is a drug that produces a stuporous, sleep-like state and may or may not relieve pain; thus it is not a precise term. In addition, the term **opiate** is also used sometimes to refer to these compounds. Opiates are defined as compounds isolated from the opium poppy (**morphine** and **codeine**) that act at opioid receptors, whereas opioids are compounds of any structural type that interact with the opioid receptors and include peptides as well as fully synthetic small organic molecules; however, these terms are often used interchangeably. Opioid analgesics include morphine and its synthetic analogs, partial agonists, mixed-acting agonist-antagonists, pure antagonists, and peptides found in brain and other tissues. Although the mixed-acting agonist-antagonists and many of the endogenous peptides do not always resemble morphine in their actions, the term **opioid** is used to refer to the entire group of drugs.

The non-opioid analgesics include the **nonsteroidal antiinflammatory drugs** (NSAIDs) typified by **aspirin**

Abbreviations

CNS	central nervous system
COX	cyclooxygenase
GI	gastrointestinal
5-HT	serotonin
IV	intravenous
MAO	monoamine oxidase
NAPQI	*N*-acetyl-p-benzoquinoneimine
NSAID	nonsteroidal antiinflammatory drug
PG	prostaglandin

and **acetaminophen.** These compounds relieve mild-to-moderate pain and have **antipyretic** and **antiinflammatory** (except acetaminophen) properties. They are used to treat pain arising from integument structures, such as headache and myalgia, dysmenorrhea, and some types of postoperative pain. They are also used to treat fever and inflammatory disorders, such as osteoarthritis and rheumatoid arthritis, which are characterized by inflammation, pain, and subsequent tissue damage. Although NSAIDs do not affect the causative factors or prevent the progression of arthritic disorders, they can provide welcome relief from the associated pain and inflammation and improve the mobility of bone joints, thereby improving quality of life.

It is now apparent that aspirin and other NSAIDs have therapeutic value for indications other than pain, fever, and inflammation. A low dose of aspirin inhibits platelet aggregation, and when taken prophylactically, lowers the incidence of myocardial infarction and stroke in patients at high risk for ischemic cardiovascular events. More recent findings indicate that chronic treatment with aspirin or other NSAIDs reduces the incidence of colorectal and certain other cancers.

The third group of analgesics includes compounds that do not relieve pain from tissue damage (i.e., **nociceptive pain**) but can provide relief in specific pain syndromes such as neuropathic pain, gout, and migraine headache. **Neuropathic pain** results from changes in sensory neurons that render them hyperactive, even in the absence of nociceptive stimuli. It is often a chronic condition that is impervious to standard analgesic drugs. However, neuropathic pain is ameliorated by tricyclic antidepressants and compounds used to treat seizure disorders, drugs that are not thought of as primary analgesic agents.

Gout, or gouty arthritis, is the most common cause of inflammatory joint disease in men over age 40. Caused by deposition of urate crystals in bone joints accompanied by increased blood uric acid concentrations, it is treated symptomatically with NSAIDs, **corticosteroids,** or **colchicine** to decrease inflammation and with specific drugs to correct the underlying hyperuricemia.

Migraine, one of three primary types of headache, afflicts as many as 10% of the population. In addition to causing pain and suffering, it has a large economic impact from direct healthcare costs and lost productivity. Migraine is treated with the NSAIDS, ergot derivatives, and the serotonin (5-HT) receptor agonists ("triptans"), the latter often the most effective for aborting a migraine headache.

The principal uses of the opioids, NSAIDs, and acetaminophen are listed in the Therapeutic Overview box.

THERAPEUTIC OVERVIEW

Opioids

Relief of most types of moderate-to-severe visceral or somatic pain
Symptomatic treatment of acute diarrhea
Cough suppression
Treatment of opiate addiction and alcoholism
Anesthetic adjunct
Reversal of opioid overdose by opioid-receptor antagonists

NSAIDs and acetaminophen

Relief of mild-to-moderate somatic pain including headache, toothache, myalgia, and arthralgia
Relief in inflammatory disorders including rheumatoid arthritis, osteoarthritis, gout, and ankylosing spondylitis (except acetaminophen)
Reduce fever
Prophylaxis of myocardial infarction and stroke

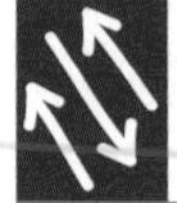

Mechanisms of action

Neurophysiology of pain

Sensations of pain are modulated by both ascending and descending pathways in the central nervous system (CNS). Noxious or nociceptive stimuli activate highly developed endings on primary afferent neurons, termed **nociceptors** (pain receptors). These stimuli give rise to action potentials that are transmitted along afferent neurons into the dorsal horn of the spinal cord. *A-delta* (Aδ) fibers are small, myelinated, rapidly conducting afferent neurons that terminate in lamina I of the spinal cord. They have a relatively high threshold for activation by mechanical and thermal stimuli and mediate sharp and localized pain, often termed **somatic pain.** C-fibers are even smaller unmyelinated afferent neurons and hence are slower conducting. They are polymodal and are activated by mechanical, thermal, or chemical stimuli. They terminate in lamina II of the spinal cord *(substantia gelatinosa)* and mediate dull, diffuse, aching, or burning pain sometimes called **visceral pain** (see Fig. 30-5). Aδ and C-fibers release excitatory amino acids in the dorsal horn; C-fibers also release neuropeptides such as substance P. These neurotransmitters activate secondary neurons that form the ascending spinothalamic pathway, which projects to supraspinal nuclei in the thalamus and then to the limbic system and cerebral cortex (Fig. 31-1, *A*).

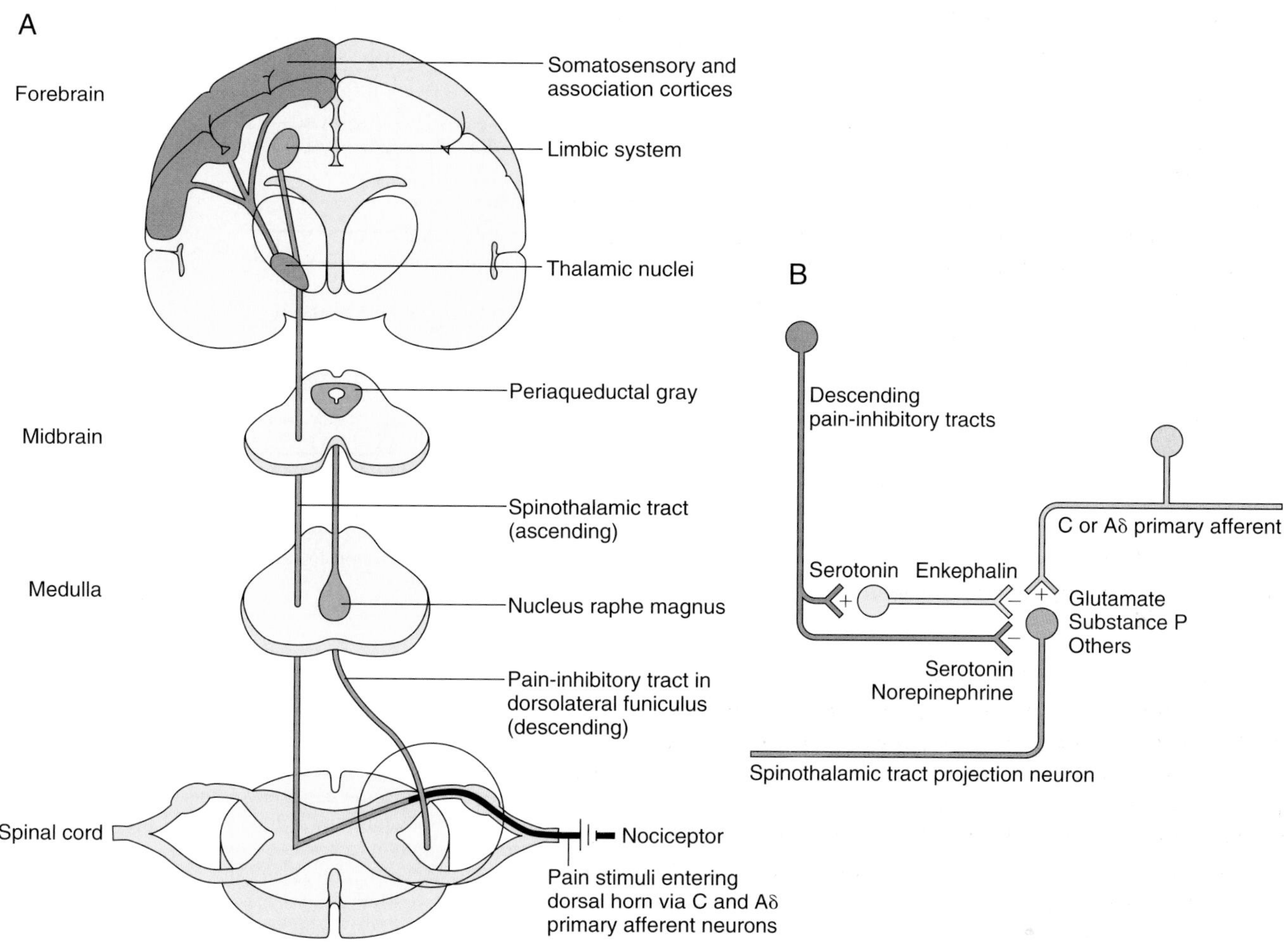

Figure 31-1 **A,** Ascending spinothalamic tract pain-transmitting pathway and descending pain-inhibitory pathway originating in the midbrain. **B,** Possible synaptic connections in the dorsal horn and mediators that may influence the transmission of pain stimuli.

Descending pain-inhibitory systems originate in the periaqueductal gray region of the midbrain and from several nuclei of the rostroventral medulla oblongata and project downward to the dorsal horn. These descending systems release norepinephrine, 5-HT, and other neurotransmitters and thereby inhibit the activity of the ascending pain pathways, either through direct synaptic contacts or indirectly by activating inhibitory interneurons. These pathways are illustrated in Figure 31-1, *B*.

Opioids

Three major families of **opioid peptides** have been identified: the enkephalins, endorphins, and dynorphins. They are derived from precursor molecules encoded by separate genes—proenkephalin, proopiomelanocortin, and prodynorphin, respectively. Although found primarily in the CNS, some opioid peptides, notably the enkephalins, also exist in peripheral tissues such as nerve plexuses of the gastrointestinal (GI) tract and the adrenal medulla (Table 31-1).

Enkephalinergic interneurons in the dorsal horn produce presynaptic inhibition of primary afferent neurons and postsynaptic inhibition of secondary neurons in ascending pathways. Shorter-chain products of prodynorphin, notably dynorphin A(1-8), like the enkephalins, occur in interneurons distributed widely throughout the CNS and are prevalent in laminae I and II of the spinal cord.

β-Endorphin and longer-chain **dynorphins**, such as dynorphin A(1-17), have a more limited distribution in the CNS and may not influence pain processing directly. Rather, they may have hormonal roles in responses to stress and fluid homeostasis, respectively. The structures of the three classical families of opioid peptides are shown in Figure 31-2.

Three major **opioid receptors** have been identified by pharmacological means and molecular cloning, and

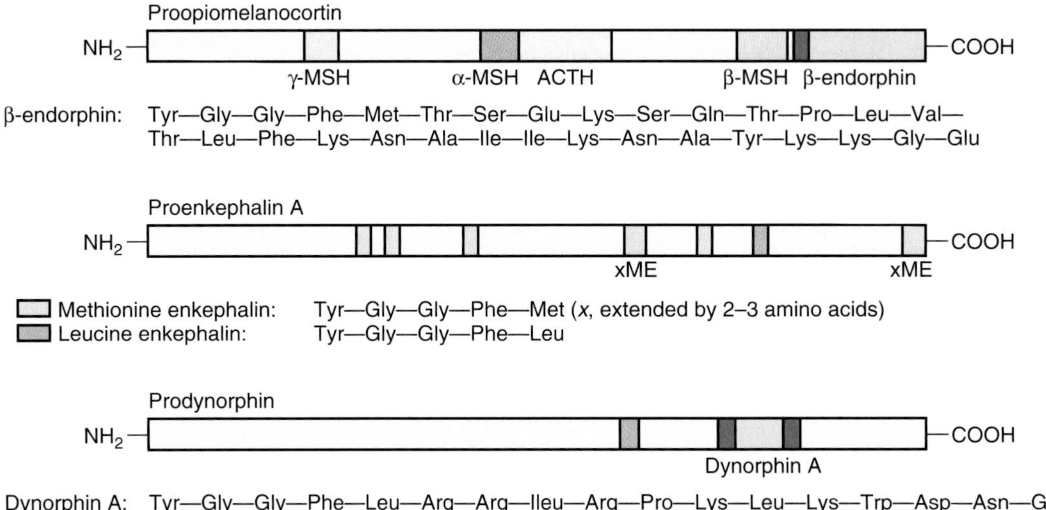

Figure 31-2 The major families of opioid peptides—endorphins, enkephalins, dynorphins—are derived from distinct precursor molecules—proopiomelanocortin, proenkephalin A, prodynorphin—and are encoded by three distinct genes.

Table 31-1 Principal endogenous opioid peptides

Opioid Family	Precursor	Distribution
Enkephalins	Proenkephalin	Widely throughout the CNS, especially in interneurons, including those associated with pain pathways and emotional behavior; also found in some peripheral tissues
Endorphins	Proopiomelanocortin	β-Endorphin in hypothalamus, nucleus tractus solitarius, and anterior lobe of the pituitary where it is co-released with adrenocorticotrophin in response to stress
Dynorphins	Prodynorphin	Dynorphin A(1-17) in the magnocellular cells of the hypothalamus and posterior lobe of the pituitary gland where it co-localizes with vasopressin; Shorter-chain dynorphins distributed widely in the CNS, some associated with pain pathways, especially in the spinal cord

are designated μ, κ, and δ (Table 31-2). They are also referred to by either their International Union of Pharmacology nomenclature (OP_3, OP_2, and OP_1, respectively) or their molecular biological nomenclature (MOP, KOP, and DOP, respectively). All three receptors belong to the superfamily of G-protein–coupled receptors with the characteristic seven transmembrane-spanning regions (see Chapter 2). Activation of these receptors decreases synthesis of cyclic adenosine monophosphate, increases K^+ conductance, and decreases Ca^{2+} conductance, effects illustrated in Figure 31-3. Because changes in K^+ and Ca^{2+} conductances inhibit neuronal activity, activation of any of the three opioid receptors usually results in decreased neuronal transmission.

Table 31-2 Opioid receptors and their ligands

Receptor	Endogenous Ligand	Drug Ligands
μ (mu) Receptor (OP_3/MOP)	Enkephalins β-endorphin endomorphins(?)	morphine buprenorphine methadone meperidine fentanyl
κ (kappa) Receptor (OP_2/KOP)	Dynorphins	butorphanol pentazocine
δ (delta) Receptor (OP_1/DOP)	Enkephalins β-endorphin	none to date

The selectivity of opioid receptors for endogenous and drug ligands is shown in Table 31-2. The anatomical distribution of opioid receptors is consistent with the actions of the opioids–that is, they are found prominently among structures of the ascending and descending pain-modulatory pathways. All clinically important effects of morphine and morphine-like drugs are mediated by μ receptors. κ-Receptors appear to mediate some of the effects of mixed-action opioids, including analgesia at the level of the spinal cord, sedation, and the dysphoria that occurs at high doses. With the exception of the opioid antagonists, there are currently no therapeutic agents that interact with δ receptors in a clinically meaningful way. In cases in which opioids can be resolved into optical isomers, the levorotatory isomer usually has a considerably higher affinity for opioid

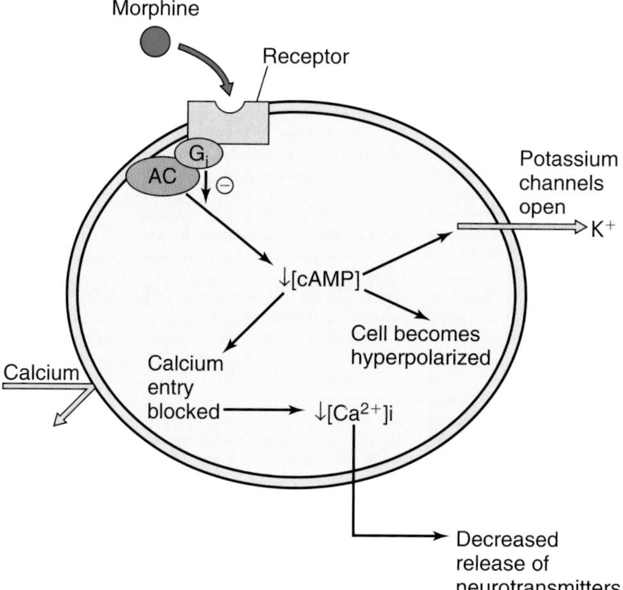

Figure 31-3 Mechanism of action of opioids on neurons. Opioid receptors μ, δ, and κ are coupled negatively to adenylyl cyclase *(AC)* by G-proteins *(G_i)*. Activation of an opioid receptor by an agonist decreases activity of adenylyl cyclase, resulting in a decrease in the production of cyclic adenosine monophosphate *(cAMP)*. This leads to an increase in the efflux of K^+ and cellular hyperpolarization, and a decrease in the influx of Ca^{2+} and lower intracellular concentrations of free calcium. The overall consequence is a decrease in the neuronal release of neurotransmitters. Opioid receptors also may be coupled by G-proteins to intracellular second messengers other than cAMP.

receptors than does its dextrorotatory counterpart. The structures of morphine and representative agonist/antagonist compounds are shown in Figure 31-4.

NSAIDs and acetaminophen

The mechanism of action, all of the therapeutic effects, and many of the side effects of the NSAIDs are due to **inhibition of cyclooxygenase (COX)**, an enzyme involved in the metabolism of the eicosanoids. The eicosanoids are derivatives of arachidonic acid synthesized by one of two families of enzyme, the lipoxygenases and the cyclooxygenases, producing the leukotrienes, and the **prostaglandins (PGs)** and thromboxanes, respectively (see Chapter 17). Two distinct COXs have been identified. **COX-1** is constitutively expressed and is involved in "housekeeping tasks" in cells. **COX-2** occurs constitutively in some tissues but is largely inducible, and induction results in a marked increase in the rate of synthesis and release of COX products, particularly the PGs. Aspirin acetylates both COX enzymes, inhibiting their activity irreversibly, whereas other nonselective NSAIDs inhibit the COX enzymes reversibly. The COX-2 inhibitors are 8- to 35-fold more selective for COX-2 relative to COX-1 and inhibit COX-2 irreversibly in a time-dependent manner. The functional consequences of inhibition of COX-2 relative to COX-1 are depicted in Figure 31-5. Structures of aspirin, acetaminophen, and the COX-2 inhibitor celecoxib are shown in Figure 31-6.

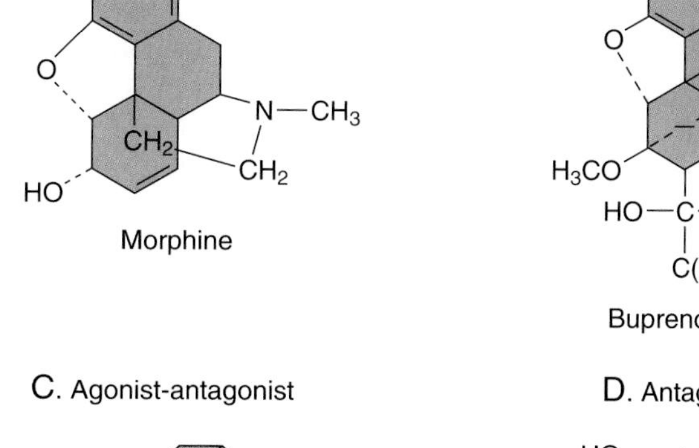

Figure 31-4 Structures of morphine and representative partial-agonist, agonist-antagonist, and antagonist opioid drugs.

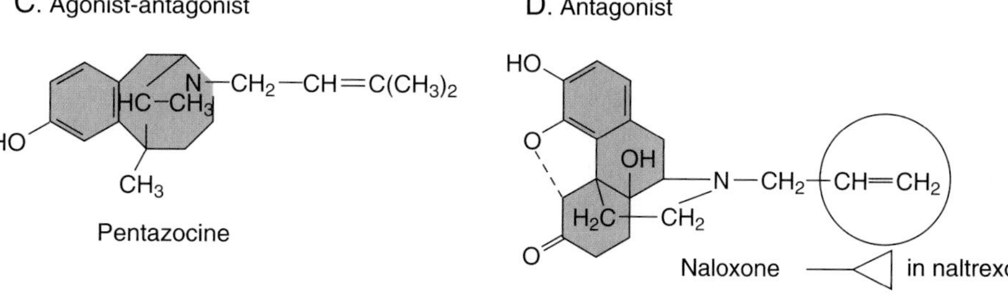

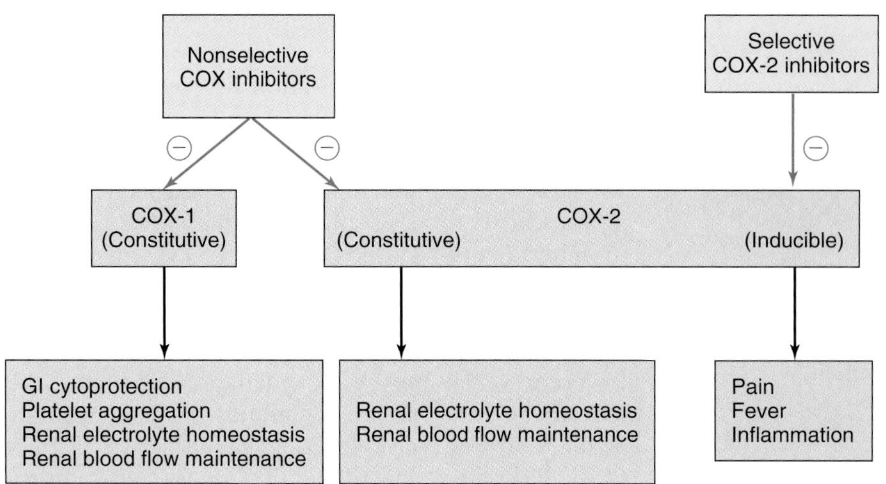

Figure 31-5 NSAIDs produce their therapeutic effects and many side effects by inhibiting the cyclooxygenase *(COX)* enzymes. Drugs that inhibit COX-2 selectively produce fewer adverse side effects than do those that inhibit both isoforms of the enzyme.

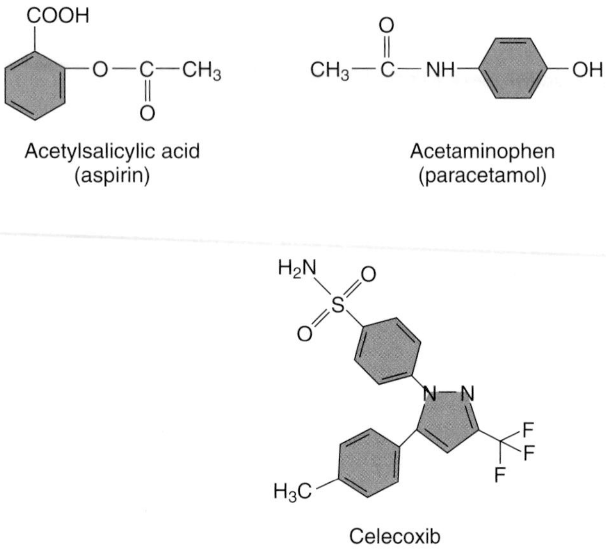

Acetylsalicylic acid (aspirin)

Acetaminophen (paracetamol)

Celecoxib

Figure 31-6 Structures of aspirin, acetaminophen, and celecoxib.

At the site of injury, PGs sensitize nociceptors to many chemical mediators of pain, including bradykinin, cytokines, and certain amino acids and neuropeptides, as well as to mechanical and thermal stimuli. In addition, PGs and prostacyclin (PGI_2) promote blood flow to injured tissues, resulting in leukocyte infiltration. These effects, together with leukotriene-induced increases in vascular permeability and attraction of polymorphonuclear leukocytes, lead to edema and inflammation. Peripheral inflammation also is associated with an increased expression of COX-2 in the dorsal horn of the spinal cord. Viruses and bacterial endotoxins, through a chain of events, induce COX-2 in the preoptic nuclei of the hypothalamus, the thermoregulatory center of the body. Prostaglandin E_2, in particular, is a potent pyrogen that raises the set-point of the thermoregulatory center, resulting in elevated body temperature. Thus, inhibition of COX-2 can be an effective treatment for certain types of pain, inflammation, and fever.

Drugs for specific pain syndromes

Neuropathic pain is the result of injury to peripheral sensory nerves and is different from the nociceptive pain caused by tissue damage, in which sensory nerves are activated by chemical mediators of pain. There are many causes of nerve injury, including physical trauma, metabolic and autoimmune disorders, viral infection, chemotoxicity, and chronic inflammation. Nearly half of all diabetic patients experience peripheral neuropathies eventually. Neuropathic pain states often are associated with **hyperalgesia** (increased sensitivity to normally painful stimuli) and **allodynia** (pain caused by stimuli that are not normally painful; e.g., touch).

In neuropathic pain, primary afferent neurons are hyperactive, discharging spontaneously (in the absence of an identifiable noxious stimulus), and there is a cascade of changes to neurons in dorsal root ganglia and in the dorsal horn of the spinal cord. These changes present multiple targets for pharmacological intervention, among which are increases in the expression and activity of sodium channels. Several drugs introduced to treat seizure disorders, such as carbamazepine and lamotrigine, inhibit voltage-dependent sodium channels (see Chapter 27) and have been shown to be effective in the treatment of neuropathic pain. Tricyclic antidepressants (see Chapter 23) have also been shown to be effective for this condition.

As mentioned, **gout** is an inflammatory disease caused by increased uric acid in the blood and the deposition of uric acid crystals in bone joints. Uric acid is a waste product formed from the catabolism of purines and normally dissolves in blood and is excreted by the

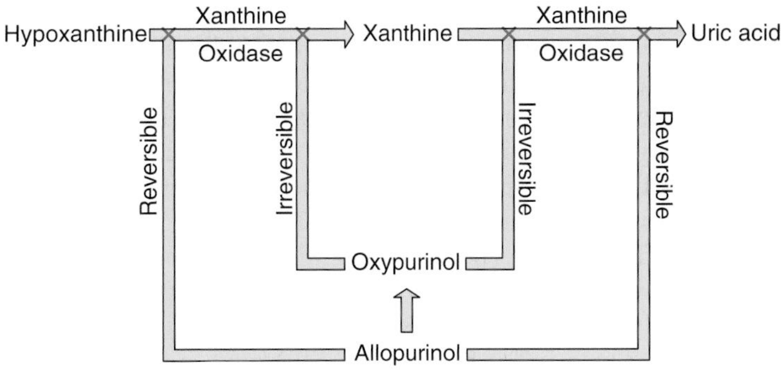

Figure 31-7 Blockade of uric acid synthesis by allopurinol and its oxidated metabolite, oxypurinol.

kidneys. However, if too much uric acid is formed or too little excreted, urate crystals precipitate. Crystals in the joints and surrounding tissue attract leukocytes, which attempt to phagocytose them, releasing inflammatory mediators in the process. In classical acute gout, the big toe is the body part most often the site of the inflammatory response and associated pain. Gout occurs in approximately 0.6% of men and 0.1% of women, primarily after menopause.

Drugs from several pharmacological classes are used to treat or prevent gout. The NSAIDs and the corticosteroids (see Chapter 33) attenuate inflammatory responses to urate crystals and the associated pain. Colchicine also reduces the inflammatory response, but through a different mechanism. Colchicine binds to tubulin in leukocytes, causing microtubules to disaggregate. This affects the structure of the cells, inhibiting their migration into the inflamed area and reducing phagocytic activity. Specific drugs are used to correct the underlying hyperuricemia in gout. **Allopurinol**, a structural analog of the purine hypoxanthine, inhibits the enzyme xanthine oxidase (Fig. 31-7), blocking the metabolism of hypoxanthine and xanthine to uric acid and lowering blood urate concentrations. Normally, about 90% of filtered urate is resorbed and only 10% is excreted. The uricosuric agents **probenecid** and **sulfinpyrazone** increase urate excretion by competing with uric acid for the renal tubular acid transporter so less urate is resorbed.

Migraine is a neurovascular syndrome characterized by throbbing unilateral headache and often a premonitory prodrome and/or aura, nausea, vomiting, photophobia, blurry vision, and GI and other unpleasant symptoms. Almost 3 times more women than men suffer from migraine. Although many triggers of migraine episodes have been identified, the pathophysiology of the disorder is not clear. Migraine may involve release of monoamines and vasoactive peptides from trigeminal neurons and structures in the brainstem, which first cause cerebral vasoconstriction, and then vasodilation, the latter associated with neurogenically induced inflammation and increased expression of COX-2 in some brain areas. 5-HT appears to be involved in migraine episodes, possibly by facilitating neuronal release of vasoactive substances, directly affecting the tone of cerebral vessels, or activating cranial nociceptors.

Migraine episodes can be aborted or lessened in intensity in most patients by drugs that activate 5-HT$_1$ receptors. The triptans are relatively selective agonists at 5-HT$_{1B/D}$ receptors, whereas ergot derivatives are partial agonists at 5-HT$_1$ and other 5-HT receptors, as well as at some catecholamine receptors. The mechanism of action of these drugs is uncertain but may involve direct constriction of intracranial arterioles, reversing the abnormal cerebral vasodilation that occurs in migraine. It has also been suggested that activation of presynaptic 5-HT$_1$ autoreceptors reduces neuronal release of vasoactive substances into the perivascular space.

The NSAIDs also bring relief from migraine episodes in many patients. They are presumed to attenuate the neurogenically-induced inflammatory response through inhibition of COX-2. Other drugs are also used as preventive therapy, including tricyclic antidepressants, especially amitriptyline (see Chapter 23) and the β-adrenergic receptor blockers propranolol and timolol (see Chapter 10).

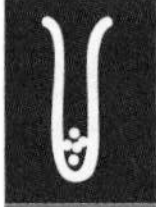

Pharmacokinetics

Opioids

Many opioids are administered parenterally, even though they are well absorbed from the GI tract. However, some opioids, such as morphine and the antagonist naloxone, undergo extensive first-pass metabolism in the liver, greatly reducing their bioavailability and therapeutic efficacy after oral administration. Although morphine often is administered orally for management of chronic pain, oral administration is much less potent compared with parenteral administration. Drugs with greater lipophilicity, including fentanyl and buprenorphine, are well absorbed through the nasal and buccal mucosa. The most lipophilic of opioids, including fentanyl, are absorbed transdermally as well. Serum protein binding ranges from approximately 30% for morphine to 80% to 90% for fentanyl and its derivatives. The pharmacokinetic profile of an opioid is a major determinant of its therapeutic use.

Because of their physicochemical properties, the speed of onset and duration of action of opioids do not always correlate with their plasma concentrations or elimination half-lives. For example, the rise in plasma concentrations of morphine long precedes the onset of analgesia because this hydrophilic drug penetrates the blood-brain barrier very slowly. In contrast, plasma concentrations of fentanyl closely parallel its therapeutic effect. Because of the rapid redistribution of lipophilic fentanyl from brain to lean body mass, its short duration of action is not predictable from its elimination half-life, which exceeds that of the longer-acting morphine. Opioids with relatively long elimination half-lives can accumulate in the body upon repeated dosing, thereby prolonging their duration of action. Remifentanil, a fentanyl analog ester, is so rapidly metabolized by plasma esterases that its plasma half-life is only 10 to 20 minutes. It does not accumulate upon repeated or slow continuous administration.

Opioids are metabolized mainly in the liver, usually to more polar and less active or inactive compounds. The mechanisms involved include *N*-dealkylation, conjugation of hydroxyl groups, and hydrolysis. However, metabolites account for most of the opioid activity of codeine (3-methoxymorphine) and its analogs, heroin (3-,6-diacetylmorphine) and tramadol, which have weak affinity for the μ-opioid receptor and have little activity themselves. The two hydroxyl groups of morphine are conjugated with glucuronic acid to produce two metabolites. Morphine-3-glucuronide is inactive, but morphine-6-glucuronide has a higher affinity for the μ-opioid receptor and is a more potent analgesic than morphine. Morphine-6-glucuronide accumulates during long-term morphine treatment, and measurable amounts are found in cerebrospinal fluid. However, morphine-6-glucuronide is relatively polar and penetrates the blood-brain barrier poorly. Thus, the extent to which it contributes to the analgesic effect of morphine administered acutely is unknown.

The accumulation of normeperidine, the *N*-demethylated product of meperidine, can result in convulsions. Significant amounts accumulate in patients receiving multiple large doses of meperidine over a relatively short time, in patients with renal insufficiency, and in people taking drugs that interfere with its metabolism, including monoamine oxidase (MAO) inhibitors.

The pharmacokinetic parameters of opioid drugs are summarized in Table 31-3.

NSAIDs and acetaminophen

All of the antipyretic analgesics have good oral bioavailability, ranging from 80% to 100%, and are distributed throughout the body. Some are also formulated as rectal suppositories and have good bioavailability by that route as well, and some are applied topically. Ketorolac often is administered parenterally; bioavailability is essentially 100%.

Aspirin (acetylsalicylic acid) has a low pK_a and is well absorbed from the acidic environment of the stomach and duodenum, the part of the GI tract that accounts for much of the absorption of the NSAIDs. Aspirin has a plasma half-life of only 15 minutes because it undergoes rapid hydrolysis to salicylic acid, which has therapeutic effects similar to those of the parent drug. The half-life of salicylic acid ranges from 2 to 3 hours at doses used to treat pain and fever to as high as 12 hours at doses sometimes used to treat inflammatory disorders. Approximately 75% is conjugated with glycine in the liver to form the inactive salicyluric acid, which is excreted by the kidneys, along with glucuronide conjugates and 10% free salicylic acid. At alkaline pH, up to 30% of a dose may be excreted as free salicylic acid, which is why sodium bicarbonate is administered to alkalinize the urine in treating toxic concentrations. The limited hepatic pool of glycine and glucuronide available for conjugation results in elimination of salicylate by first-order kinetics at low doses and by zero-order kinetics at higher doses. This accounts for the increasing half-life with increasing dose.

Other NSAIDs are metabolized by cytochrome P450 enzymes as well as other pathways in the liver, usually to inactive compounds. Some drugs, such as naproxen and indomethacin, are demethylated before being conjugated and excreted. Piroxicam and fenoprofen are hydroxylated, whereas ibuprofen and meclofenamate are hydroxylated and carboxylated before they are conjugated with glucuronic acid and excreted. Sulindac is somewhat unique in that it is metabolized to an active sulfide and undergoes extensive enterohepatic cycling, accounting for its relatively long elimination half-life. Nabumetone, like sulindac, is a prodrug; approximately 35% undergoes rapid hepatic metabolism to the active compound 6-methoxy-2-naphthylacetic acid.

Half of the NSAIDs now in clinical use are cleared from the body rapidly and have an elimination half-life

Table 31-3 Pharmacokinetic parameters of opioids

Drug	Route	Duration of Action (hrs)	Elimination Half-Life (hrs)	Active Metabolites
MORPHINE-LIKE				
Alfentanil	Parenteral*	0.5	1.5	No
Codeine	Oral, parenteral	4-6	3	Yes
Fentanyl	Parenteral, transdermal	0.5-1	3.7	No
Hydrocodone	Oral	4-5	3.8	Yes
Hydromorphone	Parenteral, oral	4-5	2.6	No
Levorphanol	Parenteral, oral	4-5	11	No
Meperidine†	Parenteral, oral	3-4	3	Yes
Methadone	Oral, parenteral	4-5	23	No
Morphine	Parenteral, oral	4-5	2.3	Yes
Oxycodone	Oral	3-5	3	Yes
Oxymorphone	Parenteral, rectal	4-5	1.5	No
Propoxyphene	Oral	4-5	9	Yes
Remifentanil	Parenteral	0.25	0.2	No
Sufentanil	Parenteral	0.5	2.7	No
Tramadol	Parenteral, oral	3-5	6	Yes
PARTIAL AGONISTS AND MIXED-ACTING				
Buprenorphine	Parenteral, sublingual	4-6	5	No
Butorphanol	Parenteral, intranasal	3-4	3	No
Dezocine	Parenteral	3-4	2.5	No
Nalbuphine	Parenteral	4-5	5	No
Pentazocine	Parenteral, oral	3-5	4	No
ANTAGONISTS				
Nalmefene	Parenteral‡	9-11§	10	No
Naloxone	Parenteral	1-2§	1	No
Naltrexone	Oral	24§	4	Yes

*Parenteral refers to administration by injection.
†Pethidine in many countries.
‡Taken orally for treatment of alcoholism.
§Duration of antagonist activity.

<6 hours. Others have a longer duration of action, with half-lives in excess of 8 hours. Because of the key roles of the liver and kidneys in inactivating (or activating) and excreting NSAIDs, drug doses should be adjusted and some drugs avoided entirely in patients with impaired hepatic function or renal failure. Most NSAIDs are highly bound to plasma proteins, especially albumin. This creates the potential for interactions with other drugs that also bind extensively to plasma proteins. The binding of some NSAIDs is saturable, and free drug concentration rises at higher doses.

Acetaminophen (paracetamol in many countries), like the NSAIDs, is a weak acid that is almost completely absorbed from the GI tract and the rectum. Peak plasma concentration is achieved within 1 hour, and distribution is relatively uniform throughout the body. Acetaminophen is converted almost completely to inactive metabolites in the liver. A small proportion is oxidatively metabolized via cytochrome P450 enzymes to N-acetyl-p-benzoquinoneimine (NAPQI), which is conjugated with glutathione and excreted. NAPQI is highly reactive with sulfhydryl groups and binds covalently to them. If the glutathione content of the liver is depressed by disease or fasting, or is depleted by high concentrations of the intermediate metabolite, NAPQI interacts with sulfhydryl-containing hepatocellular proteins, which can lead to hepatic necrosis. Glutathione-depleting concentrations of NAPQI occur following acute overdose with acetaminophen and can also occur after high doses (>4 gm/day) in patients taking drugs that induce cytochrome P450s.

The pharmacokinetic parameters for the NSAIDs and acetaminophen are shown in Table 31-4.

Antigout drugs

All drugs used primarily for the treatment of gout have good oral bioavailability. Colchicine and allopurinol also come in injectable forms; however, it is best not to inject colchicine because of its toxicity. Following metabolism in the liver, colchicine undergoes biliary excretion.

Allopurinol is oxidized to oxypurinol (alloxanthine), which, like the parent compound, is an inhibitor

Table 31-4 Pharmacokinetic parameters of NSAIDs and acetaminophen

Drug	Hours to Peak Plasma Level*	Elimination Half-Life (hrs)	Plasma Protein Binding (%)	COX-2 : COX-1 Ratio§
Acetaminophen†	0.5-1	2-4	25	3.7¶
Aspirin	—‡	0.25	60-80	0.3
Celecoxib	3	10-12	97	7.6
Diclofenac	1	1-2	99	2.8
Diflunisal	2-3	8-12	99	4.5
Etodolac	1.5-2	6-7	99	10
Fenoprofen	2	2-3	99	—
Flurbiprofen	1-2	2-3	99	—
Ibuprofen	2	2-4	90-99	0.1
Indomethacin	2	4-5	99	0.1
Ketoprofen	1.2	2-2.5	99	0.3
Ketorolac	1	2-9	99	1.8
Mefenamic acid	2-4	2	>90	—
Meloxicam	4-5	15-20	99	11.2
Nabumetone	—‡	22-30	99	1.5
Naproxen	2-4	12-16	99	0.1
Oxaprozin	1.5-3.5	≥40	99	0.4
Piroxicam	3-5	50	99	0.1
Sodium salicylate	1-2	2-12	60-80	—
Sulindac	—‡	8	93-98	0.1
Tolmetin	0.5-1	1-5	99	0.4
Valdecoxib	3	8-11	98	28

*For regular-release tablet or capsule taken orally without food in the stomach.
†Paracetamol in many countries.
‡Converted rapidly to an active metabolite.
§Determined in whole blood.
¶Low affinity for both isoforms of COX.

of xanthine oxidase (see Fig. 31-7) and is largely excreted by the kidneys. Inhibition of xanthine oxidase by oxypurinol is irreversible and accounts for most of the therapeutic effects of allopurinol.

Probenecid inhibits the renal tubular secretion of weak acids and can elevate plasma concentrations of weakly acidic drugs taken concomitantly—for example, many NSAIDs. This is used to advantage in situations in which it is necessary to maintain high plasma levels of cephalosporins, penicillin, and other β-lactam antibiotics (see Chapter 45).

Antimigraine drugs

Sumatriptan is administered orally, subcutaneously, or intranasally. Oral bioavailability is 15%, and peak plasma concentrations are reached in 1.5 to 2 hours. In contrast, subcutaneous administration results in 97% bioavailability and peak plasma concentrations in 10 to 20 minutes. Protein binding is low, and the elimination half-life is 2 to 2.5 hours. Sumatriptan is metabolized in the liver by MAO-A. After subcutaneous administration, approximately 60% of a dose is excreted renally (20% unchanged) and the rest by the biliary-fecal route. Relief from pain of severe migraine begins within 10 minutes of injection, and half of patients experience relief within 30 minutes. The onset of action is slower when given orally, with peak relief in more than half of patients occurring within 2 hours (Fig. 31-8).

The newer triptans have better oral bioavailability, ranging from 40% (zolmitriptan) to 60% to 75% (almotriptan, naratriptan) and are taken only by this route. They are metabolized 25% to 50% in the liver by MAO-A (except naratriptan, which is metabolized by microsomal enzymes), and metabolites and unchanged drug are excreted in urine and bile. Among the available drugs, only zolmitriptan has an important active metabolite; it is more potent than the parent compound and probably contributes to the therapeutic effect. Elimination half-lives range from 2 to 6 hours.

Ergotamine and dihydroergotamine are absorbed erratically and undergo significant first-pass metabolism. Ergotamine is available as a sublingual tablet and dihydroergotamine as a nasal spray and a solution for intramuscular or intravenous (IV) injection. Both are metabolized in the liver and excreted in the bile. The

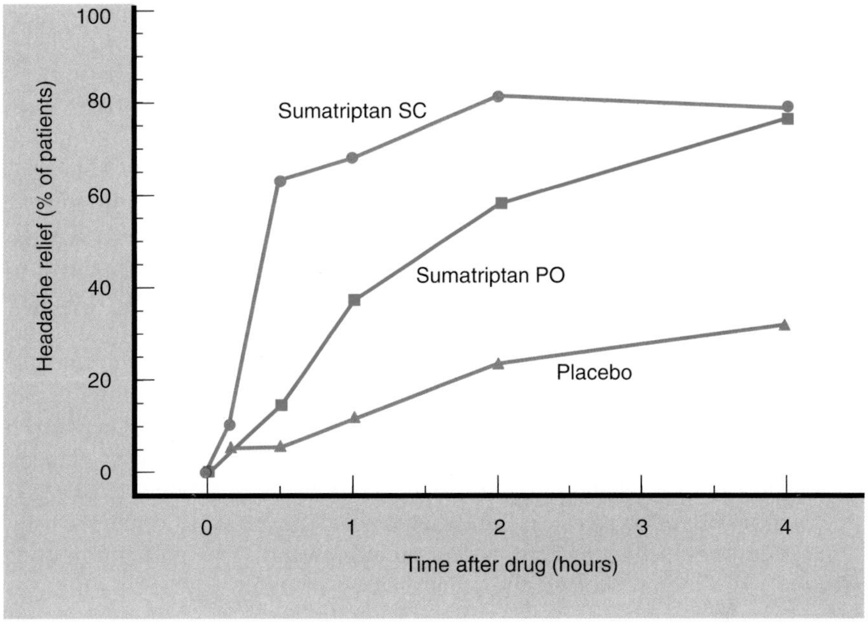

Figure 31-8 Time course of headache relief during a migraine attack following administration of a placebo or sumatriptan by either the oral (PO, 100 mg) or subcutaneous (SC, 6 mg) route. The ordinate indicates the percentage of patients who reported no headache or only mild headache at the corresponding time point. The graph is based upon data obtained from the U.S. Food and Drug Administration and from GlaxoSmithKline.

onset of relief ranges from 5 minutes after IV dihydroergotamine to 0.5 to 2 hours after sublingual ergotamine.

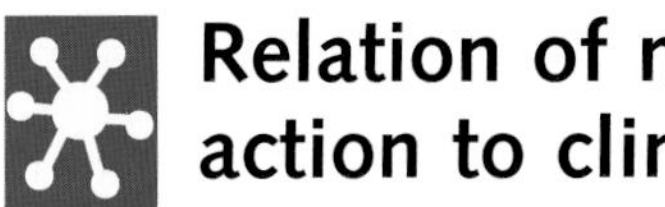

Relation of mechanisms of action to clinical response

Opioids

The experience of pain involves transduction, transmission, and perception of nociceptive stimuli, as well as the subsequent emotional reaction. Opioid analgesics affect both transmission of nociceptive information and its perception and also modify the reactive component of the experience. Transmission of nociceptive stimuli along ascending spinothalamic pathways is reduced when μ- and κ-opioid receptors on presynaptic and postsynaptic neurons in the spinal cord and brain are activated. Opioids also inhibit ascending pathways indirectly by activating descending pain-inhibitory pathways. The overall effect is an elevation of the pain threshold, which is the minimum intensity at which a stimulus is perceived as painful.

Pathological pain elicits emotional responses that include anxiety, fear, and a general state of suffering, which are accompanied by changes in autonomic and endocrine functions. Opioid analgesics blunt these emotional effects, probably by actions on receptors in the limbic system. The ability to tolerate pain increases as emotional effects are blunted, even in the absence of large changes in pain threshold. Thus, the emotional reaction to pain may be reduced even when pain perception remains unaltered. Opioids are unique among analgesics in this regard.

Analgesia In general, all morphine-like drugs are equally effective in alleviating pain except for codeine, propoxyphene, and tramadol, which are less effective. A particular drug is often chosen based on its speed of onset, duration of action, and oral bioavailability. Fentanyl and its derivatives, with rapid onsets and short durations of action, are used almost exclusively IV in anesthesiology to manage pain during and immediately after surgery (see Chapter 28). Virtually all opioids exert their analgesic effects through μ-receptors in brain and spinal cord. Tramadol is an exception, being a racemic mixture with enantiomers having complementary actions. The *d*-isomer is a μ-receptor agonist (especially its metabolite) and inhibits the neuronal reuptake of 5-HT, whereas the *l*-isomer inhibits norepinephrine reuptake.

Opioid analgesics are most effective in the management of dull, diffuse, continuous pain, with adequate doses relieving even sharp, localized, intermittent pain. A standard dose produces satisfactory relief in about 90% of patients with mild-to-moderate postoperative pain and in 65% to 70% of patients with moderate-to-severe postoperative pain. The degree of relief may decline after several days or more of frequent administration, as tolerance develops. Within limits, tolerance is overcome by increasing the dose and restoring the analgesic response. The pain relief conferred by opioids is often accompanied by drowsiness, mental clouding, and an elevated mood (i.e., euphoria). Although the euphoria is associated with a potential for abuse, in pain patients it is more likely to be a secondary consequence of pain relief.

Codeine and propoxyphene by themselves are not suitable for treating severe pain. To increase their effectiveness, they (and other opioids) are sometimes administered in combination with a non-opioid antipyretic analgesic, especially aspirin or acetaminophen. Because the sites and mechanisms of action of opioid and antipyretic analgesics differ, the combination usually results in a greater analgesic effect than that achieved with maximally effective doses of either drug alone.

Several newer delivery systems for opioids are now available. A fentanyl transdermal patch is used to treat patients with chronic pain, and fentanyl administered intranasally is used to relieve acute pain. Some morphine-like opioids, especially morphine and fentanyl, are administered intrathecally and epidurally to control pain during and after surgery and to treat otherwise intractable pain. Patient-controlled analgesia allows patients to deliver opioids on demand within preset limits by activating a microprocessor-controlled pump that delivers a bolus dose through an IV or epidural catheter. Because patients can self-medicate whenever the need arises, the quality of pain control is usually better than that provided by doses administered at predetermined intervals. When high drug concentrations need to be maintained over long periods, as in certain chronic pain syndromes and in pain associated with cancer and other terminal illnesses, there are sustained-release oral formulations of morphine and oxycodone.

Cough suppression The sites of cough-suppressant (**antitussive**) action are areas in the brainstem that mediate the cough reflex. Codeine and hydrocodone are opioids commonly used for cough suppression. **Dextromethorphan** is a widely used antitussive found in many over-the-counter medications; it is the *d*-isomer of the opioid agonist levomethorphan. Dextromethorphan has negligible affinity for opioid receptors and does not produce analgesia. Its antitussive effect appears to be mediated by other mechanisms in the brainstem.

Antidiarrheal effect Morphine-like drugs also are used for symptomatic treatment of diarrhea because they have prominent effects on GI motility. Morphine delays gastric emptying and causes spasmodic increases in intestinal smooth muscle tone, decreasing propulsive movements and allowing more time for water resorption. Morphine also reduces intestinal secretions, drying and solidifying the stool, and increases anal sphincter tone. These effects are mediated largely by μ-receptors located on nerve plexuses in GI smooth muscle. Since they produce their constipating and antidiarrheal effects locally, loperamide and diphenoxylate are used exclusively to treat diarrhea. These drugs produce few side effects and have little potential for abuse because they do not enter the CNS readily.

Partial-agonist opioids are characterized by intermediate to high affinity for μ-opioid receptors but lower efficacy for μ-receptor activation as compared with morphine. Therefore, under appropriate conditions, they can antagonize the effects of higher-efficacy μ-opioid agonists. **Mixed-action** opioids also bind to κ-receptors, which mediate at least some of their effects. Both groups of drugs are usually as efficacious as morphine in relieving pain of moderate intensity but may be less effective when pain is severe.

The pure **opioid antagonists** bind with high affinity and selectivity to opioid receptors but lack intrinsic activity and do not activate the receptors. Naloxone, the prototype (see Figure 31-4), is used clinically chiefly to reverse the respiratory depressant effect of opioid agonists. Administered IV, naloxone rapidly restores normal respiration and reverses virtually all effects of the agonist. If naloxone is administered before or along with an agonist, the effects of the agonist are blocked. Naloxone must be re-administered periodically because of its short half-life. Its affinity for μ-receptors is significantly greater than its affinity for κ- or δ-receptors. Therefore, higher doses are required to reverse the effects of mixed-action opioids (mediated at κ-receptors).

Naloxone and other antagonists can precipitate a full-blown withdrawal syndrome in people who are physically dependent on an opioid (Chapter 32). If there is a possibility of physical dependence in an overdosed patient, it is recommended that he or she be started on a low dose of naloxone. The dose can be increased gradually to reverse respiratory depression and restore consciousness while minimizing withdrawal intensity.

Naloxone is a specific opioid antagonist and is of little value in treating overdoses of drugs that do not act at opioid receptors. In addition, it will not exacerbate effects of non-opioids, and its pharmacological specificity can be useful in differential diagnosis of comatose patients.

Naltrexone has the same pharmacological characteristics as naloxone but has a longer duration of action and superior oral bioavailability. High doses taken orally produce prolonged blockade of opioid receptors, an effect used to advantage in therapy of some abusers. Naltrexone and nalmefene are also approved adjuncts in treatment of alcoholism (see Chapter 25). They are thought to work by blocking the role of endogenous opioids in alcohol craving.

NSAIDs and acetaminophen

Although selecting a drug to relieve pain or fever is relatively simple, choosing a drug to treat one of the several arthritic disorders is more complex. Selection is based on the patient's response over time and considerations such as duration of action and cost. Adequate symptom relief must be balanced with untoward side effects, both of which are variable, even with the same drug. Combinations of two or more NSAIDs, or of NSAIDs and acetaminophen, are available for treating pain, but their use is rarely justified. Since antipyretic analgesics have similar mechanisms of action, the maximum effect of a drug combination is unlikely to be greater than the effect of an optimal dose of a single drug.

Analgesia Aspirin, the prototype NSAID, remains one of the most commonly used and effective agents for treating headache and mild-to-moderate pain arising from muscles, tendons, joints, and soma. A dose of 650 to 1000 mg produces acceptable relief in 60% to 80% of patients. Aspirin is far less effective in providing relief of severe pain and pain from visceral organs, which usually require an opioid. However, unlike the opioids, aspirin and other NSAIDs do not cause analgesic tolerance or physical dependence and are not abused. Some of the major differences between aspirin and morphine, the prototype opioid analgesic, are listed in Table 31-5.

Other NSAIDs have analgesic effects similar to those of aspirin. Ibuprofen and naproxen, which are available over-the-counter, have become popular alternatives and might be slightly more effective in treating dysmenorrhea. Ketorolac most often is used to treat postoperative pain because it can be administered parenterally. It was originally thought to be as effective as morphine in relieving severe postoperative pain, but subsequent experience has shown that its analgesic efficacy is comparable with other NSAIDs. Selective COX-2 inhibitors are approved for the treatment of acute pain in adults and primary dysmenorrhea. Their greatest value appears to be in relieving pain secondary to chronic inflammatory conditions, such as osteoarthritis and rheumatoid arthritis.

Table 31-5 Comparison of analgesic effects of morphine and aspirin

Parameter	Morphine	Aspirin
Type of pain relieved	Visceral, somatic	Somatic
Intensity of pain relieved	Moderate to severe	Mild to moderate
Site of action	CNS	Local
Tolerance development	Yes	No
Physical dependence development	Yes	No
Abuse potential	High	None

Acetaminophen is also a popular alternative to aspirin for treating pain, especially by patients who are discomforted by aspirin's side effects. It is has analgesic potency and efficacy similar to aspirin. However, because it has little antiinflammatory activity, it may be less effective in treating pain secondary to inflammation. The mechanism of the analgesic effect of acetaminophen has been something of a mystery. It shares analgesic and antipyretic activity with the NSAIDs but lacks other actions associated with inhibition of COX. It is possible that its analgesic effect, like its antipyretic effect, is mediated via an action on the CNS. Interestingly, COX-3, a splice variant of COX-1, was recently discovered in brain and spinal cord and is weakly inhibited by acetaminophen. This finding raises the possibility that acetaminophen acts through another, as-yet-unknown variant or isoform of COX.

Antipyresis The current approach to fever is to treat it only if it is debilitating and lowering the elevated temperature will make the patient feel better. The NSAIDs and acetaminophen are antipyretic at the same doses that produce analgesia. By lowering the hypothalamic thermoregulatory set-point, they promote autonomic reflexes that cause loss of body heat, notably peripheral vasodilation and sweating. However, they are effective only in instances where elevated body temperature is due to the increased synthesis of PGs such as in infectious disease and autoimmune disorders.

Although a causal relationship has yet to be established, there is a significant epidemiological relationship between the use of aspirin in children with certain viral infections (e.g., influenza, chickenpox) and the occurrence of Reye's syndrome. It is not known if similar relationships exist for other NSAIDs. Because of these uncertainties, acetaminophen has become the drug of choice for treating fever in children.

Antiinflammation The term *arthritis* encompasses dozens of conditions affecting body joints and connective tissue that afflict 10% to 15% of the population. Osteoarthritis, the most common arthritic disorder, affects at least 20 million Americans, and rheumatoid arthritis, an autoimmune disorder, 2 million more. The doses of NSAIDs needed to treat these and other inflammatory disorders often are higher than analgesic doses. Because many inflammatory disorders are chronic, drug selection is influenced by side effects and cost. For example, aspirin has a long and successful history of treating rheumatoid arthritis. However, many patients cannot tolerate the GI or other side effects of daily doses as high as 4 to 6 grams. The range and incidence of side effects with high daily doses of other NSAIDs that inhibit both COX-1 and COX-2 are more-or-less similar to those of aspirin. Nevertheless, the severity of side effects as well as the adequacy of the therapeutic effect varies, and one NSAID may be preferred over another. Selective COX-2 inhibitors are as effective as the older NSAIDs in treating inflammatory disorders but have a lower incidence of side effects, notably GI, associated with chronic administration.

Inhibition of platelet aggregation Low doses of aspirin are used prophylactically by patients at high risk for serious vascular events, such as myocardial infarction or stroke (see Chapter 19).

Antitumor NSAIDs including aspirin, celecoxib, and sulindac have been found to lower the risk for and/or the extent of colorectal cancer in patients with a familial history of adenomatous polyps or who have been previously treated for colorectal cancer.

Drugs for neuropathic pain

Neuropathic pain syndromes are caused by many factors, some yet to be identified, and are difficult to manage. They are largely unresponsive to NSAIDs and only occasionally respond to opioid analgesics. Opioids can be used in responsive patients, although the side effects associated with chronic administration, including tolerance, must be addressed. However, neuropathic pain often can be alleviated by drugs ineffective in treating acute nociceptive pain. Notable among these are antiepileptic drugs and tricyclic antidepressants.

Carbamazepine and gabapentin currently are the antiepileptic drugs used most often to treat neuropathic pain (see Chapter 27). Carbamazepine has well-documented efficacy in the treatment of trigeminal neuralgia and may be beneficial in several other neuropathic pain syndromes. Gabapentin is approved for the treatment of postherpetic neuropathy and appears to reduce pain associated with a variety of syndromes, including phantom-limb pain, Guillain-Barré syndrome, and diabetic neuropathy. Because gabapentin seems to improve measures of mood and quality of life and has a relatively favorable profile of side effects, it is becoming the antiepileptic drug of choice for treating a range of neuropathies. Lamotrigine, a newer antiepileptic drug, also gives evidence of efficacy in several neuropathic pain syndromes (see Chapter 27).

Clinical studies have demonstrated the efficacy of tricyclic antidepressants for pain relief in diabetic and postherpetic neuropathies as well as in several other syndromes. Presumably, the drugs act via descending pain-inhibitory pathways, which contain noradrenergic and serotonergic neurons (see Fig. 31-1). Indeed, tricyclic antidepressants that inhibit reuptake of both norepinephrine and 5-HT (see Chapter 23), such as amitriptyline, appear to be more effective than drugs that selectively block reuptake of only one neurotransmitter. Their analgesic effect is probably independent of their antidepressant effect, since onset of pain relief occurs more rapidly and at lower doses.

Antigout drugs

Colchicine, the oldest gout-specific drug, reduces the inflammation and pain from acute gouty arthritis within 12 hours. It is used in lower doses, sometimes combined with probenecid, to treat chronic gout that is complicated by recurrence of acute attacks.

NSAIDs also provide symptomatic relief from the inflammation and pain of acute gout. Indomethacin is used most often, although ibuprofen, naproxen, sulindac, and piroxicam are also effective. Corticosteroids are efficacious antiinflammatory agents (see Chapter 33), and when used appropriately for short-term treatment of acute gout, are a safe alternative.

Allopurinol, which inhibits production of uric acid, is used in therapy of chronic gout and in hyperuricemias that develop secondary to other treatments, such as chemotherapy or radiation therapy. Uricosuric agents can also provide effective therapy of chronic gout in patients with normal renal function. However, they can exacerbate acute gouty arthritis and should not be administered until the acute attack has abated.

Antimigraine drugs

The frequency of migraine episodes may range from one to two per year to more than one per week and the severity from mild to intense. A migraine usually lasts for several hours but can extend into days. Treatment of acute migraine depends on the characteristics of the headache and the concurrent existence of other medical conditions, such as cardiovascular disease and pregnancy.

NSAIDs are first-line drugs for treating mild-to-moderate migraine if not accompanied by nausea and vomiting and severe migraine in patients whose headaches have responded well to NSAIDs in the past. There is considerable evidence supporting the effectiveness of aspirin, ibuprofen, and naproxen, especially when taken at the first indication of a migraine episode.

Ketorolac is sometimes administered parenterally to abort moderate-to-severe episodes. Acetaminophen by itself is ineffective, but the combination of acetaminophen, aspirin, and caffeine can bring relief to some patients. With the exception of intranasal butorphanol, opioids are not recommended for treating migraine because therapeutic efficacy has not been documented.

Triptans are the drugs of choice for aborting severe migraine or mild-to-moderate migraine that is unresponsive to NSAIDs. All clinically available triptans are, for the most part, equally effective; 60% to 80% of patients experiencing migraine report no headache or only mild headache 2 to 4 hours after taking a maximum dose. However, a patient may respond better to one drug than to another. Because sumatriptan is formulated for intranasal and subcutaneous administration, it is often preferred when nausea and vomiting are prominent components of the migraine episode. The awkwardness of giving oneself a subcutaneous injection, as opposed to swallowing a tablet, is offset by its more rapid onset of action. Advent of the triptans has led to a decline in the use of ergots, which are generally less effective than triptans and take longer to bring relief, especially if they are not taken right at the start of a migraine episode. Dihydroergotamine is the most widely used ergot. Drugs used to abort migraine are not used prophylactically, owing largely to unacceptable side effects with prolonged administration.

Side effects, clinical problems, and toxicity

Opioid analgesics

Respiratory depression This is the most serious side effect of opioid analgesics and is the principal cause of death from overdose. Opioids decrease the sensitivity of chemoreceptors in the brainstem to carbon dioxide, a normal stimulus of ventilatory reflexes. The result is a blunting of the ventilatory response to increases in the carbon dioxide tension (Pco_2) in blood and cerebrospinal fluid (see Fig. 28-9). At equally effective analgesic doses, most opioids, including partial agonists and mixed-acting drugs, produce a similar degree of respiratory depression, as indexed by elevation of blood Pco_2. Depression of respiration increases with increasing dose, but partial agonists and mixed-action opioids produce proportionately smaller changes in respiration than do morphine-like drugs. The respiratory depressant effect of opioids is at least additive, if not super-additive, with that produced by other CNS depressants such as general anesthetics, sedative-hypnotics, and alcohol. Tolerance tends to parallel analgesic tolerance but does not protect against the respiratory depressant effect of non-opioid drugs.

The mild respiratory depression produced by therapeutic doses of opioids is normally of little clinical consequence. However, opioid analgesics must be used cautiously in patients with traumatic head injuries because increased Pco_2 causes cerebral vasodilation, which increases intracranial pressure. Caution must also be exercised when treating patients with a lowered respiratory reserve, such as patients with emphysema or those who are morbidly obese.

Constipation Constipation is a troublesome side effect when opioids are used to treat pain and is made worse by the fact that little or no tolerance develops. Patients treated long-term with opioid analgesics often require laxatives. Mixed-action opioids produce less constipation than morphine-like opioids. By constricting the sphincter of Oddi, opioids may exacerbate the pain of biliary colic and are contraindicated in patients with suspected gallbladder disease.

Nausea Opioid analgesics stimulate the chemoreceptor trigger zone in the area postrema. Nausea, sometimes with vomiting, is a common side effect, particularly of agents administered parenterally. The incidence of vomiting is highest in ambulatory patients, indicating a vestibular component. Tolerance to the emetic effect develops rapidly in many patients.

Endocrine effects Opioids have few significant endocrine effects. Activation of μ-opioid receptors in the hypothalamus inhibits the release of gonadotropin-releasing hormone. This lowers the plasma concentration of luteinizing hormone and testosterone, which can cause menstrual cycle irregularities and male sexual impotence. Activation of μ-receptors inhibits diuresis, whereas activation of κ-receptors increases diuresis by inhibiting the release of antidiuretic hormone.

Miosis Most opioids cause pupillary constriction by stimulating the Edinger-Westphal nucleus of the oculomotor nerve. Constriction of the pupil is used clinically to gauge the adequacy of pain relief. Because miosis is apparent even in a person tolerant to most other drug effects, it is an aid in the diagnosis of overdose. Hypoxia can, however, mask the miotic effect.

Cardiovascular effects The cardiovascular system is relatively unaffected by opioid analgesics. High IV doses of morphine and some related drugs cause a decrease in peripheral resistance and a decline in blood pressure. These effects are rarely clinically significant in supine patients. Some opioids cause a vagally mediated reflex bradycardia, which can be blocked with atropine. Morphine, meperidine, and several other opioids can release histamine from mast cells in peripheral tissues upon IV administration, resulting in transient vasodilation, hypotension, and itching (see Chapter 54). Histamine release is one of the few effects of opioid drugs not mediated by opioid receptors and prevented by naloxone. Pentazocine and butorphanol have mild sympathomimetic effects, causing minor increases in heart rate and blood pressure.

Immunosuppression Animal studies have shown that opioid analgesics suppress the immune system, including natural killer cell activity. Some immunosuppressive effects occur at the level of cells of the immune system, whereas others are mediated centrally and are blocked by opioid antagonists. The mechanisms and clinical significance of immunosuppression remain unclear.

Tolerance Tolerance develops to most effects of the opioids. With repeated drug administration, larger doses are necessary to produce the original response. Tolerance develops rapidly to emetic effects; more gradually to analgesic, endocrine, and respiratory depressant effects; and virtually not at all to constipating and miotic effects. A point may be reached in highly tolerant patients where further dose increases no longer achieve pain relief. Tolerance also develops to the effects of mixed-action opioids, but at a slower rate.

Pharmacologically specific cross-tolerance is observed with the opioids—that is, a person tolerant to the analgesic and respiratory depressant effects of morphine will also be tolerant to those effects of other morphine-like drugs. The extent of cross-tolerance is a function of efficacy. Thus, an opioid with higher efficacy than morphine, such as methadone or fentanyl, may relieve pain that is no longer controlled by morphine or other lower-efficacy drugs. There is no cross-tolerance between opioid and non-opioid drugs.

Physical dependence and abuse Continuous exposure to an opioid analgesic results in development of physical dependence, a state in which the body has adapted to the presence of the drug and requires it for normal function. When administration is terminated or an antagonist is administered, withdrawal symptoms occur as discussed in Chapter 32. The major clinical problems associated with use of opioids are listed in the Clinical Problems box.

CLINICAL PROBLEMS

Opioids

Respiratory depression
Drowsiness
Nausea, vomiting
Constipation*
Endocrine disturbances
Tolerance to analgesic effect
Physical dependence
Abuse potential
Interactions with CNS-depressant drugs

NSAIDs

GI tract disturbances
Renal dysfunction
Prolonged bleeding time*
Hypersensitivity reactions
Salicylism
Interactions with highly plasma-protein-bound drugs

Antigout drugs

GI disturbances
Blood dyscrasias
Dermatological abnormalities
Hypersensitivity reactions

Antimigraine drugs

Cardiovascular disturbances
Chest tightness
Nausea, vomiting
Interactions with MAO-A inhibitors

*Also can be a therapeutic effect.

NSAIDs and acetaminophen

GI effects Epigastric distress is the most common side effect of the NSAIDs and the one most likely to cause a patient to stop taking a drug. It is produced by all nonselective COX inhibitors. Symptoms include nausea, dyspepsia, heartburn, and abdominal discomfort. A single analgesic dose of aspirin can cause occult bleeding, and four doses taken over 24 hours can cause minute lesions of the gastric mucosa. These effects are not clinically significant. However, antiinflammatory doses taken chronically result in peptic ulcers in 15% to 25% of patients and major upper GI events such as ulceration, bleeding, and perforation in 2% to 5% of patients.

The adverse GI side effects are due to two distinct actions. The first, a physical interaction between the drug and the gastric mucosa, can be reduced by taking the medication with meals and with adequate amounts of fluids to facilitate complete dissolution of tablets. The second is due to COX-1 inhibition and the resulting loss of cytoprotective eicosanoids (see Chapter 17). Because they largely spare COX-1, selective COX-2 inhibitors produce a lower incidence of significant upper GI complications than do nonselective NSAIDs.

Acetaminophen produces minimal GI side effects, even with prolonged administration, and is a good alternative for patients who require an analgesic but cannot tolerate the GI effects of NSAIDs. Indeed, acetaminophen produces none of the side effects associated with the NSAIDs. Its primary clinical problem is hepatic dysfunction.

Renal effects Eicosanoids have only a modest role in renal homeostasis under normal physiological conditions—that is, PGE_2 inhibits Na^+ and K^+ resorption, and NSAIDs have little effect on renal function in healthy individuals; transient fluid retention and edema is the most common side effect. However, in patients who have either actual or effective circulatory volume depletion (e.g., congestive heart failure, renal insufficiency), renal perfusion is maintained largely by PGI_2. These patients are at greater risk to develop edema and other NSAID-induced renal side effects such as hyperkalemia, hypertension, interstitial nephritis, and rarely, renal failure. Side effects are for the most part dose-dependent and reversible. The kidney is one of several tissues where COX-2 is expressed constitutively; thus, renal side effects also occur with COX-2-selective NSAIDs.

Cardiovascular effects Aspirin and other nonselective NSAIDs prolong bleeding time by inhibiting COX-1 in platelets, preventing synthesis of thromboxane-A_2. Clinical manifestations of this effect are usually negligible because thromboxane-A_2 is only one of several mediators of platelet aggregation. Upper GI bleeding is the most common spontaneous bleeding event associated with the use of nonselective NSAIDs. However, NSAIDs pose a more serious risk in patients with impaired hemostasis and in those taking other drugs that inhibit clotting. Because nonselective NSAIDs increase the risk of postoperative bleeding and of post-parturition hemorrhage, their use should be avoided prior to surgical procedures and during the peripartum period. Selective COX-2 inhibitors do not inhibit platelet aggregation or prolong bleeding time because COX-2 does not occur in platelets. On the other hand, selective COX-2 inhibitors can increase the incidence of major cardiovascular events (e.g., myocardial infarction) in high-risk patients because they prevent the production of PGI_2, which inhibits platelet aggregation, in vascular epithelial cells, without the benefit of blocking thromboxane-A_2 production in platelets. Indeed, rofecoxib (Vioxx) has been withdrawn from the market for this reason.

CNS effects Aspirin can cause **salicylism,** a syndrome characterized by tinnitus, hearing loss, dizziness, confusion, and even headache. Salicylism is dose-dependent and reversible. It is usually associated with high doses, but sensitive individuals may experience it after a single analgesic dose.

Hypersensitivity Hypersensitivity to aspirin occurs in a small percentage of the population and is manifest by an anaphylactoid reaction that can include rhinitis, urticaria, flushing, hypotension, and bronchial asthma. Middle-aged patients with asthma, nasal polyps, or urticaria are at a higher risk for aspirin hypersensitivity than is the general population. The mechanisms are unknown but may be due to increased levels of lipoxygenase products formed by diversion of arachidonic acid metabolism. Patients with aspirin hypersensitivity also are hypersensitive to other nonselective NSAIDs. Although there is no evidence for hypersensitivity to selective COX-2 inhibitors yet, these drugs are not recommended for use in patients with known NSAID hypersensitivity.

Acute overdose Acute overdose with aspirin or acetaminophen results in effects not seen at therapeutic doses. The syndrome produced by each drug is unique. Among the events in acute aspirin intoxication are ventilatory changes, metabolic acidosis, nausea, vomiting, hyperthermia, and stupor (Table 31-6). Treatment depends upon the severity of intoxication, which can be determined by measuring plasma salicylate levels, and

Table 31-6 Relationship between blood salicylate level and therapeutic and toxic effects

Blood Salicylate Level (μg/ml)	Effect	Consequence
50-100	Analgesia, antipyresis	
150-300	Antiinflammatory	
200-350	Salicylism	Tinnitus, dizziness, nausea
≤350	Hyperventilation	Respiratory alkalosis
450-800	Disrupted carbohydrate metabolism, sweating, vomiting, uncoupled oxidative phosphorylation, depressed respiration, increasing acidosis and body temperature	Metabolic acidosis, dehydration, hyperthermia, respiratory acidosis, delirium, convulsions, coma

is largely supportive: gastric lavage, alkalinizing the urine, cooling the body, and IV fluids containing bicarbonate and glucose. Acute aspirin overdose is a leading cause of accidental poisoning in children.

In high doses, acetaminophen is converted by cytochrome P450 enzymes to hepatotoxic amounts of NAPQI. Symptoms that occur within the first 24 hours of ingestion are relatively nonspecific and include lethargy, nausea, and anorexia. Indicators of abnormal liver function appear gradually over the next few days. These are followed by jaundice, coagulation defects, and other signs of hepatic necrosis and finally hepatic failure. Hepatotoxicity can occur after a single dose of 10 to 15 grams of acetaminophen and after a lower dose under conditions that increase the amount of acetaminophen that undergoes oxidative metabolism. Overdose is treated with *N*-acetylcysteine, which has a sulfhydryl group that attracts NAPQI. Early treatment is essential to prevent or minimize damage.

Antigout drugs

All of the drugs used primarily to treat gout produce side effects that range in severity from discomforting to life-threatening. Mild GI symptoms occur in a small percentage of patients taking probenecid, whereas more severe GI disturbances including nausea and vomiting, abdominal pain, and diarrhea occur in a high percentage of patients taking colchicine. With long-term administration, colchicine can depress bone marrow, resulting in agranulocytosis and aplastic anemia. The most frequent adverse response to allopurinol is a skin rash, which can be severe and is often indicative of a hypersensitivity reaction. Because the kidney is involved in clearing antigout drugs and is a site of action of some, they must be used with caution and are sometimes contraindicated in patients with impaired renal function.

Antimigraine drugs

Triptans cause few side effects when used for acute treatment of migraine. Some side effects appear to be due to the rapid onset of action of subcutaneously injected sumatriptan, including heaviness in the chest and throat and paresthesias of the head, neck, and extremities. Triptans alter vascular tone and can cause arterial vasospasms and hypertension and are contraindicated in patients with ischemic cardiac, cerebrovascular, or peripheral vascular disease or uncontrolled hypertension. Triptans metabolized by MAO-A (all but almotriptan) are contraindicated in patients who are taking MAO-A inhibitors or who have discontinued them within the past 2 weeks. Since liver and kidneys are the main organs involved in clearance, patients with hepatic or renal disease must use these drugs cautiously.

Side effects of ergots are more pervasive. They include nausea and vomiting from stimulation of the chemoreceptor trigger zone, pressure in the chest, numbness of extremities, and tingling of toes and fingers. Like triptans, their use is contraindicated in patients with coronary artery or peripheral vascular disease or uncontrolled hypertension. Ergots are oxytocic and contraindicated in pregnant women. Patients with impaired hepatic or renal function are at heightened risk for toxicity.

New horizons

New agents for managing pain are likely to come from multiple approaches. One is fine-tuning existing classes of analgesic agents to improve therapeutic efficacy and in particular to reduce undesirable side effects. After centuries of use, morphine is still unsurpassed for control of moderate-to-severe pain, but its therapeutic use (and that of other opioids) is limited by undesirable side effects including respiratory depression, tolerance, and abuse potential. Results of studies on animals indicate that activation of δ-opioid receptors can suppress responses to noxious stimuli, with little concomitant effect on respiration. New drugs that target δ-opioid receptors with a suitable bioavailability could prove useful in management of pain, either alone or in combination with a morphine-like opioid. It may also be feasible to use natural opioid peptides for pain control. Peptides are rapidly degraded by proteolysis, and drugs that inhibit enkephalinase activity increase tissue concentrations of these peptides and decrease responses to painful stimuli in animals.

Recently, two additional opioid-related peptide families were discovered. The first, a 17-amino-acid peptide with the cumbersome name nociceptin/orphanin FQ (N/OFQ), has sequence homology to dynorphin A(1-17), although its credentials as a member of the opioid family are uncertain. N/OFQ binds to a separate receptor with the designations NOP or OP_4. Administration of N/OFQ to animals produces either an increase or decrease in reactivity to painful stimuli, depending upon whether it is administered spinally or supraspinally. Its physiological roles in processing of nociceptive signals and the actions of endogenous opioid peptides are unclear.

The second peptide family comprises two tetrapeptides, endomorphin-1 and endomorphin-2. Although opioid in nature, little is known about how they are formed or their functional effects.

The advent of selective COX-2 inhibitors has improved the treatment of chronic inflammatory disorders by minimizing troublesome GI side effects. Further precision in targeting enzymes in the arachidonic acid cascade could yield additional benefits. For example, mutant mice that lack prostaglandin synthase, the enzyme that converts prostaglandin endoperoxide into PGE_2, have increased resistance to experimentally induced inflammation and reduced sensitivity to acute pain that accompanies an inflammatory response.

Improved targeting of receptors not currently associated with the management of pain might also give rise to new compounds. The acetylcholine receptor is a good example. Both nicotinic and muscarinic cholinergic mimetic drugs have centrally mediated antinociceptive effects in animals, but prominent activation of the autonomic nervous system precludes their clinical use as analgesics. However, drugs selective for muscarinic or nicotinic cholinergic receptors that occur only in the CNS are devoid of effects on the autonomic nervous system but retain analgesic activity; some of these drugs are in clinical trials.

TRADE NAMES

In addition to generic and fixed-combination preparations and the drugs listed in the Major Drugs box, the following trade-named materials are some of the important compounds available in the United States.

Opioid agonists

Alfentanil (Alfenta)
Fentanyl (Sublimaze, Duragesic)
Hydrocodone (Hycodan)
Hydromorphone (Dilaudid)
Levorphanol (Levo-Dromoran)
Loperamide (Imodium)
Meperidine (Demerol)
Methadone (Dolophine)
Morphine (MS Contin, Oramorph, Astramorph PF)
Oxycodone (OxyContin, Roxicodone)
Oxymorphone (Numorphan)
Propoxyphene (Darvon)
Remifentanil (Ultiva)
Sufentanil (Sufenta)
Tramadol (Ultram)

Opioid partial agonists and agonist-antagonists

Buprenorphine (Buprenex, Subutex)
Butorphanol (Stadol)
Dezocine (Dalgan)
Nalbuphine (Nubain)
Pentazocine (Talwin)

Opioid antagonists

Nalmefene (Revex)
Naloxone (Narcan)
Naltrexone (ReVia, Depade)

NSAIDs

Celecoxib (Celebrex)
Diclofenac (Voltaren)
Diflunisal (Dolobid)
Etodolac (Lodine)
Fenoprofen (Nalfon)
Flurbiprofen (Ansaid)
Ibuprofen (Advil, Motrin, Nuprin)
Indomethacin (Indocin)
Ketoprofen (Orudis)
Ketorolac (Toradol)
Mefenamic acid (Ponstel)
Meloxicam (Mobic)
Nabumetone (Relafen)
Naproxen (Aleve, Anaprox, Naprosyn)
Oxaprozin (Daypro)
Piroxicam (Feldene)
Sodium salicylate (Uracel)
Sulindac (Clinoril)
Tolmetin (Tolectin)
Valdecoxib (Bextra)

Antigout

Allopurinol (Lopurin, Zyloprim)
Colchicine (Colchicine)
Probenecid (Benemid)
Sulfinpyrazone (Anturane)

Antimigraine

Almotriptan (Axert)
Dihydroergotamine (Migranal)
Ergotamine (Ergomar)
Naratriptan (Amerge)
Rizatriptan (Maxalt)
Sumatriptan (Imitrex)
Zolmitriptan (Zomig)

FURTHER READING

Christoph T, Buschmann H. Cyclooxygenase inhibition: From NSAIDs to selective COX-2 inhibitors. In Buschmann H, Christoph T, Friderichs E, et al, editors. *Analgesics: From Chemistry and Pharmacology to Clinical Application.* Weinheim, Wiley-VCH, 2002.

Dworkin RH et al. Advances in neuropathic pain: Diagnosis, mechanisms, and treatment recommendations. *Arch Neurol* 2003; 60:1524-1534.

Rott KT, Agudelo CA. Gout. *JAMA* 2003; 289:2857-2860.

Snow V et al. Pharmacologic management of acute attacks of migraine and prevention of migraine headache. *Ann Intern Med* 2002; 137:840-849.

Self-assessment questions

1. Naloxone (Narcan):

a. Increases the threshold for pain.
b. Antagonizes respiratory depression induced by barbiturates.
c. Causes constipation.
d. Antagonizes respiratory depression induced by opioid drugs.
e. Has a longer duration of action than morphine.

2. Respiration is depressed by an analgesic dose of:

a. Morphine.
b. Pentazocine (Talwin).
c. Meperidine (Demerol).
d. Methadone.
e. All of the above.

3. Compared with morphine, an opioid with mixed agonist and antagonist properties, such as butorphanol (Stadol):

a. Depresses respiration proportionately less with each dose increment.
b. Relieves severe pain more effectively.
c. Produces greater physical dependence.
d. Produces effects that are more easily reversed by naloxone (Narcan).
e. Does all of the above.

4. A patient who develops tolerance to the analgesic effect of a fixed dose of morphine:

a. Will *not* be equally tolerant to all effects of that dose of morphine.
b. Probably will be tolerant to the analgesic effect of methadone.
c. Probably will be tolerant to the analgesic effect of meperidine (Demerol).
d. Often can be relieved of pain if the dose of morphine is increased.
e. All of the above.

5. Aspirin:

a. Does not change normal body temperature at therapeutic doses.
b. Is the drug of choice for treating fever in children with influenza.
c. Blocks prostaglandin receptors in the hypothalamus.
d. Has all of the above characteristics.
e. Has none of the above characteristics.

6. The combination of aspirin and which of the following drugs is likely to relieve pain better than a maximum analgesic dose of aspirin alone?

a. Acetaminophen
b. Ibuprofen
c. Codeine
d. Naproxen
e. Celecoxib

CHAPTER 32

Drug and substance abuse

John R. Traynor

Major Drugs

TREATMENT OF:

Opioid dependence
Buprenorphine (Subutex)
Buprenorphine + Naloxone (Suboxone)
Levomethadyl Acetate (LAAM, ORLAAM)
Nalmefene (Revex)
Naloxone (Narcan)
Naltrexone (ReVia)
Pentazocine + naloxone (Talwin Nx)

Benzodiazepine dependence
Flumazenil (Mazicon, Romazicon)

Nicotine dependence
Bupropion (Zyban)
Nicotine gum (Nicorette)
Nicotine patch (Habitrol, NicoDerm, Nicotrol, PROSTEP)

Therapeutic overview

Substance abuse is defined as a destructive pattern of drug use leading to significant social, occupational, or medical impairment. Typically, abused substances are categorized according to pharmacological class. However, they may be defined by their use or source. Thus, **club drugs** are taken at rave and trance events and include γ-hydroxybutyrate (GHB), ketamine, flunitrazepam, and methylenedioxymethamphetamine (MDMA). **Prescription drug abuse** involves illicit use of opioids (prescribed for pain), barbiturates and benzodiazepines (prescribed for anxiety and sleep disorders), and stimulants (prescribed for attention deficit disorder and narcolepsy). **Designer drugs** are chemical modifications to currently abused drugs and often become available before they are subject to legal control. These include heroin-like fentanyl derivatives (e.g., "China White") and analogs of the dissociative anesthetic phencyclidine (PCP).

Drug abuse does not require development of dependence on the drug or tolerance to its effects, although these often occur. **Tolerance** refers to a reduced effect with repeated use and a need for higher doses to produce the same effect. Because tolerance does not occur to the same extent for all effects of a single drug, people who take increasing amounts of drug risk an increase in effects for which less tolerance develops. For example, chronic heroin abusers may die from respiratory depression. **Dependence** is characterized by physiological or behavioral changes after discontinuation of drug use, effects that are reversible on resumption of drug administration. **Psychological dependence** is characterized by intense craving and compulsive drug seeking behavior. Abused substances often possess reinforcing effects accompanied by intense euphoria and feelings of well being that foster their continued use. This is particularly true of stimulants such as cocaine and amphetamine. **Physical dependence** is associated with characteristic withdrawal signs when drug taking stops. The **withdrawal syndrome** is similar for drugs within a pharmacological class but differs between classes. Its time course varies according to the rate of elimination of the drugs or their active metabolites.

Abbreviations

CNS	central nervous system
DA	dopamine
GABA	γ-aminobutyric acid
GHB	γ-hydroxybutyrate
5-HT	serotonin
IV	intravenous
LSD	D-lysergic acid diethylamide
MDMA	methylenedioxymethamphetamine
NMDA	*N*-methyl-D-aspartate
PCP	phencyclidine
THC	tetrahydrocannabinol

Withdrawal from long-acting drugs has a delayed onset, is relatively mild, and occurs over many days or weeks (Fig. 32-1, *A*), whereas withdrawal from more rapidly inactivated or eliminated drugs is more intense but of shorter duration (Fig. 32-1, *B*). Typically, physical dependence occurs when substances are used over extended times—usually days, weeks, or months. With repeated use, dependence becomes increasingly severe. Normally, occasional drug use does not result in clinically significant withdrawal. **Spontaneous withdrawal** occurs on cessation of drug taking. **Precipitated withdrawal** occurs when an antagonist is administered to displace the drug from its receptors, causing more rapid and severe effects (Fig. 32-1, *C*). An example is the administration of the opioid antagonist naltrexone to heroin-dependent individuals. The various approaches used in the treatment of drug abuse and addiction are summarized in the Therapeutic Overview box.

Different drugs in the same class often can maintain physical dependence produced by other drugs in the same class, termed **cross-dependence**. Thus, heroin withdrawal can be prevented by administration of other opioids, part of the rationale for the use of methadone in treatment. Alcohol, barbiturates, and benzodiazepines show cross-dependence with each other but not with opioids; thus benzodiazepines are effective in suppressing symptoms of alcohol withdrawal. **Cross-tolerance** is similar to cross-dependence, in that people tolerant to a

THERAPEUTIC OVERVIEW

Pharmacological approaches to opioid dependence and toxicity

Oral, Long-Acting Opioid Agonists
- Detoxification and maintenance therapy

Opioid Antagonists
- Maintenance therapy after detoxification
- Opioid toxicity

Pharmacological approaches to stimulant and hallucinogen toxicity

Antipsychotics for toxic-induced psychoses

Pharmacological approaches to depressant toxicity

Benzodiazepine antagonists

Pharmacological approaches to nicotine dependence

Replacement therapy (nicotine-containing transdermal patches, gum, inhaler, nasal spray)

Antidepressants

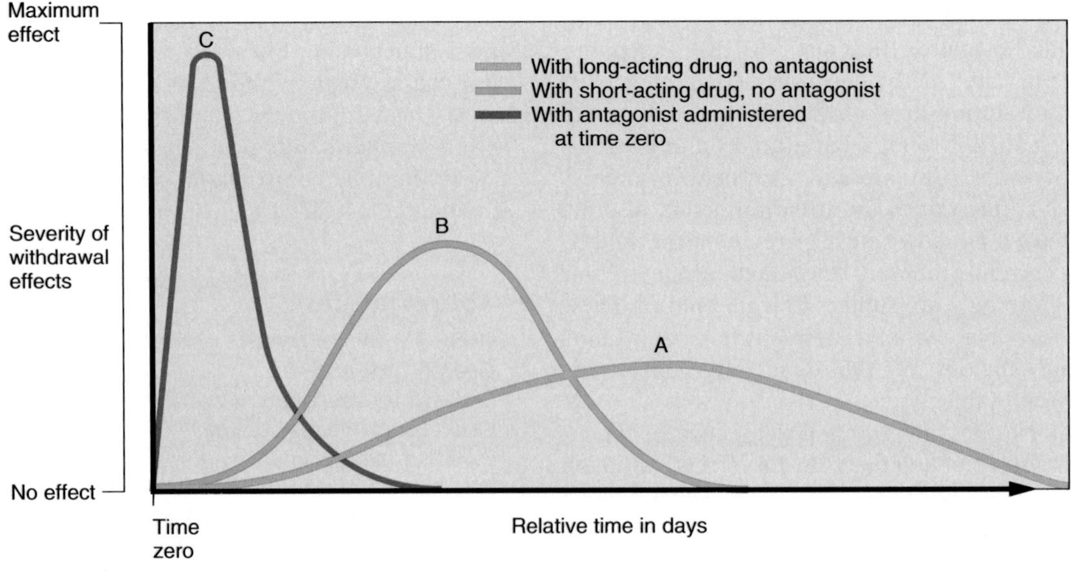

Figure 32-1 The course of severity of withdrawal effects from dependence on drugs with long *(A)* and short *(B)* durations of action or after administration of a specific receptor antagonist *(C)*.

Table 32-1 Most commonly abused substances

Class	Compound
Opiates and opioids	Heroin, morphine, codeine, meperidine, hydromorphone, hydrocodone, oxycodone
Stimulants	Cocaine, amphetamine, methamphetamine, methylphenidate
Depressants	Barbiturates, non-barbiturate sedatives (meprobamate), benzodiazepines, alcohol, GHB
Cannabinoids	Marijuana, hashish
Hallucinogens	LSD, mescaline, MDMA
Dissociative compounds	PCP, ketamine, dextromethorphan
Inhalants	Volatile solvents (e.g. toluene), gases (e.g. nitrous oxide), nitrites (e.g. amyl nitrite)
Anabolic steroids	Testosterone, nandrolone, oxandrolone, oxymetholone, and stanozolol
Nicotine	Nicotine

drug in one class will usually be tolerant to other drugs in the same class but not to drugs in other classes.

Problems associated with drug abuse include treatment of acute overdose and withdrawal, as well as consequent medical conditions. Although primary caregivers provide diagnoses, referral and short-term treatment, long-term treatment of substance abuse is increasingly the province of specialized, multidisciplinary programs that use several strategies. **Maintenance therapy** involves use of a drug such as methadone to continue opioid dependence, while psychological, social and vocational therapies are used to help deal with craving. **Detoxification** is used to treat physical dependence and consists of abruptly or gradually reducing drug doses.

The major compounds used for treatment of drug dependence are listed in the Major Drugs box. The major drugs and substances that are abused, grouped by pharmacological class, are listed in Table 32-1.

Mechanisms of action

Opioids and opiates

Opiates are compounds isolated from the opium poppy that act at opioid receptors, whereas opioids are any synthetic or natural compounds that interact with opioid receptors; however, these terms are often used interchangeably. The effects of abused opioids, including their reinforcing actions, are mediated by μ-opioid receptors in the central nervous system (CNS), particularly in brain areas concerned with antinociception and reward (see Chapter 31). The two principal naturally occurring opiates are morphine and codeine; morphine is chemically converted into heroin (3,6-diacetylmorphine), the most commonly abused opioid (Fig. 32-2). Other synthetic opioids are widely available and abused, often as diverted prescription medications. Heroin ("H" or "smack") is about 3 times more potent than morphine, but the two have very similar effects. In fact, heroin is metabolized to 6-acetylmorphine and morphine to exert its effects. Codeine is also demethylated to the more potent morphine by cytochrome P450 enzymes (see Chapter 3). The isoform involved is genetically polymorphic, and persons with mutated forms are unresponsive to codeine.

The biological mechanisms underlying physical dependence on opioids are poorly understood. The most consistent indication of dependence is the increased sensitivity to precipitated withdrawal by administration of an opioid antagonist. This may begin with the first opioid dose, because under laboratory conditions, high doses of an antagonist can precipitate a withdrawal syndrome within a few hours after a single dose of morphine.

Stimulants

The stimulant drugs are sympathomimetic amines that act on the CNS by enhancing norepinephrine and dopamine (DA) neurotransmission. Cocaine ("coke," "snow," "blow," or "crack" for the free base; Fig. 32-2) is the active ingredient of the South American coca bush. Amphetamines are structurally related to catecholamine neurotransmitters and ephedrine (see Chapter 10) and include amphetamine, *N*-methylamphetamine (methamphetamine known as "speed," "meth," or "ice"), and others such as methylphenidate.

Reinforcing effects of stimulants arise from enhanced neurotransmission at dopaminergic synapses in the ascending mesolimbic and mesocortical pathways (Fig. 32-3). Cocaine binds to DA transporters and blocks reuptake of DA, increasing its synaptic concentration. Amphetamines also act on DA transporters to enhance DA release and may increase its concentrations by inhibiting destruction by monoamine oxidase. Amphetamines may also directly activate postsynaptic receptors. The pathways activated by stimulant drugs also have important roles in reinforcement processes for many legitimate activities.

Depressants

CNS depressants such as barbiturates, non-barbiturate sedatives, and benzodiazepines enhance inhibitory

Opioids

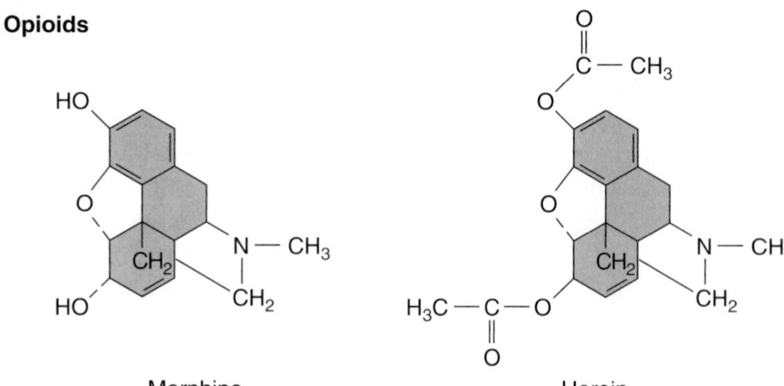

Stimulants

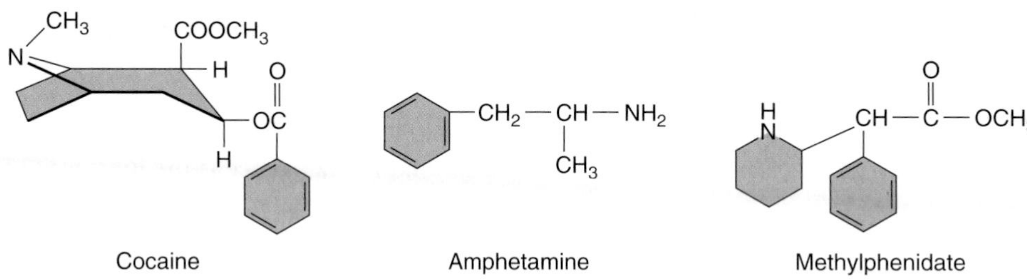

Depressants

D. Cannabinoids

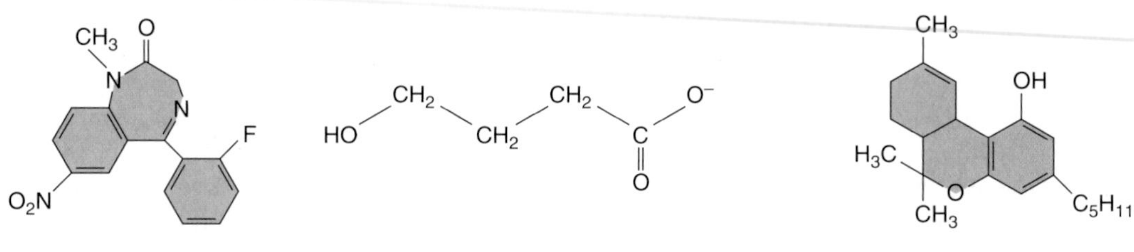

Hallucinogens

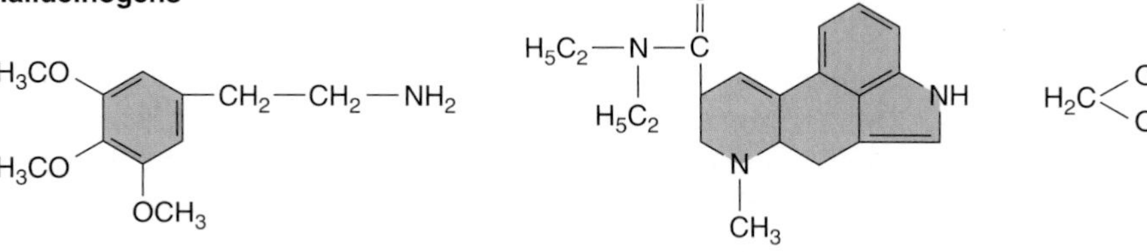

Dissociative compounds

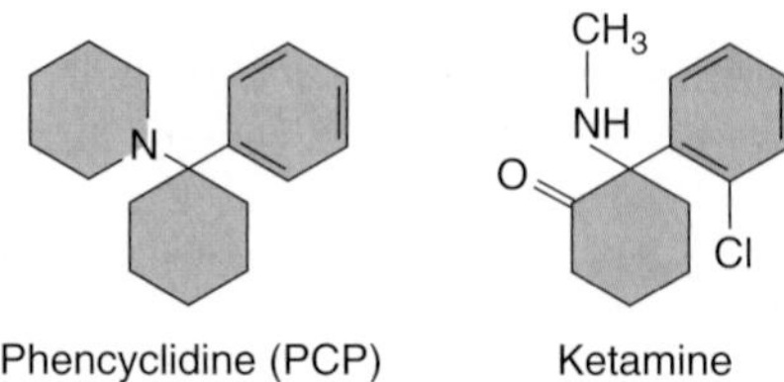

Figure 32-2 Structures of some commonly abused drugs.

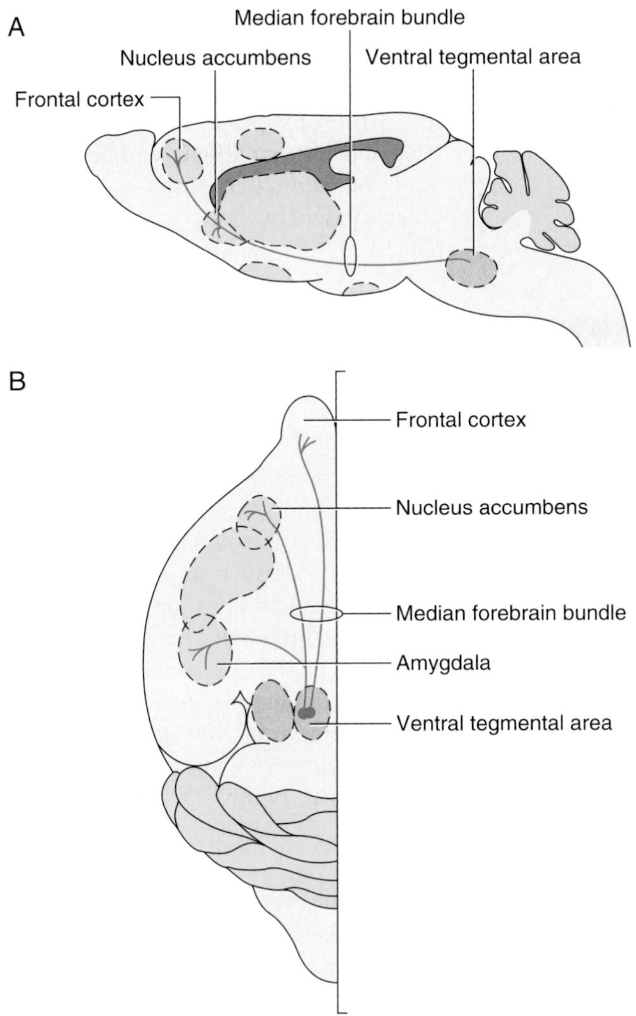

Figure 32-3 Ascending dopaminergic pathways in rat brain believed to mediate the reinforcing effects of cocaine and amphetamines. **A,** Sagittal, or side, view. **B,** Coronal, or top, view.

γ-aminobutyric acid (GABA) transmission (see Chapter 24). A particularly notorious benzodiazepine is flunitrazepam, known as "roofies" or "rophies." An additional drug in this group is GHB (see Fig. 32-2). GHB occurs naturally at low levels in the brain, is a precursor of GABA, and interacts with specific GHB receptors in many brain regions. At high doses, GHB also acts at GABA receptors, either directly or after metabolism to GABA. GHB induces anterograde amnesia, with increased doses causing drowsiness and sleep leading to general anesthesia, coma, respiratory and cardiac depression, seizures, and death. GHB is marketed for the treatment of cataplexy in patients with narcolepsy. Illicit GHB is commonly called "liquid ecstasy," "G," "grievous bodily harm," or "Georgia Home Boy."

A discussion of alcohol and its abuse is in Chapter 25.

Cannabinoids

Marijuana (cannabis) is the dried leaf material, buds, and flowering tops from the common hemp plant *Cannabis sativa*. It has a variety of names including "pot," "weed," "grass," and "maryjane"; hashish is the dried resinous material exuded by mature plants. Cannabis is the most commonly abused illegal drug in the U.S. Its major active chemical is Δ^9-tetrahydrocannabinol (Δ^9-THC; Fig. 32-2). Δ^9-THC and related molecules are termed cannabinoids and exert effects by binding to specific CB_1 and CB_2 cannabinoid G protein coupled receptors (see Chapter 2). CB_1 receptors are expressed in the brain and CB_2 receptors in the periphery and immune system. CB_1 receptors are responsible for the psychoactive properties of marijuana and are found in high levels in the cerebellum (coordination of movement), cerebral cortex (cognitive functions), hippocampus (learning and memory), nucleus accumbens (rewarding effects), and basal ganglia (control of movement). The endogenous ligand is anandamide, a long-chain arachidonic acid derivative.

Cannabinoids are effective antiemetics and appetite stimulants and have some analgesic actions. Synthetic Δ^9-THC (dronabinol) is approved for treatment of anorexia associated with weight loss in AIDS patients and to treat emesis caused by cancer chemotherapy in patients who do not respond to conventional antiemetics. Many also argue for use of smoked marijuana in treating chronic pain, improving appetite in AIDS patients, and suppressing spasticity in multiple sclerosis and spinal injury.

Hallucinogens

Hallucinogens produce changes in sensory perception such that colors, sounds, and smells are intensified, and they also produce changes in mood and thought. They are therefore called **psychedelic** or **psychotomimetic.** They have no recognized medical uses. Abused hallucinogens fall into two chemical classes, the substituted phenethylamines and the indoleamines. Mescaline is the prototype substituted phenethylamine, and D-lysergic acid diethylamide (LSD) is the prototype indoleamine (see Fig. 32-2). Others include psilocybin (from mushrooms) and dimethyltryptamine. The unique effects of hallucinogens appear to result from modulation of serotonergic neurotransmission, in particular activation of serotonin 5-HT_2 receptors. Serotonin (5-HT) is a major neurotransmitter involved in regulation of mood, sleep, pain, emotion, and appetite. 5-HT_2 receptors in the cerebral cortex—a region involved in mood, cognition, and perception—and in the locus coeruleus, an area concerned with response to external stimuli, are probably involved. The drugs also have sympathomimetic effects, producing tachycardia and increased blood pressure, probably because of enhanced catecholaminergic neurotransmission.

MDMA ("ecstasy" or "XTC") is a substituted amphetamine (see Fig. 32-2) and has properties of both a hallucinogen and a stimulant. MDMA acts to increase release of DA and particularly 5-HT. Methylenedioxyamphetamine is a related compound.

Dissociative compounds

PCP ("angel dust") and ketamine ("K" or "special K") were originally developed as anesthetics (see Fig. 32-2). Ketamine is still used for changing burn dressings, for anesthesia in children, and for short-duration anesthesia in veterinary medicine (see Chapter 28). PCP is not used therapeutically because of the severity of emergence delirium in patients. Ketamine and PCP produce a "dissociative" anesthesia—that is, amnesia and profound analgesia although the patient is not asleep and respiration and blood pressure are unaltered. This is different from anesthesia produced by inhalation and intravenous (IV) anesthetics (see Chapter 28). Dextromethorphan ("DXM" or "robo") is an over-the-counter cough suppressant (see Chapter 31) and when taken in high doses, produces effects similar to those of PCP and ketamine. PCP, ketamine, and high-dose dextromethorphan act by inhibiting NMDA glutamate receptors (see Chapter 2).

Inhalants

Inhalants comprise:

- Volatile solvents and aerosols
- Gases, including nitrous oxide
- Aliphatic nitrites

Inhalants other than nitrites produce their effects in the same way as alcohol; they are CNS depressants, producing initial excitation, disinhibition, lightheadedness, and agitation. In sufficient amounts, they can produce anesthesia. Nitrites (e.g., amyl nitrite in ampules known as "poppers" or "snappers") are abused for their vasodilating properties.

Anabolic steroids

Anabolic steroids are synthetic substances related to androgens, male sex hormones. They promote growth of male sexual characteristics and have important clinical uses (see Chapter 36). However, steroid abuse is widespread in body-building and sports for enhancement of skeletal muscle growth. Abused steroids include testosterone itself as well as synthetic compounds such as nandrolone, oxandrolone, oxymetholone, and stanozolol.

Nicotine

Nicotine acts primarily through stimulation of CNS nicotinic cholinergic receptors to release DA from the nucleus accumbens. At levels produced by smoking tobacco, nicotine also acts at sympathetic and parasympathetic ganglia and the adrenal medulla to produce effects on the cardiovascular and gastrointestinal systems (see Chapter 9).

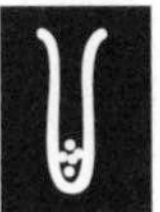

Pharmacokinetics

Abused substances represent many compounds whose pharmacokinetics depend on their structures and methods of use. A rapid effect is sought by opioid and stimulant abusers, and methods such as smoking or IV injection are preferred. Smoking allows the drug to pass rapidly from the lungs into the blood and brain. This is not true for slower-acting depressants such as alcohol or GHB or longer-lasting compounds such as LSD. The difference in degree of euphoria and the length of stimulant action for cocaine given by different routes of administration is shown in Figure 32-4.

Opioids

Heroin and morphine have poor oral bioavailability because of first-pass metabolism in the liver, although this is not true for codeine (see Chapter 31). Heroin is usually snorted, smoked ("chasing the dragon"), or injected and provides a rapid feeling of euphoria in 7 to 8 seconds when taken IV or 10 to 15 minutes when snorted or smoked. Its effects last about 4 to 6 hours, depending on dose. This very rapid euphoria makes it so addictive.

Stimulants

Pure cocaine is used as a water-soluble salt or as a free base. Cocaine salt is a bitter-tasting, white, crystalline material that is generally snorted or injected IV. Crack (free base cocaine), sold as small hard pieces or "rocks," is volatilized and inhaled. It is rapidly absorbed and provides an almost instantaneous action. IV cocaine takes a few seconds to take effect, while snorted cocaine takes 5 to 10 minutes but lasts longer. Oral cocaine is slowly absorbed (see Fig. 32-4) and produces a less-intense effect. The effect of IV or inhaled cocaine generally lasts only 30 minutes, and re-dosing is common in an attempt to maintain intoxication. Cocaine is rapidly metabolized by blood and liver esterases, with urinary metabolites found for up to a week after use. Some *N*-demethylation occurs in the liver, with metabolites

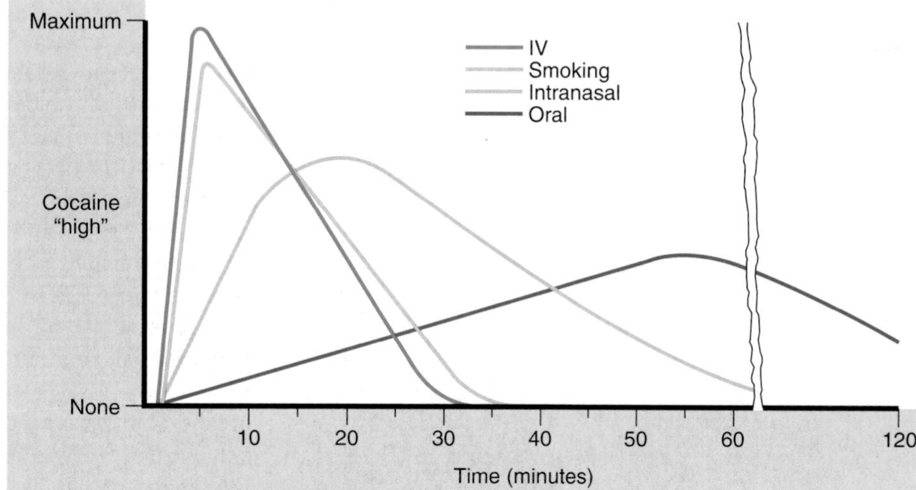

Figure 32-4 The intensity and time course (in minutes) of cocaine intoxication at equivalent doses by different routes of administration.

excreted in urine. Measurement of urinary cocaine metabolites is an important basis for establishing recent usage.

Amphetamines and similar stimulants such as methylphenidate are usually taken orally but may be snorted. Oral methamphetamine produces effects within 15 to 20 minutes but within 3 to 5 minutes when snorted. Effects last for several hours. A smokable form of methamphetamine ("ice") is used in a manner similar to crack cocaine and is an increasing problem.

Depressants

CNS depressants are taken orally, with rapid-acting barbiturates such as secobarbital and pentobarbital more widely abused than those with a slower onset such as phenobarbital and benzodiazepines. The pharmacokinetics of the benzodiazepines are discussed in Chapter 24. GHB is rapidly absorbed and readily penetrates the CNS, producing effects within 15 to 30 minutes and lasting 2 to 3 hours. Oral flunitrazepam shows effects after 30 minutes and lasting up to 8 hours.

Cannabis

Marijuana and hashish are usually smoked in cigarettes ("joints" or "reefers") or in pipes or "bongs" (water pipes) but are also taken orally. Effects begin almost immediately, peak in 15 to 30 minutes, and last for 1 to 3 hours. If taken orally, lower blood levels of Δ^9-THC are obtained because of a combination of extensive first-pass metabolism (which forms an active metabolite, 11-OH-Δ^9-THC, as well as inactive metabolites) and high lipid solubility. When ingested orally, effects begin in 1 hour and last up to 4 hours. Because of their high lipophilicity, cannabinoids remain in the body for weeks and accumulate with repeated use. Therefore it is not possible to determine recent use of cannabinoids based on urinary concentrations.

Hallucinogens

LSD is usually taken orally as capsules, tablets, or on small paper squares but can also be injected or smoked. Effects begin in 30 to 90 minutes and last up to 12 hours. MDMA is usually taken orally. Effects last up to 6 hours, but more drug is often taken when effects start to fade.

Dissociative compounds

For a rapid onset of action, PCP is generally mixed with plants (dried parsley, tobacco, or marijuana) and smoked but may also be snorted. However, effects of oral PCP occur within minutes and last for several hours. Ketamine has a shorter duration of action (30-60 minutes). For illicit use, injectable ketamine (often diverted from veterinarian's offices) is dried, powdered, and snorted or converted into pills. Dextromethorphan is taken orally in cough suppressant preparations at 6 to 10 times the antitussive dose.

Inhalants

Inhalants are sniffed or snorted from containers or bags into which aerosols have been sprayed, are sprayed directly into the nose or mouth, or are inhaled from balloons as gases. They are quickly absorbed, producing intoxication within minutes. However, effects last only a few minutes, and repeated administration is needed for a prolonged high. Nitrous oxide produces a short-lived intoxication similar to early stages of anesthesia.

Anabolic steroids

Anabolic steroids are taken orally, applied to the skin in gel formulations, or administered by intramuscular injections. Their pharmacokinetics are discussed in Chapter 36.

Nicotine

Nicotine is absorbed from the lungs in cigarette smoke and is readily absorbed through the mouth if tobacco is chewed. Greater than 90% of nicotine in lungs passes into blood. It is widely distributed and rapidly metabolized to inactive products. Serious smokers maintain nicotine in the body day and night.

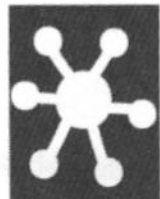

Side effects, clinical problems, and toxicity

Problems associated with drug abuse are summarized in the Clinical Problems box.

CLINICAL PROBLEMS

Societal

Loss of productivity; missed work
Constant drug seeking; criminal activity

Personal

Tolerance; need for increasing drug doses
Dependence; requirement for continuous exposure
Social; development of sociopathies and loss of personal relationships

Medical

Overdoses
Abscesses at injection sites, thrombophlebitis
Pregnancy complications and babies born dependent
Possibilities for subsequent infections:
- HIV
- Bacterial endocarditis
- Hepatitis and hepatic dysfunction
- Tuberculosis
- Pneumonia
- Septic pulmonary embolism
- Tetanus

Opioids

Opioids are widely abused and represent serious consequences for the users, their families, and the community. Abused opioids are listed in Table 32-1. The administration of heroin IV causes a surge of intense euphoria, a "rush" accompanied by a warming of the skin, dry mouth, and heavy feelings in arms and legs. The rush subsides after a few minutes, and the user feels relaxed, carefree, and somewhat dreamy but able to carry on many normal activities. Users who are not physically dependent recover readily. Unlike a person intoxicated with alcohol or other CNS depressants, opiate abusers are difficult to detect by observable behaviors.

Overdose leads to unconsciousness, respiratory depression, and extreme miosis, although the latter is not always apparent because asphyxia can result in pupillary dilation. Deaths are due to respiratory failure. IV injection of an opiate antagonist, such as naloxone or nalmefene, can reverse all effects immediately and produce rapid recovery. However, it is important not to administer too large a dose, since severe withdrawal could be precipitated in a physically dependent patient. The duration of action of naloxone is shorter than that of opioid agonists, and patients should be observed to ensure severe intoxication does not re-emerge. Nalmefene has a longer duration of action.

Heroin users often begin by smoking, but many eventually progress to IV injection because of the increased rapidity of effect. This leads to many medical problems. Particularly dangerous is sharing of needles and other injection paraphernalia, which dramatically increases blood-borne infections, including human immunodeficiency virus (HIV) and hepatitis. Street heroin is not pure but is "cut" with several compounds including sugar, starch, powdered milk, quinine, and strychnine, which causes convulsions. These substances are also dangerous because they can block small arteries to vital organs. Long-term effects of IV heroin use include collapsed veins, infection of heart linings and valves, abscesses, and pulmonary complications.

Most abusers only gradually become physically dependent. Some take opiates for years at intervals insufficient to produce dependence. Initial users are generally confident that they can control their use and only dimly aware of their gradual dependence. Taking multiple daily doses of heroin or other opioids usually results in significant dependence within a few weeks.

The significance of physical dependence is in the inexorable appearance of the withdrawal syndrome, beginning about 6 hours after the last heroin injection. Many signs and symptoms are opposite to the effects of acute administration. In withdrawal, the positive reinforcing effects are amplified by instant alleviation of withdrawal sickness. Many dependent abusers are tolerant to the positive reinforcing effects, and continued drug use provides only relief from withdrawal. If a person is not treated, withdrawal reaches peak severity in about 24 hours and ceases in 7 to 10 days. This rarely constitutes a medical emergency and is considerably **less dangerous** than withdrawal from alcohol or barbiturates.

Opioids cross the placental barrier, and a newborn of an opioid-dependent mother will undergo withdrawal within 6 to 12 hours of birth. The long-term consequences of prenatal opioid dependence are poorly understood, but it may be best to maintain the mother on methadone and treat the infant with opioids rather than withdraw the mother before parturition. Otherwise, she may leave treatment and resume opioid abuse without adequate prenatal care.

Cross-dependence occurs among all full opioid agonists. Hydromorphone, meperidine, oxycodone, and others can reverse withdrawal and at appropriate doses can produce a heroin-like intoxication in addicts. Less-efficacious agonists such as codeine and dextropropoxyphene also show cross-dependence. A major problem is that heroin abusers often exhibit convincing symptoms that require prescription of analgesics, which are then used to treat withdrawal.

Mixed opioid agonist-antagonists and partial agonists such as pentazocine, butorphanol, nalbuphine, and buprenorphine (see Chapter 31) are less abused than full agonists, although each has a slightly different profile. Except for buprenorphine, they show little cross-dependence with heroin and can exacerbate withdrawal; thus they offer little attraction for addicts.

Stimulants

IV administration or inhalation of cocaine produces a rapid-onset rush with intense positive reinforcing effects. Cocaine and other stimulants produce increased alertness, feelings of elation and well-being, increased energy, feelings of competence, and increased sexuality. Athletic performance has been reported to be enhanced in athletes who use stimulants, particularly in sports requiring sustained attention and endurance. Although these effects are small, they provide a significant advantage. Thus, all sympathomimetic drugs, including over-the-counter medications such as pseudoephedrine, are banned by most athletic associations.

Stimulant overdose results in excessive activation of the sympathetic nervous system. The resulting tachycardia and hypertension may result in myocardial infarction and stroke. Cocaine can cause coronary vasospasm and cardiac dysrhythmias. CNS symptoms in cocaine users include anxiety, feelings of paranoia and impending doom, and restlessness. Users exhibit unpredictable behavior and sometimes become violent. Adrenergic receptor-blocking drugs alleviate some of these symptoms, although they are often ineffective.

An important component of stimulant intoxication is the "crash" that occurs as drug effects subside. Dysphoria, tiredness, irritability, and mild depression often occur within hours after stimulant ingestion. Abuse of cocaine by snorting may lead to irritation of the nasal mucosa, sinusitis, and a perforated septum. Cocaine salts are often cut with inert substances, with other local anesthetics similar in appearance and taste, or with other stimulants. IV administration of stimulants is associated with the same problems as IV heroin.

A dangerous pattern of stimulant abuse is the extended, uninterrupted sequences referred to as "runs." Runs result from attempts to maintain a continuous state of intoxication, to extend the pleasurable feeling, and to postpone the postintoxication crash. Acute tolerance can occur, particularly in those taking the substance IV, resulting in a need for increasingly larger doses. This spiral of tolerance and increased dose is often continued until drug supplies are depleted or the person collapses from exhaustion. During runs, drug taking and drug-seeking behavior take on a compulsive character, making treatment intervention difficult.

Another typical abuse pattern begins with self-medication. Stimulants are used by some people to achieve sustained attention (long distance truckers or students) or to make tasks appear easier (housework). These patterns lead to increased doses and frequency of use, producing tolerance, and further dose increases. Alcohol or depressant drugs are frequently used to counteract the resultant anxiety and insomnia, establishing a cycle of "uppers and downers."

Dependence on stimulants is characterized principally by uncontrolled compulsive episodes of use, a phenomenon referred to as **psychological dependence.** Various sequences of mood and behavior changes have been observed after cessation of use. The most notable are fatigue and depression, which often result in drug craving and relapse. Sleep disturbances, hyperphagia, and brain abnormalities have also been noted. These psychological sequelae are important in fostering continued abuse and are important treatment targets.

Personality changes often occur in stimulant abusers and include delusions, preoccupation with self, hostility, and paranoia. A toxic psychosis can develop. Often difficult to distinguish from paranoid schizophrenia, severe amphetamine and cocaine psychoses require psychiatric management. Antipsychotic medication can be useful (see Chapter 22).

Cocaine use during pregnancy may be associated with complications including abruptio placentae, premature birth, lower birth weight, and neurobehavioral impairment of the newborn.

Depressants

Dose-response curves for abused CNS depressant drugs are essentially the same as those for ethanol, except that they usually have shallower slopes. If one considers that blood ethanol concentrations of 0.1% are 25% the lethal concentration (see Chapter 25), the therapeutic index for alcohol would be among the poorest of any legal drug. In contrast, gram quantities of benzodiazepines may not be lethal, resulting in much larger therapeutic indices. Like ethanol, barbiturates, non-barbiturate sedatives, and GHB have dose-response curves with slopes much steeper than slopes of dose-response curves for benzodiazepines (Fig. 32-5).

Barbiturates and non-barbiturate sedatives can produce an ethanol-like intoxication and are sometimes abused for this purpose. Flunitrazepam is a highly efficacious, high-potency benzodiazepine that causes sedation, psychomotor impairment, and amnesia. It is tasteless and odorless and has achieved notoriety as a "date rape" drug.

GHB is used for its ability to cause euphoria, relaxation, and lack of inhibition. Like flunitrazepam, it has been used as a "date-rape" drug because of its short-lived hypnotic effects. It is also abused by body-builders for its purported anabolic properties and is taken by alcoholics to reduce alcohol craving. γ-Butyrolactone and 1,4-butanedione are industrial solvents that are abused because they are metabolized to GHB *in vivo*.

After an overdose with depressant drugs, patients are unresponsive, pupils are sluggish and miotic, respiration is shallow and slow, and deep tendon reflexes are absent or attenuated. There are no known antagonists for barbiturates, nonbarbiturate sedatives, or GHB, whereas the competitive benzodiazepine antagonist flumazenil can completely reverse benzodiazepine intoxication. Although benzodiazepines are rarely lethal when taken alone, they enhance the effects of other depressants taken concurrently, including alcohol.

Repeated use of depressants produces physical dependence, and cross-dependence occurs among barbiturates, non-barbiturate sedatives, benzodiazepines, and alcohol. Signs and symptoms of withdrawal are often opposite to their acute effects. Occasional convulsions and delirium make depressant withdrawal a **medical emergency.** Long-acting benzodiazepines or phenobarbital can be used as substitution therapy to treat alcohol and barbiturate withdrawal.

The withdrawal symptoms following abrupt discontinuation of depressants and a comparison with those associated with opioid withdrawal are summarized in Box 32-1.

Cannabis

Marijuana produces an initial euphoric feeling of well-being, followed by drowsiness, sedation, and increased appetite. Thought processes, judgment, and time estimation are altered, and there is heightened sensitivity to music and other activities. Users have a reduced ability to form memories, although recall of previously learned facts is unaltered. Marijuana has little effect on psychomotor coordination, although altered perception and judgment can impair performance, including driving. Because of the prevalence of its use, accidents and injury are important concerns. High doses can induce personality changes, while physiological effects include tachycardia and reddening of conjunctival vessels. Death from acute overdose is extremely rare. Heavy smokers of marijuana will experience respiratory problems, including bronchitis and emphysema.

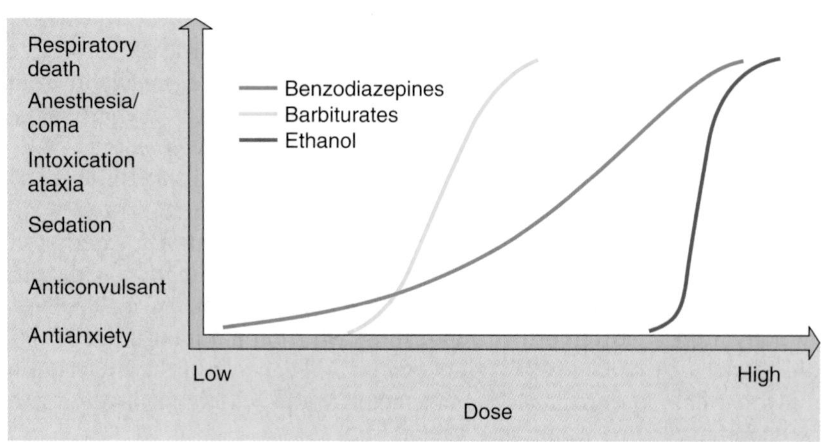

Figure 32-5 Comparison of dose-response relationships for the acute effects of ethanol, barbiturates, and benzodiazepines.

Box 32-1 Comparison of opioid and depressant withdrawal

Opioid withdrawal	Depressant withdrawal*
Anxiety and dysphoria	Anxiety and dysphoria
Craving and drug-seeking behavior	Craving and drug-seeking behavior
Sleep disturbance	Sleep disturbance
Nausea and vomiting	Nausea and vomiting
Lacrimation	Tremors
Rhinorrhea	Hyperreflexia
Yawning	Hyperpyrexia
Piloerection and gooseflesh	Confusion and delirium
Sweating	Convulsions
Diarrhea	Possible death
Mydriasis	
Abdominal cramping	
Hyperpyrexia	
Tachycardia and hypertension	

*Alcohol, barbiturates, or benzodiazepines.

Tolerance to marijuana develops following heavy use, and withdrawal causes irritability and restlessness. Addiction can develop with long-term use.

Hallucinogens

The unique psychological effects of hallucinogens include:

- Lability of mood
- Altered thought processes
- Altered visual, auditory, or somatosensory perception
- Experience of having enhanced insights into events and ideas
- Impaired judgment

Mood swings can range from profound euphoria to anxiety and terror. Panic states ("bad trips") are symptoms that most commonly lead abusers to seek assistance. Generally, bad trips are not caused by overdoses, although they are more common with larger doses. Rather, they result from the propensity of the drug experience to be rapidly transformed, since it is highly dependent on environmental context. Unexpected or frightening events can transform it dramatically. People on bad trips usually respond to calm reassurance and removal from a threatening environment until the drug wears off. Medication is rarely needed, although antipsychotic treatment may be useful. Nearly all hallucinogens produce varying degrees of sympathomimetic effects, and psychomotor stimulation may be evident. These effects are more common in people who use substituted amphetamines such as MDMA, particularly at higher doses.

Although acute overdose is not a common problem with hallucinogens, there are other hazards. The most significant is the risk of injury stemming from impaired judgment. In addition, even occasional use of hallucinogens may precipitate a psychiatric illness in predisposed subjects that is exacerbated by repeated use. A poorly understood aspect is the "flashback," in which previous users re-experience aspects of intoxication while drug-free. Flashbacks also may occur in those who have used marijuana or PCP. They may be no more than *déjà vu* experiences or they may be episodes that reflect an emerging psychopathological condition. LSD does not produce withdrawal symptoms or the intense craving caused by other drugs of abuse. However, strong tolerance occurs, with cross-tolerance to other hallucinogens, and increasingly higher doses may be used, leading to unpredictable consequences.

MDMA has cardiovascular risks similar to cocaine and amphetamine. In high doses, it produces hyperthermia and liver, kidney, and cardiovascular failure. Another potential danger is neurodegeneration resulting from severe depletion of DA or 5-HT, although whether this occurs in humans is still unknown. Effects on fetal development are poorly understood.

In addition to hallucinogens, other psychoactive drugs can also dramatically alter consciousness and perception. Some are used as adulterants or substitutes in "street drugs" and are frequently misrepresented as LSD or other drugs. The most notable class is antimuscarinics (see Chapter 9), which may be diverted from medical sources. Atropine and scopolamine are present in many plants and mushrooms, and certain groups of Native Americans and Central Americans practice their ritual use to produce profound alterations in consciousness. Antimuscarinic intoxication can be accompanied by signs of poisoning, and in severe cases, appropriate treatment is the cholinesterase inhibitor physostigmine (see Chapter 9).

Dissociative compounds

PCP produces a unique profile of effects and combines aspects of the actions of stimulants, depressants, and hallucinogens. The subjective experience of PCP intoxication is unlike that of other hallucinogens. Perceptual effects are not as profound and relate more to somesthesia. Distortions of body image are common, and one of the motivations for PCP abuse is to enhance sexual experience. PCP users have impaired judgment and may behave in bizarre and violent ways. PCP intoxication often includes motor incoordination and cataleptic behavior accompanied by nystagmus; high doses may result in a blank stare. PCP intoxication after smoking typically lasts 4 to 6 hours. Behavior may be more disrupted when PCP is taken with depressant drugs, including alcohol. Major dangers are risk-taking behavior and development of progressive personality changes culminating in a toxic psychosis. PCP overdose is rarely lethal but may require careful management because of severe incapacitation. No PCP antagonist is available, but an antibody is being developed.

Ketamine is basically a less-potent version of PCP. Ketamine is abused because of its ability to induce a dream-like state, vivid images, and hallucinations with possible delirium. The "K-hole" is a frightening, almost complete sensory detachment.

High-dose dextromethorphan produces dissociative effects similar to PCP and ketamine. It is often taken in combination cough medications that contain decongestants that increase its risks. Dextromethorphan is particularly abused by teenagers and young adults.

Inhalants

Inhalants are especially abused by young children, with abuse peaking at 8th grade. They represent a cheap entry into drug abuse.

Volatile solvents are toluene-containing materials including paint thinners and sprays, correction fluids, and plastic adhesives; solvents and cleaners contain alkylbenzenes and chlorinated hydrocarbon cleaners and degreasers. Aerosol propellants include ethyl chloride and chlorofluorocarbon-containing compounds. The most abused gas is nitrous oxide. Gases are also found in household products such as whipped cream dispensers and butane and propane sources. Motor performance deficits similar to those produced by alcohol and depressant drugs occur in those who abuse solvents. Prolonged use can lead to arrhythmias, heart failure, and death, especially with butane, propane, and aerosols. Death may also occur because of suffocation, asphyxiation, choking, and accidents while intoxicated. Inhalants are highly toxic, and chronic use can cause damage to the central and peripheral nervous systems, including well-defined axonopathies. In addition, chlorofluorocarbons are cardiotoxic. Treatment of acute toxicity is supportive to stabilize vital signs. There is no antidote or treatment for chronic exposure.

Amyl nitrite ampules are diverted from medical supplies. Other organic nitrites are available in specialty stores as room "odorizers." Nitrites are vasodilators, and dizziness and euphoria result from the hypotension and cerebral hypoxia secondary to peripheral venous pooling. Nitrites are often abused in conjunction with sexual activity and are popular among homosexual men for their ability to enhance orgasms, probably as a result of penile vasodilation. Nitrite use can result in accidents related to syncope.

Anabolic steroids

Steroids are abused largely by body-builders and athletes to improve performance. However, they are also used by others to improve muscle size and reduce body fat and by adolescents who partake in high-risk behaviors. Athletes and body-builders often "stack" steroids, taking different combinations of two or more compounds in cycles of weeks or months in the belief that this improves effects. Since amounts taken are far in excess of natural hormone levels, they result in negative feedback and prevent production of natural hormones. This often results in testicular atrophy, reduced sperm production, and gynecomastia. Steroids in high doses also increase irritability and aggression and produce depression on withdrawal. Many users report that steroids make them feel good and are addictive. Dietary supplements including dehydroepiandrostenedione and androstenedione (see Chapter 7) are also abused and are converted to anabolic steroids in the body. The use of steroids and steroid supplements is banned by governing bodies of most sports.

Nicotine

Cigarette smoking is the preferred source for 98% of nicotine users. Nicotine is highly addictive and produces an intense and long-lasting craving. Tolerance to the effects of nicotine develops rapidly, and there is withdrawal on cessation producing symptoms including anxiety, dysphoria, irritability, and insomnia. Tar from cigarettes is important in causing lung cancer, bronchitis, and emphysema. The carbon monoxide produced leads to cardiovascular disorders.

Pharmacotherapies for substance abuse

In considering treatment, it is important to remember that substance abuse is a chronic, relapsing disease. Treatment can be very effective, especially if one accepts reduction in drug use and its resultant harm as an important goal. Complete cessation of drug use can also be achieved, but may require multiple attempts.

Thus, repeated treatment of drug abuse should be considered in a similar light as treatment of other chronic diseases. It is important to distinguish physically dependent from nondependent abusers, because treatment strategies differ considerably. Unfortunately, most treatment programs are for "hard-core" dependent abusers. Strategies for preventing escalation from occasional use would be desirable but are rare.

There are no drugs to treat stimulant dependence, although antipsychotics can be useful in treating overdoses and toxic psychoses. There are also no medications to treat dependence on CNS depressants, marijuana, hallucinogens, dissociative compounds, inhalants, or anabolic steroids. However, progress in pharmacotherapy for opioid and nicotine addiction is increasing.

Opiates

Detoxification of patients receiving opioids for pain relief is accomplished by tapering the dose of a prescribed opioid or by substituting methadone or another longer-acting drug. Only rarely does such iatrogenic dependence lead to illicit opioid use, and development of dependence should not be a consideration in providing adequate relief of terminal pain.

Medications play an important role in treatment of opioid abuse but are adjuncts to psychosocial and educational interventions. Simple detoxification alone is not usually sufficient to prevent relapse. Most abusers undergo detoxification numerous times, either medically or as a result of interrupted drug supply or incarceration. Nondrug detoxification can be used, or alternatively, abusers can be stabilized on a long-acting oral medication such as methadone. The daily dose is gradually decreased over about 30 days (inpatient) or 180 days (outpatient). Withdrawal signs are mild, although the patient will be uncomfortable for most of the withdrawal period. Another approach is to terminate opioids abruptly and treat symptoms of withdrawal, many of which reflect stress and sympathetic nervous system activation. Medications such as clonidine have been used successfully, particularly in mildly dependent subjects. Antianxiety agents may also be useful.

Maintenance therapies are based on cross-dependence. Methadone is used because it has good oral bioavailability and a long duration of action. Methadone maintenance patients receive single, daily oral doses chosen to prevent withdrawal but not large enough to produce significant intoxication. Urinalysis to detect continued illicit drug use is important. Methadone maintenance is effective and has many proven benefits. It breaks the destructive pattern of continued drug abuse and lessens criminal behavior and is also attractive to abusers who would not otherwise seek treatment. It also provides an opportunity for other interventions to be implemented and has dependence-producing properties that help ensure continued patient participation. Take-home medications and other clinic privileges can be used to reinforce positive changes in behavior. The long-acting methadone analog L-methadyl acetate, which is given 3 times per week, reduces the need for daily clinic visits and may provide some advantages. The partial agonist buprenorphine (or buprenorphine with naloxone) is now available for treatment of dependence. When buprenorphine is substituted in dependent heroin abusers, it can prevent withdrawal. Also, eventual discontinuation may be accompanied by less-significant withdrawal, perhaps because of its slow rate of dissociation from its receptor. Buprenorphine is intended to allow office-based physicians to treat heroin dependence.

In theory, opioid antagonists could also be used for treatment of abuse. After a sufficient oral dose of naltrexone, positive reinforcement from opioids can be prevented for up to 24 hours. However, patients given naltrexone must be detoxified first, or precipitated withdrawal will occur. Naltrexone does not produce dependence; thus patient compliance is less assured. However, a patient must plan ahead to obtain opioids, making spontaneous relapse less likely.

Nicotine

Nicotine products used in replacement therapy include gum, patches, nasal sprays, and inhalers. The antidepressant drug bupropion decreases the craving for nicotine and reduces some symptoms of withdrawal. It may act by weak blockade of DA and norepinephrine reuptake and is also a nicotinic receptor antagonist (see Chapter 23).

New horizons

Increasing knowledge of the mechanisms of action of abused drugs could lead to medications that stabilize the user in the same way as methadone and buprenorphine do for opioid addicts, or even allow for abstinence. In a similar way, "substitute agonists" for the DA transporter, the site of action of cocaine and amphetamine, have been synthesized and shown to prevent self-administration of cocaine in non-human primates but themselves may be rewarding. Because presumed long-term alterations in dopaminergic function result from stimulant abuse, which may be a factor in relapse, research is focused on the use of compounds that alter dopaminergic pathways. Nonselective antagonists that act at D_1 and D_2 receptors block the reinforcing effects of cocaine and amphetamine in animal models. Compounds with high efficacy at D_1 receptors decrease cocaine-induced subjective effects. However, a D_3 receptor partial agonist inhibits cocaine-seeking behavior in mice, suggesting D_3 receptors may be important targets in treatment of addiction. Other compounds under study for stimulant abuse include NMDA and GABA antagonists and opioid mixed agonist-antagonists, for example, κ agonists that decrease DA release. Antidepressants that may ameliorate stimulant abstinence and depression and reduce craving are also under investigation.

Because of the widespread problems of stimulant abuse and the lack of pharmacotherapies, this is a priority of the National Institute on Drug Abuse. New techniques such as brain imaging, knock-out animal models, and microarray analysis to study gene expression in addiction, together with information from the Human Genome Project, should open up new approaches.

TRADE NAMES

All of the important drugs available in the United States for treatment of drug abuse are listed in the Major Drugs box.

FURTHER READING

George TP, O'Malley SS. Current pharmacological treatments for nicotine dependence. *Trends Pharmacol Sci* 2004; 25:42-48.

Kreek MJ, LaForge KS, Butelman E. Pharmacotherapy of addictions. *Nat Rev Drug Discov* 2002; 1:710-726.

National Institute for Drug Abuse. Principles of Drug Addiction Treatment: A Research Based Guide. Available from National Institute on Drug Abuse Web site. http://www.nida.nih.gov.

Wong CGT, Gibson KM, Snead, OC. From the street to the brain: neurobiology of the recreational drug γ-hydroxybutyric acid. *Trends Pharmacol Sci* 2004; 25:29-34.

Self-assessment questions

1. A person who has been taking one drug chronically and experiences a withdrawal syndrome upon discontinuing it finds relief from these symptoms by taking a second drug. This is an example of:
   a. Craving.
   b. Psychological dependence.
   c. Cross-dependence.
   d. Tolerance.
   e. Drug addiction.

2. Which of the following drugs most likely results in a life-threatening withdrawal?
   a. Cocaine
   b. Pentobarbital
   c. Heroin
   d. LSD
   e. Methamphetamine

3. Relative to barbiturates, the dose-effect curves for benzodiazepines are:
   a. Steep.
   b. Shallow.
   c. Parallel.
   d. Biphasic.
   e. Inverted.

4. Which of the following is NOT a common symptom of opioid withdrawal?
   a. Convulsions
   b. Lacrimation and rhinorrhea
   c. Nausea and vomiting
   d. Abdominal cramps
   e. Piloerection

5. The problems of cocaine abuse are most similar to those of:
   a. Heroin abuse.
   b. Marijuana abuse.
   c. Amphetamine abuse.
   d. Alcoholism.

6. Barbiturate withdrawal symptoms are similar to the withdrawal symptoms from:
   a. Heroin.
   b. Alcohol.
   c. Phenothiazines.
   d. Benzodiazepines.
   e. More than one of the above.

PART V

Drugs affecting endocrine systems

THE ENDOCRINE SYSTEM IS a complex communication system that is responsible for maintaining homeostasis throughout the body. The system consists of a diverse group of ductless glands that secrete chemical messengers called **hormones** into the circulation. The secreted hormones are transported in the bloodstream to target organs, where they act to regulate cellular activities. For a hormone to elicit a response, it must interact with specific receptors on the cells of the target organ, much like the interaction between neurotransmitters and receptors involved in the process of neurotransmission in the central and peripheral nervous systems (see Chapters 8 and 20). Receptors play a key role in the mechanisms of action of endocrine hormone systems; key receptor mechanisms pertinent to endocrine systems are summarized in Chapter 2.

In general, all endocrine systems share several common features, typically referred to as essential components of the endocrine system. These components are depicted in Figure V-1. At the uppermost level, the secretion of each hormone is controlled tightly by input from higher neural centers in response to alterations in plasma levels of the hormone or other substances. The second component is the gland itself, where hormone synthesis and secretion occur in specialized cells. Following synthesis, hormones are typically packaged and stored for later release, as needed. Signals from the nervous system or special releasing hormones or both, bring about secretion of stored hormone.

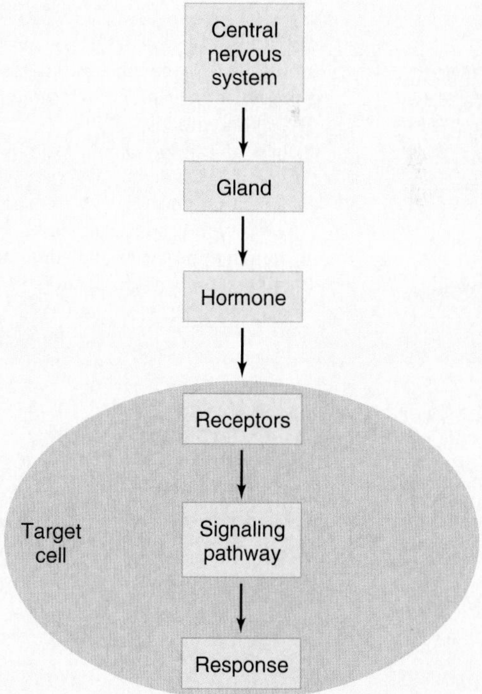

Figure V-1 Essential components of the endocrine system.

Although hormones are metabolized, their metabolism is not regulated as extensively as their synthesis and release. Hormones exert their effects by binding to and activating receptors on target cells. These receptors can be located on the cell surface as for peptide hormones, or within the cell as in the case of steroids and thyroid hormones. Following receptor activation, signaling pathways are propagated and responses are elicited.

The endocrine hormones affect the activities of most organs and many types of cells. These actions occur by means of extremely intricate pathways, including positive- and negative-feedback control loops and sequences involving hormones from endocrine glands that act to control hormones secreted by other glands. A given hormone typically exerts multiple actions, and a given function typically is influenced by several different hormones.

The endocrine hormones can be divided into three main classes based on chemical composition, viz., the amino acid analogs, the peptides, and the steroids. The amino acid analogs, often termed amine hormones, are all derived from tyrosine and include epinephrine and the iodothyronines or thyroid hormones. The peptide hormones are subclassified on the basis of size and glycosylation state, and may be single or double chain peptides. The steroid hormones are all derived from cholesterol and may be subclassified as adrenal steroids or sex steroids, the former synthesized primarily in the adrenal cortex, and the latter synthesized in the ovaries or testes.

Pharmacological interventions for treatment of endocrine malfunction or disease generally take one of three approaches: (1) a hormone is given to replace or supplement the natural hormone; (2) a hormone is used to obtain a specific response; or (3) drugs are used to modify the concentration or action of a specific hormone.

The major endocrine glands and their associated hormones are listed in Table V-1. The chapter in which each hormone is discussed is also indicated.

Table V-1 Major endocrine systems

Gland	Hormone	Chapter
Adrenal	Cortisol, corticosterone, aldosterone	33, 34
Ovaries, testes	Estradiol, progesterone, testosterone	35, 36
Thyroid	Thyroid hormones	37
Pancreas	Insulin, glucagon, somatostatin, pancreatic polypeptide	38
Pituitary	Antidiuretic hormone, oxytocin, adrenocorticotropic hormone, thyroid-stimulating hormone, luteinizing hormone, follicle-stimulating hormone, growth hormone, prolactin, gonadotropin-releasing hormone, luteinizing-hormone–releasing hormone, thyrotropin-releasing hormone, prolactin-inhibiting factor	39, 40
Parathyroid	Parathyroid hormone, calcitonin	41

CHAPTER 33

Glucocorticoids and mineralocorticoids

Helmy M. Siragy
George P. Chrousos
Margaret A. Shupnik

Major Drugs

Dexamethasone (Decadron, Hexadrol)
Fludrocortisone (Florinef)
Hydrocortisone, Cortisol (Cortef, Hydrocortone)
Methylprednisolone (A-MethaPred, Medrol)
Prednisone (Deltasone, Meticorten, Orasone)
Triamcinolone (Aristocort, Kenalog)

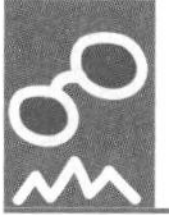

Therapeutic overview

Cortisol (also called compound F and hydrocortisone) is the main endogenous glucocorticoid in humans. It is synthesized in the adrenal cortex and exerts a wide range of physiological effects. Cortisol is involved in regulation of intermediary metabolism, the stress response, some aspects of central nervous system function, and immunity. Thus, cortisol is necessary for maintenance of life; because of its pivotal biological significance, its synthesis and secretion are tightly regulated. The hypothalamic-pituitary-adrenal (HPA) axis is very sensitive to negative feedback by circulating cortisol or synthetic glucocorticoids. High plasma concentrations of glucocorticoids suppress HPA activity, resulting in decreased cortisol biosynthesis, and thus lower concentrations of circulating cortisol. During prolonged exposure to exogenous or endogenous glucocorticoids, suppression of the HPA axis persists for long periods. Thus, abrupt cessation of a synthetic glucocorticoid that has been administered long-term or removal of tumors causing excessive cortisol production may result in a lack of endogenous glucocorticoids, and serious morbidity and even mortality. It may take a long time to taper off exogenously administered glucocorticoids because the HPA system needs up to a year to recover fully (i.e., to secrete cortisol at a normal rate).

Aldosterone is the major mineralocorticoid in humans. It is synthesized in the adrenal cortex and is regulated primarily by the renin-angiotensin system, potassium and ACTH. It is responsible for maintaining sodium and potassium concentrations in the extracellular fluid.

The main therapeutic uses of the glucocorticoids are: (1) as a **replacement** for cortisol in patients with adrenal insufficiency (i.e., inadequate endogenous production of cortisol); (2) as an **antiinflammatory/ immunosuppressant** agent; and (3) as an **adjuvant** in the treatment of myeloproliferative diseases and other malignant conditions. The major therapeutic use of the mineralocorticoids is as a replacement for aldosterone in patients with primary adrenal insufficiency or isolated aldosterone deficiency. See the Therapeutic Overview box for a summary of therapeutic issues.

Abbreviations

ACTH	adrenocorticotropic hormone
AVP	arginine vasopressin
cAMP	cyclic adenosine monophosphate
CRH	corticotropin-releasing hormone
HPA	hypothalamic-pituitary-adrenal
MSH	melanocyte-stimulating hormone
POMC	proopiomelanocorticotropin
StAR	steroidogenic acute regulatory protein

THERAPEUTIC OVERVIEW

Glucocorticoids

Replacement therapy in adrenal insufficiencies
Antiinflammatory and immunosuppressive action
Myeloproliferative diseases

Mineralocorticoids

Replacement therapy in primary adrenal insufficiencies
Hypoaldosteronism

Steroid synthesis inhibitors

Adrenocortical hyperfunction

Steroid receptor blockers

Glucocorticoid excess
Mineralocorticoid excess

Mechanisms of action

Glucocorticoids

Biosynthesis of corticoids Cholesterol is the main precursor for both cortisol and aldosterone. Cholesterol is taken up from the circulation rather than synthesized *de novo* in the adrenal cortex, though the cortex is capable of *de novo* cholesterol biosynthesis. Plasma cholesterol is carried by both low-density and high-density lipoproteins, and the adrenal cortex has receptors for these lipoproteins. In humans, low-density lipoproteins are the major source of adrenal cholesterol. Uptake of circulating cholesterol and *de novo* synthesis of cholesterol by the adrenals are interchangeable sources; thus, blockade of one or the other does not significantly decrease cortisol or aldosterone biosynthesis.

Adrenocortical cholesterol is esterified and stored in cytoplasmic lipid droplets. Esterified cholesterol is hydrolyzed by cytoplasmic cholesterol ester hydrolase and transported into the mitochondria by a sterol carrier protein, where it is converted to **pregnenolone**. This conversion requires nicotinamide adenine dinucleotide phosphate (reduced), oxygen, and the cytochrome P450 mixed-function oxidase system. It involves removal of a portion of the side chain of cholesterol and addition of a double-bonded oxygen. The synthesis of the major glucocorticoids and mineralocorticoids is shown in Figure 33-1. Figure 33-2 shows the structure of corticosterone highlighting sites for enzymatic action.

Pregnenolone is transferred from the mitochondria to the smooth endoplasmic reticulum, where most of it is hydroxylated into **17α-hydroxypregnenolone**, which in turn is converted to **17α-hydroxyprogesterone** by the 3β-hydroxysteroid dehydrogenase-Δ5-isomerase enzyme complex. A small percentage of pregnenolone is first converted by this enzyme complex to **progesterone** and then hydroxylated to 17α-hydroxyprogesterone. 17α-Hydroxyprogesterone is a strategically located steroid that undergoes two successive hydroxylations in the zona fasciculata. First, it is hydroxylated by the 21-hydroxylase enzyme in the endoplasmic reticulum, resulting in **11-deoxycortisol** (also called compound S). Compound S is then hydroxylated by the 11β-hydroxylase enzyme inside the mitochondria to cortisol. There is no 17α-hydroxylase in the zona glomerulosa, and thus all available pregnenolone is transformed to progesterone, which in turn follows the pathway for the synthesis of the mineralocorticoid aldosterone.

Regulation by ACTH Cortisol synthesis and secretion are regulated physiologically by the pituitary hormone ACTH. ACTH is synthesized in the corticotrope cells of the anterior pituitary as part of a large precursor called proopiomelanocorticotropin (POMC), which is proteolytically cleaved to form ACTH, β-endorphin, and melanocyte-stimulating hormone (MSH). β-Endorphin has opioid effects that reduce pain perception, whereas MSH acts on the melanocytes that confer skin pigmentation. The hyperpigmentation that is often associated with the overproduction of ACTH is thought to arise as a result of the associated overproduction of MSH. The POMC gene is also transcribed in the posterior pituitary, where it is differentially cleaved to form several different endorphins and MSH, but no ACTH. ACTH is secreted from the anterior pituitary in an episodic fashion, and these pulses are superimposed physiologically on larger fluctuations in ACTH defined by circadian rhythms. In general, pulses of greater frequency and magnitude are noted in the early morning and pulses of lower frequency and magnitude in early afternoon. Pulses of ACTH secretion are followed closely by bursts of cortisol secretion in plasma. These secretory bursts are characterized by a sharp rise in plasma concentrations followed by a slower decline, with approximately eight to ten major bursts of cortisol secretion occurring daily (Fig. 33-3).

ACTH secreted into the peripheral circulation binds to ACTH receptors on the surface of cells in the adrenal cortex. Ligand-bound receptors activate adenylyl cyclase to increase intracellular cyclic adenosine monophosphate (cAMP). Increased adrenal cAMP triggers stimulation of several processes, leading to

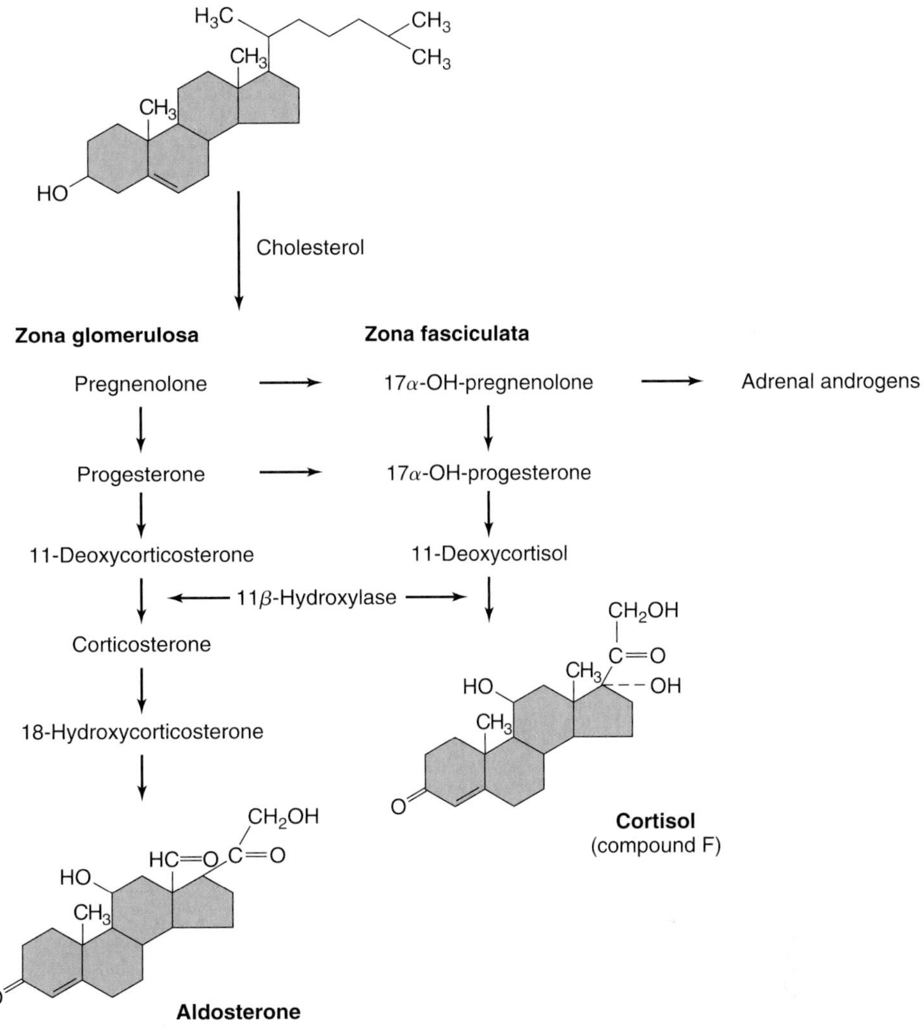

Cholesterol

Zona glomerulosa | **Zona fasciculata**

Pregnenolone → 17α-OH-pregnenolone → Adrenal androgens

Progesterone → 17α-OH-progesterone

11-Deoxycorticosterone | 11-Deoxycortisol

← 11β-Hydroxylase →

Corticosterone

18-Hydroxycorticosterone

Aldosterone

Cortisol
(compound F)

Figure 33-1 Synthesis of the major glucocorticoid (cortisol) and major mineralocorticoid (aldosterone) by the adrenal cortex. Both are 21-carbon steroids derived from cholesterol.

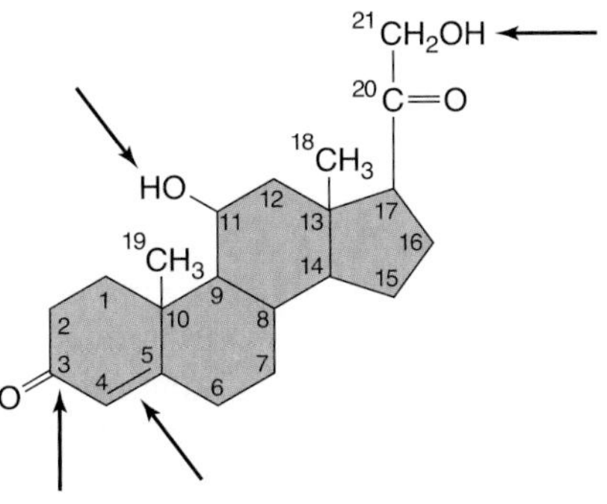

Figure 33-2 Structure of corticosterone showing sites for bioactivation and inactivation.

increased cortisol synthesis and secretion. The first step is delivery of the cholesterol substrate from cellular stores and the outer mitochondrial membrane to the inner mitochondrial membrane, where the enzymatic processes leading to steroid synthesis are initiated. This transport step through the outer mitochondrial membrane is the true rate-limiting step in overall steroid synthesis and requires the steroidogenic acute regulatory protein (StAR). StAR synthesis is rapidly stimulated by ACTH in the adrenals and by gonadal hormones in the testes and ovaries and results in increased cholesterol transport and steroid synthesis. Mutations in StAR have been identified in some patients with congenital lipoid adrenal hyperplasia (lipoid CAH), an autosomal recessive disorder where affected infants suffer from deficiencies of adrenal and gonadal hormones and die from salt loss, hyperkalemic acidosis, and dehydration unless treated with adrenal steroids.

The rate-limiting enzymatic step in steroid synthesis is the conversion of cholesterol to pregnenolone by the P450 side-chain cleavage enzyme located on the inner mitochondrial membrane. ACTH-stimulated increases in cAMP result in accelerated transcription rates of the gene coding for this enzyme as well as most other enzymes in the cortisol biosynthetic pathway. In addition, ACTH acts as a growth factor for the adrenal

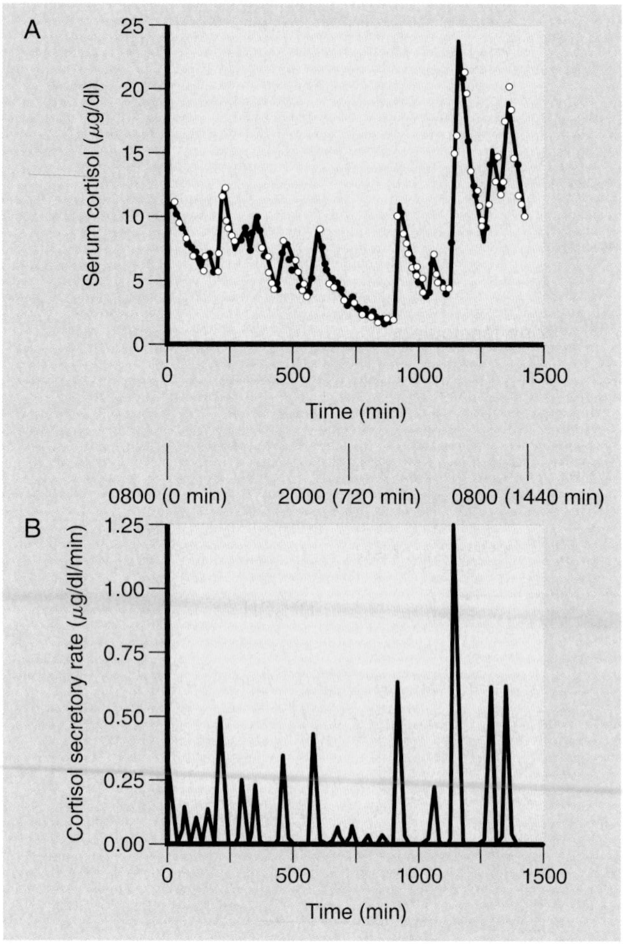

Figure 33-3 Serum cortisol concentrations in a healthy man. Serial blood samples collected at 10-minute intervals were assayed for cortisol. **A,** Concentrations plotted, with the continuous line calculated using a special multiple parameter model of combined secretion and clearance of cortisol. **B,** Calculated rates of cortisol secretion as a function of time. Zero minutes = 0800 = start of experimental period. (Modified from Veldhuis JD, Iranmanesh A, Lizarralde G, et al. Am J Physiol 1989; 257:E6)

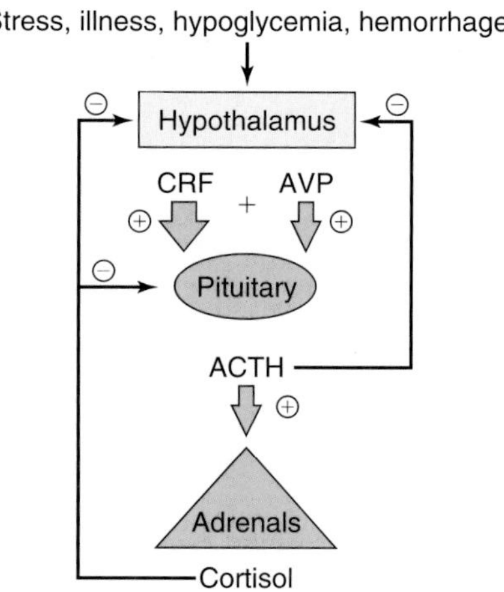

Figure 33-4 Regulatory feedback mechanisms in the HPA. *ACTH,* Adrenocorticotrophic hormone; *AVP,* arginine vasopressin; *CRF,* corticotropin-releasing hormone.

cortex. Thus, lowering plasma ACTH concentrations results not only in decreased cortisol synthesis and secretion, but also in gradual atrophy of the adrenal cortex.

Modulation of ACTH release Serum concentrations of ACTH are modulated by integrated stimulatory signals from hypothalamic releasing peptides and by inhibitory feedback from circulating cortisol (Fig. 33-4). Physiologically, serum ACTH concentrations are increased in response to stress, including severe trauma, illness, burns, hypoglycemia, hemorrhage, fever, exercise, and psychological stresses such as anxiety and depression. It is thought that this results in a physiological change by altering the release of hypothalamic factors, and thus ACTH. Two hypothalamic peptides, including CRH and to a lesser extent arginine vasopressin (AVP, also known as antidiuretic hormone), act on the pituitary to stimulate ACTH release. Both peptides bind to distinct membrane receptors on the corticotrope. CRH exerts its effect primarily via cAMP-dependent pathways, whereas AVP stimulates phosphatidylinositol hydrolysis and stimulates protein kinase C. CRF is the most important physiological stimulating factor and can be used in a pharmacological test to screen for appropriate corticotrope function. CRF may also increase POMC gene transcription and processing, thus increasing available peptide stores for subsequent release.

Feedback control mechanisms Pituitary production of ACTH is extremely sensitive to suppression by cortisol at both the pituitary and hypothalamic levels. Cortisol acts directly on the pituitary to decrease POMC gene transcription and ACTH secretion, as well as to suppress the pituitary response to CRF. It also acts on the hypothalamus to suppress CRF release. Results of this negative feedback can endure for weeks after cessation of glucocorticoid therapy. Chronic administration of high doses of glucocorticoids can result in adrenocortical atrophy and impaired steroid biosynthesis. Thus, glucocorticoid therapy and its cessation must be approached with utmost caution. Lower doses of exogenous steroid may need to continue to be administered until the physiological axis recovers from feedback inhibition. High concentrations of ACTH may also suppress CRF release from the hypothalamus.

Receptors All natural and synthetic glucocorticoids act by binding to specific cytoplasmic glucocorticoid receptors. There are two forms of the glucocorticoid receptor, type I (also known as the mineralocorticoid receptor) and type II. The receptors are closely related in their DNA and ligand-binding domains but differ considerably in the N-terminal antigenic region. Both receptors have similar binding affinities for glucocorticoids, and many cell types contain these receptors including liver, muscle, adipose tissue, bone, lymphocytes, and pituitary. The receptors are proteins consisting of about 800 amino acids, which can be divided into functional domains similar to those for other steroid receptors (see Chapter 2). The glucocorticoid-binding domain is located at the carboxy-terminus of the molecule whereas the DNA-binding domain is located in the middle of the protein and contains nine cysteine residues. This region folds into a "two-finger" structure stabilized by zinc ions that bind to specific sites on DNA, termed **glucocorticoid-responsive elements,** which influence transcription of specific genes. The zinc fingers represent the basic structure by which the DNA-binding domain recognizes specific nucleic acid sequences. The amino-terminal domain of the receptor is highly antigenic and evidence suggests that phosphorylation of this region, as a consequence of glucocorticoid binding, is involved in receptor translocation and its subsequent interaction with chromatin.

The inactive form of the glucocorticoid receptor is located in the cytoplasm as a heteromer associated with other proteins, one of which is heat shock protein 90. Binding of a glucocorticoid to its receptor results in dissociation of the hormone-receptor complex from this protein, thus freeing the DNA-binding domain of the receptor to interact with DNA. This sequence of events is generally called **glucocorticoid receptor activation.** The activated glucocorticoid-receptor complex enters the nucleus (translocation), where two molecules of activated receptor associate to form a homodimer that binds to glucocorticoid response elements near the promoter region of specific genes, resulting in altered transcription (see Chapter 2).

Metabolic effects Glucocorticoids have several metabolic effects. These include increased hepatic gluconeogenesis as a consequence of stimulating the synthesis of phosphoenolpyruvate carboxykinase and glucose-6-phosphatase, and increased amino acid degradation as a consequence of stimulating the synthesis of tyrosine aminotransferase and tryptophan oxygenase. In striated muscle, glucocorticoids act in concert with other hormones to influence protein synthesis and degradation. Cortisol has little or no effect on protein turnover in the presence of insulin and in well-fed people. However, during fasting or when the insulin concentration is low, cortisol stimulates the breakdown of muscle protein and decreases the uptake of amino acids. Thus, the presence of high concentrations of circulating glucocorticoids for long periods can lead to muscle wasting. In adipose tissue, cortisol stimulates lipolysis, resulting in the release of free fatty acids and glycerol. Other lipogenic hormones are required for the full lipolytic response to occur. Thus, overall, cortisol stimulates both protein and lipid catabolism. Glucocorticoids also regulate growth and development, particularly in fetal tissues. One of their critical actions on the fetus is to induce surfactant synthesis in the lungs prior to birth. Cortisol can be administered to lessen the severity of respiratory distress syndrome resulting from a failure of sufficient surfactant secretion.

Mineralocorticoids

Aldosterone is the major mineralocorticoid produced by the adrenal cortex and acts primarily at the distal portion of the convoluted renal tubule to promote reabsorption of sodium and the excretion of potassium (see Chapter 13). Adrenal secretion of aldosterone is controlled by the renin-angiotensin system and the concentration of potassium. ACTH plays a secondary role in the regulation of aldosterone secretion.

Receptors for mineralocorticoids (type I glucocorticoid receptors) are present in high concentrations in the renal collecting ducts, as well as in other tissues. The receptor has a similar affinity for both aldosterone and glucocorticoids. However, mineralocorticoid-responsive tissues such as the kidney, also contain high concentrations of the enzyme 11-β-hydroxysteroid dehydrogenase, which inactivates cortisol to cortisone. Cortisone has a much lower affinity for the mineralocorticoid receptor, and thus tissues with 11-β-hydroxysteroid dehydrogenase activity inactivate cortisol and permit aldosterone to bind to and activate the mineralocorticoid receptor. This is critical for an appropriate biological response because aldosterone-activated mineralocorticoid receptors recognize and stimulate different genes than those stimulated by the glucocorticoid type II receptor.

The structures of the principal glucocorticoids and mineralocorticoids are shown in Figures 33-1 and 33-5.

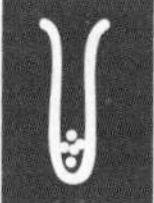

Pharmacokinetics

Pharmacokinetic parameters for clinically used glucocorticoids and mineralocorticoids are summarized in Table 33-1. Most glucocorticoids are absorbed rapidly and readily from the gastrointestinal tract as a result of their **lipophilic** character. Glucocorticoids are also

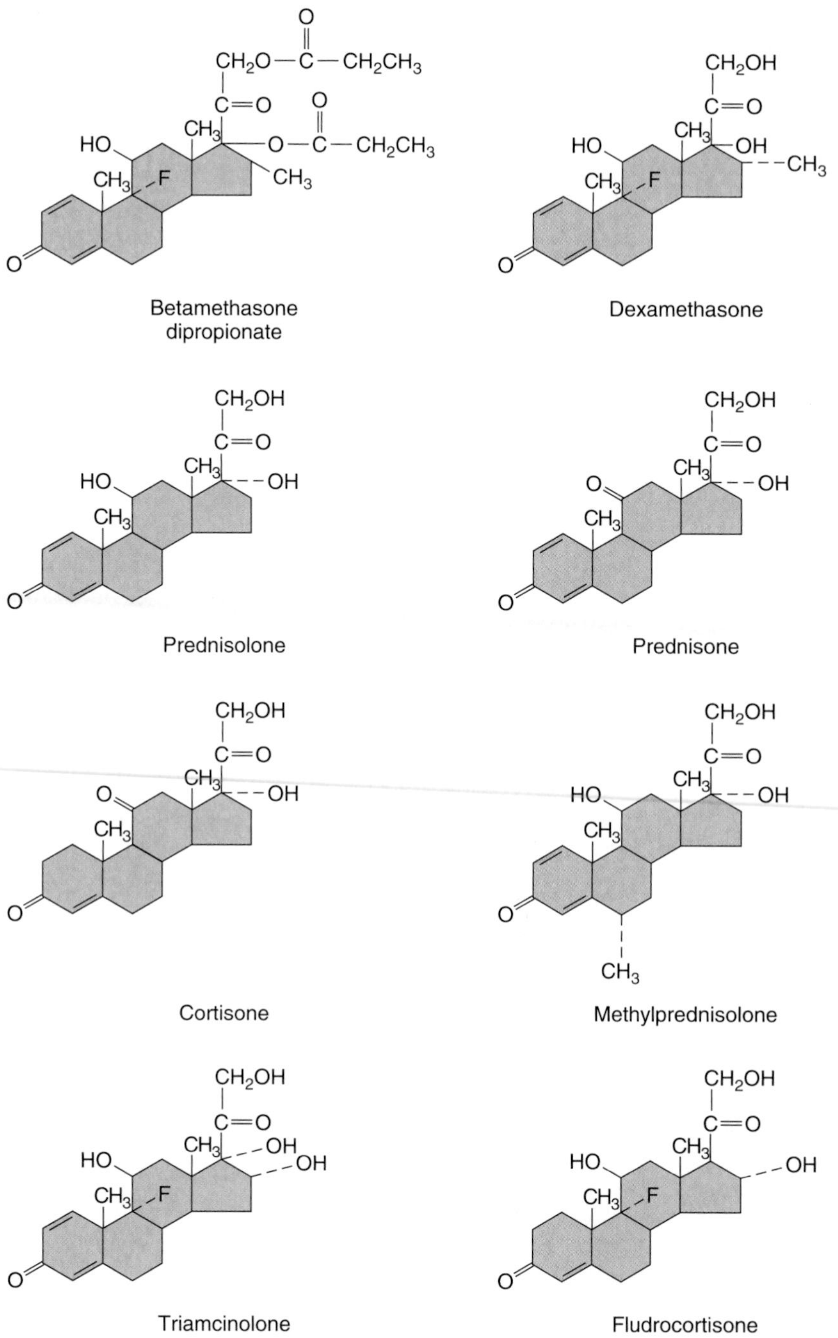

Betamethasone dipropionate

Dexamethasone

Prednisolone

Prednisone

Cortisone

Methylprednisolone

Triamcinolone

Fludrocortisone

Figure 33-5 Structures of representative glucocorticoids and mineralocorticoids.

absorbed readily from the synovial and conjunctival spaces, but are absorbed very slowly through the skin. The long-term use of steroids by nasal spray for the control of seasonal rhinitis can lead to nasal and pulmonary epithelial atrophy. Consequently, topical administration of glucocorticoids is often used only briefly to produce a local action. However, excessive and prolonged local application may result in sufficient absorption to cause systemic effects. The presence of a hydroxyl group at position 11 confers glucocorticoid activity on both cortisol and prednisolone. Cortisone and prednisone must be hydroxylated by 11β-hydroxylase to become active (see Fig. 33-2). This hydroxylation takes place primarily in the liver, therefore administration of 11-ketocorticoids to patients with abnormal liver function should be avoided. For the same reason, topical application of 11-ketocorticoids on the skin is ineffective.

Most circulating cortisol is bound to plasma proteins; 80% to 90% with high affinity to cortisol-

Table 33-1 Pharmacokinetic parameters

Drugs	Route of Administration	Half-Life
GLUCOCORTICOIDS		
Cortisol*	IM, IV, oral†	Short
Cortisone	Oral, IM, IV	Short
Prednisone	Oral	Intermediate
Prednisolone	IM, IV	Intermediate
Methylprednisolone	IM, IV, oral†	Intermediate
Dexamethasone	IM, oral,† topical, IV	Long
Betamethasone	Oral, topical, inhaled	Long
Triamcinolone	Intraarticular, topical, inhaled	Long
MINERALOCORTICOIDS		
Fludrocortisone	Oral	Intermediate
Aldosterone (for reference)	—	Short
Desoxycorticosterone acetate	IM	Long

Short, 10-90 minutes; *intermediate,* several hours; *long,* 5 hours or more.
*Same as hydrocortisone.
†Intralesional, intraarticular, nasal, and inhaled; collectively this is referred to as compartmentalized administration.
All drugs are eliminated primarily through metabolism.

binding globulin (also called transcortin) and 5% to 10% loosely bound to albumin. The free (bioactive) fraction is approximately 3–10%. The cortisol-binding globulin can also bind synthetic glucocorticoids such as prednisone and prednisolone, but not dexamethasone. As a consequence, almost 100% of plasma dexamethasone is in the bioactive form; thus, circulating dexamethasone concentrations lower than those of the natural glucocorticoids can have similar biological effects. Because estrogens increase biosynthesis of cortisol-binding globulin in the liver, in conditions where estrogen is elevated, such as during contraception or pregnancy, the concentration of cortisol-binding globulin is elevated, resulting in increased plasma cortisol concentrations.

Addition of a fluorine atom at position 9 and a methyl group at position 16, as present in betamethasone and dexamethasone (Fig. 33-5), enhances glucocorticoid receptor activation and prolongs the half-life of these compounds.

The liver and kidney are the major sites of glucocorticoid inactivation. Pathways leading to inactivation include: (1) reduction of the double bond at position 4/5, (2) reduction of the keto group at position 3, and (3) hydroxylation at position 6. Approximately 30% of inactivated cortisol is metabolized to tetrahydrocortisol-glucuronide and tetrahydrodeoxycortisol-glucuronide and excreted in the urine. As mentioned, in the kidneys, cortisol is inactivated by **11β-hydroxysteroid dehydrogenase** to cortisone which does not bind to the renal mineralocorticoid receptor and thus, does not exert a salt-retaining effect. A rare genetic clinical syndrome called Apparent Mineralocorticoid Excess has been observed in which this enzyme complex does not function efficiently, resulting in salt retention, hypokalemia and hypertension. Glycyrrhizic acid, a component of licorice, inhibits this enzyme and causes an iatrogenic syndrome.

Box 33-1 Effects of glucocorticoids

Metabolic

Increased glycogenolysis and gluconeogenesis
Increased protein catabolism and decreased protein synthesis
Decreased osteoblast formation and activity
Decreased calcium absorption from the gastrointestinal tract
Decreased thyroid-stimulating hormone secretion

Antiinflammatory

Local and systemic effects, including:
- Decreased production of prostaglandins, cytokines, and interleukins
- Decreased proliferation and migration of lymphocytes and macrophages

Established inducers of hepatic drug metabolism such as rifampin, phenobarbital and phenytoin may accelerate hepatic biotransformation of glucocorticoids. Thus, administration of these drugs may necessitate an increase in dose of glucocorticoids. Hypothyroidism may decrease metabolism of glucocorticoids.

Aldosterone does not bind to a specific plasma protein, but binds weakly to several different plasma proteins from which it dissociates rapidly. The half-life of aldosterone is very short (a few minutes) and without ongoing secretion from the adrenals, its rapid clearance from plasma effectively limits its biological effects.

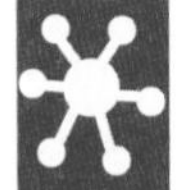

Relation of mechanisms of action to clinical response

Glucocorticoids

Glucocorticoids affect glucose, protein and bone metabolism, and possess antiinflammatory and immunosuppressant actions. Glucocorticoids influence the immune system at multiple levels affecting leukocyte movement, antigen processing, eosinophils, and lymphatic tissues (Box 33-1).

Within hours after administration of glucocorticoids, the number of circulating neutrophils increases. This neutrophilia may result from a glucocorticoid-induced decrease in neutrophil adherence to the vascular endothelium and the inability of neutrophils to egress towards bone marrow or inflammatory sites. In addition, glucocorticoids inhibit antigen processing by macrophages, suppress T-cell helper function, inhibit synthesis of mediators of the inflammatory response (i.e., interleukins, other cytokines, and prostanoids), and inhibit phagocytosis. Glucocorticoids also induce eosinopenia and lymphopenia. The latter may be attributable to a modification in cell production, distribution, or lysis and is more profound on T lymphocytes than on B lymphocytes. This explains the beneficial effect of glucocorticoids for treatment of certain leukemias, such as acute lymphoblastic leukemia of childhood.

Therapeutically, the most important effect of the glucocorticoids is inhibition of accumulation of **neutrophils and monocytes** at sites of inflammation and suppression of the phagocytic, bactericidal, and antigen-processing activity of these cells. However, these effects compromise the immune system and thus predispose the patient to infection by several common and uncommon pathogens and to saprophytic sepsis. This condition represents the single most dangerous complication of long-term glucocorticoid treatment.

Mineralocorticoids

The endogenous mineralocorticoid aldosterone is not used therapeutically because its biological action is very brief. Thus, synthetic fludrocortisone (9α-fluorohydrocortisone) is indicated for the treatment of primary adrenocortical insufficiency, aldosterone insufficiency, salt-losing congenital adrenal hyperplasia, and idiopathic orthostatic hypotension.

Selection of drugs

Cortisol and cortisone are used only for replacement therapy in patients with adrenal insufficiency, i.e., diminished production of endogenous glucocorticoids. They do not have any use in antiinflammatory therapeutic regimens because of their relatively high mineralocorticoid activity.

Prednisone, prednisolone, and methylprednisolone, on the other hand, have considerable antiinflammatory activity, intermediate plasma half-lives, and relatively low mineralocorticoid activity. These characteristics render them first-choice drugs for long-term antiinflammatory and immunosuppressant regimens. Indeed, prednisone and its derivatives are the most commonly used glucocorticoids for treatment of several autoimmune diseases, including collagen diseases (systemic lupus erythematosus and polymyositis-dermatomyositis), vasculitis syndromes (polyarteritis nodosa, giant cell arteritis, and Wegener's granulomatosis), gastrointestinal inflammatory diseases (Crohn's disease and ulcerative colitis), and renal autoimmune diseases (glomerulonephritis and the nephrotic syndromes). Intermediate-acting glucocorticoids are also used for treatment of bronchial asthma and chronic obstructive pulmonary disease.

Dexamethasone and betamethasone exhibit minimal mineralocorticoid activity and maximal antiinflammatory activity, have prolonged plasma half-lives, and pronounced growth-suppressing properties. They represent the best choice for patients who need maximal acute antiinflammatory therapy (e.g., septic shock or brain edema). Because of their prolonged action and growth suppression and bone demineralization properties, they are not first-choice drugs for long-term therapy.

Recently, a new regimen of glucocorticoid administration has been used in which glucocorticoids are administered every other day, instead of daily. This alternate-day regimen has both advantages and disadvantages. The antiinflammatory effects of glucocorticoids with an intermediate duration of action persist longer than their suppressive effects on the HPA axis and bone growth rate. Therefore, by administering prednisone or prednisolone every other day, there is less suppression of the HPA axis and bone growth while achieving a beneficial antiinflammatory effect. However, there are two potential problems. First, in some patients, insufficient control of inflammation is observed. Second, abruptly switching from a daily dosing schedule to an alternate-day regimen may precipitate symptoms of clinical hypocortisolism (i.e., a sense of being tired, nausea, vomiting, hypotension) on days between doses.

Side effects, clinical problems, and toxicity

Clinical syndromes associated with glucocorticoid and mineralocorticoid production include those resulting from lesions in the adrenal (primary) or pituitary (secondary) gland, as well as some instances of ectopic (inappropriate) ACTH production. Clinical problems most commonly encompass enzyme deficiencies, autoimmune diseases, and inappropriate or unrelated ACTH secretion from tumors.

Exposure to excessive levels of glucocorticoids

Cushing's syndrome is associated with excessive exposure to glucocorticoids. Its clinical manifestations include hypertension, truncal obesity, diabetes, hirsutism, acne, ecchymoses, proximal muscle weakness, wide purple stria over the skin, and psychiatric manifestations. The syndrome results most commonly from exogenous administration of glucocorticoids. However, there are also endogenous causes, including pituitary ACTH-dependent Cushing's syndrome, ectopic ACTH syndrome, ectopic corticotropin-releasing hormone syndrome, cortisol-secreting adrenal adenomas, and rarely, adrenal carcinoma (Fig. 33-6). To diagnose Cushing's syndrome, the presence of increased cortisol production must be confirmed by: (1) an increased urinary free cortisol concentration, and (2) failure of serum cortisol concentrations to be suppressed to less than 5 μg/dl in response to a low dose of dexamethasone. A patient with an increased cortisol production not suppressed by a low dose of dexamethasone should undergo further testing to distinguish among the different causes of Cushing's syndrome. In most cases, a high-dose dexamethasone suppression test can be used to differentiate between pituitary ACTH-dependent Cushing's disease and other causes of Cushing's syndrome. For this test, serum cortisol concentrations are determined prior to and after administration of oral dexamethasone for 3 days. If plasma cortisol concentrations decrease to less than 50% of baseline, a pituitary site is indicated; if not, an adrenal tumor or ectopic ACTH syndrome is indicated.

Many cases of pituitary Cushing's syndrome result from corticotropin- or ACTH-secreting adenomas that are constantly stimulating the adrenal glands and are only partially responsive to steroid feedback suppression. Successful removal of the adenoma can often relieve the symptoms. However, many of these tumors

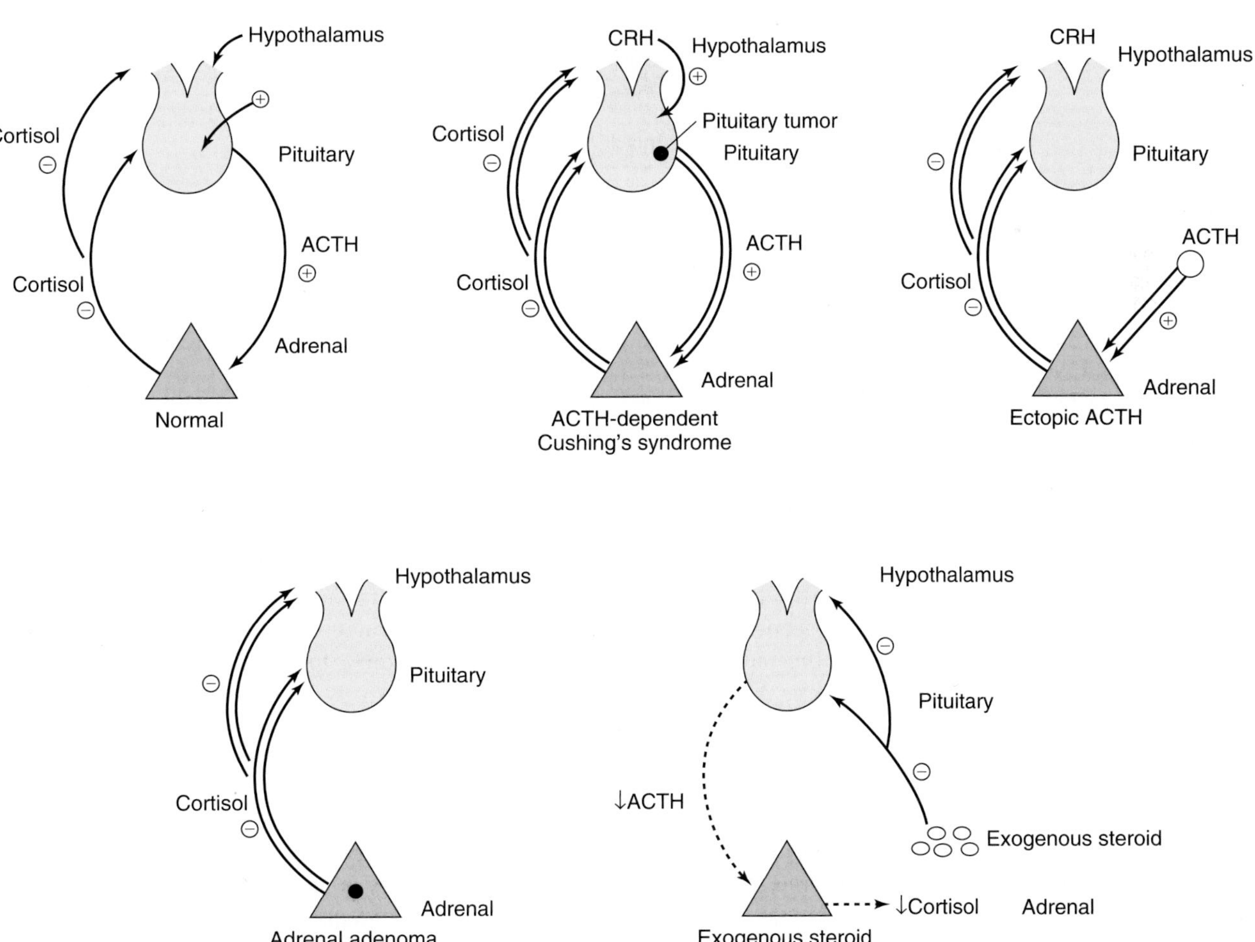

Figure 33-6 Hypercortisolemia and its impact on normal feedback mechanisms in Cushing's syndrome, ACTH-dependent Cushing's syndrome, ectopic ACTH syndrome, adrenal adenoma, and exogenous steroid administration. +, Stimulation; –, inhibition.

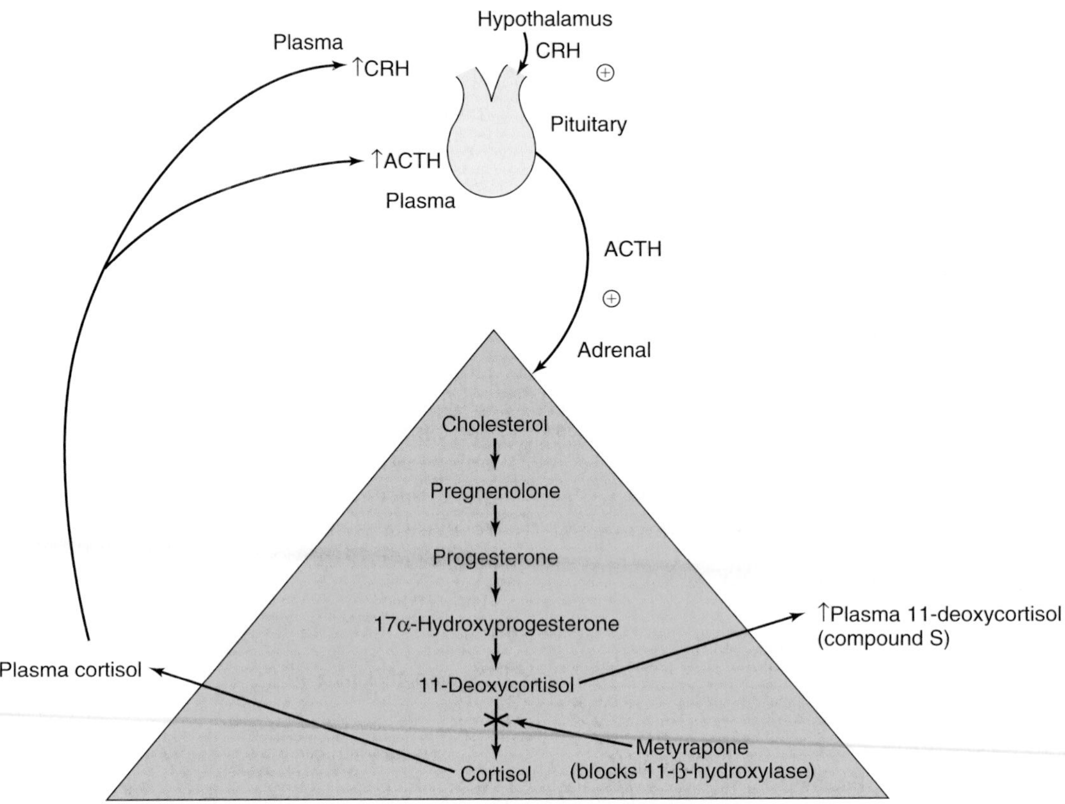

Figure 33-7 The basis of the metyrapone test to evaluate pituitary responsiveness to lowering plasma cortisol concentrations.

are microadenomas and difficult to isolate and remove. To evaluate patients with hypercortisolemia, metyrapone is administered and plasma ACTH, cortisol and 11-deoxycortisol concentrations in the plasma and urine are measured the following day. Metyrapone is a competitive inhibitor of the 11-hydroxylase enzyme involved in cortisol synthesis, thus leading to a reduced plasma cortisol concentration and an increased production of 11-deoxycortisol. A decrease in the concentration of cortisol and an increase in concentrations of 11-deoxycortisol and ACTH following the metyrapone test are indicative of a positive response (Fig. 33-7). Failure to respond to this test indicates a lesion in hypothalamic-pituitary function.

Surgical removal is the best treatment for excess cortisol (or aldosterone) secretion by an adrenal tumor. Treatment with biosynthetic inhibitors such as aminoglutethimide, ketoconazole, mitotane, or steroid receptor antagonists such as mifepristone may be useful in cases in which surgical treatment does not sufficiently reduce elevated steroid concentrations (see New Horizons).

A primary adrenal excess of mineralocorticoids occurs occasionally in patients with adrenal tumors, producing a syndrome of hypertension, hypokalemia and metabolic alkalosis, and slight hypernatremia. Both plasma and urinary aldosterone concentrations are elevated in the patient after high sodium intake. In the absence of a surgical cure, an important inhibitor is spironolactone, which is also used clinically as a diuretic and an antihypertensive agent. Spironolactone binds to the mineralocorticoid receptor and acts as a competitive antagonist to aldosterone.

Disorders associated with decreased cortisol production

Decreased cortisol production is associated with either primary or secondary adrenal insufficiency. Primary adrenal insufficiency is most commonly secondary to an autoimmune polyendocrine deficiency syndrome. Other causes are tuberculosis, adrenal hemorrhage, granulomatous diseases, amyloidosis, metastatic neoplasia, and congenital unresponsiveness to corticotropin. The secondary causes of adrenal insufficiency include adrenal suppression occurring after the administration of glucocorticoids (very common) or after treatment of Cushing's syndrome and diseases of the hypothalamus or pituitary gland leading to ACTH deficiency.

Plasma cortisol concentrations should be measured in patients with suspected acute adrenal insufficiency, and if low, patients should be treated immediately with intravenously administered hydrocortisone. A further test is required to confirm a diagnosis in patients with suspected chronic adrenal insufficiency, in which ACTH is administered intravenously. If the problem lies at the secondary or pituitary level (low ACTH secretion), a response will be obtained; failure to respond indicates a primary adrenal insufficiency. In either case, cortisol replacement should be initiated.

Congenital adrenal hyperplasia

Congenital adrenal hyperplasia can result from alterations in any of the steps in steroid synthesis leading to diminished cortisol secretion and consequent stimulation of synthesis and release of ACTH. Depending on the site of the abnormality, the steroidogenesis pathway in the adrenal gland is shifted, resulting in an imbalance of specific hormones, such as an excess secretion of androgens. The cornerstone for treatment of patients with congenital adrenal hyperplasia is administration of glucocorticoids to suppress ACTH secretion, thereby decreasing stimulation of the adrenal gland and inappropriate steroid synthesis (see Clinical Problems box).

CLINICAL PROBLEMS

Side effects caused mainly by high concentrations maintained for a long time

Most common side effects:

- Development of cushingoid habitus (truncal obesity, moon facies, buffalo hump), salt retention, and hypertension (i.e., iatrogenic Cushing's syndrome)
- Suppression of the immune system (rendering the patient vulnerable to common and opportunistic infections)
- Osteoporosis (rendering the patient vulnerable to fractures)
- Peptic ulcers (resulting in gastric hemorrhages or intestinal perforation)
- Suppression of growth in children
- Behavioral problems
- Reproductive problems
- Prolonged suppression of the HPA axis after drug discontinuation

Glucocorticoids and the HPA axis

Suppression of the HPA axis is the most common side effect of long-term glucocorticoid therapy, and can appear within days after initiation of treatment. Patients receiving glucocorticoids in doses equivalent to 5 mg or more of prednisone daily for more than 2 weeks should be considered as having a suppressed HPA axis. The time needed for recovery depends on the type of glucocorticoid given, the dose and frequency of administration (i.e., daily versus alternate days), and the length of treatment. In cases of prolonged administration, it may take up to a year or longer to recover. The short ACTH test is used to assess recovery.

Glucocorticoids and bone

A major side effect of glucocorticoids, especially when given for prolonged periods, is their detrimental action on bone. Patients at highest risk of acquiring glucocorticoid-induced osteoporosis are children and postmenopausal women. This osteoporosis involves bone trabeculae, the most metabolically active site. Glucocorticoids cause osteoporosis by disrupting the regulation of calcium metabolism at several levels: (1) by decreasing intestinal absorption and renal reabsorption of calcium; (2) by exerting a direct antianabolic and catabolic action on bone; and (3) by blocking the protective effect of calcitonin.

Glucocorticoids increase the 1α-hydroxylation of 25-hydroxyvitamin D to its active 1,25-dihydroxyvitamin D form, which facilitates intestinal calcium absorption. However, glucocorticoids also block the biological effect of active vitamin D, so the absorption rate of calcium decreases despite high concentrations of circulating 1,25-dihydroxyvitamin D. The parathyroid gland responds to the resulting hypocalcemia by secreting more parathyroid hormone, which catabolizes bone in an attempt to increase calcium concentrations in the extracellular fluid.

Glucocorticoids also affect bone directly by inhibiting osteoblastic activity. Furthermore, glucocorticoids may stimulate osteolysis by accelerating transformation of precursor cells to osteoclasts resulting in increased bone resorption. This is documented by increased concentrations of hydroxyproline in urine as an index of increased bone collagen catabolism. Finally, glucocorticoids block the bone-sparing effect of calcitonin, a peptide synthesized by the parafollicular cells of the thyroid gland that inhibits osteoclastic bone resorption (see Chapter 41).

Glucocorticoids and glucose

Glucocorticoids acquired their name from their role in glucose metabolism. They increase plasma glucose concentration by:

- increasing gluconeogenesis and glucose secretion by the liver
- increasing liver sensitivity to the gluconeogenic action of glucagon and catecholamines
- decreasing glucose uptake and utilization by peripheral tissues
- increasing the substrate for gluconeogenesis (increasing proteolysis and inhibiting protein synthesis in muscles)

As a consequence, the long-term administration of glucocorticoids may lead to hyperglycemia and diabetes mellitus in susceptible subjects.

Other side effects

Long-term administration of glucocorticoids also increases the risk for developing peptic ulcers. It has been proposed that glucocorticoids cause peptic ulcers by increasing gastric acid output and inhibiting synthesis of mucopolysaccharides that protect gastric mucosa from acid. Because even short-term treatment (<1 month) with glucocorticoids may cause gastric irritation or ulcers, some physicians prescribe antacids or H_2-histamine receptor blockers with glucocorticoids (see Chapter 55).

The main acute effect of glucocorticoids in the central nervous system is promotion of arousal and general euphoria. However, prolonged treatment may cause depression, sleep disturbances, and in some cases, true psychotic ideation.

Glucocorticoids can suppress the synthesis and secretion of gonadotropins and their effects on the gonads. Long-term glucocorticoid treatment in men may cause hypogonadism associated with decreased plasma testosterone concentrations. In women, anovulation, oligomenorrhea, or dysfunctional uterine bleeding may occur.

In most children, linear growth rate is impaired with long-term glucocorticoid therapy. Although long-term administration causes a decreased secretion of growth hormone from the anterior pituitary, the inhibitory effect of glucocorticoids on growth is thought to be due to inhibition of the effects of insulin-like growth factor-I (formerly known as somatomedin C).

New horizons

Much effort has been expended on identifying drugs for treating symptoms of hypercortisolemia, including specific glucocorticoid receptor antagonists. The steroid hormone antagonist mifepristone (RU 486) has a high affinity for both human progesterone receptors and glucocorticoid receptors, and weakly binds to androgen receptors. Mifepristone can antagonize the actions of glucocorticoids and suppress the negative feedback of endogenous cortisol. It has been used to treat endometriosis and breast cancer, to interrupt pregnancy through release of prostaglandins and increased uterine contractile sensitivity to prostaglandins, and to initiate labor. In addition, it can be used as a contraceptive drug to inhibiting follicle maturation, ovulation, and egg implantation. Currently, mifepristone is approved for the termination of intrauterine pregnancy, not for the management of glucocorticoid excess.

TRADE NAMES

In addition to generic and fixed-combination preparations and the drugs listed in the Major Drugs box, the following trade-named materials are some of the important compounds available in the United States.

Aminoglutethimide (Cytadren)
Betamethasone (Celestone)
Cortisone (Cortone)
Ketoconazole (Nizoral)
Mifepristone, RU-486 (Mifeprex)
Mitotane (Lysodren)
Prednisolone (Prelone)
Spironolactone (Pldactone)

FURTHER READING

Arnaldi G, Angeli A, Atkinson AB, et al. Diagnosis and complications of Cushing's syndrome: A consensus statement. *J Clin Endocrinol Metab* 2003; 88(12):5593-5602.

Axelrod L. Corticosteroid therapy. In Hung W, Kahn CR, Loriaux DL, et al, editors: *Principles and practice of endocrinology and metabolism*, 3rd ed. Philadelphia, Lippincott Williams & Wilkins, 2001.

Walsh JP, Dayan CM. Role of biochemical assessment in management of corticosteroid withdrawal. *Ann Clin Biochem* 2000; 37 (Pt 3):279-288.

Self-assessment questions

1. Which is the best test to assess the recovery of the hypothalamus-pituitary-adrenal axis in patients withdrawing from exogenous glucocorticoids?

a. Morning serum cortisol
b. Evening serum cortisol
c. Morning plasma ACTH
d. Insulin-tolerance test
e. ACTH stimulation test

2. Which moiety confers glucocorticoid activity on the corticoid molecule?

a. The hydroxyl group at carbon 17
b. The hydroxyl group at carbon 11
c. The keto group at carbon 3
d. The keto group at carbon 11
e. The hydroxyl group at carbon 20

3. All the following are the advantages of the alternate-day glucocorticoid therapy *except:*

a. Minimizes the clinical manifestations of hypercortisolism (Cushing's syndrome).
b. Facilitates the recovery of the hypothalamus-pituitary-adrenal axis.
c. Beneficial in the treatment of adrenocortical insufficiency.
d. Lessens growth suppression in children.
e. Does not compromise the antiinflammatory effects of glucocorticoids.

4. Each of the following is an indication for mineralocorticoid treatment *except:*

a. Primary adrenocortical insufficiency (Addison's disease).
b. Diabetic hyporenin-hypoaldosteronism.
c. Autoimmune glomerulonephritis.
d. Salt-losing congenital adrenal hyperplasia.

5. The most common cause of Cushing's syndrome is:

a. ACTH-dependent pituitary Cushing's disease.
b. Ectopic ACTH production.
c. Administration of exogenous steroids.
d. Adrenal adenoma.

CHAPTER 34

Drugs to treat asthma and chronic obstructive pulmonary disease

Lynn M. Crespo

Major Drugs

Albuterol* (AccuNeb, Proventil, Ventolin)	Terbutaline (Brethine, Bricanyl, Brethaire)
Cromolyn† (Intal, NasalCrom)	Theophylline (Slo-bid, Slo-Phyllin, Uniphyl, Theo-24, Theo-Dur)
Ipratropium (Atrovent)	Tiotropium (Spiriva)
Montelukast (Singulair)	Zafirlukast (Accolate)
Nedocromil (Tilade)	Zileuton (Zyflo)
Salmeterol (Serevent)	

*In the UK and Japan the drug name is salbutamol.

†In the UK the drug name is sodium cromoglycate; in Japan the drug name is cromoglycate sodium.

Therapeutic overview

Asthma is a chronic inflammatory disorder of the large airways in which many different cellular elements play a role. A characteristic feature of asthma is obstruction of the airways (predominantly in the third to seventh generation of the bronchi) that is reversible with time or in response to treatment. Even when patients have a normal airflow (which for mild asthmatics is much of the time), their lungs are hyperreactive to a variety of stimuli that occur naturally (e.g., cold air, exercise, chemical fumes) or are used to test pulmonary function (e.g., methacholine, histamine, cold air). **Bronchial hyperreactivity (BHR)** correlates with inflammation of the bronchi, which includes damage to the epithelium and eosinophil infiltration. Other characteristics of asthma include airway mucosal edema, mucus hypersecretion, and remodeling of the airways. Symptomatically, patients experience chest tightness, wheezing, shortness of breath, or coughing. Mild forms of the disease occur in up to 10% of the population, but asthma requiring regular treatment affects about 2% of the population.

In comparison to asthma, **chronic obstructive pulmonary disease (COPD)** is defined by the Global Initiative on Obstructive Lung Disease as "A disease state characterized by airflow limitation that is not fully reversible. The airflow limitation is usually progressive and associated with an abnormal inflammatory response of the lungs to noxious particles and gases." COPD includes chronic obstructive bronchiolitis with fibrosis and obstruction of small airways, emphysema with enlargement of airspaces and destruction of lung parenchyma, loss of lung elasticity, and closure of small airways. The majority of patients with COPD experience a triad of symptoms, including:

- Chronic obstruction
- Emphysema
- Mucus plugging

Smoking is by far the primary cause of COPD; other risk factors include occupational dust and

Abbreviations

BHR	bronchial hyperreactivity
cAMP	cyclic adenosine monophosphate
CNS	central nervous system
COPD	chronic obstructive pulmonary disease
EIB	exercise-induced bronchospasm
FEV_1	forced expiratory volume in 1 second (liters)
GCs	glucocorticoids
GI	gastrointestinal
IV	intravenous
LTs	leukotrienes
LTMs	leukotriene modulators
MDI	metered-dose inhaler
PEF	peak expiratory flow

chemical exposures, environmental exposure (second hand smoke) and genetic predisposition (primarily α_1 antitrypsin deficiency). Currently, COPD is the fourth leading cause of death in the United States.

Normal bronchial smooth muscle tone is controlled by vagal innervation (see Chapter 9). Cholinergic activity or sensitivity is often increased in asthmatics, and increased cholinergic tone is the primary reversible component of COPD. However, most patients with asthma also have increased adrenergic activity (see Chapter 10), which manifests as increased wheezing, if patients are treated with β-adrenergic blocking drugs (e.g., propranolol). A variety of agents can contribute to the **inflammation** of asthma; however, immediate hypersensitivity to **common allergens** is the most common cause. It is estimated that 80% of children and 50% of adults with asthma are allergic. The common allergens include seasonal outdoor allergens (e.g., ragweed pollen, grass pollen, and the fungus *Alternaria*) or the year-round indoor allergens (dust mites, cockroaches, and domestic animals). Although allergens cause release of the preformed granule mediator histamine, which can trigger bronchospasm, antihistamines are relatively ineffective in treatment of asthma, suggesting that other factors are involved. Indeed, numerous "newly generated" inflammatory mediators have been recognized as being increased in asthmatic patients, including the arachidonic acid metabolites and cytokines (Fig. 34-1). In recent years, studies have focused on the role of the **leukotrienes (LTs)** as primary bronchoconstrictors (primarily LTD_4). Agents that inhibit the synthesis or action of the LTs, known as **leukotriene modulators (LTMs)**, have been approved for and are prescribed as second line agents for treatment of asthma.

The inflammatory component of COPD differs from that of asthmatics in that COPD patients demonstrate increased neutrophil as opposed to eosinophil activity. In COPD, macrophage activation, resulting from exposure to noxious substances, releases neutrophil chemotactic factors, including interleukin-8 and LTB_4. Additionally, proteases are released that destroy connective tissues in the lung parenchyma, and oxidants capable of direct tissue damage are produced. These

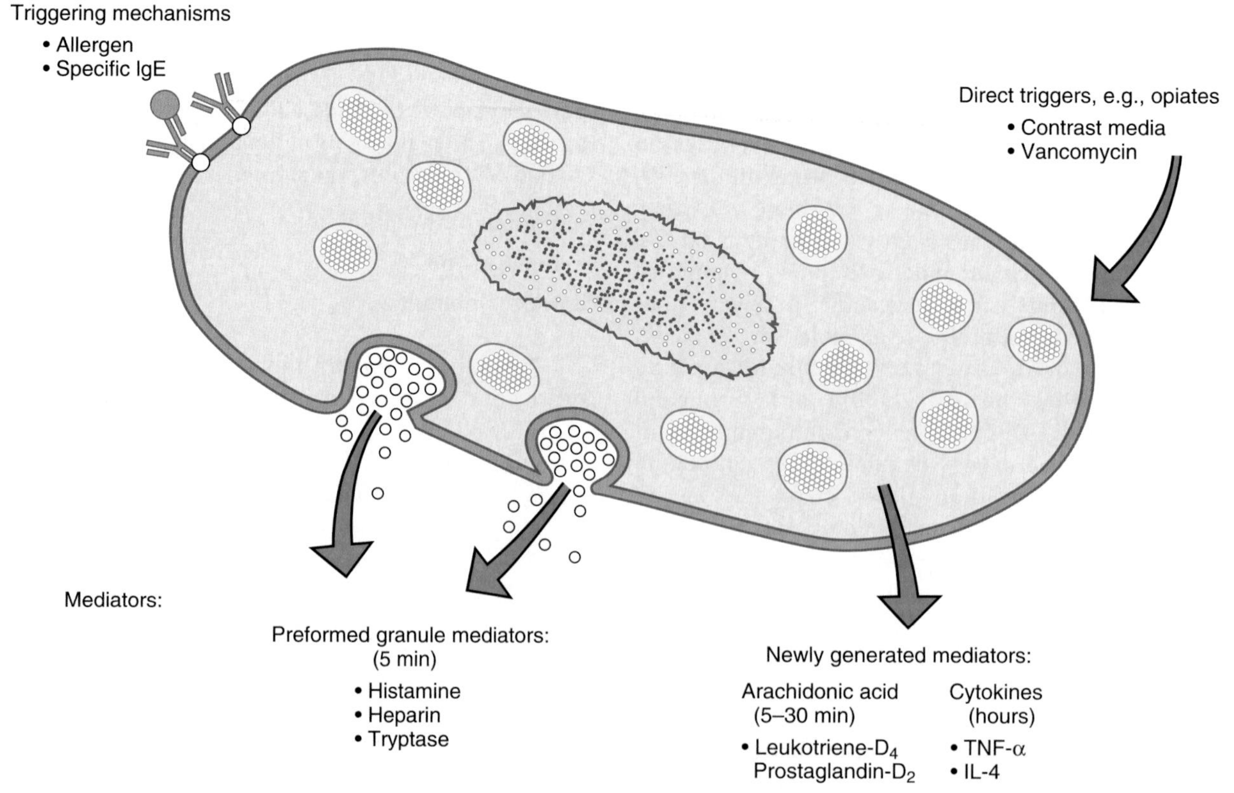

Figure 34-1 Mast cell mediator release. Some mediators are also produced by basophils. *TNF-α*, Tumor necrosis factor-alpha; *IL-4*, interleukin-4.

events lead to the small airway pathology and increased mucus secretion characteristic of COPD. The resulting chronic inflammation causes fibrosis and a proliferation of smooth muscle. As the airways progressively narrow, airflow is severely limited, and function declines.

Asthma is treated using three main approaches. The first is avoidance of the causative factors, when possible, particularly for patients sensitive to indoor allergens. The second is the use of antiinflammatory drugs, including the chromones, glucocorticoids (GCs) (see Chapter 33), and LTMs. If used regularly, these drugs can reduce the signs and symptoms of BHR. Last, drugs that can reverse or inhibit the development of bronchoconstriction are important; these compounds include methylxanthines, epinephrine and selective β_2-adrenergic agonists (see Chapter 10), and the muscarinic receptor antagonists (see Chapter 9).

The current therapeutic approaches for treatment of COPD are similar to those for asthmatics with three exceptions. First, the cessation of smoking is essential to prevent development of COPD and to slow its progression. Second, of the antiinflammatory drugs, only GCs are currently used in the treatment of acute exacerbations of COPD; long-term use of these compounds for management of COPD is not recommended. Last, although β_2 receptor agonists are used as bronchodilators for COPD patients, muscarinic antagonists result in better improvement, and the combination of a β_2-agonist and a muscarinic receptor antagonist may be used.

The goals in treatment of pulmonary disease are to reverse acute episodes, control recurrent episodes, and reduce bronchial inflammation and associated hyperreactivity. Three general considerations must be kept in mind:

- The inhaled route of drug administration is very important and has special requirements.
- The pharmacokinetics of pulmonary drugs are based primarily on lung-function response; blood concentrations are relevant only for the xanthines.
- The most commonly encountered side effects of respiratory medications are the short-term side effects of the xanthines and the cumulative side effects of orally administered GCs.

However, because of the many patients using inhaled steroids or β_2-adrenergic receptor agonists, the relatively infrequent side effects of these drugs may also be important. A summary of the therapeutic considerations for the treatment of asthma and COPD are presented in the Therapeutic Overview box.

THERAPEUTIC OVERVIEW

Antiinflammatory agents

Chromones for controlling mediator release from mast and other cells and for their generalized membrane-stabilizing effects

Glucocorticoids, local or systemic, for controlling transcription of mediator genes, and for controlling edema, mucus production, and eosinophil infiltration

Leukotriene modulators to decrease inflammatory mediator synthesis or antagonize inflammatory mediator receptors

Bronchodilators

Methylxanthines for reducing the frequency of recurrent bronchospasm

β_2-Adrenergic receptor agonists for relaxing bronchial smooth muscle and decreasing microvascular permeability

Muscarinic receptor antagonists for inhibiting the bronchoconstrictor effects of endogenous acetylcholine

Mechanisms of action

Treatment of asthma and COPD involves the use of drugs with mechanisms that affect different aspects of these diseases. Table 34-1 summarizes these drugs and their mechanisms of action.

Chromones (cromolyn and nedocromil)

Cromolyn sodium, purified from the umbelliferous plant *Amnii visagna*, has several important actions. Cromolyn was originally shown to inhibit the release of histamine from mast cells *in vitro*. Subsequently, it was demonstrated that inhaled cromolyn could inhibit exercise-induced bronchospasm (EIB), progressively decrease BHR, and inhibit seasonal rises in BHR in patients allergic to grass pollen. Studies have demonstrated that cromolyn and nedocromil alter the function of delayed chloride channels, thus inhibiting cellular activation. This effect on chloride channels in the nerves innervating the bronchial airways explains the ability of these drugs to inhibit cough. These compounds also inhibit degranulation of mast cells in response to antigen challenge and inhibit the eosinophil-mediated antigen-

Table 34-1 Mechanisms of action of drugs to treat asthma and COPD

Beneficial Effect	Drug Class	Cellular Mechanisms
Decreased inflammation	Chromones	Prevent the release of inflammatory mediators Alter chloride ion channel function
	Glucocorticoids (GCs)	Regulate gene expression
	Leukotriene modulators (LTMs)	Decrease leukotriene (LT) synthesis or prevent LT receptor activation
	Antihistamines	Prevent activation of histamine receptors
Bronchodilation	Methylxanthines	Increase cAMP Antagonize the actions of adenosine (?)
	β-Adrenergic receptor agonists	Increase cAMP
	Muscarinic antagonists	Block activation of muscarinic receptors by endogenous acetylcholine

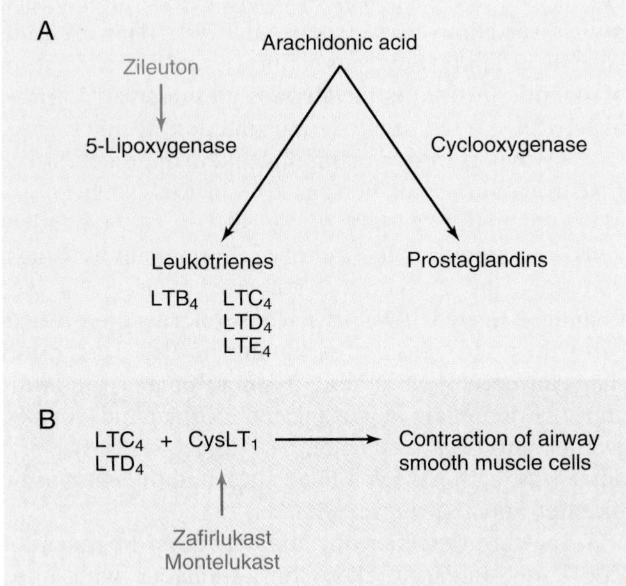

Figure 34-2 Newly generated lipid mast cell mediators depicting the sites of action of the leukotriene modulators *(LTMs)*. Zileuton inhibits 5-lipoxygenase, thereby inhibiting the synthesis of the leukotrienes, whereas zafirlukast and montelukast are antagonists at the $CysLT_1$ receptor. The inhibitory actions of the LTMs are shown in red.

induced inflammatory response. Cromolyn and nedocromil are active only on the lung when given by the inhaled route and have no direct bronchodilator effect.

Glucocorticoids

The GCs have multiple actions that decrease inflammation in asthma, which is key to improving asthmatic symptoms and preventing exacerbations. In controlling the inflammation of asthma, the primary effect of the GCs is to alter gene expression. The GCs, through activation of GC receptors (see Chapter 33), suppress the expression of genes for many inflammatory proteins. Inflammation is mediated by the increased expression of multiple inflammatory proteins, including cytokines, chemokines, adhesion molecules, and inflammatory enzymes and receptors. The expression of most of these inflammatory proteins is regulated by increased gene transcription, which is controlled by proinflammatory transcription factors. The GCs are believed to switch off only inflammatory genes and do not suppress all activated genes because of the selective binding to coactivators that are activated by proinflammatory transcription factors.

In addition to suppressing the synthesis of inflammatory mediators, the GCs also induce the transcription of several antiinflammatory proteins, including lipocortin, neural endopeptidase, and inhibitors of plasminogen activator. Lipocortin inhibits the activity of phospholipase A_2, thus decreasing the release of free arachidonic acid from phospholipids, and reducing the subsequent production of leukotrienes and prostaglandins.

GCs also have effects on eosinophils. They decrease bone marrow production of eosinophils and enhance their removal from the circulation by mediating their adherence to capillary walls (margination). GCs also reduce the local accumulation of eosinophils by inhibiting the release of eosinophil chemotactic factors, such as leukotriene B_4 and cytokine tumor necrosis factor–α. The effect of the GCs on neutrophils is opposite to that on eosinophils. By inhibiting margination and stimulating bone marrow production, GCs lead to an increase in circulating neutrophils.

Leukotriene modulators

The LTs are potent inflammatory mediators that are generated from the metabolism of arachidonic acid through the lipoxygenase pathway (Fig. 34-2). These compounds, along with prostaglandins and related compounds, belong to a group of substances termed the eicosanoids (see Chapter 17). The LTs are synthesized in many inflammatory cells in the respiratory system, including eosinophils, mast cells, macrophages and basophils, and are responsible for mediating numerous asthmatic effects through stimulation of specific LT receptors. LTB_4 is a potent neutrophil chemotactic agent whose actions result from stimulation of members of the BLT receptor family. Similarly, LTC_4 and LTD_4 cause bronchoconstriction, mucus hypersecretion and mucosal edema, and increase bronchial reactivity through activation of the CysLT receptor family. The effects of the LTs can be modulated either by inhibiting LT biosynthesis or by blocking the activation of LT receptors. Synthesis of LTs can be blocked by inhibition of the 5-lipoxygenase enzyme by the drug zileuton, whereas activation of the $CysLT_1$ (formerly known as the LTD_4) receptor can be antagonized by the "kast" compounds, such as zafirlukast and montelukast. These drugs are considered second-line agents in control of asthma. They are less effective antiinflammatory agents than the corticosteroids but are considered equally effective in reducing the frequency of acute episodes.

Methylxanthines

Theophylline is a methylxanthine, similar to caffeine. It has generally been thought that theophylline caused bronchodilation by acting on smooth muscle cells to inhibit catabolism of cyclic adenosine monophosphate (cAMP) through inhibition of phosphodiesterase. Although an increase in cAMP leads to bronchodilation, the clinical significance of phosphodiesterase inhibition is questionable because concentrations of theophylline required to inhibit this enzyme exceed those achieved with usual doses. More recent studies have suggested that the primary effects of theophylline may be due to its actions as an adenosine receptor antagonist in bronchial smooth muscle and other tissues. Inhalation of adenosine causes bronchoconstriction in patients with asthma but does not affect nonasthmatics. Adenosine also causes contraction of isolated airway smooth muscle and an increase in histamine release from lung cells. The proposed adenosine receptor antagonist mechanism of theophylline, however, does not explain why enprofylline, another xanthine derivative without adenosine receptor antagonist properties, is a more potent bronchodilator than theophylline. It has also been proposed that theophylline may act by altering intracellular Ca^{2+} transport, but there is limited evidence for this action. Thus, the molecular mechanisms of action of theophylline remain unclear.

β_2-Adrenergic receptor agonists

Stimulation of β_2-adrenergic receptors raises cAMP concentrations and inhibits smooth muscle contraction (see Chapter 10). Physiologically, bronchial smooth muscle relaxes, and the release of some mast cell derived bronchoconstricting substances is inhibited. Additionally, these drugs decrease microvascular permeability and suppress parasympathetic ganglionic activity (see Chapter 9). There is no evidence for an antiinflammatory effect of adrenergic agents, or for any beneficial effect on BHR.

Several β_2 agonists have been used therapeutically for the treatment of asthma. Epinephrine and isoproterenol are highly effective but are reserved for special circumstances due to their non-selective activity, leading to β_1-mediated cardiac stimulation. Short-acting selective β_2 agonists include albuterol,* terbutaline, metaproterenol, bitolterol, and pirbuterol. Formoterol (not available in the United States) and salmeterol have been developed as highly lipid soluble long-acting agents ($t_{1/2}$~12 hours).

Muscarinic receptor antagonists

Bronchial smooth muscle is innervated mainly by the parasympathetic nervous system, and its activation causes bronchoconstriction (see Chapter 8). Prior to the development of modern pharmacology, stramonium leaves containing certain belladonna alkaloids were smoked as a treatment for asthma. The muscarinic antagonist atropine can be used as a bronchodilator and to reduce secretions, but its use is limited by toxicity in the central nervous system. Ipratropium bromide is a quaternary nitrogen derivative of atropine that does not cross the blood-brain barrier but competitively inhibits muscarinic acetylcholine receptors in bronchial smooth muscle (see Chapter 9). Ipratropium is used as an inhaled preparation. Tiotropium is a long-acting antimuscarinic bronchodilator that has been developed and shows benefit specifically for COPD patients.

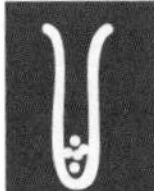

Pharmacokinetics

General considerations

The pharmacokinetics of the drugs used for the treatment of asthma are complicated as a consequence of the routes of absorption and differences in the rates of response. Because blood concentrations are irrelevant for all drugs except the xanthines, mean pulmonary function response times are generally used as an indicator of pharmacokinetic profiles. Response rates vary significantly from patient to patient, presumably

*In the UK and Japan the drug name is salbutamol.

reflecting differences in the specific pathological state of the obstruction in the lung.

Chromones

Both cromolyn and nedocromil act on inflammatory cells and neurons in the bronchial epithelium and are active only when inhaled. Thus, as mentioned, blood concentrations are largely irrelevant. Cromolyn is very poorly absorbed from the gastrointestinal (GI) tract and has few systemic side effects because it is rapidly excreted. Although cromolyn has no direct bronchodilator activity and should not be used to treat an acute attack, it can be used to control EIB if administered 10 to 15 minutes before the onset of physical activity. In contrast to its rapid effect in controlling EIB, long-term treatment with cromolyn or nedocromil requires several days or even weeks to produce an optimal antiinflammatory effect.

Glucocorticoids

The pharmacokinetics for the GCs are presented in Chapter 33. When used for the treatment of asthma or COPD, responses to inhaled or oral steroids can occur within 4 hours but may take as long as 2 weeks, depending on the nature of the underlying lung disorder.

Leukotriene modulators

The LT receptor antagonists, montelukast and zafirlukast, as well as the lipoxygenase inhibitor zileuton are all orally administered, which is advantageous for treatment of children and other patients who have difficulty with or are noncompliant with inhaled therapies. Zileuton has the disadvantage of requiring dosing four times per day. However, montelukast and zafirlukast have similar pharmacokinetic profiles and may be administered once (montelukast) or twice (zafirlukast) daily. Zileuton is also an inhibitor of hepatic *CYP3A* enzymes and will lead to increased serum theophylline levels, if the two drugs are administered concurrently.

Methylxanthines

Theophylline clearance is influenced by food, smoking, age, disease, and other drugs metabolized by the liver (Table 34-2). Monitoring serum theophylline concentrations is necessary for any patient taking more than a minimal dose orally because of the multiple factors that influence blood concentrations and because the range of safe therapeutic concentrations is narrow. The therapeutic range is 5 to 15 μg/mL, and serious toxicity is increasingly likely at blood concentrations above 20 μg/mL.

Table 34-2 Factors influencing blood concentrations of theophylline

	Blood Concentrations	Half-Life (hrs)
Normal adults	—	6-7
Neonates	Increased	8-24
Children (1-16 years)	Decreased	3-7
Mature subjects (>50 years)	Increased	—
Cigarette smokers	Decreased	4-5
Drugs Affecting Metabolism		
Cimetidine Ciprofloxacin Erythromycin Propranolol Oral contraceptives Zileuton	Increased	Prolonged
Phenytoin Rifampin	Decreased	Decreased
Diseases		
Hepatic disease Congestive heart failure COPD Fever	Increased	Prolonged

When administered intravenously, theophylline can act rapidly on the lungs as a bronchodilator. However, this requires large bolus doses, which are only used occasionally because of toxicity. It is easier to maintain therapeutic blood concentrations by the oral route using delayed-release preparations.

β_2-Adrenergic receptor agonists

A general comparison of the pharmacokinetic profiles for these compounds is presented in Table 34-3. As is evident, the bronchodilation that occurs in response to inhaled β_2-adrenergic receptor agonists is fairly consistent with an onset between 5 to 30 minutes. Tightness of the chest will abate in most patients with asthma within 10 minutes after an injection of epinephrine. An optimal effect usually occurs within an hour and may last for 2 to 4 hours. In most circumstances, β_2-agonists are effective for approximately 4 to 6 hours. Prolonged, repeated use of short-acting β_2-agonists, however, can cause a significant increase in heart rate in a small proportion of patients due to systemic absorption and concomitant stimulation of cardiac β_1-receptors. With the development of a longer-acting β_2-agonist (salmeterol), which lasts for more than 12 hours, this problem may be partially resolved. However, unlike the short-acting β-agonists, salmeterol is not effective in treating acute

Table 34-3 Comparison of the pharmacokinetics of β_2-adrenergic receptor agonists and muscarinic receptor antagonists

	Receptor Selectivity	Route of Administration	Bronchodilator Response		
			Onset (min)	Peak (hrs)	Duration (hrs)
ADRENERGIC AGONISTS					
Epinephrine	None	Inhalation*	3-5	—	1-2
		Subcutaneous	6-15	0.5	1-3
Metaproterenol	β_2	Inhalation	5-10	1-2	3-4
		Oral	15-30	0.5	6-8
Albuterol	β_2	Inhalation	5-10	1-2	4-6
		Oral	15-30	2-3	6-8
Terbutaline	β_2	Inhalation	5-10	—	4-8
		Injected	5-10	0.5	1-2
		Oral	15-30	—	6-8
Salmeterol	β_2	Inhaled	15-30	22	12+
MUSCARINIC ANTAGONISTS					
Ipratropium	None	Inhaled	15-20	1-2	3-6
Atropine	None	Inhaled	5-20	1-2	1-4
Tiotropium	M_3 (?)	Inhaled	5	1.5-3	24

*Represents average values for administration via both nebulizer and metered-dose inhaler (MDI).

episodes. Its major uses are in controlling nocturnal asthma and some cases of EIB.

Muscarinic receptor antagonists

Ipratropium bromide is poorly absorbed and has few systemic side effects. The peak bronchodilator effect occurs 1 to 2 hours after inhalation, with a duration of action of 3 to 5 hours (Table 34-3). The newer agent, tiotropium, which may exhibit selectivity at M_3 muscarinic receptors (see Chapter 8), has a duration of action of 24 hours. Both of these agents are used for management of the bronchoconstrictive component of COPD.

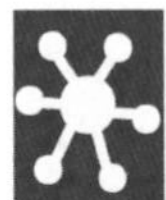

Relation of mechanisms of action to clinical response

The central problem in managing asthma is that the symptoms range from occasional tightness in the chest after exercise (which may require no treatment) to continuous airway obstruction. Assessment of pulmonary function by spirometry (to measure forced expiratory volume [FEV_1]) or a portable peak flow meter (to measure peak expiratory flow [PEF]) is essential to monitor baseline pulmonary function, correlate changes in airway obstruction with symptoms, and determine the patient's response to treatment. The patient should be encouraged to record peak flow values for a 2-week period to establish a baseline, assess the severity of episodes, and determine his or her individual response to treatment. An FEV_1 or a PEF less than 80% of the predicted value is considered a mild obstructive episode. The predicted value is determined from the patient's age, gender, race, and height, based on a healthy population. Alternatively, the patient's best recorded PEF baseline value can be used as the predicted value. An FEV_1 or PEF less than 60% of predicted values indicates moderate obstruction, and an FEV_1 or PEF less than 40% of predicted values indicates severe obstruction. Most patients will show a 15% to 20% increase in FEV_1 or PEF 15 to 20 minutes following administration by metered dose inhaler (MDI) of a bronchodilator, such as a β_2 agonist or a muscarinic antagonist. Less than a 12% increase indicates inadequate acute bronchodilator response, and further treatment will be necessary.

Reduced allergen exposure, inhaled cromolyn sodium or nedocromil, inhaled GCs, or oral LTMs are antiinflammatory treatments that are each capable of reducing BHR to help manage the problem. The chromones are used prophylactically only and are most effective for treating extrinsic asthma in children and young adults as well as EIB.

Although the mechanism of action of the xanthines is not clear, regular treatment can be very effective in controlling symptoms. The xanthines prevent episodes of airway obstruction. Theophylline administered intravenously (IV) is active within minutes, but when taken orally, 1 to 2 hours are required before its effects occur. Its duration of action depends on absorption and metabolism but correlates well with blood concentrations.

Systemic GCs are the most effective treatment for both moderately severe and severe asthma and are used for treatment of acute exacerbations of COPD. However, these compounds lead to development of side effects following chronic administration (Chapter 33). The indication for oral corticosteroids is ongoing airway obstruction that is not relieved by other medicines within 1 to 2 days. Only a very small percentage of asthmatics (0.1%) become dependent on steroids, but this may represent as many as 10 patients per 100,000; thus, it is a very important cause of iatrogenic disease.

For acute, severe episodes, corticosteroids, such as methylprednisolone may be administered IV. Although the GCs have no direct bronchodilator effects, and 6 hours are required to achieve maximal effects, peripheral blood eosinophil counts decline within 2 hours and significant effects on lung function and symptoms can be observed within 4 hours of systemic administration. Thus, the early use of systemic steroids has become a mainstay of treatment in the management of acute asthma and COPD, both in outpatient practice and in the hospital. In some cases, high doses of inhaled steroids can be used to abort an attack. However, in severe cases, mucus impaction and poor ventilation of the lungs prevent the effective delivery of inhaled steroids, and, therefore, oral or IV administration is urgently required.

Outpatient treatment of asthma

In a patient with occasional wheezing, a diagnosis must be established by demonstrating a reversible airway obstruction and having the patient use a peak-flow meter at home for 2 weeks. Treatment involves using a β_2-agonist, two puffs by MDI when necessary. In a patient with EIB, it is imperative to show that breathlessness after exercise is associated with airway obstruction. Recommended treatments to prevent EIB are an inhaled β_2-agonist, two puffs 5 to 10 minutes before exercise, or two puffs of cromolyn sodium by MDI 10 to 20 minutes before exercise, or one puff of salmeterol by MDI 30 to 60 minutes prior to exercise. Inadequate control requires identifying the causes of the BHR. Leukotriene antagonists are currently under investigation for the treatment of EIB.

In a patient who is suffering more frequent symptoms, including nocturnal asthma, or using a short-acting β_2 receptor agonist more than three times per week, documentation of reversible airway obstruction is of paramount importance. This can be achieved by: (a) measuring changes in PEF or FEV_1 before and after administration of the bronchodilator; (b) demonstrating a 15% to 20% increase in PEF or FEV_1 after bronchodilator administration; or (c) demonstrating hyperreactivity to inhaled histamine, methacholine, or cold air. Skin tests should be used to identify relevant sensitivities to allergens. If a patient has positive skin test results, then education relevant to decreasing exposure to the specific allergens is a first step in management. These patients may benefit from the combination of a long-acting β_2 agonist, in combination with a leukotriene antagonist. Short-acting bronchodilators should be reserved for the reversal of acute episodes.

Inhaled corticosteroids, cromolyn or nedocromil, taken on a regular basis, should be prescribed for any patient who continues to have symptoms necessitating bronchodilator therapy more than three times weekly. If symptoms persist and spirometry confirms obstruction, the dose of the antiinflammatory agent should be increased, and an oral delayed-release theophylline preparation, 200 to 300 mg twice or three times a day should be considered. After 4 days, the theophylline blood concentrations should be between 5 to 14 μg/mL.

For acute asthmatic episodes, doses of inhaled steroids should be increased to four puffs four times a day and theophylline added as needed. A short course of oral steroids (60 mg of prednisone reduced to zero over 6 to 8 days) may also be necessary. In the clinic or emergency room, a nebulized β_2-agonist is the first line of treatment, which can be repeated three times at 20-minute intervals, and then hourly thereafter. Patients not responding to nebulizer treatment should receive steroids (60 mg of prednisone or 125 mg of methylprednisolone IV).

Patients with unresponsive persistent symptoms may be treated with regular-dose, inhaled steroids four puffs four times a day, theophylline up to a maximum therapeutic range, and additional drugs, including cromolyn or nedocromil sodium, a β_2-agonist delivered by nebulizer, or an LTM. Courses of oral steroids (6-30 days) and other agents may also be considered. The physician should reinforce education on allergen avoidance and consider other factors, such as diet, fungal infections, drug reactions, sinusitis, and gastroesophageal reflux.

Antihistamines are generally not recommended for treatment of asthma. However, many allergic patients with rhinitis and asthma use antihistamines with no apparent harmful effects. Sedative antihistamines should not be used in patients with acute bronchospasm. Antibiotics are commonly recommended for management of an exacerbation of asthma because of sputum production but should be reserved for those patients with bronchial infiltrates, fever, or sinusitis.

Allergen avoidance

Exposure to allergens, particularly those found indoors, is well recognized as an important cause of asthma. Identification of sensitivity and education about measures necessary to decrease exposure are an important part of antiinflammatory treatment. For control of dust mites, enclosing the mattress and pillows in dust mite–proof covers, washing all bedding in boiling water, and removing carpets are important measures. Removing cats or dogs from the environment may be helpful; however, it will take weeks or months for the associated allergen levels to decrease. Cockroach eradication may be important for inner-city homes, in particular, and should involve such measures as enclosing all food, sealing gaps around pipes, and the use of poisonous bait. Special issues related to asthma are discussed in Box 34-1.

Side effects, clinical problems, and toxicity

The side effects of drugs used with asthma are summarized in the Clinical Problems box.

CLINICAL PROBLEMS

Cromolyn/nedocromil

Less potent than steroids; may produce coughing during inhalation

Inhaled steroids

Low doses induce Candidiasis; high doses cause growth retardation and other systemic effects

Oral steroids

High doses can cause GI problems and CNS disturbances

Leukotriene antagonists

Rare hepatotoxicity and eosinophilia

Theophylline

Narrow therapeutic index, nausea and vomiting, seizures, cardiac dysrhythmias

β_2-Adrenergic receptor agonists

Tachycardia, tremors

Antimuscarinic agents

Dry mouth

Box 34-1 Special issues

Asthma in young children

There are special issues concerning side effects and the delivery of antiasthmatic drugs in children. Children can be treated with a nebulizer and face mask from infancy; by age 7, they can usually use an MDI with a spacer. Inhaled cromolyn is the antiinflammatory drug of choice because it has no serious side effects and is available for use in a nebulizer. In young children, total daily doses of inhaled steroids as low as 400 μg have been reported to reduce growth. Long-term oral theophylline treatment (taken as sprinkles on food) is effective and well tolerated in many children. However, hyperactivity and/or learning difficulties are potential problems. Allergen avoidance should be recommended for any child who requires more than occasional treatment and has positive skin test results.

Pregnancy

Management of asthma in pregnancy is similar to that used for adults. Risks of uncontrolled asthma to the fetus outweigh the possible risks of drug therapy. Inhaled chromones, inhaled steroids, β_2-adrenergic receptor agonists, delayed-release theophylline, antibiotics for sinusitis associated with asthma, and short courses of steroids are given in normal adult doses.

COPD

A reactive airway often develops in patients with COPD as their disease progresses. Although these patients are generally not allergic, drug treatment of this condition has many features in common with asthma treatment in adults. Thus, theophylline, β_2-adrenergic receptor agonists, steroids, and nebulized cromolyn are commonly used. Special issues include oxygen supplementation and monitoring blood gases in respiratory compromised patients. Responses to muscarinic receptor antagonists in patients with COPD are better than with β_2-agonists, whereas the converse is true in asthmatics.

Chromones

The side effects of cromolyn and nedocromil are restricted to the irritant effects of inhaling the drugs. There is very little convincing evidence for short-term or long-term drug toxicity and no recognized blood concentration that is toxic. Occasional cases of dermatitis, gastroenteritis, and myositis that are apparently associated with cromolyn use have been reported but are very unusual.

Glucocorticoids

The side effects of systemic corticosteroids are discussed in Chapter 33 and are mentioned here briefly in the context of pulmonary disease. The most important issue is the difference between short- and long-term use. Treatment with high-dose steroids, even short-term, can cause hypertension, diabetes, GI bleeding, and central nervous system (CNS) disturbances. Elevations in blood glucose concentration and emotional changes are common but are usually easy to manage. Long-term steroid use produces a wide range of severe side effects, including thinning of the skin (striae, bruising), osteoporosis with rib fractures and vertebral compression, aseptic necrosis of the femoral head, which usually presents with pain, diabetes with complications, GI discomfort, ulceration and bleeding, and CNS disturbances, including frank psychosis. Prolonged oral use of steroids causes profound suppression of adrenal function. If patients are taking oral steroids for more than 7 days, the dose should be gradually reduced because abrupt withdrawal can result in life-threatening adrenal insufficiency. Patients must be made fully aware of the harmful effects of long-term orally administered steroids.

When they were initially introduced, there was great concern that inhaled steroids would produce serious side effects, either locally in the lungs or systemically. There were concerns that even low-dose inhaled steroids might accelerate cataract formation, influence bone formation, or delay recovery of the adrenal axis. In general, these fears were not borne out. The major side effects of inhaled steroids (e.g., beclomethasone dipropionate) have been oral Candidiasis and occasionally irritation triggered by the use of an MDI. In all patients, but especially those with COPD, yeast infection of the mouth (thrush) is common and requires local treatment. The efficacy of chronic use of inhaled steroids in patients with COPD is not well established, because the possibility exists that inhaled steroids might encourage fungal colonization in patients with a severe fixed obstruction, i.e., $FEV_1 < 40\%$ predicted.

In contrast, large doses of inhaled corticosteroids have significant effects on the adrenal axis and bone growth in children. Inhaled steroids are all active locally, and their systemic side effects depend on both absorption and metabolism. There is some evidence that budesonide and flunisolide have fewer systemic effects because their metabolites are inactive.

Leukotriene modulators

Adverse effects of the leukotriene antagonists zafirlukast and montelukast are minimal, and, generally, the drugs are well tolerated. However, rare cases of hepatotoxicity and eosinophilic vasculitis have occurred. The clinical features of the vasculitis are consistent with Churg-Strauss syndrome, a life-threatening condition typically treated with systemic corticosteroid therapy. The occurrence of the vasculitis syndrome appears to be linked with the decrease or withdrawal of oral corticosteroid therapy. Therefore, the patient and the physician need to be acutely aware of symptoms related to eosinophilia, vasculitic rash, worsening of pulmonary symptoms, cardiac complications, and developing neuropathies.

Zileuton can produce elevated liver enzymes, typically in the first few months of therapy. It also inhibits hepatic *CYP3A* enzymes, which metabolize many drugs, including theophylline. Considering the correlation of serum levels of theophylline to therapeutic and toxic effects, patient monitoring is necessary, if the two drugs are used concurrently.

Methylxanthines

The most common side effects of theophylline that can occur within the normal therapeutic range are either GI (e.g., heartburn, abdominal pain, nausea, vomiting) due to an increase in gastric acidity or are related to their effects in the CNS. These include headache, anxiety, tremor, and insomnia (similar to those reported with excess use of caffeine). Side effects occur with concentrations as low as 5 μg/mL but increase greatly in frequency and severity when the blood concentrations of theophylline exceed 15 μg/mL (the recommended upper limit). When blood concentrations exceed 20 μg/mL, seizures and cardiac dysrhythmias are possible and become common when blood concentrations exceed 35 μg/mL. Seizures can result in significant mortality; thus, elevated theophylline concentrations are treated as an emergency with gastric lavage, oral charcoal, and even dialysis. Considerable attention has been given to CNS symptoms in children receiving methylxanthines, including poor attention and insomnia, with resultant poor school performance.

β_2-Adrenergic receptor agonists

The primary side effects of adrenergic agonists are cardiac stimulation, hypertension, tremor, and restlessness (see Chapter 10). The use of β_2-selective agonists decreases the risk of some of these effects. Inhaled β_2-agonists generally produce fewer side effects than oral preparations. Nonetheless, tachycardia and muscle tremor still occur. Continued use of these agents may result in the desensitization of β receptors (see Chapter 2); however, GC therapy can prevent or partially reverse this phenomenon. Epinephrine can ameliorate severe life-threatening asthma attacks when administered subcutaneously. However, there are very few indications for this form of treatment in older patients or in those with underlying cardiovascular disease.

It was once believed that chronic use of short-acting β_2 receptor agonists would worsen asthma and increase the risk of asthma-related deaths. These concerns were based on early studies when isoproterenol, a nonselective β receptor agonist, was administered via MDI. More recent studies on the effects of the selective β_2 receptor agonists on asthma do not support these conclusions.

Muscarinic receptor antagonists

Inhaled ipratropium or tiotropium may give rise to drying of the mouth and upper airways. Because these drugs are administered via inhalation, systemic antimuscarinic side effects, such as those associated with atropine, are unusual (see Chapter 9).

New horizons

As our understanding of the role of inflammation and the immune response in chronic respiratory disease increases, novel approaches to modify these pathways are being developed. DNAse has now been approved for the treatment of pulmonary symptoms in cystic fibrosis. This disease is characterized by a significant inflammatory cell burden in the lung, high cell turnover, and DNA survival. DNAse acts to hydrolyze the residual DNA, destroying the inflammatory infiltrate, and alleviating some of the symptoms of the disease. Clinical trials are also underway to assess the effectiveness of DNAse in chronic bronchitis.

LTB_4 is a potent neutrophil chemotactant and is increased in the sputum of COPD patients. Specific BLT receptor antagonists are currently being developed for management and treatment of COPD. A potential adverse effect of such drugs is compromising the patient's immune defenses.

Tumor necrosis factor-α can induce interleukin-8, stimulate proinflammatory cells, and stimulate production of proteases that destroy tissue. Currently, antibodies to tumor necrosis factor-α are being used for the treatment of rheumatoid diseases and may be of benefit in the management of COPD. Their limitations include the need for repeated injections.

Different immunosuppressive treatments have been used in patients with severe or steroid-dependent asthma, including gold, IV gamma globulin, troleandomycin, cyclosporine, and methotrexate. The most promising results have been seen for methotrexate. Other immunosuppressive drugs are being evaluated, including FK-506, which appears to be able to inhibit the transcription of interleukin-2 and other T-cell activation genes.

Many patients with late-onset asthma have chronic colonization of their skin, nails, or mucosal surfaces with fungi (e.g., *Trichophyton* or *Aspergillus* species) or yeast (e.g., *Candida* or *Torulopsis* species). In some cases these patients also have immediate hypersensitivity to antigens derived from the colonizing organism. The treatment of fungi on skin or mucosal surfaces constitutes part of the overall treatment of some asthmatics. Recent evidence has indicated that treatment with systemic antifungals (fluconazole or itraconazole, see Chapter 50) may be helpful for asthma in some cases.

TRADE NAMES

In addition to generic and fixed-combination preparations and the drugs listed in the Major Drugs box, the following trade-named materials are some of the important compounds available in the United States.

Inhaled steroids

Beclomethasone (Beclovent, Vanceril)
Budesonide (Pulmicort)
Flunisolide (AeroBid)
Fluticasone (Flovent)
Triamcinolone acetonide (Azmacort)

Methylxanthines

Oxtriphylline (Choledyl)

β_2-Selective adrenergic receptor agonists

Bitolterol (Tornalate)
Metaproterenol (Alupent, Metaprel)
Pirbuterol (Maxair)

FURTHER READING

Barnes PJ, Adcock IM. How do corticosteroids work in asthma? *Ann Intern Med* 2003; 139(5):359.

Corless JA, Paracha M. The use of leukotriene modifying drugs in asthma and other respiratory diseases. *Inflamm Allergy* 2002; 1(3):271-275.

Faulkner MA, Hilleman DE. Pharmacologic treatment of chronic obstructive pulmonary disease: Past, present, and future. *Pharmacotherapy* 2003; 23(10):1300-1315.

Self-assessment questions

1. An 11-year-old child experiences wheezing and difficulty breathing when exercising. Which of the following drugs would be recommended to prevent these symptoms?
   a. Albuterol
   b. Cromolyn
   c. Fluticasone
   d. Ipratropium
   e. Zafirlukast

2. A 74-year-old patient with a 50-year history of smoking presents to the emergency room with an acute exacerbation of his COPD. Which of the following classes of drugs would be most effective at relieving the bronchoconstrictive component of his disease?
   a. Antimuscarinic agents
   b. Corticosteroids
   c. Leukotriene modulators
   d. Oxygen
   e. β_2-adrenergic receptor agonists

3. An essential component in the treatment and management of pulmonary disease is control of the inflammatory process. Which of the following agents will reduce the recruitment of eosinophils?
   a. Albuterol
   b. Flunisolide
   c. Ipratropium
   d. Nedocromil
   e. Zafirlukast

4. Desensitization of the β_2-adrenergic receptor is a documented consequence of overuse of these drugs. Of the following inhaled β_2 agonist bronchodilators, which would reduce the risk of this effect due to its long half-life?
   a. Albuterol
   b. Metaproterenol
   c. Salmeterol
   d. Bitolterol

CHAPTER 35

Estrogens and progestins

Michael K. Fritsch
Fern E. Murdoch

Major Drugs

Estrogens	Inhibitors of steroidogenesis and aromatase
Progestins	
Combination estrogen and progestin	
Estrogen/progesterone receptor ligands	

Therapeutic overview

The two major classes of female sex hormones are the **estrogens** and the **progestins.** Together they serve important functions in the development of female secondary sex characteristics, control of pregnancy and the ovulatory-menstrual cycle, bone homeostasis, and modulation of many metabolic processes. Their roles in cardiovascular health and cognitive function remain controversial.

Estrogens

There are three endogenous estrogens in humans:

- **17β-Estradiol,** the principal ovarian estrogen
- **Estriol,** the principal placental estrogen
- **Estrone,** a metabolite of 17β-estradiol and a major ovarian and postmenopausal estrogen

Estrogens coordinate systemic responses during the ovulatory cycle, including regulation of the reproductive tract, pituitary, breasts, and other tissues. They also play a role in the progression of some tumors. The hypothalamic-pituitary-ovarian axis is depicted in Figure 35-1, *A,* and target organs for hormone action are shown in Figure 35-1, *B.* Estrogens are also responsible for mediating development of secondary sex characteristics when a female enters puberty, including progressive development of the fallopian tubes, uterus, vagina, and external genitalia. Upon estrogen stimulation, more fat is deposited in the breast, buttocks, and thighs, leading to the characteristic female habitus. Estrogens also: (a) initiate breast development by increasing ductal and stromal growth; (b) contribute to accelerated body growth at puberty; (c) stimulate closure of the epiphyses in the shafts of the long bones; (d) stimulate synthesis and secretion of prolactin from pituitary lactotrophs; (e) accelerate cellular proliferation of uterine endometrium and stroma in the absence of progesterone, as occurs in the follicular phase of the menstrual cycle; (f) induce RNA and protein synthesis in cells; (g) generate thickening of the vaginal mucosa and thinning of cervical mucus; (h) aid in maintaining bone mass, as evidenced by substantial but preventable (with estrogen replacement therapy) bone loss in postmenopausal women; and (i) stimulate hepatic produc-

Abbreviations

ACTH	adrenocorticotropic hormone
CBG	corticosteroid-binding globulin
ERα	estrogen receptor α
ERβ	estrogen receptor β
FSH	follicle-stimulating hormone
GI	gastrointestinal
GnRH	gonadotropin-releasing hormone
HDL	high-density lipoprotein
HRE	hormone responsive element
IM	intramuscular
IUD	intrauterine devices
LDL	low-density lipoprotein
LH	luteinizing hormone
SERM	selective estrogen receptor modulator
SHBG	sex hormone-binding globulin

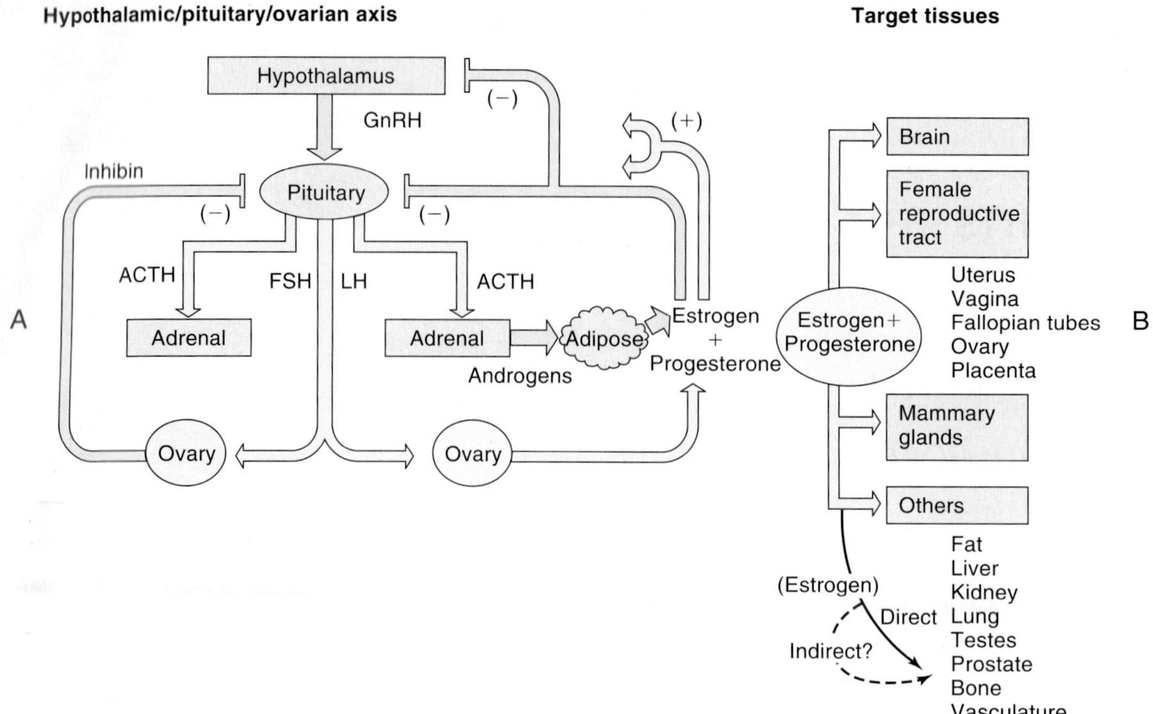

Figure 35-1 Feedback loops and target tissues. **A,** Negative and positive feedback action of estrogens and progesterone on the hypothalamic-pituitary-ovarian axis. **B,** Other target tissues for these steroid hormones.

tion of sex hormone–binding globulin (SHBG), thyroid-binding globulin, blood-clotting factors (VII to X), plasminogen, and high-density lipoprotein (HDL), but inhibit antithrombin III and low-density lipoprotein (LDL) formation. Estrogens also increase retention of sodium and water, occasionally causing edema. Estrogens can also decrease bowel motility. Estrogens may play a direct role in the progression of some endometrial tumors, and lifetime exposure to estrogens is the greatest risk factor for breast cancer. Continuous exposure of the uterus to unopposed estrogen can result in endometrial hyperplasia, episodes of breakthrough bleeding, and an increased risk of endometrial cancer.

Progestins

The important endogenous progestin is **progesterone,** but 17α-, 20α-, and 20β-hydroxyprogesterones have weak progestational activities as well. Estrogen priming is necessary for progesterone receptor expression in almost all progesterone-responsive tissues, including the uterus. Progesterone concentrations rise rapidly in the luteal phase of the menstrual cycle, resulting in a modulation of estrogen's action on the uterus. Progesterone opposes estrogen-induced proliferation in the uterus and initiates secretory changes in preparation for embryo implantation. In the absence of pregnancy, plasma progesterone concentrations decrease, resulting in sloughing of the endometrial lining. Progesterone is responsible for causing the increased basal body temperature observed in the luteal phase. A variety of menstrual cycle disorders are treated with estrogens, progestins, or both. Progesterone is important in mammary glandular development and, unlike in the uterus, probably stimulates cellular proliferation in the breast. Progesterone also aids in the maintenance of pregnancy, inhibits uterine contraction, can alter carbohydrate metabolism, may foster decreased HDL and increased LDL concentrations, and increases sodium and water elimination by competing with aldosterone for binding to mineralocorticoid receptors.

Combined effects

Progesterone and estrogen coordinate the events associated with the luteal phase of the ovulatory cycle and pregnancy. In females with primary ovarian failure, estrogens and progestins are administered to optimize normal development of secondary sex characteristics. An important pharmacological use of estrogens and progestins is as **contraceptives.** In this regard, estrogens and progestins act predominantly at the pituitary-hypothalamic axis to decrease production of the gonadotropins, follicle-stimulating hormone (FSH), and luteinizing hormone (LH). Inhibition of the midcycle LH surge prevents ovulation. A combination oral contraceptive formulation is also approved for the treatment of severe acne in females over age 15 years (acne vulgaris). Interestingly, antiestrogens have been developed that aid in **treatment of infertility** by inducing an increase in circulating FSH, which leads to ovulation. Estrogen and progestin replacement therapy has been extensively used in treatment of symptoms arising at menopause.

The major therapeutic uses of estrogens, progestins, their synthetic agonists and antagonists, and inhibitors of estrogen biosynthesis are summarized in the Therapeutic Overview box.

THERAPEUTIC OVERVIEW

Fertility control

Combination contraception (estrogens plus progestins)
Progestin-only contraception
Emergency contraception (estrogens plus progestins, progestins)
Contragestation (antiprogestin)

Infertility treatment

Ovulation induction (SERMs)

Replacement therapy

Acute symptoms of menopause (estrogens plus progestins, estrogens)
Prevention of osteoporosis (SERMs, estrogens)
Ovarian failure (estrogens plus progestins)
Dysfunctional uterine bleeding (progestins, estrogens plus progestins)
Luteal phase dysfunction (progestins)

Cancer chemotherapy

Breast cancer adjuvant treatment (SERMs, aromatase inhibitors, steroidogenesis inhibitors)
Advanced breast cancer (aromatase inhibitors, SERMs)
Advanced endometrial cancer (progestins)
Advanced prostate cancer (estrogens)
Breast cancer prevention (SERMs)

Others

Endometriosis (estrogens plus progestins, progestins, progesterone analog, progestin plus GnRH analog)
Dysfunctional uterine bleeding (progestins, estrogens plus progestins)
Luteal phase dysfunction (progestins)

Mechanisms of action

Biosynthesis of estrogens and progestins

Estrogens and progestins are produced by **steroidogenesis** in various tissues (see Fig. 35-1, *A*). The ovary is the predominant source of these steroids in nonpregnant, premenopausal women. A significant amount of estrogen is also produced by skeletal muscle, liver, and adipose tissue through the conversion of circulating androgens to estrone. Certain brain areas in males and females may produce estrogens through the conversion of circulating androgens by the enzymatic activity of aromatase. Small amounts of estradiol are produced in the male testes.

The rate-limiting step for the ovarian production of steroid hormones is the conversion of cholesterol to pregnenolone by cytochrome P450 side-chain cleavage enzymes (Fig. 35-2). Pregnenolone can then be converted directly to progesterone or 17α-hydroxypregnenolone. Through additional metabolic processes, these intermediates are converted to the androgenic steroids, **androstenedione** and **testosterone.** These androgens can be converted to estrone and 17β-estradiol, respectively, by the **aromatase** enzyme. Aromatase in the ovaries and peripheral tissues is responsible for catalyzing aromatization of the A ring and loss of the C19 methyl group, producing a molecule with estrogenic properties. Aromatase is the target molecule for **aromatase inhibitors,** which are used to lower estrogen levels in patients with estrogen responsive breast cancer. Estriol can be produced in the liver as an oxidation product derived mainly from estrone; some estriol is also made from estradiol. During pregnancy, the fetal-placental unit produces large amounts of estrogens (primarily estriol) and progesterone.

Progesterone is readily synthesized in the placenta, but direct placental conversion of cholesterol to estrogen does not occur. Maternal cholesterol is converted to dehydroepiandrosterone sulfate in fetal adrenals and then hydroxylated to the 16α-hydroxy derivative in fetal liver. In the placenta, which is rich in sulfatase and aromatase enzymes, the 16α-hydroxy derivative is then converted to estriol, whereas dehydroepiandrosterone sulfate is converted to estrone. The quantities of the various steroids produced in the adrenals, testes, ovaries, and placenta are probably regulated by the availability of key steroidogenesis enzymes in each particular cell type.

During the **menstrual cycle,** the pituitary gonadotropins FSH and LH regulate the synthesis and release of estrogen and progesterone from the ovary.

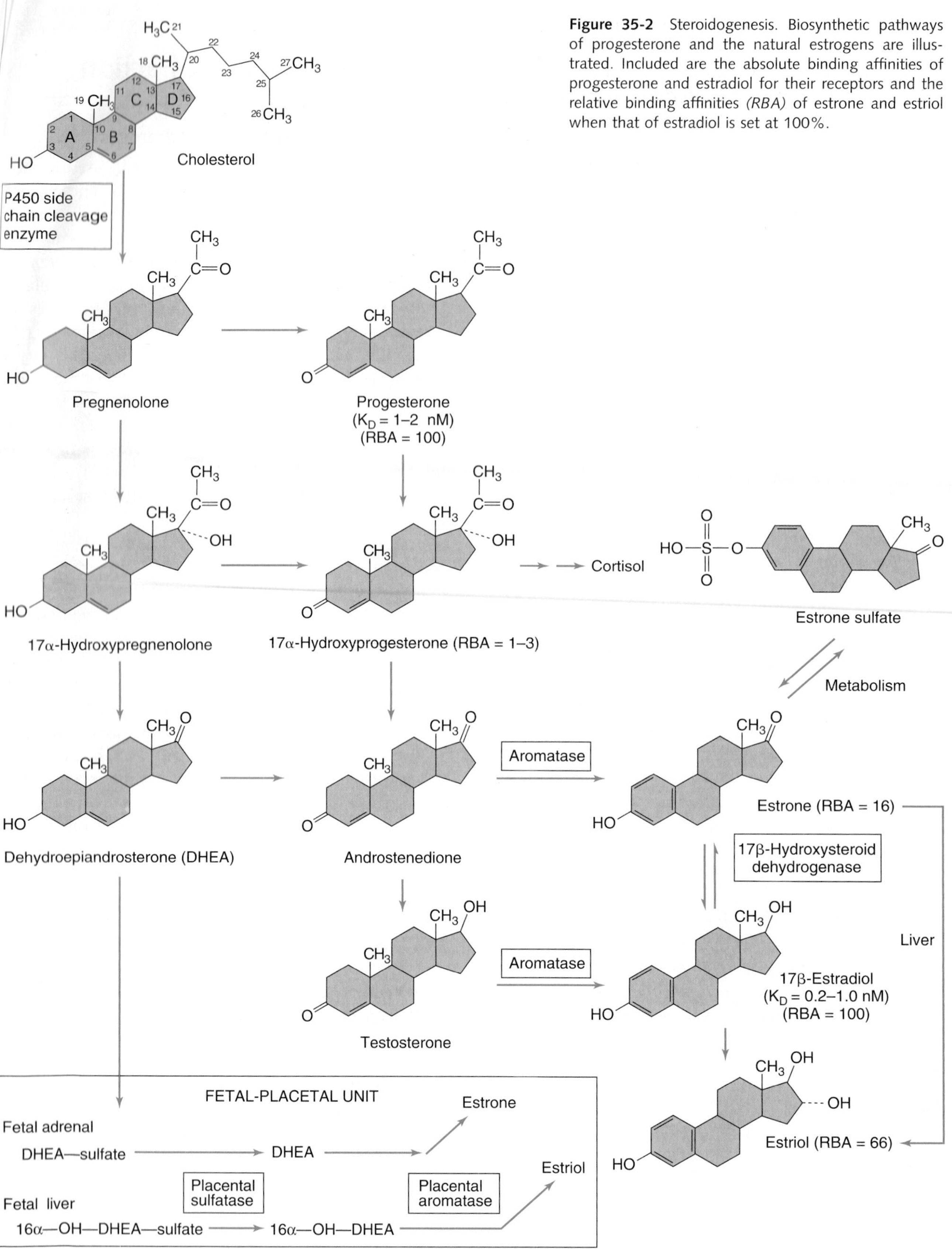

Figure 35-2 Steroidogenesis. Biosynthetic pathways of progesterone and the natural estrogens are illustrated. Included are the absolute binding affinities of progesterone and estradiol for their receptors and the relative binding affinities *(RBA)* of estrone and estriol when that of estradiol is set at 100%.

The pulsatile release of hypothalamic gonadotropin-releasing hormone (GnRH), in turn, regulates FSH and LH synthesis and release. GnRH concentrations are regulated through negative and positive feedback by the steroid hormones. Estrogens and progestins also act directly on the pituitary gonadotrophs to decrease FSH and LH concentrations. In addition, an ovarian protein, inhibin, negatively affects FSH synthesis. The pathways for the integrated control of hormone regulation are shown in Figure 35-1, *A*.

A normal ovulatory-menstrual cycle lasts 25 to 35 days. The steps in the ovarian and endometrial cycles are shown in Figure 35-3. The ovarian cycle is divided into the follicular (preovulatory) phase, which is predominantly concerned with the maturing follicle, and the luteal (postovulatory) phase, which is controlled by the corpus luteum. The follicle is the basic reproductive unit of the ovary and consists of an oocyte surrounded by granulosa cells, which are separated by a basement membrane from the theca cells. During follicular development, both the cell layers and a follicular cavity containing fluid (the antrum) enlarge. After ovulation, the remnants of the antral fluid, granulosa cells, and theca cells make up the corpus luteum. At the beginning of a menstrual cycle, FSH stimulates several follicles to accelerate maturation. FSH does this by binding to its cell-surface receptor on granulosa cells, leading to increased aromatase activity and conversion of androgens to estradiol. One follicle becomes dominant, whereas the others undergo atresia. By days 8 to 10 FSH concentrations are decreasing, but the dominant follicle has an increased number of FSH receptors and becomes more sensitive to circulating gonadotropin concentrations. LH concentrations rise slightly during this time. Circulating estradiol concentrations rise rapidly in the late follicular phase, initiating the mid-cycle LH surge (16-24 hours before ovulation) through positive feedback on the hypothalamic-pituitary axis. The LH surge leads to follicular production of progesterone, prostaglandin $F_{2\alpha}$, proteolytic enzymes, and, ultimately, to follicular rupture and ovulation.

The length of the follicular phase can vary, but the luteal phase is consistently about 14 days. The corpus luteum produces predominantly progesterone; its concentration rises throughout the first half of the luteal phase (peak concentrations of 10-20 ng/mL). The estrogen concentrations reach 0.2 ng/mL. These high concentrations feed back negatively on the hypothalamic-pituitary axis to keep concentrations of FSH and LH low. Unless pregnancy occurs, progesterone

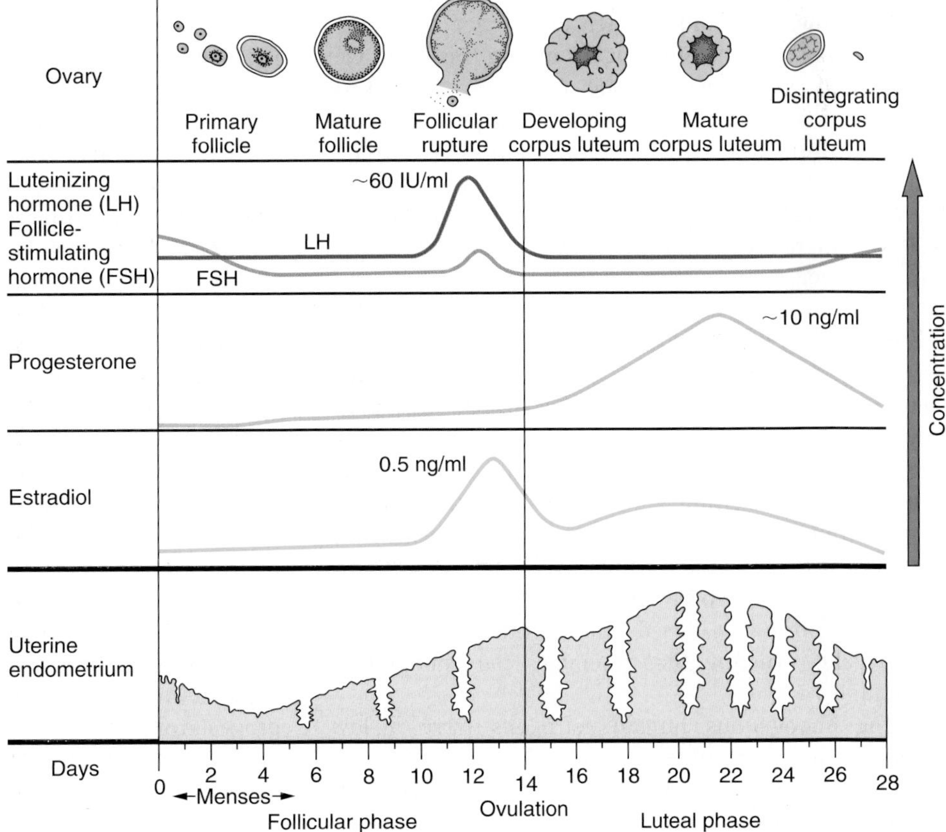

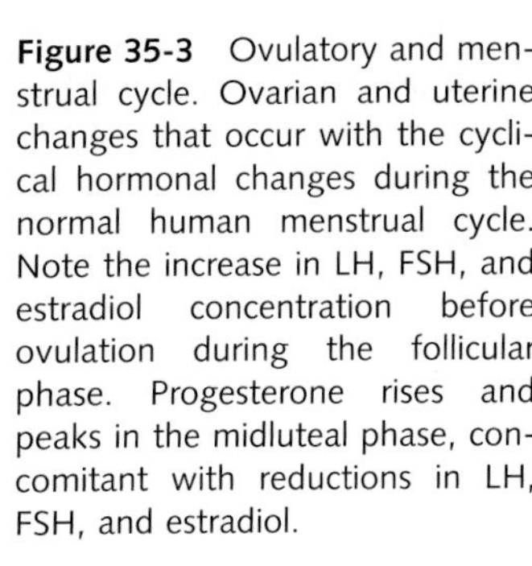
Figure 35-3 Ovulatory and menstrual cycle. Ovarian and uterine changes that occur with the cyclical hormonal changes during the normal human menstrual cycle. Note the increase in LH, FSH, and estradiol concentration before ovulation during the follicular phase. Progesterone rises and peaks in the midluteal phase, concomitant with reductions in LH, FSH, and estradiol.

and estrogen concentrations decline and luteolysis occurs, leading to menses (steroid withdrawal bleeding) and the beginning of a new cycle. The negative-feedback effect of high concentrations of estrogens and progestins is exploited in hormonal contraceptives, which inhibit the FSH and LH peaks and thereby prevent follicular maturation and ovulation.

In the event of **pregnancy**, the placenta secretes chorionic gonadotropin into the maternal circulation. The chorionic gonadotropin concentration rises rapidly after implantation and peaks about 6 to 8 weeks into pregnancy. Chorionic gonadotropin maintains the corpus luteum and stimulates progesterone production, which helps maintain pregnancy. The fetal-placental unit eventually becomes the major source of circulating progesterone and estrogens, especially estriol, sometime after the fifth week of pregnancy.

As women age, the number of follicles in the ovaries diminishes, predominantly because of atresia. Eventually, no follicles remain and the normal menstrual cycles cease **(menopause).** This lack of follicles means that estrogen and progesterone can no longer be made in the ovary. Without these two steroid hormones to feed back on the hypothalamic-pituitary axis, FSH and LH rise to very high concentrations. Adrenal androgens, predominantly androstenedione, are still produced and can be converted by aromatase to estrone in peripheral tissues. However, circulating estrogen concentrations are low and many women experience symptoms related to the absence of estrogens during this time. The major acute symptoms include vasomotor instability (hot flushes and sweats) and vaginal atrophy, resulting in discomfort, dyspareunia, and urethral syndrome. Other symptoms possibly related to decreased estrogen levels include loss of concentration, loss of libido, weight gain, depression, thinning hair, joint discomfort, and disrupted sleep.

Ligand structure

Estrogens can be classified structurally as either steroidal or nonsteroidal, with steroidal estrogens further divided into natural and synthetic compounds. The natural estrogens and progestins are steroids with structures derived from cholesterol. The structures of progesterone, the three endogenous human estrogens (estradiol, estrone, and estriol), and their biosynthetic pathways are shown in Figure 35-2. In general, the synthetic hormones used therapeutically have a heterocyclic structure that resembles the endogenous compounds.

The endogenous human estrogens have a low potency when administered orally because they are poorly absorbed and rapidly inactivated by first pass metabolism in the liver. Estradiol is the most potent of the three. The conjugated estrogens are coupled at C3, predominantly to sulfate but occasionally to glucuronic acid. Water-soluble conjugated estrogens have virtually no estrogenic activity and must be activated (hydrolyzed at C3) to be able to bind to the estrogen receptor. The endogenous estrogen pool is the result of active metabolic interconversions between the three naturally occurring estrogens and conjugated forms. Estradiol is the primary form in premenopausal women, whereas estrone sulfate predominates postmenopausally.

The synthetic estrogens include the steroidal agonists **ethinyl estradiol** and **mestranol,** used predominantly in combination oral contraceptives. These compounds have an ethinyl group at C17, which protects them against inactivation by the liver when taken orally. Mestranol is inactive until converted to ethinyl estradiol in the liver. A growing number of nonsteroidal, synthetic compounds that bind the estrogen receptor have been synthesized and are termed **selective estrogen receptor modulators (SERMs).** The activity of these compounds is highly tissue dependent, showing agonist effects in some tissues and antagonist effects in others. The prototypical SERM is **tamoxifen,** a nonsteroidal triphenylethylene derivative. Tamoxifen is an estrogen antagonist in breast and is used clinically for treatment, and more recently, prevention of breast cancer. A clinically important, though originally unanticipated, benefit of tamoxifen is its agonist activity in bone and the prevention of osteoporosis. The major clinical problem with tamoxifen is the significantly increased risk of endometrial cancer related to its estrogen-like (agonist) activity in the uterus. **Raloxifene** is a SERM used for treatment and prevention of osteoporosis in postmenopausal women. It has agonist activity in bone but displays no estrogen-like activity in breast or uterus. Clomiphene citrate is a racemic mixture of two stereoisomers and has both agonist and antagonist properties. It is used to induce ovulation. Considerable research is directed at identification of new SERMS with tissue specific agonist and antagonist properties for each therapeutic goal.

The progestin derivatives are classified on the basis of their structure at positions C21 or C19 (19-nortestosterone). The C21 derivatives include the natural progestins, progesterone and 17α-hydroxyprogesterone, which utilize the same carbon backbone as pregnenolone, from which they are derived. The synthetic C21 compounds are derivatives of 17α-hydroxyprogesterone and include medroxyprogesterone acetate, megestrol acetate, and hydroxyprogesterone caproate. The presence of an acetate ester in medroxyprogesterone acetate and megestrol acetate helps protect these compounds from being inactivated in the liver and allows their oral use.

this. The two active isomers of clomiphene reach peak plasma concentrations within 3 to 6 hours after an oral dose. However, the trans isomer (enclomiphene) has a shorter plasma elimination half-life (4-10 hours) than the cis isomer (zuclomiphene—>18 hours). Tamoxifen is administered orally, and absorption is somewhat slow with extensive metabolism. The major metabolites of tamoxifen include N-desmethyltamoxifen, which binds only weakly to estrogen receptors but is present in greater concentrations than tamoxifen itself, and 4-hydroxytamoxifen, which binds much more tightly to estrogen receptors but is present in low concentrations. The antiestrogen action of tamoxifen is probably aided by its metabolites. Conjugated metabolites of tamoxifen are primarily excreted by the biliary route into the feces. The enterohepatic recirculation of the metabolites, their binding to serum albumin, and their high-affinity binding to tissues all contribute to their long half-life of 7 days. Raloxifene is administered orally and is rapidly absorbed but is extensively conjugated to glucuronides by first pass metabolism in the liver. Raloxifene and its metabolites are interconverted with a mean plasma half-life of about 30 hours. Elimination is primarily in the feces. Orally administered danazol is rapidly absorbed and metabolized but takes 7 to 14 days to reach a steady-state concentration. Metabolites are excreted in both urine and feces.

Inhibitors of steroidogenesis and aromatase

Aminoglutethimide is rapidly absorbed after oral administration, with maximum circulating concentrations reached in 1.5 hours. Twenty percent to 35% of the drug is bound to plasma proteins, and 35% to 50% excreted unchanged in the urine; only 4% to 15% is excreted as acetyl aminoglutethimide. None of the observed metabolites block steroidogenesis. Anastrozole is rapidly absorbed after oral administration, with maximum circulating concentrations reached in 2 hours. Approximately 40% is bound to plasma proteins. It is extensively metabolized and excreted primarily in the urine.

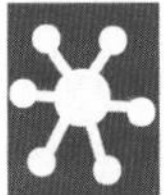

Relation of mechanisms of action to clinical response

Fertility control

Combination oral contraception The most common use for administered combination estrogens and progestins is oral contraception. Oral contraceptives are one of the most effective, reversible ways to prevent pregnancy. The failure rate in users of combination oral contraceptives is less than 1 per 100 women-years, and serious risks are rare. Combination oral contraceptives currently available in the United States contain one of two synthetic estrogens with one of several synthetic progestins. The estrogen component is usually ethinyl estradiol or, less commonly, mestranol. The progestins include norethindrone, norgestrel, and its active isomer levonorgestrel, desogestrel, ethynodiol diacetate, and drospirenone. The present low-dose (50 µg or less) estrogen contraceptives are associated with a decreased incidence of adverse side effects and have prevented pregnancy at rates equal to those of earlier higher-dose formulations. The most commonly used oral contraceptives consist of a combination preparation taken for 21 days followed by 7 days without any steroids to induce withdrawal bleeding, but many other dosing regimens are also available. The dose and type of progestin vary the most between formulations. If the estrogen and progestin are given at a fixed dose throughout the cycle, the oral contraceptive is referred to as monophasic. Altering the dose of progestin during the cycle more closely mimics endogenous progesterone levels, and the progestin level can be altered twice (biphasic) or varied more frequently (triphasic). In addition, there have been four "generations" of progestins created for use in oral contraceptives. The major differences are in their side effects (usually androgenic).

Combination oral contraceptives prevent pregnancy by inhibiting ovulation, presumably as a result of the effects of estrogen and progestin on the hypothalamic-pituitary axis to suppress gonadotropin synthesis and release. The increased FSH concentrations in the early follicular phase and the midcycle peaks of FSH and LH are not observed in patients taking combination oral contraceptives. The lower concentration of FSH results in decreased ovarian function with minimal follicular development. In addition, lower concentrations of endogenous steroids are secreted during both phases of the menstrual cycle. Oral contraceptives also act directly on the cervix and uterus. The cervical mucus of oral contraceptive users is usually thick and less abundant than that normally seen in the postovulatory phase. This may also aid in preventing pregnancy by inhibiting sperm penetration. In addition, the endometrium may be prevented from developing into the appropriate state for implantation. The risk of pregnancy is substantially increased, if two or more doses are missed during a cycle. Therefore, a high compliance rate is needed to ensure adequate contraception, especially with low-concentration estrogen preparations.

Combination oral contraceptives confer several well-documented health benefits beyond the control of fertility, including a decreased risk of ovarian and endometrial cancers. The relative risk of ovarian malignancy, which carries a relatively high mortality, is about half that in long-term oral contraceptive users (>5 years), as compared to nonusers. This protective effect continues for 10 to 15 years after discontinuance of oral contraceptives. Endometrial cancers are associated with a relatively low mortality but are more common in women than ovarian cancer. A causal link between an increased incidence of endometrial cancer and the use of sequential oral contraceptives (estrogen alone for 14-16 days, then 5-6 days of estrogen plus progestins, and then 7 days without steroid) led to the cessation of their use in 1976. Early studies with combination oral contraceptives containing higher estrogen doses showed as much as a 40% decrease in the risk of endometrial cancer. This effect appeared after as little as 1 year of use and lasted for 10 to 15 years after discontinuing the contraceptive. The mechanism is thought to be related to the use of daily progestin to oppose the proliferative actions of estrogens on the endometrium. More recent studies with current formulations are limited, but some benefit is expected. Other benefits of long-term combination oral contraceptive use include a 25% decrease in the risk of fibroadenomatosis and fibrocystic breast disease and up to a 50% reduction in the risk of pelvic inflammatory disease. A reduction in the severity of acne is also observed, presumably by decreasing the concentration of free testosterone. Increased menstrual cycle regularity, a decreased incidence of dysmenorrhea and functional ovarian cysts, and decreased blood loss during menses are other benefits.

Combination contraception—other delivery Combination estrogen and progestin contraception is also available in formulations for nonoral delivery. A vaginal ring containing ethinyl estradiol and etonogestrel is inserted for 3 weeks then removed for 1 week to allow withdrawal bleeding. The advantage of this method is the local delivery of low dose steroids. The failure rate is 1 to 2 per 100 woman-years. An injectable formulation containing estradiol cypionate and medroxyprogesterone acetate is used monthly with a failure rate of 1 per 100 woman-years. Patches for the transdermal delivery of estradiol and a synthetic progestin are also available. Patches are changed weekly with no patch worn the fourth week to allow withdrawal bleeding. The failure rate is 1 per 100 woman-years.

Progestin-only contraception Progestin-only formulations of hormonal contraceptives were developed to avoid the adverse side effects of estrogens in combination oral contraceptives. Major problems with this approach are a slightly higher failure rate and a much higher incidence of menstrual disturbances ranging from frequent, occasionally heavy, irregular bleeding to amenorrhea, often leading to discontinuation of the medication.

Progestin only contraception has a variety of delivery methods. A progestin-only oral contraceptive (the mini-pill) is taken daily and contains one of the synthetic progestins, norgestrel or norethindrone. Failure rates of 1 to 3 per 100 woman-years have been observed. To avoid the inconvenience of taking a daily pill and to try to obtain lower continuous doses of steroid to minimize side effects, alternative methods of progestin-only administration have been developed such as silastic capsules containing levonorgestrel that are placed subdermally, usually in the arm. The major benefits of this form of contraception are that it is effective for up to 5 years, and much lower doses of steroid are released. Failure rates are less than 1 per 100 woman-years. Problems include irregular uterine bleeding and the need for surgical insertion and removal. Medroxyprogesterone acetate in microcrystals is given as an IM injection at a dose of 150 mg every 3 months. Failure rates are 0.3 to 1 per 100 woman-years. Another benefit is that normal menstrual cycles return very quickly following removal. Progestin-releasing intrauterine devices (IUD) deliver low, continuous doses of the steroid locally, instead of systemically. The progestin-induced endometrial atrophy decreases bleeding, which is a significant problem of the nonsteroid-containing IUD. Failure rates of 0.1 to 2 per 100 woman-years have been reported for these devices.

Progestin-only medication suppresses FSH and LH concentrations and ovulation to variable degrees; however, these actions cannot be the only explanation for the observed high success rate of the agent. Scant, thick cervical mucus preventing sperm penetration, endometrial atrophy (which could prevent implantation), and bleeding that is quite variable in duration likely contribute to prevention of pregnancy as well.

Emergency contraception Large doses of estrogens alone, progestins alone, or estrogens in combination with progestins, may prevent pregnancy after unprotected coitus. However, to prevent pregnancy, these compounds must be taken within 72 hours of coital exposure and are currently recommended only in cases of rape, incest, failure of a barrier method, or unprotected intercourse. The high doses probably act by inhibiting ovulation and implantation by making the endometrium nonreceptive to the blastocyst. Two formulations have been specifically approved in the United States: Preven Emergency Contraceptive Kit and Plan

B. Preven is a combination of levonorgestrel and ethinylestradiol. Plan B is levonorgestrel alone. The first dose is taken within 72 hours of unprotected coitus and a second dose is taken 12 hours later. Several existing combination oral contraception formulations can also be used for emergency contraception by using a specified number of pills per dose. An 80% reduction in the risk of pregnancy is observed. Emergency contraception requires a prescription at this time in the United States.

Contragestation Mifepristone (RU 486) is a synthetic, potent antiprogestin that acts as a contragestational agent when taken within 50 days of the last menses. It acts by binding to progesterone receptors, thereby preventing binding by endogenous progesterone. It also binds weakly to androgen receptors and tightly to glucocorticoid receptors. Mifepristone causes pregnancy termination directly at the level of the endometrium. It blocks progesterone action leading to endometrial shedding (progesterone withdrawal bleeding) and prostaglandin release within 2 to 4 days. The conceptus is then detached from the uterine wall and human chorionic gonadotropin concentrations decline, resulting in luteolysis. The most effective dosage is a single dose of 600 mg given on the day of expected menses. Mifepristone alone is successful in less than 10% of women at 48 hours. The remainder receive prostaglandin E_1 48 hours after administration of mifepristone, leading to at least a 96% success rate. Follow-up examination is at 14 days to confirm pregnancy termination. Surgical termination is recommended, if medical termination has not occurred. Mifepristone has decreased effectiveness after 5 weeks of pregnancy, because the placenta probably produces enough local progesterone to overcome its antiprogestin effects.

Ovulation induction

About 20% to 30% of cases of infertility result from an anovulatory condition. Agents that induce ovulation in these patients include gonadotropins, GnRH, and clomiphene citrate. Clomiphene citrate, a SERM with both agonist and antagonist properties, is used to treat ovulatory failure in women desiring pregnancy whose mates are fertile and potent. This agent may act as an antiestrogen in the hypothalamus relieving estrogen-induced negative feedback on GnRH release. After clomiphene administration, the pulse frequency (but not amplitude) of LH release increases significantly, possibly because of an increase in the pulse frequency of GnRH release. Clomiphene is most effective in women with normal concentrations of estrogen before therapy and is not useful in women with primary ovarian or pituitary dysfunction. This agent can cause multiple ovulations resulting in a 6% to 12% incidence of multiple gestation.

Replacement therapy

Menopause Menopause, the natural cessation of menses, results from ovarian failure after depletion of functional ovarian follicles. Decreased estrogen and progesterone production ensue, and this leads to physiological and psychological changes. The increased risk of vasomotor symptoms, genitourinary atrophy, osteoporosis, and cardiovascular disease in postmenopausal women has long been presumed to result from the loss of estrogen. This view is supported by the substantial decrease in vasomotor symptoms, genitourinary atrophy, and osteoporosis in women who begin estrogen replacement therapy during menopause. However, results from recent clinical trials have forced a complete reexamination of the role of estrogen and progestin in prevention of cardiovascular disease. The role of estrogens and progestins in maintenance of cognitive function in postmenopausal women is also unclear but of intense interest. There is considerable controversy regarding patient selection and treatment regimens in the use of hormone replacement therapy, and guidelines have recently changed dramatically. A large number of questions remain on the adverse effects of specific replacement regimens with regard to their use in specific patient subpopulations. Guidelines for the use of replacement therapy can be expected to continue to evolve as additional data become available.

Estrogen replacement in postmenopausal women remains the most effective treatment for the acute symptoms of menopause. It is used for treatment of moderate to severe symptoms of vulvar and vaginal atrophy and moderate to severe vasomotor symptoms, such as hot flushes (also termed "hot flashes") and night sweats. It is currently recommended that the use of estrogens for postmenopausal replacement be for the shortest time and at the lowest dose possible to relieve acute symptoms. A progestin is added to the treatment for women with an intact uterus to oppose the proliferative actions of estrogen on the endometrium. The most commonly used preparation is a mixture of conjugated estrogens taken orally. Transdermal and vaginal delivery is also available. Vaginal delivery is recommended when treatment is only for symptoms of genitourinary atrophy. Estrogen replacement is also very effective at reducing the risk of osteoporosis. However, if the only clinical goal is prevention of postmenopausal osteoporosis, alternative treatments are available.

Raloxifene is a SERM that is an agonist in bone but does not show estrogenic effects in uterus or breast. Raloxifene is approved for prevention of postmenopausal osteoporosis. There are also other drugs for prevention and treatment of osteoporosis (see Chapter 41).

For many years, estrogen was believed to reduce the risk of cardiovascular disease in women. Before menopause the incidence of coronary artery disease is lower in women than in men of the same age, but after menopause the incidence increases with age and is eventually the same as that in men. The increased risk may be associated with changes in lipoproteins, in that, ordinarily, HDL concentrations decrease and LDL concentrations increase after menopause. In men these changes have been correlated with an increased risk of coronary artery disease. Estrogen replacement therapy increases HDL and lowers LDL concentrations. In the mid-1990s, data from observational studies suggested that the risk of atherosclerotic cardiovascular disease was reduced by up to half in postmenopausal women who used estrogen replacement therapy with or without a progestin. These data spurred the design and funding of randomized, placebo controlled, clinical trials to determine benefits and risks. To the great surprise of the medical community, the estrogen plus progestin randomized trials from the Heart and Estrogen/Progestin Replacement Study, and Women's Health Initiative showed no benefit, and possibly an increase, in the risk of cardiovascular disease. The estrogen-only trial is ongoing. These results have prompted a complete reevaluation of the use of estrogen-replacement therapy for the long-term prevention of cardiovascular disease. The beneficial effects of estrogen replacement on vasomotor symptoms and prevention of osteoporosis are not in doubt. Current recommendations are outlined in earlier text but will evolve as additional data become available.

Other uses of replacement therapy Hormone replacement therapy is useful in treatment of ovarian failure (primary or premature), dysfunctional uterine bleeding, and luteal phase deficiency. Estrogen therapy initiated near the time of puberty may help stimulate normal sexual development in girls with primary ovarian failure from multiple causes. Dysfunctional uterine bleeding occurs during irregular menstrual cycles and is often characterized by prolonged bleeding. High-dose progestin therapy can be used to stop an episode of prolonged bleeding but should be followed by long-term cyclic therapy with an orally administered progestin to ensure occurrence of regular withdrawal bleeding. Luteal phase deficiency results from insufficient progesterone. Ovulation is normal, but the corpus luteum functions subnormally, with insufficient progesterone produced to maintain pregnancy. The most popular method of treating this is natural progesterone supplementation.

Cancer chemotherapy

Approximately one-third of patients with advanced breast cancer who undergo therapy that decreases estrogen production or action will exhibit tumor regression, a prolongation of disease-free survival, or both. An overall response rate of 30% to 40%, with few adverse effects, is observed in women with breast cancer receiving adjuvant treatment with tamoxifen. Tamoxifen is a SERM showing antagonist effects in the breast, while being an agonist in uterus and bone. Tamoxifen acts in the breast by competition with endogenous estrogen and preventing estrogen receptor activation. Tamoxifen has also been approved for use as a breast cancer preventative based on clinical trials with women who were at high risk. Factors used to assess high risk include age, family history of breast cancer, and others. The studies showed a 49% decrease in the risk of developing breast cancer in women taking tamoxifen compared to those taking placebo. The results are consistent with earlier studies that showed a 50% reduction in the risk of developing a new tumor in the opposite breast in women with breast cancer who took tamoxifen. Raloxifene, another SERM, is currently in clinical trials for prevention of breast cancer.

A reduction in estrogen production in postmenopausal women as a means of preventing breast cancer recurrence can be achieved by inhibition of adrenal steroidogenesis or peripheral aromatization of adrenal androgens. Aminoglutethimide acts by inhibiting two enzymes. One is the cholesterol side-chain–cleaving enzyme, which converts cholesterol to pregnenolone, and the other is the aromatase enzyme, which converts adrenal androstenedione to estrone, and testosterone to estradiol (Fig. 35-2). Glucocorticoid replacement therapy is needed in such patients, mainly to inhibit the compensatory rise in adrenocorticotropic hormone, which can override the action of aminoglutethimide. Several drugs are now available that specifically inhibit the aromatase enzyme and not the cholesterol side-chain–cleaving enzyme. Adrenal steroidogenesis is not inhibited, avoiding the need for glucocorticoid replacement. Circulating estrogen concentrations are effectively suppressed. These compounds include anastrozole, letrozole, and exemestane. Clinically they are used in the adjuvant treatment of breast cancer but also as first-line treatment in advanced disease. Recent clinical studies have shown that the sequential use of tamoxifen for 5 years followed by an aromatase inhibitor reduced the risk of breast cancer recurrence compared to tamoxifen use alone.

Progestin therapy is used as an adjuvant and palliative treatment of advanced endometrial carcinoma. Several synthetic progestins can be used and likely act through the progesterone receptor to down-regulate the estrogen receptor and induce formation of 17β-hydroxysteroid dehydrogenase to increase estradiol metabolism. In addition, it may have direct cellular actions, leading to decreased cell division. High progesterone receptor concentrations in endometrial tumors correlate with increased survival.

High doses of estrogens can be used as an adjuvant and palliative treatment for advanced prostate cancer. High dose estrogen therapy is associated with a high incidence of adverse cardiovascular events, predominantly thromboembolic. The use of the synthetic non-steroidal estrogen, diethylstilbestrol, has been replaced with newer therapies using a combination of steroidal estrogens that have a somewhat lower incidence of side effects. The benefit of high dose estrogen is presumed to be due to its suppression of testosterone production.

Other uses

Endometriosis results from implantation of ectopic endometrial cells outside the uterus. These cells continue to respond to steroid hormones but may show subtle differences in estrogen and progesterone receptor concentrations and function. Clinically, patients experience dysmenorrhea and sometimes dyspareunia. The goal of therapy in endometriosis is to induce an estrogen-poor environment to inhibit the growth of implants and thereby alleviate symptoms. The compounds used in the United States to treat endometriosis are a combination oral contraceptives, danazol, progestins, and GnRH analogs. These hormone regimens may function by binding to the progesterone receptor and opposing estrogen action or inhibiting the LH-FSH surge. Danazol can interact with both androgen and progesterone receptors.

Side effects, clinical problems, and toxicity

Potential problems associated with some of the important drugs are briefly summarized in the Clinical Problems box.

CLINICAL PROBLEMS

Estrogens

Endometrial cancer, venous thromboembolism/pulmonary embolism, gallbladder disease, myocardial infarction (high dose), stroke (high dose), thrombophlebitis (high dose), menstrual disorders, GI disturbances, headache, breast discomfort and enlargement, weight gain, mood changes

Progestins

Ectopic pregnancy, menstrual disorders, drug interactions leading to contraceptive failure, GI disturbances, headache, breast discomfort, adverse changes in lipoprotein levels, abnormal glucose tolerance

Combination estrogen-progestin

Contraception—Venous thromboembolism, myocardial infarction (with other risk factors), stroke (with other risk factors), breast cancer, drug interactions leading to contraceptive failure

Replacement therapy—Venous thromboembolism, stroke, myocardial infarction/coronary heart disease, breast cancer

Antiestrogens/SERMs/progesterone receptor ligands

Clomiphene—Multiple gestations, vasomotor symptoms, ovarian enlargement and cysts, ovarian hyperstimulation syndrome, GI disturbances, breast discomfort

Tamoxifen—Endometrial cancer, stroke, deep vein thrombosis, thromboembolism, vasomotor symptoms, GI disturbances

Raloxifene—Thromboembolism, deep vein thrombosis, vasomotor symptoms

Mifepristone—Menstrual disturbances, uterine cramping

Danazol—Androgenic effects in women, antiestrogen-like effects, adverse changes in lipoprotein concentrations

Inhibitors of steroidogenesis/aromatase

Aminoglutethimide—GI disturbances, CNS disturbances

Anastrozole—Hot flashes, nausea

Estrogens

The more serious, long-term side effects occasionally encountered with estrogen usage include endometrial cancer, thromboembolic disorders, and gallbladder disease. The incidence of endometrial cancer is increased as much as 24-fold in those exposed to prolonged (>5 years) unopposed estrogens, but this increased risk can be completely eliminated by using a progestin in combination. The risk of venous thromboembolism increases twofold to threefold with estrogens. The incidence of thromboembolic disorders is greatest among smokers. High dose estrogen used in prostate cancer treatment is associated with an increased risk of nonfatal myocardial infarction, stroke, pulmonary embolism, and thrombophlebitis. A twofold to fourfold increase in the risk of gallbladder disease is seen in estrogen users. A substantial increase in blood pressure, that has been reported in a small number of women, appears to be an idiosyncratic response to estrogens not seen in large clinical trials. An increased risk of ovarian cancer has been seen in some studies but not others. Studies on estrogen-only therapy show no, or only a small, increased risk of breast cancer, and any increased risk was associated with prolonged use and higher doses. The trial by the Women's Health Initiative is ongoing and should provide more definitive data.

Some less serious, more acute adverse effects of estrogen therapy include changes in vaginal bleeding patterns, nausea, occasional vomiting, abdominal cramps, bloating, diarrhea, appetite changes, fluid retention, dizziness, headache, breast discomfort, weight gain, mood changes, ocular changes, allergic rash, and changes in some serum proteins. Most of these effects are related to dose. High dose therapy in men is associated with gynecomastia and impotence.

An etiological role for diethylstilbestrol, a nonsteroidal estrogen agonist, in the development of clear-cell adenocarcinoma of the vagina and cervix, is based on epidemiological data from the 1950s when it was used to prevent miscarriage. An increased incidence of rare cancers of these types has been noted in women exposed to diethylstilbestrol *in utero,* and it is no longer used in the United States.

Progestins

Progestin-only implant and oral contraception is associated with an increased incidence of ectopic pregnancy upon contraceptive failure. The occasional and less serious side effects of progestin-only therapy include breakthrough bleeding, spotting, changes in menstrual flow, amenorrhea, edema, weight changes, nausea, bloating, headache, allergic rash, mood changes, and changes in lipoprotein concentrations (HDL, decreased; LDL, increased). Glucose tolerance test results are abnormal in 4% to 16% of women receiving high-dose progestin. Plasma glucose concentrations should be monitored in diabetic women and in those with a prior history of glucose intolerance taking oral contraceptives. A progestin, at as low a dose and with as low a potency as possible, should be used in such women. The most common side effects of intramuscular medroxyprogesterone acetate and Norplant used for contraception are menstrual abnormalities, characterized by irregular bleeding early in the treatment, followed by amenorrhea in 50% to 70% of patients after 2 years of treatment. In addition, the surgical insertion and removal of Norplant-2 silastic rods can be associated with patient discomfort and possible infection.

Combination oral contraceptives

Despite more than 40 years of oral contraceptive use, some controversy remains concerning the risks. However, several factors must be considered to put this controversy into perspective. First, the hormone doses used in many of the early studies that associated oral contraceptive use with specific side effects were much higher than those used currently. Fewer adverse effects have been noted in recent studies with the use of low-dose oral contraceptives. Second, the design of several early studies was criticized because subgroups were not identical in makeup. Finally, restricting oral contraceptive use in certain high-risk patient subgroups has led to a decrease in the incidence of cardiovascular side effects.

A number of clinical studies show an association between combined oral contraceptive use and thromboembolic disease in the absence of other predisposing factors. The risk of venous thromboembolism is twofold to sixfold greater in those who use combined oral contraceptives than in nonusers. The increased risk is dependent on the type of progestin used. The increased risk of thromboembolic events is greater in women who smoke, in older women (over 35), and with higher doses of estrogen. Women who use oral contraceptives should not smoke. The risk of thromboembolic disease rapidly returns to normal after use is discontinued and should be stopped at least 2 to 4 weeks before elective surgery and not restarted until at least 2 weeks after surgery. Combination oral contraceptives can cause a small increase in both systolic and diastolic blood pressure in some patients, and their use is contraindicated in patients with moderate to severe hypertension.

An increased risk of stroke and myocardial infarction are not definitively correlated with combination oral contraceptive use in women with no other risk factors. Nearly all recent studies have shown no increased risk of myocardial infarction or ischemic stroke without other major risk factors. However, compared to nonusers, there is a substantial increased risk of myocardial infarction and ischemic stroke in women who use combination oral contraceptives and also have one or more of these risk factors: smoking, uncontrolled hypertension, diabetes, hypercholesterolemia; and the risks increase with age.

Multiple studies have shown no change in the incidence of breast cancer in women who take combination oral contraceptives, though a few studies showed an increased risk. Given the relatively small number of breast cancer patients in the age group of women using contraception, the number of increased cases is actually small. The association of breast cancer with oral contraceptive use continues to be an area of uncertainty. Women who are positive for human papilloma virus and use oral contraceptives may be at increased risk for cervical cancer, if they have used these drugs for more than 5 years.

Oral contraceptives are contraindicated in women with a current or past history of thrombophlebitis or thromboembolic disorders; cerebrovascular or coronary artery disease; a known or suspected pregnancy; undiagnosed abnormal genital bleeding; a known or suspected carcinoma of the breast, uterus, cervix, vagina, or other estrogen-dependent neoplasm; hepatic adenoma or carcinoma; and cholestatic jaundice of pregnancy or jaundice following prior oral contraceptive use. Oral contraceptives should be used with caution in patients with liver or renal disease, asthma, migraine headaches, diabetes, hypertension, or congestive heart failure, and in patients receiving medications that can interfere with its effectiveness. Women who smoke and use oral contraceptives should be advised to use alternative methods of birth control after 35 years of age. The metabolism of oral contraceptives can be increased by a number of drugs, reducing their effectiveness and raising the risk of contraceptive failure. Examples of such drugs include barbiturates, rifampin, phenylbutazone, phenytoin, carbamazepine, oxcarbazepine, topiramate, ampicillin, and tetracyclines.

Combination replacement therapy

Our understanding of the risks and benefits of estrogen plus progestin replacement therapy in postmenopausal women with an intact uterus has been strongly influenced by the results of the Women's Health Initiative randomized, placebo-controlled clinical trial published in July 2002. The strengths of this trial were its randomized design, large numbers (16,608 women enrolled), and over 5 years detailed follow-up. The limitations include the use of only one replacement formulation (0.625 mg/day conjugated equine estrogens, plus 2.5 mg/day medroxyprogesterone acetate), inclusion of a broad age range with many women several years past the initial cessation of menses (average age 63), and a high rate of patient withdrawal from the study. The results have fueled extensive debate on the use of replacement therapy and significantly changed recommendations.

The most serious risks observed in this study for users of estrogen plus progestin replacement therapy were an increase in venous thromboembolic disease, stroke, nonfatal myocardial infarction and fatal coronary heart disease, and breast cancer. The overall rates of cardiovascular disease were low, but up to a twofold increase in venous thromboembolism, a 41% increase in stroke, and a 29% increase in coronary heart disease were observed. Much of the increased risk of cardiovascular disease was seen in the first year. A 26% increase in breast cancer was observed, with the difference between the replacement and placebo groups being evident only after 4 years. A decreased risk of ovarian cancer was not observed. Rather, an increased number of ovarian cancers was observed in the replacement group, although the increase over the placebo group was not statistically significant.

Current recommendations for use of estrogen plus progestin combination therapy is for treatment of acute symptoms of menopause for the shortest duration possible. Use is contraindicated in women with abnormal genital bleeding, a history of breast cancer or other estrogen-dependent neoplasia, venous or arterial thromboembolic disease, or liver dysfunction. The treatment of individual patients should be governed by the particular patient's risk profile.

Antiestrogens, SERMs, and progesterone receptor ligands

The frequency and severity of the adverse effects of clomiphene citrate are dose-related and include vasomotor symptoms that resemble those in menopausal patients. Visual problems occur occasionally and have been correlated with an increase in total dose. Other high-dose side effects include ovarian enlargement or cyst formation, ovarian hyperstimulation syndrome, abdominal discomfort, nausea and vomiting, abnormal uterine bleeding, breast tenderness, headache, dizziness, depression, allergic dermatitis, and urinary frequency. There is a 6% to 12% incidence of multiple gestations, particularly twins, in women taking clomiphene, as compared with a 1% incidence in the general population. Clomiphene is contraindicated in patients with ovarian cysts, pregnancy, a history of liver disease, abnormal uterine bleeding, and with thyroid or adrenal dysfunction.

The serious side effects of tamoxifen include a twofold increased risk of endometrial cancer, a threefold increased risk of pulmonary thromboembolism, a 59% increased risk of deep vein thrombosis, and a 40% increased risk of stroke. Less serious side effects seen in some women include vasomotor symptoms, nausea, and vomiting. Pregnancy should be avoided in women taking tamoxifen, because, although the teratogenic effects of this drug in humans are unknown, numerous defects have been demonstrated in animals. Tamoxifen is contraindicated in women using anticoagulation therapy, or with a history of deep vein thrombosis or pulmonary embolus.

The serious side effects of raloxifene include an increase in the risk of pulmonary thromboembolism and deep vein thrombosis. The most common, less serious side effect seen in some women is vasomotor symptoms. Raloxifene is contraindicated in women who are lactating, pregnant, or have a history of venous thromboembolic events.

Mifepristone is well tolerated and associated with only occasional prolonged uterine bleeding. Less serious, but common side effects, include uterine cramping, abdominal pain, back pain, headache, and GI disturbances.

The use of danazol is fraught with multiple antiestrogen-like and androgenic side effects, including weight gain, muscle cramps, decreased breast size, deepening of the voice, edema, amenorrhea, emotional lability, flushing, sweating, acne, mild hirsutism, oily skin and hair, altered libido, nausea, headache, dizziness, insomnia, rash, increased LDL and decreased HDL concentrations, and increased hepatic enzyme activities. Most of these are reversed upon cessation of the drug. Danazol is contraindicated in pregnant women or in breastfeeding mothers.

The most frequent reversible side effects of aminoglutethimide include drowsiness, rash, nausea, anorexia, fever, dizziness, and ataxia, but these usually diminish with continued use. Reported adverse effects of anastrozole include fatigue, nausea, headache, hot flashes, pain, and back pain.

TRADE NAMES

In addition to generic and fixed-combination preparations, the following trade-named materials are some of the important compounds available in the United States.

Steroidal estrogens

Conjugated equine estrogens (Premarin)
Estramustine (Emcyt)
Estradiol (Estraderm, Climara, Estrace)
Estradiol cypionate (Depo-estradiol Cypionate, Depogen)
Estropipate (Ogen)
Esterified estrogens (Estratab, Menest)
Synthetic, conjugated steroidal estrogens (Cenestin)

SERMs

Clomiphene (Clomid, Serophene)
Fulvestrant (Faslodex)
Raloxifene (Evista)
Tamoxifen (Nolvadex, Valodex)
Toremifene (Fareston)

Progestins

Levonorgestrel (Norplant System, Plan B)
Medroxyprogesterone (Depo-Provera, Provera)
Norethindrone (Micronor)
Norgestrel (Ovrette)

Antiprogestins, progestin analogs

Danazol (Danocrine)
Mifepristone, RU 486 (Mifeprex)

Inhibitors of steroidogenesis/aromatase

Aminoglutethimide (Cytadren)
Anastrozole (Arimidex)
Exemestane (Aromasin)
Letrozole (Femara)

Combinations of oral contraceptives

Ethinyl estradiol, desogestrel (Mircette, Ortho-Cept, Desogen)
Ethinyl estradiol, drospirenone (Yasmin)
Ethinyl estradiol, levonorgestrel (Trivora, Tri-Levlen, Alesse, Levora-28, Aviane, Preven)
Ethinyl estradiol/norgestimate (Ortho Tri-Cyclen)
Ethinyl estradiol/norgestrel (Lo Ovral, Cilest)
Ethinyl estradiol/norethindrone (Ortho-Novum, Loestrin, Norlestrin, Ortho-Novum 7/7/7)
Mestranol/norethindrone (Necon 1/35)

Replacement therapy

Conjugated estrogens/medroxyprogesterone (Prempro, Premphase)

New horizons

The development of estrogen receptor ligands that target specific tissues, with minimal effects on other tissues, continues to be a focus of intense research. These compounds, the SERMs, offer the promise of matching desired benefits of estrogen to specific clinical goals. The ideal agent for postmenopausal women would be an estrogen antagonist in breast and uterus, but an agonist in bone, with no increased cardiovascular risks. The development of new SERMs for the adjuvant treatment as well as prevention of breast cancer is in progress. The combined and sequential use of SERMs with aromatase inhibitors for cancer chemotherapy is also under investigation.

Recent results from the Women's Health Initiative and Heart and Estrogen/Progestin Replacement Study trials showing a lack of cardiovascular benefit, and even increased risk, in postmenopausal women using replacement therapy were unexpected. Many questions were not addressed in these studies, including the relationship of cardiovascular risk to the dose and type of hormones used. Another major issue is whether timing of initiation of replacement therapy (at the time of menses cessation versus years later) affects the risk profile. Additional clinical trials may address some of these questions.

The potential role of exogenous estrogens in maintenance of cognitive function remains controversial. Some studies suggest that estrogen replacement therapy might reduce the risk or severity of Alzheimer's disease. Some studies have also shown a beneficial effect on cognitive function in women on estrogen replacement therapy. However, the Women's Health Initiative study did not observe any protection against cognitive impairment in women taking estrogen plus progestin compared to placebo.

FURTHER READING

Jensen EV, Jordan VC. The estrogen receptor: A model for molecular medicine. *Clin Cancer Res* 2003; 9:1980-1989.

Petitti DB. Combination estrogen-progestin oral contraceptives. *N Engl J Med* 2003; 349:1443-1450.

Rossouw JE, Anderson GL, Prentice RL, et al. Risks and benefits of estrogen plus progestin in healthy postmenopausal women: Principal results from the Women's Health Initiative randomized controlled trial. *JAMA* 2002; 288:321-333.

Self-assessment questions

1. What enzyme is directly responsible for the conversion of testosterone to 17β-estradiol and is therefore a target for both aminoglutethimide and anastrozole?
   a. Cytochrome P450 side-chain cleavage enzyme
   b. Placental sulfatase
   c. Aromatase
   d. Megestrol acetate
   e. None

2. Which compound is not an estrogen?
   a. 17β-Estradiol
   b. Estriol
   c. Levonorgestrel
   d. Mestranol
   e. Estrone

3. Unopposed estrogens cause a significantly increased risk of all of the following *except:*
   a. Endometrial cancer.
   b. Breast cancer.
   c. Thromboembolic disorders.
   d. Gallbladder disease.

4. Estrogen plus progestin postmenopausal replacement therapy causes a significantly increased risk of all of the following *except:*
   a. Stroke.
   b. Endometrial cancer.
   c. Thromboembolic disorders.
   d. Breast cancer.
   e. Myocardial infarction.

5. The ethinyl side chain at the carbon 17 position is added to several synthetic estrogens and progestins to alter:
   a. Metabolism of the compound and decrease its half-life.
   b. The receptor-binding specificity of the compound.
   c. The affinity of the ligand for the receptor.
   d. The metabolism of the compound and prolong its half-life.
   e. The molecular weight of the compound.

CHAPTER 36

Androgens and antiandrogens

Stephen J. Winters

Major Drugs	
Androgens	Androgen antagonists
Antiandrogens	

Therapeutic overview

Androgens are produced by the testis, ovary, and adrenal glands. **Testosterone** is the most important androgen in males. It stimulates **virilization** and is an important **spermatogenic** hormone. Within the ovary, testosterone and androstenedione are precursor steroids for estradiol production (see Chapter 35). In both sexes, androgens stimulate body hair growth, positive nitrogen balance, bone growth, muscle development, and erythropoiesis. The mechanism of action of testosterone at its target organs is similar to that of other steroid hormones (see Chapter 2). The major use of androgens in clinical medicine is for **replacement therapy** in men whose production of testosterone is impaired. Testosterone synthesis inhibitors and **antiandrogens** are used to limit the effects of androgens in patients with androgen-dependent disorders, such as prostatic cancer, hirsutism, and precocious puberty.

Testosterone is required for the normal development of the internal ducts of the **male reproductive tract.** Its 5α-reduced product, **dihydrotestosterone (DHT),** is responsible for stimulating the development of male external genitalia during the first trimester of fetal life. Therefore, when the fetal synthesis of androgen is insufficient (e.g., due to an inborn enzymatic error) or the action of androgen is ineffective at its target tissues (e.g., androgen receptor mutation), the genital phenotype may be female or ambiguous.

An increase in circulating androgen concentrations at puberty in males stimulates the expression of adult secondary sex characteristics. The scrotum darkens and becomes rugated; beard and body hair growth are stimulated; sebaceous glands are stimulated; the phallus, prostate, seminal vesicles, and larynx enlarge; and the voice deepens. Muscle mass, skeletal development, and linear growth increase. Finally, androgens affect the brain to stimulate libido. These processes are incomplete if the synthesis or actions of androgen are impaired.

Testosterone is also an important spermatogenic hormone. Both Sertoli and myoid cells contain **androgen receptors (AR)** and appear to be androgen target cells. Thus, androgen deficiency is associated with

Abbreviations

AR	androgen receptor
DHEA	dehydroepiandrosterone
DHT	dihydrotestosterone
FSH	follicle-stimulating hormone
GnRH	gonadotropin-releasing hormone
hCG	human chorionic gonadotropin
IM	intramuscular
LH	luteinizing hormone
SHBG	sex hormone–binding globulin
StAR	steroidogenic acute regulatory protein

hypospermatogenesis, and hypogonadal men are often infertile. The principal therapeutic considerations pertaining to the androgens and related compounds are summarized in the Therapeutic Overview box.

THERAPEUTIC OVERVIEW

Androgens

Primary testicular insufficiency
Hypogonadotropic hypogonadism
Constitutional delay of growth and adolescence
Osteoporosis, anemia
Male contraception

Antiandrogens and androgen antagonists

Virilization in women
Precocious puberty in boys
Prostate cancer

Mechanisms of action

Testosterone synthesis

Testosterone, a 19-carbon steroid hormone, is synthesized from cholesterol in the Leydig cells of the testis, the adrenal cortex, and the theca cells of the ovary, following the pathways shown in Figure 36-1. In the adult gonads, the principal regulator of testosterone synthesis and secretion is **luteinizing hormone (LH)**, which is produced by the anterior pituitary gland (see Chapter 40). The precursor **cholesterol** is itself synthesized in the Leydig cells from acetate and stored as cholesterol esters in lipid droplets. A cholesterol ester hydrolase mobilizes free cholesterol from the lipid droplets, which, in turn, is transferred to the inner mitochondrial membrane. Stimulation of this transfer represents a major action of LH and is mediated by the **steroidogenic acute regulatory (StAR) protein.** The mitochondrial oxidation of cholesterol occurs at positions C20 and C22, followed by lyase cleavage of the C–C bond between positions 20 and 22, resulting in the production of pregnenolone, a reaction catalyzed by the cytochrome P450 enzyme system (Fig. 36-1).

Pregnenolone, a 21-carbon steroid with a double bond in the 5-6 position, is converted to a 21-carbon androgen by two pathways, as discussed in Chapter 35 and depicted again in Figure 36-1. One pathway is through 17α-hydroxypregnenolone to dehydroepiandrosterone (DHEA), and the second is through progesterone to 17α-hydroxyprogesterone and androstenedione. DHEA is readily oxidized to androstenedione, and the microsomal enzyme 17β-hydroxysteroid dehydrogenase catalyzes conversion of androstenedione to testosterone. Leydig cells also convert a small fraction of testosterone to estradiol (see Chapter 35). Each of the enzymes in this synthetic pathway is upregulated by LH.

Unlike the peptide hormones, there is little intracellular storage of steroid hormones before secretion. The content of testosterone in the human testis is approximately 300 ng/g of wet tissue. Because one adult human testis weighs about 15 g, the total testicular content of testosterone in an adult is approximately 9 μg. This represents about 0.1% of the usual daily production of testosterone in normal adult men (5-7 mg).

Testosterone synthesis begins during the first trimester of pregnancy. The human fetal testis is stimulated by human chorionic gonadotrophin (hCG) of placental origin to produce the testosterone required for male sexual differentiation because gonadotrophs are not present in the fetal pituitary until the end of the first trimester. In the second trimester, gonadotrophs begin to function, and the principal stimulus to the fetal gonadotroph, as in the adult, is **gonadotropin-releasing hormone (GnRH).** Gonadotropin secretion and sex steroid production decline late in fetal life, followed by a prominent postnatal surge that lasts 2 to 3 months. By 3 or 4 months of age, little testosterone is secreted. At puberty, gonadotropin secretion increases and reawakens the Leydig cell to produce testosterone. The neurotransmitters GABA, neuropeptide Y, and kisspeptins (ligands of the orphan G-protein–coupled receptor GPR54) have each been proposed to influence puberty by regulating GnRH.

Gonadotropin secretion exhibits a striking diurnal rhythm in early puberty, with elevated concentrations of LH and testosterone at night. In adult men it is more difficult to demonstrate a diurnal rhythm for LH, although testosterone concentrations are approximately 25% higher in the early morning than in the late afternoon. LH secretion also fluctuates every 1 to 2 hours in adults as a result of the intermittent stimulation of gonadotrophs by GnRH. GnRH secretory episodes in turn are coupled to excitatory discharges of a neural oscillator system. Intermittent GnRH secretion is required for the pituitary to function normally, and testosterone is released into the circulation in pulses in response to the pulsatile stimulation of Leydig cells by LH.

Androgen production by the adrenal glands

Glucocorticoids and mineralocorticoids are the principal products of the adult adrenal gland. However, the

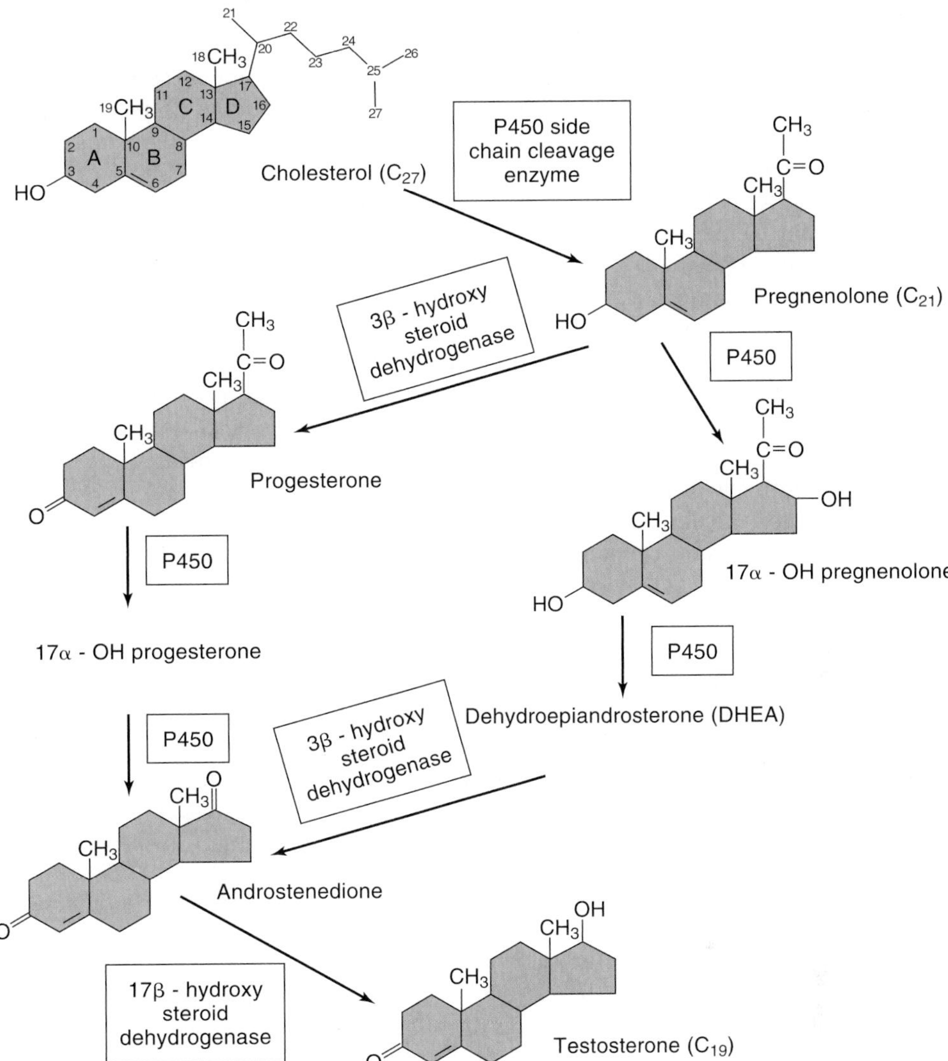

Figure 36-1 Pathways of testosterone synthesis in the Leydig cell. Also shown are structures of intermediates and the numbering system for steroid rings (*A, B, C, D*).

adrenal glands also secrete DHEA, androstenedione, and testosterone, as well as some DHEA sulfate and estrone. The concentrations of DHEA, DHEA sulfate, and androstenedione in the circulation increase between 7 to 10 years of age. This process has been termed *adrenarche,* to distinguish it from puberty or *gonadarche,* which refers to the onset of adult gonadal function. Because adrenocorticotropin stimulates the adrenal to secrete cortisol as well as sex steroids, and there is no concomitant increase in cortisol secretion in children at this age, a selective mechanism exists to produce adrenal androgens. Adrenal androgen secretion declines in the elderly and during severe illness.

Control of testosterone synthesis and secretion

The major regulator of testosterone synthesis and secretion is LH. Leydig cells have cell-surface receptors for LH, which stimulate adenylyl cyclase. The steroidogenic response also requires intracellular Ca^{2+} and the Ca^{2+}-binding protein calmodulin. Like other protein hormones, the action of LH may also involve activation of phospholipase C (see Chapter 2). The acute effect of LH involves rapid stimulation of testosterone production (within minutes) and is thought to be mediated by the StAR protein. LH also has more chronic actions on Leydig cells, which include up-regulation of messenger RNAs for steroidogenic hormones. Other hormones that may influence testosterone synthesis include prolactin, cortisol, insulin, insulin-like growth factors, estradiol, activin, and inhibin. There is a growing awareness that multiple factors produced within the seminiferous tubules by germ cells and Sertoli cells or peritubular myoid cells can also regulate testosterone synthesis. Together these factors maintain the concentration of testosterone in adult men at 300 to 1000 ng/dL (10-30 nM). During illness, LH production declines and cytokines suppress testosterone production.

Sertoli cells are somatic cells within the seminiferous tubules. Tight junctions between these cells at the base of seminiferous tubules form a blood-testis barrier, which prevents circulating proteins from entering the tubular compartment. Sertoli cells secrete many types of proteins. Some enter the tubular lumen and are important in spermatogenesis. Others are secreted through the basal end of the cell and enter the circulation. Among these proteins are the androgen-binding protein, transferrin, and inhibin-B. Follicle-stimulating hormone (FSH) is the major regulator of Sertoli cell function. The FSH receptor is also membrane bound and acts through both cyclic adenosine monophosphate and Ca^{2+}. Insulin and insulin-like growth factors, testosterone, vitamin A, and β-endorphins also influence Sertoli cell function.

The hormones of the hypothalamus, pituitary, and testes form an internally regulated unit (Fig. 36-2), which is discussed further in Chapter 40. Not only are the testes stimulated by pituitary gonadotropins, but the testes also regulate LH and FSH secretion through negative-feedback mechanisms. Testosterone suppresses gonadotropin secretion by slowing the pulsatile release of GnRH. Estradiol, which is synthesized from testosterone in the testes, adipose tissue, liver and brain, inhibits gonadotropin release through effects on both the hypothalamus and pituitary. Inhibin-B selectively reduces FSH synthesis and secretion.

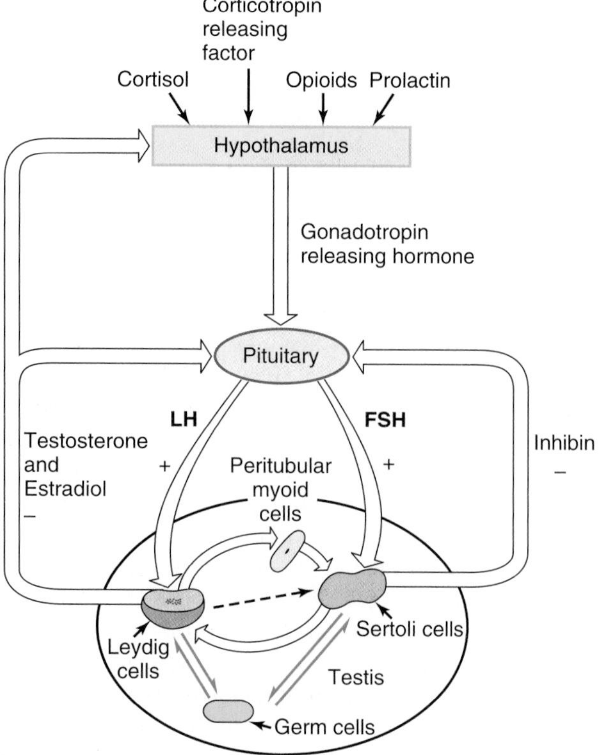

Figure 36-2 Hormonal control of testicular function. See the text for further information.

Normal women produce approximately 0.25 mg/day of testosterone, compared with the 5 to 7 mg/day for adult men. Most testosterone circulating in women is derived from the peripheral conversion of androstenedione secreted by the ovaries and adrenals (see Chapter 35). Benign and malignant tumors of the adrenal and ovary, congenital steroidogenic enzyme defects, and disturbances of gonadotropin secretion can be associated with increased androgen production in women.

Androgen action

Endogenous testosterone or exogenous testosterone derivatives are transported to their target tissues through the blood. Circulating testosterone is bound tightly to a serum glycoprotein of hepatic origin, called sex hormone binding–globulin (SHBG), and weakly to albumin. Approximately 1% to 3% of circulating testosterone is generally unbound. However, binding to albumin is of such low affinity that it is functionally equivalent to unbound testosterone. Together the free and weakly bound testosterone, which account for approximately 50% of the testosterone found in adult male serum, can enter target tissues.

There is some evidence that SHBG binds androgen target cells and may play a role in the action of testosterone. Estrogens and thyroxine increase, and androgens, growth hormone, and insulin decrease SHBG production. As a result, the concentrations of SHBG are twofold to threefold greater in women than in men, and are increased in hyperthyroidism. Obesity is associated with low concentrations of SHBG, perhaps because of hyperinsulinemia.

Once testosterone enters the target cell, it may be converted to other compounds or interact directly with ARs (Fig. 36-3). When testosterone enters the prostate gland, nearly 90% of it is metabolized to DHT by 5α-reductase enzymes. There are two 5α-reductase enzymes encoded by separate genes; 5α-reductase type I is expressed in liver, skin, sebaceous glands, most hair follicles, and prostate, whereas 5α-reductase type II predominates in genital skin, beard and scalp hair follicles, as well as prostate. The presence of ambiguous genitalia in patients with inactivating mutations of the 5α-reductase type II gene underscores the importance of this enzyme in normal development of male external genitalia.

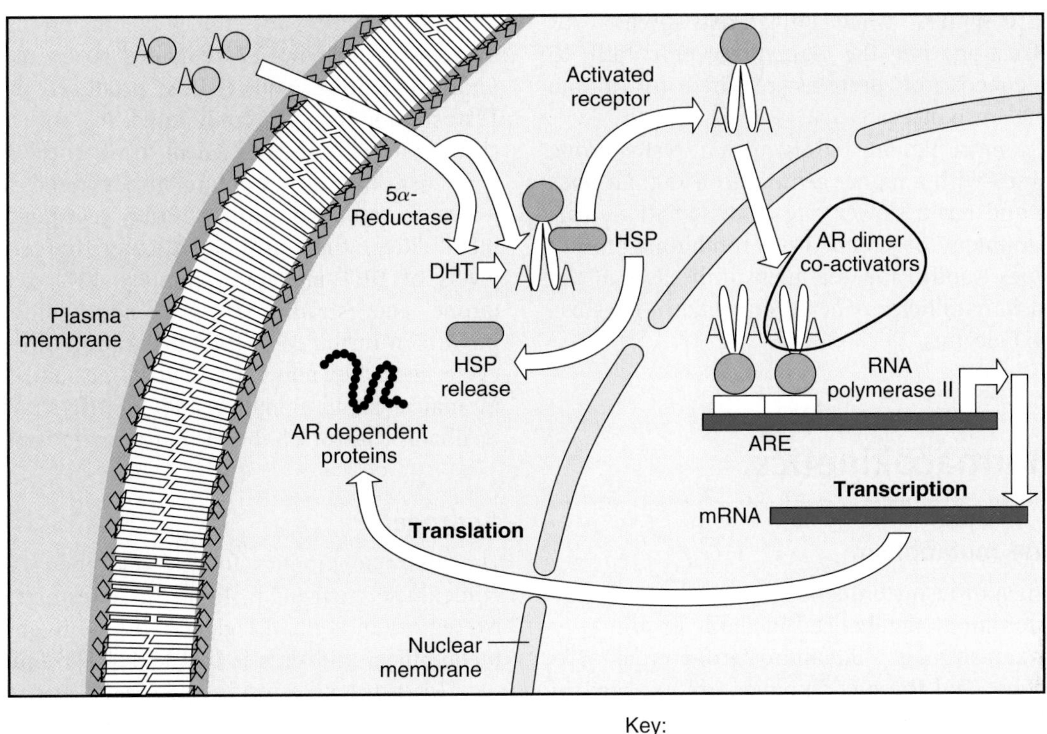

Key:
HSP Heat shock protein complex
ARE Androgen response element
A Androgen (T or DHT)
SHBG
Androgen bound to SHBG
Androgen receptor (AR)

Figure 36-3 Androgen action at target cells. See the text for further information.

Androgen binding to ARs and the postreceptor events that follow are similar to those of other steroid hormones (see Chapter 2). The AR is encoded by a gene on the X chromosome and is expressed in most tissues. When a ligand binds to the AR, the conformation of the receptor is altered, it binds to DNA response elements, multiple coactivator proteins are recruited, and the transcription of messenger RNAs for tissue-specific proteins ensues. Although most actions of androgens are mediated by transcriptional activity of the receptor, others are mediated through second messengers, such as the mitogen-activated protein kinase pathway.

Androgen regulation of target tissues may be positive, as in the stimulation of androgen-dependent proteins within the prostate, or negative, as in the inhibition of pituitary α-subunit gene expression and GnRH release by the hypothalamus. Negative regulation is less well understood, but in certain cases has been explained by AR binding to, and interfering with, the actions of stimulatory transcription factors.

Antiandrogens and androgen antagonists

Antiandrogens act by blocking the synthesis of endogenous testosterone, whereas androgen antagonists bind to ARs. Spironolactone and ketoconazole decrease testosterone production by reducing the activity of cytochrome P450 in testicular microsomes responsible for converting progesterone to androstenedione. These drugs are substrate analogs and compete with the natural substrates for binding to the active site of the enzyme.

Androgen antagonists exert their effects by competing with testosterone and DHT for the ligand binding site on ARs. Antagonists may be either steroidal or nonsteroidal. Steroidal antiandrogens may act as weak agonists in the absence of androgens and bind to other receptors, such as progesterone receptors. Nonsteroidal antiandrogens are more specific. Although dissimilar from testosterone in structure, they undergo sufficient folding to allow them to bind to the receptor to form an inactive complex. Some antagonists permit AR nuclear trafficking, but the bound receptor fails to recruit the coactivator proteins required to initiate transcriptional responses.

DHT is a more potent androgen than testosterone because it binds with a higher affinity to ARs than does testosterone and has a slower rate of dissociation. This led to development of competitive inhibitors of 5-α reductase types I and II for treatment of diseases of the prostate and hair follicles, where conversion of testosterone to DHT occurs.

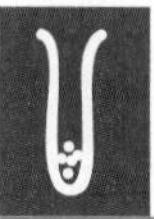

Pharmacokinetics

Testosterone metabolism

The metabolism of testosterone is summarized in Figure 36-4. Testosterone is metabolized in the liver primarily to the 17-ketosteroids, 5α-androsterone and 5β-etiocholanolone, and these compounds are excreted in the urine. However, these compounds constitute only a small fraction of the 17-ketosteroids found in urine. Most urinary 17-ketosteroids are metabolites of androstenedione and DHEA produced by adrenals. Testosterone is also conjugated to sulfuric and glucuronic acids and excreted in urine and bile.

DHT and estradiol are also formed from testosterone metabolism. Although they represent minor (5%) metabolites, they are biologically active. Circulating levels of DHT are approximately 10% that of testosterone, and estradiol levels in men approximate those in women in the early follicular phase of the menstrual cycle. Estradiol plays a role in bone matrix regulation in males, as in females, and contributes to negative feedback control of GnRH and gonadotropins.

Androgens

The pharmacokinetics for the androgens available for clinical use are listed in Table 36-1. Testosterone administered orally is rapidly cleared by the liver by first pass metabolism, and thus is ineffective for clinical use.

Testosterone esterified at the 17-hydroxyl position and contained in an oil suspension is used for intra-

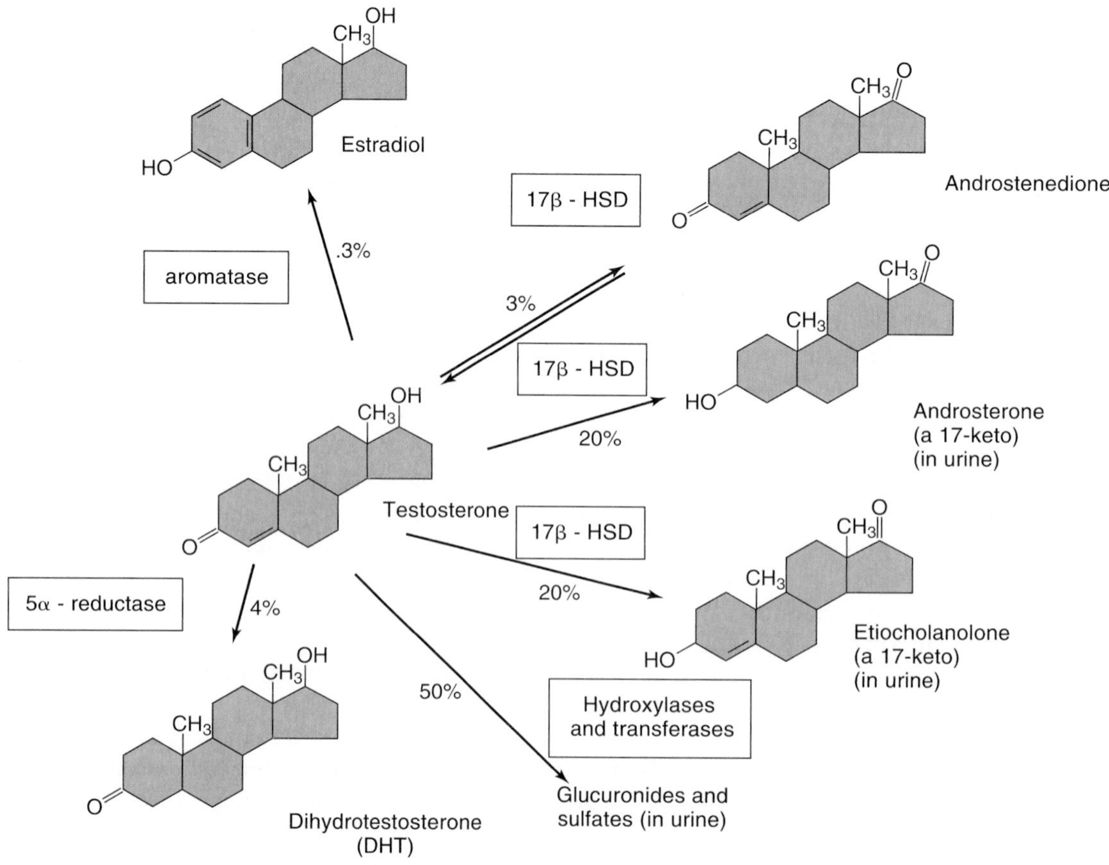

Figure 36-4 Metabolism of testosterone. *17β-HSD*, 17β-Hydroxysteroid dehydrogenase.

Table 36-1 Pharmacokinetic parameters

Drug	Route of Administration	Duration (peak levels, trough levels)	Disposition
Testosterone propionate	IM	Short-acting (1 day, 2-3 days)	M
Testosterone cypionate	IM	Long-acting (1-2 days, 10-14 days)	M
Testosterone enanthate	IM	Long-acting (1-2 days, 10-14 days)	M
Methyltestosterone	Oral, buccal	Short-acting (1-2 hours, 4-5 hours)	M
Fluoxymesterone	Oral	Short-acting (—, —)	M
Danazol	Oral	Short-acting (2 hours, —)	M
Nandrolone	IM	Long-acting (—, —)	M

M, Metabolized.

muscular (IM) injection. Esterification increases the lipid solubility of testosterone and decreases hepatic metabolism, prolonging its action. The esters are converted to free testosterone in the circulation. Testosterone propionate has a relatively short duration of action (1-2 days). When the cypionate or enanthate esters are administered by IM injection, testosterone levels peak in the first few days and then decline towards baseline over 10 to 21 days. The high levels of testosterone and estradiol in the days following injection may produce acne, polyhemia, and gynecomastia, and are associated with mood swings in some patients.

A transdermal method of delivering testosterone was developed in an effort to produce stable physiological drug concentrations. However, the early products had several problems, including suboptimal skin adherence, limited patient acceptability, and frequent production of skin reactions at the application site. Recent developments include testosterone gels and a buccal tablet containing testosterone that forms a gel after it is placed on the surface of the gum.

Testosterone implants in pellet form are inserted subcutaneously using a trocar cannula to lie on top of the rectus sheath in subcutaneous fat. Although popular in some countries, the need for surgical implantation and the tendency for the pellets to extrude through the skin has limited their use in the United States. Another method of testosterone delivery being tested is the IM injection of biodegradable microspheres containing drug.

The synthetic androgens, methyltestosterone and fluoxymesterone, are less extensively metabolized by the liver than testosterone, and are available for sublingual or oral use. Methyltestosterone and fluoxymesterone have relatively short durations of action.

Danazol is only weakly androgenic and interacts with progesterone as well as androgen receptors. It inhibits the pulsatile release of gonadotrophin, with a subsequent decline in serum concentrations of estradiol and estrone in women. Danazol undergoes extensive hepatic metabolism, and peak concentrations occur within 2 hours after oral administration, with a half-life of 4.5 hours. The anabolic steroid nandrolone exhibits high interindividual variability in its metabolic and excretion kinetics.

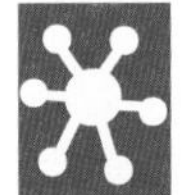

Relation of mechanisms of action to clinical response

Testosterone deficiency may result from a disorder intrinsic to the testis or from insufficient stimulation of the testes by pituitary gonadotropins. The former condition is termed *primary testicular failure,* and the latter, *hypogonadotropic hypogonadism.* Either type may be congenital or acquired. The goal of therapy is to stimulate body and beard hair growth, phallic enlargement, muscle and bone development, voice deepening, and stimulation of libido and potency. Although testosterone treatment stimulates expression of secondary sex characteristics in men with primary testicular failure, they remain infertile.

A decline in testicular function begins in middle age. As men age, Leydig cell volume decreases, and less testosterone is produced. Although the primary defect is in Leydig cells, GnRH secretion is also modified. Because many signs of aging are similar to those of hypogonadism, healthy middle-aged and older men are sometimes treated with testosterone. However, the benefits and risks of androgen replacement for healthy older men are not well understood.

Testosterone is also used in boys to treat congenital microphallus. Most boys with a small phallus will ultimately prove to be hypogonadal as adults. Presumably, the phallus fails to develop normally as a result of impaired androgen production *in utero* or a resistance to androgen action. Treatment is usually begun with intermittent small doses of testosterone, and the patient is monitored carefully to make sure unwanted virilization does not occur.

Androgen replacement is used to stimulate sexual development and increase the height of short teenagers with constitutional delay of puberty. Often human growth hormone is also prescribed. Short stature and delayed puberty are psychologically important. At low doses, testosterone can hasten pubertal growth and adolescent development without compromising adult height. However, premature closure of the epiphyseal plates with resultant growth arrest, and unacceptable virilization may occur if treatment is not carefully monitored.

Androgen levels also decrease in women after menopause and are reduced in women with ovarian failure or hypopituitarism. Accordingly, various androgen preparations have been used to increase libido and sexual function, mood, and well being in women. Although studies suggest benefit, side effects of acne and hirsutism occur.

Anabolic steroids in normal men

Androgens known as anabolic steroids are used by athletes to increase muscle mass and physical performance, and are used therapeutically in children to promote growth. These drugs are believed to be more anabolic than androgenic. This conclusion is based on studies in immature male rats, where increased levator ani muscle weight occurred at lower doses than those that stimulated growth of seminal vesicles and prostate. Interpretation of these data has been criticized, however, because the levator ani is not a typical skeletal muscle, but a sexual dimorphic muscle of the reproductive tract. Whether the mechanisms by which anabolic steroids act differ from androgens is controversial because ARs in skeletal muscle are not known to differ from those in seminal vesicles and prostate. However, prostate contains 5α-reductase, whereas skeletal muscle does not. Although this enzyme amplifies the action of testosterone, it does not influence the potency of most testosterone derivatives and may reduce the potency of 19-nortestosterone. Thus, local metabolism may influence the potency of various androgens differently, and this effect may vary among target tissues. Coactivators recruited to ARs may be ligand-dependent and also contribute to tissue-specific responses. Drugs commonly used for their anabolic activity include nandrolone, oxandrolone, oxymetholone, and stanozolol.

Other androgen uses

Patients of both sexes with wasting resulting from chronic disease or malnutrition are often androgen deficient. For example, plasma testosterone concentrations are often reduced in men with AIDS, among whom testosterone replacement increases muscle mass and strength, although there is no evidence that androgens prolong survival.

The erythropoietic effect of androgens is well established, as shown by the fact that the hemoglobin concentration is 1 to 2 g/dL higher in men than in women or children, and mild anemia is common in hypogonadal men. Polycythemia may occur as an unwanted effect of androgen therapy.

Androgens have been shown to stimulate erythropoiesis by increasing renal erythropoietin production (see Chapter 19). Androgens also have a direct effect on erythrocyte maturation. Because 5β-androgens (which bind weakly to ARs) are more effective than 5α-androgens, this may constitute a novel mechanism explaining the direct effect of androgens on bone marrow cells. Androgens may be used to treat patients with aplastic anemia, although responses vary. Danazol is an androgen derivative that has been used for the treatment of endometriosis, fibrocystic disease of the breast, and premenstrual tension syndrome. Danazol is used in women, rather than testosterone, because it is weakly androgenic. Danazol is also used to prevent attacks of hereditary angioneurotic edema, a disorder characterized by recurrent edema of the skin and mucosa. These patients lack the function of the inhibitor of the activated first component of complement, and androgens increase serum concentrations of this protein.

Androgens have also been used for treatment of inoperable breast cancer, postpartum breast pain, and engorgement. The mechanisms by which androgens affect the normal breast and modify growth of breast cancer cells are uncertain. The rate of positive responses in women with breast cancer, which average 30%, is less than that seen for other hormonal therapies.

Antiandrogens and androgen antagonists

Blockade of the synthesis or actions of androgen is used as a treatment for female hirsutism, alopecia, acne, precocious puberty in males, benign prostate tumors, and other diseases. In addition, several gonadotropin suppressants that inhibit testosterone production, including leuprolide, buserelin, nafarelin, and goserelin, have been approved for use in the United States. Although the role of androgens in the pathogenesis of benign and malignant prostate disease remains uncertain, patients with disseminated prostate cancer are treated by decreasing testosterone production and impeding androgen action, because the symptoms of bone pain are lessened and survival is prolonged somewhat in such patients.

Finasteride is a competitive inhibitor of 5α-reductase type II that blocks conversion of testosterone to 5α-DHT in tissues containing this enzyme but has little activity against 5α-reductase type I. Finasteride reduces prostate DHT content by 80%, decreasing prostate size, and is used to treat benign prostatic hyperplasia. It is less effective in improving urine flow than are α_1-adrenergic receptor antagonists (see Chapter 10), and its onset of action is much slower. Finasteride may be used concomitantly with α_1-adrenergic receptor antagonists when symptoms progress. Finasteride has little effect in treating established prostate cancer. In a large multicenter primary prevention trial, finasteride prevented or delayed the appearance of prostate cancer (6.3% vs. 8.7% of men followed developed cancer), but, unexpectedly, the risk of high-grade prostate cancer was increased. Consequently, it is not recommended for prevention of prostate cancer. Finasteride at a reduced dose of 1 mg/day is also approved to treat male pattern baldness. After 12 months of therapy, visible improvement occurs in about 50% of treated men.

Dutasteride is a competitive inhibitor of both types of 5α-reductase. It was developed for treatment of men with moderate to severe lower urinary tract symptoms secondary to benign prostatic hyperplasia.

Spironolactone is a synthetic steroid used primarily as an aldosterone antagonist in the treatment of primary and secondary hyperaldosteronism, as an antihypertensive agent, and as a treatment for heart failure (see Chapters 12 and 15). In addition to occupying aldosterone receptors, spironolactone interacts with ARs. Further, spironolactone reduces the concentration of cytochrome P450s in testicular microsomes, resulting in a decline in testosterone synthesis. Progesterone concentration increases because its further metabolism is inhibited. However, a decrease in serum androgen concentration in men produces an increase in gonadotropin secretion, which may return serum testosterone concentrations to normal. Because of its ability to block testosterone synthesis and impede androgen action, spironolactone is used in treatment of hirsute women.

Ketoconazole is a broad-spectrum antimycotic agent used in treatment of systemic fungal infections (see Chapter 50). It inhibits the synthesis of ergosterol in fungi, resulting in altered membrane permeability. It also inhibits the synthesis of cholesterol and interferes with the action of cytochrome P450s in several mammalian cell types, including Leydig cells. The result is a dose-dependent decline in circulating testosterone concentrations in adult men and a rise in serum 17α-hydroxyprogesterone concentrations. Serum LH and FSH concentrations rise because of the decline in testosterone negative feedback. This action of ketoconazole has prompted its investigational use in treatment of prostate cancer and gonadotropin-independent precocious puberty in boys. However, the extent to which it suppresses testosterone synthesis in men is highly variable. Ketoconazole also inhibits cortisol biosynthesis and is used as an adjunct therapy in patients with Cushing's syndrome. Gynecomastia may develop in ketoconazole-treated men.

Megestrol acetate is a progestin with antiandrogenic activity. It is used as an appetite stimulant in patients with cancer anorexia/cachexia and as a treatment for metastatic breast cancer in postmenopausal women. Cyproterone acetate, a synthetic steroid derived from 17α-hydroxyprogesterone, is a steroidal antiandrogen that is not available for clinical use in the United States. Both megestrol and cyproterone activate the glucocorticoid receptor and suppress the hypothalamic pituitary axis. In combination with estrogen, these drugs suppress gonadotropin secretion, inhibit ovulation, and reduce circulating testosterone concentrations.

Flutamide, nilutamide, and bicalutamide are nonsteroidal androgen antagonists approved for immediate and adjuvant treatment of prostate cancer. These drugs are used in combination with GnRH analogs to offset their initial stimulatory effect on LH secretion and thereby testosterone production. These drugs are also used to treat hirsutism in women, but use in healthy women is limited by potential hepatotoxicity. Flutamide is rapidly and extensively metabolized, with a hydroxylated derivative responsible for mediating its antiandrogenic effects.

The histamine receptor antagonist cimetidine, used to decrease gastric acid secretion in treatment of peptic ulcer disease and esophagitis (see Chapter 54), also acts as an antiandrogen. Thus, it has been reported to produce gynecomastia when given in large doses, such as those used in the treatment of patients with Zollinger-Ellison syndrome. Gynecomastia occurs in less than 1% of patients treated with the doses used in peptic ulcer disease. Cimetidine interacts with ARs about 0.01% as effectively as testosterone and has been used to treat hirsutism in women with limited effectiveness.

Side effects, clinical problems, and toxicity

The potential problems associated with some of the important drugs are summarized in the Clinical Problems box. Many side effects of androgens are dose-related and occur when target tissues are stimulated excessively. These include priapism (sustained erection), acne, polycythemia, and prostatic enlargement. Androgens in high doses also decrease high-density lipoprotein concentrations and may be atherogenic. Weight gain and sodium retention may occur during androgen therapy, though the mechanism is unclear. Long-term androgen treatment suppresses gonadotropin secretion, decreases testis size, and depresses spermatogenesis. For this reason, testosterone has been evaluated as a male contraceptive. Occasionally, gynecomastia develops in patients treated with testosterone, which may result from bioconversion to estradiol. Obstructive sleep apnea has been reported to be exacerbated in susceptible men treated with testosterone. Androgens should not be used in men with suspected prostate or breast cancer.

Other side effects of androgens are drug specific. The 17α-methylated androgens may disturb hepatic function, which appears to be an idiosyncratic response. Serum transaminase concentrations may rise, and jaundice develops in 1% to 2% of patients as a result of intrahepatic cholestasis. Peliosis hepatitis and hepatocellular carcinoma have both been observed in a few patients treated with very high doses of alkylated androgens. The 17α-methylated androgens produce greater suppression of high density lipoprotein cholesterol concentrations than testosterone because of their oral route of administration, thereby exposing the liver to high drug concentrations, and because they are not bioconverted to estrogens.

Danazol may produce acne, oily skin, decreased breast size, hirsutism, and decreased high density lipoprotein cholesterol in treated women.

Professional and amateur athletes often use multiple androgens in doses that far exceed physiological concentrations. These androgens, like testosterone, suppress gonadotropin secretion and reduce testicular function, including spermatogenesis. Recovery of normal function may take several years. These drugs also cause increased concentrations of low density lipoprotein cholesterol and decreased high density lipoprotein synthesis and concentrations. This may increase the risk of atherosclerosis in these men. Long-term, high-dose androgen treatment may also increase risk of benign prostatic hyperplasia and cause prostate cancer when these men age.

The testosterone precursor, androstenedione, is available as a nutritional supplement in the United States (see Chapter 7) and is used by amateur and professional athletes as a performance-enhancer. The ingestion by young men of 100 mg of androstenedione three times daily did not increase total serum testosterone levels, but did increase androstenedione, free testosterone, estradiol, and DHT. Most of the orally administered androstenedione is metabolized to testosterone glucuronide and other metabolites.

CLINICAL PROBLEMS

Growth acceleration in children
Priapism
Masculinization in women
Jaundice
Edema
Acne
Hypertension
Weight gain
Suppression of spermatogenesis
Lipid disturbances
Fetal masculinization during pregnancy

Finasteride is associated with a slightly increased risk of sexual dysfunction. Finasteride is not approved for use in women and is contraindicated in women who may become pregnant because it may cause abnormal genital developmental in the male fetus.

Antiandrogens block the actions of androgens. They stimulate gonadotropin secretion by blocking testosterone negative feedback, and the rise in LH increases estradiol production. Together these effects cause gynecomastia with breast pain in as many as 50% of men treated with spironolactone. Libido may decline, and impotence may also occur. Amenorrhea and breast tenderness occur in women. Steroidal antiandrogens tend to be weak agonists and bind to other steroid receptors. Megestrol binds to progesterone and glucocorticoid receptors and may cause edema and nausea and reduce adrenocorticotropin and cortisol levels. Cyproterone acetate has similar side effects and disrupts cyclic menstrual bleeding. The nonsteroidal antiandrogen, flutamide, may produce serious hepatotoxicity. Rarely, hepatic damage has evolved to fulminating liver failure and death. Diarrhea occurs in 20% of men. Both hepatotoxicity and diarrhea are much less frequent with bicalutamide.

New horizons

Testosterone gels that contain 1% testosterone have quickly become the most frequently prescribed method for testosterone replacement. The skin acts as a reservoir and slowly releases testosterone into the circula-

TRADE NAMES

In addition to generic and fixed-combination preparations, the following trade-named materials are some of the important compounds available in the United States.

Androgens

Danazol (Danocrine)
Fluoxymesterone (Halotestin)
Methyltestosterone (Android, Metandren, Testred, Virilon)
Nandrolone (Deca-Durabolin, Durabolin)
Oxandrolone (Anavar)
Oxymetholone (Anadrol)
Stanozolol (Winstrol)
Testosterone cypionate (Depo-testosterone, Virilon IM)
Testosterone gel (Andro Gel, Testim)
Testosterone enanthate (Delatestryl)
Transdermal testosterone (Androderm, Testoderm)

Antiandrogens and androgen antagonists

Finasteride (Proscar)
Flutamide (Eulexin)
Spironolactone (Aldactone)

tion. Gels produce a dose-dependent rise in circulating testosterone that lasts for over 24 hours. The usual daily dose for adult men is 5 to 10 gm of gel applied daily (50–100 mg testosterone). The pain from injections and the peaks and troughs in serum testosterone levels that occur following IM administration of testosterone esters do not occur with gels. This difference in pharmacokinetic properties reduces the likelihood of dose-dependent side effects, such as polycythemia and mood swings. Some patients experience drying and flaking of the skin at the application site with gels, but most do not. There is some concern over transfer of testosterone to female partners and children, so close contact is discouraged for 30 minutes after application. Gels containing testosterone have been available through compounding pharmacists for some time.

Because androgens suppress gonadotropin secretion and spermatogenesis, they have been investigated as hormonal male contraceptives for over 30 years. Within 6 months of weekly IM injections of 200 mg testosterone enanthate, severe oligospermia (less than 3 million sperm per milliliter of ejaculate) was observed in 98% of 357 men in a worldwide study. Although a low sperm count (oligospermia) reduces the chance of impregnation, azoospermia (the absence of sperm in the ejaculate) is the ultimate goal of a male contraceptive. Because progestins work synergistically with androgens to reduce LH and FSH secretion, much interest has focused on combining testosterone with an oral progestin, especially levonorgestrel. A second approach to suppressing LH and FSH secretion is to combine a GnRH antagonist with testosterone replacement, but these peptides are expensive and must be injected subcutaneously.

FURTHER READING

Bagatell CJ, Bremner WJ. *Androgens in Health and Disease.* Towata, NJ, Humana Press, 2003.

Singh SM, Gauthier S, Labrie F. Androgen receptor antagonists (antiandrogens): Structure-activity relationships. *Curr Med Chem* 2000; 7(2):211–247.

Winters SJ. Clinical disorders of the testis. In DeGroot LJ, editor. *Endocrinology,* 4th ed. Philadelphia, WB Saunders, 2001.

Self-assessment questions

1. Gynecomastia may occur during treatment with all of the following *except:*
   a. Spironolactone.
   b. Testosterone.
   c. Finasteride.
   d. Cimetidine.
   e. Flutamide.

2. All of the following statements about anabolic steroid use are true *except:*
   a. LH and FSH secretion are suppressed.
   b. Spermatogenesis is inhibited.
   c. SHBG concentrations decline.
   d. HDL cholesterol concentration is increased.
   e. Hypertension may occur.

3. All of the following inhibit testosterone biosynthesis *except:*
   a. Ketoconazole.
   b. Spironolactone.
   c. Cimetidine.
   d. Estradiol.
   e. Leuprolide.

4. An androgen-deficient adult man with a pituitary adenoma may be treated with:
   a. Testosterone propionate.
   b. Testosterone cypionate.
   c. GnRH.
   d. Danazol.
   e. Flutamide.

5. All of the following increase LH and FSH secretion *except:*

a. Clomiphene.
b. GnRH.
c. Spironolactone.
d. Flutamide.
e. Danazol.

6. All of the following statements about dihydrotestosterone are true *except* that it:

a. Is the major androgen in the prostate.
b. Is the major androgen in the circulation of adult men.
c. Is secreted by the testis.
d. Binds to sex hormone–binding globulin.
e. Is metabolized in the liver.

CHAPTER 37

Thyroid and antithyroid drugs

Stephen W. Spaulding

Major Drugs	
Hormones	Recombinant human TSH (Thyrogen)
Levothyroxine (Levoxyl, Synthroid)	Thyroglobulin (Proloid)
Liothyronine (Cytomel, Triostat)	**Antithyroid drugs**
Liotrix (T_4 plus T_3) (Euthyroid, Thyrolar)	Methimazole (Tapazole, Thiamazole)
	Propylthiouracil (generic)

Therapeutic overview

The thyroid, like most endocrine glands, can secrete too much or too little hormone, producing **hyperthyroidism** or **hypothyroidism,** respectively. Hypothyroidism most commonly results from the end stages of autoimmune thyroid disease (Hashimoto's thyroiditis), in which autoantibodies destroy the thyroid gland. Other causes include familial goiter and surgical removal of the thyroid. Irrespective of the cause, hypothyroidism can be treated with thyroid hormone, either **thyroxine (T_4 or tetraiodothyronine)** or **triiodothyronine (T_3).**

Treatment for hyperthyroidism is more complex. The most common causes of hyperthyroidism are **Graves' disease** (another thyroid autoimmune disease) and **toxic nodular goiter.** In Graves' disease, autoantibodies directed at thyroid-stimulating hormone (TSH) receptors in the thyroid membrane stimulate overproduction of thyroid hormone. The optimal therapy would be to block the immunological stimulation, but this approach is currently impractical. Rather, antithyroid drugs, radioactive iodine, or surgery are used to block the synthesis or effects of excess thyroid hormone. Various treatments for hypothyroidism and hyperthyroidism are summarized in the Therapeutic Overview box.

THERAPEUTIC OVERVIEW

Hypothyroidism

Thyroxine (T_4) or triiodothyronine (T_3)

Hyperthyroidism

Thioureylene drugs for controlling circulating levels of thyroid hormone

β-Adrenergic receptor blockers to ameliorate sympathetic nervous system activity

Glucocorticoids

Radioactive iodine

Surgery

Abbreviations

DIO	deiodinase
DIT	diiodotyrosine
MIT	monoiodotyrosine
PTU	propylthiouracil
rT_3	reverse T_3
T_3	triiodothyronine
T_4	thyroxine, tetraiodothyronine
TBG	thyroxine-binding globulin
Tg	thyroglobulin
TRH	thyrotropin-releasing hormone
TSH	thyroid-stimulating hormone, thyrotropin

Mechanisms of action

Thyroid hormones

Thyroid hormone biosynthesis The two major thyroid hormones are the L-isomers of T_4 and T_3 that represent tetra- and tri-iodinated tyrosine molecules (Fig. 37-1). All T_4 in the body comes from the thyroid, but only a small fraction of T_3 is produced there. The majority of T_3 in the circulation is produced by peripheral tissues, which remove an iodide from the outer ring of T_4, producing T_3.

Within the thyroid, T_3 and T_4 are synthesized by follicular cells **(thyrocytes)** through iodination of the glycoprotein precursor **thyroglobulin (Tg)**. The thyroid gland has an extracellular compartment known as the follicular lumen, in which Tg is stored and processed. The steps involved in synthesis of T_3 and T_4 in the thyroid are depicted in Figure 37-2. The thyrocytes synthesize and process Tg, transport it to the apical membrane, and store it in the follicular lumen until needed.

The thyrocytes take up iodide from the circulation via a symporter present on their basolateral surface that admits sodium down its electrochemical gradient. This sodium/iodide symporter, which is also present in salivary glands, breast and stomach, can transport other anions, such as pertechnetate and perchlorate, which can competitively inhibit iodide transport. Once iodide enters the thyrocyte, it is transported to the follicular lumen by an anion transporter in the apical membrane termed **pendrin.** As iodide reaches the follicular lumen, it is oxidized by a mechanism involving thyroperoxi-

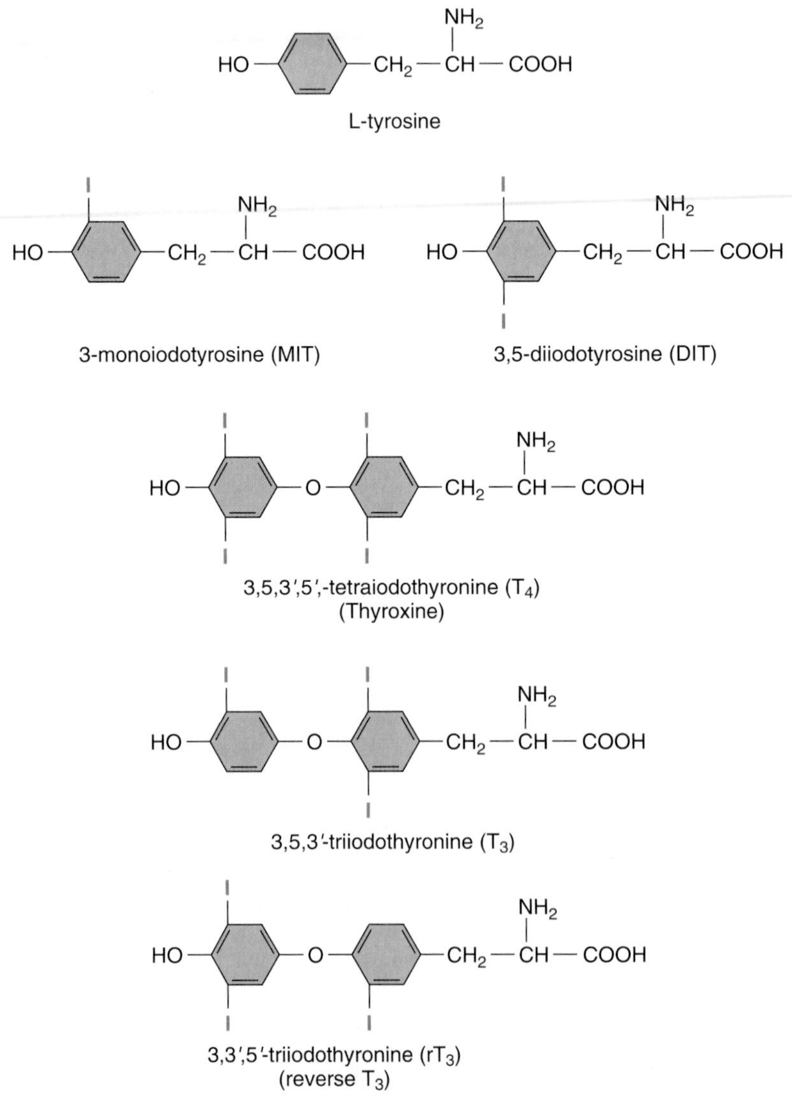

L-tyrosine

3-monoiodotyrosine (MIT)

3,5-diiodotyrosine (DIT)

3,5,3′,5′-tetraiodothyronine (T_4)
(Thyroxine)

3,5,3′-triiodothyronine (T_3)

3,3′,5′-triiodothyronine (rT_3)
(reverse T_3)

Figure 37-1 Structures of tyrosine and its iodinated derivatives.

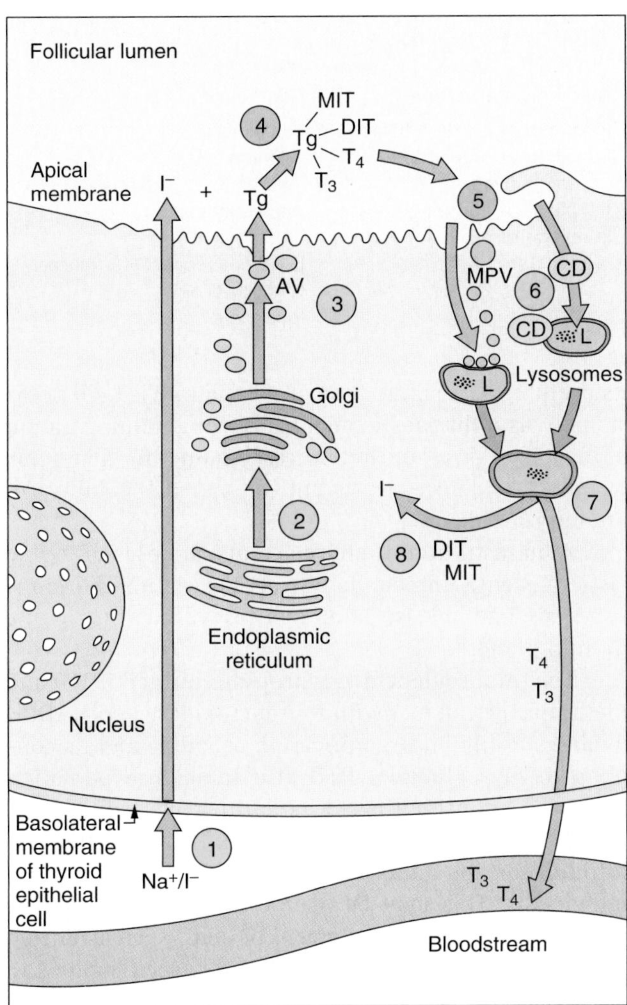

Figure 37-2 Intrathyroidal synthesis and processing of thyroid hormones. *(1)* Iodide is taken up at the basolateral cell membrane and transported to the apical membrane. *(2)* Polypeptide chains of Tg are synthesized in the rough endoplasmic reticulum, and posttranslational modifications take place in the Golgi. *(3)* Newly formed Tg is transported to the cell surface in small apical vesicles *(AV)*. *(4)* Within the follicular lumen, iodide is activated and iodinates tyrosyl residues on Tg, producing fully iodinated Tg containing MIT, DIT, T_4 and a small amount of T_3 (organification and coupling), which is stored as colloid in the follicular lumen. *(5)* Upon TSH stimulation, villi at the apical membrane engulf the colloid and endocytose the iodinated Tg as either colloid droplets *(CD)* or small vesicles *(MPV)*. *(6)* Lysosomal proteolysis of the droplets or vesicles hydrolyzes Tg to release its iodinated amino acids and carbohydrates. *(7)* T_4 and T_3 are released into the circulation. *(8)* DIT and MIT are deiodinated, and the iodide and tyrosine are recycled.

dase, H_2O_2, and two NADPH oxidases. Activated iodide forms covalent links with specific tyrosyl residues on thyroglobulin, producing the thyroid hormone precursors **monoiodotyrosine (MIT)** and **diiodotyrosine (DIT).** This process is called the **organification** of iodide. Some of the iodotyrosyl residues formed donate their iodinated phenolic rings to acceptor iodotyrosyl residues on

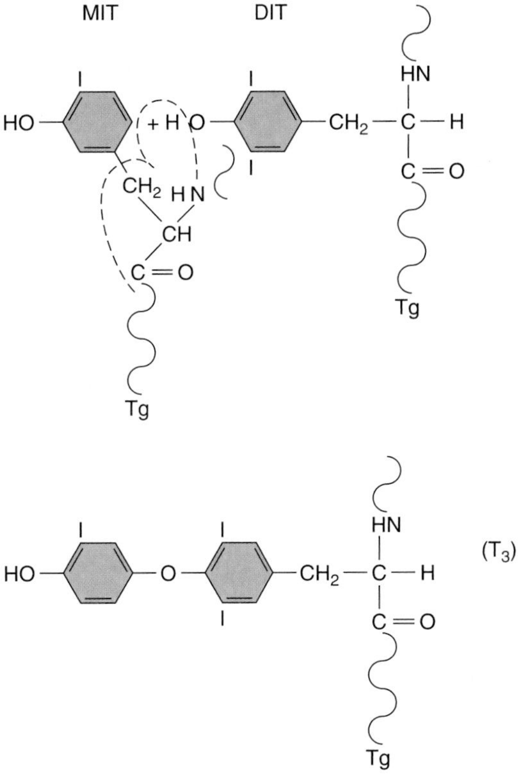

Figure 37-3 Formation of 3,5,3′-triiodothyronine (T_3) by coupling of an "acceptor" diiodotyrosine residue with a "donor" monoiodotyrosine residue, with loss of the alanine side chain of the latter. T_4 is formed in the same manner by coupling of two diiodotyrosine residues.

the thyroglobulin backbone by forming an ether linkage with the acceptor phenolic ring. This process is called **coupling** and is illustrated in Figure 37-3. When thyroid hormone is needed by the body, the newly iodinated thyroglobulin is taken back into follicular cells by endocytosis, where it undergoes proteolysis, releasing T_3 and T_4 to enter the circulation. The MIT and DIT released are deiodinated, and the released iodide is reutilized.

If the circulating level of iodide is elevated persistently, it may cause the thyroid to overproduce thyroid hormone. Thyrocytes utilize several mechanisms to maintain iodide homeostasis to prevent hormone overproduction from occurring. Initially, high levels of iodide cause thyrocytes to shut down organification and coupling, an inhibitory response referred to as the **Wolff-Chaikoff effect.** With continued iodide elevations, this inhibitory effect diminishes. However, the activity of the sodium/iodide symporter decreases in response to elevated iodide levels, preventing overproduction of thyroid hormone. In some patients with thyroiditis or in the fetus, the thyroid does not escape from the Wolff-Chaikoff effect, and persistently high iodine levels can cause goiter or hypothyroidism.

Hormone synthesis in thyrocytes is regulated by TSH released from the pituitary. If the circulating level of thyroid hormone is too high, the pituitary reduces its sensitivity to **thyrotropin-releasing hormone (TRH)** secreted by the hypothalamus into the pituitary portal blood; this results in decreased production of TSH. Pituitary portal blood also carries counter-regulatory compounds that inhibit TSH release, including dopamine and somatostatin (see Chapter 40).

If levels of circulating thyroid hormone are too low, the pituitary becomes more sensitive to pulses of TRH from the hypothalamus, stimulating TSH secretion, and causing thyrocytes to release more thyroid hormone.

Thyroid hormone receptors Thyroid hormones exert their major effects by binding to nuclear thyroid hormone receptors (see Chapter 2). Two genes encode thyroid hormone receptors, and each can be transcribed into several alternatively spliced products. The relative proportions of each isoform expressed in a given cell vary according to its stage of development. One thyroid receptor splice variant (TRα2) does not bind hormone but does bind thyroid hormone response elements in DNA. If TRα2 is expressed at high levels, a tissue's sensitivity to thyroid hormone can be reduced. Thyroid hormone receptors can homodimerize but are generally present as heterodimers, most commonly with the receptor for 9-cis-retinoic acid, but also with other nuclear hormone receptors.

Thyroid hormone receptors associate with DNA as part of a complex of transcription factors, even in the absence of thyroid hormone. When T_3 binds to its receptor, the interactions of the receptor with transcription co-repressors and co-activators change, and local chromatin structure is modified by changes in histone acetylation. Binding of T_3 increases transcription of some genes and decreases the transcription of others. Thyroid hormones also regulate the processing of RNA transcripts, the stability of specific mRNAs, and have other nonnuclear actions.

Antihyperthyroid drugs

As indicated in Table 37-1, antithyroid drugs can inhibit the synthesis, release and metabolism of thyroid hormone, as well as alter its peripheral actions.

Drugs that inhibit thyroid hormone production As depicted in Figure 37-2, thyroid hormone synthesis involves uptake, organification and coupling of iodide, each of which can be inhibited by specific compounds. **Perchlorate** decreases thyroid hormone production by competing with iodide for the sodium/iodide symporter. Although perchlorate can be used briefly as a clinical antithyroid agent, cases of aplastic anemia have limited its usefulness. A single dose of perchlorate is used occasionally as a diagnostic agent following administration of a tracer dose of radioactive iodine to determine whether a defect exists in a patient's ability to organify iodide.

Table 37-1 Antithyroid drugs

Mechanism of Action	Compound
Inhibition of iodide transport	Perchlorate
Inhibition of organification and coupling	Thioureylenes
Inhibition of hormone release	Iodide, lithium
Inhibition of deiodination of T_4 to T_3	Thioureylenes
	β-Adrenergic receptor blockers
	Glucocorticoids
	Iopanoate

Administration of pharmacological doses of **iodide** also transiently inhibits iodide uptake, thyroid hormone synthesis and release, and reduces vascularity of the thyroid gland.

The **thioureylene** drugs **propylthiouracil (PTU)** and **methimazole** interact with thyroperoxidase and NADPH oxidases to inhibit organification of iodide and its coupling to thyroglobulin. PTU also inhibits deiodination of T_4 to T_3, contributing to its antithyroid activity.

Thyroid hormone release can be inhibited by **lithium**, causing goiter or even hypothyroidism in some individuals. This may be a problem in patients maintained on lithium for prolonged periods, such as during treatment of manic-depressive disorder (see Chapter 23).

Drugs that affect the action of thyroid hormones Some symptoms of hyperthyroidism, such as tachycardia, mimic overactivity of the sympathetic nervous system, whereas the bradycardia commonly seen in hypothyroid patients resembles the action of **β-adrenergic receptor blocking drugs.** Thyroid hormones can act on pathways that are also affected by catecholamines, particularly pathways regulated by cyclic AMP. Thyroid hormone affects cyclic AMP responses to catecholamines at several levels. Thyroid hormone alters the density of β-adrenergic receptors, affects the expression of G-protein subunits, alters the activities of adenylyl cyclases or phosphodiesterases, and promotes expression of proteins that are both T_3-responsive and cyclic AMP-responsive, such as uncoupling protein 1, which is involved in thermogenesis. In addition to suppressing sympathetic symptoms, β-adrenergic receptor blockers have some direct antithyroid effect as a consequence of their ability to inhibit the conversion of T_4 to T_3. Therefore, β-adrenergic receptor blockers are sometimes used in hyperthyroidism to ameliorate clinical symptoms, such as tremor and tachycardia, but are not used as a principal therapy.

Table 37-2 Selected pharmacokinetic parameters of thyroid hormones

Drug	Route of Administration	Oral Absorption	Half-Life (euthyroid state)	Disposition	Plasma Protein Binding
Thyroxine (T_4)	Oral, IV	Fair (50%-80%)	7 days	Metabolism, enterohepatic circulation	>99%
Triiodothyronine (T_3)	Oral	Good	24 hours	Metabolism, enterohepatic circulation	>99%
Propylthiouracil	Oral	Good	2 hours	Metabolism	82%
Methimazole	Oral	Good	8-12 hours	Metabolism	8%

Glucocorticoids are often included in acute therapy of severe hyperthyroidism. Although there is no convincing evidence that patients with hyperthyroidism have clinical adrenal deficiency, hyperthyroidism increases delta-4 steroid reductase activity, which enhances the rate of cortisol degradation. In addition, the glucocorticoids inhibit deiodinases, decreasing catabolism of T_4 to T_3. In severe hyperthyroidism, glucocorticoids may have an antipyretic effect.

Several iodine-rich oral agents developed for radiological visualization of the gall bladder (cholecystography) are potent inhibitors of all three deiodinases. One of these compounds, **iopanoic acid**, has been used clinically as an adjunct in the treatment of severe hyperthyroidism, although this is not an approved indication. It must be kept in mind that these compounds provide a source of iodide that could exacerbate hyperthyroidism, unless the patient has been pretreated with a thioureylene drug to inhibit organification.

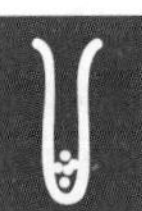

Pharmacokinetics

The pharmacokinetic parameters for thyroid hormones and representative antithyroid drugs are listed in Table 37-2.

Thyroid hormones

The absorption of orally administered T_3 is virtually complete with a half-life of 24 hours in euthyroid subjects. Thus, blood levels rise and fall appreciably after each dose. In contrast, oral absorption of T_4 is incomplete and variable. Because T_4 has a half-life of approximately 7 days in euthyroid subjects, its blood levels do not display substantial variations following a daily dose. Oral absorption of T_4 can be impeded by several compounds, including dietary constituents such as ferrous sulfate, calcium, and soy flour. Conjugated thyroid hormone metabolites are secreted in the bile, and there is substantial enterohepatic recirculation, which can be blocked by ingestion of drugs like cholestyramine (see Chapter 18).

T_4 and T_3 are almost completely protein-bound in the blood, and of the plasma proteins, **thyroxine-binding globulin (TBG)** has highest affinity for them, binding approximately 70% of circulating hormones. Transthyretin (thyroxine-binding prealbumin or TBPA) binds 15% of circulating hormones, whereas albumin, which has a lower affinity but massive binding capacity, accounts for 10% to 15%. Several drugs inhibit binding of thyroid hormones to plasma proteins, including salsalate, salicylate, and phenytoin. Acute illness can decrease the levels of TBG and TBPA, thus reducing total blood levels of thyroid hormone. Sex hormone levels also influence expression of TBG; a rise in estrogen increases hepatic production of TBG, whereas a rise in androgen decreases TBG production. When levels of binding proteins change, the total level of thyroid hormones measured in the blood also change. Thus, it is important to measure serum TSH levels when assessing a patient's thyroid status. The effective level of binding proteins can be assessed by measuring the amount of tracer-labeled T_3 that binds to a resin, or by measuring free hormone level by dialysis.

T_4 is metabolized peripherally primarily by deiodination. Removal of an iodide from the outer ring of T_4 produces T_3, which is more biologically active than T_4. However, removing an iodide from the inner ring of T_4 (see Fig. 37-1) produces **reverse T_3 (rT_3)**, which is biologically inactive. Similarly, removing an iodide from either ring inactivates T_3.

The metabolism and excretion of the iodothyronines are increased by sulfation or glucuronidation. Because rT_3 is more susceptible to sulfate conjugation than either T_3 or T_4, it is metabolized faster. The alanine side chain of the amino acids on T_3 and T_4 can also be metabolized to form the thyroacetic acids, TRIAC and TETRAC, which have very short half-lives.

Three **iodothyronine deiodinases**, which are intrinsic membrane selenoproteins, remove iodide from thyroid hormones. Deiodinase 1 (**DIO1**) removes iodide from both rings, **DIO2** selectively deiodinates the outer ring, whereas **DIO3** selectively deiodinates the inner ring. DIO1 is most active in removing iodide from the inner ring of T_3 sulfate and less active on T_4; it is even less active in removing iodide from the outer ring of T_3. DIO1 is the major deiodinase present in liver, kidney, and thyroid. Thyroid hormone levels regulate DIO1 in some tissues. DIO2 is the "activating" enzyme, selectively deiodinating the outer ring of T_4, converting it to T_3. DIO2 is the major enzyme in brown fat, heart, skeletal muscle, pituitary and pineal, and thyroid hormone levels and adrenergic agents regulate DIO2 in some tissues. DIO3 deiodinates the inner ring of iodothyronines selectively, inactivating both T_4 and T_3. It is the major isoform in brain, fetal liver, and placenta.

In hyperthyroidism, transcription of DIO1 and DIO3 increases in some tissues, whereas transcription of DIO2 is reduced and its degradation is increased. In contrast, in hypothyroidism, DIO2 activity increases in some tissues, increasing conversion of T_4 to T_3.

Many factors influence the metabolism of thyroid hormones. Prolonged fasting reduces peripheral conversion of T_4 to T_3 by half, while doubling the amount of T_4 converted to rT_3. The composition of a patient's diet or nonthyroidal illness can also influence metabolism of thyroid hormones. Turnover of thyroid hormones is increased in hyperthyroidism and is slowed in hypothyroidism. Of the drugs that affect thyroid hormone metabolism, the iodine-rich antiarrhythmic agent amiodarone is the most egregious (see Chapter 14). It inhibits 5′-deiodinase activity, thus increasing serum T_4 and rT_3 levels, while decreasing the level of T_3. However, amiodarone has direct effects on the thyroid, promoting thyroiditis, and can cause hyperthyroidism or hypothyroidism as it releases iodide. One tablet of amiodarone contains 75 mg iodine.

Iodide

Daily intake of about 150 µg iodide is considered normal, and doses up to 500 µg do not affect thyroid function appreciably. Large doses of iodine can exacerbate hyperthyroidism, induce hypothyroidism, or cause a goiter to grow, depending upon the underlying pathology. Two solutions of iodine are used therapeutically, Lugol's solution (which contains 5% KI and 5% elemental iodine, or about 6 mg per drop) and saturated solution of potassium iodide (which contains 1 gm/mL KI or about 40 mg per drop). Surgeons often administer 30 mg iodine twice/day for a few days or weeks prior to surgery to inhibit hormone release and reduce thyroid vascularity in patients with Graves' disease. In general, iodine preparations should only be administered after blocking organification, to prevent iodide from being incorporated into thyroid hormones.

Thioureylenes

Gastrointestinal absorption of thioureylenes is nearly complete. About 80% of PTU is bound to plasma proteins, yet its serum half-life is only 1 to 2 hours; thus, it must be administered every 8 hours. In contrast, methimazole is not bound appreciably to plasma proteins, yet its serum half-life is 8 to 12 hours. Methimazole is concentrated substantially by the thyroid, and its turnover in the thyroid is slow; thus, it is effective administered once a day. Because the thioureylenes act primarily by inhibiting thyroid hormone synthesis, many weeks of administration may be required before thyroid hormones become depleted and euthyroidism is achieved. Both agents are metabolized by oxidation and conjugation.

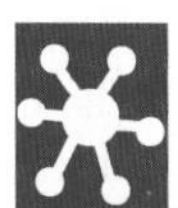

Relation of mechanisms of action to clinical response

Hyperthyroidism

Initial treatment of most patients with hyperthyroidism involves a thioureylene drug. Once the levels of thyroid hormone and TSH begin to normalize, the dose is usually reduced, reflecting the slower metabolism of thyroid hormone in euthyroid subjects. To avoid the risk of hypothyroidism once hormone levels return to normal, a small dose of T_4 may be added.

Long-term therapy for hyperthyroidism includes radioiodine, surgery or continued treatment with thioureylene drugs. In North America, the therapy used most commonly for the definitive treatment of hyperthyroidism is radioactive iodine. Most patients treated with [^{131}I] will become hypothyroid eventually, so it is common to administer a dose that will ablate thyroid function, rather than try to tailor the dose to the percent of radioiodine taken up and the size of the gland.

In selected patients, surgery can offer definitive therapy, but, even so, the patient is usually rendered euthyroid with thioureylenes beforehand. If this is impossible, the risk of a thyroid crisis may be reduced by use of β-adrenergic blocking drugs, glucocorticoids, and iodide.

If hyperthyroidism is due to Graves' disease, which has an immune etiology, a remission sometimes occurs. After maintaining euthyroidism with a thioureylene for 1 to 2 years, the drug can be discontinued, and the patient is monitored to determine whether disease recurs. Patients who have had the disease for a short time, or who have relatively small goiters, are more likely to experience remission. The percentage of patients likely to exhibit permanent remission varies but is less common (~20%) in areas where iodine intake is relatively high, such as in North America. If hyperthyroidism is due to autonomous thyroid nodules, spontaneous remission is very unlikely.

Hypothyroidism

Levothyroxine (T_4) is the hormone preparation used most commonly for hypothyroidism, but liothyronine (T_3), as well as combinations of T_4 plus T_3, desiccated thyroglobulin, and even thyroid extract, are also available. To treat most hypothyroid patients, the thyroid hormone dose is gradually increased while monitoring the patient's symptoms, as well as serum levels of TSH. Because T_4 has a long half-life in euthyroid individuals, which is even longer in hypothyroidism, it can take several months to establish the appropriate replacement dose for an individual patient. Furthermore, that dose can change. If a patient has a functioning remnant of thyroid tissue initially, that remnant can either hypertrophy or atrophy, affecting the replacement dose. In addition, the dose will change, if drugs that alter thyroid hormone absorption or metabolism are prescribed or discontinued. Thus, symptoms and TSH levels should be periodically monitored in hypothyroid patients.

To reduce the risk of precipitating or worsening angina, particularly in older hyperthyroid patients, the dose of thyroid hormone should be increased gradually. However, more aggressive replacement is required occasionally in myxedema stupor/coma, despite the increased risk of precipitating acute cardiac disease.

Side effects, clinical problems, and toxicity

Potential problems associated with some of the important drugs are summarized in the Clinical Problems box.

Common side effects of thioureylene drugs include pruritus, rash, and drug fever. Some patients on PTU complain of a bitter taste. Worrisome but rare side effects include agranulocytosis (0.2%-0.5%) and hepatic dysfunction (1%). Side effects can occur at any time during therapy, so it is important to warn the patient that, if she develops a persistent fever or other symptoms of infection, she must stop taking the drug, until it has been established that the white blood count is not depressed. PTU and methimazole both cross the placenta, so the doses used in pregnant women should be minimized. Both agents are also secreted in breast milk.

Acute side effects of a large oral dose of iodine include gastrointestinal upset and rash, whereas longer exposure can cause swelling of the lachrymal or salivary glands, with persistent tearing and salivation as well as sore gums and teeth (iodism).

CLINICAL PROBLEMS

Thyroid hormones

Acute over-replacement
- Angina, arrhythmias, or myocardial infarction

Chronic over-replacement
- Accelerate osteoporosis or alter metabolism of other drugs

Chronic under-replacement
- Bradycardia, sleepiness, hypercholesterolemia and coronary artery disease

Iodide

- Goiter, hyperthyroidism, hypothyroidism, iodism (swollen salivary and lachrymal glands)

Thioureylene drugs

- Skin rash, granulocytopenia, serum sickness, hepatic toxicity

New horizons

Recent data indicate that different thyroid receptor isoforms can mediate different functional responses. **Synthetic thyroid analogs** with receptor-specificity are currently being developed, such as GC-24, which binds relatively selectively to the β isoform. In GC-24, methyl groups replace the iodides on the inner ring, a phenylmethyl group replaces the iodide on the outer ring, a methylene bridge replaces the ether link between inner and outer rings, and oxoacetate takes the place of the acetate in TRIAC. Such agents could be used potentially to selectively modulate certain thyroid hormone-responsive genes in certain tissues.

If the level of serum Tg becomes undetectable after a thyroid cancer has been resected, then Tg levels can be monitored for development of recurrent disease. Although it is very expensive, **recombinant human TSH** is commercially available and can stimulate a poorly functioning metastasis to produce enough Tg to be detectable. Recombinant human TSH can also increase the amount of radioiodine taken up by poorly functioning thyroid cancer, enhancing its therapeutic effect.

TRADE NAMES

All of the important compounds available in the United States are listed in the Major Drugs box.

FURTHER READING

Duncan Bassett JH, Harvey CB, Williams GR. Mechanisms of thyroid hormone receptor-specific nuclear and extra nuclear actions. *Mol Cell Endocrinol* 2003; 213:1-11.

Shi YB, Ritchie JWA, Taylor PM. Complex regulation of thyroid hormone action: Multiple opportunities for pharmacological intervention. *Pharmacol Ther* 2002; 94*(3)*:235-251.

Self-assessment questions

1. A reliable hypothyroid young woman who had been on a stable dose of 75 µg of T_4 presented with symptoms suggesting mild hypothyroidism. Her serum TSH was 5.5 (normal 0.4-4 µIU/ml and her serum free T_4 was in the lower range of normal. Which is the likely cause of this change?
   a. A change in the manufacturer of the T_4.
   b. The patient had begun taking calcium and iron supplements along with the T_4.
   c. The patient had some residual thyroid function tissue that has now atrophied.
   d. All are possible.

2. Which one of the following is the best reason to choose T_4 over T_3 for the treatment of hypothyroid patients?
   a. T_4 acts more rapidly.
   b. T_4, by being converted to T_3, allows the body some control over hormone delivery to tissues.
   c. T_4 is better absorbed.
   d. T_4 has selective actions on the heart and liver that are more effective than those of T_3.
   e. T_3 causes more allergic reactions than T_4.

3. Which of the following statements is *not* true? β-Adrenergic receptor blockers are useful in treating hyperthyroidism because they:
   a. Block peripheral conversion of T_4 to T_3.
   b. Do not interfere with radioiodine therapy.
   c. Promptly relieve the cardiovascular features of hyperthyroidism.
   d. Do not interfere with thioureylene therapy.
   e. Provide permanent control of hyperthyroidism.

CHAPTER 38

Insulin and drugs used in the therapy of diabetes mellitus

John C. Lawrence, Jr.

Major Drugs	
Insulin	Meglitinides
Biguanides	Sulfonylureas
α-Glucosidase inhibitors	Thiazolidinediones

Therapeutic overview

Diabetes mellitus encompasses a heterogeneous group of disorders characterized by elevated blood glucose and caused by defects in the secretion and/or actions of the pancreatic hormone insulin. Such disorders have been diagnosed in approximately 4.5% of the general population, although the actual incidence is believed to be close to 6.3%. Complications of diabetes mellitus are the leading causes of new blindness in adults, renal failure, and limb amputations, and diabetes is a major risk factor for heart disease and stroke.

Normally, blood glucose is maintained within a relatively narrow range (80-100 mg/dl, or 0.44-0.55 mM). Insulin inhibits hepatic glucose output and stimulates glucose uptake into skeletal muscle and adipose tissue. When insulin action becomes inadequate for any reason, blood glucose levels rise. A diagnosis of diabetes mellitus is indicated when plasma glucose is equal to or above 200 mg/dl (11 mM) at any time in an individual exhibiting other diabetic symptoms, 126 mg/dl (7 mM) after an 8-hour fast, or 200 mg/dl (11 mM) at the 2-hour point in an oral glucose tolerance test (Fig. 38-1). There are two major types of diabetes mellitus, and pharmacological strategies for treating the two types differ in important ways.

Type 1 **diabetes mellitus** results from autoimmune destruction of the pancreatic β cells that produce insulin. It is the more serious of the two types and accounts for approximately 5% to 10% of total cases. There is a genetic predisposition, although other factors are also involved, since the incidence of type 1 diabetes in homozygous twins is only about 50%. The stimulus that prompts the immune system to attack the β cells remains a mystery. The disease has an abrupt onset clinically, although there is evidence that the process actually occurs over a period of years. Onset usually occurs in childhood or early adulthood and is associated with polyuria, polydipsia, and polyphagia. The increased urine volume is caused by osmotic diuresis resulting from increased concentrations of glucose, and ultimately ketone bodies, in urine. Thirst and hunger are compensatory responses. Weight loss is a hallmark of the untreated disease, as is premature cessation of growth in children in whom diabetes develops.

Abbreviations	
GI	gastrointestinal
GLUT	glucose transporter
Hb	hemoglobin
IRS	insulin receptor substrate
IV	intravenous

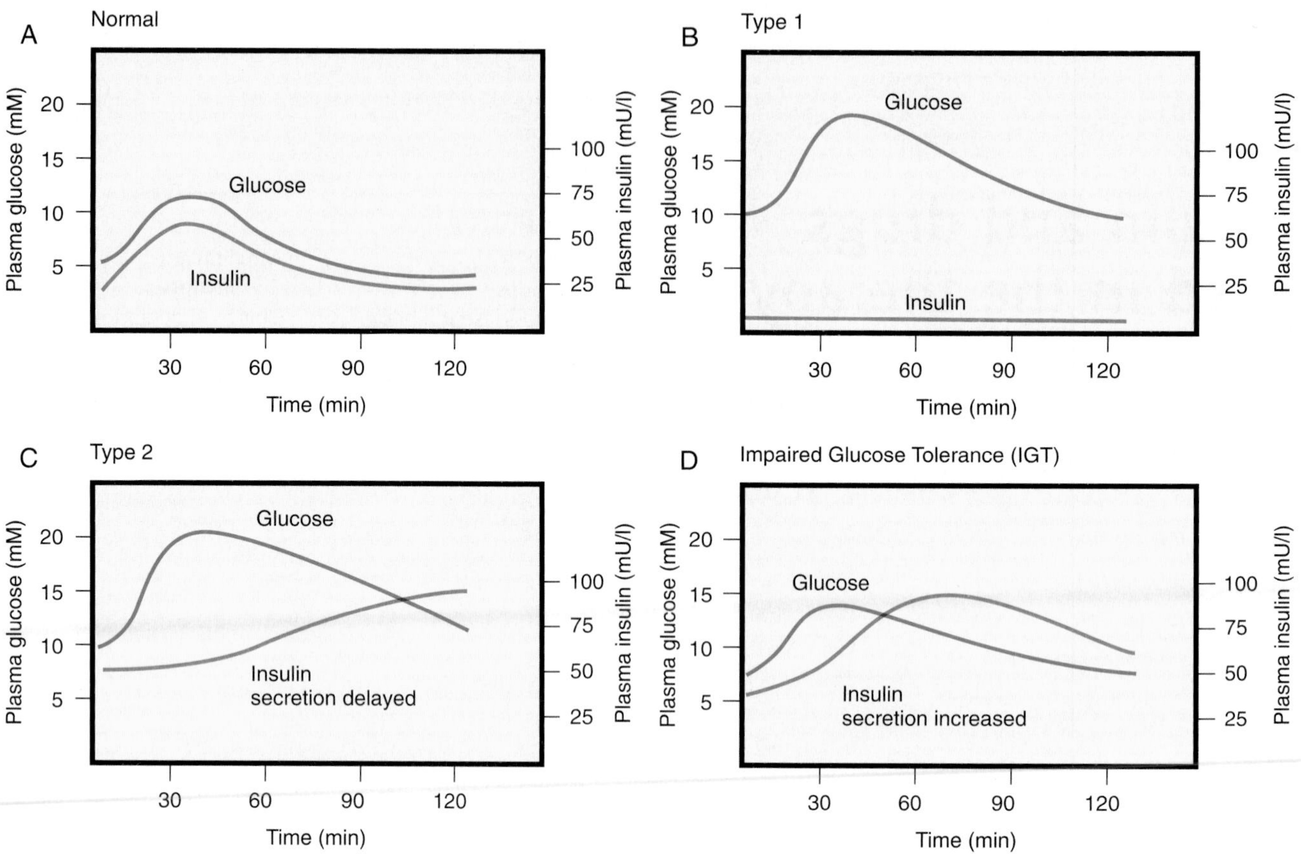

Figure 38-1 Plasma glucose and insulin concentrations in oral glucose tolerance tests in diabetic and control subjects. Nondiabetic subjects **(A)**, type 1 diabetics **(B)**, type 2 diabetics **(C)**, and individuals with impaired glucose tolerance **(D)** were fasted for 8 hours. Plasma glucose concentrations were determined at increasing times after subjects had consumed a drink containing 75 gm of glucose dissolved in water. In nondiabetic individuals the plasma glucose concentration reaches a peak by 30 minutes and returns to normal in 90 to 120 minutes. The insulin concentration rises and returns to normal during the same time period. In type 1 patients, the plasma glucose is greatly elevated at all time points, and plasma insulin is essentially nondetectable. In type 2 diabetes mellitus, the plasma glucose concentration is elevated at all time points and the increase in plasma insulin is delayed and prolonged. The insulin released is insufficient to overcome the insulin resistance. In early type 2 diabetes (glucose intolerance), the plasma glucose concentration is somewhat higher than normal at 30 to 60 minutes and may or may not return to normal at 120 minutes. Because of β cell compensation, the plasma insulin concentrations are higher than normal, both in the fasting state and after glucose is administered.

There may be a detectable, although lower than normal, concentration of serum insulin at the time of onset. However, the concentration declines to negligible values as the disease progresses, and if insulin is not supplied, metabolic acidosis (ketosis) ensues, followed by diabetic coma and death. Thus all type 1 diabetics must be treated with insulin. Restoring glucose levels to near normal is an important goal, since tight control of blood glucose in type 1 diabetics delays or prevents the onset of long-term diabetic complications.

Type 2 diabetes mellitus usually develops after 35 years of age, but it can occur at any age. Indeed, there has been a disturbing increase in the incidence of type 2 diabetes in children. As with type 1, there is a genetic predisposition, but the risk of developing the disease is strongly influenced by environmental factors. Major risk factors are obesity and sedentary life style.

Metabolic abnormalities that lead to type 2 diabetes are inevitably present for some time before overt symptoms appear. Individuals destined to develop diabetes go through a prediabetic phase of variable duration in which insulin levels are elevated but fasting blood glucose concentrations are nearly normal (see Figure 38-1, *D*). The major mechanisms involved are insulin resistance and β cell compensation. In pharmacological terms, insulin resistance simply means that the dose-response curves for insulin in its target tissues are shifted to the right. Thus, insulin is able to stimulate glucose uptake in insulin-resistant tissues, but higher than normal concentrations are required. Nondiabetic insulin-resistant individuals maintain blood glucose within the normal range by releasing more insulin, a phenomenon known as β cell compensation. Even after the onset of diabetes, insulin continues to be synthesized and released in significant quantities, although the diabetic individual is hyperglycemic because the amount of insulin released is insufficient to overcome resistance.

Because only a small amount of insulin is needed to prevent ketone body formation, ketosis and diabetic coma rarely develop in type 2 diabetics. However, a related condition, hyperosmolar coma, can occur. It is most often observed in elderly patients and is usually preceded by an illness or other stressful situation that increases the requirement for insulin. Under these circumstances, the insulin present becomes insufficient to prevent glucosuria. Fluid loss is compounded when vomiting is associated with the precipitating illness. As dehydration becomes severe, urinary output decreases despite the high urinary concentration of glucose. Thus, renal excretion of glucose declines, and blood glucose and serum osmolarity increase to extremely high concentrations, leading to loss of consciousness. Like diabetic coma, hyperosmolar coma is life-threatening, particularly in older diabetics with compromised cardiovascular function.

At onset, type 2 diabetes is usually not life-threatening. Moreover, because symptoms may develop slowly, the type 2 diabetic may be experiencing little discomfort at the time of diagnosis. Nevertheless, it is important to attempt to correct the hyperglycemia in such individuals. Maintaining blood glucose concentrations near the normal range by using either insulin or oral agents has been proven to prevent or delay development of long-term complications in type 2 diabetics. Weight reduction and exercise are proven ways to increase insulin sensitivity, and in many cases type 2 diabetes can be effectively treated by such approaches. However, most type 2 diabetics find it too difficult to adhere to weight reduction and exercise programs, and drug therapy is required. Ultimately, about half will need to go on insulin.

The oral agents that are used to treat type 2 diabetes can be divided into the following two categories (Therapeutic Overview box):

- **Oral hypoglycemic agents,** which include the **sulfonylurea** and **meglitinide** classes of drugs
- **Antihyperglycemic agents,** which include **metformin, thiazolidinediones,** and **α-glucosidase inhibitors.**

THERAPEUTIC OVERVIEW

Type 1 diabetes mellitus

Insulin
Insulin plus thiazolidinedione (when insulin resistance is severe)
Diet
Exercise

Type 2 diabetes mellitus

Diet and weight reduction
Exercise
Metformin
Oral hypoglycemic agent (sulfonylurea or meglitinide)
Thiazolidinedione
α-Glucosidase inhibitor (in combination with one of the above)
Combination of metformin plus thiazolidinedione or sulfonylurea
Insulin

Mechanisms of action

Insulin

When administered as a drug, insulin lowers blood glucose by mimicking effects of the endogenous hormone. Insulin is synthesized in the β cells of the islets of Langerhans. It is a relatively small acidic protein composed of an A chain and a B chain, which are covalently joined by two inter-chain disulfide bonds (Fig. 38-2). The chains are formed by proteolysis of proinsulin, a larger single-chain precursor, by removal of an intervening sequence of amino acids referred to as the C peptide. The conversion of proinsulin to insulin occurs in the secretory granule of the β cell, where most of the insulin undergoes crystallization with Zn^{2+}. Approximately equimolar amounts of insulin and C peptide are stored in the granule, along with a much smaller amount of proinsulin. Insulin release is modulated by many factors (Box 38-1) but is primarily controlled by glucose. A rise in blood glucose stimulates exocytosis of the granules, releasing insulin and other components into the circulation. Insulin inhibits hepatic glucose output and stimulates glucose uptake by skeletal muscle and adipocytes, thereby limiting the rise in blood glucose.

The cellular effects of insulin are initiated after insulin binds to a plasma membrane receptor (Fig. 38-3).

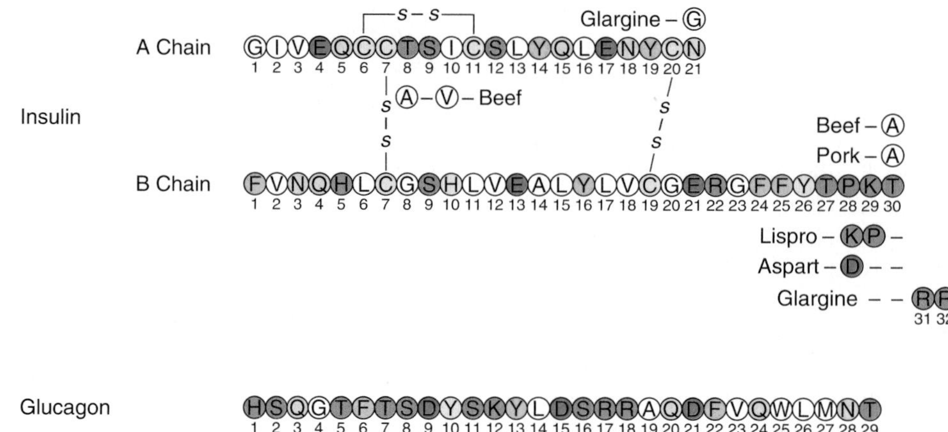

Figure 38-2 Primary structures of insulin and glucagon. The amino acid sequences of the 21 amino acid A chain and the 30 amino acid B chain of human insulin, and the 29 amino acids in human glucagon, are denoted by single letter code. The two interchain disulfide bridges and the intrachain disulfide in the A chain are indicated. Residues in beef or pork insulins that differ from those in human insulin are shown above or below the A and B chain sequences. Also depicted are the amino acids in glargine insulin, lispro insulin, and aspart insulin that differ from those in unmodified insulin.

Box 38-1 Some factors that control the release of endogenous insulin

Stimulate

Nutrients
- Glucose
- Amino acids
- Fatty acids
- Ketone bodies

Hormones
- Secretin
- Glucagon
- Pancreozymin
- Gastrin
- Vasoactive intestinal peptide
- Gastric inhibitory polypeptide

Drugs
- β-Adrenergic agonists
- Cholinergic agonists
- Sulfonylureas and meglitinides

Inhibit

Somatostatin
α-Adrenergic agonists

This interaction generates signals that are transmitted to the inside of the cell to trigger activation of various anabolic pathways and inhibition of catabolic processes. The insulin receptor is a **tyrosine kinase** composed of two α-subunits and two β-subunits. Insulin binding to the α-subunit activates the kinase, which resides in the β-subunit. The major substrates for the insulin receptor are insulin receptor substrate (IRS)-1 and IRS-2. Phosphotyrosine residues in the IRS proteins serve as binding sites for elements involved in several signal transduction pathways. Perhaps the best defined of these pathways involves the small GTP-binding protein Ras and leads to cell growth, differentiation, or both. However, most important acute metabolic effects of insulin are mediated by phosphatidylinositol-3-kinase, which is activated when it binds to phosphorylated IRS proteins. The phospholipid products generated by phosphatidylinositol-3-kinase promote activation of isoforms of the protein kinases Akt and PKC. These kinases then phosphorylate effectors that lead to activation of glucose transport and glycogen synthase as well as to increased synthesis of triglyceride and protein.

Stimulation of glycogen synthesis is very important in the action of insulin to lower the blood glucose concentration, as most glucose taken up in response to insulin is deposited as glycogen in skeletal muscle. Activation of glucose transport and glycogen synthase contributes to the overall effects of insulin on glycogen synthesis. Increasing glucose transport allows more glucose to enter the muscle fiber, and activation of glycogen synthase directs the glucose into glycogen. Both covalent and allosteric mechanisms are involved in the control of glycogen synthase (Fig. 38-4). Glycogen synthase is inactivated when it is phosphorylated by the protein kinase GSK-3 and activated when dephosphorylated by the protein phosphatase PP1G. GSK-3 is inhibited when it is phosphorylated by Akt. Thus, by activating Akt, insulin decreases GSK-3 activity, thereby tipping the balance to favor PP1G and

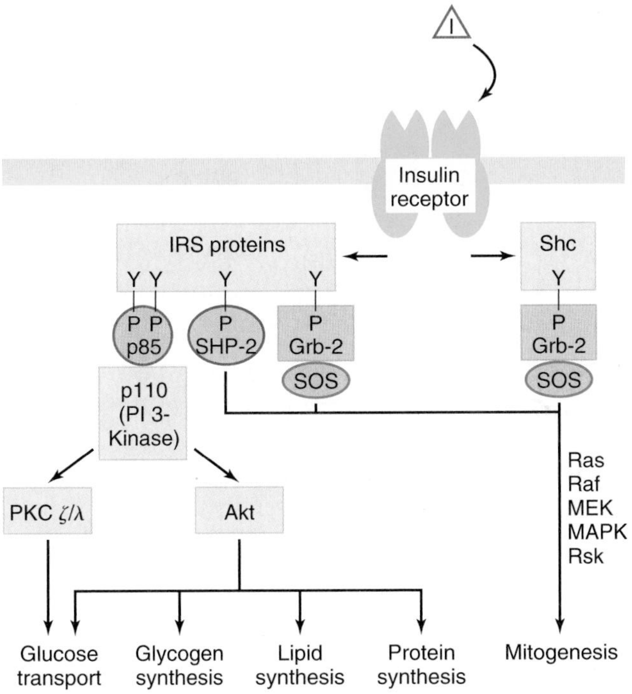

Figure 38-3 Major signal transduction pathways that mediate insulin action. Insulin *(I)* binding to its receptor results in increased tyrosine phosphorylation of the adapter proteins, Shc and insulin receptor substrate *(IRS)* proteins 1 and 2. This creates docking sites for downstream effectors, which bind to phosphotyrosine-containing sites. One such effector is the Grb-2/mSOS complex, which is activated when it binds to either Shc or IRS proteins. Grb-2/mSOS activates Ras, which triggers the sequential phosphorylation and activation of the following kinases: Raf, MEK, mitogen-activated protein kinase *(MAPK)*, and Rsk. This pathway is involved in the proliferative response of cells to insulin and several growth factors. The MAPK pathway is also activated by the protein tyrosine phosphatase SHP-2, which is recruited to IRS proteins in response to insulin. Phosphatidylinositol-3-kinase *(PI 3-kinase)* utilizes two SH domains in its p85 regulatory subunit to bind phosphorylated IRS proteins. Binding activates the p110 catalytic subunit of PI 3-kinase, generating phospholipid products that activate several downstream protein kinases, including Akt and isoforms of protein kinase C *(PKC)*. These downstream kinases then phosphorylate regulatory proteins in the cell, leading to the activation of glucose transport and to increases in the rates of synthesis of glycogen, lipid, and protein.

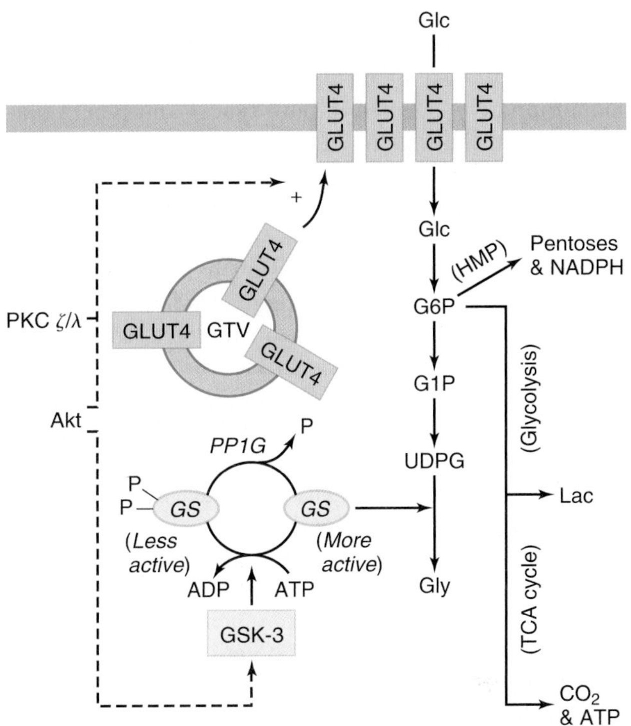

Figure 38-4 Stimulation of glycogen synthesis by insulin involves activation of both glucose transport and glycogen synthase. Insulin stimulates glucose transport by promoting movement of GLUT4-containing vesicles *(GTV)* to the plasma membrane. Translocation of the vesicles occurs in response to activation of Akt and/or PKC. After the vesicles fuse with the membrane, the number of glucose transporters at the cell surface is increased. Glucose *(Glc)* is then able to cross the membrane more rapidly, and in the cell it is phosphorylated to glucose 6-phosphate *(G6P)*. A portion of the G6P is metabolized by the hexose monophosphate pathway *(HMP)*. This pathway, which is stimulated by insulin generates pentoses for nucleotide synthesis and reducing equivalents for fatty acid synthesis. Another portion of G6P enters the glycolytic pathway. Pyruvate generated from glycolysis enters the tricarboxylic acid *(TCA)* cycle and is metabolized to CO_2, resulting in the generation of ATP. The bulk of the glucose that enters a muscle fiber in response to insulin is converted to glycogen *(Gly)*. The G6P is isomerized to glucose 1-phosphate *(G1P)*, which is converted to uridine diphosphoglucose *(UDPG)*, the substrate for glycogen synthase *(GS)*, the enzyme that synthesizes glycogen. Insulin activates GS by increasing the activity of Akt, which phosphorylates and inactivates GSK-3. This allows the protein phosphatase, *PP1G*, to predominate, thereby increasing the fraction of glycogen synthase that is in the dephosphorylated, active form.

allowing accumulation of active glycogen synthase. In addition, by stimulating glucose transport, insulin increases the concentration of intracellular glucose 6-phosphate, an allosteric activator of glycogen synthase. Insulin stimulates glucose transport in skeletal muscle and adipocytes by causing the glucose transporter GLUT4 to be relocated from intracellular vesicular compartments to the plasma membrane. Glucose transport increases because the number of transporters at the cell surface increases. Signals arising from Akt and/or PKC cause vesicles containing GLUT-4 to move to the plasma membrane (Fig. 38-4).

Glucagon Glucagon is a single-chain polypeptide with a molecular weight of about 3500 (see Fig. 38-2). It is synthesized in the α cells of the pancreatic islets through processes involving enzymatic cleavage of specific bonds in proglucagon, a large precursor. A related molecule, glycentin, is formed from proglucagon in the stomach and gastrointestinal (GI) tract. Glucagon is sometimes referred to as a **counter-regulatory hormone,** because its action of increasing blood glucose is counter to that of insulin. Glucagon levels may be inappropriately elevated in both type 1 and type 2 diabetics, contributing to the hyperglycemia in these diseases.

The major physiological role of glucagon is to maintain blood glucose during times of fasting. Glucagon secretion is inhibited by hyperglycemia and is stimulated in response to hypoglycemia or an increase in certain amino acids. Glucagon interacts with a specific receptor on the outer surface of sensitive cells, leading to activation of adenylyl cyclase and phospholipase C and increases in intracellular cyclic AMP and inositol 1,4,5-trisphosphate. In the liver, these second messengers increase glucose output by increasing glycogenolysis and gluconeogenesis.

Glucagon is sometimes used as a drug to increase blood glucose concentrations in seriously hypoglycemic patients who are unable to take glucose orally. Its chief use, however, is in radiology. When administered with a radiopaque substance, it relaxes GI smooth muscles, allowing better visualization of tumors and other GI disorders. Glucagon also stimulates lipolysis in adipocytes, and it has both chronotropic and inotropic effects in the heart. It is occasionally used to stimulate cardiac function following an overdose of a β-adrenergic receptor antagonist.

Oral hypoglycemic agents

Oral hypoglycemic agents refer to a category of drugs that decrease blood glucose levels by **promoting release of insulin** from pancreatic β cells. As their name implies, these agents have the potential to decrease blood glucose to subnormal levels. There are two classes of oral hypoglycemic agents, the sulfonylureas and the meglitinides (Fig. 38-5).

Sulfonylureas Tolbutamide, tolazamide, acetohexamide, and chlorpropamide are first generation sulfonylureas. Glyburide, glipizide, and glimepiride are second-generation agents. The second-generation drugs are effective at 10 to 100 times lower concentrations, but all of the drugs promote insulin release by binding to SUR1, a subunit of $K_{IR}6.2$, an inwardly rectifying ATP-sensitive K^+ channel (Fig. 38-6). Binding inhibits channel conductance, resulting in partial depolarization of the membrane and activation of voltage-sensitive Ca^{2+} channels. The resulting increase in cytosolic Ca^{2+} promotes exocytosis of the secretory granules that contain insulin. Glucose also promotes insulin release by inhibiting $K_{IR}6.2$, but in this case, the channel is inhibited by the increase in the ATP/ADP ratio resulting from glucose metabolism. It is clear that insulin

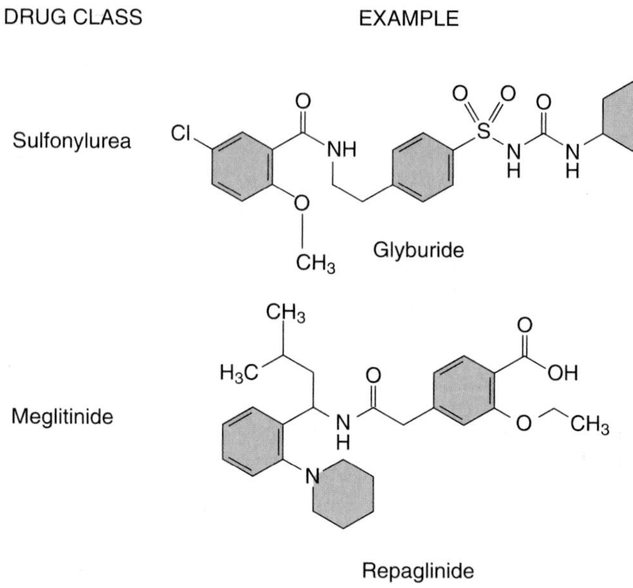

DRUG CLASS | EXAMPLE

Sulfonylurea — Glyburide

Meglitinide — Repaglinide

Figure 38-5 Structures of representative hypoglycemic agents. The chemical structures of the sulfonylurea, glyburide, and the meglitinide, repaglinide, are shown.

release is essential for the hypoglycemic actions of sulfonylureas. However, after long-term treatment with sulfonylureas, the concentrations of insulin return to pretreatment values even though the hypoglycemic effect persists. Thus, sulfonylureas seem to increase insulin sensitivity, apparently by enhancing the effect of insulin on stimulating glucose uptake into muscle and fat cells.

Meglitinides Two members of this class have been approved for use in the United States, repaglinide and nateglinide. These agents are structurally unrelated to sulfonylureas but have a similar mechanism of action. Meglitinides inhibit K^+ conductance by $K_{IR}6.2$. Although the meglitinides bind to a site distinct from that occupied by sulfonylureas, the end result is the same—membrane depolarization and insulin release (see Fig. 38-6).

Antihyperglycemic agents

Antihyperglycemic agents refer to a category of drugs that are capable of lowering elevated levels of blood glucose but which have relatively little potential to produce hypoglycemia. The drugs act by mechanisms that are fundamentally different from oral hypoglycemic agents, because none of them promote insulin release. Currently, three classes of antihyperglycemic agents are used in treating diabetes mellitus (Fig. 38-7).

Metformin Metformin is a biguanide that decreases hepatic glucose output, inhibits absorption of glucose from the gut, and increases glucose uptake by muscle

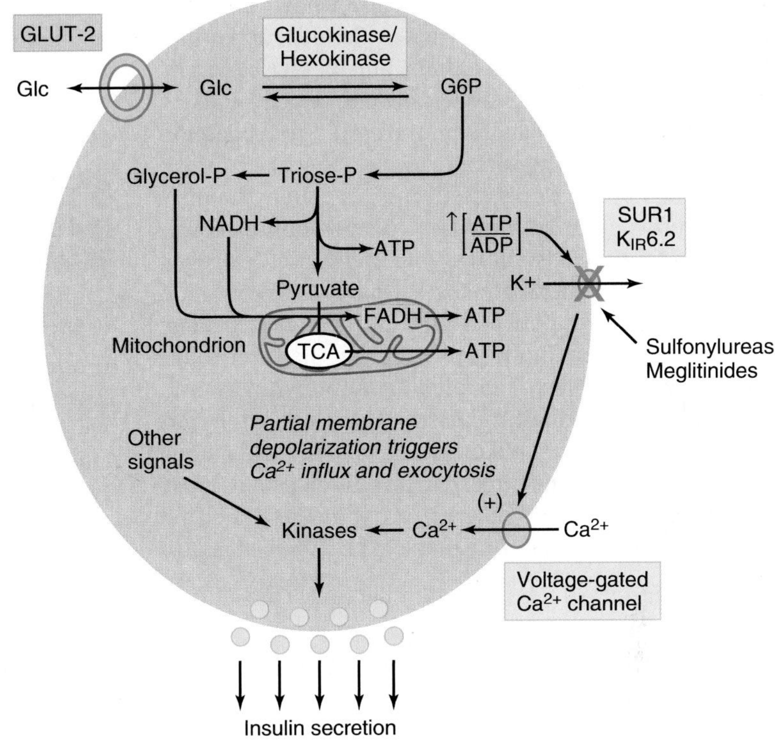

Figure 38-6 Stimulation of insulin secretion by glucose and oral hypoglycemic agents involves partial depolarization of the β cell plasma membrane. Following an increase in blood glucose (Glc), more Glc enters the β cell via the glucose transporter, GLUT2. The Glc is phosphorylated by glucokinase to G6P, which is subsequently metabolized via glycolysis and the TCA cycle, increasing intracellular ATP and decreasing ADP. The resulting increase in the ATP/ADP ratio results in inhibition of the inwardly rectifying K^+ channel, $K_{IR}6.2$. The decrease in K^+ permeability partially depolarizes the β cell plasma membrane, triggering activation of voltage-gated Ca^{2+} channels. The rise in intracellular Ca^{2+} stimulates exocytosis of secretory granules containing insulin. The sulfonylurea and meglitinide oral hypoglycemic agents bind to sites in the SUR1 subunit of $K_{IR}6.2$ and inhibit channel conductance. This also leads to membrane depolarization and insulin secretion.

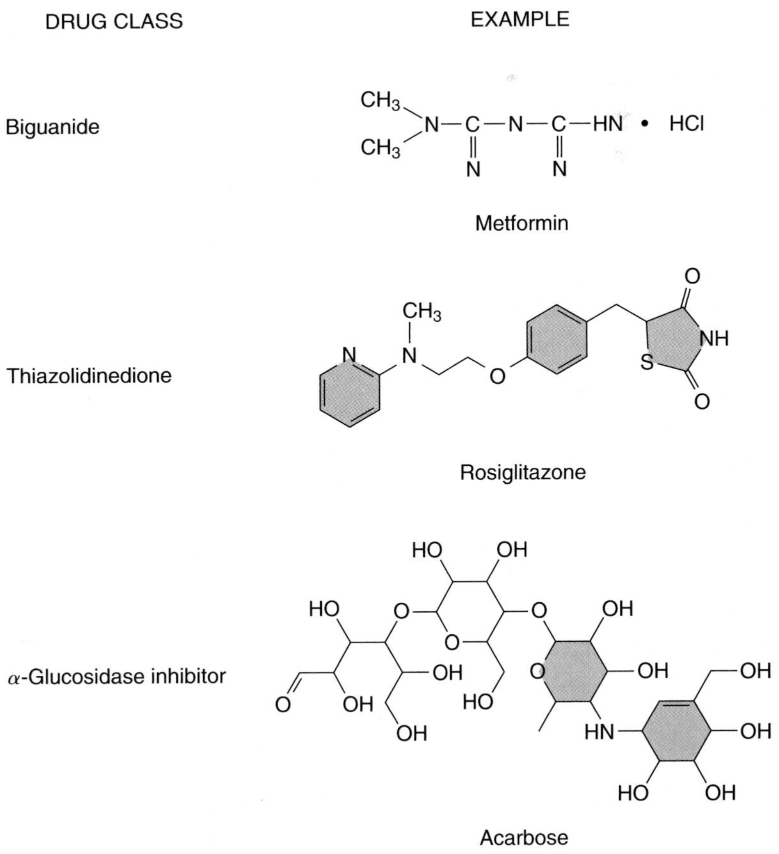

DRUG CLASS	EXAMPLE
Biguanide	Metformin
Thiazolidinedione	Rosiglitazone
α-Glucosidase inhibitor	Acarbose

Figure 38-7 Structures of representative antihyperglycemic agents. The chemical structures of the biguanide, metformin, the thiazolidinedione, rosiglitazone, and the α-glucosidase inhibitor, acarbose, are shown.

and fat cells. The mechanisms involved have not been fully characterized but appear to involve activation of cyclic AMP-dependent protein kinase. Activation of this kinase in skeletal muscle and adipocytes leads to increased glucose transport by promoting translocation of GLUT4 to the cell surface.

At therapeutic doses, metformin is usually comparable in efficacy to sulfonylureas in maintaining lower levels of blood glucose in the type 2 diabetic. However, the acute effect of a single dose of metformin on blood glucose is less pronounced than an oral hypoglycemic agent such as repaglinide. Nevertheless, metformin has the advantage when compared to sulfonylureas and meglitinides of having little potential for causing hypoglycemia. Moreover, unlike insulin, oral hypoglycemic drugs and thiazolidinediones, metformin does not cause weight gain. For this reason metformin is often the first choice drug in treatment of obese type 2 diabetics.

Thiazolidinediones The thiazolidinediones are a new class of antihyperglycemic agents that lower blood glucose by **increasing insulin sensitivity.** Two drugs in this class, rosiglitazone and pioglitazone, are currently approved for use in the U.S. A related agent, troglitazone, was withdrawn from the market when its use was connected with serious hepatotoxicity.

By increasing insulin sensitivity, thiazolidinediones allow insulin to produce a more pronounced decrease in blood glucose. The thiazolidinedione receptor is the ligand-activated transcription factor PPAR-γ. Binding of thiazolidinediones activates PPAR-γ, thereby increasing the expression of mRNAs encoding enzymes and proteins required for optimal insulin sensitivity. Since thiazolinediones attack insulin resistance, the primary defect of type 2 diabetes, the drugs would seem to be ideal for treating this disease. When used alone, however, they are generally somewhat less effective than sulfonylureas in lowering blood glucose levels. On the other hand, rosiglitazone and pioglitazone synergize with sulfonylureas and insulin in decreasing blood glucose in type 2 diabetics; therefore the thiazolidinediones are most commonly used in **combination** therapy. Thiazolidinediones are completely ineffective if used without insulin for the treatment of type 1 diabetes; however, the drugs may be useful in combination therapy with insulin in treating type 1 diabetes when insulin resistance is a problem.

α-Glucosidase inhibitors Acarbose and miglitol inhibit α-glucosidases, which are enzymes in the GI tract involved in degradation of complex carbohydrates. By preventing generation of monosaccharides, which are more readily absorbed than complex carbohydrates, these inhibitors blunt the rise in blood glucose concentrations after a meal. The reduction in blood glucose produced with these inhibitors is relatively small, and α-glucosidase inhibitors are most often used in combination with another antihyperglycemic agent or with an oral hypoglycemic agent.

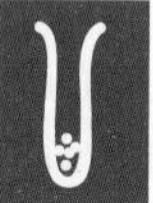

Pharmacokinetics

Insulin

If administered orally, insulin is destroyed by the proteases in the GI tract before it can be absorbed. Except in emergency treatment of diabetic coma, insulin is administered subcutaneously. Regular insulin injected IV acts within minutes but is cleared within an hour. When injected SC, insulin has an onset of action of approximately 1 hour and a duration of about 6 hours. The delay in the absorption of the insulin from the site of SC injection is the reason the duration of action is extended relative to that of insulin injected IV. The half-life of circulating insulin is approximately 8 minutes. Insulin is degraded by proteolytic systems in a variety of tissues, with the liver being the most prominent. In fact, almost half of the insulin released from the pancreas into the portal vein is destroyed by the liver before it can gain access to the general circulation.

Insulin preparations Before 1982, all insulin preparations were extracted from the pancreases of slaughterhouse animals. Almost all preparations now contain recombinant human insulin. Porcine insulin is still available for individuals unable to tolerate recombinant human insulin.

Insulin preparations with differing onsets and durations of action have been generated by altering its solubility, either by genetic manipulation of the insulin protein or by adding modifying agents. These preparations can be divided into four categories (Table 38-1):

- Rapid-acting
- Short-acting
- Intermediate-acting
- Long-acting

Rapid- and short-acting preparations are commonly used in combination with one of the extended-action preparations to obtain a prompt rise in insulin following a meal while maintaining a baseline level of insulin between meals. Several premixed formulations of such preparations are available (see Trade Names Box).

Regular insulin is classified as a short-acting preparation. Insulin has a strong tendency to dimerize, and dimeric insulin is absorbed less rapidly than

Table 38-1 Pharmacokinetic parameters of selected insulin preparations

Insulin Preparation	Species	Onset (hrs)	Peak (hrs)	Duration (hrs)
RAPID (ULTRA-SHORT) ACTING				
Lispro insulin	Human	0.25	0.5-1.5	3-5
Aspart insulin	Human	0.25	0.5-1.5	3-5
SHORT-ACTING				
Regular Insulin	Human, pork	0.5-1	1-2	6-8
INTERMEDIATE-ACTING				
NPH insulin	Human, pork	1-3	4-8	10-16
Lente insulin	Human, pork	1-3	4-8	10-16
LONG-ACTING				
Ultralente Insulin	Human	2-8	None	20-30
Glargine Insulin	Human	1-2	None	24

monomeric insulin. Two rapid-acting preparations, lispro insulin and aspart insulin, have been developed by modifying the insulin protein to prevent dimerization. In lispro insulin, the lysine and proline residues at positions 28 and 29 in the B chain are interchanged (see Fig. 38-2), while in aspart insulin, proline 28 is replaced with arginine. Rapid-acting preparations have an onset of action of 15 minutes but a short duration of action.

In extended-action preparations, the insulin is either in a precipitated state or forms a precipitate after injection, which can be absorbed only after dissolving in the interstitial fluid. A prolonged duration of action is achieved by forming a depot from which the drug is slowly released. The extended action preparations must not be injected IV.

NPH insulin is an intermediate-acting preparation containing the modifier protein protamine. When insulin is mixed with protamine, the two proteins form an insoluble complex, delaying absorption and onset and extending the duration of action. NPH insulin has a neutral (N) pH, contains protamine (P), and was developed by Hagedorn (H). NPH insulin has an onset of 1 to 3 hours and a duration of action of 10 to 16 hours. Lente insulin is another intermediate-acting preparation that is a mixture of precipitated forms that occur when insulin is mixed with Zn^{2+}. Lente insulin has an onset and duration of action comparable to NPH insulin but does not contain a protein modifier.

There are two long-acting insulin preparations. Ultralente insulin is a suspension of large insulin-Zn^{2+} crystals that dissolve slowly at the site of injection. Its onset of action of is variable (2-8 hours), and its duration of action is 20 to 30 hours. Glargine insulin was developed by engineering two additional arginines at the COOH terminus of the B chain and a glycine in place of the aspargine at position 21 in the A chain (see Fig. 38-2). The additional arginines increase the charge and decrease the solubility of the protein at neutral pH; thus preparations must be mildly acidic to maintain solubility. Arginine 21 was replaced with glycine to prevent desamidation, a process accelerated by acidic pH. Glargine insulin also precipitates at the site of SC injection, creating a depot that dissolves slowly and produces a stable baseline level of circulating drug.

Oral hypoglycemic agents

The **sulfonylureas** are all rapidly and completely absorbed from the GI tract and highly bound to plasma proteins. The first-generation drugs typically bind by ionic interactions and may be displaced by other drugs utilizing such interactions. The second-generation drugs are bound by nonionic interactions and are less readily displaced. Most sulfonylureas are metabolized in the liver, and the metabolites are excreted by the kidney.

Pharmacokinetic parameters of some sulfonylureas are summarized in Table 38-2. Tolbutamide has the shortest half-life of all the agents and is rapidly metabolized in the liver to inactive products. In some cases the metabolites are active as hypoglycemic agents and extend the duration of action. Tolazamide, the most slowly absorbed, is metabolized to mildly hypoglycemic products, which are rapidly excreted. Although extensively metabolized by the liver, chlorpropamide has the longest half-life of the first-generation drugs and is administered once daily. The half-lives of the second-generation drugs–glipizide, glyburide, and glimepiride–range from 3 to 7 hours with glipizide to 10 to 16 hours with glyburide. The durations of actions of these drugs are such that they are administered as a single daily dose. The drugs are metabolized to inactive or weakly active products by the liver.

The **meglitinides**, repaglinide and nateglinide, have more rapid onsets and shorter durations of action than the sulfonylureas. Hypoglycemic actions with the meglitinides may occur as early as 20 minutes following an oral dose. Consequently, these drugs are generally taken immediately before meals so that the effect on

Table 38-2 Pharmacokinetic properties of oral hypoglycemic agents

Drug	Administration	T ½ (hrs)	Plasma Protein Binding	Duration (hrs)	Metabolite Activity	Elimination
FIRST-GENERATION SULFONYLUREA						
Tolbutamide	Oral	3-5	>90%	6-12	None	95% M, R
Tolazamide	Oral	7	>90	12-14	Weak	90% M, R
Chlorpropamide	Oral	24-48	>90%	Up to 60	Moderate	90% M, R
SECOND-GENERATION SULFONYLUREA						
Glipizide	Oral	3-7	>90%	24	None	90% M, R
Glyburide[1]	Oral	10-16	>90%	24	None	50% M, R
Glimepiride	Oral	5-9	>99%	24	Weak	99% M, R
MEGLITINIDE						
Repaglinide	Oral	1-2	>98%	2-3	None	99% M, F
Nateglinide	Oral	1.5-2	>98%	2-3	Weak	85% M, R

M, Metabolized; *R*, renal excretion; *F*, feces.

Table 38-3 Pharmacokinetic properties of antihyperglycemic agents

Drug	Administration	T ½ (hrs)	Plasma Protein Binding	Metabolite Activity	Elimination
BIGUANIDE					
Metformin	Oral	2-4	Negligible	None	R
THIAZOLIDINEDIONE					
Rosiglitazone	Oral	3-4	>99%	Weak	99% M, R
Pioglitazone	Oral	3-7 16-24	>99%	Moderate	M, F, R
α-GLUCOSIDASE INHIBITOR					
Acarbose	Oral	NA	None	None	F
Miglitol	Oral	2	None	None	R

NA, Not absorbed; *R*, renal excretion; *M*, metabolized; *F*, feces

enhancing insulin release coincides with the increase in blood glucose. Half-lives of meglitinides are 1 to 2 hours, with durations of action of 2 to 3 hours. They are highly bound to plasma proteins but not readily displaced by other drugs. Repaglinide is metabolized by oxidation and conjugation with glucuronic acid to products eliminated in the feces. Nateglinide is metabolized in the liver to products excreted in the urine.

Antihyperglycemic agents

Pharmacokinetic properties of antihyperglycemic agents are summarized in Table 38-3.

Metformin is administered orally and has a half-life of 2 to 4 hours. Binding to serum proteins is negligible and the drug is excreted unchanged in the urine.

The **thiazolidinediones** are rapidly and completely absorbed after oral administration and highly bound to serum proteins. The half-life of rosiglitazone is 3 to 4 hours, and essentially none of the drug is excreted in an unchanged form. It is metabolized to inactive products in the liver, followed by glucuronidation and sulfation. The half-life of pioglitazone is 3 to 7 hours. Pioglitazone is also extensively metabolized, and a significant fraction of metabolites is conjugated with glucuronic acid or sulfate. Several metabolites are active and accumulate to higher levels in the blood than the unmodified drug, thus increasing the duration of action. The circulating half-life of total pioglitazone is 16 to 24 hours. Most drug and its metabolites are excreted in the bile.

The amount of **acarbose** absorbed systemically is negligible. **Miglitol** is absorbed, although there is no evidence that the circulating drug contributes to its actions. The half-life of circulating miglitol is 2 hours, and almost all the drug is eliminated unchanged in the urine.

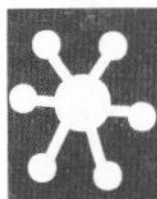

Relation of mechanisms of action to clinical response

Sustained elevation of blood glucose, as occurs in both type 1 and type 2 diabetes mellitus, is damaging to the **microvasculature.** The damage is believed to result from nonenzymatic glycation of proteins in the vessel wall and generation of other reactive products, as a result of the abnormal metabolism of glucose and lipids. Measurements of blood glucose provide an indication of the risk of developing long-term complications. An increase in the incidence of retinopathy is first detected when fasting blood glucose reaches a sustained level of 126 mg/dl, a primary reason this value was selected as the critical point for diagnosing diabetes mellitus. Therapy with insulin and/or oral agents that reduce blood glucose to near-normal levels clearly reduces the vessel damage that underlies diabetic retinopathy, nephropathy, and neuropathy.

Glycosylated hemoglobin (Hb)A1c values are routinely used to assess treatment efficacy. HbA1c undergoes nonenzymatic glycation in red blood cells at a rate directly proportional to glucose concentration. The glycosylated fraction provides an index of the blood glucose concentrations over the previous 8-week period. Values between 4% and 6% are found in nondiabetic individuals. Reducing blood glucose sufficiently to maintain glycosylated HbA1c below 7% is the goal for diabetics. It is important to recognize that it is not desirable to reduce glycosylated HbA1c values to the normal range if doing so results in hypoglycemic episodes.

Insulin

Effects of insulin that contribute to uptake and storage of glucose are summarized in Box 38-2. Insulin stimulates transport of glucose by facilitated diffusion into muscle and fat cells by promoting translocation of GLUT-4 to the cell surface. Insulin does not stimulate translocation of glucose transporters in liver. Glucose transport in hepatocytes is mediated by GLUT-2, which is in the plasma membrane even in the absence of insulin. However, insulin does inhibit glycogenolysis and gluconeogenesis in hepatocytes, decreasing glucose output. Although the effects of insulin on gluconeogenesis are restricted to the liver, the hormone affects activity of many intracellular enzymes involved in energy storage in all major insulin-sensitive tissues. As a result, glucose is efficiently converted to glycogen, triglyceride, and protein.

Elevated blood lipids increase the risk of atherosclerosis, and insulin has several actions that decrease serum lipid concentrations (see Box 38-2). Lipids are transported in blood primarily as particles containing cholesterol esters complexed with proteins (see Chapter 18). Before the fatty acids can be taken up into cells, the cholesterol esters must be hydrolyzed by lipoprotein lipase, which is stimulated by insulin. Insulin also stimulates fatty acid synthesis, although the concentration of free fatty acids in the circulation decreases because insulin decreases lipolysis and accelerates fatty acid esterification. Stimulation of glucose transport into fat cells increases the supply of glycerol phosphate used in esterification.

Box 38-2 Actions of insulin

Carbohydrate metabolism

Increases glucose transport
Increases glycogen synthesis
Increases glucose oxidation
Decreases gluconeogenesis

Lipid metabolism

Increases fatty acid transport
Increases triglyceride synthesis (includes fatty acid synthesis and esterification)
Decreases lipolysis

Protein metabolism

Increases amino acid transport
Increases protein synthesis (including messenger RNA transcription and translation)
Decreases protein degradation

Type 2 diabetes is frequently associated with hypercholesterolemia and hypertension, and when present together the three disorders define a condition referred to as **metabolic syndrome.** The significance of this association with respect to the underlying causes of type 2 diabetes, hypercholesterolemia, and hypertension is unclear. However, it is important to recognize that type 2 diabetics often have other disorders that place them at risk of developing atherosclerosis. Aggressively treating hypertension and hyperlipidemia in such individuals is important to decrease the risk of cardiovascular disease.

Effects of insulin on lipid metabolism are also critical in preventing **ketoacidosis.** Ketone bodies are synthesized from acetyl coenzyme A, and production of ketone bodies during fasting is a normal activity in the liver, which releases ketones into the circulation for transport to heart, skeletal muscle, and other tissues for use as an energy source. The term ketone body, used to describe the compounds that produce ketosis, is a misnomer because the major ketone body produced during diabetes or fasting in humans, β-hydroxybutyrate, is not a ketone. Except for acetone, all ketone bodies are organic acids, explaining why decreased blood pH is associated with their production. Because acetone is volatile, it is excreted to some extent by the lungs, accounting for the "fruity" acetone breath of people with severe ketosis. When insulin concentrations are decreased, as occurs in diabetes or fasting, production of ketone bodies is favored. Severe ketosis does not develop in nondiabetic individuals, however, because only a small amount of insulin is needed to reduce fat cell lipolysis. This reduces the supply of fatty acids, which are a major source of acetyl coenzyme A in the liver.

The later stages of diabetic ketoacidosis are associated with severe fluid depletion, partly because of the osmotic diuresis caused by increased glucose and ketone bodies in the urine. Fluid loss also occurs with vomiting. Unconsciousness, referred to as diabetic coma, followed by cardiovascular collapse and death, occurs if appropriate therapy is not instituted. Treatment involves administration of insulin and rehydration, with careful monitoring to establish and maintain electrolyte balance and to prevent hypoglycemia.

Muscle wasting is a consequence of untreated type 1 diabetes that is corrected by therapy with insulin. Insulin increases protein synthesis in various cells by stimulating several steps in the synthetic pathway, including transcription, rate of amino acid transport, and translation of messenger RNA into protein. Insulin also potently slows proteolysis.

Oral hypoglycemic agents

Oral hypoglycemic agents lower blood glucose by promoting release of insulin from pancreatic β cells, and the drugs may also enhance insulin action in target tissues. Thus the clinical response to oral hypoglycemic agents results indirectly through the actions of insulin.

Antihyperglycemic agents

Metformin acts in part by enhancing insulin sensitivity but also has direct effects on inhibiting hepatic glucose output and increasing glucose transport that are independent of insulin. Metformin decreases blood glucose elevated in type 2 diabetics and has been proven to decrease the incidence of long-term diabetic complications.

Rosiglitazone and pioglitazone increase insulin sensitivity in muscle, liver, and adipose tissue, enhancing insulin action on glucose, as well as lipid and protein metabolism. By decreasing the amount of insulin that needs to be released to control blood glucose, the thiazolidediones may also exert protective effects on β cells.

α-Glucosidase inhibitors only delay glucose absorption, which blunts excursions in postprandial blood glucose levels. These agents do not affect fasting blood glucose.

Side effects, clinical problems, and toxicity

Problems in controlling blood glucose

A major problem in treating diabetes mellitus is that control of blood glucose cannot be achieved with a fixed concentration of insulin. Insulin release is subject to complex regulation by many factors (see Box 38-1), and circulating concentrations change dramatically in nondiabetic subjects to maintain glucose levels within the normal range. Matching insulin concentrations to the glucose load is a major challenge in insulin therapy, particularly since insulin sensitivity may vary greatly among individuals. Too little insulin results in hyperglycemia, while too much causes hypoglycemia and insulin shock. The general strategy is to inject a short-acting insulin preparation to produce a peak in insulin that coincides with the rise in blood glucose that follows a meal. An extended-action preparation is used to establish a baseline concentration to prevent hyperglycemia between meals and during the overnight period. Administering insulin with variable-rate infusion pumps provides a more flexible means to control circulating insulin. There is evidence that tighter control of the blood glucose concentration is possible with these devices, although hypoglycemic episodes are also more frequent. Careful monitoring of blood glucose levels is essential.

Any of several factors can cause insulin sensitivity to change, foiling even conscientious attempts at control. A change in dietary pattern is frequently the cause of episodes of hyperglycemia or hypoglycemia. Exercise or ethanol intake can greatly increase insulin sensitivity, decreasing the hormonal requirement. Stress, pregnancy, or drugs, including thiazide diuretics and β-adrenergic antagonists, decrease insulin sensitivity and exacerbate signs and symptoms of diabetes mellitus.

Insulin

Hypoglycemia is the most serious complication of insulin therapy. Among the causes are mistakes in calculating dose or injecting the hormone, changes in eating patterns, increased energy expenditure, or an increase in sensitivity. The brain and nervous tissue have an absolute requirement for glucose, and severe hypoglycemia can cause loss of consciousness, convulsions, brain damage, and death. Symptoms of hypoglycemia are often caused by increases in epinephrine secretion, abnormal functioning of the central nervous system, or both. When the blood glucose concentration declines rapidly, epinephrine is released as a compensatory measure to stimulate hepatic glucose production and mobilization of energy reserves. Rapid heart rate, headache, cold sweat, weakness, and trembling are characteristic responses to epinephrine (see Chapter 10). The extent to which these symptoms are observed varies considerably, depending on the individual and the rate of fall of the blood glucose concentration. Impaired neural function leads to blurred vision, an incoherent speech pattern, and mental confusion. At this point, an experienced diabetic may be able to recognize his or her hypoglycemic state and take corrective action. However, the mentally disoriented person is likely to need assistance. A glucose tablet or other source of rapidly absorbed glucose may be given to a conscious person.

The unconscious hypoglycemic state induced by an overdose of insulin is referred to as **insulin coma.** Because of the risk of choking, one should never attempt to administer food or drink to an unconscious person. In this case, glucose should be administered IV. Insulin coma is sometimes confused with diabetic coma, but the two have opposite causes and the therapeutic interventions are fundamentally different. Diabetic coma results from an insulin deficit and involves ketoacidosis, electrolyte imbalance, and dehydration. This usually develops over hours or days, whereas a patient in insulin coma may be well one minute and seriously debilitated a few minutes later. Thus a rapid onset implicates insulin coma, particularly if the subject has recently received insulin. Even when diabetic coma is suspected, it is good practice to first administer glucose, because administering insulin to a patient in insulin coma could easily cause death. Giving glucose to a patient in diabetic coma will do no harm, particularly since the subject may actually be hypoglycemic because of the depletion of energy stores. A hypoglycemic patient will recover as soon as blood glucose is increased, provided there is no brain damage.

Insulin has relatively few other side effects. Temporary visual disturbances may result from changes in the refractile properties of the lens brought about by decreasing osmolarity as glucose is brought under control. Localized fat accumulation can occur if insulin is repeatedly administered at the same site. This is caused by the stimulation of triglyceride accumulation in fat cells surrounding the injection site. Curiously, lipoatrophy also sometimes occurs at the injection site. Both of these problems are usually easily remedied by rotating injection sites, a practice now routinely encouraged. Injecting insulin preparations can cause localized allergic reactions leading to pain and itching. These reactions are usually not severe and may disappear with time. Systemic allergic reactions, which may trigger anaphylaxis, occur much less frequently.

Oral hypoglycemic agents

For many years the use of sulfonylureas in the treatment of type 2 diabetes was controversial, as a result of the University Group Diabetes Program, a large long-term clinical trial involving 12 university medical centers. The original goal was to determine whether insulin therapy or orally administered hypoglycemic agents were of any benefit in delaying the onset of diabetic complications. Several years into the study, some participants, notably elderly women treated with tolbutamide, appeared to be dying of cardiovascular disease at a higher rate than those in the control groups, and tolbutamide was withdrawn from the trial. If sulfonylureas were known to place patients at increased risk of death, their use could not be justified, particularly since other treatments are available. However, questions casting serious doubt on the validity of these findings have been raised. For example, the patients assigned to the tolbutamide group appeared to have had more risk factors (e.g., high blood pressure or elevated serum cholesterol concentration). Such issues prompted the American Diabetes Association to withdraw its support of the University Group Diabetes Program's stance on tolbutamide. More recently the United Kingdom Prospective Diabetes Study detected no increase in the incidence of cardiovascular death, myocardial infarction, or sudden death with sulfonylurea (glimepiride or chlorpropamide) therapy. Thus the consensus is that sulfonylureas may be safely used to treat type 2 diabetes.

Weight gain, related to the increase in insulin action on triglyceride synthesis, occurs in most diabetics treated with oral hypoglycemic agents. A more serious complication is hypoglycemia, which may be brought on by an overdose, increased insulin sensitivity, change in dietary pattern, or increased energy expenditure. If the response is mild, it can be corrected by decreasing the dose of the drug. However, severe cases may persist for days and require infusion of glucose.

The activity of the meglitinides may be complicated by drugs that induce or inhibit the cytochrome P450 system. Drugs that induce the system—such as rifampin, barbiturates, and carbamazepine—decrease the concentration of repaglinide. Accumulation of repaglinide is increased by erythromycin, ketoconazole, and miconazole, which inhibit *CYP*3A4. Gemfibrozil markedly enhances repaglinide action and should not be co-administered.

GI disturbances, allergic reactions, dermatological problems, and transient leukopenia can be expected in a small percentage of patients taking oral hypoglycemic agents. A disulfiram type of response (i.e., flushing, nausea, headache) caused by inhibition of aldehyde dehydrogenase is sometimes a problem if sulfonylureas are taken with alcohol, particularly with chlorpropamide. Chlorpropamide also causes fluid retention, resulting from release of antidiuretic hormone.

Contraindications

Oral hypoglycemic agents are contraindicated in patients who do not have a proven pancreatic reserve of insulin. Attention must be given to the metabolism and route of excretion of the drugs before beginning sulfonylurea therapy in patients with impaired hepatic or renal function. Treatment with insulin may be the best choice in these cases. Although no teratogenic effects have been reported, the drugs should not be administered to pregnant or lactating women. Clinical problems are summarized in the Clinical Problems box.

CLINICAL PROBLEMS

Insulin

Hypoglycemia
Visual disturbances
Peripheral edema
Local or systemic allergic reactions

Sulfonylureas

Hypoglycemia
Gastrointestinal disturbances
Hematological disturbances
Ethanol intolerance
Contraindicated in patients with hepatic or renal insufficiency
Drug interactions

Metformin

Lactic acidosis (very infrequent and most likely in patients with renal insufficiency in whom the drug can accumulate)
Gastrointestinal problems

Thiazolidinediones

Weight gain
Edema
Possible hepatic toxicity

α-Glucosidase inhibitors

Abdominal pain
Diarrhea
Flatulence

Antihyperglycemic agents

The antihyperglycemic agents rarely produce hypoglycemia. However, each class of antihyperglycemic agents has different complications and side effects, which are described below.

Metformin Some form of GI distress occurs in over half of the individuals receiving metformin. These side effects are at least partly due to inhibition of nutrient absorption and may include diarrhea, nausea, vomiting, and flatulence. The severity usually diminishes with time, and only about 6% of individuals are ultimately unable to tolerate metformin. GI symptoms are less frequent with an extended-release preparation.

Phenformin, a biguanide related to metformin, was withdrawn from the market when it was clearly demonstrated that the drug had serious side effects, including lactic acidosis, which resulted in death in about half of the cases. Metformin has also been linked to lactic acidosis, although the incidence is very low. Those at highest risk appear to be elderly diabetic patients with impaired renal function. Thus, metformin is indicated for use only in patients having normal renal function, and renal function should be monitored frequently in elderly patients. Excessive consumption of ethanol is contraindicated, because ethanol potentiates effects of metformin on lactate metabolism.

Thiazolidinediones Weight gain is experienced by most patients treated with rosiglitazone or pioglitazone. As PPARγ agonists, thiazolidinediones increase fat cell proliferation and insulin sensitivity, thereby enhancing accumulation of triglycerides. Thiazolidinediones also cause fluid retention, which contributes to the increase in body weight. Edema can complicate therapy with antihypertensives and diuretics. No evidence of hepatotoxicity has been obtained in clinical studies with rosiglitazone and pioglitazone. Nevertheless, troglitazone, a structurally related compound, has been associated with idiosyncratic hepatotoxicity. Therefore, liver enzymes should be monitored before treatment and periodically during therapy.

α-Glucosidase inhibitors Acarbose and miglitol disrupt the normal metabolism of complex carbohydrates in the GI tract, and side effects relating to carbohydrate malabsorption may be as high as 70%. The incidence and/or severity of these side effects, which include abdominal pain, diarrhea, and flatulence, generally diminish with continued treatment. Nevertheless, α-glucosidase inhibitors are contraindicated in inflammatory bowel disease, colonic ulceration, partial intestinal obstruction, or any other intestinal disease or condition that could be exacerbated by the increased formation of gas in the intestine.

New horizons

Successful transplantation of human islets has been achieved, although the immunosuppression required to prevent rejection limits its widespread use, and the supply of islets is insufficient to allow transplantation in all type 1 diabetics. There is great interest in determining whether stem cells can be stimulated to differentiate into functioning β cells for transplantion. Treatments to prevent onset of type 1 diabetes are also being investigated. Several candidate autoantigens that may be involved in islet β-cell destruction have been identified, and trials of antiinflammatory and immunosuppressive interventional therapy in at-risk populations are being designed.

The insulin resistance in type 2 diabetes is related chiefly (70% to 80%), but not exclusively, to defects in nonoxidative glucose disposal. Genetic links to subsets of type 2 diabetes have been established. Mutations in the insulin receptor, glucokinase, and mitochondrial genes have been observed in specific families with type 2 diabetes. These mutations account for a relatively small percentage of the total cases of type 2 diabetes, and efforts to identify the important genes continue.

The mechanisms underlying the connection between obesity and insulin resistance are being elucidated. It is now clear that adipose tissue is an endocrine organ, releasing hormones that affect appetite and insulin sensitivity. Several factors are released by adipocytes to act in skeletal muscle and liver to either increase (adiponectin) or decrease (free fatty acids, TNFα) insulin sensitivity.

With the increasing appreciation of the central role of obesity in insulin resistance, hypertension, and cardiovascular disease, many approaches are being taken to develop drugs to treat metabolic syndrome. These approaches include neuropeptide Y antagonists for control of appetite; low-dose bromocriptine to improve glycemic control; β_3-adrenergic receptor agonists to control obesity; adenosine A_1 receptor agonists to control lipolysis; and inhibitors of IκB kinase, which enhance insulin sensitivity.

TRADE NAMES

In addition to generic and fixed-combination preparations, the following trade-named materials are some of the important compounds available in the United States.

Insulin

Rapid Acting
- Lispro insulin (Humalog)
- Aspart insulin (NovoLog)

Short-Acting
- Regular human insulin (Humulin R, Novolin R, Velosulin)
- Regular porcine insulin (Iletin II regular)

Intermediate acting
- Human Lente insulin (Humulin-L, Novolin L)
- NPH human insulin (Humulin NPH, Novolin N)
- NPH porcine insulin (Iletin II NPH)

Long-acting
- Ultralente human insulin (Humulin-U)
- Glargine human insulin (Lantus)

Combinations

- Mixture 50% NPH insulin, 50% regular insulin (Humulin 50/50)
- Mixture of 75% lispro insulin protamine suspension and 25% lispro insulin (Humalog Mix 75/25)
- Mixture of 70% insulin aspart protamine suspension and 30% insulin aspart (NovoLog Mix 70/30)

Sulfonylureas

- Chlorpropamide (Diabinese)
- Acetohexamide (Dymelor)
- Glimepiride (Amaryl)
- Glipizide (Glucotrol)
- Glyburide (Micronase, DiaBeta)
- Tolazamide (Tolinase)
- Tolbutamide (Orinase)

Meglitinides

- Repaglinide (Prandin)
- Nateglinide (Starlix)

Biguanides

- Metformin (Glucophage)
- Metformin extended release (Glucophage XR)

Thiazolidinediones

- Rosiglitazone (Avandia)
- Pioglitazone (Actos)

α-Glucosidase inhibitors

- Acarbose (Precose)
- Miglitol (Glyset)

Drug combinations containing metformin

- Rosiglitazone plus metformin (Avandamet)
- Glyburide plus metformin (Glucovance)
- Glipizide plus metformin (Metaglip)

FURTHER READING

Charpentier G. Oral combination therapy for type 2 diabetes. *Diabetes Metab Res Rev* 2002; Suppl 3:S70-S76.

Pessin JE, Saltiel AR. Signaling pathways in insulin action, Molecular targets of insulin resistance. *J Clin Inv* 2000; 106:165-320.

Zangeneh F, Kudva YC, Basu A. Insulin sensitizers. *Mayo Clin Proc* 2003; 78:471-479.

Self-assessment questions

1. Insulin action involves all of the following *except:*

a. Stimulation of glycogen synthesis in muscle fibers.
b. Inhibition of lipolysis in the adipocyte.
c. Stimulation of fatty acid synthesis in the hepatocyte.
d. Inhibition of protein breakdown in muscle fibers.
e. Stimulation of gluconeogenesis in the hepatocyte.

2. All of the following are true *except:*

a. Lispro insulin has a more rapid onset of action than that of NPH insulin.
b. Glargine insulin has the longest duration of action of various insulin preparations.
c. Lente insulin contains the protein modifier, protamine.
d. Aspart insulin has a very rapid onset of action.
e. Regular human insulin is used to treat ketoacidosis and diabetic coma.

3. All of the following are true *except:*

a. Acetohexamide is metabolized to a compound with more of a hypoglycemic action than that of the parent compound.
b. Chlorpropamide causes ADH release.
c. Pioglitazone acts to decrease insulin resistance.
d. Glimepiride causes hyperpolarization of the β-cell plasma membrane.
e. Lactic acidosis is a very infrequent side effect of metformin.

4. All of the following are true *except:*

a. metformin is useful in treating type 1 diabetes.
b. meglitinides stimulate insulin release from the β cells of the islets.
c. glyburide is sometimes used in combination therapy with metformin to treat type 2 diabetes.
d. with continued therapy, sulfonylureas can lose their efficacy in a proportion of patients.
e. nateglinide can cause hypoglycemia as a side effect.

5. All of the following are true *except:*

a. Insulin-stimulated glucose transport involves the translocation to the cell membrane and activation of a specific glucose transporter, GLUT-4, in insulin-sensitive tissues such as muscle and fat.
b. Insulin activates glycogen synthase, the enzyme that utilizes UDP glucose to make glycogen.
c. GLUT-4, the insulin-sensitive glucose transporter, is responsible for glucose entry into hepatocytes.
d. The insulin receptor is a tyrosine kinase.
e. The lipid kinase, phosphatidylinositol-3-kinase, has an important role in mediating the cellular actions of insulin.

CHAPTER 39

Drugs affecting uterine motility

B. F. Mitchell

Major Drugs

Uterine stimulation	Uterine relaxation
Oxytocin (Syntocinon, Pitocin)	Ritodrine (Yutopar)
Prostaglandin $F_{2\alpha}$ (Dinoprost)	Terbutaline (Bricanyl, Brethine)
Prostaglandin E_2 (Dinoprostone, Cervidil)	Indomethacin (Indocid, Indocin)
Ergot alkaloids (Ergotrate, Ergometrine)	Celecoxib (Celebrex)
Mifepristone (RU486, Mifeprex)	Nicardipine (Cardene)
Misoprostol (Cytotec)	Progesterone (Prometrium)
	17-Hydroxyprogesterone (Delalutin)

Therapeutic overview

Disorders associated with abnormal uterine motility range from relatively minor aggravations to life-threatening emergencies. The principal goals of drug therapy may be to either **stimulate** or **relax** uterine motility. Since the effects of these drugs are often based on empirical observations rather than on well-designed, controlled studies, their potential benefits must be weighed against possible adverse effects to the woman or her fetus.

Uterine stimulants

There are three clinical uses for uterine stimulants:

- To induce **abortion** in the first half of pregnancy
- To **induce or augment labor** in late gestation
- To prevent or arrest **postpartum hemorrhage**

Use of drugs to terminate early pregnancy is increasingly replacing surgical procedures and their attendant complications. Development of **oxytocic** drugs to prevent or treat postpartum hemorrhage represents a major advance and has largely eliminated this important cause of maternal mortality. These drugs have also reduced markedly dangers associated with the induction of labor.

Although treatment goals are similar for each of these situations, the specific drugs used differ, because of subtle differences in uterine environment and physiological status. Uterine contractions are naturally **phasic**, allowing for resumption of normal utero-fetal-placental hemodynamics between contractions in pregnancy. However, for post-partum hemorrhage, stimulation of **tonic** contractions is necessary to avert excessive blood loss. Changes in plasma **estrogen** and **progesterone** concentrations through the menstrual cycle or during pregnancy can significantly alter uterine responses. This may occur through alterations in receptor density, coupling to effector mechanisms, or other processes.

Abbreviations

COX	cyclooxygenase
IM	intramuscular
IV	intravenous
MLC	myosin light-chain
MLCK	myosin light-chain kinase
MLCP	myosin light-chain phosphatase
NSAID	nonsteroidal antiinflammatory drug
NO	nitric oxide
OT	oxytocin
PG	prostaglandin

In general there are four groups of compounds used clinically to stimulate uterine motility. The most potent and specific is **oxytocin (OT),** which is commonly used to induce or augment labor in late gestation. It is much less useful in early gestation, however, when the uterus responds poorly to OT. The second group consist of the **prostaglandins (PGs)** of the E or F families. Because the uterus is always responsive to PGs, they can stimulate contractions at any stage of gestation (see Chapter 17). They are used in combination with mifepristone to induce early abortion. They are also commonly used in late gestation and can ripen the cervix as well as cause myometrial contraction. The third group is the **ergot alkaloids** (see Chapter 10). These compounds cause intense tonic myometrial contractions, which are undesirable for stimulating labor but useful for treating postpartum hemorrhage. They are rapidly being replaced by analogs of OT or PGs. The final group is the **progesterone receptor antagonists,** of which **mifepristone** is the most widely used (see Chapter 35). These are particularly useful for termination of early pregnancy when uterine quiescence is dependent principally on progesterone. They have also recently been used to induce labor in late gestation.

Uterine relaxants

There are four clinical uses for uterine relaxants:

- To prevent or arrest **preterm labor**
- To reverse **inadvertent overstimulation**
- To facilitate **intrauterine manipulations,** such as conversion of a fetus from a breech to a cephalic presentation, surgical procedures, or postpartum replacement of an inverted uterus
- To relieve painful contractions during menstruation, referred to as **dysmenorrhea.**

The most important disorder of uterine motility is preterm labor (delivery before 37 weeks of gestation). Although this occurs in only 6% to 10% of births in the United States, it is associated with about 75% of deaths and disabilities arising from birthing. In addition to the human loss and emotional costs, health care associated with neonatal intensive care of premature newborns costs billions of dollars each year. Resulting neurodevelopmental problems, or other chronic illnesses, contribute to an even greater loss of human potential.

In contrast to uterine stimulants, the effectiveness of uterine relaxants is controversial. There are several groups of agents used to stop uterine contractions, referred to as **tocolytics,** during late pregnancy when the fetus may be too premature to thrive outside the uterus. They are most commonly administered between 20 and 35 weeks of gestation. Most tocolytic drugs are nonspecific and also cause relaxation of other smooth muscle beds, including blood vessels. Cardiovascular side effects often limit their clinical usefulness.

Because there is no evidence clearly supporting the superiority of any one tocolytic, their use varies markedly. **β_2-Adrenergic receptor agonists** (see Chapter 10), usually ritodrine or terbutaline, have often been prescribed, but their use is declining because of maternal side effects. The **nonsteroidal antiinflammatory drugs (NSAIDs)** and **PG synthesis inhibitors** (see Chapter 31) have also been used, although there are concerns about potential adverse effects on the fetus. **Magnesium sulfate** has become frequently used as a tocolytic agent despite the lack of evidence of effectiveness from well-designed trials. Similarly, **calcium-channel blockers** (principally nifedipine) are used increasingly, but their efficacy has not been proven. The more recently developed **OT antagonist,** atosiban, has demonstrated efficacy but may be associated with fetal adverse effects and has not been approved for use as a tocolytic in the United States. Limited research supports the use of nitroglycerin as a **nitric oxide (NO) donor** to enhance uterine quiescence, and there has been a resurgence of interest in the use of **progesterone supplementation** in early pregnancy to prevent preterm labor in high-risk women.

Dysmenorrhea is caused by uterine spasms secondary to release of PGs at the time of endometrial breakdown associated with menstruation. Several NSAIDs will relieve the discomfort associated with uterine cramps around the time of menstruation (see Chapter 31).

A summary of the therapeutic considerations for the use of drugs that affect uterine motility is presented in the Therapeutic Overview box.

THERAPEUTIC OVERVIEW

Uterine stimulation

Pregnancy termination
Cervical ripening
Induction of labor
Augmentation of labor
Postpartum uterine atony

Uterine relaxation

Arrest of preterm labor
Facilitation of intrauterine manipulation
Reversal of pharmacological uterine hyperstimulation
Relief of dysmenorrhea

Mechanisms of action

Though similar in many ways to other organs containing smooth muscle, the uterus is unique. Its physiological and pharmacological characteristics change constantly in response to changes in estrogen and progesterone throughout the **menstrual cycle** and more so during **pregnancy**. Most unique are the massive anatomical and physiological changes that transform it during pregnancy. Not surprisingly, the factors regulating uterine contractility, and the effectiveness of drug therapy, change remarkably during the menstrual cycle, early and late pregnancy, and around parturition.

At first glance, the uterus appears anatomically simple (Fig. 39-1). There is a body (**fundus**) and an outflow tract (**cervix**) through which the fetus and placenta must pass during parturition. The fundus is composed principally of smooth muscle (**myometrium**) surrounding the uterine cavity, which is lined with a specialized **endometrium** containing stromal cells and glandular epithelium. In pregnancy the myometrium undergoes massive hypertrophy and hyperplasia, predominantly under the influence of estrogen. The endometrium is also is a target for estrogen and progesterone, changing dramatically throughout the menstrual cycle. In pregnancy, stromal cells enlarge, whereas glandular epithelial cells become less prominent. The pregnant endometrium is termed the **decidua.** As pregnancy progresses, the fetus grows in a gestational sac composed of two types of fetal tissue—the inner **amnion**, a single layer of cuboidal epithelial cells with a loose connective tissue matrix, and the outer **chorion**, which is a continuation of placental trophoblasts that extends from the edge of the placenta and surrounds the entire developing conceptus. As the fetus grows, the amniochorial layer becomes fused with the maternal decidua. Near the time of parturition, the decidua is invaded by cells of the immune system. The timing of parturition is a complex and coordinated event involving fetal tissues as well as the maternal decidua, myometrium, and immune system. It appears that there are several redundant pathways for initiation of labor.

It is important not to view labor simply as the onset of myometrial contractions. For successful parturition, the cervix must also undergo dramatic changes, called **ripening.** In this process, collagen and glycosaminoglycans of the cervix are broken down and the content of water and hyaluronic acid increases, probably by matrix metalloproteinases. As a result, the cervix is transformed from a rigid structure that keeps the products of conception confined to the uterus into a soft and pliable structure. During ripening the cervix becomes thin (**effacement**) and then begins to open (**dilation**). Active labor contractions then ensue to continue the process of dilating the cervix and bringing the fetal presenting part through the maternal pelvis. These processes must be well coordinated to ensure normal progressive labor.

Parturition can be considered as an evolution from the quiescent, relatively unresponsive uterus of pregnancy to a sensitive contractile organ at the onset of labor, involving two distinct phases, **activation** and **stimulation.** During activation, the myometrium acquires an increased number of receptors for

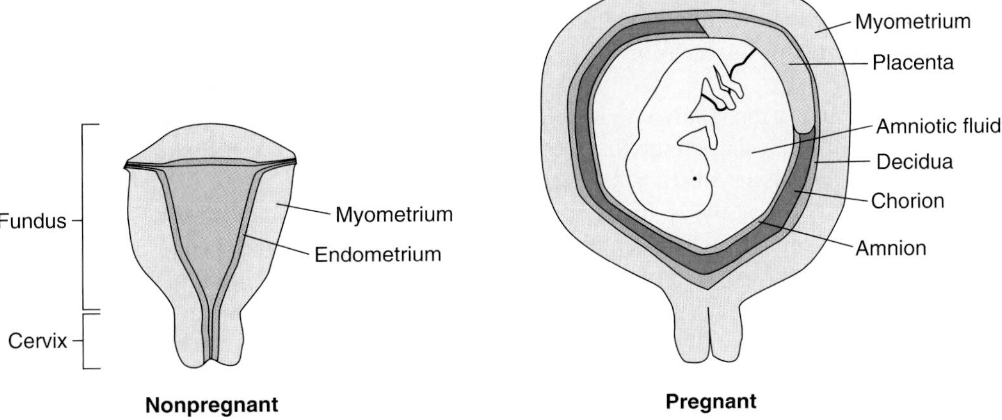

Figure 39-1 Anatomy of the nonpregnant and pregnant uterus. Uterine contractility in the nonpregnant uterus depends on circulating hormonal factors, particularly estrogen and progesterone, and to a lesser extent on interactions between the endometrium and myometrium. There is growing evidence that in late pregnancy, paracrine interactions involving the fetal membranes (amnion and chorion), endometrium (decidua), and myometrium may be the major regulators of uterine activity.

stimulants, particularly OT, an increased number of ion channels, and an increased number of gap junctions. Gap junctions are important in efficient cell-to-cell signal transmission essential to generation of a strong, coordinated contraction characteristic of active labor. The stimulation phase occurs with the arrival of a stimulant to the now-responsive myometrium. Increasing evidence supports an important role for OT or PGs produced locally within an intrauterine paracrine system in this event.

Regulation of myometrial contractility

Although the processes regulating the myometrium and other smooth muscles are similar in some respects (see Chapters 8, 11, and 16), there are unique aspects to control of the myometrium that determine its responsiveness to drugs. Much of our understanding of this process is derived from animal models, particularly **sheep**. In this species, the signal for parturition is mediated through the fetus. In the days preceding the onset of labor, the **fetal adrenal** secretes more **cortisol**, and the resulting increased fetal serum cortisol concentrations induce synthesis of **placental 17-hydroxylase**, which catalyzes conversion of placental progesterone to estrogen. The resulting large increase in the maternal **serum estrogen/progesterone ratio** stimulates increased uterine contractility and labor onset. In most species, this "progesterone withdrawal" is thought to be a critical step in transformation of the uterus from its quiescent state during pregnancy into an active state during parturition.

In humans, however, there appears to be no major increase in fetal serum cortisol concentration and no significant change in the estrogen/progesterone ratio in maternal serum before labor onset. In addition, administration of cortisol does not induce labor. Thus, many investigators have concluded that the mechanisms regulating parturition in humans differ from those in animal models.

Recently, however, it has been shown that fetal membranes and decidua synthesize and metabolize both estrogen and progesterone, and also synthesize OT, suggesting the possible existence of a **paracrine system** within the pregnant human uterus. Other evidence suggests an increase in the estrogen/progesterone ratio in these tissues and an increase in local synthesis of OT at the onset of human labor. Thus, human hormonal mechanisms may be similar to those in animals but occur in a more localized manner. At term, there is also an influx of **immune** cells into the decidua, including pro-inflammatory cytokines (tumor necrosis factor, interleukin-1, and interleukin-6). It is now thought that interactions between the intrauterine paracrine system and the maternal immune system may be important regulators of human parturition.

The actions of estrogen and progesterone on the uterus are not well understood. As in other tissues (see Chapter 35), expression of some uterine genes may be increased while others are decreased through interactions with nuclear receptors. The reproductive effects of estrogen appear to utilize **estrogen receptor α**, while effects of progesterone are mediated primarily through the **progesterone receptor** B isoform (see Chapter 35). In human pregnancy, it has been speculated that a **"progesterone withdrawal"** may be caused by increased expression of the progesterone receptor A isoform, reversing effects of progesterone receptor B activation.

The molecular mechanism of myometrial contraction is similar in most respects to that of other smooth muscle (see Chapter 16). The final focal point of the contractile response is the interaction of phosphorylated **myosin light chains** (MLCs) with actin. Phosphorylation of MLCs is regulated by the balance of activity between MLC kinase **(MLCK)** and MLC phosphatase **(MLCP)**, which is regulated by Ca^{2+}-calmodulin (Fig. 39-2). The most important uterine stimulants (OT, $PGF_{2\alpha}$) activate specific G-protein coupled membrane receptors that activate G_q and membrane phospholipase C (see Chapter 2), leading to the release of Ca^{2+} from the sarcoplasmic reticulum and the influx of Ca^{2+} through **L-type Ca^{2+} channels**. The resultant increase in intracellular Ca^{2+} increases MLCK activity and uterine contraction.

Uterine stimulants

The most potent and specific uterine stimulant is **OT** (Fig. 39-3). This nonapeptide hormone is synthesized in the hypothalamus and stored in the posterior pituitary. It has been used for many decades to stimulate uterine contractions, which are indistinguishable from normal labor. However, its role in the physiological regulation of parturition is not yet completely clear. There is a marked increase in the concentration of OT receptors in the uterus at the time of parturition, suggesting that OT plays an important functional role in mediating this event.

The other major uterine stimulants are the PGs, principally **PGE_2 and $PGF_{2\alpha}$** (see Chapter 17). The rate of intrauterine synthesis of PGs increases several-fold at parturition; however, the role of this process in normal labor is controversial. PGs are known to stimulate uterine activity at any time during gestation and for this reason are used as abortifacients (see Chapter 17). PGE_2 also appears to be important in stimulating processes that result in ripening of the cervix.

The mechanism of action of the **ergot alkaloids** in the uterus is unclear. Most evidence suggests their

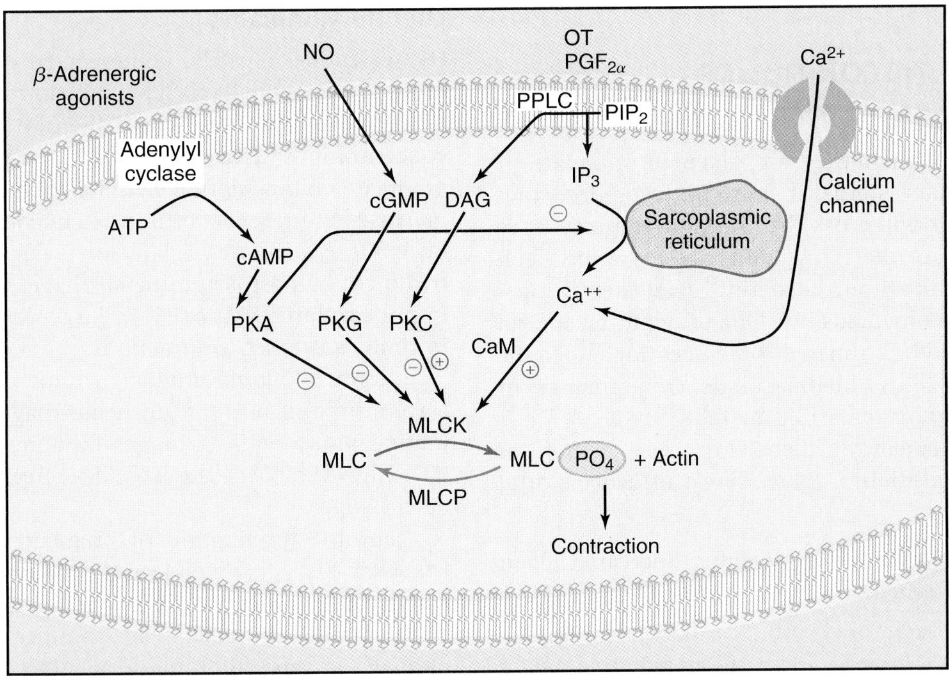

Figure 39-2 Regulation of uterine contractility. The major uterine stimulants are OT and $PGF_{2\alpha}$, which have specific G-protein coupled receptors on the cell surface linked to membrane phospholipase C *(PPLC)*, which hydrolyzes membrane phosphatidylinositol-4,5-bisphosphate (PIP_2) to produce inositol trisphosphate (IP_3) and diacylglycerol *(DAG)*. IP_3 stimulates release of Ca^{2+} from the sarcoplasmic reticulum, followed by influx of Ca^{2+} through L-type calcium channels. The increased intracellular Ca^{2+} binds to and activates calmodulin *(CaM)*, which then activates myosin light chain kinase *(MLCK)*. This enzyme phosphorylates myosin light chains *(MLC)*, and this stimulates the myosin-actin interaction that results in contraction. DAG stimulates protein kinase C *(PKC)*, which may contribute to the activation of MLCK. Inhibition of uterine contractions may be attempted by pharmacologically inhibiting any of the steps in this pathway. Uterine relaxation may result from stimulation of β_2-adrenergic receptors, which results in the production of cyclic AMP *(cAMP)*. This activates protein kinase A *(PKA)*, which may phosphorylate and inactivate MLCK. The cAMP also increases reuptake of the Ca^{2+} into the sarcoplasmic reticulum. Nitric oxide *(NO)* stimulates soluble guanylyl cyclase, which stimulates protein kinase G *(PKG)*, and this may have an effect similar to PKA. Stimulation of these pathways may promote uterine quiescence.

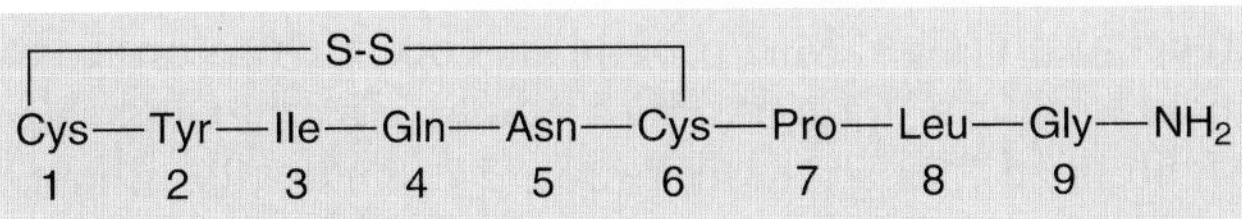

Figure 39-3 Structure of oxytocin.

contractile effects are mediated by interaction with α_1-adrenergic receptors (see Chapter 10), but they also bind to serotonin and dopamine receptors. The use of these drugs is rapidly being replaced by OT or PG agonists.

The finding that administration of **progesterone receptor antagonists** during pregnancy caused cervical ripening and uterine contractions supports a role for progesterone in the maintenance of uterine quiescence. The molecular mechanisms are poorly understood.

Uterine relaxants

As in many other smooth muscles, **β_2-adrenergic receptor** stimulation causes relaxation (see Chapters 10, 16 and 34), an effect mediated by activation of adenylyl cyclase and inhibition of MLCK activity (see Fig. 39-2). **NSAIDs** inhibit PG synthesis by inhibiting cyclooxygenase (see Chapters 17 and 31). Both cyclooxygenase isoforms (COX-1 and COX-2) catalyze PG generation in the pregnant uterus, but the increased PG generation noted at parturition appears to result predominantly from increased COX-2. However, selective inhibitors of COX-2 have not shown a decreased incidence of unwanted side effects, as originally expected. Although **magnesium sulfate** is a commonly used tocolytic drug in North America, its mechanism of action is unclear but may be related to its actions as a divalent cation and competition with Ca^{2+} in myometrial cells.

Ca^{2+}-channel blockers would be expected to inhibit uterine contractions because of their ability to limit Ca^{2+} influx by blocking L-type Ca^{2+} channels in smooth muscle cells (see Chapter 16). Although early studies in animals showed that Ca^{2+}-channel blockers produce metabolic acidosis in the fetus, they are increasingly used as tocolytic agents.

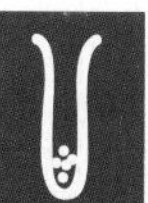

Pharmacokinetics

Regardless of whether they are given to stimulate or relax the pregnant uterus, it must be recognized that most compounds will **cross the placenta** and may have adverse effects on the fetus. Many agents affect fetal cardiovascular function, rendering fetal heart rate–based monitoring methods invalid and requiring special vigilance to avoid detrimental outcomes for either the mother or the fetus. Pharmacokinetic parameters of selected drugs are summarized in Table 39-1.

During pregnancy, there are five important **maternal adaptations** that can influence drug pharmacokinetics:

- Absorption may be increased due to increased blood flow or more efficient mucosal absorption.
- The initial volume of distribution may be increased due to the 40 to 50% increase in maternal blood volume.
- There is increased blood flow to maternal liver and kidney that may increase drug metabolism and/or excretion.
- There is an increased concentration of plasma binding proteins that may decrease metabolism and excretion.
- The placenta may be a site of drug metabolism or maternal drug disposal secondary to fetal transfer, which can be later transferred back into the maternal compartment.

Table 39-1 Selected Pharmacokinetic Parameters

Drug	Route	Metabolic Half-Life	Disposition
Oxytocin	IV, IM	1-6 min	M
PGE_2	Intracervical, intravaginal, IV	Variable	M
Misoprostol	Oral, rectal, intravaginal	30 min	—
Ergonovine	Oral, IM, IV	approx 2 hr	—
Mifepristone	Oral	20-30 hr	M, E
Ritodrine	IV or oral	2 hr	—
Indomethacin	Oral, rectal	4-5 hr	R, B
Magnesium sulfate	IV or IM	—	R

IV, Intravenous; *IM,* intramuscular; *M,* metabolized; *E,* excreted, *B,* Biliary; *R,* renal.

Uterine stimulants

OT, a peptide, must be administered parenterally. It is given intravenously (IV) by infusion pump to induce or augment labor with a half-life of 1 to 6 minutes. In concentrations used to induce or augment labor, OT produces clonic uterine activity. The infusion rate is increased at intervals until the frequency and amplitude of contractions are satisfactory. For prophylaxis or treatment of postpartum hemorrhage, OT can be given intramuscularly (IM) or IV in large doses, which result in tonic, sustained contractions.

Ergot alkaloids produce a tonic contraction ideal for controlling postpartum hemorrhage resulting from uterine atony, with a longer duration of action than OT. However, because of side effects, their use is decreasing.

For the termination of pregnancy in the second trimester, **$PGF_{2\alpha}$** is given into the amniotic fluid. Uterine activity often does not occur for up to 12 hours, indicating an indirect mechanism. In other protocols, $PGF_{2\alpha}$ or PGE_2 is infused through a catheter placed in the cervix.

PG preparations now are used extensively in late gestation to ripen the cervix before induction of labor or to induce labor. PGE_2 is usually administered as a gel into the cervix or vagina or as a solid vaginal suppository with little systemic absorption and few side effects. For the gel preparations, it may be difficult to remove the drug from the vagina in cases of hyperstimulation, and gels should be used only when cervical ripening is required. Once the cervix is ripe, it is common to switch to IV OT. However, OT should not be given for at least 6 hours after the last administration of a PG to avert hyperstimulation. **Misoprostol** has been given orally to induce labor at term. It appears to be effective and safe. Methylated PGs are more resistant to metabolism, more efficacious, and have longer actions. There is increasing evidence of efficacy and effectiveness for induction of labor at any stage of pregnancy.

The antiprogestin **mifepristone** is increasingly used for early (<8 weeks gestation) termination of pregnancy. It is most effective when used in concert with a PG analogue (usually misoprostol).

Uterine relaxants

Ritodrine was the first **β_2-adrenergic receptor agonist** approved for use as a tocolytic agent in late pregnancy. To arrest active labor, it is administered by an IV infusion pump, with the dose carefully titrated to uterine activity. The infusion must be increased slowly and maternal and fetal cardiovascular and metabolic parameters carefully monitored to avert the predictable side effects of these agents. Terbutaline and other β_2-

agonists have also been used as tocolytics (see Chapter 10). These drugs often lose their effectiveness as a result of **tachyphylaxis.** Although oral forms of these agents have been used for prophylaxis, the best evidence indicates they are not effective when administered by this route.

Results of early studies indicated that birth could be delayed for 48 hours through use of the **NSAIDs.** However, the prototype drug indomethacin caused the fetal ductus arteriosus to be constricted (see Chapter 17), because PGE_2 is necessary to maintain ductal patency, reducing their use. However, recently there has been a resurgence in the use of indomethacin by rectal suppository, often followed by oral maintenance therapy. Recent trials have evaluated intravenous infusions of selective COX-2 inhibitors such as **celecoxib.**

Magnesium sulfate is administered IV and excreted by the kidney, so its dose must be closely monitored in patients with impaired renal function. High infusion rates are required to achieve effective tocolysis, and significant side effects are common at these rates. Recent studies have evaluated the tocolytic effects of **progesterone** (as vaginal suppositories) or 17-hydroxyprogesterone caproate (IM).

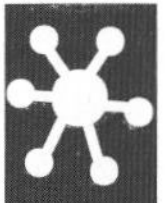

Relation of mechanisms of action to clinical response

Induction/augmentation of labor

Induction of labor must include **ripening of the cervix,** if this has not occurred naturally. Oxytocic drugs stimulate contractions but often must be administered for a prolonged time if the cervix is unripe. Pre-induction use of **PGE_2** preparations will facilitate labor in such instances. Whereas the uterine contractile effects of OT are immediate, it takes several hours for cervical ripening by PGE_2. **Mechanical devices** are also used to ripen the cervix, and their effects may be partially mediated by induction of PGE_2 synthesis. The use of progesterone antagonists for cervical ripening has been reported but is not commonly used.

In the presence of a ripe cervix, infusion of **OT** IV is the best way to stimulate or augment contractions. In general, induction of contractions requires more OT than augmentation. Induction at term usually requires less OT than preterm, which is a result of increased OT receptors at term.

Care must be taken to avoid **overstimulation,** and two types of stimulants should generally not be used together. At least 4 to 6 hours should elapse from the most recent use of PGE_2 before beginning OT infusion.

Early pregnancy termination

There are few OT receptors in the myometrium in early pregnancy, and OT is of little use in stimulating activity at this time. The **antiprogestin** mifepristone can disrupt embryonic and placental development. However, given alone, there is a high rate of incomplete abortion that may still require surgical completion. When given in combination with a **PG** analog, mifepristone is very successful in inducing abortion in pregnancies at less than 8 weeks' gestation. Surgical abortion is usually preferred beyond 8 weeks' gestation. However, administration of PGs locally is also efficacious, particularly after 18 weeks' gestation.

Treatment of preterm labor

Our lack of understanding of the mechanisms involved in initiation of parturition has hindered development of effective tocolytic drugs. The drugs currently used often result in increased myometrial relaxation at the cost of systemic side effects, since none of them has specific effects on uterine smooth muscle. Vascular relaxation, subsequent decreases in blood pressure, and tachycardia are the most common side effects, as discussed below. Along with the development of tachyphylaxis, these limit the duration of successful treatment with many currently available drugs.

Treatment of dysmenorrhea

Painful menstruation is very expensive in terms of productivity and quality of life. The most common form of dysmenorrhea is **primary** dysmenorrhea, consisting of uterine spasm without underlying pathology. The spasm results from the release of PGs from degenerating endometrial cells. NSAIDs have been extremely effective in preventing or ameliorating this condition (see Chapters 17 and 31). They are generally administered a few hours before expected menstruation, or at the first sign of bleeding, and taken 1 to 2 days thereafter. An alternative approach is to use oral contraceptives to inhibit ovulation, reducing synthesis of PGs in the endometrium and resulting in less uterine spasm during menstruation.

Side effects, clinical problems, and toxicity

Clinical problems are summarized in the Clinical Problems box.

CLINICAL PROBLEMS

Uterine stimulants	Maternal	Fetal
Oxytocin	Uterine hypertonus, rupture, hypotension, H_2O intoxication	Hypoxia
Prostaglandins	Uterine hypertonus, rupture, vomiting, diarrhea, fever, bronchospasm	Hypoxia
Mifepristone	None	None
Uterine relaxants	**Maternal**	**Fetal**
β-Adrenergic receptor agonists	Hypotension, tachycardia, palpitations, dysrhythmias, pulmonary edema, hyperglycemia, hypokalemia	Tachycardia Hyperglycemia
NSAIDs	Gastrointestinal bleeding, nausea, headaches, myelosuppression	Constriction of ductus arteriosus, oligohydramnios
Magnesium sulfate	Skin flushing, palpitations, headaches, depressed reflexes, respiratory depression, impaired cardiac conduction	Muscle relaxation, CNS depression (rare)
Progesterone	None	None

Uterine stimulants

The major side effect of uterine stimulants is **hyperstimulation.** This is usually easy to recognize by the appearance of frequent (<2 minute interval) contractions, or of a prolonged tetanic contraction usually accompanied by maternal pain and often fetal bradycardia. Hyperstimulation produced by IV OT is easily reversed by reducing the infusion rate or discontinuing it altogether. Because OT has a short half-life, normal uterine tone returns within a few minutes. Hyperstimulation resulting from **PG gel** insertion into the cervix or vagina may be a greater problem, but in severe cases, saline can be used to wash out the PG. If there is no reduction in tone or continued fetal bradycardia, it may be necessary to administer β_2-adrenergic agonists IV. In rare instances, emergency cesarean section may be necessary. Induction of labor should only be performed when necessary, and always in settings with adequate facilities.

Because of the low density of OT receptors in the myometrium in early pregnancy, very high doses of **OT** are required to stimulate contractions. Such high concentrations can result in cross-stimulation of vasopressin receptors, which can cause **water intoxication** with severe hyponatremia. A similar problem can occur with treatment of post-partum hemorrhage.

As discussed above, uterine stimulants should never be given in **combination** during pregnancy, because of the risk of hyperstimulation and adverse maternal and fetal outcomes. At least 6 hours should elapse after insertion of a PG gel before OT or additional PG is administered. If IV OT has been used, at least 2 hours should elapse before PG preparations are given. Conversely, combinations of uterine stimulants are often **beneficial** in the management of postpartum hemorrhage due to uterine atony that is resistant to single agents.

PGE_2 preparations for cervical ripening may be associated with an increased incidence of uterine rupture during labor in women who have had a previous cesarean section. Other side effects of PG preparations include gastrointestinal and pulmonary problems (see Chapter 17). However, these very infrequently result from local application of a PG gel.

Ergot alkaloids were commonly used to control postpartum hemorrhage. However, because they act on all smooth muscle, a serious risk is **hypertension.** Myocardial ischemia and infarction also have been reported. From the few studies available, it appears that the progesterone receptor antagonist **mifepristone** has very few systemic side effects.

Uterine relaxants

Most tocolytic agents lack specificity for the uterus and produce predictable side effects stemming from their actions on other tissues. Selective **β_2-adrenergic** receptor agonists are available, but they still stimulate all β-adrenergic receptors to some degree. As a result, **cardiovascular** or **metabolic** complications may occur in the mother or fetus. β-Adrenergic receptor agonists cause vasodilation, which commonly results in hypotension. Maternal tachycardia arises as a compensatory mechanism and also results from a direct action of the drug on the heart. These effects are a source of significant discomfort in patients. β-Adrenergic agents also increase hepatic glycogenolysis, resulting in maternal hyperglycemia, stimulating the secretion of insulin. As glucose is driven into cells by insulin, K^+ is also accumulated intracellularly, resulting in maternal hypokalemia. The cardiovascular side effects, particularly in the face of hypokalemia, may trigger cardiac dysrhythmias, which can lead to heart failure. Infusion of β-adrenergic agonists IV, especially in combination with glucocorticoids (which have salt-retaining properties), may cause excessive fluid retention, which can result in a potentially fatal pulmonary edema. Fluid balance should be monitored closely when these drugs are used in pregnant women. Tachycardia, as well as hyperglycemia and hyperinsulinemia, may also develop in the fetus. Neonatal hypoglycemia may result from prolonged hyperinsulinemia.

Concern has been raised about the use of **indomethacin** to arrest preterm labor because of the adverse effect this may have on constriction of the fetal ductus arteriosus (see Chapter 17). Although this effect may be greater in term fetuses, it can be seen throughout the third trimester. Fetal renal toxicity is also frequent and commonly manifests as a reduction in fetal urine output resulting in reduced amniotic fluid volume (oligohydramnios). It is not clear whether these disturbances are associated with adverse fetal outcomes, but this is a serious concern in light of increasing evidence regarding the fetal origins of adult disease. Also, findings from retrospective studies have shown that there is an increased incidence of intracranial hemorrhage, patent ductus arteriosus, and necrotizing enterocolitis in neonates receiving indomethacin, although some were treated with higher doses for longer periods than are currently recommended. Prospective randomized trials are clearly required to evaluate the risk-benefit ratios of NSAIDs for arresting preterm labor.

High doses of **magnesium sulfate** may cause obtundation, a loss of deep tendon reflexes, respiratory depression, and myocardial depression. Despite the lack of evidence for efficacy, magnesium sulfate is often the tocolytic drug of choice because of its low toxicity when given at low infusion rates.

There is much controversy about tocolytic drugs, particularly concerning their effectiveness and cost-benefit ratio. Many clinical studies have not included a placebo control group, limiting their conclusions without knowledge of potential placebo effects. Although most trials measure prolongation of pregnancy as the primary outcome, the important outcome is the eventual health of the newborn and the mother. In addition, there is no consensus as to the criteria used to exclude treatment in clinical trials. In addition, although there is a consensus that administration of glucocorticoids to the mother for 24 to 48 hours before birth will accelerate fetal pulmonary maturation and reduce the incidence of neonatal respiratory distress syndrome, randomized, placebo-controlled studies have not shown that use of tocolytic drugs increases the chance of completing a course of glucocorticoid therapy. Further, the extensive use of artificial surfactant treatment in preterm neonates may reduce the benefit of glucocorticoids administered *in utero*. Finally, in most regions of the United States and Canada, tocolytic therapy is the standard of care in preterm labor. Thus the medico-legal climate often dictates that some form of tocolytic therapy be attempted, despite the lack of strong supportive evidence.

New horizons

Possible novel tocolytic agents include competitive **antagonists of OT receptors**. The clinical utility of these agents depends on the role of OT in initiating or propagating preterm labor. One large clinical trial reported significant efficacy for an OT antagonist (atosiban) in delaying delivery, but with a questionable increase in neonatal mortality resulting in failure of the drug to be approved for use in the United States. However, there is interest in developing other compounds, since oxytocic activity is specific to uterine smooth muscle, and specific OT receptor antagonists should produce few side effects. Similarly, new PG analogs such as misoprostol will be investigated for use in pre-induction ripening of the cervix. As further studies with mifepristone are performed and other progesterone receptor blockers are developed, a therapeutic niche in the management of early and late pregnancy complications may be created. The effects of NO in animals include relaxation of the uterus, similar to effects on other smooth muscles (see Chapter 16). Clinical trials currently are underway to evaluate its use as a tocolytic, although its lack of specificity is likely to be a problem. Recent clinical trials and meta-analyses have brought renewed interest in the use of **progesterone** supplementation to prevent preterm labor in women at high risk.

Another approach is the development of isoform-specific PG receptor blockers, which might allow the optimal benefit of blocking effects of maternal $PGF_{2\alpha}$ without accompanying adverse fetal effects, which are probably associated with PGE_2. There is also increasing evidence that the immune system plays an important role in labor onset, and immunomodulators may eventually be used to stimulate or relax the uterus. Future research should lead to a better understanding of the regulation of parturition, which will facilitate development of new drugs.

TRADE NAMES

All of the important compounds available in the United States are listed in the Major Drugs box.

FURTHER READING

Keelan JA, Blumenstein M, Helliwell RJA, et al. Cytokines, prostaglandins and parturition–a review. *Placenta* 2003; 24(Suppl A):S33-S46.

Lopez-Bernal A. Mechanisms of labour–biochemical aspects. *Br J Obstet Gynecol* 2003; 110(Suppl 20):39-45.

Mitchell BF, Olson DM. Prostaglandin endoperoxide H synthase inhibitors and other tocolytics in preterm labour. *Prostaglandins Leukot Essent Fatty Acids* 2003; 70:167-187.

Self-assessment questions

1. Stimulation of a myometrial cell by OT results in all of the following intracellular events *except:*

a. Stimulation of phospholipase C.
b. Stimulation of protein kinase C.
c. Stimulation of adenylate cyclase.
d. Release of Ca^{2+} from sarcoplasmic reticulum.
e. Influx of extracellular Ca^{2+}.

2. Drugs commonly used to cause uterine relaxation include all of the following *except:*

a. Ritodrine.
b. Terbutaline.
c. Nicardipine.
d. Misoprostol.
e. Indomethacin.

3. The mechanism of action of indomethacin includes:

a. Stimulation of adenylate cyclase.
b. Inhibition of cyclooxygenase.
c. Stimulation of β-adrenergic receptors.
d. Blockade of the PGF receptor.
e. Inhibition of myosin light chain kinase.

4. Significant maternal side effects of β-adrenergic agonists include all of the following *except:*

a. Hypertension.
b. Tachycardia.
c. Hypokalemia.
d. Hyperglycemia.
e. Palpitations.

5. A pregnant patient at term presents for induction of labor. The best pharmacological approach would be:

a. Administration of PGE_2 vaginal gel until the women is in active labor.
b. Administration of PGE_2 vaginal gel with concurrent intravenous OT through an infusion pump.
c. Administration of OT intramuscularly.
d. Administration of PGE_2 vaginal gel until the cervix has ripened followed in 6 hours by intravenous OT through an infusion pump if active labor has not occurred.
e. Intravenous administration of ergotamine.

6. Which of the following is characteristic of OT?

a. It readily crosses the placenta, where it can cause harmful side effects in the fetus.
b. It is the drug of choice for cervical ripening.
c. The plasma half-life is a few minutes.
d. In early pregnancy the uterus is more sensitive to this drug than to PGs.
e. The drug can be administered orally.

CHAPTER 40

Hypothalamic-pituitary hormones

Gordon M. Wotton
Wende M. Kozlow
William S. Evans

Major Drugs

Hypothalamic hormones and analogs	Pituitary hormones and analogs

Therapeutic overview

The hypothalamus and pituitary gland work in concert to regulate the endocrine systems throughout the body. Peptides and biogenic amines, synthesized and secreted by specialized neurons within the hypothalamus, are transported by the **hypothalamic-hypophyseal portal circulation** to the anterior pituitary, where they act through specific receptors to stimulate or inhibit hormone secretion (Fig. 40-1). **Anterior pituitary hormones** trigger the production of hormones by peripheral endocrine organs. Hormones originating from peripheral endocrine organs have their own functions and provide feedback at the hypothalamic or pituitary level (or both) to modulate the synthesis and release of their particular tropic hormone. **Hypothalamic gonadotropin-releasing hormone** (GnRH; also called **luteinizing hormone releasing hormone** or LHRH) stimulates the secretion of **luteinizing hormone** (LH) and **follicle-stimulating hormone** (FSH) by the pituitary. LH and FSH promote **gametogenesis** and gonadal hormone production by the testes and ovaries (see Chapters 35 and 36). **Thyrotropin-releasing hormone** stimulates secretion of thyroid-stimulating hormone, which in turn controls thyroid function. **Corticotropin-releasing hormone** stimulates the secretion of **adrenocorticotropic hormone**, which promotes the secretion of cortisol by the adrenal cortex (see Chapter 33). **Growth hormone–releasing hormone** stimulates and **somatostatin** inhibits the production of growth hormone (GH), which has numerous effects on growth and metabolism. Hypothalamic dopamine functions to tonically inhibit secretion of prolactin, the hormone primarily responsible for lactation. The posterior pituitary (or **neurohypophysis**) secretes **oxytocin** and **arginine vasopressin** (AVP), also known as antidiuretic hormone. Unlike the anterior pituitary, which is under hypothalamic control, the neurohypophysis is made up of neurons with cell bodies in the hypothalamus. These cells synthesize and secrete oxytocin and AVP, which are transported by carrier proteins (neurophysins) through axons to the posterior pituitary, where

Abbreviations

AVP	arginine vasopressin, antidiuretic hormone
DI	diabetes insipidus
FSH	follicle-stimulating hormone
GH	growth hormone
GnRH	gonadotropin-releasing hormone
hCG	human chorionic gonadotropin
hMG	human menopausal gonadotropin
IGF-1	insulin-like growth factor–1
IM	intramuscular
IV	intravenous
LH	luteinizing hormone
SC	subcutaneous

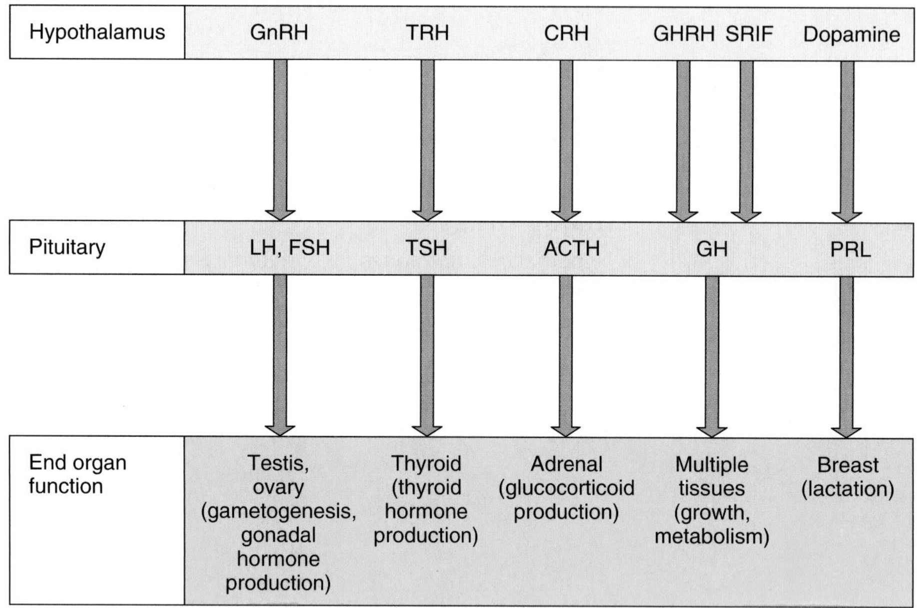

Figure 40-1 Relationships among hypothalamic releasing and inhibiting hormones, the anterior pituitary hormones controlled by hypothalamic hormones, and their respective target organs or tissues. *ACTH,* Adrenocorticotropic hormone; *CRH,* corticotropin-releasing hormone; *FSH,* follicle-stimulating hormone; *GH,* growth hormone; *GHRH,* growth hormone–releasing hormone; *GnRH,* gonadotropin-releasing hormone; *LH,* luteinizing hormone; *PRL,* prolactin; *SRIF,* somatotropin-release inhibiting factor (somatostatin); *TRH,* thyrotropin-releasing hormone; *TSH,* thyroid-stimulating hormone.

THERAPEUTIC OVERVIEW

Hypothalamic hormones

GnRH
- Replacement therapy for idiopathic hypogonadotropic hypogonadism

GnRH Analogs
- Prostate and breast cancer
- Idiopathic precocious puberty
- Endometriosis
- Contraception

Dopamine Agonists
- Pathological hyperprolactinemia
- Acromegaly
- Parkinson's disease

Somatostatin and Analogs
- Acromegaly
- Carcinoid and vasoactive intestinal peptide-secreting tumors

Pituitary hormones

LH and FSH
- Infertility in women
- Infertility in men with hypogonadotropic hypogonadism

GH
- Adult GH deficiency
- Growth failure

AVP
- Diabetes insipidus

they are stored and released directly into the systemic circulation.

GH-releasing hormone, thyrotropin-releasing hormone, corticotropin-releasing hormone, thyroid-stimulating hormone, and adrenocorticotropin are used mostly for **diagnostic** purposes and are not discussed further. The hypothalamic hormones (or their analogs) GnRH, dopamine, and somatostatin; the anterior pituitary hormones GH and LH/FSH; and the posterior pituitary hormone AVP are used therapeutically and discussed in this chapter. The pharmacology of oxytocin is discussed in Chapter 39. An overview of hypothalamic and pituitary hormones is presented in the Therapeutic Overview box.

Mechanisms of action

Hypothalamic hormones

Most **GnRH**-positive neurons in humans are located in the medial basal hypothalamus between the third ventricle and the median eminence. Projections from these neurons terminate in the median eminence, in contact with the capillary plexus of the hypothalamic-hypophyseal portal circulation. This allows GnRH to reach the circulation without passing through a blood-brain barrier. GnRH is formed by processing of a larger prohormone, preproGnRH, and transported in secretory granules to nerve terminals for storage, degradation, or release into pituitary portal blood vessels.

At the target, GnRH binds to receptors and initiates secretion of LH and FSH. The GnRH receptor gene consists of a 327-amino acid protein with seven transmembrane domains but without the typical intracellular C-terminus of a G protein–coupled receptor. Microaggregation stimulates upregulation of GnRH receptors and is followed by internalization of the hormone-receptor complex (see Chapter 2). Receptor activation results in increased intracellular Ca^{2+}.

GnRH is released in a pulsatile manner by the so-called "hypothalamic GnRH pulse generator." This pattern of intermittent bursts is essential for normal function. Continuous administration of GnRH will initially produce an increase in serum gonadotropin concentrations. However, this is followed by a decrease in gonadotropin secretion secondary to pituitary GnRH receptor downregulation, a decrease in expression of GnRH receptors, and desensitization of pituitary gonadotrophs. GnRH analog agonists and antagonists have been synthesized through selective substitution of amino acids in the GnRH peptide (Figure 40-2). These GnRH analogs have greater receptor binding and reduced susceptibility to enzymatic degradation, resulting in prolonged biological activity.

GnRH secretion is increased by norepinephrine, epinephrine, neuropeptide Y, galanin, and *N*-methyl-D-aspartic acid and decreased by endogenous opioids, progesterone and prolactin. Estradiol inhibits GnRH secretion except for a brief period of stimulation, which results in the midcycle LH surge.

Secretion of GH is regulated by two opposing hypothalamic hormones: GH-releasing hormone and somatostatin (Fig. 40-3). **Somatostatin** is a cyclic peptide that is processed from a preprohormone into two molecular forms: somatostatin-14 and somatostatin-28. The 14 amino acid sequence at the carboxyl terminal of somatostatin-28 is identical to somatostatin-14. In addition to its presence in the hypothalamus, somatostatin is widely distributed throughout the central nervous system, the gastrointestinal tract, pancreas, thyroid, thymus, heart, skin, and eye. Somatostatin has multiple actions including inhibition of gastrointestinal hormone secretion (e.g., gastrin, vasoactive intestinal peptide, motilin, secretin), pancre-

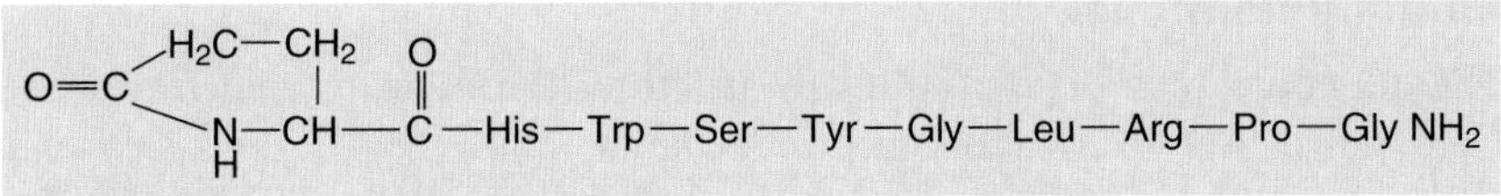

Figure 40-2 Structure of gonadotropin-releasing hormone *(GnRH)*.

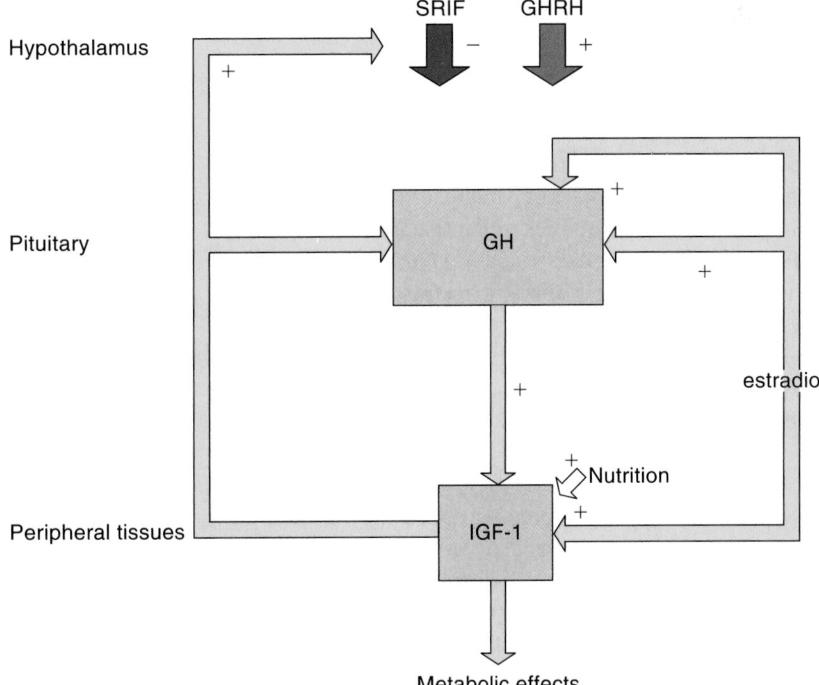

Figure 40-3 Regulation of growth hormone secretion in humans. Growth hormone–releasing hormone *(GHRH)* and somatostatin *(SRIF)* are the primary stimulatory and inhibitory peptides, respectively. *IGF-1*, Insulin-like growth factor 1.

atic exocrine secretion (e.g., gastric acid, pepsin, pancreatic bicarbonate), pancreatic endocrine secretion (e.g., insulin, glucagon), intestinal motility, gastric emptying, and gallbladder contraction. Somatostatin also decreases gastrointestinal absorption and mesenteric blood flow. In the central nervous system, somatostatin acts as both a neurotransmitter and a neuromodulator.

There are five somatostatin receptor subtypes: SSTR1 through SSTR5. They are G protein-coupled receptors that differ in tissue distribution and post-receptor signaling pathways. Somatostatin-14 and somatostatin-28 bind all five receptor subtypes. Binding of somatostatin to SSTR2 and SSTR5 suppresses GH secretion and the secretion of TSH.

Dopamine is synthesized in the tubero-infundibular neurons of the hypothalamus and transported to the anterior pituitary gland via the hypothalamic-hypophyseal portal system. Dopamine acts at its receptor (D_2) on the pituitary lactotrophs to inhibit prolactin secretion. Prolactin is the only anterior pituitary hormone under tonic inhibition by a hypothalamic hormone.

Pituitary hormones

The gonadotropins **LH** and **FSH** are structurally similar, each consisting of two polypeptide chains linked by hydrogen bonds, with internal cross-linking accomplished by disulfide bonds. LH and FSH are composed of an identical 89–amino acid α-chain and a 115–amino acid β-chain unique to each hormone. The β-chain is responsible for specificity. Two complex carbohydrate side chains are attached to specific locations on the α-subunit, two to the FSH–β-subunit, and one to the LH–β-subunit. The α- and β-chains are synthesized separately and appear to combine before carbohydrate addition. A terminal sialic acid is found on approximately 5% and 1% of FSH and LH carbohydrate molecules, respectively. Sialic acid prolongs the metabolic clearance of glycoproteins and results in a longer half-life for FSH than for LH. There is no evidence that other molecular forms of LH and FSH, such as prohormones and fragments, circulate in the plasma. The pituitary gonadotropes secrete LH and FSH.

Gonadotropins bind to high-affinity membrane receptors in the testes and ovaries. The LH and FSH receptors are glycoproteins encoded by homologous genes and are characterized by seven transmembrane-spanning domains. A large N-terminal region forms the binding site for the specific gonadotropin. Both LH and FSH receptors exhibit distinctive Ca^{2+} signaling properties, in addition to activating adenylyl cyclase. Cyclic adenosine monophosphate triggers activation of its protein kinase and phosphorylation of proteins necessary for steroidogenesis.

In addition to regulating estrogen production, gonadotropins have multiple effects on ovarian follicles. FSH directly stimulates follicular growth and maturation and enhances granulosa cell responsiveness to LH. LH is essential for the breakdown of the follicular wall, resulting in ovulation, and for the subsequent resumption of oocyte meiosis.

By contrast, testicular steroidogenesis requires only LH. The Leydig cells, which constitute about 10% of testicular volume, are stimulated to produce testosterone by the binding of LH to surface receptors. FSH binds to Sertoli cells and, with testosterone, is essential for mediating cellular maturation and spermatid differentiation, the first step of spermatogenesis. The Sertoli cell is necessary for maintenance of seminiferous tubule function and germ cell development.

GH is a 191–amino acid polypeptide belonging to a family of structurally similar hormones, including prolactin and chorionic somatomammotropin (also known as human placental lactogen). GH is synthesized by somatotropes of the anterior pituitary. The major product is a peptide with two disulfide bonds. The precise signaling mechanism by which GH exerts its intracellular effects likely involves its interaction with specific plasma membrane receptors and activation of the JAK family of intracellular tyrosine kinases and the STAT family of nuclear transcription factors (see Chapter 2). Additionally, GH binds to proteins in both the cytosol and plasma. The specificity of the circulating binding protein is similar to that of the GH receptor.

The majority of actions of GH are mediated through the stimulation of **insulin-like growth factor-1** (IGF-1) produced in the liver, cartilage, bone, muscle, and kidney. Other direct effects of GH on tissue include DNA and RNA synthesis, plasma protein synthesis and amino acid transport and incorporation into proteins.

AVP, also known as antidiuretic hormone, is a polypeptide that functions as the primary antidiuretic hormone in humans (Fig. 40-4). Synthesized primarily in the magnocellular neuronal systems of the supraoptic and paraventricular nuclei of the hypothalamus, the AVP precursor molecule contains a signal peptide, a neurophysin, and a glycosylated moiety, in addition to the AVP sequence. Following translation of the mRNA to form a preprohormone (166 amino acids), the signal peptide is cleaved, forming a prohormone. The prohormone is stored in neurosecretory granules that travel down the supraoptico-hypophyseal tract to the posterior pituitary. The primary stimuli for AVP release are hyperosmolarity, as measured by osmoreceptors found in the supraoptic and paraventricular nuclei, and volume depletion, detected by baroreceptors in the vascular bed and the heart. Nausea, emesis, and hypoglycemia may also stimulate release of AVP.

AVP acts via V1 and V2 receptors found in smooth muscle and renal collecting tubules, respectively. V1 receptors mediate vasoconstriction, while V2 receptors mediate antidiuretic effects. Specifically, AVP binding to V2 receptors activates adenylyl cyclase and a subsequent cascade resulting in fusion of the water channel, aquaporin-2, with the luminal membrane, thereby allowing water reabsorption.

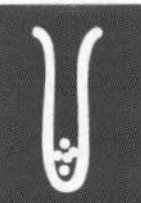

Pharmacokinetics

The pharmacokinetic parameters for the hypothalamic and pituitary hormones and analogs are summarized in Table 40-1.

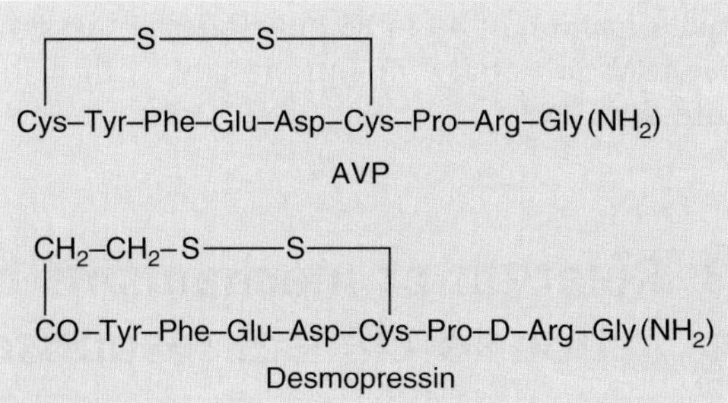

Figure 40-4 Amino acid sequences of arginine vasopressin *(AVP)* and 1-desamino-8-D-arginine-vasopressin (desmopressin, DDAVP).

Hypothalamic hormones

GnRH Synthetic GnRH is administered by intravenous (IV) or subcutaneous (SC) routes. Continuous SC infusions of GnRH in hypogonadotropic patients result in steady-state concentrations that are one third less than those achieved with the IV route. Therefore, SC administration results in delayed and prolonged absorption and lower serum concentrations. In patients receiving SC pulsatile GnRH therapy, these characteristics cause plasma GnRH concentration peaks to be significantly dampened. The lack of a pulsatile GnRH concentration waveform may diminish pituitary responsiveness and explain the lower success rate for induction of ovulation associated with SC as compared with IV administration.

Initially, GnRH analog agonists were administered daily either intranasally or by SC injection. More recently, long-acting depot formulations have been developed. Leuprolide, a GnRH agonist, can be administered SC daily or intramuscularly (IM) every 1, 3, or 4 months depending on dose. Leuprolide acetate can be administered through an osmotic pump enclosed in a titanium cylinder (the Viadur system) placed subcutaneously in the inner area of the upper arm. The pump releases 120 μg of leuprolide acetate SC every day for 1 year. Goserelin, a GnRH analog with agonist activity, is administered as a subcutaneous implant every 28 days. There is also a pellet administered every 12 weeks, indicated only for treatment of advanced prostate cancer. Triptorelin, a GnRH analog with agonist activity, can be administered as a short-acting SC injection or as a long-acting IM formulation in biodegradable polymer microspheres. The microspheres last for a month. Nafarelin, a GnRH analog with agonist activity,

Table 40-1 Pharmacokinetic Parameters

Drugs	Administration	Absorption	Half-Life	Disposition
HYPOTHALAMIC HORMONES AND ANALOGS				
GnRH	IV, SC	—	2-8 min	R, M
GnRH agonists	SC, intranasal	—	3 hr	—
Bromocriptine	Oral	Fair (28%)	6 hr*	M, B
Octreotide	SC	—	80-90 min	—
PITUITARY HORMONES AND ANALOGS				
LH/FSH	IM	Good	30-60 min	M
FSH	IM	Good	4-5 hr	—
GH	IM, SC	—	19 min	—
Vasopressin	IM, SC	Good	3-15 min	M
Vasopressin tannate	IM	Erratic	—	M
Desmopressin	IV, SC, oral, intranasal	Good	75 min	M
Clomiphene	Oral	Good	5 days	B (main)

M, Metabolized; *R,* renal excretion as unchanged drug; *B,* excreted in bile.
*90% bound to serum albumin.

is administered intranasally. GnRH antagonists are administered by SC injection.

GnRH is not significantly bound to plasma proteins. The primary route of excretion is renal, and in the setting of renal insufficiency the overall clearance rate is significantly lengthened. Moderate abnormalities of hepatic function do not affect GnRH clearance.

Somatostatin and analogs IV administration of native somatostatin results in a prompt decline in serum GH concentrations. Somatostatin is rapidly inactivated by peptidase enzymes and cannot be administered orally. It must be administered by continuous IV infusion, making it unsuitable for therapeutic use.

There are two cyclic octapeptide somatostatin analogs, octreotide and lanreotide. Lanreotide is currently only available in Europe. As compared to somatostatin, octreotide and lanreotide are more potent inhibitors of GH, glucagon, and insulin secretion. Octreotide is administered by SC injection three times a day. A long-acting release formulation of octreotide, dispersed in microspheres of a biodegradable polymer, is administered IM once a month.

Dopamine agonists Dopamine, in addition to being a neurotransmitter, is a sympathomimetic and is commonly used in the treatment of cardiogenic shock, septic shock, acute myocardial infarction, and renal failure. Because of its vasoconstrictor properties, it cannot be administered SC or IM. It has a short half-life (two minutes) and must be administered by continuous IV infusion. Therefore, it is not used in treatment of hyperprolactinemia, although it does effectively decrease serum prolactin levels.

Bromocriptine is a long-acting dopamine agonist (see Chapter 21). After oral administration, approximately 28% of bromocriptine is absorbed, producing peak plasma levels in 1 hour. Women who experience nausea can place the tablets in the vagina and still effectively lower plasma prolactin concentrations. Bromocriptine is metabolized in the liver, has a half-life of approximately 6 hours, and must be administered at least twice daily.

Cabergoline is a long-acting dopamine agonist with a high affinity for D_2 receptors. It is extensively metabolized by the liver, although cytochrome P-450 mediated metabolism is minimal. The elimination half-life is 63 to 69 hours, therefore it can be administered just twice weekly.

Pituitary hormones

LH and FSH The gonadotropins LH and FSH may be administered IM or SC. The absorption characteristics and subsequent metabolism of the gonadotropins have not been elucidated, but the liver appears to be the major source of glycoprotein clearance after the enzymatic removal of sialic acid. The estimated half-life of LH is between 30 and 60 minutes. FSH has higher sialic acid content and consequently a longer half-life because of decreased hepatic uptake. The clearance of LH is about 30 ml/min in women and 50 ml/min in men. The clearance of FSH is approximately 15 ml/min in women and has not been determined in men.

GH GH is administered via SC and IM routes. GH produced from recombinant DNA is metabolized in both liver and kidney. The mean half-life of GH administered SC or IM is 3.8 and 4.9 hours, respectively.

Vasopressin AVP, vasopressin tannate, and desmopressin circulate unbound to plasma proteins. All are metabolized in liver and kidney and may be initially inactivated by cleavage of the C-terminal glycinamide. A small amount of AVP is excreted intact in urine.

The durations of action of the three preparations are different. When administered SC, AVP is effective for only 2 to 8 hours. After IM administration, vasopressin tannate is often absorbed erratically, with a duration of action of 48 to 96 hours. Desmopressin may be given IV, SC, orally, or intranasally, with a longer half-life than AVP.

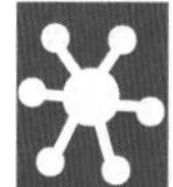

Relation of mechanisms of action to clinical response

Hypothalamic hormones

GnRH and analogs The approved and potential indications for therapy with GnRH and analogs can be divided into two categories:

- Replacement therapy in disorders characterized by isolated abnormal function of the hypothalamic pulse generator
- Promotion of pituitary desensitization, thus producing a functional orchiectomy or ovariectomy

GnRH has been used for ovulation induction in women with primary hypothalamic (or central) amenorrhea. This disorder is characterized by abnormal function of the GnRH pulse generator, resulting in inadequate gonadotropin secretion, failure of ovarian follicular development, and amenorrhea. The pituitary, however, is intrinsically normal and will release LH and FSH in response to GnRH. Pulsatile administration of GnRH IV every 90 minutes by a portable infusion pump can compensate for the underlying defect and frequently results in LH, FSH, estradiol, and progesterone profiles indistinguishable from those observed in normal spontaneous menstrual cycles. Clomiphene and human menopausal gonadotropin are also used for treatment of central amenorrhea. These methods are clearly successful in inducing ovulation but are associated with two major complications:

- Ovarian hyperstimulation syndrome
- Increased incidence of multiple gestation pregnancies

The incidence of complications may be less for pulsatile GnRH therapy because it maintains the integrity of the pituitary-ovarian axis and more accurately reproduces the physiology of the normal menstrual cycle. GnRH agonists and antagonists administered as SC injections are frequently used in *in vitro* fertilization to prevent premature LH surges in women undergoing controlled ovarian hyperstimulation.

Faulty GnRH secretion in men is referred to as idiopathic hypogonadotropic hypogonadism. Long-term pulsatile administration of GnRH was tested in a small number of men for at least 3 months. Significant increases in serum testosterone concentrations and testicular size were noted. Mature spermatogenesis may be achieved in 50% of patients, and linear growth may occur in men with unfused epiphyses. Idiopathic or surgically induced hypogonadotropic hypogonadism is now treated with testosterone (see Chapter 36) to promote masculinization and to preserve bone mineral density. Human chorionic gonadotropin and human menopausal gonadotropin are used to promote spermatogenesis and restore fertility in male hypogonadotropic hypogonadism.

The observation that orchiectomy causes prostate cancer to regress led to the development of approaches to decrease serum androgen concentrations in men with metastatic prostate cancer. Methods to induce androgen deprivation include orchiectomy, estrogen therapy, GnRH analogs, and antiandrogens (see Chapter 36). Combined androgen blockade, in which orchiectomy or GnRH analogs are combined with an antiandrogen, is also used in treating metastatic hormone-dependent prostate cancer.

Orchiectomy is an effective and relatively safe procedure to lower testosterone levels by 90%. The psychological impact of orchiectomy, however, has made it unpopular among men with metastatic prostate cancer. Estrogens decrease serum androgen levels by suppressing LH secretion from the pituitary and competing with androgens for their receptors. However, estrogen therapy has been associated with venous thromboembolic disease, cardiovascular disease, and gynecomastia.

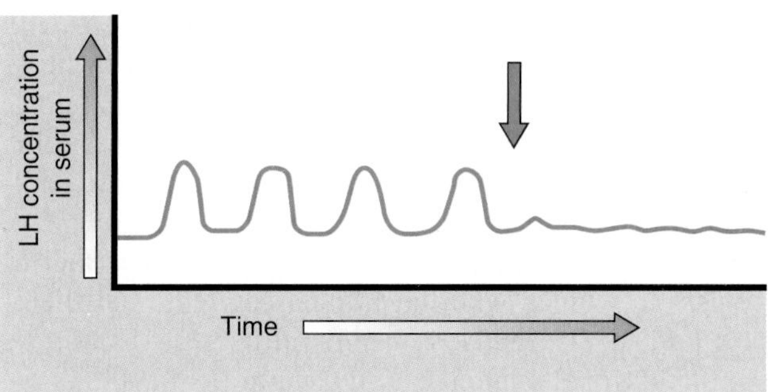

Figure 40-5 Luteinizing hormone *(LH)* serum concentration profile in a normal subject, showing initial LH pulses resulting from gonadotropin-releasing hormone *(GnRH)* pulse generator. Administration of a long-acting GnRH agonist (*red arrow*) down-regulates receptors and leads to decreased LH secretion.

Long-acting GnRH agonists can be used to down-regulate pituitary gonadotropin receptors and suppress release of LH (Figure 40-5), resulting in reduction of serum testosterone concentrations equal to that seen with orchiectomy. However, continuous GnRH agonist therapy will initially increase LH secretion from the pituitary, causing a transient increase in serum testosterone. This occurs approximately 72 hours after initiating therapy and can exacerbate symptoms of metastatic prostate cancer, such as bone pain and ureteral obstruction. Co-administration of the antiandrogen flutamide with a GnRH agonist can prevent these negative effects. Pituitary gonadotroph desensitization occurs 1 to 2 weeks after starting the GnRH agonist, with castrate levels of testosterone seen in 2 to 4 weeks.

GnRH antagonists can also dramatically reduce serum testosterone. Unlike agonists, GnRH antagonists immediately suppress pituitary gonadotrophs, thereby avoiding the undesired transient increases in LH secretion and serum testosterone concentrations and obviating the need for co-administration of an antiandrogen.

GnRH agonists and antagonists have also been used in premenopausal women with hormone-dependent metastatic breast cancer as an alternative to oophorectomy to decrease serum estrogen to menopausal levels. Breast cancer "flare" reactions have occurred in some women treated with continuous GnRH agonists, and are likely related to a transient increase in gonadotropin secretion from the pituitary. Comparison of the GnRH agonist goserelin with ovariectomy in premenopausal women with estrogen-receptor positive or progesterone-receptor positive metastatic breast cancer showed that response rates, failure-free survival, and overall survival were equivalent.

GnRH analog therapy is approved as a means of obtaining a medical oophorectomy for treatment of endometriosis and uterine leiomyomas. Treatment with GnRH agonists for 6 months has been shown to be as effective as danazol in reducing the size of endometrial implants and decreasing clinical symptoms, including pelvic pain, dysmenorrhea, and dyspareunia. In addition, GnRH agonists have been used for treatment of hirsutism and other manifestations of hyperandrogenism in women who have failed conventional therapies (oral contraceptives or antiandrogens). Histrelin, a synthetic GnRH analog, is also used to treat acute intermittent porphyria associated with menses. Idiopathic precocious puberty has been treated successfully with GnRH agonists.

Somatostatin and analogs The short half-life and requirement for continuous IV administration limit the usefulness of somatostatin. There are many uses, however, for the analogs octreotide and lanreotide. They are commonly used to treat patients with excessive GH secretion. **Gigantism** occurs if GH hypersecretion is present before epiphyseal closure during puberty, and **acromegaly** occurs if hypersecretion develops after puberty. Excessive GH secretion has many deleterious effects as a result of tissue growth stimulation and altered glucose and fat metabolism.

Generally, patients with gigantism or acromegaly are treated by transsphenoidal resection of the GH-secreting adenoma. Some patients, however, cannot be surgically cured and receive adjuvant treatment with irradiation and/or medical therapy. Medical therapy for treatment of acromegaly includes dopamine agonists, pegvisomant (a GH receptor antagonist), or somatostatin analogs. Somatostatin analogs bind to the pituitary somatostatin receptors and block GH secretion. Somatostatin receptors SSTR2 and SSTR5 are the main receptors found in GH-secreting pituitary tumors and are the receptors for which octreotide and lanreotide have the highest affinity. Several studies show that long-acting somatostatin analogs are useful in acromegaly as adjunctive therapy. Improvement in symptoms can be seen even without normalization of serum GH and IGF-1 levels, most likely because even small reductions in GH secretion will result in a clinical response. Such therapy can also lead to tumor shrinkage in 30% of patients treated for acromegaly.

Somatostatin analogs have also been approved for use in the treatment of carcinoid syndrome and vasoactive intestinal peptide tumors. In addition, because most neuroendocrine tumors express somatostatin receptors, radiolabled somatostatin analogs have been used to image these tumors (scintigraphy) and to deliver isotopes to the tumors to inhibit their growth.

Dopamine agonists Physiological hyperprolactinemia normally occurs during pregnancy, lactation, nipple stimulation, and stress. Pathologic hyperprolactinemia is most commonly caused by a prolactin-secreting pituitary adenoma. Other causes of pathologic hyperprolactinemia include lactotroph hyperplasia, caused by decreased dopamine inhibition of prolactin secretion, and decreased clearance of prolactin. Hyperprolactinemia can result in galactorrhea in both women and men. More importantly, hyperprolactinemia results in suppression of gonadotropin secretion, with resulting sex steroid deficiency. Women with hyperprolactinemia commonly present with oligomenorrhea or amenorrhea and/or infertility. Men with hyperprolactinemia commonly present with decreased libido, erectile dysfunction, and other signs of low testosterone, including osteoporosis.

Dopamine agonists are used to treat hyperprolactinemia caused by both prolactinomas and lactotroph hyperplasia. Dopamine agonists bind to the dopamine receptors on the lactotrophs, resulting in decreased prolactin synthesis and secretion. Decreases in prolactin concentration can be seen within 2 to 3 weeks of initiating therapy. Dopamine agonists also result in decreased size of the lactotroph, leading to shrinkage of the prolactinoma. Signs and symptoms of intracranial tumor expansion show an extraordinary abatement within a few days. Decrease in tumor size can be detected by imaging within 6 weeks of starting the dopamine agonist. Prolactinomas are the only type of pituitary adenoma in which medical therapy, as opposed to transsphenoidal resection, is first-line treatment. With reduction of the serum prolactin concentration to normal, galactorrhea is abolished and gonadal function is restored.

Patients who do not respond to one dopamine agonist may respond to another. Cabergoline, however, may be more effective than bromocriptine. In a study of 455 patients treated with cabergoline for hyperprolactinemia, prolactin concentrations normalized in 86% of patients, including 41 of 58 patients (70%) who were initially resistant to bromocriptine.

Dopamine agonists also inhibit GH secretion and can be used in the treatment of acromegaly. Bromocriptine is less effective than cabergoline. The combination of a dopamine agonist with a somatostatin analog may be effective when neither agent alone is adequate.

Women with pathological hyperprolactinemia requiring treatment with a dopamine agonist who desire pregnancy should be treated with bromocriptine. There has not been a reported increased incidence of birth defects in infants of mothers who took bromocriptine during pregnancy. It is not known whether cabergoline is safe in pregnancy; therefore, women taking cabergoline who desire pregnancy should be switched to bromocriptine.

See Chapter 21 for the use of dopamine agonists in Parkinson's disease.

Pituitary hormones

LH and FSH The first report of pregnancy resulting from treatment with human urinary gonadotropin occurred in 1962. Today, **human menopausal gonadotropins** (hMG), purified urinary FSH and recombinant FSH, are used for induction of ovulation. hMG consists of a purified preparation of LH and FSH extracted from the urine of postmenopausal women. Given either SC or IM, hMG is indicated for ovulation induction in women with amenorrhea secondary to hypogonadotropic hypogonadism (including hypothalamic amenorrhea) or normogonadotropic amenorrhea, including women with polycystic ovary syndrome who have failed to ovulate with clomiphene. More recently, purified forms of urinary FSH and recombinant FSH have become available. In a recent study, the use of gonadotropins for ovulation induction in women with polycystic ovary syndrome was successful in about 70% of patients, with 40% achieving pregnancy. Multiple gestation births occur in approximately 10% to 15% of patients receiving gonadotropins.

The gonadotropins, both urinary and recombinant, are used to induce spermatogenesis in treatment of male-factor infertility. Men with hypogonadotropic hypogonadism as a result of hypothalamic or pituitary disease are candidates for treatment with **human chorionic gonadotropin** (hCG) and/or hMG. hCG contains the biologic activity of LH, thereby stimulating testosterone production from Leydig cells and eventual spermatogenesis. If the onset of hypogonadism occurs after puberty, Sertoli cells will have already been primed with FSH, and hCG alone may be effective. Onset before puberty will likely require FSH in addition to LH, and treatment with hMG (containing both) is indicated.

Clomiphene Clomiphene belongs to a class of compounds with both estrogenic and antiestrogenic activity and is indicated for women with normogonadotropic anovulation (see Chapter 35). In comparison to gonadotropins, clomiphene results in lower rates of multiple gestation births, which occurs in approximately 4% to 6% of patients.

Growth hormone GH promotes linear growth by causing generation of IGF-1 and influences all aspects of metabolism. This hormone is described as anabolic, lipolytic, and diabetogenic. Replacement of GH in children with GH deficiency stimulates the incorporation of amino acids into muscle protein, as indicated by decreased serum amino acid concentrations and decreased urinary nitrogen excretion. Treatment of GH deficiency with GH does not result in severe glucose intolerance or diabetes mellitus, however, as seen with the excessive serum GH concentrations in gigantism and acromegaly. Long-term administration of GH to GH-deficient adults causes a decrease in adipose mass and an increase in muscle mass.

Treatment of GH deficiency dates back to the 1950s, when children were treated with human GH derived from human cadaver pituitary glands. This was halted in 1985 after cases of spongiform encephalopathy in association with human GH treatment were reported. In 1985, recombinant human GH became available for treatment of GH deficiency. While GH replacement is an accepted practice in children with GH deficiency, treatment of adult-onset GH deficiency remains controversial.

Vasopressin Three forms of AVP are approved for clinical use: native AVP, vasopressin tannate, and desmopressin. Clinical indications include diabetes insipidus (DI), gastrointestinal variceal hemorrhage, nocturnal enuresis, bleeding diatheses, and cardiac arrhythmia.

Central (or neurogenic) DI is characterized by polyuria and polydipsia and results from inadequate secretion of AVP from the posterior pituitary (see Chapter 38). Nephrogenic DI results from failure of the kidney to respond to secreted AVP. The diagnosis of DI is confirmed by using AVP during a water deprivation test. The water deprivation test is also used to distinguish between central and nephrogenic DI. During water deprivation and subsequent elevation of plasma osmolality, patients with DI exhibit inability to retain water or concentrate their urine. Patients with central DI will show an increase in urine osmolality following administration of AVP. Little to no response is seen in nephrogenic DI after AVP administration.

AVP is also used for treatment of certain bleeding disorders, such as mild hemophilia A and mild-to-moderate von Willebrand's disease. AVP increases circulating concentrations of factor VIII (antihemophilic factor; see Chapter 19), perhaps by stimulating its release from cells in the vascular endothelium. Desmopressin is used for treatment of acute bleeding in patients with platelet dysfunction due to uremia and is preferred to AVP because of its lack of vasopressor activity.

Side effects, clinical problems, and toxicity

Clinical problems are summarized in the Clinical Problems box.

Hypothalamic hormones

GnRH is generally well tolerated, but occasionally nausea, light-headedness, headache, and abdominal discomfort are reported. SC administration is associated with antibody formation in a few patients. GnRH agonist and antagonist therapy is associated with hot flashes/flushes, decreased libido, fatigue, and decreased bone mineral density.

Gastrointestinal side effects such as nausea, vomiting, diarrhea, and abdominal cramps have been reported after treatment with native somatostatin. Hyperglycemia, hypoglycemia, and hypothyroidism, secondary to somatostatin inhibition of TSH, may be seen. In addition, after discontinuing an IV infusion of somatostatin, rebound hypersecretion of GH, insulin, and glucagon can occur. Side effects of somatostatin analogs are similar to those of the native peptide. In addition, patients may develop gallbladder sludge or cholelithiasis.

When a dopamine agonist is first administered, patients may experience nausea, vomiting, dizziness, or orthostatic hypotension. These effects can be minimized if therapy is begun in low doses and the drug is taken with food and at bedtime, with a gradual increase in frequency to a full-dose regimen. A few patients experience headache, fatigue, abdominal cramping, nasal congestion, drowsiness, or diarrhea.

CLINICAL PROBLEMS

Hypothalamic hormones and analogs

GnRH	Adverse reactions infrequent Occasional nausea, headache, abdominal discomfort Anaphylaxis (rare) with IV use Localized problems at injection site
Dopamine agonists	Nausea, orthostatic hypotension initially Confusion, hallucinations in Parkinson's disease
Somatostatin analogs	Hyperglycemia, loose stools, gallstones

Pituitary hormones and analogs

LH and FSH	Multiple gestation pregnancy Gynecomastia in men Occasional febrile reactions
GH	Antibodies Misuse in athletes
AVP	Nausea, vertigo, headache Anaphylaxis Angina, myocardial infarction

Drug interactions

Bromocriptine	Phenothiazine or butyrophenones: prevents dopamine agonist action
Vasopressin analogs	Carbamazepine, chlorpropamide, clofibrate, fludrocortisone, tricyclic antidepressants: potentiate action Lithium, heparin, alcohol: inhibit action

Pituitary hormones

The major adverse reactions of **hMG** are multiple gestation pregnancy and the ovarian hyperstimulation syndrome. Potentially a life-threatening condition, it is characterized by ovarian enlargement and extravascular accumulation of fluid resulting in ascites, pleural and pericardial effusions, renal failure, and hypovolemic shock. Classified as mild, moderate, or severe, it can potentially lead to massive ovarian enlargement of greater than 12 cm. Fortunately, the incidence of severe disease is less than 2%.

Administration of recombinant human GH can result in formation of anti-GH antibodies. Additional adverse effects include hyperglycemia, peripheral edema, arthralgias, paresthesias, and carpal tunnel syndrome. Benign intracranial hypertension (pseudotumor cerebri) has rarely been associated with children receiving GH therapy.

Nonspecific adverse reactions to AVP that may occur include nausea, vertigo, headache, and anaphylaxis. Other signs and symptoms may relate directly to specific pressor and antidiuretic effects. Vasoconstriction may occur and cause relatively mild problems, such as skin blanching or abdominal cramping, or more serious effects such as angina or myocardial infarction. All preparations should be used with caution in patients with coronary artery disease, but desmopressin has lower pressor effects and may be the drug of choice. All vasopressins may cause water retention and hyponatremia. Signs and symptoms of hyponatremia include drowsiness, listlessness, weakness, headaches, seizures, and coma, requiring close supervision.

Several drugs, if administered simultaneously, potentiate or inhibit the effects of AVP. Potentiators include carbamazepine, chlorpropamide, clofibrate, fludrocortisone, and tricyclic antidepressants. Inhibitors include lithium carbonate, heparin, and alcohol.

New horizons

GnRH receptors have been found in human prostate cancer, and there has been recent work to develop cytotoxic GnRH analogs as an additional therapy. GnRH agonist therapy has been investigated as a means of female and male contraception. Successful results have been seen in preliminary studies in women, but further trials are required to test for long-term side effects (e.g., osteoporosis). GnRH antagonists, in combination with testosterone, are being investigated for use as male contraception.

TRADE NAMES

In addition to generic and fixed-combination preparations, the following trade-named materials are some of the important compounds available in the United States.

Hypothalamic hormones and analogues

GnRH Agonists

Buserelin (Suprefact)
Gonadorelin (Factrel)
Goserelin (Zoladex)
Histrelin (Supprelin)
Leuprolide (Lupron, Lupron Depot, Viadur)
Nafarelin (Synarel)
Triptorelin (Trelstar Depot, Trelstar LA)

GnRH Antagonists

Abarelix (Plenaxis)
Cetrorelix (Cetrotide)
Ganirelix (Antagon)

Dopamine Agonists

Bromocriptine (Parlodel)
Cabergoline (Dostinex)

Somatostatin Analogue

Octreotide (Sandostatin, Sandostatin LAR)

Pituitary hormones and analogues

Clomiphene (Clomid, Milophene, Serophene)
Desmopressin (DDAVP, Stimate)
Human chorionic gonadotropin (Ovidrel)
Human recombinant GH (Genotropin, Humatrope, Norditropin, Nutropin, Protropin, Saizen, Serostim)
LH-FSH (Pergonal, Repronex,)
Urofollitropin (Bravelle, Fertinex, Follistim, Gonal-F, Metrodin)
Vasopressin (Pitressin)

FURTHER READING

Schally AV. Luteinizing hormone-releasing hormone analogs: their impact on the control of tumorigenesis. *Peptides* 1999; 20:1247-1262.

Schonbrunn A. Somatostatin receptors: present knowledge and future directions. *Ann Oncol* 1999; 10:S17-S21.

Abs, R, Verhelst J, Maiter D, et al. Cabergoline in the treatment of acromegaly: a study in 64 patients. *J Clin Endocrinol Metab* 1998; 83:374-378.

Self-assessment questions

1. The release of which of the following is *not* under hypothalamic control?
   a. LH
   b. FSH
   c. TSH
   d. Adrenocorticotropin
   e. GH
   f. AVP

2. Of the vasopressin–vasopressin analog family available for clinical use, the agent(s) having excellent antidiuretic effects but minimal pressor effects is/are:
   a. AVP.
   b. AVP tannate.
   c. Desmopressin.
   d. *a* and *b*.
   e. None of the above.

3. Patients treated with the somatostatin analog octreotide are at risk for:
   a. Peptic ulcer disease.
   b. Gallstone formation.
   c. Rash.
   d. Hyperthyroidism.

4. GH is currently approved for treatment of:
   a. Short children.
   b. GH-deficient children.
   c. The elderly.
   d. GH-deficient adults.
   e. Athletes.
   f. *a* and *b*.
   g. *b* and *d*.

Calcium-regulating hormones and other agents affecting bone

Paula H. Stern

Major Drugs

Alendronate (Fosamax)	Paricalcitol (Zemplar)
Calcitonin (Calcimar)	Raloxifene (Evista)
Calcitriol (Rocaltrol)	Risedronate (Actonel)
Ergocalciferol* (Calciferol, Drisdol)	Teriparatide (Forteo)

*In Canada the drug name is Ostoforte.

Therapeutic overview

The calcium concentration in plasma is maintained normally within narrow limits, approximately 8.5 to 10.4 mg/dl. Approximately 45% of the plasma calcium is bound to plasma proteins, and about 10% is complexed with anions. When the ionized calcium concentration falls outside the narrow physiological range, the functions of many tissues are affected. **Hypocalcemia** can lead to increased neuromuscular excitability and tetany and impairment of mineralization of the skeleton. **Hypercalcemia** can result in life-threatening cardiac dysrhythmias, kidney stones, and central nervous system abnormalities. In addition, there are disorders of the skeleton such as **osteoporosis** and **Paget's disease** of bone that cause loss of the normal structure. These changes in bone integrity result in increased susceptibility to fracture.

The sites at which various compounds act to produce effects on calcium metabolism include the kidney, gastrointestinal (GI) tract, and bone (Fig. 41-1). Normally, 10% to 20% of dietary calcium is absorbed in the GI tract. Absorption is impaired in the absence of **vitamin D** and augmented in the presence of excess vitamin D. **Renal tubular reabsorption** normally recovers 99% of the 10 to 20 g of calcium filtered per day, and diuretics can alter reabsorption of calcium. Bone is the major storehouse and contains approximately 1 kg in a 70 kg human. Of this, more than 99% is in a stable pool, and 1% is in an exchangeable pool that turns over at a rate of approximately 20 g/day; turnover is a passive physicochemical process.

Diseases of calcium metabolism or bone, and compounds used to treat them, are listed in Table 41-1. **Hypocalcemia** and rickets (inadequate bone mineralization during development) or **osteomalacia** (inadequate bone mineralization in adults) result from inadequate vitamin D intake or resistance to its action and are treated with vitamin D and calcium. Disorders that lead to **hypercalcemia** are more diverse in nature and cause. Therapy for these disorders is determined by the cause of the disease and its severity and the need for rapid correction. Various compounds including bisphosphonates, calcitonin, glucocorticoids, antiinflammatory agents, diuretics, and anticancer drugs are employed to treat hypercalcemia. There are also disorders of bone turnover not usually associated with abnormal serum calcium and phosphate concentrations

Abbreviations

EDTA	ethylenediaminetetraacetic acid
GI	gastrointestinal
OPG	osteoprotegerin
PTH	parathyroid hormone
RANK	receptor activator of nuclear factor-κB
RANKL	receptor activator of nuclear factor-κB ligand
SERM	selective estrogen receptor modulator

that are amenable to therapy. **Paget's disease of bone** is a localized disorder that is characterized by both excessive formation and resorption occurring in an irregular manner in one or more bones; it is treated with the antiresorptive agents bisphosphonates and calcitonin. **Osteoporosis** is a systemic skeletal disorder characterized by compromised bone strength predisposing to an increased risk of fracture; it is treated mainly with antiresorptive agents. Recently, anabolic treatment for osteoporosis has become available and provides another treatment option.

The therapeutic considerations for calcium-regulating hormones and other agents affecting bone are summarized in the Therapeutic Overview box.

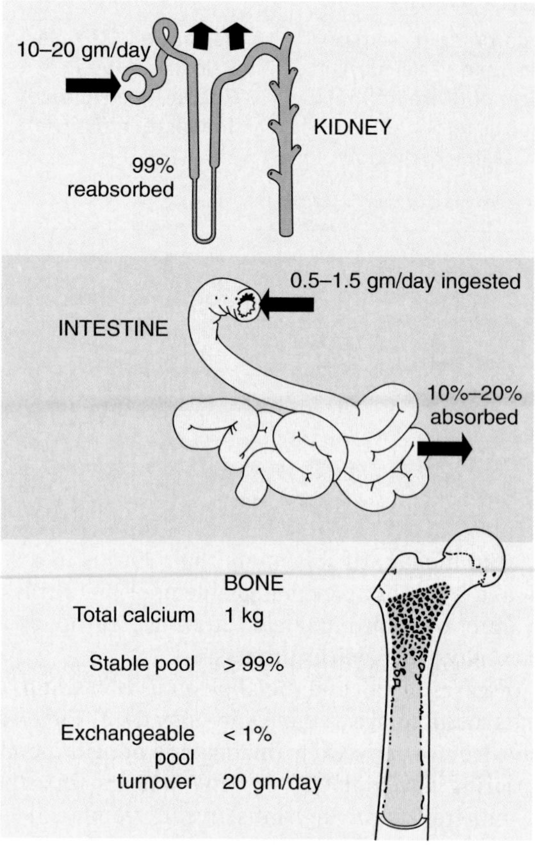

Figure 41-1 Sites of calcium regulation. Bone is the primary storage site, containing approximately 1 kg of calcium.

THERAPEUTIC OVERVIEW

Vitamin D, vitamin D metabolites, and vitamin D analogs

Rickets
Osteomalacia
Hypocalcemia
Hypoparathyroidism
Psoriasis

Parathyroid hormone

Osteoporosis

Calcitonin

Paget's disease of bone
Osteoporosis

EDTA, furosemide, ethacrynic acid, glucocorticoids, plicamycin

Hypercalcemia

Calcium, estrogen, SERMS, bisphosphonates, calcitonin

Osteoporosis

Table 41-1 Disorders of bone and calcium metabolism

Type of Disorder	Examples	Treatment
Hypocalcemic	Inadequate dietary calcium and/or vitamin D intake	Vitamin D compounds and calcium
	Malabsorption caused by defective activation of or end-organ resistance to vitamin D	
	Hypoparathyroidism	
	Pseudohypoparathyroidism	
	Renal failure	
Hypercalcemic	Hyperparathyroidism	Bisphosphonates, calcitonin, glucocorticoids, antiinflammatory agents, loop diuretics, fluids, low calcium diet, sulfate, plicamycin
	Hypervitaminosis D	
	Sarcoidosis	
	Neoplasia	
	Hyperthyroidism	
	Immobilization	
Bone remodeling	Paget's disease of bone	Bisphosphonates, calcitonin
	Osteoporosis	Bisphosphonates, calcitonin, estrogen (female), SERMs supplemented with calcium and vitamin D

Mechanisms of action

Vitamin D, metabolites, and analogs

Vitamin D is a secosteroid, a steroid in which the B ring is cleaved and the A ring rotated (Fig. 41-2). Vitamin D_3, cholecalciferol, is the natural form of vitamin D and is synthesized from cholesterol in the skin in response to the ultraviolet rays from the sun. Vitamin D_2, ergocalciferol, is the plant-derived form of vitamin D; both vitamins D_2 and D_3 are present in the diet.

Vitamin D is not biologically active but is metabolized to active products by the liver and kidney (see

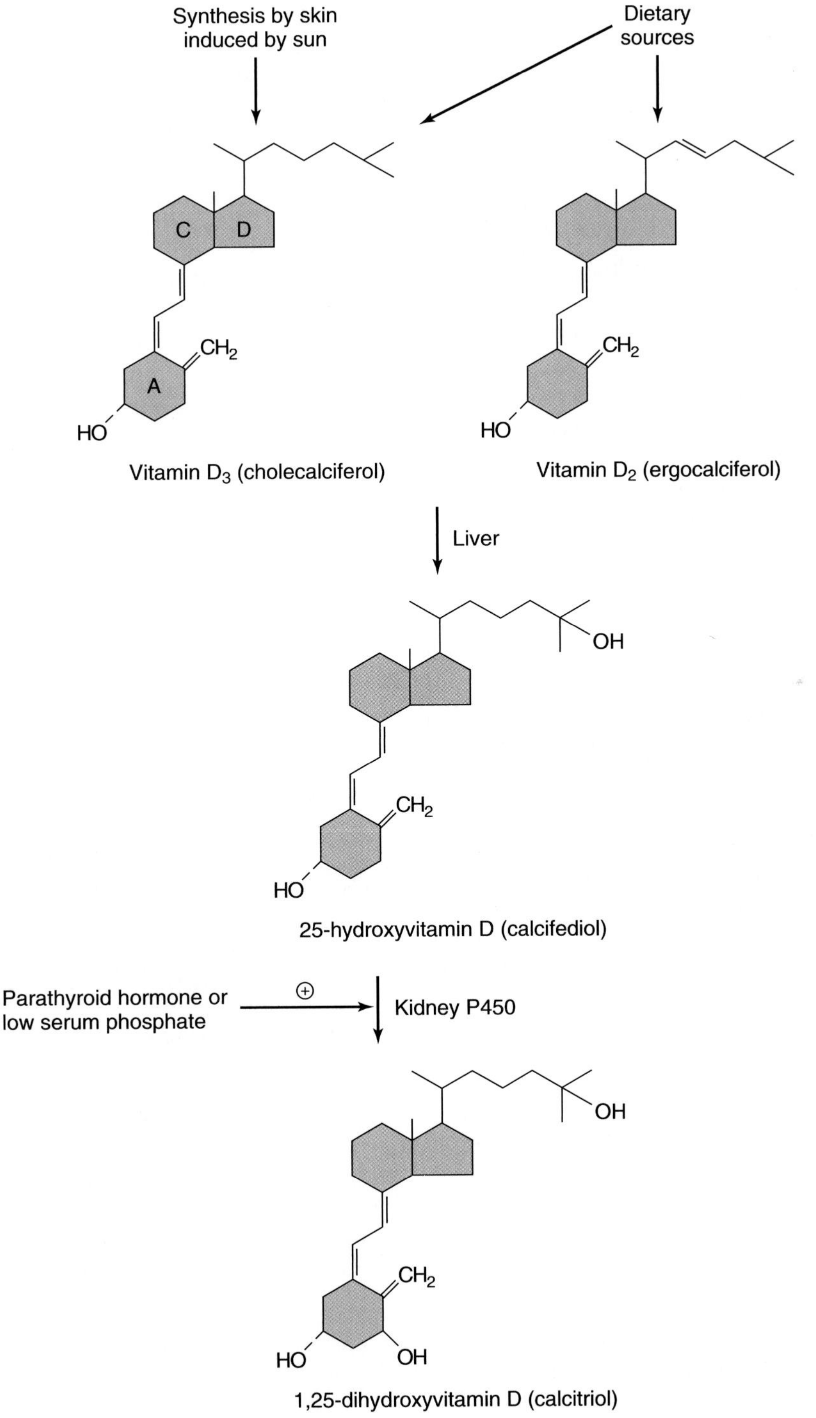

Figure 41-2 Sources, structure, and metabolism of vitamin D.

Fig. 41-2). In the endoplasmic reticulum and mitochondria of the liver, vitamin D is hydroxylated to form 25-hydroxyvitamin D (calcifediol), which is active. In addition, 25-hydroxyvitamin D can be α-hydroxylated by mitochondrial P450 in the kidney to 1,25-dihydroxyvitamin D (calcitriol). This hydroxylation is feedback regulated and stimulated by parathyroid hormone (PTH) and low plasma phosphate concentrations.

Active vitamin D metabolites bind primarily to receptors in the nucleus of target cells. These act through a mechanism similar to that of other steroid hormones, binding to response elements on genes and initiating synthesis of specific proteins (see Chapter 2). Among the protein products resulting from actions of vitamin D on the intestine are two high-affinity calcium-binding proteins, the **calbindins,** which play a role in stimulation of intestinal calcium transport. Vitamin D metabolites increase absorption of dietary calcium and phosphate by stimulating uptake across the GI mucosa, leading to an increase in serum calcium concentration (Fig. 41-3). The antirachitic effect of vitamin D on bone mineralization is an indirect result of this increased calcium and phosphate absorption, which also results in deposition of more mineral in bone.

Vitamin D metabolites, especially at higher concentrations, can also stimulate release of calcium from bone. They increase synthesis of a membrane-associated cytokine, receptor activator of nuclear factor-κB ligand **(RANKL),** which interacts with receptor activator of nuclear factor-κB **(RANK)** receptors on osteoclasts to stimulate osteoclast differentiation, survival, and activity, resulting in release of calcium (Fig. 41-4). A decoy receptor, **osteoprotegerin (OPG),** is produced by bone marrow stromal cells and can inhibit the effects of RANKL. Increased RANKL is a general mechanism by which many factors, including PTH, prostaglandins, and inflammatory cytokines, stimulate bone resorption. Vitamin D metabolites inhibit PTH synthesis and secretion. Vitamin D also affects differentiation of other cell types, including keratinocytes.

Several synthetic vitamin D analogs have unique clinical utility. 1α-Hydroxyvitamin D2 and dihydrotachysterol (in which the A ring is not rotated) are active even in the absence of the renal 1α-hydroxylase. 19-Nor-1α, 25-hydroxyvitamin D2 (paricalcitol), and calcipotriene have less action on calcium metabolism and can therefore be used for other therapeutic indications with less risk of hypercalcemia. Paricalcitol is used to suppress elevated PTH secretion in chronic renal disease, and calcipotriene is used to promote normal skin cell differentiation in psoriasis.

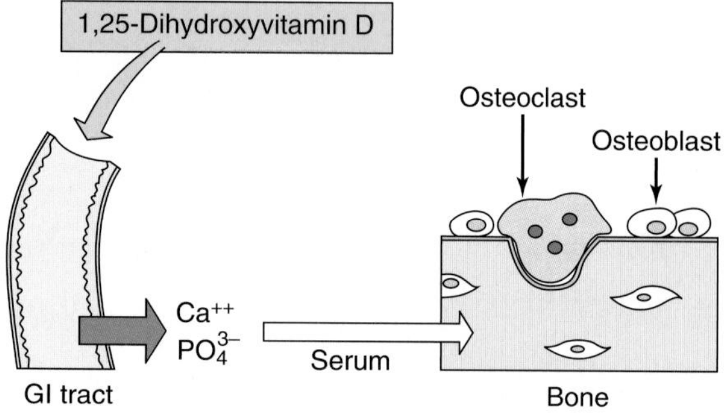

Figure 41-3 Mechanism of the antirachitic effect of 1,25-dihydroxyvitamin D. 1,25-dihydroxyvitamin D increases calcium and phosphate absorption from the intestine increasing serum concentrations. The ions deposit in bone, increasing bone mineralization.

Parathyroid hormone

PTH is an 84 amino acid polypeptide that is formed from the cleavage of larger precursors in the parathyroid gland. The first 34 amino acids of PTH (PTH 1-34) retain the full activity of the peptide on bone and calcium metabolism. PTH secretion is regulated by calcium in a negative feedback manner mediated through a specific

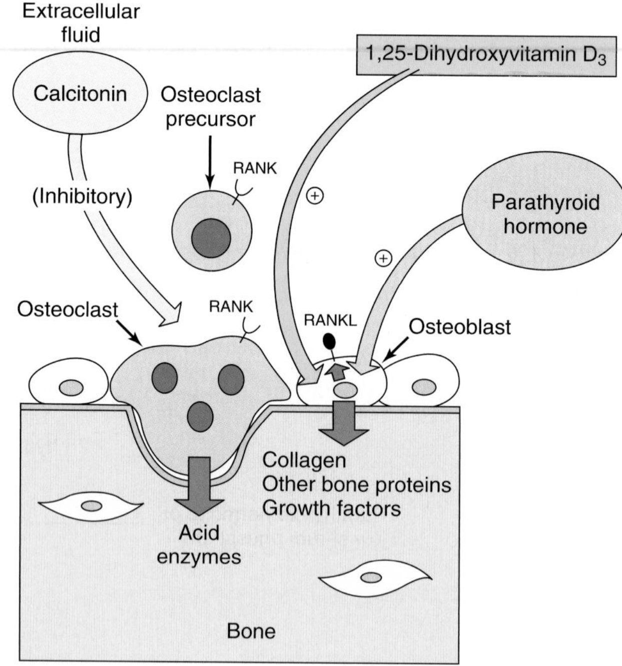

Figure 41-4 Effects of 1,25-dihydroxyvitamin D, PTH, and calcitonin on osteoblast and osteoclast activity. Osteoblasts stimulate osteoclast formation, survival, and activity by a membrane-associated cytokine, RANKL, that binds to receptors on osteoclast precursors and osteoclasts. Osteoblasts also stimulate bone formation and produce bone growth factors. Osteoclasts secrete acid and proteolytic enzymes and resorb the bone matrix. Active vitamin D metabolites and PTH increase the expression of RANKL in osteoblasts, resulting in activation of osteoclasts and resorption of bone. Calcitonin inhibits osteoclast activity via interaction with a G-protein-coupled receptor.

calcium receptor, which is a G-protein linked membrane receptor.

PTH binds to receptors in target cells and stimulates protein phosphorylation by both protein kinase A and specific protein kinase C isozymes. PTH has multiple effects that influence calcium and phosphate metabolism and bone (Fig. 41-5). PTH acts directly on the kidney to decrease renal tubular reabsorption of phosphate and increase renal tubular reabsorption of calcium, resulting in decreased serum phosphate and increased serum calcium concentrations. On bone, PTH interacts with receptors on osteoblasts, and like vitamin D metabolites, increases production of RANKL, stimulating resorption and increasing serum calcium concentrations (Fig. 41-4). When PTH is administered intermittently, an anabolic effect on bone is apparent with increased bone formation, an action that may involve growth factors such as insulin-like growth factor-1. This anabolic effect is the basis for the recent introduction of PTH 1-34 as a treatment for severe osteoporosis for patients in whom antiresorptive agents have failed to prevent recurrent fractures. PTH enhances calcium absorption indirectly by stimulating formation of 1,25-dihydroxyvitamin D (see Fig. 41-2). A recently discovered protein, the PTH-related protein, has significant amino acid sequence homology to PTH at the N-terminal region of the molecule. PTH-related protein is produced by several types of tumors, is important in malignancy-related hypercalcemias, in normal calcium metabolism in mammary gland and placenta, and in chondrocyte differentiation.

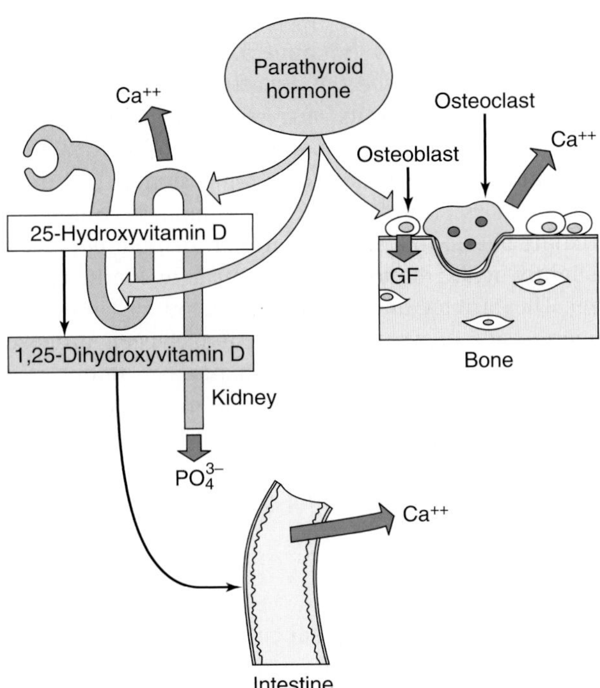

Figure 41-5 Direct and indirect effects of PTH on calcium metabolism. Renal tubular reabsorption of phosphate decreases and that of calcium increases. Hormone-stimulated osteoblast activates osteoclast to release calcium into extracellular fluid. Intermittent stimulation of osteoblasts by PTH has anabolic effects mediated by growth factors *(GFs)*.

Calcitonin

Calcitonin is a 32-amino acid polypeptide secreted by the parafollicular cells of the thyroid. It decreases postprandial absorption of calcium; increases excretion of calcium, sodium, magnesium, chloride, and phosphate; and inhibits the activity of osteoclasts by direct actions on G-protein-linked receptors in these cells (see Fig. 41-4). The inhibition of osteoclast activity results in a decrease in both serum calcium and phosphate. The ability of calcitonin to decrease hypercalcemia diminishes with continued use. Calcitonin is effective in treatment of Paget's disease of bone and is also approved for treatment of osteoporosis. Calcitonin and the neuronal calcitonin gene-related peptide arise from differential splicing in the parafollicular cells and in neural tissue.

Estrogens and selective estrogen receptor modulators

Estrogens (see Chapter 35) inhibit bone resorption and prevent fractures. The mechanism appears to involve decreased production of interleukins that activate and promote survival of osteoclasts. Consistent with this protective effect, inhibition of estrogen production, such as by the long-acting gonadotropin-releasing hormone agonists, can produce osteoporosis. Estrogens are used in hormone replacement therapy after menopause for the prevention of osteoporosis, although their use has declined following problems observed in studies from the Women's Health Initiative (see Chapter 35). Other studies have shown that low doses of conjugated estrogens and micronized estradiol are effective in maintaining bone mineral density. The selective estrogen receptor modulators (SERMs), such as raloxifene, have estrogenic effects on bone and are used for prevention and treatment of osteoporosis. However, SERMs generally antagonize the effects of estrogen on the mammary gland, possibly because of differential interactions with stimulatory and inhibitory co-factors present in different tissues.

Bisphosphonates

Bisphosphonates are small molecules having a geminal bisphosphonate backbone. Bisphosphonates inhibit osteoclast activity, decrease bone resorption, and prevent fractures. Bisphosphonates are useful in treatment of hypercalcemia, osteoporosis, and Paget's disease of bone. There appear to be several mechanisms involved. Some of them are metabolized to an ATP analog that promotes osteoclast apoptosis, while others inhibit synthesis of isoprenyl groups through an effect on the mevalonate pathway and inhibit activation of proteins required for osteoclast activity. Two bisphosphonates that are used in the treatment of osteoporosis are alendronate and risedronate.

Fluoride

Fluoride can stimulate osteoblast activity and increase bone formation. It is also incorporated into bone matrix, resulting in formation of fluoroapatite in place of hydroxyapatite, making the bone denser. However, fluoride use has also been associated with an increased incidence of fractures, suggesting that it may cause formation of weaker bone, at least at some doses.

Additional agents used in the treatment of hypercalcemia

Sodium sulfate and the **chelating agent ethylenediamine tetraacetic acid** (EDTA) form poorly dissociable calcium salts and increase calcium excretion. The loop diuretics **ethacrynic acid** and **furosemide** increase both calcium and sodium excretion, whereas the benzothiadiazide diuretics decrease calcium excretion. **Plicamycin,** an antitumor agent that inhibits RNA synthesis (see Chapter 42), inhibits bone resorption by inducing apoptosis of osteoclasts and has been used to lower calcium in hypercalcemia of malignancy at one tenth the antineoplastic dose; however, it is still much more toxic than other antiresorptive agents, and its use is declining. **Glucocorticoids** (see Chapter 33) can lower serum calcium, largely by decreasing absorption. However, long-term exposure to glucocorticoids has deleterious effects on bone. Glucocorticoids decrease the synthesis of collagen and the formation of bone by decreasing protein synthesis in osteoblasts. They also increase RANKL and decrease OPG in osteoblasts. These direct effects on bone, together with the decreased calcium absorption and resultant increased PTH secretion, are probably the mechanisms mediating glucocorticoid-induced osteoporosis. **Nonsteroidal antiinflammatory agents** may be effective in inhibiting resorption caused by increased prostaglandins, such as in inflammatory conditions that can cause local bone loss. Table 41-2 summarizes the mechanisms of action of compounds affecting calcium and bone metabolism.

Table 41-2 Mechanisms of action of agents altering bone and calcium metabolism

Mechanism	Agents
Increase intestinal calcium absorption	Vitamin D metabolites PTH (indirect)
Increase renal calcium excretion	Sodium sulfate, EDTA Loop diuretics Calcitonin
Increase bone reabsorption	PTH Vitamin D metabolites
Increase bone formation	PTH (intermittent) Fluoride
Decrease intestinal calcium absorption	Glucocorticoids Calcitonin (postprandial)
Decrease renal calcium excretion	PTH Benzothiadiazide diuretics
Decrease bone resorption	Bisphosphonates Calcitonin Estrogens SERMs Plicamycin

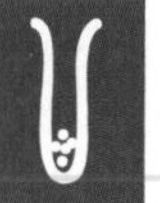

Pharmacokinetics

Vitamin D

Vitamin D, 25-hydroxyvitamin D, and 1,25-dihydroxyvitamin D are absorbed rapidly after oral administration (Table 41-3). Bile salts are required, however, and absorption is impaired in patients with biliary cirrhosis. Absorption is also decreased during steatorrhea or an excessive loss of fat in the feces. Vitamin D compounds circulate bound to a specific vitamin D-binding protein, a slightly acidic monomeric glycoprotein synthesized in liver. They are metabolized to inactive glucuronides and undergo side-chain metabolism. It has been proposed that 24,25-dihydroxyvitamin D may have unique mineralization properties, although this is not well established. Clearly, 1,24,25-trihydroxyvitamin D is less active than its precursor, 1,25-dihydroxyvitamin D. Vitamin D is stored for long periods in liver, fat, and muscle.

Parathyroid hormone

PTH 1-34 is administered subcutaneously. Plasma concentrations peak at 30 minutes in normal individuals and are cleared with a mean half-life of 75 minutes.

Calcitonin

Calcitonin is administered intramuscularly, subcutaneously, or intranasally. It is weakly bound to plasma

Table 41-3 Pharmacokinetic parameters

Agent	Route of Administration	Half-Life	Disposition
Vitamin D	Oral*	14 days	B**
1,25-dihydroxy vitamin D (calcitriol)	Oral*	1-3 days	M, R
PTH	SC	30 min	M, R
Calcitonin	SC, IM, nasal	20 min	M, R
Bisphosphonates	Oral	—	R
Fluoride	Oral or topical	—	R, sweat, milk, GI tract

*Bile salts needed.
**Binds to a special protein.
M, Metabolized; *R,* renally excreted.

proteins, has a plasma half-life of 20 minutes, and is metabolized rapidly in liver and kidney.

Estrogens and SERMs

The estrogens used for prevention of osteoporosis include conjugated estrogens and micronized estrogen. Their pharmacokinetics and those of the SERMs are discussed in Chapter 35.

Bisphosphonates

Bisphosphonates are typically administered orally, poorly absorbed (1% to 6%), and not metabolized. About 50% of absorbed drug is excreted by the kidneys in 72 hours, while the remainder is bound to hydroxyapatite in bone and retained in the body for years.

Fluoride

Fluoride is well absorbed after oral administration. However, calcium and nonabsorbable antacids can interfere with its absorption. Fluoride is concentrated in skeletal tissues, and excretion is largely renal.

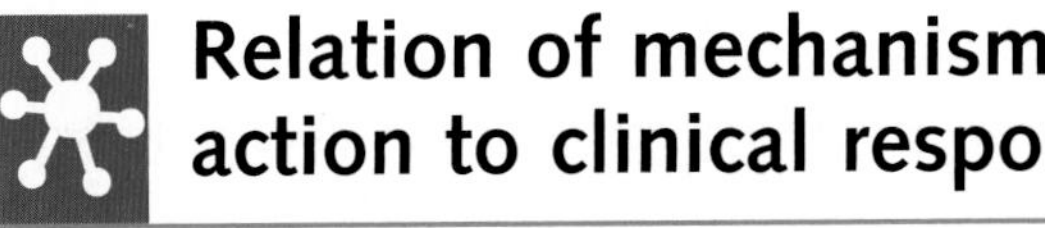

Relation of mechanisms of action to clinical response

Vitamin D and metabolites

Vitamin D and its active metabolites are used primarily in treatment of rickets, osteomalacia, and hypocalcemia. The actions of vitamin D compounds in increasing calcium absorption form the basis for their antirachitic activity. Their effects on calcium release from bone probably contribute to the hypercalcemic effect. Use of the metabolites 25-hydroxyvitamin D and 1,25-dihydroxyvitamin D is logical if this disorder results from a defect in formation of these metabolites. Alternatively, larger doses of the precursor can be given to produce sufficient concentrations of active metabolites to increase serum calcium. Therefore, doses of vitamin D more than 10 times greater than those used for simple replacement therapy are used to treat hypoparathyroidism or vitamin D-resistant rickets. Calcipotriol, applied topically, can promote keratinocyte differentiation without affecting calcium metabolism and is used in treatment of psoriasis. 19-Nor-1α,25-dihydroxyvitamin D2 can suppress the parathyroid glands with minimal hypercalcemic effects. It is used to inhibit PTH secretion in treatment of renal osteodystrophy, where impaired renal function and hydroxylation of vitamin D results in secondary hyperparathyroidism.

Parathyroid hormone

PTH 1-34, administered once daily, has an anabolic effect on bone and leads to an increase in bone density and a decrease in fractures. PTH 1-34 is used for treatment of severe osteoporosis when initial therapy with antiresorptive drugs has not been effective.

Calcitonin

Calcitonin inhibits osteoclast activity and thus is an antiresorptive agent. It is used in treatment of Paget's disease of bone to inhibit abnormal bone turnover. Calcitonin is also used to treat osteoporosis; however, it is less effective than estrogen or the bisphosphonates. Although used in treatment of hypercalcemia of malignancy, its effects in this setting are somewhat delayed and less dramatic than those of other agents.

Estrogens and SERMs

Estrogens and SERMs inhibit osteoclast activity by inhibiting of the expression of local inflammatory interleukins and other cytokines, and produce inhibition of bone resorption and increased bone density. Estrogen treatment started at the time of menopause prevents bone loss and decreases fractures. These compounds are used for the prevention and treatment of osteoporosis.

Bisphosphonates

Bisphosphonates are highly effective inhibitors of osteoclast activity and are used in the treatment of osteoporosis, Paget's disease of bone, and hypercalcemia.

Other agents used to treat hypercalcemia

Sodium sulfate and EDTA form complexes with calcium and accelerate its elimination. The loop diuretics, furosemide and ethacrynic acid, increase calcium excretion concomitantly with sodium excretion. Glucocorticoids decrease calcium absorption and increase excretion. Plicamycin inhibits osteoclast activity; by preventing bone breakdown it can decrease serum calcium.

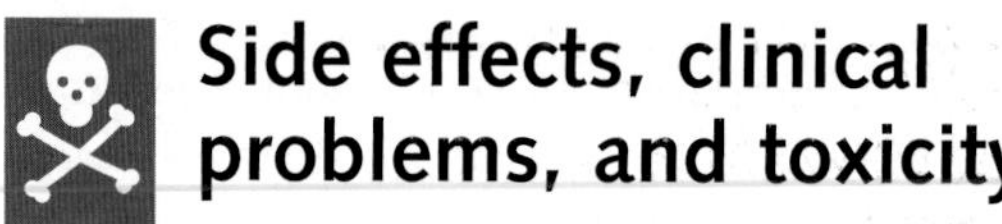

Side effects, clinical problems, and toxicity

The clinical problems are summarized in the Clinical Problems box.

CLINICAL PROBLEMS

Vitamin D and metabolites

Hypercalcemia (benzothiadiazides can increase risk of hypercalcemia)

Parathyroid hormone

Hypercalcemia (uncommon with intermittent dosing)

Calcitonin

Local hypersensitivity, loss of effectiveness

Bisphosphonates

GI side effects, osteomalacia, bone pain

Fluoride

GI side effects including nausea, musculoskeletal pain, joint swelling, mottled teeth enamel, dose-related bone fracture

Vitamin D

Excess vitamin D and its metabolites can lead to hypercalcemia, a potentially fatal side effect. The immediate risk of this is greatest for 1,25-dihydroxyvitamin D because this metabolite bypasses the enzyme that is feedback regulated, viz., the renal 1α-hydroxylase. However, because 1,25-dihydroxyvitamin D has the shortest half-life, hypercalcemia and the risk of cumulative effects are potentially less than for the other metabolites. There is an increased risk of toxicity in patients with impaired renal function. Serum calcium concentrations must be monitored in patients receiving vitamin D, and it must be discontinued if hypercalcemia occurs. Benzothiadiazide diuretics, which decrease calcium excretion, can increase the risk of hypercalcemia from vitamin D. Drug interactions can occur with phenobarbital, phenytoin, and glucocorticoids, all of which interfere with vitamin D activation, as well as actions of metabolites on target tissues.

Parathyroid hormone

Hypercalcemia is a potential side effect of PTH because the hormone stimulates bone resorption. The risk is less when it is given intermittently, as in therapy of osteoporosis.

Calcitonin

Local hypersensitivity reactions including rashes, other allergic reactions, and nausea have been noted in patients receiving calcitonin. Although calcitonin could elicit hypocalcemia, this is not common. A potential problem with calcitonin is a loss of effectiveness with prolonged use.

Bisphosphonates

Upper GI tract side effects, including pain on swallowing and heartburn, have been reported with bisphosphonates. Etidronate decreases bone mineralization and has been reported to cause osteomalacia and bone pain.

Fluoride

Fluoride has GI side effects including nausea. Musculoskeletal pain and joint swelling have been reported, and there is a possible dose-related risk of increased fractures.

The side effects of diuretics, glucocorticoids, estrogens, and SERMs are discussed in other chapters.

New horizons

The importance of the RANKL-RANK interaction in stimulating osteoclast differentiation, survival, and activity has resulted in interest in the decoy receptor, **OPG,** as a potential therapeutic agent. Recognition of the role of the calcium receptor in the parathyroid gland as a critical regulator of PTH secretion has led to the development of **calcimimetics,** compounds that mimic the effects of calcium, as well as **calciolytics,** which inhibit the calcium receptor. The use of these compounds to decrease or increase PTH will likely have therapeutic application. Because PTH most likely elicits its anabolic effects through increased expression of growth factors in bone such as **insulin-like growth factors, transforming growth factor β, and bone morphogenetic proteins,** these could potentially be used to promote bone formation. The **statins,** which, like the bisphosphonates, decrease the production of isoprenyl groups through inhibitory effects on the mevalonate pathway, can increase bone through increased bone morphogenetic protein-2. The challenge is to develop a means to target systemic growth factors or statins specifically to bone. **Benzothiadiazide diuretics,** which decrease calcium excretion and are useful in the prevention of nephrolithiasis (renal stones), may also be useful in diminishing bone loss. Finally, osteoclasts have unique organelles and metabolic processes that can provide new targets for treatments to reduce bone resorption. The ability of vitamin D analogs to promote differentiation makes them potential treatments for certain malignancies.

TRADE NAMES

In addition to generic and fixed-combination preparations and the drugs listed in the Major Drugs Box, the following trade-named materials are some of the important compounds available in the United States.

Vitamin D, metabolites, and analogs

Calcifediol (Calderol)
Calcipotriene (Dovonex, MC903)
Dihydrotachysterol (DHT, Hytakerol)
Doxercalciferol (Hectorol)

Bisphosphonates

Etidronate (Didronel)
Ibandronate (Boniva)
Pamidronate (Aredia)
Tiludronate (Skelid)
Zoledronic acid (Zometa)

FURTHER READING

Akesson K. New approaches to pharmacological treatment of osteoporosis. *Bull World Health Org* 2003; 81:657-664.

Holick MF: Vitamin D. A millenium perspective. *J Cell Biochem* 2003; 88:296-307.

Martin KJ, Gonzalez, EA. Vitamin D analogs for the management of secondary hyperparathyroidism. *Am J Kidney Dis* 2001; 38:1430-1436.

Self-assessment questions

1. Which one of the following is true with regard to renal calcium and phosphate metabolism?
   a. Approximately 10 g of calcium is filtered per day and 1% of that is reabsorbed.
   b. Furosemide and ethacrynic acid stimulate Na-linked calcium reabsorption.
   c. Thiazide diuretics can prevent nephrolithiasis by increasing calcium excretion.
   d. PTH decreases renal phosphate reabsorption.
   e. High phosphate stimulates the renal [25-hydroxyvitamin D]1-α-hydroxylase.

2. Which one of the following statements is true of PTH?
   a. PTH acts through a nuclear receptor.
   b. PTH stimulates 25-hydroxylation of vitamin D.
   c. PTH inhibits bone resorption.
   d. Intermittent PTH has anabolic effects on bone.
   e. PTH inhibits intestinal calcium absorption.

3. Which one of the following statements is true of vitamin D?
   a. Vitamin D inhibits the synthesis of an intestinal calcium-binding protein.
   b. Active vitamin D metabolites inhibit cell differentiation.
   c. Vitamin D stimulates parathyroid hormone secretion.
   d. Vitamin D increases mineralization and resorption of bone.
   e. Ultraviolet light activates the vitamin D precursor in the skin by cleaving the A ring.

4. Which of the following is a SERM currently used to prevent or treat osteoporosis?
   a. RANKL
   b. Calcitonin
   c. Alendronate
   d. Raloxifene
   e. Estrogen

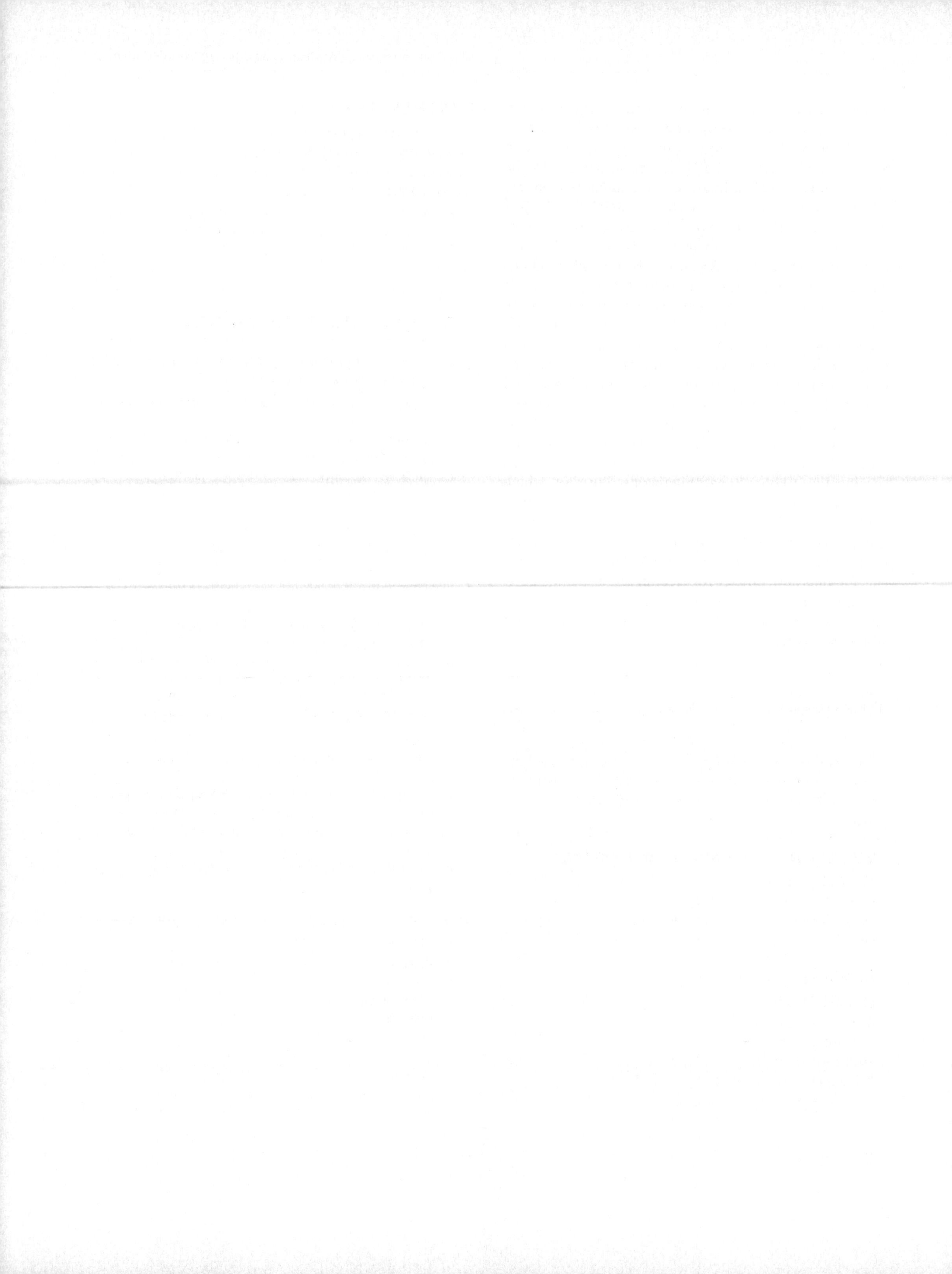

PART VI

Antineoplastic drugs

ONE OF THE FUNDAMENTAL advances made in oncology in the last few decades is the recognition that cancer is a genetic disease. This does not mean that all cancers are inherited (although numerous genetic diseases are associated with a predisposition to cancer) but that neoplastic cells have an altered genetic content. This was first recognized in leukemias, which were all found to be associated with an abnormal karyotype. Eventually it was noted that most malignant cells have chromosomal rearrangements, and even cells with apparently normal karyotypes can almost always be found to have definable abnormalities (e.g., translocations, deletions).

By definition, neoplastic cells and tissues are characterized by uncontrolled growth, usually accompanied by a loss of cellular differentiation (anaplasia). The diseased cells and tissues are described as tumors, neoplasms, or cancers and occur in benign (non-virulent) or malignant (virulent) states. Malignant neoplastic cells typically invade surrounding tissues, violating the basement membrane of the tissue of origin and eventually undergoing metastasis. Over 100 types of malignant neoplasms affect humans and are classified primarily according to their anatomical location and the type of cell involved. The advent of molecular diagnostic methods will almost certainly modify this number.

In the United States, malignant neoplasms are responsible for causing about 500,000 deaths per year (20% to 25% of total mortality), with about 1,000,000 new cases developing each year. Lung, large intestine, breast, and prostate neoplasms account for about 55% of both new cases and cancer deaths in the United States. Solid tumors arising from epithelial cells are termed *carcinomas,* whereas those originating from connective or mesenchymal tissue are termed *sarcomas.* Malignancies that arise from the hematopoietic system include the *leukemias* and *lymphomas.*

The mechanisms by which malignant neoplasms originate in humans are still not clear. Carcinogenesis (i.e., the creation of malignant neoplastic cells) appears to result from the activation of specific dominant growth genes, called **oncogenes,** or a loss of functional negative effectors, called **tumor suppressor genes.** On the basis of the findings in the best-studied tumors, it is now believed that both kinds of genetic changes are essential for development of a full malignant phenotype. Proto-oncogenes, when activated, become oncogenes, which encode modified proteins that cause cellular dedifferentiation and proliferation characteristics of the neoplastic state. Activation of protooncogenes can occur by means of several pathways that often involve the exposure of cells to chemicals, radiation, or viruses. Activation can result from a single-point mutation. The most common oncogenes found thus far in human tumors belong to the *ras* gene family, which codes for guanosine triphosphate (GTP)–binding proteins. When *ras* is converted to the activated form, it fails to dephosphorylate GTP and cells are transformed to a neoplastic phenotype. Over 100 proto-oncogenes are known to exist. Clearly, most if not all products of these variously dominantly acting oncogenes are components of cellular signaling pathways. Other genes, known as *tumor-suppressing genes,* also are present in human cells and function to suppress excessive cellular growth. Retinoblastoma (tumor of the eye) is a prototype of a malignancy caused by a genetic loss of the tumor-suppressor gene Rb. A second common tumor suppressor gene is p53, which has recently been shown to possess the important function of protecting genomic stability. Because cancer can be defined by a loss of genomic stability, it is not surprising that mutations in p53 are the single most prevalent lesion in human cancer. Tumor growth represents a balance between cell division and cell death. Recently it has become clear that, in addition to cells dying from necrosis, cells can exit the cell cycle by way of apoptosis, which is a form of programmed cell death. Apoptosis is not only important developmentally (e.g., thymic involution), but the apoptotic pathway is also an important pathway in the cellular response to DNA-damaging agents such as chemotherapy. It is now believed that all chemotherapeutic agents act via apoptosis. Indeed, the apoptotic pathway is now being targeted in the development of drugs. Interestingly, some oncogenes, namely bcl2, act by blocking apoptosis.

From the clinical standpoint, the primary difficulty in the successful control and treatment of malignant neoplasms is that by the time cancers are detected, they are relatively large, (a 1-cm^3 volume of tumor usually contains 10^9 cells) and frequently have metastasized. The chances of curing metastatic disease are small, because effective local treatments such as surgery and radiotherapy cannot remove or destroy all the malignant cells.

The generally accepted approach in the therapy of neoplastic diseases (as shown in Fig. VI-1) remains the removal or destruction of the neoplastic cells while minimizing toxic effects on non-neoplastic cells. It has been a long-standing question whether drugs effective against one type of neoplasm should be effective against all types. Clinical experience, however, has shown a wide range of drug activities among different types of tumors (sarcoma, carcinoma, leukemia, lymphoma) and among tumors in different anatomical locations (breast, colon, lung). Therefore interest has focused on treating each of the over 100 clinically important forms of cancer as distinct diseases. Some of the therapeutic approaches listed in Figure VI-1 are not available for clinical use but represent experimental approaches that are under study. For example, drugs that function specifically to return neoplastic cells to normal differentiating cells and drugs that prevent metastases are not available or are highly experimental.

The chapters in this section cover the mechanisms of action and the problems associated with the clinical use of antineoplastic drugs in humans. Individual drugs are discussed in Chapter 42, and their clinical uses, usually in multiple-drug protocols, are discussed in Chapter 43.

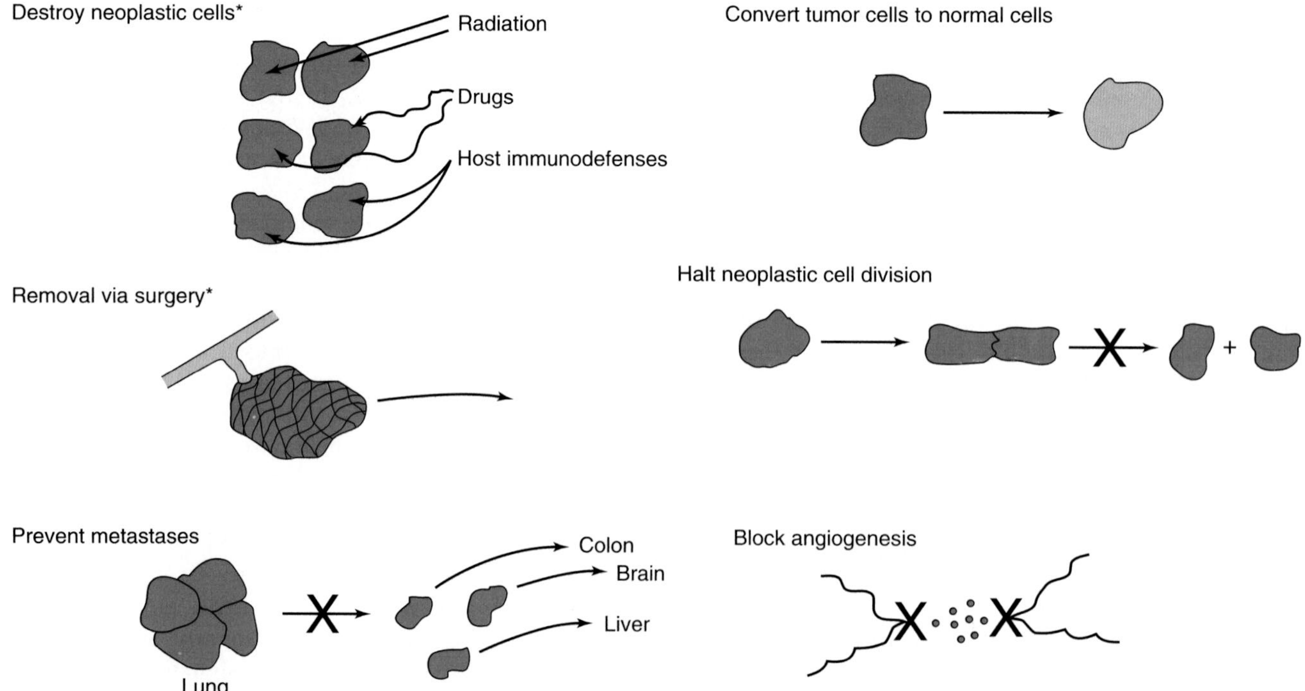

Figure VI-1 Major approaches to therapy of cancers. Tumor cells are shown in red and non-tumor cells in green. *In clinical use. Others are experimental.

CHAPTER 42

Mechanisms of action of antineoplastic drugs

James M. Larner
William W. Grosh

Major Drugs

Alkylating agents	Kinase inhibitors
Antibiotics	Plant alkaloids
Antibodies	Proteasome inhibitors
Antimetabolites	Recombinant proteins
Hormonal agents	

Therapeutic overview

Antineoplastic agents are used to treat more than 100 types of neoplastic diseases, with the goal of destroying malignant cells. Additional drugs (see Chapter 43) are used to enhance host defense mechanisms to eradicate those tumor cells not killed by the antineoplastic drugs. In clinical practice, nearly all neoplastic diseases are treated by using multiple drugs, although only individual drugs are discussed in this chapter. These form the basis for multiple-drug protocols described in Chapter 43.

The effectiveness of antineoplastic drugs varies greatly with the following:

- Type of cancer
- Biological and physiological condition of the patient
- Extent to which the tumor has grown or spread

The end point used to evaluate effectiveness (e.g., tumor response, patient survival) is also important. Most antineoplastic agents, particularly chemotherapeutic agents, are more effective in destroying cells that are progressing through the **cell cycle** (Fig. 42-1) than in destroying cells that are resting in the G_0 phase. The "growth fraction," defined in Figure 42-1, is the fraction of cells progressing through the cycle. Besides tumor cells that may be proliferating, however, there are also some non-neoplastic cells undergoing division, particularly those of hair follicles, bone marrow, and intestinal epithelium. These rapidly dividing cells are especially sensitive to antineoplastic drugs and account for many of their undesirable side effects. It is believed that most, if not all, anticancer drugs kill cells primarily through a programmed, energy-dependent process called **apoptosis** rather than through necrosis.

The number of cultured neoplastic cells that survive exposure to each drug typically shows a first-order relationship to the drug concentration (Fig. 42-2). This means that the same fraction of cells are killed with each drug dose and that a series of several doses does not kill 100% of them. This "log-cell kill" hypothesis is compatible with the clinical observation that a functional host immune system is needed for killing all

Abbreviations

ADCC	antibody dependent cell mediated cytotoxicity
Ara-C	cytarabine
ATPase	adenosine triphosphatase
EGFR	epidermal growth factor receptor
FH_4	tetrahydrofolate
5-FU	5-fluorouracil
MESNA	sodium 2-mercaptoethane sulfonate
6-MP	6-mercaptopurine
MTX	methotrexate
6-TG	6-thioguanine

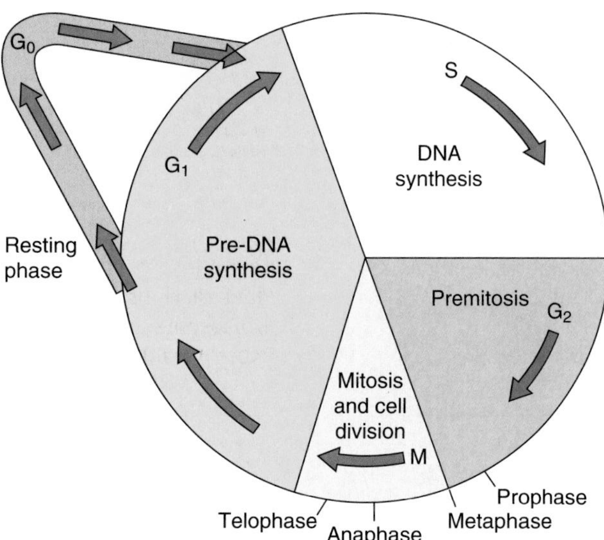

Figure 42-1 Growth cycle for mammalian cells. The cells are dormant in the G_0 (resting) phase. A variety of stimulants, often of unknown origin in clinical situations, cause cycling of cells to begin by entry into the G_1 phase (pre-DNA synthesis). Here, precursors for DNA are formed. DNA synthesis occurs in the S, or synthetic, phase. This is followed by premitotic synthesis and structural developments in the G_2 phase. Mitosis occurs in the M phase to produce two cells, each of which can continue to cycle by entry again into G_1 or can enter the resting phase, G_0. Growth fraction is defined as the total cells in the growth cycle (G_1, S, G_2, M) divided by the total cells (G_1, S, G_2, M, G_0).

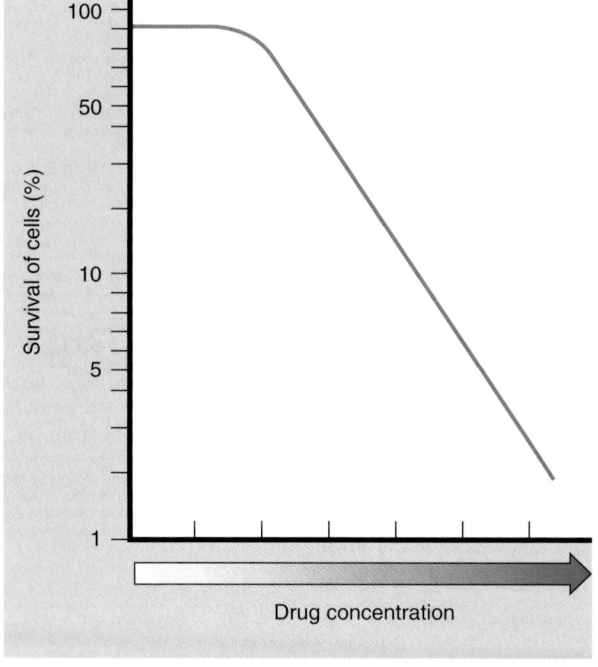

Figure 42-2 Decline in viable cells is first order with respect to drug concentration. Many antineoplastic agents and cultured tumor cells follow this relationship, thus establishing the principles of a fixed percentage of viable cells killed per concentration of drug. This same relationship appears to apply *in vivo,* although the actual situation may be more complex. A threshold concentration of drug is often required to cause a noticeable decrease in cell survival. This phenomenon, called *survival shoulder,* may reflect endogenous repair processes.

THERAPEUTIC OVERVIEW

Goal

Kill tumor cells selectively with no side effects

Uses

Treatment of systemic disease (curative and palliative)
Decrease tumor burden
Treatment of carcinomas, sarcomas, leukemias, lymphomas

Effects

Some but not all tumors respond

Considerations

Drug-delivery problems to individual cells
Cycling versus noncycling cells
Log-cell kill (same fraction of cells killed per dose)
Need for active immune system (host defenses) to eradicate remaining neoplastic cells
Problem of central hypoxic zone of tumors
Drug resistance

neoplastic cells and curing a patient. Endogenous cellular defenses, such as thiols or DNA repair enzymes, however, can necessitate a threshold of drug concentration, or "shoulder," in the survival curves of patients receiving these drugs (see Fig. 42-2).

Of the four major types of tumors, the faster-growing hematological (non-solid) types (leukemias and lymphomas) are more responsive to treatment than are the slower-growing solid types (carcinomas and sarcomas). Factors responsible for this difference are the more rapid doubling times of hematological malignancies and the greater ease of drug distribution to hematological cells than to solid tumors. The outer, more recently synthesized portions of many solid tumors are well vascularized and readily accessible to drugs, however. This is attributable in part to the growth of new blood vessels by **angiogenesis.** The inner and older portions of many solid tumors are hypoxic and often necrotic because angiogenesis is inadequate, making them poorly accessible to drugs. The necrotic inner cells may be dead or merely in the resting phase of the cell cycle and therefore still capable of returning to cycling. Delivery of drugs to inner portions of solid tumors is a major unsolved problem.

Antineoplastic drugs must enter the cell to produce their cytotoxic effects. Some drugs can pass through the membrane by passive diffusion, with the concentration gradient driving uptake. Other drugs must bind to carrier proteins that transport the drug through the membrane and release it in the cytoplasm; this is especially common with antimetabolites. Such carrier-mediated transport is an active process that is not concentration driven, and the rate of transport is often limited by the fixed number of carrier molecules available.

Once the drug enters the cell and diffuses into the nucleus or other sites, the drug can react with target molecules to disrupt key processes necessary for cell viability. These target molecules and their interactions with antineoplastic drugs are described in the next section.

Mechanisms of action

Basic approaches

The basic mechanisms by which antineoplastic drugs kill tumor cells are summarized in Figure 42-3. Only compounds that show some selectivity for neoplastic cells are used clinically. In general, **antimetabolites** inhibit DNA synthesis. **Alkylating agents, intercalators,** and **antibiotics** damage or disrupt DNA, interfere with topoisomerase activity, or alter RNA structure. Other agents, including **steroids,** interfere with transcription, whereas the several **plant alkaloids** disrupt mitosis. Agents such as **asparaginase** destroy essential amino acids needed for translation. Other drugs act through important **growth factor** signal transduction pathways. Many clinically used antineoplastic drugs must undergo either chemical or enzymatic modification to become actively cytotoxic, as discussed later in this section.

The principal classes of antineoplastic drugs are listed in the Major Drugs box.

Alkylating agents

Alkylation refers to the covalent attachment of alkyl groups to other molecules. Alkylating agents came to be used for cancer therapy as a result of observations of the effects of the mustard war gases on cell growth. Although these are too toxic for clinical use in cancer, the first effective antineoplastic agents, including mechlorethamine, were developed from related nitrogen mustard alkylating agents and are still used today.

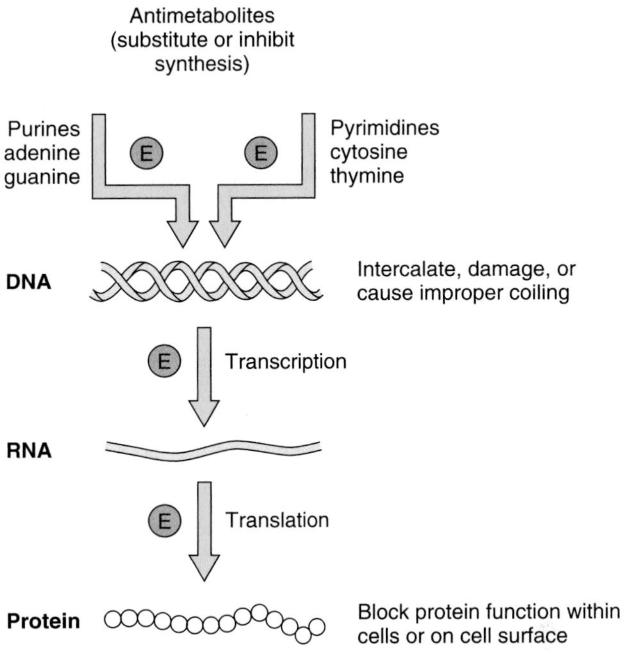

Antimetabolites
(substitute or inhibit synthesis)
Purines
adenine
guanine
E
E
Pyrimidines
cytosine
thymine
DNA
Intercalate, damage, or cause improper coiling
E
Transcription
RNA
E
Translation
Protein
Block protein function within cells or on cell surface

Figure 42-3 Basic mechanisms by which antineoplastic drugs selectively kill tumor cells. *E* stands for enzymes, some of which are inhibited by these drugs. Inhibition of DNA or RNA synthesis or replication, production of miscoded nucleic acids, and formation of modified proteins are key mechanisms of action for many of these drugs.

Alkylation takes place through chemical formation of a positively charged carbonium ion that reacts with an electron-rich site, particularly on DNA or RNA, to form modified nucleic acids. Most clinically used alkylating drugs have two active groups, which enable them to form **covalent links** between adjacent nucleic acid strands that are more difficult to repair than monofunctional adducts. These cross-links also prevent separation of the dual strands of DNA during cell cycling. For maximal kill, it is important to administer the maximally tolerated dose. The alkylation sequence for mechlorethamine (nitrogen mustard) reacting with the N-7 position of deoxyguanylate is shown in Figure 42-4. Although many other nucleophilic constituents—including RNA, proteins, and membrane components—become alkylated within cells, it is generally believed that the primary cytotoxic events occur through alkylation of DNA, especially by coupling to the N-7 position of the deoxyguanylates of either single- or double-stranded DNA.

Structures of several clinically used alkylating agents are shown in Figure 42-5. Cyclophosphamide undergoes a combination of enzymatic and chemical activation to form the active phosphoramide mustard alkylating agent (Fig. 42-6). Exposure of cells to cyclophosphamide and other alkylating agents can also lead to carcinogenesis. For example, leukemia is a well-known long-term complication in patients with Hodgkin's disease treated with a regimen including mechlorethamine.

Another group of antineoplastic alkylating agents in clinical use are the **nitrosoureas.** The structures and primary mechanisms of activation for these compounds are shown in Figure 42-7. Carbamoylation of proteins also occurs with nitrosoureas (see Fig. 42-7), and the carbamoylated proteins may play a role in cytotoxicity. The alkylation route, however, is probably the major source of cytotoxicity. Nitrosoureas are lipophilic and can cross the blood-brain barrier, so they are often used to treat brain tumors.

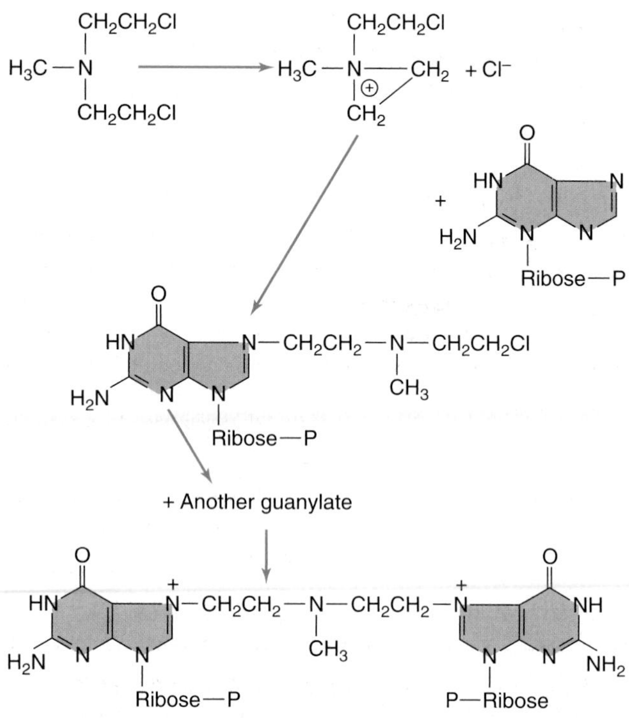

Figure 42-4 Alkylation by mechlorethamine, showing positively charged intermediate ion and its covalent attachment to the N-7 position of two deoxyguanylate nucleotides of DNA.

Temozolomide is the first new alkylating agent approved for treatment of malignant gliomas in decades. It has a structure similar to dacarbazine and is is rapidly absorbed after oral administration. Unlike many other alkylating agents, temozolomide crosses the blood-brain barrier. It methylates guanine and adenine, resulting in misincorporation of thymidine (across from the methylated guanidine), which cannot easily be corrected by the mismatch repair system. Resistance occurs by upregulation of components of the DNA mismatch repair system. Other compounds that form covalent bonds with DNA are cisplatin and the newer analog carboplatin, whose structures are shown in Figure 42-8. Cisplatin is a square planar complex of platinum with two ammonia molecules and two chloride ions at the corners of the plane. The reaction sequence of the active species is complex and not completely understood. Replacement of a chloride with a hydroxyl must occur before the platinum-nitrogen bond can interact with DNA. Subsequently, the second chloride is aquated and reacts with DNA. The stereochemistry of the complex enables the *cis* but not the *trans* isomer to form two covalent platinum-nitrogen bonds, primarily at two adjacent deoxyguanylates of DNA. This intrastrand cross-link prevents DNA replication and is cytotoxic. Cisplatin also forms interstrand cross-links and protein-DNA cross-links. Similar DNA cross-links are formed with carboplatin. Oxaliplatin is an organoplat-

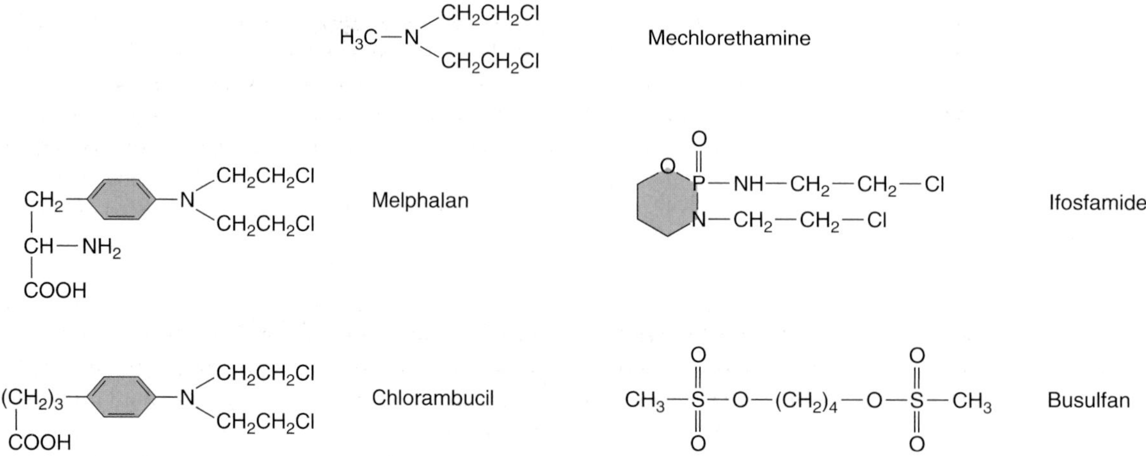

Figure 42-5 Structures of nitrogen mustards and busulfan.

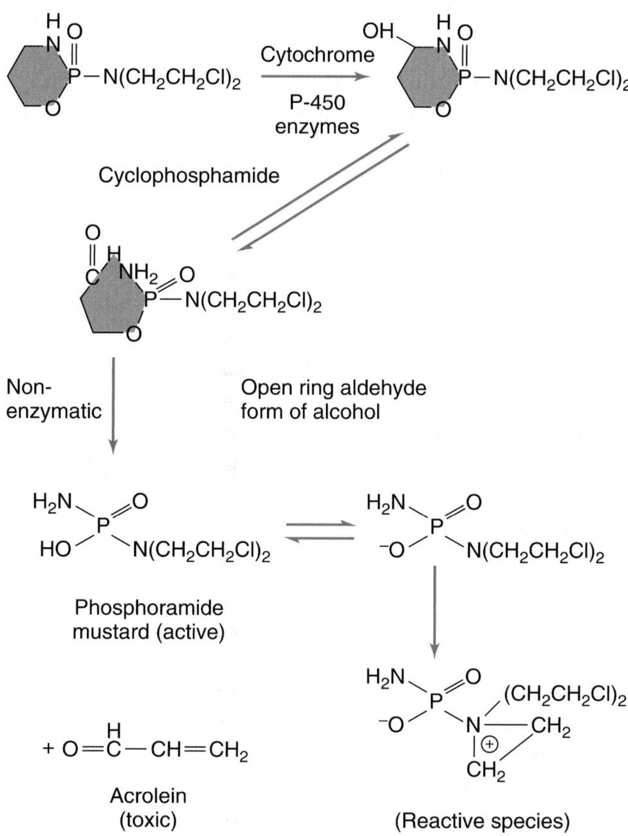

Figure 42-6 Mechanism of enzymatic and chemical activation of cyclophosphamide to form active phosphoramide mustard. Acrolein has some antitumor activity but much less than that of the phosphoramide mustard.

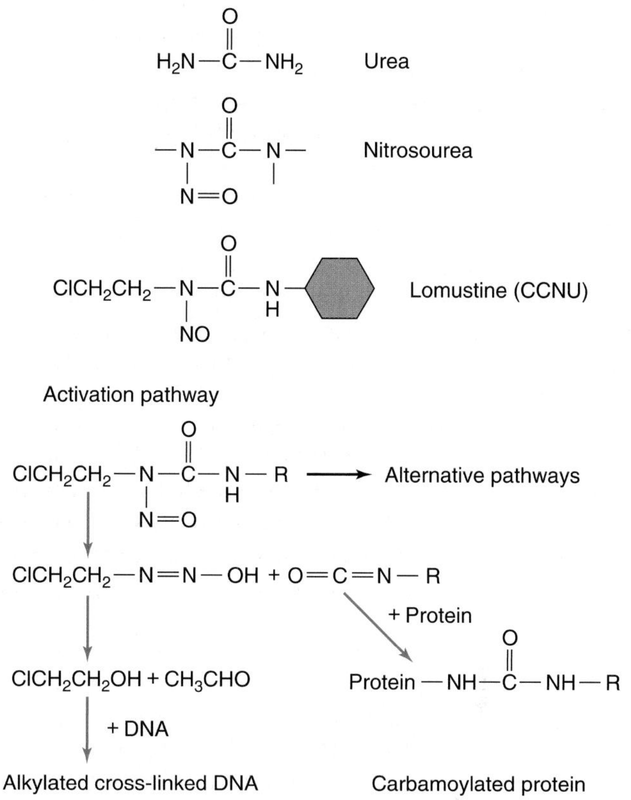

Figure 42-7 Structures and activation pathways for nitrosourea alkylating agents. Carbamoylation of proteins also occurs but is believed to be a lesser cause of cell cytotoxicity than is alkylation of DNA.

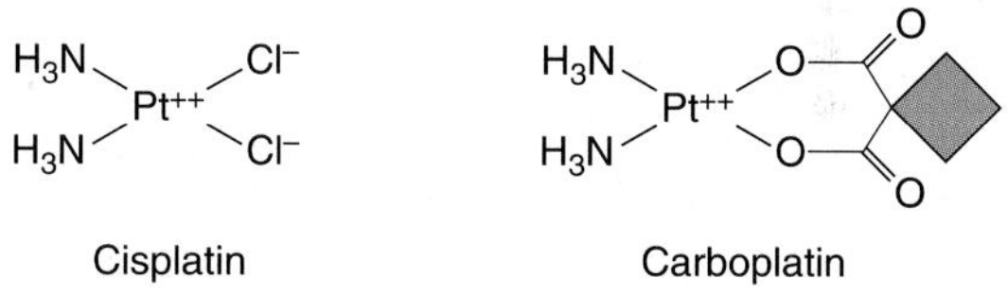

Figure 42-8 Square planar complex of *cis*-diamminedichloroplatinum (II), cisplatin, and a new platinum derivative, carboplatin.

inum compound constructed to overcome resistance to cisplatin by binding the platinum atom to 1,2-diaminocyclohexane. Oxaliplatin undergoes conversion to reactive metabolites that covalently bind to either adjacent guanines, adjacent adenine-guanines, or guanines separated by an intervening nucleotide. This creates inter- and intra-strand cross-links and inhibits DNA replication and transcription. Oxaliplatin is approved for treatment of metastatic colorectal carcinoma, has activity in lung cancer, and may have activity in breast and esophageal cancers and lymphoma.

Several other clinically useful alkylating agents include busulfan, dacarbazine, procarbazine, ifosfamide, and melphalan. The busulfan type of compounds alkylate nucleic acid bases, primarily at the N-7 of guanine, and also alkylate SH groups of glutathione and protein thiols.

The specific reaction sequences by which dacarbazine or procarbazine alkylate DNA are not well understood. Melphalan is a phenylalanine derivative and is actively transported into the cell by the carriers that transport leucine and glutamine. Melphalan is associated with induction of secondary leukemias. Chlorambucil is structurally similar to melphalan and is used primarily in treatment of chronic lymphocytic leukemia. Ifosfamide, like its analog cyclophosphamide, is activated by hepatic microsomes. Early studies with ifosfamide showed its use was associated with a significant incidence of hemorrhagic cystitis. Ifosfamide is now given with a systemic thiol, MESNA. MESNA becomes a free thiol after glomerular filtration and combines with the products responsible for causing the cystitis. Ifosfamide is active against several cancers, including small-cell lung cancer, sarcomas, lymphomas, testicular carcinoma, and gynecological cancers.

Antimetabolites

The antimetabolites are compounds that mimic the structures of normal metabolic constituents including folic acid, pyrimidines, or purines. The antimetabolites inhibit the enzymes necessary for folic acid regeneration or the pyrimidine or purine activation of DNA or RNA synthesis in neoplastic cells. Antimetabolites frequently kill cells in S phase (see Fig. 42-1). Methotrexate (MTX), 5-fluorouracil (5FU), cytarabine (Ara-C), 6-mercaptopurine (6-MP), gemcitabine, and 6-thioguanine (6-TG) are the primary antimetabolites used clinically.

Folic acid is essential for enzymatic reactions that transfer methyl and related groups during purine and pyrimidine synthesis. The antimetabolite MTX competitively inhibits the enzyme **dihydrofolate reductase,** which catalyzes the reduction of dihydrofolate to FH_4 (Fig. 42-9). This blocks regeneration of FH_4 and prevents synthesis of purines and pyrimidines. MTX is specific for cells in the S phase of the cell cycle. Intracellular addition of several glutamates to MTX greatly enhances its inhibitory activity and also prevents cellular efflux. MTX is more toxic to tumor cells than normal cells, in part because of the greater polyglutamating enzyme activity in tumor cells. Thus a higher concentration of the more active MTX covalently linked to multiple glutamates is trapped within tumor cells where it acts as an antimetabolite.

Transport of MTX is carrier mediated, and reduced MTX uptake is a prominent mechanism of tumor cell resistance. To overcome limitations of carrier uptake and enhance drug entry by passive diffusion, some investigators have infused high-dose MTX IV over several hours. When high-dose MTX is administered, it is mandatory that it be followed by a "rescue process"

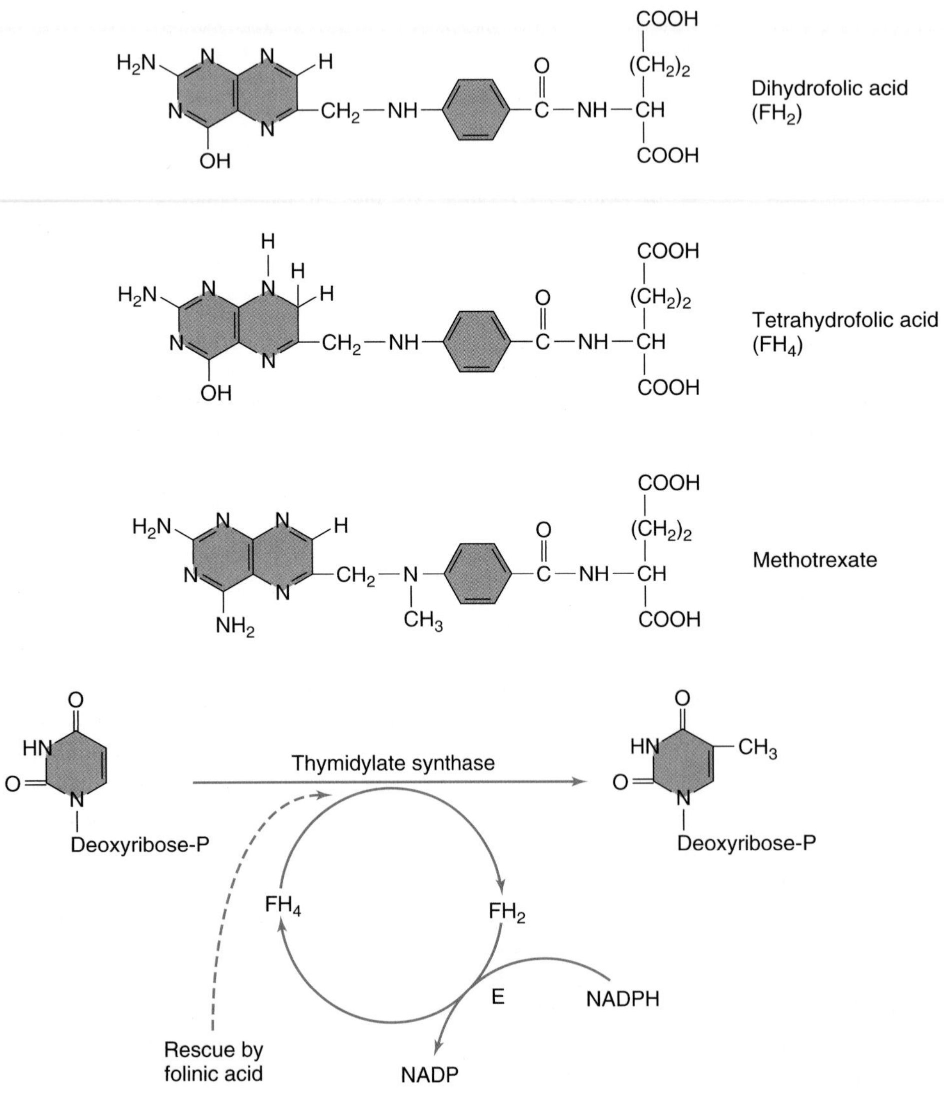

Figure 42-9 Structures of dihydrofolic acid (*FH_2*), tetrahydrofolic acid (*FH_4*), and methotrexate. The reaction shown is a pyrimidine synthesis (thymidine monophosphate from deoxyuridylic acid) catalyzed by thymidylate synthase and requiring FH_4 as cofactor. *E* is dihydrofolate reductase, which is reversibly inhibited by methotrexate, thus preventing regeneration of FH_4 from dihydrofolate (*FH_2*). The rescue path is discussed in the text. The pyrimidines are needed for DNA formation.

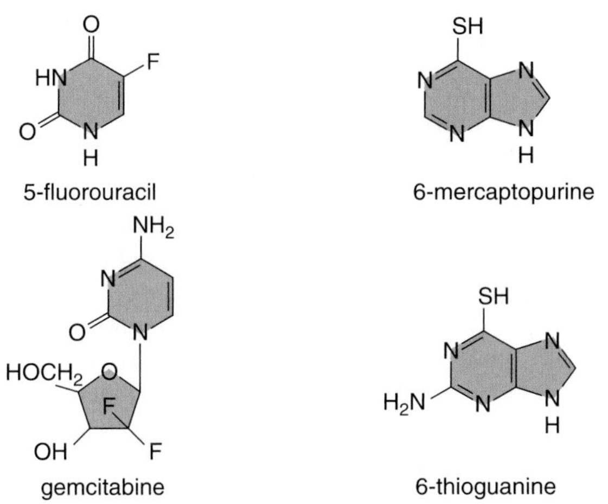

Figure 42-10 Structures of prototype purine and pyrimidine antimetabolites.

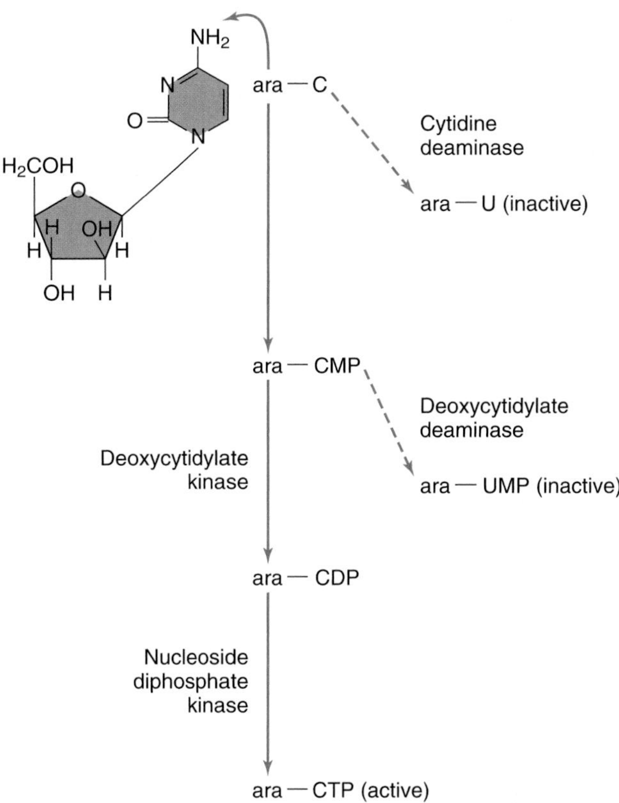

Figure 42-11 Competing activation and deactivation pathways for conversion of cytosine arabinoside to the active form that inhibits DNA polymerase.

of leucovorin (citrovorum factor of *N*6-formyl-FH_4). This is a substitute for FH_4, which is believed to enter nonmalignant cells by a carrier-mediated process, enabling purine and pyrimidine synthesis to proceed. The clinical efficacy of this high-dose MTX-leucovorin rescue approach, however, is still under debate.

Pemetrexed is an MTX analogue that inhibits several folate-dependent enzymes involved in synthesis of thymidine and purine nucleotides. Pemetrexed is preferentially converted to polyglutamate forms in malignant as compared with normal cells. Since polyglutamated metabolites have an increased half-life, pemetrexed is most active in malignant cells. It was recently approved for treatment of malignant mesothelioma in combination with cisplatin. It also appears, like MTX, to have activity in cervical and breast cancer.

Another antimetabolite, 5-FU, acts primarily by inhibiting pyrimidine synthesis and thus DNA formation. Its structure is shown in Figure 42-10. 5-FU is metabolized to the 5-fluoro analog of deoxyuridylic acid, which inhibits **thymidylate synthase** by covalent coupling. Capecitabine, an oral fluoropyrimidine, is an inactive precursor of 5-FU. It is converted to 5-FU selectively in the liver and tumor tissues. Evidence suggests that thymidine phosphorylase, the enzyme responsible for the final step in conversion to active 5-FU, is overexpressed in neoplastic tissues.

Ara-C also acts to inhibit pyrimidine synthesis but through a more complex pathway (Fig. 42-11). The drug must undergo enzymatic conversion to the active cytosine triphosphate derivative, which is incorporated into DNA. At high doses, ara-C also binds to and inhibits DNA polymerase competitively. Cytidine deaminase activity is high and deoxycytidylate kinase activity is low in some patients, resulting in considerable inactivation of the drug before conversion to its active form.

Gemcitabine is another pyrimidine antimetabolite (see Figure 42-10). It is a prodrug that, once transported into cells, must be phosphorylated by deoxycytidine kinase to an active form that inhibits DNA synthesis. Cell death most likely occurs as a result of blockade of DNA strand elongation. Gemcitabine appears to have activity against adenocarcinoma of the pancreas.

The purine analogs 6-MP and 6-TG (see Figure 42-10) also must undergo activation to form nucleotides, which then act as competitive inhibitors of several enzymes in purine synthesis pathways. The adenosine deaminase inhibitor pentostatin (2-deoxycoformycin) is highly active against hairy cell leukemia.

Antibiotics

Several antibiotics of microbial origin are very effective in treatment of certain tumors. These antibiotics include doxorubicin, daunorubicin, bleomycin, actinomycin D, and mitomycin. The anthracycline structures of daunorubicin and doxorubicin are shown in Figure 42-12.

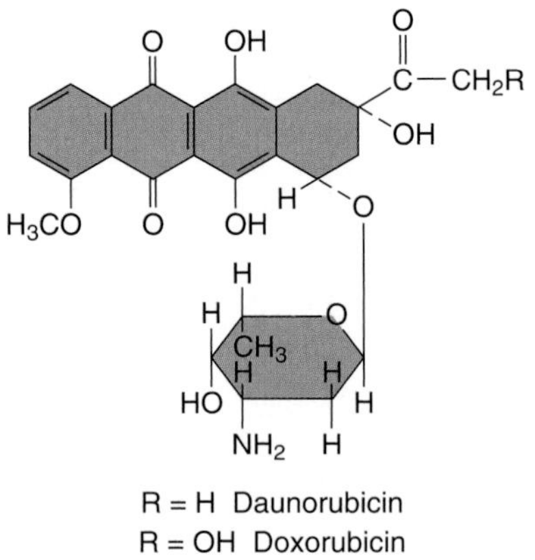

R = H Daunorubicin
R = OH Doxorubicin

Figure 42-12 Structures of daunorubicin and doxorubicin.

Bleomycin is a mixture of several basic glycopeptides, with one called A2 predominating. Among the common anticancer drugs, it has a unique mechanism of action in that it forms a tertiary complex with oxygen and iron to cause sequence-specific single- and double-stranded DNA cleavage. The double-stranded DNA cleavage that results is thought to be lethal. Doxorubicin and daunorubicin **intercalate** between the bases in double-stranded DNA, poison topoisomerase II, generate free radicals, and possibly disrupt the functioning of the cell membrane. It is generally believed that their poisoning of DNA **topoisomerase II** constitutes their major antitumor action (Fig. 42-13). DNA topoisomerase II is essential for DNA replication and catalyzes the uncoiling and breakage of both strands of double-stranded DNA to modify the number and the types of linkage twists. Doxorubicin and daunorubicin inhibit the enzyme by stabilizing a covalent complex of an enzyme-DNA intermediate, preventing the DNA breaks from rejoining and leading to cell death. Doxorubicin is the single most active agent against breast cancer; daunorubicin and idarubicin are frequently used to treat leukemias.

Actinomycin D also intercalates into DNA, thus blocking transcription, which is a major source of its antitumor activity. Actinomycin D also causes single-stranded DNA breaks, possibly through production of free radicals, and it prevents synthesis of RNA. Mitomycin undergoes chemical activation in cells, resulting in formation of a derivative that cross-links DNA by alkylation.

Plant alkaloids

The primary plant alkaloids, vincristine and vinblastine, bind avidly to **tubulin,** block microtubule polymerization, and disrupt mitotic spindle formation during mitosis at the M phase of the cell cycle (see Figs. 42-1 and 42-14). Cell death results from an inability to segregate chromosomes properly. Paclitaxel, which acts as a mitotic inhibitor, binds specifically and reversibly to tubulin, but unlike other antitubule drugs, it stabilizes microtubules in the polymerized form. Paclitaxel is active against solid tumors, including ovarian carcinomas. Etoposide is a semisynthetic derivative of podophyllotoxin that is prepared from the mandrake plant (mayapple). Etoposide and teniposide, a close analog, also inhibit topoisomerase II. Etoposide has significant activity against small-cell cancer of the lung and testicular carcinoma and is used in most first-line regimens for these diseases. Teniposide is active against acute leukemias in children.

Topotecan is a semisynthetic plant alkaloid that inhibits **topoisomerase I,** thereby leading to single-stranded DNA breaks. Topotecan is used for refractory ovarian cancer and may have activity against small-cell lung cancer.

Irinotecan, a camptothecin derivative, is a prodrug requiring hydrolysis to form an active metabolite that binds to the topoisomerase I-DNA complex. Topoisomerase I relieves strain in DNA by reversibly breaking single strands of the double-stranded DNA helix. Camptothecins are cytotoxic because they combine with the topoisomerase I-DNA complex, stabilizing the structurally protective single strand breaks induced by topo I and preventing their reconnection. This defect cannot be repaired by replication enzymes, and DNA synthesis is therefore prevented. Irinotecan is approved for treatment of metastatic colorectal carcinoma and may have activity in cervical, non-small cell lung and gastric cancer.

Hormonal agents

Steroids act by passing through the plasma membrane and binding to cytoplasmic receptors, which then enter the nucleus and interact with specific hormone-responsive elements on chromatin to induce synthesis of specific mRNAs. Translation of these mRNA species leads to formation of new proteins that alter physiological or biochemical reactions in a beneficial manner. Most of the proteins involved, however, have not yet been identified and characterized.

Hormonal drug treatment strategies for breast cancer have included:

- Attempts to eliminate estrogen production by the adrenals
- Blockade of estrogen receptors using **antiestrogen** drugs

It is not always possible to completely eliminate adrenal-produced estrogens in postmenopausal women,

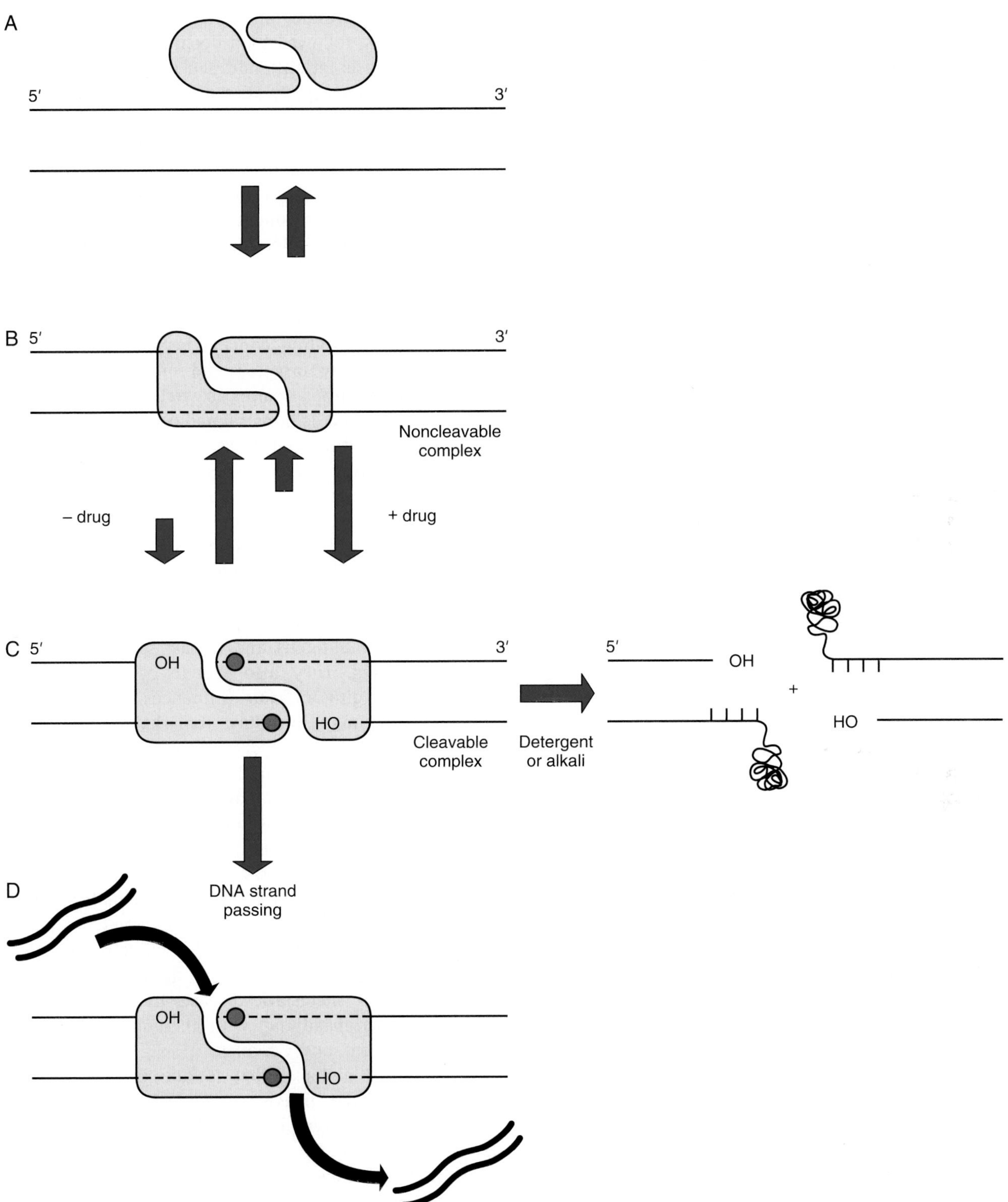

Figure 42-13 Mammalian DNA topoisomerase II mechanism and anticancer drug action. Mammalian DNA topoisomerase II forms two different types of protein-DNA complex that are in rapid equilibrium: the noncleavable complex **(B)** and the cleavable complex **(C)**. These complexes can be identified *in vitro* by the ability of detergent or alkali to separate DNA strands. The cleavable complex is transient but is stabilized by doxorubicin, daunorubicin, etoposide, and actinomycin D. In the absence of drug, DNA strand passage occurs, whereas drugs block DNA strand passage and DNA replication.

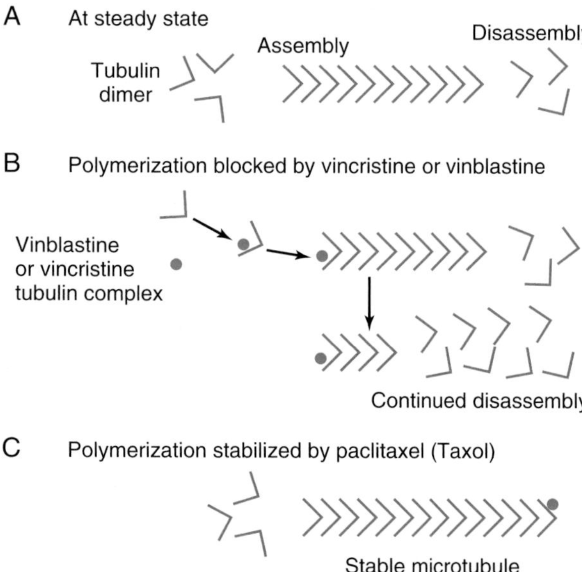

Figure 42-14 Microtubule dynamics in the presence of vincristine, vinblastine, or paclitaxel. A dynamic steady-state exists, with microtubule assembly occurring at one end and disassembly at the other **(A)**. Vincristine and vinblastine **(B)** bind to tubulin dimers and block polymerization, allowing disassembly to predominate. In contrast, paclitaxel **(C)** blocks disassembly, causing stable microtubules to form even in the absence of normally essential cofactors. Cells treated with any of these agents are blocked in mitosis.

however, because the adrenals secrete androstenedione, which undergoes peripheral conversion to an estrogen (estrone) or to testosterone. Estrone in turn is converted to estradiol.

About 70% of all postmenopausal patients whose breast tumors show the presence of estrogen receptors respond favorably to antiestrogen therapy, as opposed to only about 10% of those who show no receptors. Tamoxifen is the main antiestrogen used clinically, and it acts by binding to the estrogen receptors and blocking estrogen-dependent transcription in cells in the G_1 phase. By blocking the binding of estrogens, tamoxifen (see Chapter 35) may decrease estrogen stimulation of the production of transforming growth factor-α and secretion of associated proteins.

In metastatic prostate cancer, as in breast cancer, hormonal manipulations can produce objective responses. For prostate cancer this involves either orchiectomy or **pharmacological castration.** Testosterone concentrations can be reduced by the estrogen diethylstilbestrol or by suppression of the pituitary gonadotropic axis. Leuprolide and goserelin are analogs of gonadotropic-releasing hormones that inhibit release of gonadotropins and result in reduced testosterone concentrations. The two agents are available in depot form and can be given monthly. Both are agonists as well as antagonists of luteinizing hormone–releasing hormone. They produce an initial rise in gonadotropin concentrations, followed by a decline in 2 to 3 weeks.

Flutamide is an antiandrogen that inhibits androgen binding to receptors in the nucleus. Unlike other agents discussed, it increases concentrations of testosterone; however, the testosterone is ineffective because flutamide blocks its action. There has been recent interest in achieving total androgen blockade (both testis and adrenal) through concurrent use of flutamide and luteinizing hormone–releasing hormone analogs.

Biological therapy

Harnessing intrinsic biological systems for treatment of disease is an appealing concept because theoretically it could be highly targeted and of limited toxicity. "Biological therapy" attempts to wield our native host defense system and its humoral and cellular components as weapons to fight cancer as discussed more extensively in Chapter 53. Many of these weapons are intended to stimulate the immune system for destruction of malignant cells. The immune system involves the action of many different cell types acting in concert, particularly lymphocytes, which can be classified as either B, T, or null cells. These cells can secrete proteins including antibodies, which possess unique affinity for their conjugate antigens and impart specificity to the immune system. They also secrete cytokines, which have wide-ranging cellular influences. Utilization of these systems may introduce remarkable therapeutic target specificity at the risk of induction of autoimmunity and unique toxicities. Agents currently in use include cytokines, monoclonal antibodies, and vaccines.

Interleukin 2 (IL-2) is one of a family of soluble glycoprotein agents that is involved in direct communication between leukocytes. IL-2 is produced by activated T lymphocytes and is a growth factor for T cells. Recombinant IL-2 therapy as a single agent has activity in treatment of melanoma and renal cell carcinoma, producing durable resolution of all disease in 6% to 7% of patients with metastatic disease. IL-2 is also being investigated as an adjunct with chemotherapy, monoclonal antibodies, and vaccines.

Interferon alpha (IFNα) is one of a family of glycoproteins, the interferons, which are made by macrophages and lymphocytes that have been stimulated by mitogens, antigens, or RNA or infected by a virus. Interferons also express a wide variety of biologic activities, often making it difficult to determine which ones might be operant in a particular context. They modulate immune responses, augmenting T-cell and NK cell-mediated cytotoxicity; participate in the regulation of cellular differentiation and antigenic expression; possess anti-viral activity, hence their clinical use against hepatitis; express anti-angiogenic activity; and can interfere directly with cell proliferation. Interferon-α has clinical activity in the treatment of hairy cell leukemia, chronic myelogenous leukemia, indolent lymphoma, multiple myeloma, Kaposi's sarcoma, superficial bladder carcinoma, renal cell carcinoma, and melanoma. Benefit from adjuvant therapy with high-dose interferon-α after resection of high-risk cutaneous melanoma remains controversial.

Antibodies are products of B cells produced as a result of exposure to specific stimulating agents or antigens. Technological advances, including development of hybridoma methodologies, have allowed production of large quantities of pure antibodies specific for individual epitopes. These can be employed as an informer, identifying malignant cells as targets for attack by antibody-dependent cell-mediated cytotoxicity (ADCC). Bi-specific antibodies simultaneously and specifically target a tumor cell antigen and "trigger" molecules on neighboring effector cells, inducing cytotoxicity. Antibodies have been constructed to target and then block selected growth factor receptors and affect cellular growth. Cetuximab is an example of an antibody directed against the epidermal growth factor receptor (EGFR). Antibodies may also be used as the missile of biological "smart bombs" carrying a radiopharmaceutical or biologic toxin warhead to a specific target.

Rituximab is a chimeric IgG_1 kappa monoclonal antibody raised against the CD20 antigen, constructed with a murine light- and heavy-chain variable region and a human constant region sequence. CD20 is a transmembrane protein expressed by most B cells at various stages of development and by malignant B lymphocytes. It is found on more than 90% of B cell non-Hodgkin lymphomas but, importantly, is not expressed by hematopoietic stem cells or other normal tissues. Rituximab binds to B lymphocytes following IV administration; therefore serum concentrations vary inversely with tumor burden. Complement-dependent cytotoxicity and ADCC are both mechanisms through which this agent may cause target cell lysis. Rituximab is used in the treatment of indolent low-grade non-Hodgkin's lymphoma, where it may be used as monotherapy and in combination with CHOP chemotherapy (cyclophosphamide, doxorubicin, vincristine, and prednisone) as treatment for CD20-positive diffuse large B-cell non-Hodgkin's lymphoma. Rituximab is a component of a combination regimen employing ibritumomab tiuxetan, which will be described further and is being evaluated in the treatment of chronic lymphocytic leukemia, thrombocytopenic purpura, and Waldenström's macroglobulinemia.

I^{131} tositumomab is composed of a monoclonal murine anti-CD20 antibody (tositumomab) linked to I^{131}, which is both a beta and gamma emitter. This drug may induce apoptosis, incite complement-dependent cytotoxicity or ADCC, and can cause cell death from radiation. Prior to administration, thyroprotection is provided with potassium iodide, then unlabeled tositumomab is administered to saturate non-tumor sites. A test dose of I^{131} is given next to calculate the appropriate therapeutic dose based on the rate of clearance, terminal half-life, and volume of distribution. In patients with a high tumor burden, splenomegaly, or bone marrow involvement, clearance is faster and the volume of distribution is larger. I^{131} is excreted in the urine. This drug is not appropriate as initial therapy, as resultant cytopenias may eliminate other potential effective therapies. However, tositumomab is efficacious when administered as a single-course treatment in patients with relapsed, CD20-positive, follicular non-Hodgkin's lymphoma, with or without transformation, who are refractory to rituximab. Radiotherapeutic dosimetry must be appropriately pursued or profound and durable toxicity may result.

Y^{90} Ibritumomab tiuxetan is composed of ibritumomab, a murine anti-CD20 monoclonal antibody related to rituximab, linked to a moiety, tiuxetan, designed to chelate a radioisotope. Indium-111 is attached, creating an agent that can be used for imaging or yttrium-90 to create an agent to be used therapeutically. An initial rituximab infusion is given to clear peripheral B cells prior to treatment to permit more effective targeting, since Y^{90}-ibritumomab tiuxetan is cleared from plasma mainly by cellular or tumor binding with minimal urinary and no fecal excretion. Although there is no correlation between the pharmacokinetics of Y^{90} and severity of hematologic toxicity, the extent of baseline bone marrow involvement and level of the platelet count accurately predict hematotoxicity and indicate necessary dose adjustments when taken into account with weight. This agent is used for patients with relapsed or refractory low-grade, follicular, or transformed B-cell non-Hodgkin's lymphoma, including patients with rituximab refractory follicular non-Hodgkin's lymphoma. Further study, however, is needed to establish the role of this agent in various therapeutic regimens and to clarify its effectiveness relative to that of tositumomab.

Gemtuzumab ozogamicin is a recombinant humanized monoclonal antibody against CD33 designed to deliver calicheamicin, a chemotherapeutic, to the myeloid cell surface, where the chemotherapeutic agent can be internalized by the cell and cause cytotoxicity. Treatment with gemtuzumab ozogamicin is indicated for patients who are 60 years of age or older with no other alternatives for therapy who suffer from CD33-positive acute myeloid leukemia in first relapse.

Others

L-Asparaginase is administered to hydrolyze asparagine, required for growth in higher amounts by tumor cells than by normal cells. Depletion of asparagine shuts off protein and eventually nucleic acid synthesis. This approach is selective for neoplastic cells devoid of asparagine synthetase that are unable to synthesize the essential asparagine.

Hydroxyurea inhibits ribonucleotide reductase, which reduces ribonucleoside diphosphates to the deoxyribonucleotides required for DNA synthesis. It presumably complexes with the non-heme iron required by the enzyme for activity and is an S phase–specific agent.

The mechanism of action of arsenic trioxide remains unclear, although the cellular changes it induces suggest that it causes apoptosis. Arsenic trioxide is metabolized by arsenate reductase to trivalent arsenic, which undergoes methylation predominantly within the liver. Trivalent arsenic is excreted in the urine. Arsenic accumulates mainly in liver, kidney, heart, lung, hair, and nails and is approved for therapy of anthracycline-resistant acute promyelocytic leukemia characterized by the presence of specific markers. Arsenic trioxide also appears to have activity in multiple myeloma.

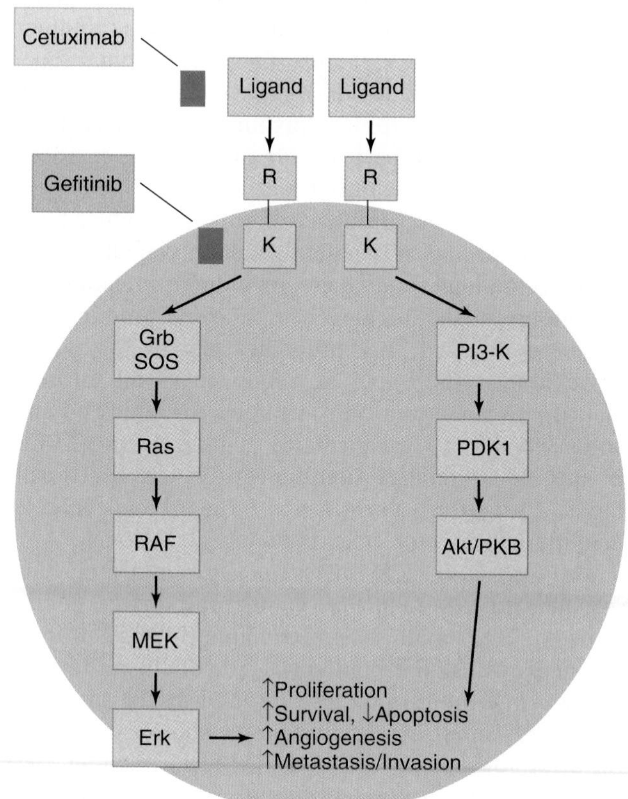

Figure 42-15 The EGFR family is a group of structurally similar growth factor receptors with tyrosine kinase activity *(K)*, which play a critical role in regulating cell cycle progression and metastasis. Upon stimulation by ligands including EGF, transforming growth factor, as well as mitogenic signals, the receptor *(R)* dimerizes and the intracellular tyrosine kinase is activated which transmits the pro-growth signal to the effector molecules as shown. The EGFR pathway can be inhibited either immunologically with the monoclonal antibody cetuximab or pharmacologically by inhibiting the tyrosine kinase ATP binding site as shown with gefitinib. Over-expression of EGFR is frequent in non–small cell lung cancers as well as head and neck cancers.

Growth factor receptors: anti-EGFR therapy

The EGFR is present on a variety of solid tumors including non-small cell lung cancer, head and neck cancer, and malignant gliomas. EGFR expression correlates with poor clinical outcome and resistance to cytotoxic agents. The EGFR receptor consists of an extracellular ligand binding domain, a hydrophobic transmembrane domain, and an intracellular domain with tyrosine kinase activity. Upon stimulation by ligand the EGFR receptor dimerizes, which initiates an intracellular pro-survival signaling cascade resulting in increased cell proliferation, metastasis, and decreased apoptosis (Fig. 42-15). The EGFR pathway can be inhibited by either blocking the extracellular domain with monoclonal antibodies or by small molecule tyrosine kinase inhibitors that block ATP binding and inhibit kinase activity.

Trastuzumab is a recombinant DNA-derived humanized monoclonal antibody that selectively binds with high affinity to the extracellular domain of the human EGFR2 protein Her2. The Her2 (or c-erbB2) protooncogene encodes a transmembrane receptor protein structurally related to the EGFR. Trastuzumab inhibits the proliferation of human tumor cells that overexpress Her2 and is approved for treatment of patients with metastatic breast cancer. As a single agent, it is indicated for treatment of patients with metastatic breast cancer whose tumors overexpress the Her2 protein and who have received one or more chemotherapy regimens for metastatic disease. It is also indicated for treatment of patients with metastatic breast cancer who are chemotherapy naive and whose tumors overexpress the HER2 protein in combination with paclitaxel.

Cetuximab is the first monoclonal antibody directed against the EGFR to be approved for treatment of colorectal cancer, either alone or in combination with irinotecan. Cetuximab is a genetically engineered version of a mouse antibody that contains both human and mouse components targeting EGFRs.

Gefitinib, an orally available small molecule tyrosine kinase inhibitor, was approved as third line treatment for non-small cell lung cancer. This was based on a 10% objective response rate and an improvement in quality of life. Several other small molecule tyrosine kinase inhibitors as well as monoclonal antibodies directed against the EGFR are in late stage clinical trials.

Inhibitors of intracellular signaling

Anti-Abl protein kinase inhibitors Imatinib is an orally available inhibitor of the Abl group of tyrosine kinases whose activity is unregulated in chronic myelogenous leukemia. The constitutively active Bcr-Abl oncoprotein results from the chromosomal translocation known as the Philadelphia chromosome, which is found in 95% of patients with chronic myelogenous leukemia. Imatinib competitively inhibits the Bcr-Abl kinase by binding to the ATP binding domain of the inactive conformation of c-Abl. Imatinib has revolutionized the treatment of chronic myelogenous leukemia by producing complete remissions in the vast majority of patients with Philadelphia-positive chronic myelogenous leukemia. Despite the success of imatinib, mutations in the Bcr-Abl kinase domain occur that lead to resistance. Imatinib also produces responses in an unusual tumor known as gastrointestinal stromal cell tumor. This tumor is known to contain a c-kit protooncogene mutation that results in increased tyrosine kinase activity.

Farnesyl transferase inhibitors Members of the Ras gene family signal transduction pathway have been implicated in several malignancies. Ras exists in an inactive GDP bound form and an active GTP bound form. Oncogenic mutations result in rendering the p21Ras GTP form insensitive to hydrolysis. For Ras to be membrane associated and active following synthesis, it requires posttranslational modification at its carboxy-terminal, requiring farnesylation of a sulfur residue. Farnesyltransferase inhibitors have shown impressive *in vivo* activity in inhibiting cellular growth and inducing apoptosis, although none are yet approved for clinical use.

Proteosome inhibitors The proteosome is a large multiprotein complex present in both the cytoplasm and nucleus of all eukaryotic cells. The 26S proteosome is a primary component of the protein degradation pathway of cells. Targeted degradation of proteins via the proteosome is key to many cellular processes including cell cycle progression and apoptosis. Proteins that are targeted for degradation are first marked with a polyubiquitin chain on specific lysine residues. The basis for proteosome inhibition as an anti-neoplastic strategy is uncertain. However, inhibition of proteosome degradation by such agents as bortezomib has been shown to be beneficial. Bortezomib is indicated for treatment of refractory multiple myeloma.

Angiogenesis inhibitors Bevacizumab is a recombinant humanized monoclonal antibody that binds to and inhibits the biologic activity of human vascular endothelial growth factor, inhibiting stimulation of new blood vessel formation. Tumor growth is slowed since a decreased blood supply results in decreased oxygen and other nutrients needed for growth. Bevacizumab is approved for the first-line treatment of metastatic colorectal cancer.

Mechanisms of resistance

Unfortunately, some patients initially respond favorably to antitumor drugs, but later the tumor may return and the same drugs may be ineffective. In other patients a drug protocol may show few positive results, even though the same protocol has proved beneficial in others. These situations are typical of resistance to antitumor drugs.

In resistant subjects, the reduced effectiveness can often be attributed to a decreased intracellular concentration of drug, repair of drug-induced damage, or a modification of drug targets. Increased expression of proteins that block the energy-dependent process of apoptosis, including oncogenes such as *bcl*2, can also cause resistance to many agents. Several mechanisms account for these differences, as indicated in Box 42-1.

Box 42-1 Possible mechanisms for the development of resistance to antineoplastic agents

Antineoplastic agent

Decreased uptake of active agent into cancer cell
Failure of agent to be metabolized to a chemical species capable of producing a cytotoxic effect
Enhanced conversion of agent to inactive metabolite
Increase in transport of agent from the cancer cell

Cancer cell (DNA, target enzyme, or other macromolecule)

Repair of drug-induced DNA damage
Gene amplification or increased gene transcription leading to greater amount of target enzyme within the cancer cell
Reduced ability of target enzyme to bind agent
Increase in concentration of sulfhydryl scavengers
Altered concentrations of target protein
Increased expression of antiapoptotic genes, such as *bcl2*

Decreased drug uptake by cells is one mechanism of resistance, especially to drugs such as MTX that require carrier proteins for transmembrane transport. Actinomycin D resistance also results from decreased uptake. Cyclophosphamide requires metabolic activation, and in the absence of this pathway, tumor cells can be resistant. Enhanced conversion of the active agent to an inactive metabolite is a third mechanism. For example, increased activity of aldehyde dehydrogenase leads to enhanced metabolism of cyclophosphamide and drug resistance.

Enhanced cellular efflux of drug is a fourth mechanism. Mammalian cells possess a large phosphoglycoprotein called ***P*-glycoprotein** that acts as an ATP-driven transmembrane transport protein. This *P*-glycoprotein functions to transport hydrophobic compounds with aromatic and basic properties out of the cell. Doxorubicin, daunorubicin, actinomycin D, etoposide, teniposide, vincristine, and vinblastine are all antitumor drugs to which cells possessing elevated concentrations of the multidrug-resistant *P*-glycoprotein are resistant. Intracellular drug concentrations are decreased because of energy-dependent removal by *P*-glycoprotein. Efforts are under way to develop compounds that can block the action of the *P*-glycoprotein pumps and circumvent multidrug resistance. Verapamil and other calcium-channel blockers block the *P*-glycoprotein pump, but only at unacceptably high doses. Analogs of cyclosporin that lack immunosuppressive properties may be more promising.

Bleomycin resistance exemplifies a fifth mechanism of resistance, in which cells rapidly repair the DNA breaks caused by this drug. DNA repair mechanisms may also be a source of resistance to other DNA-directed antitumor drugs. Intracellular targets are a sixth mechanism, and MTX is an example. In one example, cells have increased intracellular concentrations of dihydrofolate reductase as a result of gene amplification. A seventh mechanism is the presence of an altered enzyme that is still enzymatically active but has a lower binding affinity for MTX. For example, MTX is not conjugated with polyglutamates and is therefore not retained within the tumor cell. A higher unconjugated MTX concentration is required to inhibit dihydrofolate reductase. Thus the enzyme is no longer inhibited to the same degree by the usual concentration of MTX.

Sulfhydryl compounds, including glutathione and metallothioneins, act as cellular protective groups, particularly against alkylating agents. Increased concentrations of such protective compounds scavenge highly reactive compounds and represent the eighth mechanism of resistance. In a ninth mechanism, cells can decrease the available target to produce a resistant phenotype. For example, a decrease in topoisomerase II activity leads to resistance to etoposide and teniposide. Unfortunately, cancer cells often possess multiple pathways for drug resistance that may make therapeutic efforts to block one or two pathways ineffective clinically in reversing resistance.

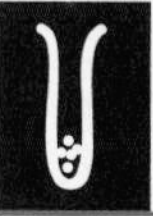

Pharmacokinetics

Numerous measurements have been performed to determine the plasma concentration decay curves for antitumor drugs. A standard compartment model is used to explain the plasma concentration versus time decay curves. It is a sum of one to three exponentials and is useful in providing guidance in planning dosing schemes that maximize drug tumor contact but minimize drug tissue contact. For antitumor agents that disappear rapidly from the plasma, continuous IV infusion rather than bolus injection often is needed to obtain a high enough concentration to achieve a therapeutic effect. The modes of administration and disposition of several antineoplastic agents are listed in Table 42-1.

6-MP undergoes enzyme-catalyzed metabolism, with xanthine oxidase as the principal enzyme. Allopurinol, a drug used in the treatment of gout, also is metabolized by the same enzyme, and a drug interaction occurs if the two compounds are given concurrently. Allopurinol also lengthens cyclophosphamide's half-life and increases myelotoxicity, possibly resulting from the decreased renal elimination of cyclophosphamide metabolites. MTX and weak organic acids such as nonsteroidal antiinflammatory agents compete for plasma binding and for renal tubular excretion, and significant increases in MTX concentrations have been noted in patients receiving these drugs.

Rituximab pharmacokinetics appear to vary with dose, but mean serum half-life following intravenous infusion of a conventional dose is about 76 hours.

The other drugs that undergo metabolism also may show interactions during multiple-drug antitumor dosing, resulting in prolonged plasma concentrations of the involved drugs.

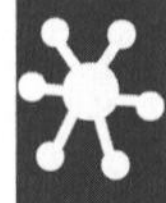

Relation of mechanisms of action to clinical response

Most antineoplastic drugs are used in multiple-agent protocols in which the cytolytic effects of the different agents interact in a complex manner. The clinical

Table 42-1 Pharmacokinetic parameters for selected drugs

Drug	Administration	Disposition	Notes
Nitrogen mustard	IV	M	—
Melphalan	Oral	M	—
Cyclophosphamide	IV, oral	M	—
Nitrosoureas	IV	M	Lipid soluble, crosses blood-brain barrier
Cisplatin	IV	R	90% protein bound
Carboplatin	IV	R	3-6 hr half-life
Oxaliplatin	Oral	R	Rapidly protein bound; ultrafilterable agent is active
Busulfan	IV, oral	M	Few-minute half-life
Methotrexate	IV	R	50%-60% plasma protein bound
Edatrexate	IV	M, R	Renal clearance 7%-55%
5-Fluorouracil	IV	M	—
Cytarabine	IV	M	Few-minute half-life
6-MP and 6-TG	Oral	M*	Large first-pass effect (10-minute half-life)
Doxorubicin	IV	M	—
Daunorubicin	IV	M	—
Bleomycin	IV	R (50%), M	—
Arsenic trioxide	IV	R	No pharmacokinetic data
Asparaginase	IV, IM	—	—
Vincristine	IV	M, B	Minimal entry into CSF
Vinblastine	IV	B	—
Etoposide	IV, oral	R (main), M, B	97% plasma protein bound
Irinotecan	IV	—	6-12 hr half-life; disposition not fully known
Tamoxifen	Oral	M (main)	Enterohepatic cycling
Interferon-α	IV, SC	R	—
Interleukin 2	IV, SC	R	Rapid clearance by renal excretion and metabolism

M, Metabolized; *R*, renal excretion; *B*, biliary excretion.
*See text for drug interaction.

use of combination chemotherapy is discussed in Chapter 43.

Side effects, clinical problems, and toxicity

Typical undesirable side effects of many anti-tumor drugs are listed in Table 42-2. Many of these side effects reflect effects of the drug on populations of rapidly proliferating normal cells. Nausea and vomiting are quite common and can be attributable to effects on both cycling and noncycling cells. Strategies for ameliorating these effects are available (see Chapter 43).

Combinations of different drugs are generally designed on the basis of the nonoverlapping, dose-limiting toxicities such as those listed in the Clinical Problems box. These toxicities are unrelated to rapidly proliferating populations of normal cells.

Nephrotoxicity, peripheral neuropathy, and ototoxicity remain the major side effects of cisplatin, although the severity of the renal toxicity can be reduced through hydration of the patient and administration of mannitol (see Chapter 13). Renal damage arises from the toxic effects of cisplatin on renal tubules, resulting in decreased glomerular filtration rates and increased reabsorption. Nephrotoxicity does not develop until a week or two after treatment is begun and may be worsened if nephrotoxic agents are

Table 42-2 Typical undesirable side effects of antineoplastic drugs in humans*

Tissue	Undesirable Effects
Bone marrow	Leukopenia and resulting infections Immunosuppression Thrombocytopenia Anemia
GI tract	Oral or intestinal ulceration Diarrhea
Hair follicles	Alopecia
Gonads	Menstrual irregularities, including premature menarche; impaired spermatogenesis
Wounds	Impaired healing
Fetus	Teratogenesis (especially during first trimester)

*Many of these effects are caused by drug action on nontumor cells that usually are growing (i.e., cycling).

CLINICAL PROBLEMS

Arsenic trioxide: Cytopenia, nausea, vomiting, diarrhea, hepatotoxicity, prolongation of the QT interval, cardiac arrhythmias including torsades de pointes and complete heart block, acute promyelocytic leukemia differentiation syndrome and sudden death
Bleomycin: Pulmonary fibrosis ("bleomycin lung")
Busulfan: Pulmonary fibrosis ("busulfan lung")
Doxorubicin: Cardiotoxicity
Edatrexate: Stomatitis, nausea, vomiting, diarrhea, hepatotoxicity, pulmonary toxicity and rash
Cisplatin: Nephrotoxicity and peripheral neuropathy
Oxaliplatin: Peripheral neuropathy, hypersensitivity, pulmonary fibrosis (rare) and abdominal pain
Cyclophosphamide: Hemorrhagic cystitis
Vincristine: Neurotoxicity
Interferon α: Flu-like symptoms; cytopenias; anorexia and weight loss; fatigue; depression; and intensification or induction of autoimmune and inflammatory disorders
Interleukin 2: Flu-like symptoms; cytopenias; hypotension; capillary leak syndrome; acute kidney failure; adult respiratory distress syndrome; intensification or induction of autoimmune and inflammatory disorders
Irinotecan: Diarrhea (early and late), nausea and vomiting, cholinergic syndrome, myelosuppression
Cytarabine: Cerebral damage

co-administered—for example, if an aminoglycoside is coadministered for treatment of an infection. Cisplatin-induced neuropathy occurs mainly in large sensory fibers and results in numbness and tingling, followed by loss of a sense of joint position and a disabling sensory ataxia. The toxicity is reversed upon discontinuation of the drug, but it may take a year or longer for it to resolve. Nephrotoxicity is more common in patients who receive a bolus injection of cisplatin. Fractionating the dose over several days has been observed to reduce the intensity of this toxicity. Cisplatin neuropathy is a more recently observed cumulative dose-limiting side effect. Carboplatin causes less neurotoxicity and nephrotoxicity but more pronounced myelosuppression than cisplatin.

Bleomycin and busulfan both result in drug-induced pulmonary fibrosis, but this side effect is dose limited. Fifty percent or more of bleomycin is excreted in the urine unchanged. The dose should be reduced when creatinine clearance drops below 30 ml/min (from a standard value of 120 ml/min). Bleomycin accumulates in the lungs and skin, where bleomycin hydrolase (which in other tissues actively metabolizes the drug) is present at very low activity. Continued elevated concentrations of bleomycin lead to the recruitment of lymphocytes and polymorphonuclear leukocytes in bronchoalveolar fluids. It is not known how this leads to fibrosis. Hypersensitivity pneumonitis also is observed in those who receive bleomycin therapy but is less frequent in those who receive MTX, mitomycin C, nitrosoureas, and alkylating agents.

The major side effects of Ara-C are myelosuppression and dose-limiting cerebellar damage. Ocular toxicity also has occasionally been associated with higher doses. Nausea and vomiting are seen in almost all patients receiving higher doses of Ara-C administered to overcome drug transport resistance.

Doxorubicin and daunorubicin are associated with the long-term, dose-limiting side effect of myocardial failure. Although the acute cardiac effects of hypotension, tachycardia, and dysrhythmias are usually not clinically significant, long-term effects leading to congestive heart failure can be life-threatening and necessitate discontinuance of drug therapy. The long-term effects appear after weeks to months of therapy and have been observed up to several years after the discontinuance of treatment especially in pediatric cancer patients. Thirty-five percent of patients who receive a cumulative dose of more than 600 mg/m^2 experience congestive heart failure refractory to medical management. Bone marrow and gastrointestinal toxicity vary with the plasma concentrations of doxorubicin.

Cyclophosphamide, which is metabolized to an active compound and other reactive metabolites (see Fig. 42-6), occasionally causes hemorrhagic cystitis. The risk of this can be largely eliminated through vigorous hydration of patients during treatment. As little as a single IV dose of cyclophosphamide can produce cystitis. MESNA is used as a protectant in patients receiving very high doses of IV cyclophosphamide. The cystitis appears to be caused by acrolein, which is produced as a toxic byproduct of the metabolism of cyclophosphamide. This side effect is not age or sex related and leads to a 9 to 45 times greater risk of bladder cancer. The risk of bladder cancer is not as great in those given cyclophosphamide orally as opposed to IV.

The main side effect of MTX, vinblastine, etoposide, and 5-FU is bone marrow suppression. Vinca alkaloids such as vincristine can cause peripheral neuropathy, but this is a less frequent problem with etoposide (or vinblastine) therapy.

Toxicities of IL-2, although extensive and potentially severe, are manageable and include symptoms unlike those of chemotherapy. Patients routinely develop features of inflammatory disease including flu-like symptoms with fever, chills, and myalgias; capillary leak syndrome with attendant hypotension, acute kidney failure, adult respiratory distress syndrome and rarely respiratory failure requiring intubation; diarrhea, nausea, and emesis; anorexia; confusion and seizures; sepsis; and intensification or induction of autoimmune and inflammatory disorders.

Interferon alpha toxicities are multiple and include features of inflammatory disease like those of IL-2: flu-like symptoms such as fever, chills, fatigue, and myalgia; GI toxicities such as anorexia, nausea, vomiting, and weight loss; depression; hepatotoxicity; neutropenia and thrombocytopenia; autoimmune diseases; renal toxicity; and thyroid abnormalities induced by autoimmunity.

Since rituximab is a protein, severe hypersensitivity reactions may occur. Infusion reactions may include life-threatening cardiac arrhythmias and angina. A less-severe infusion-related complex of symptoms often includes fever, chills, hypotension, nausea, urticaria, and bronchospasm. These symptoms may be attenuated by reducing the infusion rate. Tumor lysis syndrome, hemolytic anemia, and severe mucocutaneous reactions (i.e., Stevens-Johnson syndrome) have also been reported.

Adverse effects of I^{131} tositumomab are similar to those seen with rituximab, including hypersensitivity reactions and anaphylaxis; fever, rigors, hypotension, dyspnea, bronchospasm, nausea, vomiting, abdominal pain, and diarrhea. Development of human anti-murine antibodies have been reported with the use of tositumomab as with most other murine antibodies. The addition of I^{131} adds the potential for additional radiation-induced toxicities of hypothyroidism, prolonged and severe cytopenias and associated infection and bleeding, myelodysplastic syndrome, and secondary malignancies including acute leukemia. This drug is not appropriate as initial therapy, as resultant cytopenias may eliminate other potentially effective therapies.

Gemtuzumab ozogamicin causes the conventional side effects of monoclonal antibodies including infusion-related reactions, hypersensitivity reactions, hypotension, tumor lysis syndrome, and pulmonary events. Additionally this agent can cause serious and sometimes fatal hepatotoxicity, and because myeloid precursors may also be targeted, it may cause severe myelosuppression.

The most significant toxicities of trastuzumab include include cardiomyopathy, hypersensitivity reactions including anaphylaxis, infusion reactions, pulmonary events, and exacerbation of chemotherapy-induced neutropenia. Gefitinib's two most common side effects are skin rash and diarrhea. Toxicities of bortezomib include peripheral neuropathy and myelosuppression. The most common toxicities of bevacizumab are hypertension, fatigue, blood clots, diarrhea, neutropenia, headache, appetite loss, and mouth sores. Less common but more serious side effects include gastrointestinal perforations that may require surgery, impaired wound healing, and bleeding from the lungs or other organs.

Nearly all antineoplastic drugs have side effects that patients consider very objectionable.

New horizons

There have been enormous advances in our understanding of the molecular and cellular biology of cancer. As a result, a large number of new targets have become available, including targets associated with oncogenic kinases and phosphatases, growth factors, and growth factor receptors involved in signal transduction. Bioreductive alkylating agents and radiation sensitizers have become subjects of considerable interest as a result of the observation that malignant cells within the center of the tumor are hypoxic, and hypoxia is a cause of drug resistance. Compounds designed to affect angiogenesis and hormone receptors and agents targeted toward redox systems are also emerging as exciting new therapeutic approaches to cancer. Many currently available antineoplastic agents require IV administration, and considerable effort has been directed toward the development of orally active compounds that would permit patients to be treated outside of a hospital setting. Cancer vaccines and gene therapy continue to be actively investigated. The next 5 years may provide important clues concerning which of the aforementioned approaches are likely to yield effective new anticancer drugs.

TRADE NAMES

In addition to generic and fixed-combination preparations, the following trade-named materials are available in the United States.

Alkylating agents

Nitrogen mustards

- Chlorambucil (Leukeran)
- Cyclophosphamide (Cytoxan, Neosar)
- Ifosfamide (Ifex)
- Mechlorethamine (Mexate)
- Melphalan (Alkeran)

Nitrosoureas

- Carmustine (BCNU, BiCNU)
- Lomustine (CCNU, CeeNU)
- Streptozocin (Zanosar)

Others

- Busulfan (Myleran)
- Carboplatin (Paraplatin)
- Cisplatin (Platinol)
- Dacarbazine (DTIC-Dome)
- Oxaliplatin (Eloxatin)
- Procarbazine (Matulane)
- Temozolomide (Temodal)

Antimetabolites

Capecitabine (Xeloda)
Cytarabine (Cytosar-U)
Floxuridine (FUDR)
5-Fluorouracil (Efudex, Adrucil)
Gemcitabine (Gemzar)
6-Mercaptopurine (Purinethol)
Methotrexate (Mexate)
Pemetrexed (Alimta)
Pentostatin (Nipent)
Thioguanine (Thioguan tabloid)

Antibiotics

Bleomycin sulfate (Blenoxane)
Dactinomycin, actinomycin D (Cosmegen)
Daunorubicin (Cerubidine)
Doxorubicin (Adriamycin)
Mitomycin (Mutamycin)
Mitoxantrone (Novantrone)

Hormonal agents

Flutamide (Eulexin)
Goserelin (Zoladex)
Leuprolide (Lupron)
Prednisone (Deltasone)
Tamoxifen (Nolvadex)

Others

Arsenic trioxide (Trisenox)
Asparaginase (Elspar)
Hydroxyurea (Hycamtin)

Plant alkaloids

Etoposide (VePesid)
Irinotecan (Camptosar)
Paclitaxel (Taxol)
Teniposide (Vumon)
Topotecan (Hycamtin)
Vinblastine (Velban, Velsar)
Vincristine (Oncovin, Vincasar)

Antibodies

Bevacizumab (Avastin)
Cetuximab (Erbitux)
Gemtuzumab ozogamicin (Mylotarg)
Trastuzumab (Herceptin)
Y^{90} Ibritumomab tiuxetan (Zevalin IN111 or Y90)
Rituximab (Rituxan)
Tositumomab (Bexxar)

Kinase inhibitors

Gefitinib (Iressa)
Imatinib (Gleevec)

Recombinant proteins

Interferon α_{2b}, recombinant (Intron A)
Interferon α_{2a}, recombinant (Roferon-A)
Interleukin 2, aldesleukin (Proleukin)

Proteasome inhibitors

Bortezomib (Velcade)

FURTHER READING

Berdeja JG. Immunotherapy of lymphoma: update and review of the literature. *Curr Opin Oncol* 2003; 15:363-370.

Brunton VG, Workman P. Cell-signaling targets for antitumour drug statistics, 2004. *CA Cancer J Clin* 2004; 54:8-29.

Swanton C. Cell-cycle targeted therapies. *Lancet Oncol* 2004; 5(1):27-36.

Self-assessment questions

1. All of the following antineoplastic agents are antimetabolites *except:*

a. Cisplatin.
b. Methotrexate.
c. Cytarabine.
d. Thioguanine.

2. A 28-year-old man is being treated for testicular carcinoma, and severe and irreversible pulmonary fibrosis develops. Which of the following drugs are most likely responsible for causing this adverse effect?

a. Vinblastine
b. Cisplatin
c. Doxorubicin
d. Bleomycin

3. Most antineoplastic agents kill malignant cells by:

a. Zero-order kinetics.
b. First-order kinetics.
c. Hypoxic sensitization.
d. Enzyme inhibition.
e. Oncogene suppression.

4. All of the following anticancer drugs are thought to function by blocking topoisomerase II *except:*

a. Etoposide.
b. Doxorubicin.
c. Daunorubicin.
d. Mitomycin C.

5. Of the following drugs, which functions to block ribonucleotide reductase?

a. Bleomycin
b. Hydroxyurea
c. L-Asparaginase
d. Chlorambucil

6. Antimetabolites frequently act to kill cells in which phase of the cell cycle?

a. M phase (mitotic phase)
b. G_1 phase
c. S phase (DNA synthetic phase)
d. G_2 phase
e. Phase nonspecific

CHAPTER 43

Clinical effects of antineoplastic drugs

James M. Larner
William W. Grosh

Therapeutic overview

A growing number of tumor types now respond to treatment with anti-neoplastic drugs. The types of clinical response to chemotherapy in patients of various ages with advanced-stage tumors are listed in the Therapeutic Overview box.

Chemotherapy has been very effective in the management of **leukemias** and **lymphomas**, both in children and adults, such that most cases of leukemia in children are now curable. The success of treatment for adult leukemias is somewhat less, but complete remission in response to induction therapy is often achievable. On the other hand, only a small number of **solid tumors** respond completely to chemotherapy. Choriocarcinoma, Ewing's sarcoma, and testicular carcinoma are examples of solid tumors that can be cured with chemotherapy, even if they have metastasized.

It is of interest to compare the tumor types in which therapy has been aided greatly by antineoplastic drugs with the leading causes of cancer mortality (Fig. 43-1). Unfortunately, chemotherapy is only minimally effective in management of the most common forms of neoplastic diseases. Overall, carcinoma of the lung accounts for the greatest number of cancer deaths in men and women, and although chemotherapy can produce objective responses, it is not curative in this setting. Thus, despite progress, there is still a great need for more effective chemotherapy for the major neoplastic diseases.

Drug selection and problems

The nature of the problem

One of the difficulties in treating neoplastic diseases is that the tumor burden often is excessive by the time the diagnosis is made. This is shown in Figure 43-2, where the number of cells in a typical solid tumor is shown versus time, with 10^9 cells roughly equivalent to a volume of 1 cubic centimeter, and representing the minimum size tumor that can usually be detected. It takes approximately 30 doublings for a single cell to reach 10^9 cells. On the other hand, it takes only 10 additional doublings for 10^9 cells to reach a population of 10^{12} cells, which is no longer compatible with life. The significance of a large number of cells already established at the time of detection becomes readily evident, with 10^{12} to 10^{13} tumor cells leading to death. Thus, by the time a tumor is detected, only a small number of doublings are required before it is fatal. Of course, not all tumor cells are cycling, so no meaningful predictions about longevity can be made purely on the basis of doubling times. Also, **doubling times** of human tumors vary greatly. For acute lymphocytic leukemia, the doubling time during log-phase (first-order) growth is 3 to 4 days, whereas the doubling time for lung squamous cell carcinoma is about 90 days. Thus in roughly 100 days, two lymphocytic leukemia cells in theory could keep doubling and reach 10^9 cells. Such a situation is extremely difficult to treat only with drugs and is cited here to emphasize the difficulty of the therapeutic task using

THERAPEUTIC OVERVIEW

Cancers in which complete remissions to chemotherapy are common and cures are seen even in advanced disease*

Acute lymphocytic leukemia (adults and children)
Acute myelogenous leukemia
Hodgkin's disease (lymphoma)
Non-Hodgkin's lymphoma
Choriocarcinoma
Testicular cancer
Burkitt's lymphoma
Ewing's sarcoma
Wilms' tumor
Small-cell lung cancer
Ovarian cancer
Hairy cell leukemia

Cancers in which objective responses are seen but chemotherapy does not have curative potential in advanced disease

Multiple myeloma
Breast cancer
Head and neck cancer
Colorectal carcinomas
Chronic lymphocytic leukemia
Chronic myelogenous leukemia
Transitional cell carcinoma of bladder
Gastric adenocarcinomas
Cervical carcinomas
Medulloblastoma
Soft-tissue sarcoma
Neuroblastoma
Endometrial carcinomas
Insulinoma
Osteogenic sarcoma
Non–small cell lung cancer

Cancers in which only occasional objective responses to chemotherapy are seen

Melanoma
Renal tumor
Pancreatic carcinomas
Hepatocellular carcinoma
Prostate carcinomas (hormone nonresponsive)

*Depending on tumor type, complete remission may result in cure.

currently available diagnostic timetables. In addition, by the time a tumor is clinically detectable, it already has a well-developed vascular supply and the potential for metastasis and likely has already metastasized. Mathematical models suggest that it also has a high likelihood of being resistant to cytotoxic agents that function through the same pathways.

Primary versus adjuvant therapy

The objective of chemotherapy in an individual patient may be:

- **Curative,** to obtain complete remission (e.g., Hodgkin's disease).
- **Palliative,** to alleviate symptoms but with little expectation of complete remission (e.g., carcinoma of the esophagus, with chemotherapy performed to ease the dysphagia).
- **Adjuvant,** to improve the chances for a cure or prolong the period of disease-free survival when no detectable cancer is present but subclinical numbers of neoplastic cells are suspected (e.g., chemotherapy for breast cancer after surgical resection of all known tumor).

Selection of drug regimen

Although choriocarcinoma (gestational trophoblastic disease) and hairy cell leukemia are treated by using single drugs, nearly all other neoplasms are treated with **combinations** of drugs.

The choice of drugs and dosing schedule for multiple-drug therapy has been and remains largely empirical. There are continuing efforts to try to understand why some combinations are more effective than others for the management of certain tumor types. Despite this empirical approach, several guidelines are generally applicable when selecting drug combinations:

- Use drugs that show **activity** against the type of tumor being treated. The rationale is that only rarely will a compound that shows no activity alone have an effect when used in combination. Agents employed should also not be cross-resistant, thus expanding their anti-tumor activity.
- Use drugs that have minimal or no overlapping **toxicities.** Although this may broaden the range of undesirable side effects of the drug combination, the goal is to reduce the possibility of life-threatening side effects that act in concert. For this reason, the side effects of the drugs selected should be diverse and not centered on the same organ system.
- The **dosing schedule** for each drug should be optimal, and doses should be given at consistent times. In

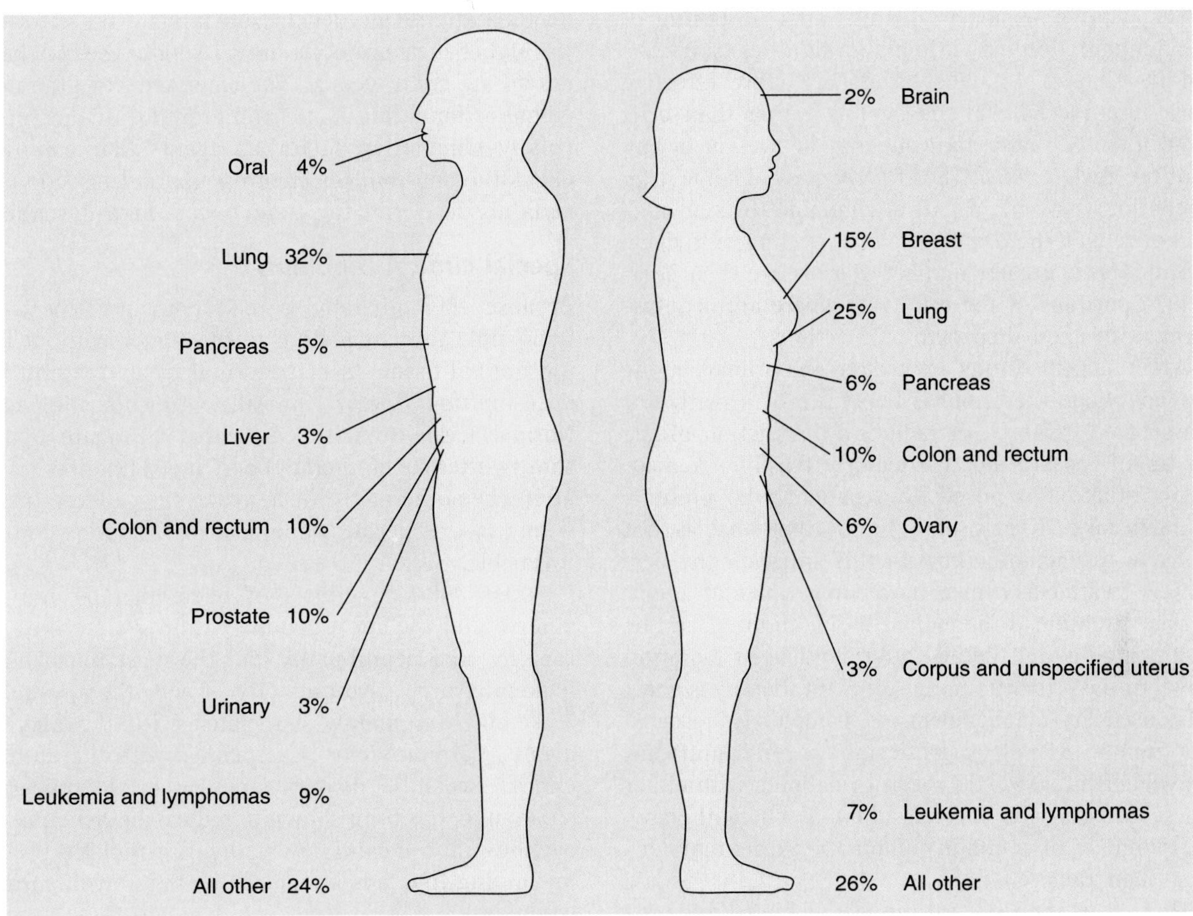

Figure 43-1 Estimated cancer deaths in the United States in 2004—percentage distribution of sites by sex. (Excludes basal and squamous cell skin cancers and carcinoma *in situ*, except bladder.) (Adapted from American Cancer Society: Cancer statistics, 2004. *CA Cancer J Clin* 2004; 54:1.)

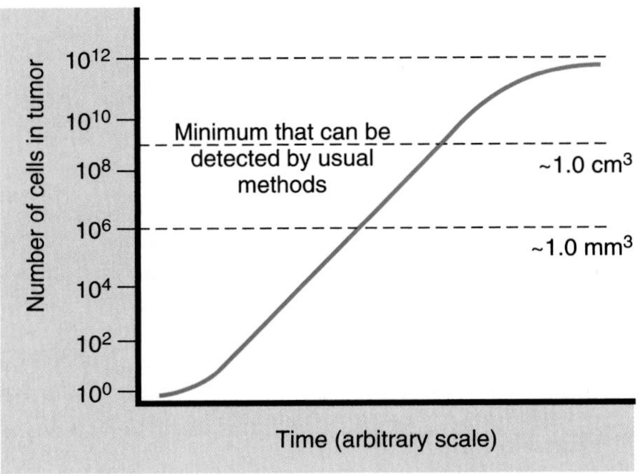

Figure 43-2 Typical tumor growth curve showing that roughly 10^9 cells are needed for the diagnosis usually to be made.

establishing the frequency of a dosing regimen, it is usual to allow sufficient time between dosage sequences to permit the most-sensitive tissues (often bone marrow) to recover.

Many sophisticated approaches have been used for selecting drugs and dosing schedules for combination chemotherapy, but the results have been disappointing. Some approaches have included drugs that have different mechanisms of action, in the hope that one mechanism would succeed where the others fail. Another goal of the multiple-mechanism approach has been the discovery of synergistic combinations. Several combinations–including sequential methotrexate-5-fluorouracil, doxorubicin-cyclophosphamide, and cisplatin-etoposide–have been found to be synergistic when tested against tumor cells cultured *in vitro*. A major problem of this approach, however, is that the observed *in vivo* clinical results often do not correlate with the *in vitro* data.

The relative sequence of drugs and the timing of drug administration may also play a significant role. As noted in Chapter 42, most drugs are more effective against tumor cells that are cycling rather than cells resting in the G_0 phase, but cells may be present in any part of the cycle *in vivo*. The effectiveness of some drug combinations may be in part attributable to their activation of cells in the G_0 phase to start cycling or to cycle more rapidly. A greater number of cells are then positioned in portions of the cell cycle where antineoplastic drugs can exert their cytotoxic actions.

Antineoplastic drugs are used as the primary mode of therapy when the tumor is known to be sensitive or when surgical removal or radiation destruction of the main tumor mass is not particularly feasible. A more difficult situation is posed by a patient who presents with metastatic disease of a tumor type that is not responsive to chemotherapy. In this situation the best option is treatment with a newer experimental agent. An easier situation is the patient in whom drugs can be used as an adjuvant therapy after surgical or radiation removal of the primary tumor. Adjuvant therapy is commonly used in management of completely resected breast cancer as well as colorectal cancer. Significant improvement in survival is seen in patients with either of these tumors who receive adjuvant chemotherapy. Some examples of common combination drug regimens are given in Table 43-1.

There is a trend toward the use of **high-dose** protocols using drugs other than methotrexate to try to push higher concentrations of drug into the tumor cells. Drugs that are rapidly degraded in plasma (e.g., cytarabine) are also being used for this. In most cases the detailed studies needed to substantiate the efficacy of the higher-dose protocols are missing or the conclusions drawn are controversial. The emergence of granulocyte colony–stimulating factor and granulocyte macrophage colony–stimulating factor as agents that can reduce chemotherapy-induced neutropenia and infections will certainly accelerate this trend toward high-dose therapy.

Special clinical problems

Because chemotherapy is a systemic treatment, it is impossible to deliver drug to the tumor without injuring normal tissue. In fact, **normal tissue toxicity** is the dose-limiting factor for all antineoplastic agents. Normal tissue toxicity can either be acute (with or shortly after chemotherapy) or delayed (months to years after chemotherapy). Most acute side effects (nausea, vomiting, alopecia, bone marrow suppression) are reversible.

Delayed side effects of chemotherapy are quite diverse and include pulmonary fibrosis, sterility, neuropathy, and nephropathy, but the most important are **leukemia** and **cardiotoxicity.** Chemotherapy-induced leukemias are mainly associated with the alkylating agents. Cardiotoxicity is associated with the anthracyclines. Recently dexrazoxane, a bisdioxopiperazine compound, has been shown to reduce the risk of anthracycline-induced cardiomyopathy. It is thought to act by preventing free radical damage by the iron-doxorubicin complex.

Nausea and **vomiting** can be expected in a high fraction of patients receiving anti-neoplastic drugs. Some of the drugs most and least likely to trigger emesis are listed in Box 43-1. Although the clinical manage-

Table 43-1 Current combination drug regimens

Terminology	Cancer	Drugs
MOPP	Hodgkin's	Mechlorethamine, vincristine, procarbazine, prednisone
ABVD	Hodgkin's	Doxorubicin, bleomycin, vinblastine, dacarbazine
CMF	Breast	Cyclophosphamide, methotrexate, 5-fluorouracil
CAF	Breast	Cyclophosphamide, doxorubicin, 5-fluorouracil
—	Acute lymphocytic leukemia	Vincristine, prednisone, asparaginase, daunorubicin
—	Acute myelogenous leukemia	Cytarabine, plus mitoxantrone or idarubicin or daunorubicin
—	Chronic myelogenous leukemia	Hydroxyurea, interferon
—	Wilms'	Actinomycin D, vincristine, doxorubicin
—	Small cell (lung)	Etoposide-cisplatin
—	Non–small cell (lung)	Cisplatin, etoposide
PVC	Anaplastic oligodendrogliomas	Procarbazine, vincristine, CCNU
BEP	Germ cell cancers	Bleomycin, etoposide, cisplatin
—	Ovary	Paclitaxel, carboplatin
CHOP	Lymphoma	Cyclophosphamide, doxorubicin, vincristine, prednisone
—	Head and neck	5-Fluorouracil, cisplatin
—	Colon/rectum	5-Fluorouracil, leucovorin

ment of nausea and vomiting can become a serious problem, the serotonin receptor antagonists ondansetron and granisetron used as antiemetics greatly decrease the severity and incidence of the problem. In addition, oral phenothiazine, dexamethasone, butyrophenone, metoclopramide, and diphenydramine are useful as antiemetics, and sedation with benzodiazepines is also possible.

Targeted therapies and biological response modifiers

Targeted therapies are becoming increasingly important in treatment of cancer. Examples include bevacizumab, which targets vascular endothelial growth factor; I^{131} tositumomab and Y-90-ibritumomab tiuxetan, which target CD20 and are used for treatment of chemotherapy-refractory non-Hodgkin's lymphoma; and gefitinib and the antibody cetuximab, which target the EGFR pathway. Biological response modifiers comprise a class of agents that stimulate the human **immune** system to destroy tumor cells. The α and β human interferons are efficacious in hairy cell leukemia and in certain skin cancers and may become aids for treating chronic myelogenous leukemia and non-Hodgkin's lymphoma. Interleukin-2 is another endogenous compound that may prove beneficial in treating lung, renal, colorectal, and several other tumor types. Still other compounds include tumor necrosis factor, human growth factors, and monoclonal antibodies (see Chapter 53).

New horizons

Although significant advances have been made in the treatment of the hematological neoplastic diseases over the past several decades, less progress has been made in the treatment of most solid tumors. During this same time there has been an explosion in our understanding of the basic science of cancer. For example, the past few decades have witnessed the description of RNA and DNA tumor viruses, oncogenes, and antioncogenes *(tumor suppressor genes)* as well as dramatic advances in our understanding of cell-cycle regulation, apoptosis, and the signaling pathways in DNA damage responses. Many gene products, involved in these pathways are new targets in the treatment of malignancies (see Chapter 42). Over the next several years many cancer treatments are certain to be devised based on our increased understanding of these basic molecular mechanisms, thereby narrowing the chasm between the molecular biology of cancer and clinical oncology. Hopefully, new agents targeted at key receptors and pathways will be more efficacious and less toxic than the classical antineoplastic agents.

Box 43-1 Tendency of antineoplastic drugs to induce nausea or vomiting

Strong tendency

Cisplatin, dacarbazine, mechlorethamine, cyclophosphamide, doxorubicin, lomustine, carmustine

Moderate tendency

Daunorubicin, actinomycin D, cytarabine, procarbazine, methotrexate, mitomycin, etoposide

Low tendency

Chlorambucil, vincristine, tamoxifen, bleomycin, hydroxyurea, fluorouracil

FURTHER READING

Workman, P. Strategies for treating cancers caused by multiple genome abnormalities: from concepts to cures? *Curr Opin Investig Drugs* 2003; 4(12):1410-1415.

Tiseo M, Loprevite M, Ardizzoni A. Epidermal growth factor receptor inhibitors: a new prospective in the treatment of lung cancer. *Curr Med Chem Anti-Canc Agents* 2004; 4:139-148.

Self-assessment questions

1. Which of the following diseases is potentially curable with combination chemotherapy even when both the liver and lung are involved by metastatic disease?
   a. Breast cancer
   b. Hodgkin's disease
   c. Colon cancer
   d. Non–small cell carcinoma of the lung
   e. Stomach cancer

2. Which of the following regimens is effective for treating Hodgkin's disease and not associated with a significant risk of secondary leukemia?
   a. CMF (cyclophosphamide, methotrexate, fluorouracil)
   b. MOPP (mechlorethamine, vincristine, procarbazine, prednisone)
   c. ABVD (Adriamycin [doxorubicin], bleomycin, vinblastine, dacarbazine)
   d. CAF (cyclophosphamide, Adriamycin, fluorouracil)
   e. BIP (bleomycin, ifosfamide, cisplatin)

3. Which of the following anti-neoplastic agents is associated with the greatest likelihood of nausea and vomiting?
   a. Vincristine
   b. Tamoxifen
   c. Methotrexate
   d. Cisplatin
   e. Fluorouracil

4. Which of the following cancers is associated with only a minimal (<20%) objective response rate to chemotherapy?
   a. Acute myelogenous leukemia
   b. Large cell lymphoma
   c. Renal cell carcinoma
   d. Small cell carcinoma of the lung
   e. Seminoma

5. When patients fail to respond to first-line chemotherapy, the likelihood of a response to a second-line regimen may be diminished because of:
   a. Tumor cell resistance caused by multidrug resistance gene.
   b. Tumor cell resistance caused by selection of resistant clones.
   c. Decreased performance status of patient.
   d. Increased tumor burden.
   e. All of the above.

PART VII

Drugs that kill invading organisms

VIRUSES, BACTERIA, OTHER UNICELLULAR organisms, and multicellular organisms existing in the environment can also live in the human body. This relationship can produce desirable as well as undesirable responses within the host. In a healthy person, normal bacteria in the GI tract have beneficial effects, assisting in production of vitamins and breakdown of foods. However, deleterious responses can occur when pathogenic organisms enter the GI tract. Pathogenic organisms can enter by oral ingestion, inhalation, trauma, surgical procedures, or any bodily opening. These unwanted host-pathogen responses (termed **infections**) can occur directly through release of toxins or antigens, or indirectly through generation of inflammation or tissue invasion. Infections arising from parasitic organisms in human hosts are the greatest cause of morbidity and mortality worldwide. In addition, many infections develop secondary to noninfectious primary diseases that diminish natural host defenses.

Table VII-1 lists the types of pathogenic organisms that invade the human body and cause unwanted biological responses. Treatment of the problems generated by these invasions is approached in two ways: (1) destruction or removal of invading organisms and (2) alleviation of symptoms. The availability of drugs for successful eradication of invading organisms varies considerably with the type and location of the organisms within the human host.

The only acellular organisms known to induce infectious diseases in humans are **viruses** and proteinaceous agents lacking nucleic acids called **prions.** Other small molecular weight acellular nucleic acids called viroids can exist in humans but probably do not contribute to disease.

Viral infections are a major source of temporary disability and loss of productivity in humans, and some viral infections are fatal. There are still only a few effective drugs available to halt proliferation of, or eliminate, clinically important viruses, although this situation is improving. Vaccines have provided effective protection against viruses, but prophylactic use of drugs may be more effective in preventing some viral infections, as described in Chapter 51.

There are many unicellular pathogenic microorganisms that are a major cause of human morbidity and mortality. Only a few species of the **mycoplasmas,** *Chlamydia,* and *Rickettsia* infect humans; however, there are many different **bacteria** that cause infectious diseases, and the pathogenicity of a bacterial species may change with time. Many approaches have been used to develop drugs to destroy specific bacteria but produce minimal adverse effects on the human host. The many antimicrobial drugs and vast variety of infectious microorganisms may seem overwhelming to the student. However, by noting common aspects in mechanisms of action or chemical structures, and the fact that some drugs are most effective in certain anatomical regions, this topic can be organized into a reasonably logical format. However, specific microbial strains of clinical relevance change with time, because new strains appear, existing strains develop **resistance,** old strains disappear, and new problems develop with old strains thought to be relatively benign. This complicates planning drug treatment, and requires the clinician to stay informed.

An overview of the classes of drugs and principles specific to the use of antimicrobial drugs is provided in Chapter 44. A large group of agents act by inhibiting

Table VII-1 Pathological organisms that can live in a parasitic invader–host relationship in humans, listed in order of increasing complexity

Cell Type	Organism	Typical Size (nm)
Acellular	Viruses	20-200
Unicellular	*Chlamydia* (P)	1000
Unicellular	*Mycoplasma* (P)	1000
Unicellular	*Rickettsia* (P)	1000
Unicellular	Bacteria (P)	1000
Unicellular	Fungi: yeasts (E)	3000-5000
Unicellular	Protozoa (E)	
Multicellular	Fungi: molds (E)	2000-10,000 and larger
Multicellular	Helminths (E)	

P, Prokaryotes (no nuclear membrane); *E,* eukaryotes (with a nucleus).

the synthesis of bacterial cell walls (see Chapter 45), while another group act at the ribosomal level to inhibit protein synthesis (see Chapter 46). Drugs acting on the bacterial tetrahydrofolate cofactor system, bacterial DNA replication inhibitors, and drugs that create pores in bacterial membranes are discussed in Chapter 47. Guidelines for use of antibacterial drugs are summarized in Chapter 48. Chapter 49 discusses those drugs used to treat mycobacterial infections, which cause tuberculosis and leprosy.

Bacteria are unicellular, nonnuclear organisms. Higher orders of size and complexity are found in unicellular, nucleated fungi (including yeast and filamentous forms) and protozoa. Major differences include the addition of a membrane-enclosed nucleus and mitochondria within the cell. More complex fungi are found in the multicellular, nucleated molds. Still higher orders of parasitic organisms are helminths (worms), which are estimated to infect 40% to 60% of the world's population and are a medical problem in both industrialized and developing countries. Drugs used to treat fungi are covered in Chapter 50; viruses in Chapter 51; protozoa and helminths in Chapter 52.

CHAPTER 44

Principles of antimicrobial use

James P. Steinberg

The development of antimicrobial therapy is considered by many to be one of the most important advances in the history of medicine. The efficacy and relative safety of these drugs has led to their widespread use and overuse, with up to 50% of antimicrobials consumed in the United States considered unnecessary. Because of their ability to alter microbial flora and lead to antibiotic-resistant microorganisms, they are fundamentally different from other types of drugs. Their misuse can lead to obsolescence, making it incumbent upon the practitioner to use them wisely. This chapter introduces the principles involved in selecting antimicrobial therapy. Because of the importance of antimicrobial resistance, this topic is discussed in a separate section later in this chapter and in the other chapters on individual drugs. Although this chapter focuses on antibacterial agents, many of the principles discussed also apply to antifungal, antiviral, and antiparasitic drugs.

Major historical events leading to the development of antimicrobial therapy are listed in Box 44-1. The term **antibiotic** traditionally refers to substances produced by microorganisms to suppress the growth of other microorganisms. The term **antimicrobial agents** is broader in meaning, because it encompasses drugs synthesized in the laboratory as well as those natural antibiotics produced by microorganisms. Some natural antibiotics originally produced by microbial fermentation are now produced by chemical synthesis. Many agents are semisynthetic; that is, the key portion of the compound is produced by microbial fermentation, and various moieties are attached synthetically. Thus the distinction between the terms antibiotics and antimicrobial agents is somewhat blurred and has little meaning today; many physicians use the terms interchangeably.

Antimicrobial agents can be classified into major groups according to the point in the cellular biochemical pathways at which they exert their primary mechanism of action (Fig. 44-1). These are:

- Inhibition of synthesis or damage to the peptidoglycan cell wall
- Inhibition of synthesis or damage to the cytoplasmic membrane
- Modification in synthesis or metabolism of nucleic acids
- Inhibition or modification of protein synthesis
- Modification in energy metabolism

Agents that inhibit the synthesis of cell walls include the β-lactams—such as penicillins, cephalosporins,

Abbreviations

CSF	cerebrospinal fluid
IM	intramuscular
IV	intravenous
MBC	minimal bactericidal concentration
MIC	minimal inhibitory concentration
MRSA	methicillin-resistant *Staphylococcus aureus*
PBP	penicillin binding proteins

Box 44-1 History of antimicrobial therapy

Early 17th century	The first recorded successful use of antimicrobial therapy involving the use of an extract from cinchona bark for the treatment of malaria.
1909	Paul Ehrlich's quest for a "magic bullet" that would bind specifically to particular sites on parasitic organisms leads to an arsenic derivative, salvarsan, with modest activity against syphilis. He also suggested that antimicrobial drugs would be most useful if the sites of action were not present in the organs and tissues of the human host.
1929	Alexander Fleming discovers penicillin.
1935	Discovery of prontosil, a forerunner of sulfonamides.
1940	Florey and Chain first use penicillin clinically.

monobactams, and carbapenems–and others, such as vancomycin. Inhibitors of cytoplasmic membranes include the polymyxins and daptomycin. In fungi, the cell wall is damaged by the polyene antifungal drugs or by the azoles. Inhibitors of nucleic acid synthesis include the quinolones, which inhibit DNA gyrase, and the RNA polymerase inhibitor rifampin. Protein synthesis is inhibited by aminoglycosides, tetracyclines, chloramphenicol, erythromycin, clindamycin, linezolid and streptogramins. These agents are usually bacteriostatic except the aminoglycosides and sometimes streptogramins, which can be bactericidal. Finally, folate antagonists such as sulfonamides and trimethoprim interfere with cell metabolism. These antimicrobial drugs are listed by their mechanisms of action in Table 44-1.

Drug selection for individual patients

Major factors to be considered when selecting an antimicrobial agent are outlined in Box 44-2. An understanding of these factors assists with rational selection

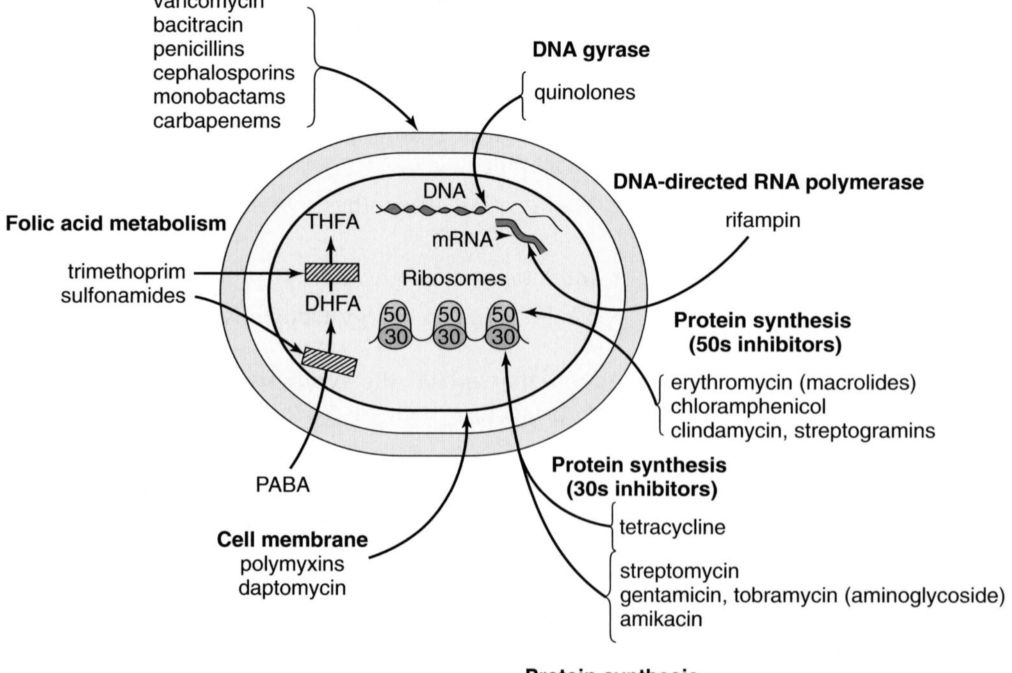

Figure 44-1 Antimicrobial sites of bactericidal or bacteriostatic action on microorganisms. The five general mechanisms comprise (1) inhibition of synthesis of cell wall, (2) damage to cell membrane, (3) modification of nucleic acid/DNA synthesis, (4) modification of protein synthesis (at ribosomes), and (5) modification of energy metabolism within the cytoplasm (at folate cycle). *PABA*, Paraaminobenzoic acid; *DHFA*, dihydrofolic acid; *THFA*, tetrahydrofolic acid.

Table 44-1 Classification of antimicrobial agents by mechanism of action

Mechanism of Action	Agent	Discussed in Chapter
Inhibition of synthesis or damage to cell wall	Penicillins	45
	Cephalosporins	45
	Monobactams	45
	Carbapenems	45
	Bacitracin	45
	Vancomycin	45
Inhibition of synthesis or damage to cytoplasmic membrane	Polymyxins	47
	Amphotericin B	50
Modification of synthesis or metabolism of nucleic acids	Quinolones	47
	Rifampin	49
	Nitrofurantoins	47
Inhibition or modification of protein synthesis	Aminoglycosides	46
	Tetracyclines	46
	Chloramphenicol	46
	Erythromycins	46
	Clindamycin	46
	Streptogramins	46
	Linezolid	46
	Mupirocin	46
Modification of energy metabolism	Sulfonamides	47
	Trimethoprim	47
	Dapsone	49
	Isoniazid	49

Box 44-2 Factors to consider when selecting antimicrobial agents for therapy in patients

- Is an antimicrobial agent necessary?
- Identification of the pathogen
- Empiric versus directed therapy
- Susceptibility of infecting microorganism
- Need for bactericidal versus bacteriostatic agent
- Pharmacokinetic and pharmacodynamic factors
- Anatomical site of infection
- Cost
- Toxicity
- Host factors
  - Allergy history
  - Age
  - Renal function
  - Hepatic function
  - Pregnancy status
  - Genetic or metabolic abnormalities
  - Host defenses, white blood cell function
- Need for combination therapy
- Antibiotic resistance concerns

of an appropriate compound. Each factor is important, but their relative importance may vary from case to case, so the order of discussion is not absolute.

Is an antimicrobial agent indicated?

About half of antimicrobial agents used in the United States are not necessary. These drugs are often given for viral infections that do not respond to antibiotics or noninfectious processes mimicking a bacterial infection. Antibiotics are often administered because of culture isolation of an organism that is **colonizing** an anatomical site and not causing an infection. In general, the clinician should resist temptation to begin antimicrobial therapy unless there is a reasonable probability that a bacterial infection is present. However, the threshold for starting antimicrobial therapy needs to be adjusted depending on the clinical setting. When the downside risk of withholding therapy is great, such as with bacterial meningitis or in clinically unstable patients, therapy should be started without delay even when the presence of a bacterial infection is uncertain. Another indication for antimicrobials is **prophylactic** therapy, which is intended to prevent illness in someone at risk of infection.

Identification of the pathogen

For many infections, an attempt should be made to determine the possible pathogen or pathogens before initiating antimicrobial therapy. Specimens for direct inspection and culture should be obtained before therapy is started, because drug therapy can decrease the yield of culture. Gram staining is the fastest, simplest, and most inexpensive method to identify bacteria and fungi. Because Gram stain can be accomplished quickly, the results can be used to guide the initial antimicrobial choice. Most body fluid that is normally sterile should be Gram stained. In addition, stains of wound exudates, sputum, and fecal material can sometimes yield information about the infecting microorganisms.

Empiric versus directed therapy

Although effort should be made to obtain material for laboratory testing, for certain infections including cellulitis, otitis media, and sinusitis it is often not possible or practical to obtain specimens for Gram stain and culture. In other infections such as pneumonia, the yield of culture material is low. When it is not possible to obtain a specimen, antimicrobial therapy is often started **empirically.** Knowledge of the antimicrobial spectrum of an agent and the likely pathogens causing infection at a particular anatomical site (see Chapter 48) can help direct therapy.

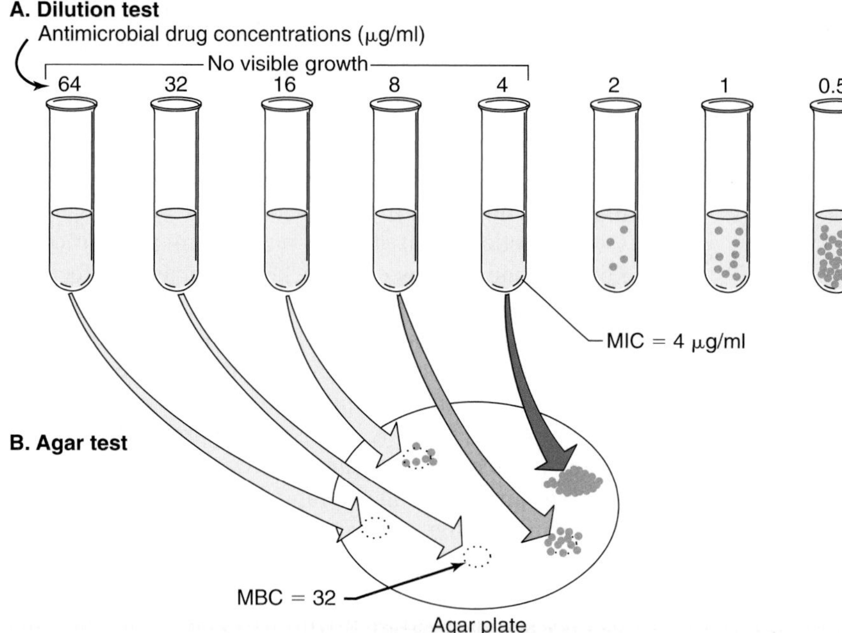

Figure 44-2 Dilution/agar tests for determination of MIC and MBC for a given drug and microorganism. **A,** Dilution test: each tube contains 5×10^5 colony-forming units (CFU) of bacteria, plus antibiotic at the concentration indicated. The MIC is the minimal drug concentration at which no visible growth of bacteria is observed (4 μg/ml in this example). This method has been adapted to automated systems by using a microtiter plate instead of test tubes. **B,** Dilution/agar test: each tube in **A** that shows no visible growth is cultured on a section of the new agar plate (no additional antibiotic is added to the agar plate). The MBC is the lowest concentration at which no growth occurs on the agar (32 μg/ml in this example).

Empiric therapy is usually broader than therapy directed at a particular pathogen or therapy based on the results of susceptibility testing. The use of agents with broad activity probably disturbs normal bacterial flora to a greater degree than **narrow spectrum** therapy and may promote the development of antibiotic-resistant pathogens. While empiric therapy is often used early in the course of therapy, the specter of antibiotic resistance and the added costs associated with broad therapy emphasize the importance of narrowing coverage if and when susceptibility testing results become available.

The setting in which an infection occurs should be considered when selecting empiric therapy. **Nosocomial infections,** those occurring in the hospital setting, are often caused by antibiotic-resistant bacteria, and the pattern of antibiotic resistance can vary from hospital to hospital. Most hospitals compile an "antibiogram" that lists the susceptibility profiles of common pathogens recovered at that institution. Knowledge of these local resistance patterns is very helpful in directing empiric therapy.

Susceptibility of infecting microorganisms

When pathogenic bacteria are isolated in culture, susceptibility to specific antimicrobial agents can be determined. The results of these tests generally are not available until 18 to 48 hours after an initial culture sample has been obtained.

Susceptibility testing is often performed by automated systems based on the broth dilution method. This method detects the lowest concentration of antimicrobial agent that prevents visible growth after an 18- to 24-hour incubation. This concentration is referred to as the **minimal inhibitory concentration (MIC).** The broth contains antibiotics in serial dilutions that encompass the concentrations normally achieved in humans. The technique is shown in Figure 44-2, *A*. Deciding whether the results show the organisms to be susceptible requires an understanding of the pharmacokinetics of the antimicrobial agent, correlations between clinical outcomes and MIC data, and knowledge of the relationship between resistance mechanisms and MICs. Detemining what MIC indicates the "cut-off" for susceptibility is often not straightforward and is the purview of an international committee. This same test procedure can be extended further to determine the minimal bactericidal concentration (MBC), or minimal concentration that kills 99.9% of cells. In this test, samples are removed from the antibiotic-containing tubes in which there is no visible microbial growth and plated on agar that contains no additional antibiotic. The lowest concentration tube from which bacteria do not grow on the agar is the MBC (see Fig. 44-2, *B*). MBC determinations are no longer used regularly in most clinical laboratories.

Another method for determining bacterial susceptibility to antibiotics is the disk diffusion method. In this method, disks impregnated with the drugs to be tested are placed on an agar plate freshly inoculated with the bacterial strain in question. After the plates have been incubated for 18 to 24 hours, bacterial growth occurs

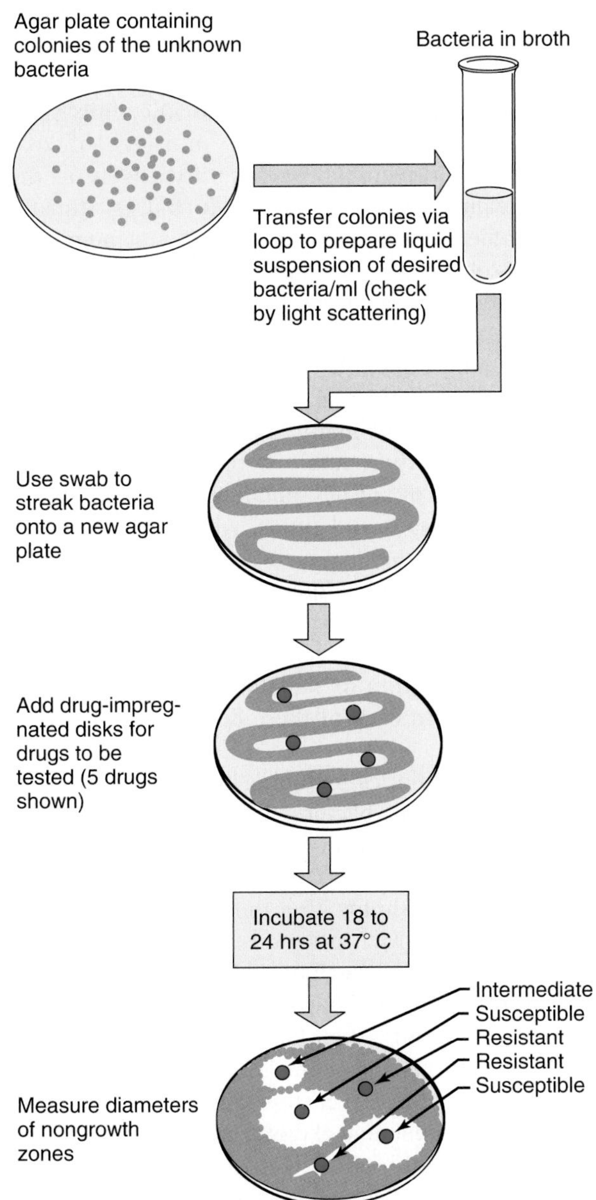

Figure 44-3 Disk diffusion method for testing bacteria for susceptibility to specific antimicrobial agents.

except near the disks where a "zone of inhibition" may be present. If sufficiently large, the zone indicates that the bacterial strain is susceptible to the antibiotic in the disk. This test is simple to perform but only semiquantitative, not useful for determining the susceptibility of many slow-growing or fastidious organisms, and has been replaced by automated broth dilution systems in many laboratories. The test procedure and typical results are shown in Figure 44-3. A newer and related method is the E-test that, instead of a disk, uses a strip containing the antibiotic in a concentration gradient along with a numerical scale. The point where the zone

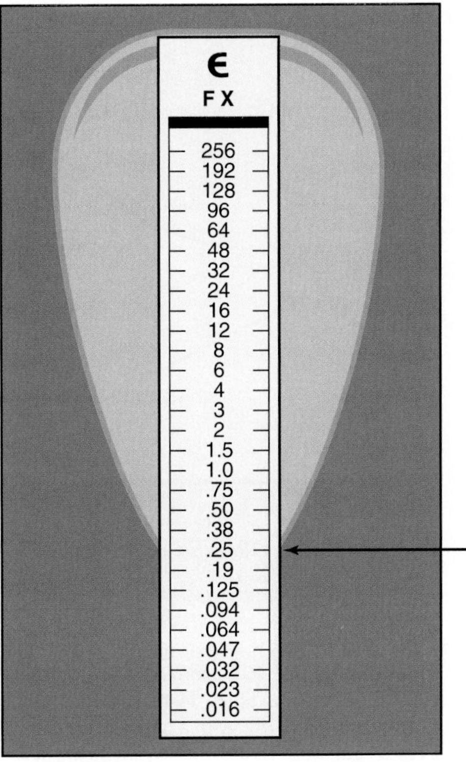

Figure 44-4 E-test method for susceptibility testing. The strip impregnated with a gradient of antibiotic is placed on a freshly inoculated agar plate. The point where the border of the zone of inhibition touches the strip defines the MIC *(arrow)*.

of inhibition touches the strip indicates the MIC (Fig. 44-4).

Because of the many antimicrobial agents available, it is difficult to test routinely all antimicrobial agents against an isolate. To circumvent this problem, laboratories often use one compound as representative of a class of compounds. It is important to recognize that susceptibility tests require interpretation, are not error-proof, and may fail to identify a resistant subset population.

Need for bactericidal versus bacteriostatic agent

Antimicrobial agents can be **bactericidal** (i.e., the organisms are killed) or **bacteriostatic** (i.e., the organisms are prevented from growing) (Fig. 44-5). A given agent may show bactericidal actions under certain conditions but bacteriostatic actions under others, depending on the concentration of drug and the target bacteria. A bacteriostatic agent often is adequate in uncomplicated infections because the host defenses will help eradicate the microorganism. For example, in pneumonococcal pneumonia, bacteriostatic agents suppress the multiplication of the pneumococci and the pneumococci are destroyed by interaction with alveolar

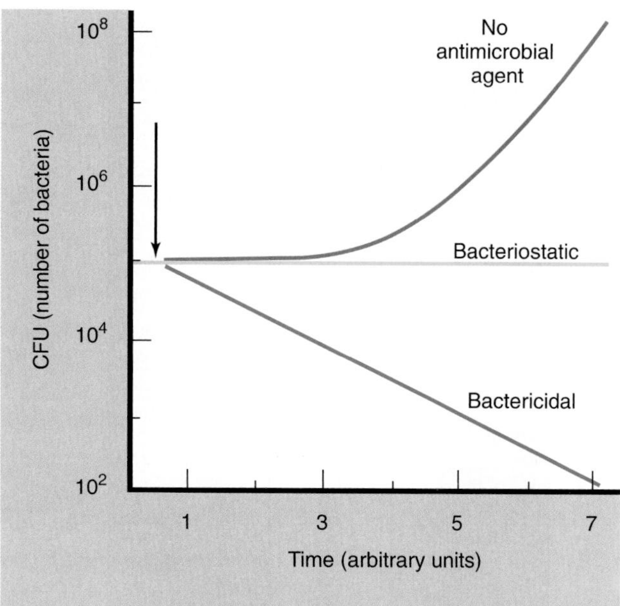

Figure 44-5 Bactericidal versus bacteriostatic antimicrobial agents. A typical culture is started at 10^5 colony-forming units (CFU) and incubated at 37° C for various times. In the absence of an antimicrobial agent, there is cell growth. With a bacteriostatic agent added, no growth occurs, but neither are the existing cells killed. If the added agent is bactericidal, 99.9% of the cells are killed during the standardized test time.

macrophages and polymorphonuclear leukocytes. For a neutropenic individual, such a bacteriostatic agent might prove ineffective, and a bactericidal agent would be necessary. Thus the status of the host influences whether a bactericidal or bacteriostatic agent is selected.

In addition, because the site of infection influences the ability of certain host defenses to effectively contend with microbes, bactericidal agents are required for management of infections in areas "protected" from host immune responses, such as endocarditic vegetations and cerebrospinal fluid (CSF). In endocarditis, treatment with bacteriostatic antibiotics such as tetracyclines or erythromycin is associated with an unacceptably high failure rate, in contrast with cure rates in excess of 95% for bactericidal agents such as penicillin. Concentrations of an antimicrobial agent 8- to 10-fold greater than the MBC must be achieved in the spinal fluid of patients with meningitis to effect a cure. Thus susceptibility is not the only criterion for efficacy.

Pharmacokinetic and pharmacodynamic factors

Antimicrobial agents are usually administered by oral, intramuscular (IM), or intravenous (IV) routes. Most agents reach peak serum concentrations 1 to 2 hours after oral administration. However, peak concentrations may be delayed if drugs are ingested with food or in patients with delayed intestinal transit such as sometimes occurs in diabetics. Peak plasma concentrations are reached in 0.5 to 1 hour after IM injections and at the end of the infusion after IV infusions of 20 to 30 minutes. Antimicrobial agents vary widely in their oral bioavailability. Some agents including trimethoprim/sulfamethoxazole, fluoroquinolones, rifampin, and metronidazole are almost completely absorbed after oral administration; these drugs can often be used orally even when a severe infection is present. That said, most life-threatening infections are treated, at least initially, with IV agents. Parenteral therapy ensures adequate serum levels, and, for many agents, higher drug levels can be achieved when administered IV.

The amount of antimicrobial agent that reaches the extravascular tissues and fluids, where the infection is usually present, depends on the concentration gradient between plasma and target tissue, degree of drug binding to plasma and tissue proteins, molecular size, degree of ionization and lipid solubility of the drug, and its rate of elimination or metabolism. There is considerable variation in each of these factors among antimicrobial agents.

Certain antibiotics including fluoroquinolones and aminoglycosides kill bacteria faster at higher concentrations, a property called **concentration-dependent killing.** These agents also continue to inhibit growth of bacteria for several hours after the concentrations of the drug fall below the MIC in the serum. This is called **post-antibiotic** effect. Agents that exhibit these two properties can often be administered less frequently than would be predicted by their half-life because drug levels do not have to be above the MIC for the bulk of the dosing interval. Most β-lactam agents do not exhibit concentration-dependent killing nor do they have a prolonged post-antibiotic effect.

Anatomical site of infection

The site of infection often influences not only the agent used but also the dose, route, and duration of administration. The desired peak concentration of drug at the site of infection should be at least 4 times the MIC. However, if host defenses are adequate, peak concentrations may be much lower and even be equal to the MIC and still be effective. When host defenses are absent or inoperative, peak concentrations 8- to 16-fold greater than the MIC may be required.

Most antimicrobial agents readily enter most body tissues and compartments, except for the CSF, brain, eye, and prostate. By using the parenteral route, concentrations adequate to treat infections of the pleural, pericardial, and joint spaces can be obtained. Certain antibiotics such as aminoglycosides and erythromycin,

Table 44-2 Ability of antibiotics to enter the cerebrospinal fluid in effective concentrations

Readily Enter CSF	Enter CSF When Inflammation Present	Do Not Enter CSF Adequately to Treat Infection
Chloramphenicol	Penicillin G	Cefazolin
Sulfonamides	Ampicillin	Cefoxitin
Trimethoprim	Piperacillin	Erythromycin
Rifampin	Oxacillin	Clindamycin
Metronidazole	Nafcillin	Tetracycline
	Cefuroxime	Gentamicin
	Cefotaxime	Tobramycin
	Ceftriaxone	Amikacin
	Ceftazidime	
	Aztreonam	
	Ciprofloxacin	
	Vancomycin	
	Meropenem	
	Cefepime	

however, may not be active in abscesses because of the low pH and the reservoir of pus and necrotic debris.

Endocarditis is difficult to treat because bacteria trapped in a fibrin matrix divide slowly, and many antibiotics are effective only on growing microorganisms. Antibiotics used in endocarditis therefore must be bactericidal, administered at high concentrations, and administered for prolonged periods so that the antibiotic diffuses into the matrix and all bacteria are killed.

Meningitis is a difficult problem, because many antimicrobial agents do not cross the blood-brain or blood-CSF barriers very well (Table 44-2). Lipid-soluble agents such as chloramphenicol easily enter the CSF, as do agents such as rifampin and metronidazole; however, aminoglycosides do not enter the CSF even in the presence of inflammation. Penicillins, aztreonam, cephalosporins, and carbapenems enter the CSF to variable degrees in the presence of meningitis, depending on the compound. Quinolones such as ciprofloxacin also enter the CSF at concentrations adequate to kill some microorganisms. Vancomycin is active against all pneumococci and, because of possible resistance to other agents, it is used routinely as part of empiric therapy for pneumococcal meningitis. Yet microbiologic failures on vancomycin have been reported because this agent does not penetrate into the CSF sufficiently to guarantee acceptable bactericidal levels.

Osteomyelitis is an infection in which prolonged therapy is required. Less than 4 weeks of drug administration is usually associated with high rates of failure, because the concentration of antibiotic in bone is often low and the bacteria are sequestered and prevented from coming into contact with the antibiotics.

Antimicrobial drug therapy frequently is ineffective in the presence of a foreign body such as an artificial joint or a prosthetic heart valve. Many microorganisms growing at a slow rate in a sessile form accumulate on the foreign surface and become covered with a glycocalyx coating. The coating protects them from attack by leukocytes and most importantly from destruction by antimicrobial agents.

Microorganisms also persist in abscesses because circulation is impaired, reducing delivery of antibody, complement, and leukocytes. Moreover, complement is destroyed in abscesses and cannot potentiate the destruction of bacteria by leukocytes. Leukocytes function less effectively in an abscess because of the absence of adequate oxygen and the acidic environment. Bacteria in an abscess frequently grow much more slowly than at other infection sites yet are not killed by antimicrobial agents that easily kill them when they are rapidly dividing. In some situations the antimicrobial agent is destroyed by enzymes induced by the microorganisms or by enzymes released when the microorganisms are killed by the antibiotic. Antibiotic therapy can rarely cure established abscesses, lesions containing foreign bodies, or infections associated with excretory duct obstruction unless these sites are drained surgically.

Some infections are caused by microorganisms that can survive intracellularly following ingestion by polymorphonuclear phagocytes or macrophages. *Mycobacterium, Legionella,* and *Salmonella* species are organisms that can survive within phagocytic cells, and antimicrobial agents that do not penetrate the phagocytic cells often are not successful in eradicating infection caused by these organisms. Compounds such as isoniazid and rifampin are successful in the treatment of *Mycobacterium tuberculosis,* because these agents enter mononuclear cells in which tubercle bacilli survive, and the antimicrobial agents kill the bacilli within the phagocytic cells.

Bacterial infections associated with obstructions of the urinary, biliary, or respiratory tracts tend to persist despite antibiotic therapy because antimicrobial agents penetrate poorly into these areas. In addition, bacteria present in the obstructed regions are in a quiescent state from which they emerge after antimicrobial therapy is discontinued, and most agents do not kill resting bacteria.

Cost

All things being equal, one should choose the least-expensive agent, and oral therapy is generally less expensive than parenteral therapy. While economic considerations are real, it is important to recognize that the cost of an antimicrobial agent is only one component of the total cost of care. Should efficacy be compromised or a less-effective therapy lead to a longer hospital stay or greater toxicity, the cost of the antimicrobial agent will likely be dwarfed by the increase in overall cost.

Toxicity

Most commonly used antimicrobial agents have favorable safety profiles, and the potential for toxicity, while always a concern, is generally not the pivotal factor driving the selection process. Because of nephrotoxicity and ototoxicity, aminoglycoside use has decreased with the development of β-lactams and fluoroquinolones with broad gram-negative activity. Unfortunately, the development of antibiotic resistance is beginning to force clinicians to use antimicrobial agents that were once discarded for less-toxic alternatives. For example, some strains of *Pseudomonas aeruginosa* and *Acinetobacter* spp. have developed resistance to all commonly used agents, which has led to the recycling of parenteral polymyxin B, an agent with considerable toxicity that had not been used by a generation of physicians.

The risk of toxicity of a given drug may be significantly influenced by one or more of the host factors discussed below.

Host factors

Allergy history

A history of an adverse reaction to an antibiotic is important because a similar reaction to other members of the same drug class may occur. It is important to characterize the reaction to distinguish an **intolerance** such as gastrointestinal upset from a true allergy and to recognize potentially life-threatening allergic reactions such as anaphylaxis or exfoliative dermatitis. When these serious reactions occur, administration of chemically related compounds should be avoided. Significant allergy appears to be more common with β-lactams, particularly penicillins, and sulfonamides. In anaphylactic reactions to penicillins, the IgE antibody is usually directed at the penicillin nucleus, so the potential for allergic reactions to other penicillins is high. For many other allergic reactions, the potential for cross-allergy to related compounds in not known.

Age

Because renal function decreases with age, the dosage or administration interval of renally cleared agents should be adjusted when used in elderly patients. The pH of gastric secretions also is affected by age, and this factor may influence selection of a drug. Certain antibiotics should not be given to children. For example, tetracyclines bind to developing teeth and bone and should be avoided in children. Similarly, sulfonamides should not be given to newborns because they displace bilirubin from serum albumin and can produce kernicterus, a central nervous system disorder. Finally, common pathogens for certain infections, such as bacterial meningitis, are age dependent and the age of the patient must be considered when selecting empiric therapy.

Renal function

The presence of reduced renal function may influence the choice of an antibiotic and the dosage used. Many antimicrobial agents are eliminated from the body by renal filtration or secretion, and some of these agents can accumulate in the body and cause serious toxic reactions unless there is a proper adjustment in dosage in the setting of reduced renal function. Antimicrobial agents that require dosage adjustment include aminoglycosides, vancomycin, certain penicillins, most cephalosporins, carbapenems, and quinolones. Failure to adjust dosage can lead to ototoxicity from aminoglycosides and neurotoxicity from penicillins, imipenem, or quinolones. Aminoglycosides can cause renal toxicity and should be used with caution in patients with preexisting renal insufficiency. Dosage adjustments for agents eliminated by glomerular filtration usually can be estimated on the basis of the patient's age, body size, and on serum creatinine concentration.

Hepatic function

Antimicrobials metabolized in the liver include chloramphenicol, erythromycin, clarithromycin, rifampin, nitroimidazoles, and some of the quinolones. It may be necessary to reduce the doses of these agents to avert toxic reactions in patients with impaired hepatic function. Chloramphenicol toxicity in newborns stems from the inability of underdeveloped livers to convert the drug to an inactive, nontoxic glucuronide.

Pregnancy

Almost all antimicrobial agents cross the placenta to some degree and may affect the fetus. With most agents, the greatest risk of teratogenic and toxic effects on the fetus is in the first trimester (Table 44-3). Metronidazole

Table 44-3 Antimicrobial agents to be used with caution or avoided during pregnancy

Agent	Potential Toxicity
Aminoglycosides	Eighth nerve damage
Chloramphenicol	Gray baby syndrome
Erythromycin estolate	Cholestatic hepatitis in mother
Metronidazole	Possible teratogenicity
Nitrofurantoin	Hemolytic anemia
Sulfonamides	Hemolysis in newborn with glucose-6-phosphate dehydrogenase deficiency; increased risk of kernicterus
Tetracyclines	Limb abnormalities, dental staining, inhibition of bone growth
Trimethoprim	Altered folate metabolism
Quinolones	Abnormalities of cartilage
Vancomycin	Possible auditory toxicity

is teratogenic in lower animals, but it is not clear if this drug poses a risk to human fetuses. Other agents such as rifampin and trimethoprim may have a teratogenic potential and should be used only when alternative agents are unavailable. Quinolones cause cartilage abnormalities in animal models. As with some other agents, it is not clear if these effects seen in animals translate to significant human health risks.

Use of tetracyclines in pregnancy should be avoided because they alter fetal dentition and bone growth. Tetracyclines have also been associated with hepatic, pancreatic, and renal damage in pregnant women. Streptomycin has been associated with auditory toxicity in children of mothers treated for tuberculosis. Sulfonamides should not be used in the third trimester of pregnancy because they may displace bilirubin from albumin-binding sites and cause central nervous system toxicity in the fetus.

Many antibiotics are excreted in breast milk and can cause the newborn's microflora to be distorted or act as a sensitizing agent to cause future allergy.

Genetic and metabolic factors

Genetic abnormalities of enzyme function may alter the toxicity of certain agents. For example, hemolysis in glucose-6-phosphate dehydrogenase–deficient people can be provoked by sulfonamides, nitrofurantoin, pyrimethamine, sulfones, and chloramphenicol. In addition, isoniazid may not be adequately inactivated in people who do not acetylate drugs well, and peripheral neuropathy can develop in such patients unless they are treated with pyridoxine. Because 50% of the U.S. population are slow acetylators, pyridoxine is usually prescribed with isoniazid.

Box 44-3 Reasons for concurrent use of more than one antimicrobial agent in a patient

To treat a life-threatening infection
To treat a polymicrobial infection
Empiric therapy when no one agent is active against potential pathogens
To achieve synergy (obtain enhanced antibacterial activity)
To prevent the emergence of resistant bacteria
To permit the use of a lower dose of one of the antimicrobial agents

Host defenses

An absence of white blood cells predisposes a patient to serious bacterial infection, and bacteriostatic agents are often ineffective in treating serious infections in neutropenic hosts. The critical white blood cell count is between 500 and 1000 mature polymorphonuclear cells/mm^3. Bactericidal agents are also required in the setting of other host defects, such as agammaglobulinemia or asplenia. The latter predisposes patients to pneumococcal or *Haemophilus* infection. The absence of complement components C_7 to C_9 predisposes patients to serious infection with *Neisseria* species. Knowledge of the organisms most frequently causing infections in patients with defects of white blood cells, complement, T cells, or immunoglobulin production aids in selection of bactericidal agents to be used when fever develops.

Antimicrobial combinations

The reasons for using antibiotic combinations are listed in Box 44-3. Although combination therapy is sometimes necessary, combinations tend to be overused. Some of the reliance of antibiotic combinations is due to a failure to identify the etiologic agent, forcing continuation of broad empiric therapy.

Antimicrobial combinations directed at a single organism are considered to elicit **indifferent** effects if the combined activity equals the sum of the separate activities. **Synergism** is present if the activity of the combined antimicrobial agents is greater than the sum of the independent activities. Combinations of antibiotics are **antagonistic** when the activity of the combination is less than could be achieved by using the agents separately. There are several laboratory methods to demonstrate synergy testing. The "kill curve" method is shown in Figure 44-6.

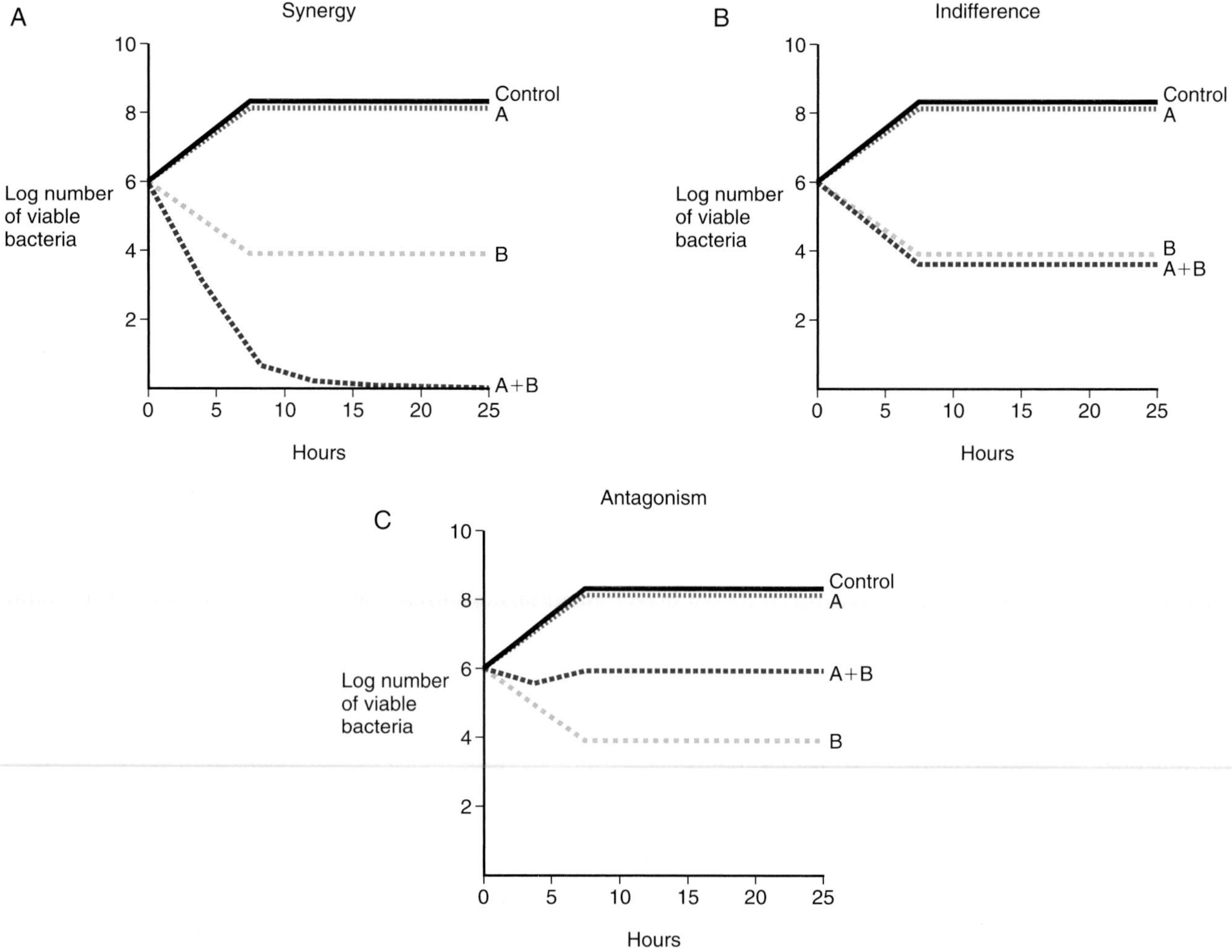

Figure 44-6 Trends in bacterial viability over time after exposure to two different antimicrobial agents (*A* and *B*) demonstrating: synergy **(A)**, indifference **(B)**, and antagonism **(C)**.

The evidence that combination antimicrobial therapy is of value in life-threatening infections has been shown, albeit not consistently, in neutropenic patients with such infections. For example, the combination of an anti-pseudomonal penicillin and an aminoglycoside yielded better survival rates in some studies of patients with *Pseudomonas* sepsis. The major disadvantages of combination therapy for serious infections are the added cost and the risk of toxicity.

Combination therapy is sometimes used for polymicrobial infections including those occurring at intraperitoneal and pelvic sites. Combination therapy is currently recommended for the empiric treatment of many patients with community-acquired pneumonia to treat both *S. pneumoniae* and atypical pathogens including *Mycoplasma, Chlamydia,* and *Legionella.*

Combination therapy is essential in treatment of tuberculosis because subpopulations of organisms intrinsically resistant to all first-line agents are present in patients with cavitary disease and a high organism burden. In this setting, the use of multiple drugs prevents the resistant organisms from surviving. The ability of combination therapy to prevent development of resistance by other bacteria is less well established.

A synergistic effect has been documented for three combinations of antimicrobials:

- The combination of an inhibitor of cell-wall synthesis with an aminoglycoside antibiotic
- The combination of agents acting on sequential steps in a metabolic pathway
- The combination of agents in which one (such as an inhibitor of β-lactamases) inhibits an enzyme that inactivates the other compound, such as clavulanate with amoxicillin

A classic example of synergy is the use of penicillin or ampicillin plus an aminoglycoside to treat enterococcal

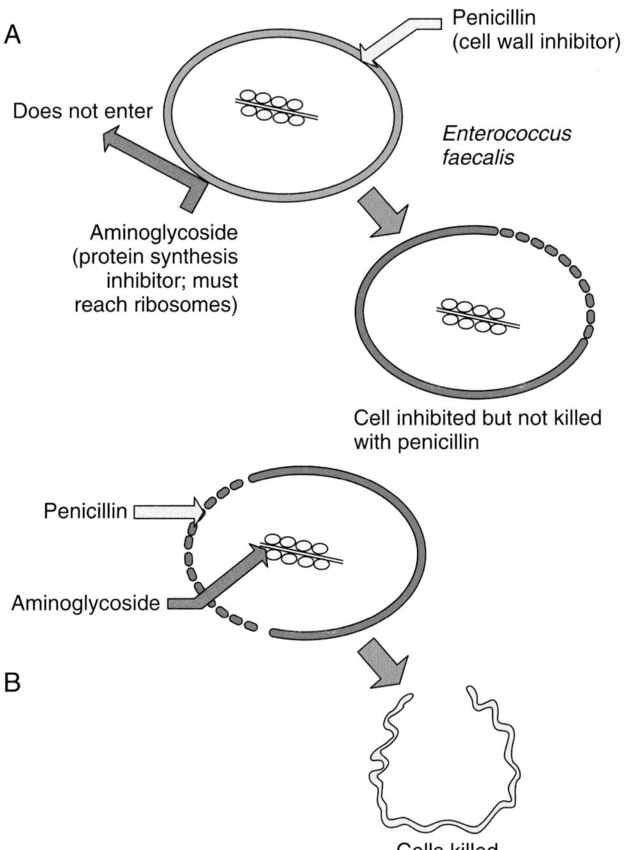

Figure 44-7 An example of synergy between two antibiotics. **A,** Penicillin or aminoglycoside is given, but not both; the cells are only inhibited. **B,** Penicillin and aminoglycoside are given concurrently; penicillin opens holes in the cell wall through which aminoglycosides can enter and reach the ribosomes and halt protein synthesis; therefore the cells are killed.

endocarditis. Although penicillins are usually bactericidal, they affect enterococci in a bacteriostatic fashion, with a large difference between the inhibitory and bactericidal concentrations. Aminoglycosides alone are inactive against enterococci because they cannot get inside the cell to reach their ribosomal target site. Penicillins alter the cell wall of enterococci, allowing the aminoglycoside to enter the bacterial cell when both drugs are administered (Fig. 44-7). The combination is bactericidal, and this synergistic effect is critically important in the treatment of enterococcal endocarditis in humans.

Antibiotic decision making after therapy has started

The need for ongoing antimicrobial therapy should be reassessed regularly as the patient's clinical course evolves. Empiric therapy should be reassessed after initial culture results return, typically in 2 days. Empiric therapy is often broad, sometimes excessively so depending on the anxiety of the treating physician and the severity of illness. The misdemeanor of overly broad empiric regimen can be forgiven if, when culture and sensitivity results return, the regimen is refined accordingly. Switching from parenteral to oral therapy is cost effective and, depending on the infection, should be done when the patient's condition allows. The optimal duration of therapy for many infections is not known. Some approximate durations are listed in Table 44-4.

Table 44-4 Approximate duration of antimicrobial therapy for common infections

Infection	Duration (days)
Streptococcal pharyngitis	10
Otitis media	5-10
Sinusitis	10
Uncomplicated urinary tract infection	3
Pyelonephritis	14
Cellulitis	3 days after inflammation resolves
Pneumococcal pneumonia	3-5 days after fever resolves
Other pneumonia	variable, often 14
Bacteremia	variable, often 10-14 days without endocarditis
Endocarditis	28-42
Meningitis	7-14
Osteomyelitis	42
Septic arthritis	21

Monitoring antimicrobial therapy

Because of the favorable safety profile of most antimicrobial agents, predictable pharmacokinetics, and the ability to achieve serum levels well above MICs, it is usually not necessary to monitor serum antibiotic concentrations. Agents for which serum levels are often obtained are aminoglycosides and vancomycin. Measuring drug concentrations of these agents can help ensure that therapeutic and not toxic concentrations are attained. This is particularly important in patients with diminished renal function, because these agents undergo renal elimination and have nephrotoxic potential.

Prophylaxis with antimicrobial agents

Prophylaxis is the use of an antimicrobial agent to prevent infection. Prophylaxis is often administered following exposure to a virulent pathogen or prior to a procedure associated with an increased risk of infection. Chronic prophylaxis is sometimes administered to persons with underlying conditions that predispose to recurrent or severe infection. Several concepts are important in determining whether prophylaxis is appropriate for a particular situation. In general, prophylaxis is recommended when the risk of infection is high or the consequences of infection are significant. The nature of the pathogen, type of exposure, and immunocompetence of the host are important determinants of the need for prophylaxis. The antimicrobial agent should be able to eliminate or reduce the probability of infection, or, if infection occurs, reduce the associated morbidity. The ideal agent should be inexpensive, orally administered in most circumstances, have few adverse effects, have minimal effect on the normal microbial flora, and have limited potential to select for antimicrobial resistance. Consequently, the choice of agents is critical and the duration of prophylaxis should be as brief as possible. Often a single dose is sufficient. The emerging crisis of antibiotic-resistant bacteria underscores the importance of rational and not indiscriminate use of antimicrobial agents.

The efficacy of prophylaxis is well-established in situations such as perioperative antibiotic administration prior to certain surgical procedures, exposure to invasive meningococcal disease, and prevention of recurrent rheumatic fever. To prevent postoperative wound infections, the antimicrobial agent must be present at the surgical site when the area is exposed to the bacteria. The antibiotic should be given immediately preoperatively and should inhibit the most common and important bacteria likely to produce infection. Prophylaxis can be effective without eradication of all bacteria so it is not essential to administer an agent with a broad activity.

Prophylaxis is accepted in other situations without supporting data. When the risk of infection is low, such as the occurrence of bacterial endocarditis following dental procedures, randomized clinical trials of prophylaxis are not feasible. However, the consequences of infection may be catastrophic, providing a compelling argument for prophylaxis despite the low risk of infection. People with valvular or structural lesions of the heart, in whom endocarditis is common, should receive antibiotic prophylaxis at the time of surgical, dental, or other procedures that may produce a transient bacteremia. Prophylaxis reduces the number of organisms that could lodge on the valvular tissue and alters the surface properties of the microorganism so they have reduced affinity for cardiac tissue. The prophylactic antibiotic should be administered just before the procedure; limiting exposure minimizes the selection of resistant bacteria. Because viridans group streptococci from the mouth or intestine and enterococci from the intestine or genitourinary tract have a propensity to cause endocarditis, prophylaxis should be directed against these organisms.

Antimicrobial prophylaxis has been advocated following other exposures, including some bite wounds; *Haemophilus* meningitis; exposure to sexually transmitted diseases; following sexual assault; influenza; and some potential agents of bioterrorism including anthrax. Prophylaxis can prevent opportunistic infections in persons with AIDS and is sometimes used to prevent postsplenectomy infections, cellulitis complicating lymphedema, and recurrent lower urinary tract infections. Tuberculosis "prophylaxis" should be considered preemptive therapy because it is typically given to persons already infected with *Mycobacterium tuberculosis* (by virtue of having a positive skin test) in an attempt to prevent clinical disease.

There are many other situations, some controversial, for which antimicrobial prophylaxis is used. When prophylaxis is advocated without data confirming efficacy, there should be a scientific rationale to support the use of a particular antimicrobial agent.

Bacterial resistance

The importance of antibiotic resistance cannot be overstated. The ability of bacteria to develop resistance to all drugs in our armamentarium threatens many of the chemotherapeutic advances of the antimicrobial era. There are several consequences of antibiotic resistance; the most obvious is that treating a patient with an ineffective drug will lead to therapeutic failure or relapse. The development of resistance also forces physicians to use newer, more-costly, and sometimes more-toxic agents. Resistant bacteria have a competitive advantage over other flora and, under the pressure of heavy antibiotic use, can spread in the hospital environment. Most ominously, because of resistance, we now face the prospects of untreatable infections more than any time in the last several decades. The drugs of choice for treating many infections have changed over the years, in large part because of expanding resistance. Knowledge of the resistance patterns of organisms in the community and in the hospital setting helps direct empiric therapy. In addition, recognizing that some bacteria have the propensity to develop resistance to certain antibiotics during a course of treatment should influence antibiotic selection even after the susceptibility profile is known.

Antibiotic resistance can be **intrinsic** or **acquired.** For example, *Pseudomonas aeruginosa* is intrinsically resistant to many antibiotics because of the inability of antibiotics to cross its outer membrane or bind to target sites. Acquired resistance can be due to mutation of existing genetic information or acquisition of new genes. Exchange of genetic information among bacteria is very common and occurs by several mechanisms (Fig. 44-8). Conjugation is the process by which two physically apposed bacteria exchange genetic information, usually contained on plasmids (extrachromosomal pieces of DNA). Resistance-conferring plasmids have been identified in virtually all bacteria. Resistance is also present on transposable genetic elements (transposons or "jumping genes") that can "jump" to plasmids or become integrated into chromosomes. Certain bacteria are naturally transformable, meaning that they can pick up exogenous DNA from the environment. A third means of genetic exchange is transduction or exchange of DNA via phages or viruses that have tropism for a particular bacterial species. This mechanism is thought to be important in resistance to *Staphylococcus aureus.*

Intensive use of antimicrobials is a major factor in development of both chromosomal and plasmid-mediated bacterial resistance. The use of antibiotics, whether in an individual patient or in a hospital with its special environment and microorganisms, permits proliferation of bacteria that are intrinsically resistant or have acquired resistance. From an epidemiological point of view, plasmid resistance is most important, because it is transmissible and may be associated with other properties that enable a microorganism to colonize and invade a susceptible host. These resistant organisms are often transferred from patient to patient on the hands of healthcare workers. Thus, a simple but unfortunately under-utilized method to prevent transmission of antibiotic resistant bacteria is proper hand hygiene before and after all patient contact.

The basic mechanisms of resistance to antimicrobial agents include:

- Development of altered receptors or targets to which the drug cannot bind
- A decrease in the concentration of drug that reaches the receptors (by altered rates of entry or removal of drug)
- Enhanced destruction or inactivation of drug
- Synthesis of resistant metabolic pathways

These are shown in Figure 44-9, and examples of each mechanism are listed in Table 44-5. Microorganisms can possess one or more of these mechanisms simultaneously.

Resistance based on altered receptors for drug

Important examples of this mechanism are the production of altered penicillin binding proteins (PBP) to which penicillins, cephalosporins, and other β-lactams cannot

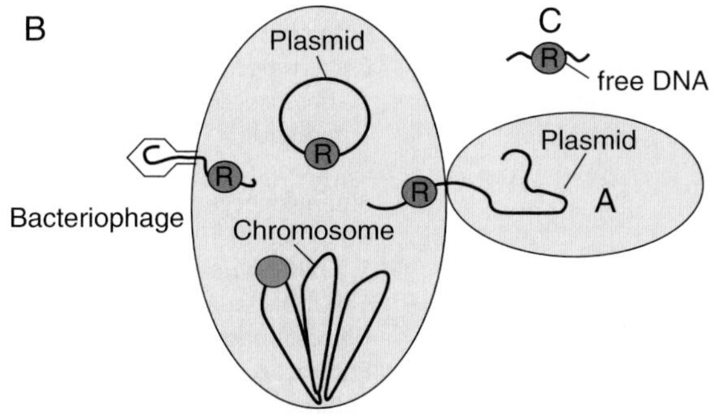

Figure 44-8 Mechanisms of genetic exchange. **A,** Bacterial **conjugation** between two physically attached bacteria with exchange of plasmid DNA containing resistance determinant R. **B, Transduction** with a virus (bacteriophage) carrying resistance determinant R to target bacteria. **C, Transformation** is the ability of certain bacteria to pick up free DNA from the environment.

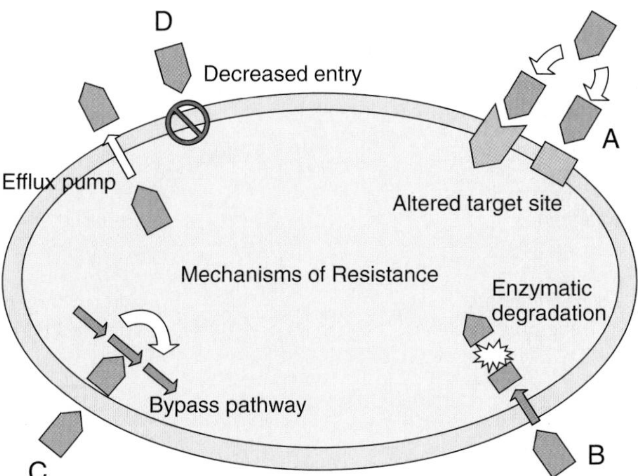

Figure 44-9 The major mechanisms of bacterial resistance to antibiotics are shown. These mechanisms include **(A)** altered receptors or targets to which the drug can not bind, **(B)** enhanced destruction or inactivation of drug, **(C)** synthesis of resistant metabolic pathways, **(D)** a decrease in the concentration of drug that reaches the receptors (by altered rates of entry or removal of drug).

Table 44-5 Resistance mechanisms of different bacteria to various antibiotics

Antibiotic(s)	Mechanisms	Pathogens with Potential for Resistance Development
β-Lactams	Altered penicillin-binding proteins	*Staphylococcus aureus*
Penicillins		Coagulase-negative staphylococci
Cephalosporins		*Streptococcus pneumoniae*
Monobactams		Enterococci
Carbapenems		*Neisseria gonorrhoeae*
		Pseudomonas aeruginosa
	Reduced permeability	*P. aeruginosa*
		Enterobacter cloacae
		Serratia marcescens
		Acinetobacter sp.
	β-Lactamase	*S. aureus*
		Coagulase-negative staphylococci
		Enterococci
		P. aeruginosa
		Enterobacteriaceae
		N. gonorrhoeae
		N. meningitidis
		Moraxella sp.
		Bacteroides sp.
		Acinetobacter sp.
Fluoroquinolones	Altered DNA gyrase	*S. aureus*
	Reduced permeability/efflux	Enterobacteriaceae
		Pseudomonas sp.
		Campylobacter
Aminoglycosides	Modifying enzymes	Enterococci
Gentamicin	Reduced uptake	Staphylococci
Tobramycin		*Pseudomonas* sp.
Amikacin		Enterobacteriaceae
		Streptococci
Macrolides/lincosamides	Methylating enzymes	Streptococci
Erythromycin		*S. pneumoniae*
Clindamycin		Staphylococci
		Enterococci
Chloramphenicol	Acetyltransferase	Staphylococci
		Streptococci
		S. pneumoniae
		Enterobacteriaceae
		Neisseria sp.
Tetracyclines	Efflux	Staphylococci
		Streptococci
		Enterococci
		Enterobacteriaceae
		Bacteroides sp.
Rifampin	Reduced DNA polymerase binding	Staphylococci
		Enterococci
		M. tuberculosis
Folate-inhibitors	Altered targets	Staphylococci
Trimethoprim/sulfamethoxazole	Reduced permeability	Streptococci
		S. pneumoniae
		Enterobacteriaceae
		Campylobacter sp.
Glycopeptides	Altered target	Enterococci
Vancomycin		Staphylococci

Modified from Neu HC: The crisis in antibiotic resistance, *Science* 1992; 257:1064.

bind and consequently are unable to inhibit bacterial cell wall synthesis. In reality, it is somewhat misleading to call these acquired proteins PBP because their virtue to the bacteria is that they resist binding by penicillins. All methicillin-resistant *S. aureus* or MRSA (a bad name because MRSA is resistant to all β-lactam agents and because methicillin is no longer used clinically) resists β-lactams because of the acquisition of a novel protein called PBP2a. MRSA previously was confined to hospitals but recently has spread to the community setting, and clusters of community-onset MRSA infection have been reported with increasing frequency. Penicillin resistance in *S. pneumoniae* is also due to altered PBPs.

With the exception of vancomycin, resistance to every major class of antibiotic was recognized before or within a few years of introduction for clinical use. Resistance to vancomycin took three decades to develop. The mechanism is complex but involves a change in the target site for the drug on the side chains of cell wall peptidoglycan. This mechanism likely evolved from the *Streptomyces* that produce glycopeptide antibiotics and is an example of resistance in pathogenic bacteria borrowed from the self-protection mechanism used by the antibiotic producing organism.

A change of only one amino acid in the β-subunit of the DNA-directed RNA polymerase can confer resistance to rifampin. For this reason, rifampin is almost always used in combination with other agents to prevent development of resistance. Resistance to quinolones is usually attributable to an altered DNA gyrase.

Decreased entry and increased efflux

Decreased uptake has been described for aminoglycosides, some β-lactams, tetracyclines, and others. Efflux pumps are the main mechanism of resistance for tetracyclines and have also been described for quinolones.

Destruction or inactivation of drug

The most widely recognized example of bacterial drug resistance is that of the β-lactamases. These enzymes catalyze the hydrolysis of penicillins, cephalosporins, and other β-lactams. When hydrolyzed, the β-lactam is unable to bind to bacterial transpeptidases and other enzymes needed for cell wall synthesis and repair. The β-lactamases are discussed in Chapter 45. Many enzymes have been described that inactivate aminoglycosides.

Synthesis by resistant metabolic pathway

Some thymidine-requiring streptococci are not inhibited by trimethoprim and sulfonamides because the microorganisms fail to undergo the thymine-less death that normally occurs when bacteria are exposed to these agents. The resistant bacteria produce adequate concentrations of thymidine nucleotides by an alternative pathway and as a result survive exposure to these drugs.

FURTHER READING

Antimicrobial prophylaxis in surgery. *Medical Lett* 2001; 43:92.

Gold HS, Moellering RC Jr. Antimicrobial-drug resistance. *N Engl J Med* 1996; 335:1445-1453.

Steinberg JP, Blass MA. Non-surgical antibiotic prophylaxis. In Schlossberg D: *Current therapy of infectious diseases*, Philadelphia, Mosby-Harcourt Health Sciences, 2000.

Self-assessment questions

1. In which of the following infections is it necessary to have a drug with bactericidal activity?

a. Bacterial exacerbation of bronchitis
b. Pneumonia
c. Meningitis
d. Urinary tract infection

2. Which of the following agents should be avoided in treating an infection in a pregnant woman?

a. Ampicillin
b. Tetracycline
c. Cephalexin
d. Erythromycin

3. The combination of ampicillin and gentamicin is an example of:

a. Indifference.
b. Synergy.
c. Antagonism.
d. Bacterial symbiosis.

4. Perioperative antimicrobial prophylaxis:

a. Should be started just before surgery to ensure adequate serum concentrations of antibiotics when the incision is made.
b. Should include antibiotics active against all possible bacterial pathogens.
c. Is indicated for all surgical procedures regardless of the infection risk.
d. Is more effective if the antibiotic is continued for >24 hours following the procedure.
e. Usually involves a penicillin derivative because of their short half-life.

5. Protein synthesis inhibitors include all *except:*

a. Erythromycin.
b. Aminoglycosides.
c. Tetraycline.
d. Fluoroquinolones.
e. Clindamycin.

6. The following antibiotics are matched with a resistance mechanism. Which one is *incorrect?*

a. Penicillin	β-lactamase production
b. Quinolone	Mutations of DNA gyrase gene
c. Vancomycin	Enzymatic inactivation
d. Sulfonamide	"Bypass" pathway in folic acid metabolism
e. Erythromycin	Altered ribosomal target

CHAPTER 45

Bacterial cell wall inhibitors

Carolyn V. Gould
James P. Steinberg

Major Drugs

Penicillins	β-Lactamase inhibitors
Cephalosporins	Vancomycin (Vancocin)
Carbapenems	Bacitracin (Baciguent, AK-Tracin)
Monobactams	

Therapeutic overview

The **β-lactam** and **glycopeptide** antibiotics act by inhibiting synthesis of bacterial cell walls. The β-lactams encompass the widely used **penicillins** and **cephalosporins,** as well as the **carbapenems** and **monobactams.** Although penicillin was first discovered in 1928, it was not until the early 1940s that penicillin was developed as a therapeutic drug. Difficulties in large-scale manufacturing were finally overcome by use of a deep-fermentation procedure, allowing for its widespread availability. The remarkable results achieved with penicillin therapy revolutionized treatment of infectious diseases.

Since its introduction, however, many strains of bacteria, particularly *Staphylococcus aureus,* have become **resistant** to penicillin through production of metabolic enzymes called β-lactamases. Resistance to penicillin led to development of semisynthetic penicillins resistant to hydrolysis by β-lactamases as well as numerous compounds with greater activity against gram-negative organisms. The development of resistance to β-lactams is an ongoing clinical problem and is increasing at a dramatic rate. β-Lactam resistance may be mediated by β-lactamases, altered **penicillin binding proteins** (PBPs), or reduced permeability or active efflux of the drugs by resistant bacteria.

β-Lactam agents are **bactericidal** under most conditions. Because they inhibit cell wall production, they have maximal activity against rapidly dividing bacteria. The clinically used β-lactams differ in the following ways:

- The organisms against which they are effective
- Their pharmacokinetics, stability, and modes of administration
- The type and extent of resistance found in specific bacteria

The glycopeptide drug **vancomycin** and the topical agent **bacitracin** are also bactericidal cell wall inhibitors but do not contain a β-lactam nucleus. Vancomycin was originally isolated from an actinomycete found in soil.

Abbreviations

CSF	cerebrospinal fluid
ESBLs	extended-spectrum β-lactamases
GI	gastrointestinal
IM	intramuscular
IV	intravenous
MIC	minimal inhibitory concentration
MRSA	methicillin-resistant *Staphylococcus aureus*
NAG	*N*-acetylglucosamine
NAM	*N*-acetylmuramate
PBPs	penicillin-binding proteins

It is primarily active against gram-positive bacteria and came into prominence for several reasons. These include the occurrence of **methicillin-resistant *S. aureus*** (MRSA), the presence of pseudomembranous colitis caused by *Clostridium difficile,* and the increasing number of organisms resistant to β-lactams. Resistance to vancomycin, however, is an increasing problem in enterococcus species. Even more alarming has been the discovery of clinical isolates of *S. aureus* with reduced vancomycin susceptibility, or even full resistance mediated by transfer of resistance genes from enterococcus species.

Therapeutic considerations are summarized in the Therapeutic Overview box.

THERAPEUTIC OVERVIEW

β-Lactam agents

Bactericidal: inhibit many gram-positive and gram-negative organisms

Agents differ by
- Organism inhibited
- Pharmacokinetics
- Bacterial resistance

Agents include
- Penicillins
- Cephalosporins
- Carbapenems
- Monobactams
- β-Lactamase inhibitors

Vancomycin

Bactericidal: inhibits many methicillin-resistant staphylococci

Bacitracin

Topical use only for gram-positive bacteria

Mechanisms of action

β-Lactams

All β-lactam antibiotics have a β-lactam ring structure (Fig. 45-1, *A*). This is a four-membered ring; a lactam is a cyclic amide, and the β indicates that the amine is on the second carbon from the carbonyl. Such a small ring is normally structurally strained with **low inherent stability,** explaining why some penicillins readily

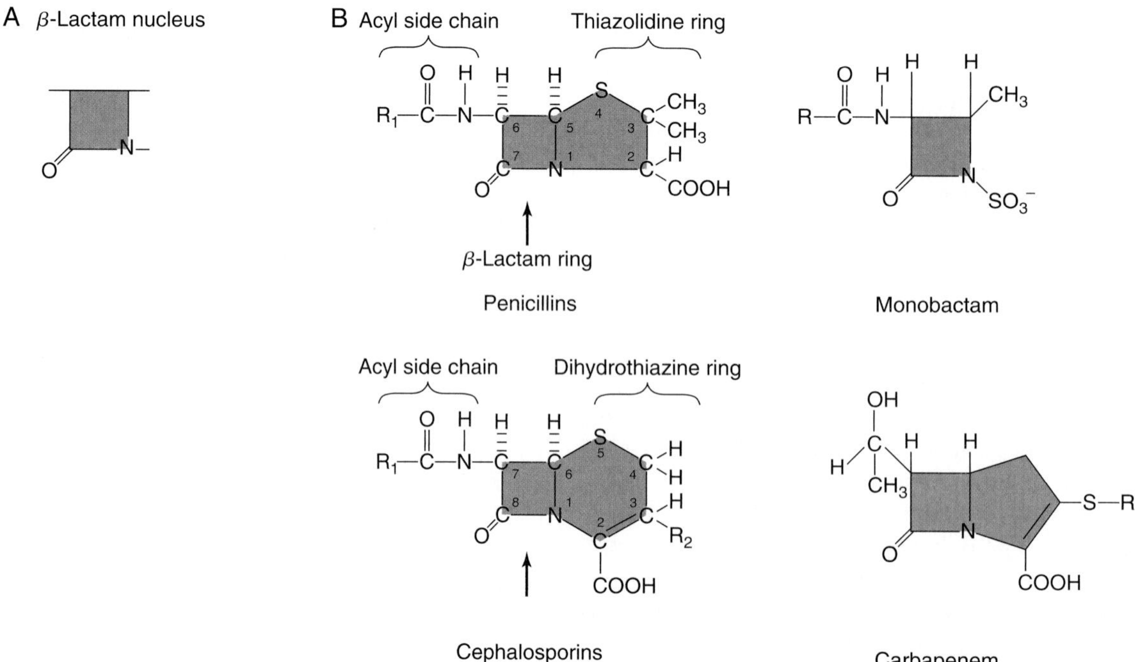

Figure 45-1 **A,** β-Lactam ring structure. **B,** General structures of the four main classes of β-lactam antibiotics. Additional variations are possible at some of the non–R-group positions. The arrow points to the bond that is broken during β-lactamase–catalyzed hydrolysis.

undergo hydrolysis and because of high stomach acidity are not effective when given orally.

The general structures of penicillins, cephalosporins, carbapenems, and monobactams are shown in Figure 45-1, *B*. All of these classes, except the monobactams, have a second ring in addition to the β-lactam ring. In penicillins, the second ring is a thiazolidine, while in cephalosporins it is a dihydrothiazine. Carbapenems have an unsaturated ring with an external sulfur. Many variations have been made by addition of different side chains, which can alter many of the properties of the antibiotic.

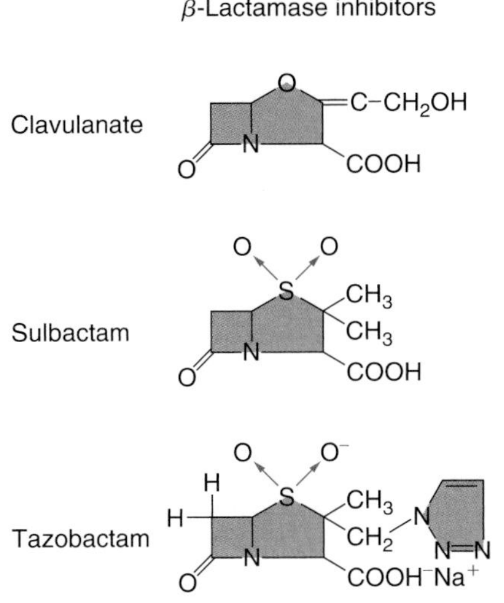

Figure 45-2 Structures of β-lactamase inhibitors.

Some penicillin derivatives are marketed in combination with β-lactamase inhibitors (Fig. 45-2), which also contain the β-lactam ring structure.

β-lactams interfere with bacterial **cell wall synthesis.** The outer cellular coverings of gram-positive and -negative bacteria differ (Fig. 45-3), but both classes have a rigid cell wall composed of a highly cross-linked peptidoglycan matrix. In gram-negative bacteria, an outer membrane of lipopolysaccharide is located exterior to a few layers of peptidoglycan. In gram-positive bacteria, the lipopolysaccharide layer is missing and many more (15-30) layers of peptidoglycan are present. The cell wall is assembled in a series of steps, originating in the cytoplasm of the bacteria and ending outside the cytoplasmic membrane.

The glycan part of the peptidoglycan is composed of repeating disaccharide units of *N*-acetylglucosamine (NAG) and *N*-acetylmuramate (NAM) connected through β-1,4-linkages. A pentapeptide is attached to the glycan (Fig. 45-4). The rigid peptidoglycan cell wall is formed by cross-linking of the glycan chains by peptide chains to form continuous two-dimensional sheets (Fig. 45-5).

The initial stages of peptidoglycan synthesis occur in the cytoplasm. A membrane carrier lipid transports the NAG and NAM-pentapeptide across the cytoplasmic membrane, and the saccharide units are then linked in sequence to form long chains of alternating disaccharides. The final stage involves a **cross-linking** reaction, which occurs outside the cytoplasmic membrane but is catalyzed by membrane-bound **transpeptidase** enzymes. It is at the final cross-linking step, during

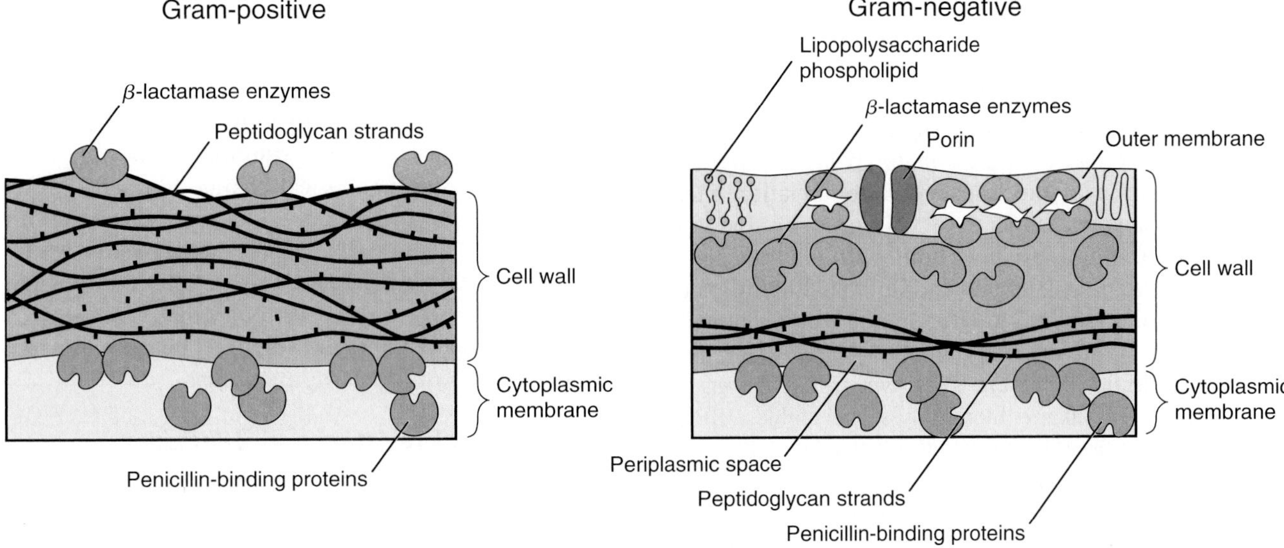

Figure 45-3 Outer coating of gram-positive (15-30 strands) and gram-negative bacteria showing a thinner (3-5 strands) rigid peptidoglycan structure but an added outer membrane for gram-negative cells. β-Lactam drugs act by inhibiting the synthesis of the rigid peptidoglycan part of the cell wall.

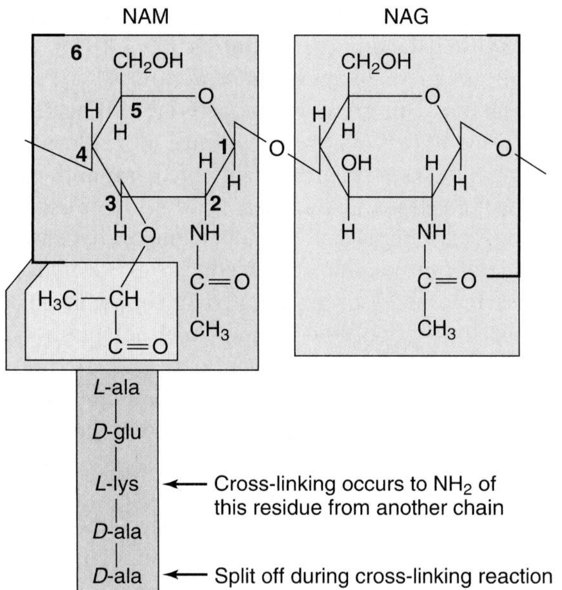

Figure 45-4 Repeating glycan portion of peptidoglycan matrix, consisting of the disaccharide *N*-acetylmuramate (NAM) plus *N*-acetylglucosamine (NAG) connected through the β-1, 4-link and with the lactyl and pentapeptide attached as shown.

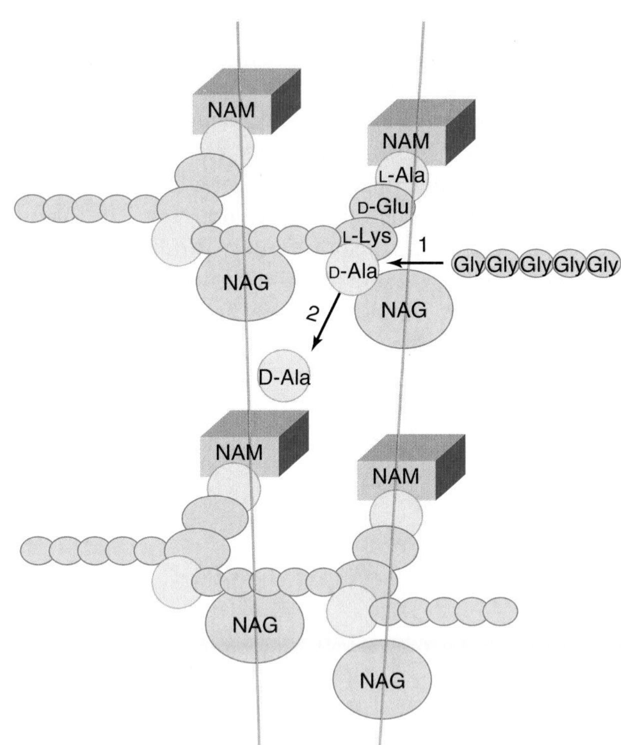

Figure 45-5 Cross-linking reaction to join strands and form sheets of peptidoglycan. 1. The D-Ala-D-Ala terminus of the pentapeptide reacts with a transpeptidase enzyme to displace the final D-Ala (2), forming a cross-link with the third residue of the pentapeptide of an adjacent chain. To prevent cross-linking, β-lactams inhibit the transpeptidase enzymes, while vancomycin binds to the terminal D-Ala-D-Ala.

synthesis of the rigid peptidoglycan matrix, that β-lactams and glycopeptide antibiotics (by different mechanisms) exert their actions.

During the cross-linking reaction to connect the peptidoglycan chains, the D-Ala-D-Ala terminus of the pentapeptide reacts with a transpeptidase to displace the final D-Ala and form an acylenzyme intermediate. This intermediate is reactive and readily couples to the free amino group of the third residue of the pentapeptide of an adjacent chain, thus completing the cross-linking and regenerating the enzyme. Molecular modeling shows that penicillins and cephalosporins can assume a conformation very similar to that of the D-Ala-D-Ala peptide, with the reactive β-lactam ring in the same position as the transpeptidase acylation site. Therefore β-lactams undergo acylation, with the β-lactam ring forming a **covalent bond** with the transpeptidase, inactivating it, and preventing cross-linking. The points of antibiotic binding in the inhibition of cell wall synthesis are summarized in Figure 45-5.

The multiple β-lactam–sensitive transpeptidases in bacterial cytoplasmic membranes are called PBPs, because they covalently bind radiolabeled penicillin G. The PBPs in a given organism are numbered in order by decreasing molecular weight. PBPs of gram-negative and -positive bacteria differ; there are usually five PBPs in gram-positive and six in gram-negative organisms. However, a particular numerical designation is not the same protein in different organisms. In addition to their transpeptidase activity, some PBPs show carboxypeptidase or endopeptidase activity and hydrolyze β-lactams.

The effects of exposure to β-lactams depend on the bacterial species and the PBP to which the drug binds. Some bacteria swell rapidly and burst. Some develop into long filamentous structures that do not divide but eventually fragment, with disruption of the organism. Others show no morphological change but cease to be viable. Lysis of gram-positive bacteria treated with β-lactams is ultimately dependent on autolysins, which are normally involved in new cell wall synthesis when cells divide. There are bacteria that lack these autolysins, which are termed "tolerant" because they are only inhibited, not killed, by β-lactams.

Mechanisms of resistance to β-lactams

There are three major mechanisms of resistance to β-lactams:

- Destruction by **β-lactamase enzymes**
- Failure to reach the target PBP
- Failure to bind to the target PBP

These mechanisms may coexist, and in some cases it takes a combination, such as decreased permeability and poor binding, within a single organism to confer resistance.

The major forms of resistance of gram-positive bacteria to β-lactams stem from β-lactamases or altered PBPs. Within two decades of the first widespread use of penicillin G, most *S. aureus* showed resistance to the drug. Currently, over 95% of staphylococci are resistant to penicillin G and ampicillin. This resistance occurs by spread of a plasmid-encoded β-lactamase, which acylates the β-lactam ring to inactivate the drug. In gram-positive species, such as staphylococci, β-lactamase expression is induced by penicillin, and they are secreted as exoenzymes.

The presence of PBPs that **bind poorly** to β-lactams, either due to intrinsic structural features or acquisition of alterations by mutation, also results in resistance to β-lactams, especially in gram-positive organisms. An important clinical example is MRSA, which poses a serious hospital and, increasingly, a community problem. These staphylococci are not inhibited by any currently available β-lactams because of acquisition of a high molecular weight PBP-2a with poor affinity for all β-lactams. The recent marked increase in penicillin resistance in *S. pneumoniae* stems from multiple changes in the structure of several PBPs. Several of these changes in more-resistant strains are associated with non-pneumococcal DNA inserted into PBP genes by homologous recombination. Enterococci are intrinsically resistant to cephalosporins, because they do not bind to enterococcal PBPs. Aztreonam also fails to bind to the PBPs of gram-positive species and does not inhibit them.

Common forms of resistance in gram-negative bacteria stem from the presence of β-lactamases and failure of the drug to reach the PBPs adjacent to the outer lipopolysaccharide membrane. The β-lactamases of gram-negative bacteria can be encoded by chromosomal or plasmid genes. A wider variety of β-lactamases are produced by gram-negative than gram-positive bacteria.

Over 300 β-lactamases have been described. Mutations that occurred in preexisting β-lactamases after introduction of new β-lactams have produced the so-called extended-spectrum β-lactamases (ESBLs), which are plasmid-encoded enzymes found mainly in *Klebsiella* spp. and *Escherichia coli.* The ESBLs confer high-level resistance to ceftazidime and aztreonam, as well as reduced susceptibility to other third-generation cephalosporins. There are several classification systems for β-lactamases based on structure, spectra of activity, and susceptibility to inhibitors. The β-lactamase inhibitors block the activity of most plasmid-mediated β-lactamases and some chromosomal β-lactamases. However, they do not inhibit the inducible ampC chromosomal β-lactamases expressed by many nosocomial gram-negative pathogens, particularly *Enterobacter cloacae* and *Pseudomonas aeruginosa.*

In gram-negative bacteria, β-lactams must pass an outer lipid membrane to reach the PBPs on the cytoplasmic membrane (see Fig. 45-3). Channels in the outer membrane, referred to as **porins,** allow β-lactams to pass through. Alterations in porin proteins that reduce the amount of drug reaching the PBPs have been observed. For example, *P. aeruginosa* can delete the porin protein through which imipenem passes and develop resistance. Some β-lactams are extremely resistant to β-lactamases but do not readily pass through porins of gram-negative outer membranes and thus fail to inhibit these bacteria.

Vancomycin and bacitracin

Vancomycin and bacitracin are two cell wall inhibitors that are structurally quite different from the β-lactam compounds and function by different mechanisms. Vancomycin is a **glycopeptide** with a high molecular weight. It binds to the free carboxyl end of the pentapeptide, sterically interfering with cross-linking of the peptidoglycan backbone. The specificity of the interaction of vancomycin with D-Ala-D-Ala partially explains the minimal resistance that has been observed with this antibiotic.

However, more than 25% of nosocomial enterococcal isolates, primarily *E. faecium,* are now vancomycin resistant. Resistance is caused by production of a new pentapeptide ending in a terminal D-Ala-D-Lac instead of D-Ala-D-Ala, which does not bind vancomycin. There are also other types of resistance to vancomycin (Table 45-1); the *vanA* cluster of genes, transferred by a transposable genetic element, is the best characterized. This is an elegant resistance mechanism that contains at least eight genes. One gene product, *van S,* functions like a transmembrane receptor, senses the presence of vancomycin, and activates the gene *van R* to upregulate expression of three additional genes. The products of these three genes cleave the terminal D-Ala-D-Ala and insert D-Ala-D-Lac. Similar resistance genes are present in streptomyces that produce glycopeptide antibiotics and probably evolved as a self-preservation strategy for the organism. Vancomycin-resistant strains of *S. aureus,* mediated by increased numbers of vancomycin binding sites in the cell wall, are also emerging. Also, the first two clinical strains of *S. aureus* isolates with high level vancomycin resistance, which acquired the *vanA* gene cluster from vancomycin-resistant enterococci, appeared in 2002.

Table 45-1 Resistance of gram-positive bacteria to vancomycin

Mechanisms	Altered Binding Sites			Increased Numbers of Binding Sites
Resistance type	VanA	VanB	VanC	
Development	Plasmid	Plasmid	Chromosomal	Chromosomal
Level of resistance	High	Low	Low	Low
Major microorganisms	*E. faecium* *E. faecalis* *S. aureus*	*E. faecium* *E. faecalis*	*E. gallinarum* *E. casseliflavus*	*S. aureus*

Table 45-2 Pharmacokinetic parameters of penicillins and β-lactamase Inhibitors

Penicillin	Route(s) of Administration	Half-Life (hrs)	Protein Bound (%)	Elimination
Penicillin G*	Oral*/IV	0.5	55	R (main), M
Benzathine penicillin	IM	14 days	55	R (main)
Penicillin V	Oral	1.0	60	R (main)
Oxacillin	Oral/IV	0.4	92	R (main), M
Dicloxacillin	Oral	0.6	97	R (main), M
Nafcillin	IV	0.5	90	R (some); mainly B
Ampicillin	IV	1.0	15	R (some); some B
Amoxicillin	Oral	1.0	15	R (main)
Ticarcillin	IV	1.2	50	R (main), M
Piperacillin	IV	1.3	50	R, M
β-LACTAMASE INHIBITORS				
Clavulanate				
(with amoxicillin)	Oral	1.0	30	R (main), M
(with ticarcillin)	IV			
Sulbactam (with ampicillin)	IV	1.0	15	R (main)
Tazobactam (with piperacillin)	IV	1.0	20	R (main), M

M, Metabolized; *B*, biliary; *R*, renal.
*Poor acid stability.

Bacitracin is a polypeptide bactericidal antibiotic. It inhibits bacterial cell wall synthesis by interfering with dephosphorylation of the lipid carrier that moves the early cell wall components through the membrane.

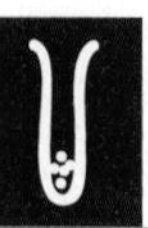

Pharmacokinetics

Penicillins

Penicillins differ greatly in oral absorption, binding to serum proteins, metabolism, and renal excretion. Most penicillins are excreted unchanged via renal tubular mechanisms, and dosages must be adjusted in patients with severely depressed renal function.

In general, penicillins are well distributed to most areas of the body, achieving therapeutic concentrations in some abscesses and in otic, pleural, peritoneal, and synovial fluids. Distribution to eye, brain, and prostatic fluid is low, whereas urinary concentrations generally are high. Concentrations of penicillins in CSF are less than 1% of plasma values in uninflamed meninges and rise to 5% during inflammation. Penicillins do not accumulate in phagocytic cells, because the drug that enters is extruded by a pump.

All β-lactam agents exhibit time-dependent killing of bacteria and have little postantibiotic effect, unlike fluoroquinolones and aminoglycosides, which function by concentration-dependent mechanisms. Consequently, efficacy of the β-lactam depends on the amount of time the concentration of the drug is above the minimal inhibitory concentration (MIC) for the organism at the site of infection.

The pharmacokinetic parameters for penicillins of clinical interest are summarized in Table 45-2.

Penicillins G and V

Penicillin G is rapidly hydrolyzed in the stomach at low pH. Decreased gastric acid production improves absorption, while food intake impairs it. Absorption is rapid, primarily in the duodenum. Unabsorbed penicillin is destroyed by bacteria in the colon. In contrast, **penicillin V** is acid-stable and well absorbed even if ingested with food.

A peak plasma concentration of penicillin G is achieved in 15 to 30 minutes after IM injection but declines quickly because of rapid removal by the kidney. Repository forms are available as **procaine** or **benzathine** salts. Procaine penicillin is an equimolar mixture of procaine and penicillin and results in concentrations of penicillin G for 12 hours to several days after doses of 300,000 to 2.4 million units. Benzathine penicillin is a 1:2 combination of penicillin and the ammonium base, is slowly absorbed, and plasma concentrations are detectable for up to 15 to 30 days.

Penicillin G is primarily eliminated by tubular secretion and renal clearance is equivalent to renal plasma flow. Excretion can be blocked by probenecid. Renal elimination is also considerably less in newborns because of poorly developed tubular function; the half-life of penicillin G is 3 hours in newborns, compared with 30 minutes in 1 year old children. Excretion declines with age, but adjustments in dose are not necessary until renal clearance decreases below 30 ml/min.

Hemodialysis will remove penicillin G from the body, but peritoneal dialysis is less efficient. A small amount is excreted in human milk and saliva, but it is not present in tears or sweat.

β-Lactamase–resistant penicillins

The β-lactamase–resistant penicillins **oxacillin, cloxacillin,** and **dicloxacillin** are acid stable and orally absorbed, but absorption is decreased in the presence of food. Peak plasma concentrations are achieved approximately 1 hour after ingestion, and they are all highly protein bound. Elimination is primarily via the kidney, with some biliary excretion and some liver metabolism. These drugs are minimally removed from the body by hemodialysis. Oxacillin is less effective orally; adequate plasma and CSF concentrations are achieved when it is administered IV. **Nafcillin** is erratically absorbed when ingested orally, and the preferred route is IV. Elimination is primarily by biliary excretion. It enters the CSF in concentrations adequate to treat staphylococcal meningitis or brain abscesses.

Ampicillin, amoxicillin, ticarcillin, and piperacillin

Ampicillin is moderately well absorbed after oral administration, but absorption is decreased in the presence of food. Its half-life can be prolonged if it is coadministered with probenecid. Ampicillin is well distributed to most body compartments, and therapeutic concentrations are achieved in pleural, synovial, peritoneal, and cerebrospinal fluids. Ampicillin is excreted in bile and undergoes enterohepatic recirculation. It is primarily removed by renal excretion. **Amoxicillin** is better absorbed than ampicillin after oral ingestion and is not influenced by food. Its distribution is similar to that of ampicillin. **Ticarcillin** is not absorbed from the gastrointestinal (GI) tract and is administered parenterally. It is excreted by renal tubules. Distribution is extensive, except that concentrations in CSF are inadequate for treating *Pseudomonas* meningitis. **Piperacillin** can only be administered IV or IM, since none is absorbed orally. It has nonlinear pharmacokinetics, with plasma concentrations not proportional to dose.

β-Lactamase inhibitor combinations

The β-lactamase inhibitors are marketed only with a penicillin derivative. In general, the paired penicillin/β-lactamase inhibitor have similar half-lives. However, clearance of the two compounds may diverge in renal insufficiency. **Clavulanate** in combination with amoxicillin or ticarcillin is available, and moderately well absorbed, with peak plasma concentrations 1 hour after ingestion. In combination with ticarcillin and administered IV, clavulanate is rapidly distributed. Clavulanate enters most body compartments, with therapeutic concentrations reached in middle ear fluid, tonsils, sinus secretions, bile, and the urinary tract. **Sulbactam** is combined with ampicillin for parenteral use. Its pharmacokinetic properties are similar to those of ampicillin, and it is widely distributed in the body, including the CSF in the presence of meningitis. It is excreted in the urine, and its half-life is increased to 6 hours in adults in renal failure and in newborns. **Tazobactam** is combined with piperacillin. Its half-life is prolonged in the presence of piperacillin, and it is excreted primarily by the kidneys.

Cephalosporins

Many cephalosporins can be administered only parenterally. Although they are distributed widely into body compartments, only a few enter the CSF in sufficient concentrations for treatment of meningitis. Cephalosporins are generally eliminated by renal excretion, and their accumulation depends on renal status. Ceftriaxone is an exception, with significant biliary excretion. All cephalosporins reach high enough urinary concentrations to treat urinary tract infections. In the absence of common duct obstruction, biliary concentrations of all cephalosporins exceed plasma concentrations.

Table 45-3 Pharmacokinetic parameters of cephalosporins

Cephalosporin	Route of Administration	Half-Life (hrs)	Protein Bound (%)	Route of Elimination	CSF Penetration*
FIRST GENERATION					
Cefazolin	IV/IM	2.0	85	R	
Cephalexin	Oral	1.0	15	R	
Cefadroxil	Oral	1.5	20	R	
SECOND GENERATION					
Cefaclor	Oral	1.0	25	R, M	
Cefprozil	Oral	1	20	R	
Loracarbef	Oral	1	25	R	
Cefuroxime	IV/IM/Oral	1.7	35	R	Yes
Cefoxitin	IV/IM	0.8	70	R	
Cefotetan	IV/IM	3.5	85	R	
Cefprozil	Oral	1.3	45	R	
THIRD GENERATION					
Cefotaxime	IV/IM	1.0	50	R	Yes
Ceftizoxime	IV/IM	1.8	30	R	Yes
Ceftriaxone	IV/IM	6-8	90	R(50%), B(60%)	Yes
Cefixime	Oral	3.7	75	R(50%), ?(other)	
Ceftazidime	IV/IM	1.8	15	R	Yes
Cefpodoxime	Oral	1.2	25	R	
FOURTH GENERATION					
Cefepime	IV/IM	2.1	20	R	Yes

R, Renal; *B*, biliary.
*Adequate for therapeutic use.

Pharmacokinetic parameters for cephalosporins of clinical interest are listed in Table 45-3.

First-generation cephalosporins **Cefazolin** can be administered IM or IV, is widely distributed, but does not adequately penetrate the CSF. **Cephalexin** and **cefadroxil** are extremely well absorbed orally to yield a wide distribution in body tissues, including bone. Dosages must be adjusted in patients with renal failure.

Second-generation cephalosporins **Cefuroxime** can be administered parenterally or as cefuroxime axetil with sufficient oral bioavailability to be clinically useful. Cefuroxime axetil is hydrolyzed into cefuroxime after oral absorption. **Cefoxitin** can only be administered IV or IM, with good distribution except for inadequate CSF concentrations. **Cefotetan** is administered IV and has a long half-life. An orally administered agent, **cefaclor,** is metabolized in addition to being eliminated renally. **Loracarbef** is similar to cefaclor but more stable.

Third-generation cephalosporins **Cefotaxime, ceftriaxone, ceftizoxime,** and **ceftazidime** enter the CSF and can be used to treat meningitis. Cefotaxime is partially metabolized to a desacetyl derivative, which has antibacterial activity less than that of cefotaxime but may act synergistically with the parent compound against many microorganisms. Ceftriaxone differs from other cephalosporins by its long plasma half-life. It is also highly protein bound, with a greater fraction of free drug present at higher total concentrations, so the drug is administered once daily. Ceftriaxone is not metabolized but is excreted in bile and by the kidneys. Dosage need not be adjusted in renal failure, but combined hepatic-renal dysfunction is likely to require dose adjustment. Ceftriaxone is not removed by hemodialysis, so does not require additional dosing after dialysis. **Cefixime** is moderately well absorbed orally, with a half-life of about 4 hours. **Cefpodoxime** is better absorbed orally but has a shorter half-life.

Fourth-generation cephalosporins **Cefepime** is administered parenterally, has a half-life of about 2 hours, and penetrates well into the CSF.

Carbapenems and monobactams

Pharmacokinetic parameters of the carbapenem antibiotics imipenem, meropenem, and ertapenem, and the only monobactam, aztreonam, are summarized in Table 45-4.

Imipenem is administered primarily IV, is widely distributed, but enters CSF only during inflammation. It has a high affinity for brain tissue. Imipenem is eliminated by glomerular filtration and tubular secretion and is inactivated by a dehydropeptidase in the renal

Table 45-4 Pharmacokinetic parameters of carbapenems, aztreonam, vancomycin, and bacitracin

Agent	Route of Administration	Half-Life (hrs)	Protein Bound (%)	Route of Elimination	Metabolized
Imipenem	IV	1.0	20	R	Yes*
Meropenem	IV	1	2	R	Yes (minor)
Ertapenem	IV	4	95	R	Yes
Aztreonam	IV	1.5-2.0	45-60	R	No
Vancomycin	IV, oral†	6‡	55	R	No
Bacitracin	Topical				

*Prevented by cilastatin.
†Used to treat *C. difficile*—associated diarrhea or colitis.
‡5-9 days in anuric patients.

tubules. To overcome this hydrolysis, imipenem is combined with a renal dehydropeptidase inhibitor, **cilastatin.** Cilastatin has no antibacterial activity and does not affect the properties of imipenem, except to prevent its hydrolysis. Minimal amounts of drug are excreted in bile, though biliary concentrations are adequate for treatment of biliary tract infections. Serum half-life increases as creatinine clearance falls and is increased in patients with renal insufficiency. **Meropenem** has a broad spectrum of action similar to imipenem, also penetrates well into most fluids and tissues as well as the CSF after IV administration. Most meropenem is excreted unchanged in the urine, so dosages must be adjusted in renal insufficiency. Meropenem is not hydrolyzed by renal dehydropeptidase. **Ertapenem** has recently been approved for IV use in the United States. Its advantage over imipenem and meropenem is its relatively long half-life, enabling once-daily dosing. It is highly protein-bound and mainly renally excreted, requiring dosage changes with severe renal impairment. It is also less susceptible to hydrolysis by renal dehydropeptidase and is not administered with cilastatin.

Aztreonam is not orally absorbed but can be administered IV or IM. It is widely distributed to all body sites and compartments, including the CSF. It is removed by glomerular filtration and tubular secretion, so doses must be reduced for renal insufficiency.

Vancomycin and bacitracin

Pharmacokinetic parameters for vancomycin and bacitracin are also summarized in Table 45-4.

Vancomycin is not absorbed and is administered IV, except for treatment of *G. difficile*-associated diarrhea or colitis, when it is administered orally and acts locally. IV vancomycin enters many body fluids, including bile and pleural, pericardial, peritoneal, and synovial fluids. It crosses the meninges during inflammation. Vancomycin is eliminated by glomerular filtration, with no metabolism, and dosage should be adjusted on the basis of renal function. Vancomycin is not removed efficiently by hemodialysis or peritoneal dialysis. Monitoring of plasma concentrations is necessary to ensure therapeutic concentrations are achieved and toxicity averted in patients with depressed renal function.

Bacitracin is applied topically and is combined in several preparations with neomycin or polymyxin.

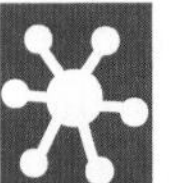

Relation of mechanisms of action to clinical response

Penicillins and cephalosporins

Penicillins Penicillins are classified by their main antibacterial activities, as follows:

- Penicillin G and penicillin V are active against gram-positive and gram-negative cocci, except organisms that produce β-lactamase or those with highly altered PBPs (such as highly resistant pneumococci). They are ineffective against the majority of *S. aureus* strains.
- β-Lactamase–resistant agents (oxacillin, nafcillin, and dicloxacillin) are effective against *S. aureus* (unless resistant to methicillin, an older agent in this class used for susceptibility testing) and are less active than penicillin G against streptococci.
- Aminopenicillins (ampicillin and amoxicillin) are active against gram-positive and gram-negative organisms and also inhibit β-lactamase–free strains of *Haemophilus influenzae, E. coli, Proteus mirabilis, Neisseria gonorrhoeae,* and *Salmonella* species.
- The carboxypenicillin ticarcillin inhibits *P. aeruginosa* and some *Enterobacter* and *Proteus* species but is destroyed by β-lactamases.
- The ureidopenicillin piperacillin inhibits ampicillin-susceptible organisms, *Pseudomonas,* some *Klebsiella*

organisms, and streptococci but is destroyed by some β-lactamases.

Penicillins G and V Although antibiotic resistance to penicillin is widespread in many bacterial species, penicillin remains the drug of choice for a variety of infections including streptococcal pharyngitis, other infections caused by β-hemolytic streptococci, and viridans streptococcal infections including endocarditis. Penicillin is also the drug of choice for all forms of syphilis, meningococcal infections, actinomycosis, and several less-common infections. Recent increases in resistance among *S. pneumoniae* militate against use of penicillin in meningeal infections unless the isolate is confirmed to be susceptible. Even moderately resistant extrameningeal pneumococcal infections (pneumonia), however, still respond to penicillin. Although *N. meningitidis* remains highly susceptible, many strains of *N. gonorrhoeae* are resistant through plasmid-mediated β-lactamase production.

Many anaerobic species, except the *Bacteroides fragilis* group, are susceptible to penicillin G, but aerobic gram-negative Enterobacteriaceae and *Pseudomonas* species are resistant.

β-Lactamase-resistant penicillins The β-lactamase–resistant penicillins are not destroyed by most β-lactamases of staphylococci. They are still used principally to treat staphylococcal infections, although strains of *S. aureus* that contain altered PBPs conferring resistance to all β-lactams (MRSA) are dramatically increasing in frequency. The β-lactamase-resistant penicillins retain sufficient activity against most streptococci to be clinically useful in treating soft tissue infections. This is important because streptococci and *S. aureus* are the major causes of cellulitis. These agents are less active against oral cavity anaerobic species than penicillin G and show no activity against gram-negative bacilli.

Aminopenicillins, carboxypenicillins, and ureidopenicillins Ampicillin and amoxicillin are inactivated by β-lactamases found with increasing frequency in many gram-positive and gram-negative bacteria. The antibacterial activity of the two compounds is similar; they possess 2 to 4 times more activity than penicillin G against enterococci and *Listeria monocytogenes*. Ampicillin and amoxicillin remain useful for treating some upper respiratory tract infections, provided the infection is not caused by β-lactamase–producing *Haemophilus* organisms.

Ticarcillin and piperacillin are active against *Pseudomonas* and certain species of *Proteus* that are resistant to ampicillin. Piperacillin is also useful for treatment of *Klebsiella* infections. Both drugs are inactivated by many β-lactamases of both gram-positive and gram-negative bacteria and are therefore ineffective against most strains of *S. aureus*, although they inhibit streptococcal and enterococcal species to varying degrees. Piperacillin has moderate activity against anaerobes and is similar to ticarcillin in its activity against *Enterobacter, Serratia*, and *Providencia* species. Because of their β-lactamase susceptibility, these drugs are often combined with aminoglycosides or β-lactamase inhibitors (see below) to treat serious infections. They act synergistically with aminoglycosides to inhibit *P. aeruginosa*.

β-Lactamase inhibitor combinations The β-lactamase inhibitors inactivate the β-lactamases of *S. aureus* and of many gram-negative bacteria, including plasmid-mediated common β-lactamases in *E. coli, Haemophilus, Neisseria, Salmonella*, and *Shigella* species and chromosomal β-lactamases in *Klebsiella, Moraxella*, and *Bacteroides* species. None of the β-lactamase inhibitors bind to the chromosomal ampC β-lactamases in *Pseudomonas, Enterobacter, Citrobacter*, and *Serratia* species. β-Lactamase inhibitors differ in relative potency, and this difference is reflected in the ratio of inhibitor to the paired penicillin. Sulbactam, the weakest inhibitor, is available in a 1:2 ratio of sulbactam to ampicillin; the ratio of tazobactam to piperacillin is 1:8; while the ratio of clavulanate to ticarcillin is 1:30. The major differences between the penicillin β-lactamase inhibitor combinations lie in the different spectra of the penicillin component. All combinations have excellent activity against anaerobes.

Clavulanate has a β-lactam ring but only minimal antibacterial activity, because it binds poorly to most PBPs. It binds irreversibly to β-lactamases and causes irreversible inhibition. Combinations of clavulanate with amoxicillin are used to treat otitis media in children and sinusitis, bacterial exacerbations of bronchitis, and lower respiratory tract infections in adults. This combination is also effective in skin infections, particularly when anaerobic as well as aerobic organisms are present. It is the drug of choice for human and animal bite wounds. The ticarcillin-clavulanate combination is effective in treating hospital-acquired respiratory tract, intraabdominal, obstetric-gynecological, and skin infections and in treating osteomyelitis when mixed bacteria are present.

Sulbactam is a penicillanic acid derivative that has extremely weak antibacterial activity against gram-positive cocci and Enterobacteriaceae but inhibits several other organisms at higher concentrations. It also irreversibly inhibits the β-lactamases inhibited by clavulanate, although it is less potent. Sulbactam is used in combination with ampicillin to treat mixed aerobic and anaerobic skin and soft tissue infections, including diabetic foot infections, mixed aerobic/anaerobic pulmonary and odontogenic infections, and intra-abdominal infections.

Tazobactam is another penicillanic acid derivative that is similar in structure to sulbactam but with a higher potency. It is used in combination with piperacillin. The main advantages of this combination over ticarcillin-clavulanate are better pseudomonal and enterococcal activity, both due to the piperacillin component. Because of the superior antipseudomonal activity of piperacillin, this combination has been used extensively to treat nosocomial infections and infections in neutropenic patients.

Cephalosporins The cephalosporins were discovered in 1945 from a fungus, *Cephalosporium acremonium,* in seawater samples near a sewage outlet in Sardinia. Compounds that possess a methoxy group at position 7 often are called **cephamycins,** but for practical purposes these agents can be considered cephalosporins. Similarly, agents in which the sulfur at position 1 has been replaced by an oxygen are **oxycephems,** and agents in which the sulfur is replaced with a carbon are called **carbacephems.** Microbiologically and pharmacologically these agents are considered cephalosporins.

Cephalosporins are classified by **generations** on the basis of their antimicrobial activity. First-generation cephalosporins have relatively good activity against gram-positive organisms and moderate gram-negative activity, inhibiting many *E. coli, P. mirabilis,* and *K. pneumoniae.* Some second-generation compounds have increased activity against *Haemophilus* and inhibit more gram-negative organisms and show less activity against staphylococci than first-generation agents. Third-generation cephalosporins have less antistaphylococcal activity and more activity against streptococci, Enterobacteriaceae, *Neisseria,* and *Haemophilus* species. Ceftazidime also inhibits *P. aeruginosa.* The third generation cephalosporins are increasingly threatened by the spread of plasmid-mediated ESBLs as well as inducible chromosomal AmpC β-lactamases of certain nosocomial gram-negative pathogens. The so-called fourth-generation cephalosporins represent a new class with expanded activity against some gram-positive cocci and improved stability in response to AmpC β-lactamases. Cefepime, the first fourth-generation cephalosporin approved for use in the U.S., also has activity against *P. aeruginosa.*

Resistance to cephalosporins is caused by the same mechanisms that cause resistance to penicillins—that is, hydrolysis by β-lactamases, failure to pass the outer wall of gram-negative bacteria, or failure to bind to PBPs. However, cephalosporins are less susceptible to β-lactamase than penicillins.

First-generation cephalosporins in clinical use are cefazolin, cephalexin, and cefadroxil. Their spectra of activity are similar, inhibiting most gram-positive cocci (except for enterococci), many *E. coli, Klebsiella* species, and *P. mirabilis* (indole-negative). Most other Enterobacteriaceae are resistant, and *Pseudomonas, Bacteroides,* and *Haemophilus* species are also not inhibited. First-generation cephalosporins are used to treat respiratory, skin, and urinary tract infections and also as prophylaxis before cardiac surgery or before orthopedic prosthesis procedures. Cefazolin has a similar antimicrobial spectrum as the oral agents, but it has slightly enhanced activity against *E. coli* and *Klebsiella* species.

Second-generation cephalosporins in clinical use include cefuroxime, cefprozil, cefaclor, loracarbef, and the cephamycins (cefoxitin and cefotetan). Cefuroxime has greater activity against *S. pneumonia* and *S. pyogenes* than first-generation cephalosporins but less activity against *S. aureus.* Cefaclor, an oral cephalosporin, has similar activity to cephalexin, with somewhat more activity against *H. influenzae, M. catarrhalis, E. coli,* and *P. mirabilis* and is used to treat upper respiratory tract infections in children. Loracarbef is a carbacephem that inhibits β-lactamase–producing *H. influenzae* and respiratory tract pathogens.

Cefoxitin is less active against gram-positive organisms than the first-generation agents but it is more stable against β-lactamase degradation by Enterobacteriaceae (but not *Enterobacter* or *Citrobacter* species) and anaerobic bacteria. Also, it is not hydrolyzed by the plasmid-mediated ESBLs that destroy cefotaxime, ceftriaxone, and ceftazidime and has been used to treat aspiration pneumonia and intraabdominal and pelvic infections. Cefotetan inhibits many β-lactamase–producing Enterobacteriaceae and most *Bacteroides* species. It is also used to treat intraabdominal and pelvic infections. However, these two agents are not as active against *B. fragilis* as the penicillin β-lactamase inhibitor combinations discussed above and not as active against gram-negative bacilli as later cephalosporins. Consequently, use of second-generation cephalosporins has declined, although they are still used for perioperative prophylaxis.

Third-generation cephalosporins include cefotaxime, ceftizoxime, ceftriaxone, cefpodoxime, and ceftazidime. Cefotaxime has excellent activity against gram-positive streptococcal species, including *S. pneumoniae,* and gram-negative *Haemophilus* and *Neisseria* species. A metabolite acts synergistically with cefotaxime, and the two compounds have better activity against *Bacteroides* species than the parent compound. The activity of ceftizoxime and ceftriaxone is similar to that of cefotaxime. These agents are used to treat lower respiratory tract infections, urinary tract infections, skin infections, osteomyelitis, and meningitis. Ceftriaxone also is used to treat gonorrhea and Lyme disease. Because of favorable pharmacokinetics allowing once daily dosing, ceftriaxone is more widely used than the other two agents.

Ceftazidime inhibits *P. aeruginosa,* most streptococci, *Haemophilus, Neisseria,* and most Enterobacteriaceae. It does not inhibit *Bacteroides* species and is inactivated by ESBL-producing organisms. It is less active against gram-positive and anaerobic organisms than other parenteral third-generation cephalosporins. Cefpodoxime inhibits streptococci, *Haemophilus, Moraxella, Neisseria* and many Enterobacteriaceae.

Fourth-generation cephalosporins have an extended spectrum of activity against some gram-positive cocci and Enterobacteriaceae. Structurally related to third-generation cephalosporins, these compounds contain a quaternary nitrogen along with the negatively charged carboxyl, rendering them zwitterions. Zwitterions have a net neutral charge but are capable of penetrating the outer membrane of gram-negative bacteria at higher rates than third-generation drugs. In addition, these compounds have a low affinity for class I AmpC β-lactamases. Cefepime, the only fourth-generation cephalosporin currently available in the United States, is active against most pathogenic gram-positive cocci (except *Enterococcus* and MRSA), Enterobacteriaceae, *P. aeruginosa, H. influenzae, N. meningitidis,* and *N. gonorrhoeae.*

Other β-lactams

Carbapenems Imipenem, meropenem, and ertapenem have high affinity for critical PBPs of a wide variety of organisms, excellent stability against most β-lactamases, and good permeability, leading to very broad antibacterial activity. They inhibit most gram-positive organisms such as the hemolytic streptococci, *S. pneumoniae,* viridans group streptococci, and *S. aureus* (not MRSA). Imipenem and meropenem have some activity against *E. faecalis* but not *E. faecium,* whereas ertapenem does not have antienterococcal activity. Most Enterobacteriaceae, *Haemophilus* species, *Moraxella* species, *Neisseria* species, and *P. aeruginosa* are also inhibited by these compounds, although ertapenem is not active against *P. aeruginosa.* These agents have extensive activity against anaerobic organisms, inhibiting most *Bacteroides* species. They also inhibit *Nocardia* species and some mycobacteria.

Imipenem and meropenem show an interesting postantibiotic effect on many gram-positive and gram-negative bacteria. After the concentration of drug decreases below MIC, the bacteria that have not been killed do not resume growth for another 2-4 hours. The carbapenems are not hydrolyzed by the β-lactamases of gram-positive or gram-negative bacteria, with the exceptions of β-lactamases from *Stenotrophomonas maltophilia* and some *Bacteroides* species. *P. aeruginosa* can develop selective imipenem resistance by deleting a porin protein that imipenem uses to traverse the outer cell membrane, as mentioned previously.

The carbapenems can be used to treat bacteremias and lower respiratory tract, intraabdominal, gynecological, bone and joint, central nervous system, and complicated urinary tract infections caused by resistant bacteria. They may also be used in febrile neutropenic patients. Because of their broad spectrum of activity, these agents are useful as single-agent therapy in mixed aerobic and anaerobic bacterial infections. Resistance in gram-negative nosocomial pathogens such as *Pseudomonas* and *Acinetobacter* is increasingly a problem, however.

Monobactams Aztreonam is a monocyclic β-lactam with a high affinity for the PBPs of certain gram-negative bacteria. It inhibits only aerobic gram-negative bacteria by binding to PBP-3 of Enterobacteriaceae and *P. aeruginosa* to produce long filamentous bacteria that ultimately lyse and die. It does not bind to PBPs of gram-positive or anaerobic species. It is not hydrolyzed by most β-lactamases, except from *Klebsiella oxytoca, S. maltophilia,* and bacteria containing plasmid encoded ESBLs. Aztreonam is effective in treatment of bacteremia, respiratory and urinary tract infections, osteomyelitis, and skin infections. Like other β-lactams, it exhibits synergy when used in combination with aminoglycosides.

Vancomycin and bacitracin

Vancomycin is active against gram-positive organisms only; it is a large molecule and cannot penetrate the outer cell membrane of gram-negative organisms. Vancomycin is weakly bactericidal against staphylococci, including MRSA and methicillin-resistant coagulase-negative staphylococci. However, β-lactam agents are more rapidly bactericidal than vancomycin against methicillin-sensitive staphylococci, and vancomycin appears to be clinically inferior to antistaphylococcal penicillins against susceptible isolates. Hemolytic streptococci such as *S. pyogenes* (group A), *S. agalactiae* (group B), viridans group streptococci and *S. pneumoniae,* including penicillin-resistant strains, are also inhibited. Vancomycin inhibits *Enterococcus faecalis, E. faecium,* and *Listeria* species, but not in a bactericidal fashion. Vancomycin-resistant enterococci, most of which are *E. faecium,* pose a serious clinical problem. A combination of vancomycin with aminoglycosides is bactericidal against susceptible enterococci. Other species that are inhibited include *Bacillus, Actinomyces,* lactobacillus, *Clostridium,* and *Corynebacterium* (diphtheroids).

Vancomycin should be used primarily in serious infections. It is also appropriate for therapy of staphylococcal infections in penicillin-allergic patients and is the drug of choice for treatment of MRSA infections. Pneumonia, endocarditis, osteomyelitis, and wound infections respond to vancomycin, and it also useful for treating infections of prosthetic valves and catheters caused by coagulase-negative staphylococci and *Corynebacterium*.

Vancomycin is also useful for penicillin-allergic patients with serious streptococcal infections (such as viridans group endocarditis) and, in combination with an aminoglycoside, is the agent of choice for the treatment of enterococcal infections in such patients.

Orally administered vancomycin is useful for treating *C. difficile*–associated diarrhea or colitis that fails to respond to metronidazole (see Chapter 52) or that is severe and potentially life-threatening. Because the use of oral vancomycin is a risk factor for colonization and infection with vancomycin-resistant enterococci, however, it is not considered the agent of choice in most cases.

Bacitracin inhibits gram-positive cocci and bacilli and some *Neisseria* species and *Haemophilus* organisms, but Enterobacteriaceae and *Pseudomonas* species are resistant. It is often applied topically but has no proven value in treatment of furunculosis, pyoderma, carbuncles, or cutaneous abscesses. Topically administered bacitracin zinc has been shown to reduce the risk of infections in patients with uncomplicated soft-tissue wounds.

Side effects, clinical problems, and toxicity

Problems associated with the clinical use of the β-lactam antibiotics are summarized in the box on clinical problems of β-lactam agents, and the frequencies of specific adverse reactions to β-lactam drugs are shown in Table 45-5. Problems associated with the use of vancomycin and bacitracin are summarized in a separate box.

CLINICAL PROBLEMS OF β-LACTAM AGENTS

Penicillin G
- IgE antibody allergic reaction (anaphylaxis or early urticaria)
- Neutropenia

Ampicillin
- Delayed hypersensitivity and contact dermatitis
- Idiopathic; skin rash and fever
- Diarrhea
- Enterocolitis

Oxacillin
- Elevated aspartate aminotransferase activity
- Neutropenia

Nafcillin
- Elevated aspartate aminotransferase activity

Imipenem
- Seizures

Amoxicillin-clavulanate
- Diarrhea

Cephalosporins
- Idiopathic; skin rash and fever
- Phlebitis; false-positive Coombs' or glucose test results

Cefixime, cefpodoxime
- Diarrhea

Cefoxitin
- Enterocolitis

Ceftriaxone
- Precipitation in gallbladder
- Diarrhea

See Table 45-5 for frequency of clinical problems.

Table 45-5 Frequency of adverse reactions to β-lactams

Reaction Type	Frequency (%)	Typical Drugs
IgE antibody allergy (anaphylaxis)	0.004-0.4	Penicillin G
Delayed-type hypersensitivity and contact dermatitis	4-8	Ampicillin
Idiopathic; rash	4-8	Ampicillin and cephalosporins
Gastrointestinal problems	2-5	Orally administered agents
Diarrhea	25	Ampicillin, cefixime, ceftriaxone, cefoxitin, β-lactamase inhibitor combinations
Enterocolitis	1	Any agent
Elevated hepatic aspartate aminotransferase	1-4	Oxacillin Nafcillin
Interstitial nephritis	1-2	Nafcillin
Hemolytic anemia, serum sickness, cytotoxic antibody, hyperkalemia, neurological seizures, hemorrhagic cystitis	Rare	Any agent

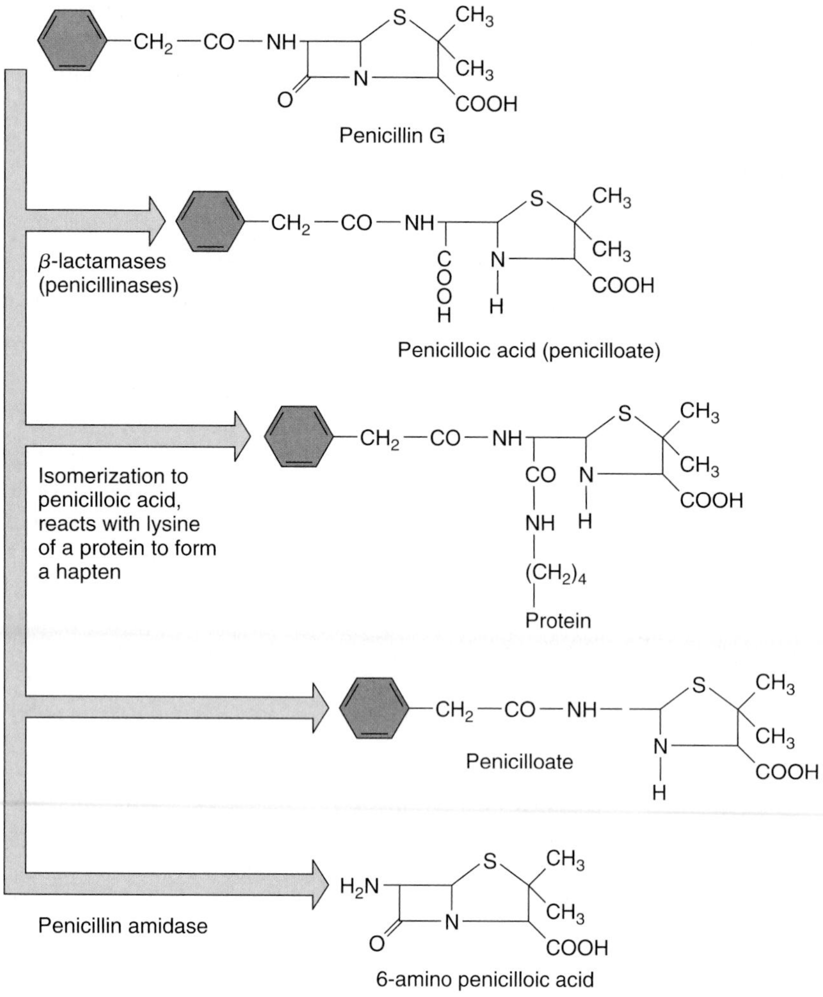

Figure 45-6 Some breakdown products of penicillin G in the presence of different enzymes and conditions.

Penicillins

Although penicillins can cause a wide variety of adverse effects, serious adverse reactions are fortunately rare. Hypersensitivity, which can be life-threatening, is the most important and includes anaphylaxis, wheezing, angioedema, and urticaria. It occurs through IgE-mediated antibody reactions, usually directed at the penicillin nucleus, which is common to all drugs of the class. Therefore, a patient who develops anaphylaxis to one penicillin should be considered allergic to them all. Penicillins also can be partially degraded to compounds with varying allergenicity. The major determinants of penicillin allergy are penicilloyl acid derivatives (Fig. 45-6), but minor components of benzylpenicillin and benzylpenicilloate are important mediators of anaphylaxis. Anaphylactic reactions to penicillins are uncommon, occurring in 0.2% of 10,000 courses of treatment. In contrast, a morbilliform skin eruption–type of allergy occurs in 3% to 5% of patients receiving penicillin. Any of the β-lactams can rarely cause Stevens-Johnson's syndrome, a life-threatening immune-complex–mediated hypersensitivity disorder of the skin and mucus membranes.

Skin testing with benzylpenicilloyl polylysine, benzylpenicillin G, and sodium benzylpenicilloate (see Fig. 45-6) is 95% successful in identifying people likely to have an anaphylactic reaction. However, a negative skin test does not exclude later development of a rash. Anaphylactic reactions to penicillins should be treated with epinephrine (see Chapter 10). There is no evidence that antihistamines or corticosteroids are beneficial. Where feasible, it is more practical to use a different type of antibiotic.

Penicillin induced neutropenia is rare but can occur as a result of the suppression of granulocyte colony-stimulating factor. All penicillins, particularly high concentrations of ticarcillin, alter platelet aggregation by binding to adenosine diphosphate receptors on the platelets. However, significant bleeding disorders are infrequent. Penicillins can also cause renal toxicity. Interstitial nephritis is uncommon but produces fever, macular rash, eosinophilia, proteinuria, eosinophiluria, hematuria, and eventually anuria. Interstitial nephritis also occurs occasionally in patients receiving nafcillin and can lead to tubular damage. Discontinuation of penicillin results in return of normal renal function.

Diarrhea is more common following oral ampicillin than amoxicillin, so the latter is generally preferred. Penicillins and almost all other antibiotics can cause *Clostridium difficile* enterocolitis. This organism can overgrow when the normal bowel flora is disrupted by antibiotic therapy and produce a cytotoxin and an enterotoxin that cause diarrhea and pseudomembrane formation. Distortion of normal intestinal flora by penicillins can also cause bowel function to be altered and cause colonization with resistant gram-negative bacilli or fungi such as *Candida*.

Hepatic function abnormalities, such as elevation of aspartate aminotransferase or alkaline phosphatase concentrations, often follow the use of high doses of antistaphylococcal penicillins or extended-spectrum antipseudomonal agents. In general, hepatic function rapidly returns to normal when agents are discontinued.

CNS-based seizures occur only in patients possessing epileptogenic foci, receiving large doses of penicillin G or other penicillins, or with impaired renal function. Penicillins do not cause vestibular or auditory toxicity.

There are no unusual reactions noted for the penicillin β-lactamase inhibitor combinations, although the incidence of diarrhea with oral amoxicillin-clavulanate is relatively high. This is not observed with the parenteral inhibitor combinations. Incidences of rash and other GI reactions are similar to those noted for use of a penicillin class drug used alone.

Cephalosporins

Cephalosporins are less likely to cause allergic reactions than penicillins. Cephalosporins can produce anaphylaxis, but the incidence is extremely low. Anaphylaxis to cephalosporins in patients with known penicillin hypersensitivity appears to be <5%. However, if other therapeutic options exist, cephalosporins should be avoided in patients who had a severe immediate hypersensitivity reaction to a penicillin. Patients who had reactions to penicillins in the form of a rash are at low risk for having a similar reaction to cephalosporins. However, maculopapular and morbilliform eruptions may occur in patients receiving cephalosporins.

About 1% of cefaclor-treated patients have a reaction consisting of fever, joint pain, and local edema. All cephalosporins sometimes produce fever, with or without rash. GI adverse effects are uncommon, though ceftriaxone may cause diarrhea. Enterocolitis from *C. difficile* can occur in association with any of the cephalosporins. Although Coombs-positive reactions occur in patients receiving high doses of cephalosporins, these agents rarely cause hemolytic anemia. Neutropenia and granulocytopenia occur infrequently. Interstitial nephritis is uncommon but may occur in patients receiving any of the cephalosporins.

Other β-lactams

Imipenem and meropenem can cause allergic reactions similar to those produced by the penicillins, and should not be administered to patients who have had anaphylactic reactions to penicillins or cephalosporins. Cutaneous eruptions and diarrhea can also occur. Rapid infusion of imipenem-cilastatin can produce nausea and emesis. Imipenem binds to brain tissue more avidly than does penicillin G and so can cause seizures, which constitute its most serious toxic reaction. Seizures have occurred in patients with decreased renal function and an underlying seizure focus; therefore imipenem should not be used to treat meningitis. In contrast, meropenem is unlikely to cause seizures and can be used safely to treat bacterial meningitis caused by susceptible organisms.

Unlike other β-lactams, aztreonam does not cross-react with antibodies against penicillin and its derivatives. Consequently, it can be used in patients with a known hypersensitivity to penicillins and most cephalosporins. Because antibodies to cephalosporins can be directed at the side chain, however, aztreonam should be used with caution in patients with anaphylaxis to ceftazidime, a drug with the same side chain off the β-lactam ring as aztreonam.

Vancomycin and bacitracin

Many of the original problems associated with the use of vancomycin have been overcome through improved purification. However, vancomycin can produce hypersensitivity reactions involving the development of macular skin rashes. Infusion of the drug often produces a "red-man" syndrome, with head and neck erythema and sometimes hypotension caused by histamine release. Slowing the infusion rate reduces the likelihood of this reaction.

The most important side effect is ototoxicity, which can occur in patients with high plasma concentrations, but this is rarely seen at concentrations below 30 μg/ml. The risk of ototoxicity is increased when vancomycin is given in combination with aminoglycosides. Nephrotoxicity is uncommon in patients receiving vancomycin alone but is noted in patients who also receive aminoglycosides (see Chapter 46). Phlebitis, which is common, can be avoided through the use of dilute solutions and slow infusion.

Hypersensitivity rarely occurs after the topical use of bacitracin. If given parenterally, bacitracin can cause severe nephrotoxicity.

CLINICAL PROBLEMS OF VANCOMYCIN AND BACITRACIN

Vancomycin

Ototoxicity
Injection site irritation
Red man syndrome—histamine release-mediated erythema, hypotension
Rash
Nephrotoxicity when combined with aminoglycosides

Bacitracin

Nephrotoxic if enters systemic circulation (thus limited to topical use)

New horizons

Since the discovery of penicillin in 1929 and its widespread availability in the 1940s, β-lactam antibiotics have been a mainstay of treatment of bacterial infections. However, their widespread use has resulted in increasing resistance through a variety of mechanisms. Inventive approaches to preventing resistance include the use of specific metabolic inhibitors, development of newer structures that are less susceptible to degradation, and the development of whole new classes of compounds. The main approaches used currently are to restrict their use unless absolutely necessary and to use the minimal durations of therapy needed. However, it is clear that new classes of compounds will be needed because most organisms eventually become resistant to these and other antibiotics. Fortunately, the ability to rapidly sequence the genomes of specific bacterial species are providing many new targets for antibiotic development and may shed new light on essential processes that can be targeted to specifically eradicate these infectious diseases. Such new targets are likely to include both metabolic and structural proteins, including those involved in synthesis and maintenance of bacterial cell walls.

TRADE NAMES

In addition to generic and fixed-combination preparations and the drugs listed in the Major Drugs box, the following trade-named materials are some of the important compounds available in the United States.

Penicillins

Amoxicillin (Amoxil, Polymox, Trimox)
Ampicillin (Principen)
Benzathine penicillin (Bicillin L-A)
Cloxacillin (Tegopen)
Dicloxacillin (Dynapen)
Nafcillin (Nallpen)
Oxacillin (Bactocill)
Penicillin G (generics)
Penicillin V (Pen-Vee K, Veetids)
Piperacillin (Pipracil)
Ticarcillin (Ticar)

Cephalosporins

First-Generation
Cefadroxil (Duricef, Ultracef)
Cefazolin (Ancef, Kefzol)
Cephalexin (Keflex)
Second-Generation
Cefaclor (Ceclor)
Cefotetan (Cefotan)
Cefoxitin (Mefoxin)
Cefuroxime (Kefurox, Zinacef)
Cefuroxime axetil (Ceftin)
Cefprozil (Cefzil)
Loracarbef (Lorabid)
Third-Generation
Cefixime (Suprax)
Cefotaxime (Claforan)
Cefpodoxime (Vantin)
Ceftazidime (Fortaz, Tazicef, Tazidime)
Ceftizoxime (Cefizox)
Ceftriaxone (Rocephin)
Fourth-Generation
Cefepime (Maxipime)

Carbapenems

Ertapenem (Invanz)
Imipenem-cilastatin (Primaxin)
Meropenem (Merrem)

Monobactams

Aztreonam (Azactam)

β-Lactam inhibitor combinations

Amoxicillin-clavulanate (Augmentin)
Ampicillin-sulbactam (Unasyn)
Piperacillin-tazobactam (Zosyn)
Ticarcillin-clavulanate (Timentin)

FURTHER READING

Craig WA. Basic pharmacodynamics of antibacterials with clinical applications to the use of β-lactams, glycopeptides, and linezolid. *Infect Dis Clin N Am* 2003; 17:479-501.

Karchmer AW. Cephalosporins. In Mandell GL, Bennett JE, Dolin R, editors: *Principles and practice of infectious diseases,* ed 5, New York, Churchill Livingstone, 2000.

Samaha-Kfoury JN, Araj GF. Recent developments in β-lactamases and extended spectrum β-lactamases. *Brit Med J* 2003; 327:1209-1213.

Self-assessment questions

1. Which of the following statements is *incorrect?*

a. Gram-negative bacteria have porin proteins that allow β-lactams to pass through the outer lipid cell membrane.
b. Gram-positive bacteria are missing a lipopolysaccharide membrane layer and have many more layers of peptidoglycan than gram-negative bacteria.
c. β-Lactam agents and vancomycin inhibit cell wall synthesis through similar mechanisms at the final cross-linking step of the peptidoglycan matrix.
d. Bacteria that lack autolysins may exhibit tolerance to bacterial cell wall inhibitors.

2. Antistaphylococcal penicillins such as nafcillin:

a. Are active against MRSA.
b. Have a bulky side chain that prevents β-lactamase hydrolysis of the β-lactam nucleus.
c. Have good gram-negative coverage, except for *Pseudomonas.*
d. Are routinely used in patients with a history of IgE-mediated penicillin reaction.
e. Are less active against susceptible strains of *Staphylococcus aureus* than vancomycin.

3. Resistance to vancomycin in enterococci is mediated by:

a. β-Lactamase enzymes.
b. Efflux mechanisms.
c. Changes in cell wall precursors, resulting in low affinity for vancomycin binding.
d. Altered binding proteins in bacterial cytoplasmic membranes.

4. Penicillin G is mainly:

a. Conjugated to inactive glucuronide.
b. Excreted in bile.
c. Excreted by kidney.
d. Deacylated by the liver.

5. Which one of the following statements is *incorrect?*

a. Aztreonam is useful in patients with a history of anaphylaxis following administration of penicillin.
b. β-Lactamase inhibitor combinations and imipenem have excellent activity against anaerobes.
c. Because imipenem has such broad activity, it can be used empirically in most settings thus eliminating the need to get specimens for culture.
d. Aztreonam is active against gram-negative aerobic organisms only.
e. Most third-generation cephalosporins have good CSF penetration.

6. Which of the following β-lactam agents could be used to treat an *Escherichia coli* infection in a patient who has had an urticaria-accelerated reaction to penicillin G?

a. Piperacillin
b. Cefazolin
c. Aztreonam
d. Imipenem

CHAPTER 46

Inhibitors of bacterial ribosomal actions

Mark D. King

Major Drugs	
Aminoglycosides	Macrolides
Spectinomycin (Trobicin)	Clindamycin (Cleocin)
Tetracyclines	Mupirocin (Bactroban)
Chloramphenicol (Chloromycetin)	Ketolides
Streptogramins	Oxazolidinones

Therapeutic overview

Some antimicrobial agents act by binding to bacterial ribosomes and interfering with protein synthesis. Some of these agents exert **bactericidal** and others **bacteriostatic** actions.

The **aminoglycosides** are effective primarily against gram-negative organisms; although they are used less commonly than some of the other agents because of their toxicity, they remain important for treatment of selected infections. They are effective against aerobic gram-negative bacteria and are often used in combination with other classes of antibiotics but are ineffective against anaerobic organisms. Because the therapeutic index of the aminoglycosides is narrow and toxicity can be serious, close attention must be paid to the pharmacokinetics of these drugs in individual patients. Renal function must be assessed, and monitoring of plasma concentrations is recommended.

Another ribosome-binding agent, **spectinomycin,** is similar to the aminoglycosides in that it is also an aminocyclitol, but the structures and actions are different. In addition, the aminoglycosides are bactericidal while spectinomycin is bacteriostatic.

The ribosome-binding sites for **macrolides** such as erythromycin, azithromycin, clarithromycin, and clindamycin are on the same 50S subunit (*S* represents the sedimentation parameter), but the structures of the drugs and the spectrum of activities differ considerably. **Tetracyclines** bind to the 30S ribosomal subunit and are effective against aerobic and anaerobic gram-positive and gram-negative organisms. Given their wide spectrum of activity, tetracyclines remain widely used for treatment of bacterial, chlamydial, rickettsial, and mycoplasmal infections, although the development of bacterial resistance has reduced their efficacy against some pathogens (Box 46-1).

Chloramphenicol was widely used at one time, but serious side effects have limited the applications for which the drug is used in the United States. **Erythromycin,** however, is relatively safe and widely used, especially for treatment of infections in children (Box 46-2). Because of the success of macrolides in treatment of pulmonary infections, these drugs continue to be used in the treatment of respiratory tract infections in adults. **Clindamycin** displays antimicrobial activity somewhat similar to that of erythromycin. The two differ structurally, however, with clindamycin displaying extensive anaerobic activity while having no activity for atypical respiratory pathogens.

The **ketolides** represent a new class of antibiotics within the macrolide-lincosamide-streptogramin B family. Ketolides are semisynthetic derivatives of erythromycin that inhibit protein synthesis via interaction with the 50S ribosomal subunit. Activity against macrolide-resistant respiratory tract pathogens is maintained in ketolides, which also demonstrate excellent activity against atypical respiratory pathogens. There-

Abbreviations	
CSF	cerebrospinal fluid
MIC	minimal inhibitory concentration
MRSA	methicillin-resistant *Staphylococcus aureus*
tRNA	transfer ribonucleic acid
VRE	vancomycin-resistant enterococci

Box 46-1 Therapeutic uses of tetracyclines

Drug of choice

Rickettsial diseases: Rocky Mountain spotted fever, typhus, scrub typhus, Q fever
Ehrlichiosis
Mycoplasma pneumoniae
Chlamydia pneumoniae
Chlamydia trachomatis
Chlamydia psittaci
Lyme disease *(Borrelia burgdorferi)*
Relapsing fever caused by *Borrelia* organisms
Brucellosis

Alternative agent

Plague
Pelvic inflammatory disease

As treatment of syndromes

Acne: low-dose oral or topical
Bacterial exacerbations of bronchitis
Malabsorption syndrome resulting from bowel bacterial overgrowth

Box 46-2 Therapeutic uses of erythromycin

Drug of choice

Mycoplasma pneumoniae
Group A streptococcal upper respiratory tract infection (penicillin-allergic patient)
Legionella infection
Bordetella pertussis
Campylobacter jejuni
Ureaplasma urealyticum
Bartonella henselae
Corynebacterium diphtheriae

Alternative agent

Lyme disease
Chlamydia infection

As treatment of syndromes

Bacterial bronchitis
Otitis media (with sulfonamide)
Acne, topical

Prophylaxis

Endocarditis (penicillin-allergic patient)
Large bowel surgery
Oral surgery

fore, ketolides may provide an additional treatment option for lower respiratory tract infections.

The **streptogramins** and **oxazolidinones** are newer classes of antibiotics that were developed primarily for the treatment of gram-positive organisms and often have activity against organisms that are resistant to β-lactams and glycopeptides. Both inhibit protein synthesis, but their structures and mechanisms of action are different. These drugs represent important agents for the treatment of multi-drug resistant gram-positive infections, but prudent use will be important to prevent the development of resistance to these agents.

Mupirocin, which interferes with tRNA synthesis, is a topical agent primarily used to treat cutaneous streptococcal and staphylococcal infection (see Therapeutic Overview box).

THERAPEUTIC OVERVIEW

Aminoglycosides

Inhibit gram-negative aerobes.
Narrow therapeutic index.
Toxicities to patient can be serious: renal, otic.
Pharmacokinetics are an important consideration.
Plasmid-mediated resistance is a problem.

Tetracyclines

Broad spectrum of organisms are inhibited.

Chloramphenicol

Kills major meningitis pathogens.
Serious toxicity in patients.

Macrolides

Inhibit *Mycoplasma, Chlamydia, Legionella.*
Inhibit gram-positive organisms.

Ketolides

Inhibit respiratory pathogens.
Active against penicillin and macrolide resistant *S. pneumoniae.*

Clindamycin

Inhibits gram-positive cocci and anaerobic species.
Clostridium difficile–associated diarrhea and colitis.

Streptogramins

Inhibit gram-positive organisms.
Active against VRE.

Oxazolidinones

Inhibit gram-positive organisms.
Active against VRE.

Mechanisms of action

The bacterial ribosomal subunit to which each of these drugs binds is given in Table 46-1, along with the bactericidal or bacteriostatic response of susceptible bacteria to the drug. The principal steps in bacterial ribosomal synthesis of proteins, as carried out by the 70S ribosomes and relevant RNAs, and the points at which the drugs act, are summarized schematically in Figure 46-1.

Aminoglycosides

Aminoglycosides consist of aminosugars linked through glycosidic bonds to an aminocyclitol. The structures of streptomycin, gentamicin, and other clinically impor-

Table 46-1 Bacterial ribosomal binding and resulting overall effect on bacterial viability

Drugs	Subunit It Binds To	Bactericidal	Bacteriostatic
Aminoglycosides	30S, 50S, 30S/50S interface	X	—
Chloramphenicol	50S	—	X*
Clindamycin	50S	—	X
Erythromycin	50S	—	X†
Ketolides	50S	—	X‡
Streptogramins	50S	—	X§
Oxazolidinones	50S	—	X
Mupirocin	Leu tRNA	X	—
Spectinomycin	30S	—	X
Tetracyclines	30S	—	X

*Bactericidal for *Streptococcus pneumoniae, Haemophilus influenzae, Neisseria meningitidis.*

†Bactericidal for *S. pneumoniae, Staphylococcus pyogenes.*

‡Bactericidal for *S. pneumoniae* and *H. Influenzae.*

§Individually, quinupristin and dalfopristin are bacteriostatic. The combination is bactericidal for *S. pneumoniae* and *S. aureus.*

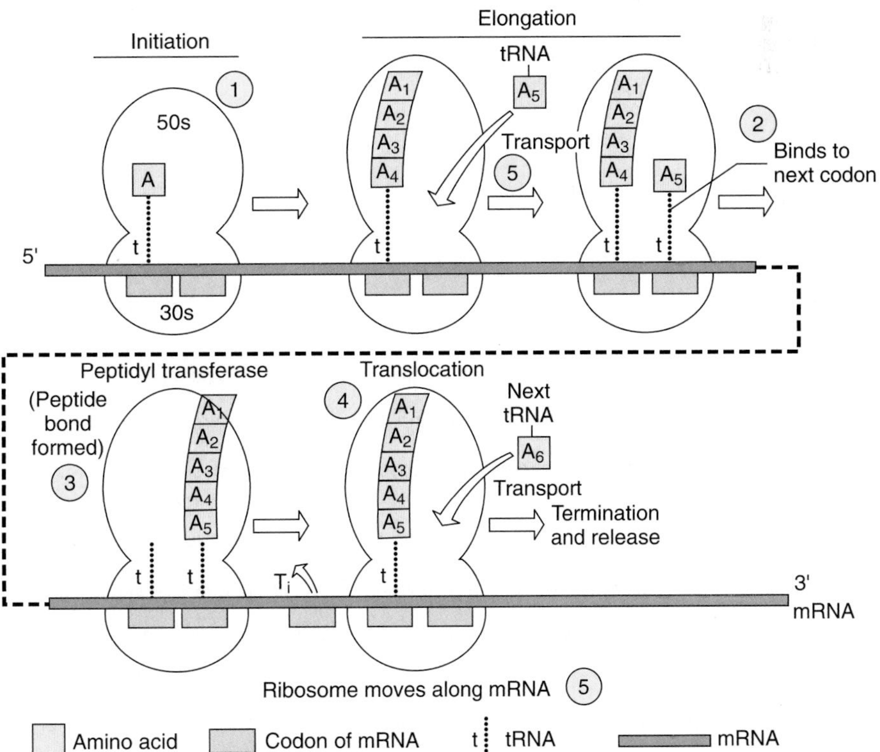

Figure 46-1 Bacterial protein synthesis and points where clinically used antibiotics act. The steps are as follows: *(1)* Streptomycin and other aminoglycosides freeze initiation, so ribosome does not progress along in mRNA and converts from polysome to monosome; oxazolidinones inhibit formation of 70S initiation complex *(2)* tetracycline and chloramphenicol prevent tRNA from binding to mRNA codon; *(3)* chloramphenicol, erythromycin, ketolides and streptogramins block peptide bond formation; *(4)* erythromycin, clindamycin and ketolides block translocation step; and *(5)* streptomycin and other aminoglycosides cause misreading of mRNA so that the wrong amino acid is added.

tant aminoglycosides are shown in Figure 46-2. The particular amino sugars and specific locations of the amino groups distinguish the compounds and are important for their antimicrobial effects and toxicity. Gentamicin consists of a mixture of three species with little difference in activities.

The aminoglycosides exert a concentration-dependent **bactericidal** action by entering the bacterial cell and **inhibiting protein synthesis.** The overall process consists of two main steps:

1. Transport through the bacterial cell wall and cytoplasmic membrane
2. Binding to ribosomal sites, thus inhibiting protein synthesis.

The aminoglycosides are more effective against **aerobic gram-negative** than against gram-positive bacteria. These drugs can cross the more complex cell membrane structures of the gram-negative bacteria. The cell membrane structures of gram-negative and gram-positive bacteria are compared in Figure 45-3.

Transport of aminoglycosides into bacterial cells involves several steps. These cationic compounds bind to anionic surfaces and penetrate **porin channels** of the outer membrane of gram-negative bacteria or the water-filled areas of the peptidoglycan wall in gram-positive bacteria. In gram-negative bacteria, aminoglycosides **disrupt the outer membrane,** enhancing their own uptake through nonporin-type channels. The aminoglycoside then binds to a molecule in the electron transport chain in the cytoplasmic membrane. The drug-transporter complex is moved across the cytoplasmic membrane by its potential gradient. The transport is an energy-requiring, aerobic step that does not occur in an anaerobic environment or at low pH. After crossing the cytoplasmic membrane, the aminoglycosides bind to

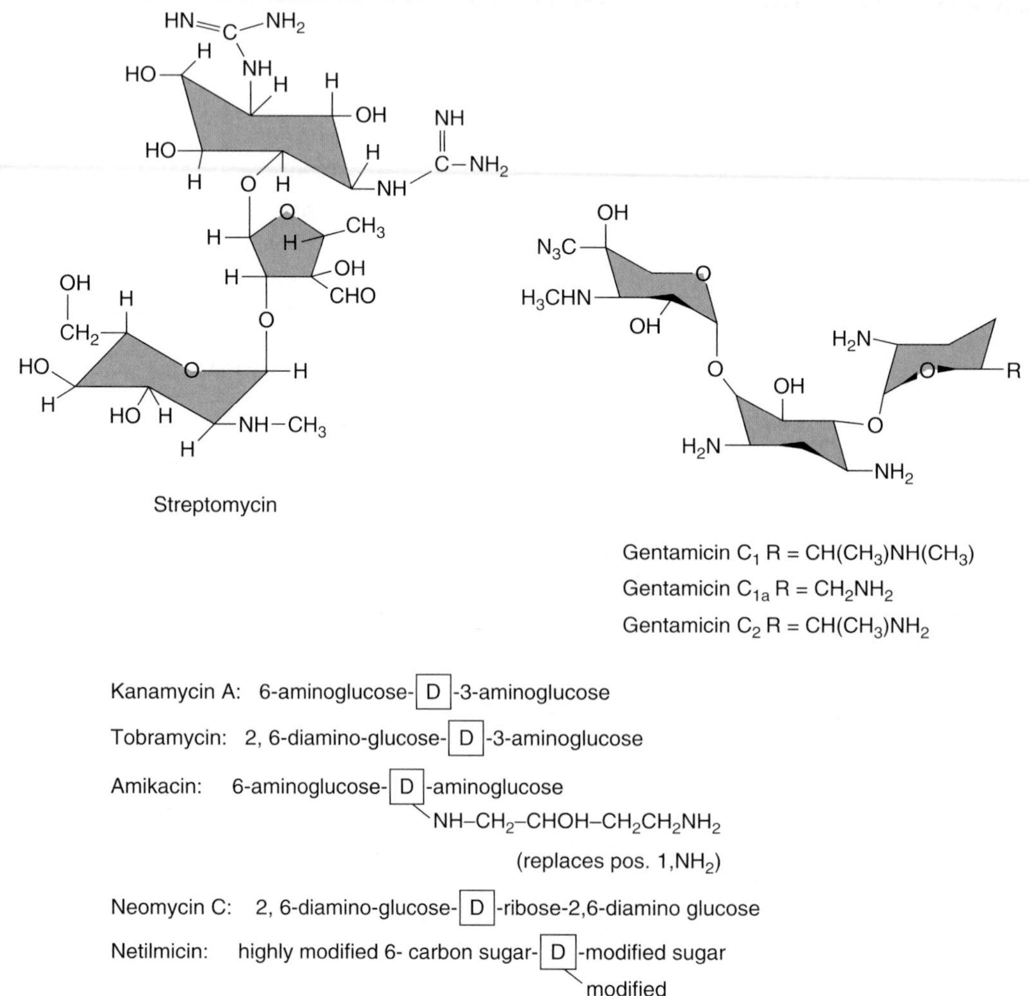

Figure 46-2 Structures of streptomycin and gentamicin and main components of other clinically used aminoglycosides. *D*, 2-Deoxystreptamine.

ribosomes, maintaining a low concentration of intracellular free drug, which facilitates continued drug transfer accumulation. This results in a loss of membrane integrity and eventual death of the bacteria. Calcium, magnesium, and other divalent ions inhibit transport of aminoglycosides into bacteria.

Binding to the ribosome leads to inhibition of protein synthesis. This takes place on the ribosomes, where messenger RNA (mRNA) acts as a template for the addition of activated amino acids attached to tRNAs. The 70S ribosomal particles move along the mRNA template, adding the appropriate amino acid (see Fig. 46-1). Aminoglycosides bind to several ribosomal sites (see Table 46-1) of the 30S and 50S subunits of the bacterial ribosome. **Streptomycin,** the most thoroughly studied, binds to the 30S subunit, although this can be altered by mutation of particular amino acids. Binding of aminoglycosides interferes with protein synthesis in two ways:

- It restricts **polysome formation.**
- It causes **mRNA to be misread.**

Disaggregation of polysomes blocks their ability to move along the mRNA and synthesize a new peptide chain. Aminoglycosides also bind to the juncture between the 30S and 50S subunits and cause distortion of codon recognition, resulting in abnormal protein production. However, the presence of miscoded proteins does not necessarily correlate with cell death, as exemplified by other protein synthesis inhibitors that are bacteriostatic, while aminoglycosides are bactericidal. The bactericidal activity of aminoglycosides likely results from a combination of impaired protein synthesis and membrane dysfunction.

Aminoglycosides also demonstrate a prolonged **postantibiotic effect,** in which suppression of bacterial growth continues after the serum concentration falls below the minimal inhibitory concentration (MIC). Higher aminoglycoside concentrations are associated with a longer postantibiotic effect. This postantibiotic effect has allowed for once-daily dosing of aminoglycosides with a lower risk of associated toxicities.

Synergistic killing has been demonstrated when aminoglycosides are combined with cell wall active agents (e.g., β-lactams, glycopeptides). The explanation for synergy is partly related to increased uptake of aminoglycosides in the presence of cell wall active agents. Clinically, aminoglycosides and cell wall active agents are combined to achieve synergistic killing against enterococci, *Staphylococcus aureus, Pseudomonas aeruginosa,* and other Enterobacteriaceae.

Bacterial **resistance** to aminoglycosides occurs and results from:

- Altered ribosomes
- Inadequate transport within the cell
- Enzymatic modification of drug.

The third mechanism is the most important clinically.

Resistance stemming from altered ribosomes is relatively uncommon. It has been found in enterococci but is uncommon in gram-negative bacteria. Resistance stemming from inadequate transport of drug across the cytoplasmic membrane is uncommon in aerobic or facultative species, but it is seen in strict anaerobes. Mutants with alterations in the electron transfer chain and in adenosine triphosphatase activity have been found, but they are very rare. The resistance of some *Pseudomonas* species to aminoglycosides may be related to failure of the drug to distort the lipopolysaccharide of the outer membrane, thus not allowing drug to enter the bacterial cell.

The most common form of resistance stems from **modification of the aminoglycoside,** which occurs through enzyme-catalyzed phosphorylation, adenylation, or acetylation. The genes for these enzymes are located on plasmids or transposons, which can be spread to many different bacterial species. Many such enzymes have been identified, some of which can inactivate only one or two compounds, while others can inactivate multiple compounds. For example, an enzyme that acetylates the amino group at position 6 of the amino hexose can inactivate kanamycin, neomycin, tobramycin, amikacin, and netilmicin but not gentamicin or streptomycin. The altered aminoglycosides do not bind as well to ribosomes, and the modified compounds do not trigger accelerated drug uptake.

Aminoglycoside resistance varies by location and local usage patterns. In one hospital there may be a low resistance to gentamicin and in another hospital, a high resistance. It is not feasible at present to predict precise resistance mechanisms. Over prolonged periods, selective use or substitution of one aminoglycoside may lead to reductions in resistance to other aminoglycosides. This was demonstrated at the Minneapolis Veterans Affairs Medical Center when repeated selective use of amikacin reduced resistance to gentamicin and tobramycin among aerobic gram-negative organisms. Amikacin is the most resistant of the aminoglycosides to inactivation by resistant organisms, and netilmicin is the second most resistant.

Spectinomycin

Spectinomycin acts by binding to the 30S ribosome subunit and inhibiting a translocation step, perhaps by interfering with movement of mRNA along the 30S subunit. Resistance to this drug stems from the transfer

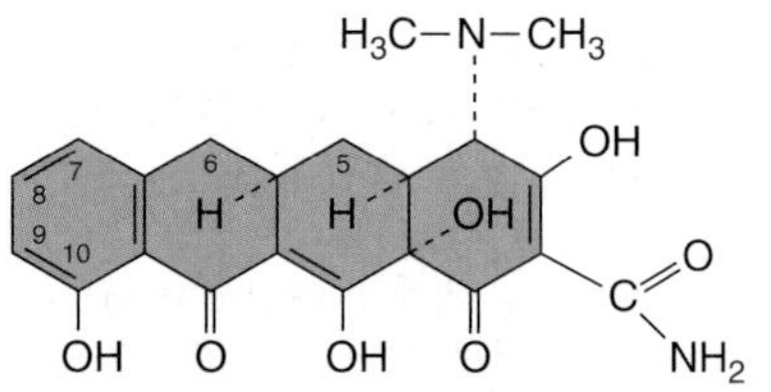

Ring position substitutions

	5	6	7
Chlortetracycline	— H	— CH; — OH	—Cl
Oxytetracycline	— OH	— CH_3; — OH	— H
Tetracycline	— H	— CH_3; — OH	— H
Demeclocycline	— H	— OH	— Cl
Doxycycline	— OH	— CH_3	— H
Minocycline	— H	— H	— $N(CH_3)_2$

Figure 46-3 Structures of tetracyclines.

of a plasmid directing synthesis of an enzyme that acetylates the compound or changes amino acids in the S5 protein of the 30S subunit.

Tetracyclines

The structures of tetracyclines are shown in Figure 46-3. They act by binding to 30S ribosomes, thereby preventing attachment of the aminoacyl-tRNA to its acceptor site. This binding prevents the addition of amino acids to the peptide chain being synthesized. Differences in activity of individual tetracyclines are related to their solubility in lipid membranes of the bacteria. These drugs enter the cytoplasm of gram-positive bacteria by an **energy-dependent process,** but in gram-negative organisms, they pass through the outer membrane by diffusion through the porins. Because minocycline and doxycycline are more lipophilic, they can enter gram-negative cells through the outer lipid membrane and through the porins. Once in the periplasmic space, the tetracyclines are transported across the inner cytoplasmic membrane by a **protein-carrier system.**

There are several mechanisms of resistance to tetracyclines. The most common mechanism, found in both gram-positive and gram-negative bacteria, is plasmid or transposon mediated and involves decreased intracellular accumulation of the drug and increased transport of the drug out of the bacterial cell (Fig. 46-4). **Drug efflux** occurs as a result of the action of a new protein, probably induced by the drug. A second mechanism appears to be alteration of outer membrane proteins resulting from mutations in chromosomal genes. In a third mechanism, the ribosomal binding site is protected as a result of the presence of a plasmid-generated protein that binds to the ribosome. Resistance to one tetracycline usually implies resistance to all these compounds. However, some staphylococci and some *Bacteroides* species are resistant to tetracycline but susceptible to minocycline and doxycycline because of the lipophilicity of these latter agents. New tetracyclines, the glycylcyclines, have been developed that inhibit bacteria previously resistant to all the commercially available tetracyclines but are not yet available for clinical use.

Chloramphenicol, macrolides, and clindamycin

Chloramphenicol, macrolides, and clindamycin are discussed as a group because they bind to the same site or sites on the ribosomal 50S subunit. Their structures are shown in Figure 46-5. They bind to bacterial 70S ribosomes but not to the 80S ribosomes of mammalian cells. Bacterial resistance is observed for all of these agents.

Chloramphenicol prevents addition of new amino acids to growing peptide chains by interfering with binding of the amino acid–acyl–tRNA complex to the 50S subunit, preventing formation of a peptide bond. Chloramphenicol displays primarily bacteriostatic activity but is bactericidal for selected pathogens including *Streptococcus pneumoniae, Neisseria meningitidis,* and *Haemophilus influenzae.* Macrolides and clindamycin bind to the same ribosomal site, causing competitive inhibition of the activity of chloramphenicol (antagonism), and should not be used concurrently. Most resistance to chloramphenicol is caused by chloramphenicol acetyltransferase. This enzyme catalyzes acetylation of the hydroxy groups of chloramphenicol, which makes it unable to bind to the 50S subunit. Less common mechanisms of resistance stem from alterations in cell wall permeability or ribosomal proteins.

Erythromycin reversibly binds to 50S ribosomal subunits causing disassociation of peptidyl transfer RNA from the ribosome and interference with peptide elongation. The newer macrolides azithromycin, clarithromycin, and dirithromycin bind to the same site. Erythromycin inhibits the binding of chloramphenicol to 50S ribosomes, but chloramphenicol does not inhibit erythromycin binding. The activity of macrolides is primarily bacteriostatic, but bactericidal activity is observed for certain organisms (see Table 46-1).

Bacterial **resistance to macrolides** occurs by several mechanisms, some of which also confer resistance to clindamycin and streptogramin type B. The most problematic forms of resistance arise either from alteration of ribosomal binding sites or drug efflux. Alteration of ribosomal binding sites occurs via a plasmid encoded enzyme that methylates the 50S ribosomal subunit. Methylation likely causes a conformational change of the ribosomal target and decreased binding. This type of resistance is associated with the *erm* (erythromycin ribosome methylation) gene and is

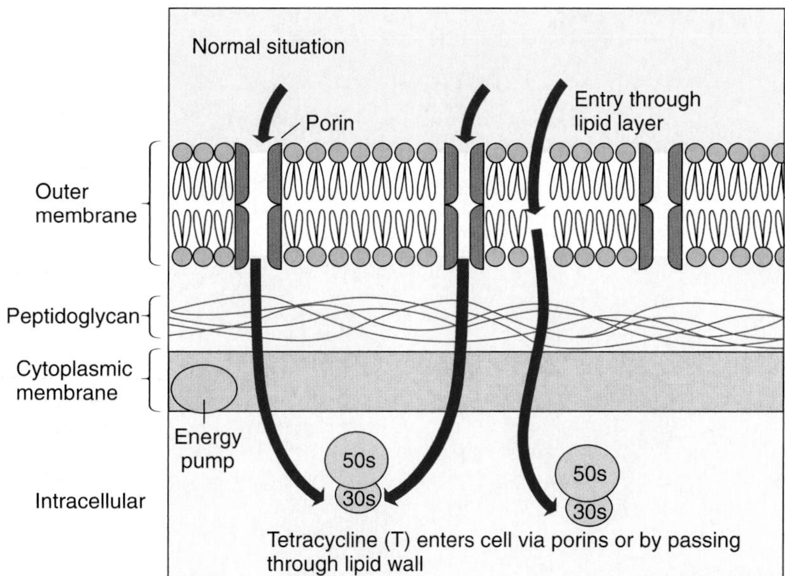

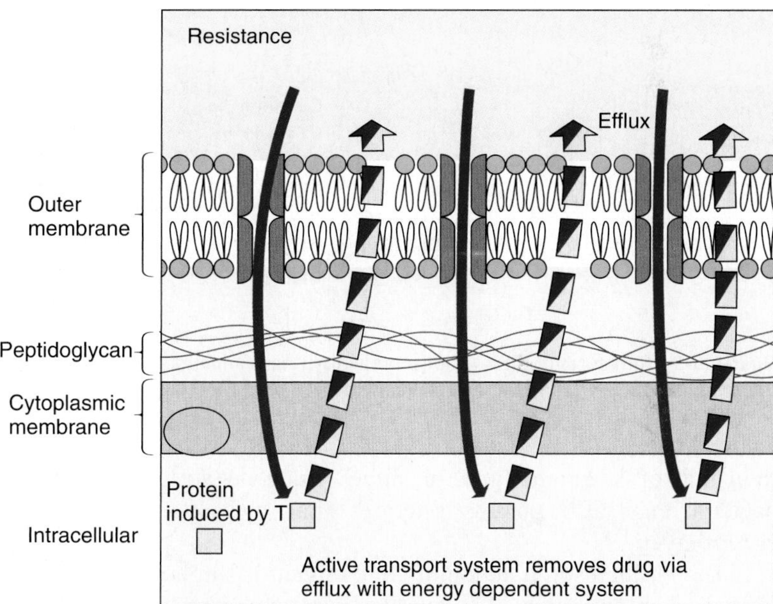

Figure 46-4 Mechanism for bacterial resistance to tetracycline *(T)* caused by efflux.

referred to as the MLS_B phenotype, since it confers resistance to macrolides, clindamycin, and streptogramin B. Both erythromycin and clindamycin also act as inducers of this enzyme, but erythromycin has greater activity. This is clinically important, because an organism resistant to erythromycin and susceptible to clindamycin can become resistant to both drugs during therapy. This applies to the treatment of infections caused by methicillin-resistant *Staphylococcus aureus,* which is often resistant to erythromycin but may appear susceptible to clindamycin. This form of resistance is present on plasmids that can pass from enterococci to streptococci and is encountered in strains of macrolide resistant *Streptococcus pneumoniae* and *Streptococcus pyogenes.* Efflux systems represent another prominent mechanism of macrolide resistance; this type of resistance is associated with *mef* genes and does not confer resistance to clindamycin or streptogramin B. For these resistance types, complete cross-resistance exists between erythromycin, clarithromycin, and azithromycin.

Although some gram-negative bacteria possess ribosomes that do not bind erythromycin or clindamycin, the common form of resistance to erythromycin is its failure to pass through the outer membrane of aerobic gram-negative bacteria. For example, 100 times less erythromycin can cross the outer membrane of gram-negative *Escherichia coli*

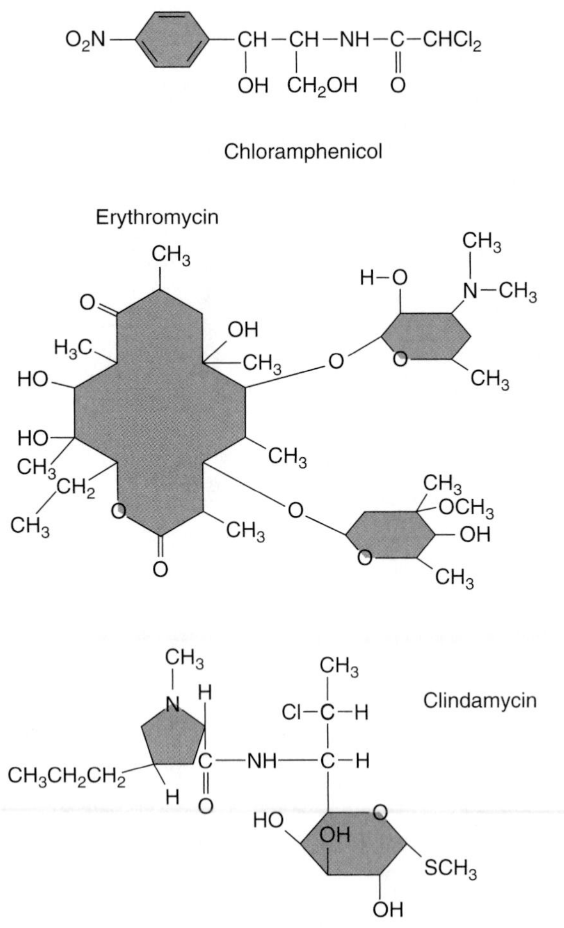

Figure 46-5 Structures of the additional protein synthesis inhibitors chloramphenicol, erythromycin, and clindamycin.

than that of *S. aureus* (gram-positive). Gram-negative bacteria may also possess esterases that hydrolyze erythromycin.

The mechanism of action of **clindamycin** is similar to that of erythromycin. The ribosomal binding site for clindamycin overlaps with that of macrolides and chloramphenicol, creating the potential for antagonism when used concurrently. Resistance to clindamycin may arise from alterations in ribosomal binding sites as described above, with a resultant MLS_B phenotype conferring resistance to both clindamycin and macrolides. This form of resistance is often plasmid-mediated and has been observed in clindamycin-resistant strains of *Bacteroides fragilis*. Intrinsic resistance to clindamycin is seen in Enterobacteriaceae and *Pseudomonas* resulting from poor permeability of the cell envelope to clindamycin.

Ketolides

Ketolides, semisynthetic derivatives of erythromycin, are part of the macrolide-lincosamide-streptogramin B (MLS_B) family of antimicrobials. The structure of the ketolides is shown in Figure 46-6. Similar to macrolides, ketolides inhibit protein synthesis at the 50S ribosomal subunit. However, ketolides demonstrate a **higher binding affinity.** Ketolides are primarily bacteriostatic but demonstrate bactericidal activity against some pathogens, including *S. pneumoniae* and *H. influenzae.*

In contrast to macrolides, ketolides retain activity against most organisms whose ribosomal binding sites have been modified via methylation (MLS_B phenotypes). In addition, ketolides do not appear to induce MLS_B resistance in streptococci but may promote constitutive expression of *erm* genes in staphylococci with an inducible MLS_B phenotype. Telithromycin-resistant strains of *S. pneumoniae* have been described in which both ribosomal modification and mutations in ribosomal proteins were present. Finally, telithromycin has retained activity against streptococci demonstrating *mef* mediated efflux pumps.

Streptogramins

Streptogramins are a family of compounds derived from *Streptomyces pristinaespiralis* whose members are classified into groups A and B based upon structure. For clinical use, two streptogramins, quinupristin from group B and dalfopristin from group A, are combined as quinupristin-dalfopristin in a 30:70 mixture. The structure of **quinupristin-dalfopristin** is shown in Figure 46-6. Bacterial protein synthesis is inhibited by sequential binding of each component to the 50S ribosomal subunit. This forms a stable drug-ribosome complex that interferes with peptide chain elongation and peptidyl transferase. The activity of each individual component is bacteriostatic, but the combination is bactericidal against some organisms. The spectrum of activity of quinupristin-dalfopristin encompasses many gram-positive organisms, but activity against gram-negative organisms is limited.

Resistance to streptogramins occurs by ribosomal modification (*erm* gene), drug efflux, or drug inactivation, with ribosomal modification being most common. *Enterococcus faecalis,* in contrast to *Enterococcus faecium,* is resistant to quinupristin-dalfopristin; resistance in *Enterococcus faecalis* is mediated by an intrinsic efflux pump for dalfopristin. Inherent resistance to quinupristin-dalfopristin occurs in Enterobacteriaceae and *Pseudomonas aeruginosa* related to cell-wall impermeability.

Oxazolidinones

Oxazolidinones inhibit protein synthesis by binding to the 50S ribosomal subunit and preventing formation of the initiation complex. The oxazolidinone available for

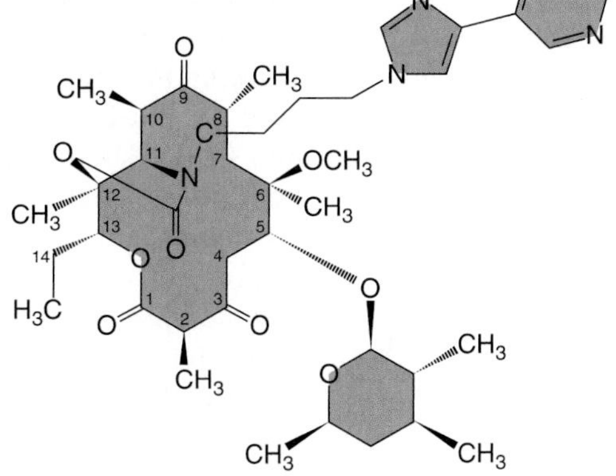

Telithromycin

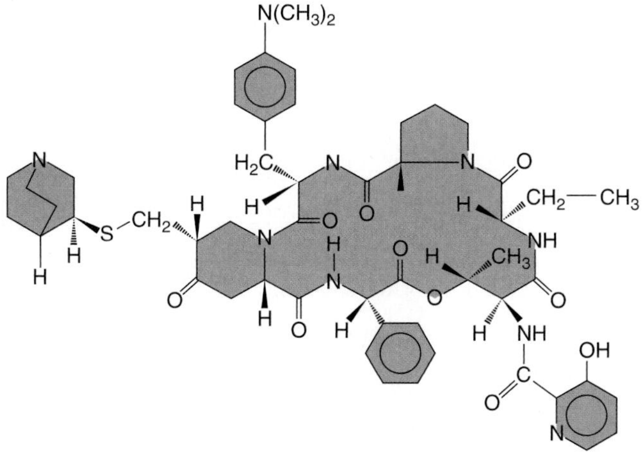

Quinupristin

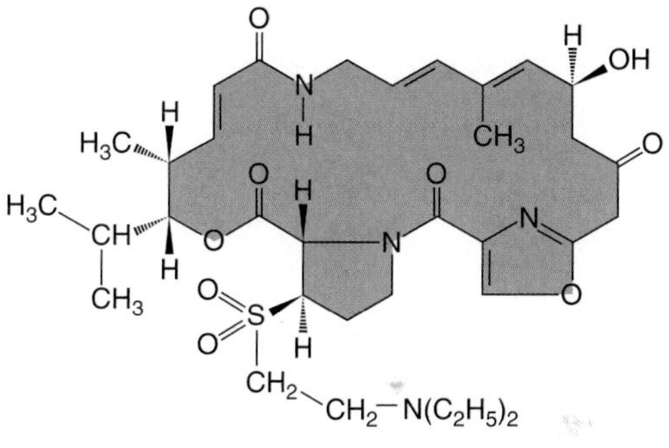

Dalfopristin

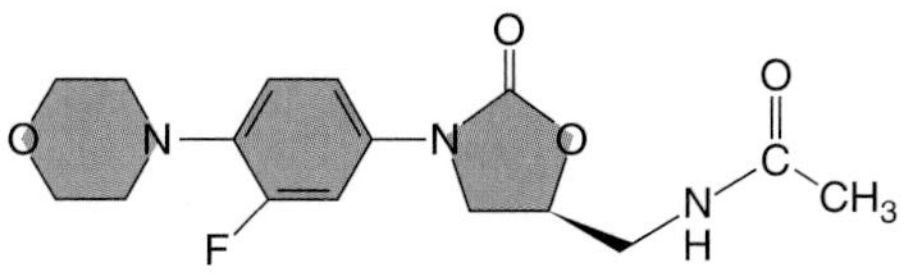

Linezolid

Figure 46-6 Structures of telithromycin, quinupristin, dalfopristin, and linezolid.

use in the United States is linezolid (see Fig. 46-6). Linezolid is bacteriostatic, with activity primarily directed against gram-positive organisms, including those resistant to other antibiotics.

The development of resistance to linezolid in gram-positive organisms has been relatively limited. Although uncommon, resistance has been observed in vancomycin-resistant enterococci and methicillin-resistant *S. aureus*. Resistance in gram-positive organisms occurs by alteration of ribosomal binding sites because of mutations in the 23S rRNA gene. Cross-resistance with other ribosomal inhibitors has not been demonstrated. Gram-negative organisms become resistant to linezolid via drug efflux.

Mupirocin

Mupirocin is a topical agent, previously known as *pseudomonic acid*, that inhibits gram-positive and some gram-negative bacteria by binding to isoleucyl-tRNA synthetase, preventing isoleucine incorporation into bacterial proteins. Mupirocin has been shown to eliminate the nasal carriage of methicillin-resistant staphylococci.

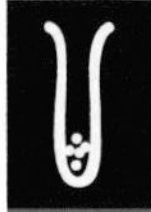

Pharmacokinetics

The pharmacokinetic parameters for the antibiotics that act by inhibiting bacterial protein synthesis are given in Table 46-2.

Aminoglycosides

Aminoglycosides are not absorbed after oral or rectal administration, except after oral use in newborns with necrotizing enterocolitis. If there is renal impairment, even the small amount of drug absorbed by the oral route may accumulate and cause toxicity in adults. Peak plasma concentrations occur in 30 to 60 minutes after IM injection, with plasma concentrations comparable to those achieved after a 30-minute infusion. Absorption from the IM site of injection is decreased in patients in shock, and thus the IM route is rarely used to treat life-threatening infections.

Topical application of aminoglycosides results in minimal absorption, except in patients with extensive cutaneous damage such as burns or epidermolysis. Such rapid absorption occurs after intraperitoneal and intrapleural instillation that toxicity may develop, but irrigation (of bladder), intratracheal, and aerosol delivery do not result in significant absorption. However, new techniques of aerosolization with correct particle size can produce concentrations of more than 100 μg/ml in the lung but only 4 μg/ml in plasma.

Table 46-2 Pharmacokinetic parameters

Drug	Administration	Absorption	Plasma Half-Life (hrs) Normal	Plasma Half-Life (hrs) Anuric	Disposition	Plasma Protein Binding (%)
AMINOGLYCOSIDES*						
Gentamicin	IV, IM	Poor	2	35-50	R (100)	<10
Streptomycin	IM	Poor	2-2.5	35-50	R (100)	35
Kanamycin	IV, IM	Poor	2-2.5	35-50	R (100)	<10
Tobramycin	IV, IM	Poor	2	35-50	R (100)	<10
Amikacin	IV, IM	Poor	2-2.5	35-50	R (100)	<10
Netilmicin	IV, IM	Poor	2	35-50	R (100)	<10
TETRACYCLINES						
Tetracycline	Oral, IM, IV, topical	75%	8	>50	R, M	55
Doxycycline	Oral, IV	93%	16	20-30	R, M, B	85
Oxytetracycline	Oral, IM	Good	9	Long	R (20-35), M	30
Minocycline	Oral, IV	95%	16	20-30	R (5%), M	75
Chlortetracycline	Oral	30%	6	>50	R, M	50
OTHER DRUGS						
Chloramphenicol	Oral, IV	Good	3	—	M (90%) R	50
Erythromycin	Oral, IV	Good but variable	1.5	4	M (90%) R	<70
Azithromycin	Oral, IV	Good[†]	10-50	—	Fecal	7-50
Clarithromycin	Oral	Good	4	—	Fecal, R	—
Dirithromycin	Oral	Good[‡]	30-44	—	M	20
Clindamycin	Oral, IM, IV	90%	2.4	6	M (90%) R	90
Spectinomycin	IM	Poor	2.5	—	R (100%)	<10
Telithromycin	Oral	57%[§]	13	—	M (70%)	70
Quinupristin-dalfopristin	IV	—	1-3	—	M, R (15%)	90
Linezolid	Oral, IV	100%	4.5-5.5	7	M, R	31

M, Metabolized; *R*, renal excretion as unchanged drug; *B*, biliary.
*Aminoglycosides have long half-lives in tissue (25-500 hr).
[†]Decreased by food.
[‡]Slightly enhanced by food.
[§]Oral absorption is 90%, with 57% bioavailable after first-pass metabolism.

Because of their high polarity, aminoglycosides do not enter phagocytic or other cells, the brain, or the eye. They are distributed into interstitial fluid, with a volume of distribution essentially that of the extracellular fluid. The highest concentrations of aminoglycosides occur in the kidney, where it concentrates in proximal tubular cells. Urine concentrations are generally 20 to 100 times greater than those in plasma and remain so for 24 hours after a single dose. These drugs enter peritoneal, pleural, and synovial fluids relatively slowly but achieve concentrations only slightly less than those in plasma.

Concentrations of aminoglycosides in CSF after IM or IV administration are inadequate for treatment of gram-negative meningitis. Intrathecal administration into the lumbar space produces inadequate intraventricular concentrations, whereas intraventricular instillation yields high concentrations in both areas. Subconjunctival injection produces high aqueous fluid concentrations but inadequate intravitreal concentrations.

Disposition of aminoglycosides occurs almost completely by **glomerular filtration.** A small amount is reabsorbed into proximal renal tubular cells. Renal clearance of aminoglycosides is approximately two thirds that of creatinine. However, these drugs can become trapped in tissue compartments, such that they have tissue half-lives of 25 to 500 hours, and aminoglycosides can be detected in urine for up to 10 days after discontinuation of treatment for a week. Dosing schedules must be adjusted in patients who have reduced renal capacity. Since clearance of aminoglycoside is linearly related to creatinine clearance, the latter can be used to calculate dosing.

Aminoglycosides can be removed from the body by hemodialysis but not so well by peritoneal dialysis.

Spectinomycin

Spectinomycin is not absorbed from the GI tract and therefore is administered IM. Elimination is primarily by glomerular filtration, with 85% to 90% removed in 24 hours.

Tetracyclines

Some tetracyclines are incompletely absorbed, while others are well absorbed when administered orally, but all attain adequate plasma and tissue concentrations. Minocycline and doxycycline are the most completely absorbed and chlortetracycline the least. Absorption is favored during fasting because tetracyclines form complexes with divalent metals, including calcium, magnesium, aluminum, and iron. Absorption of some tetracyclines is decreased when they are ingested with milk products, antacids, or iron preparations. However, food does not interfere with absorption of minocycline or doxycycline, and absorption is not reduced by H_2 receptor blockers.

The tetracyclines are **widely distributed** in body compartments. High concentrations are found in liver, kidney, bile, bronchial epithelium, and breast milk. These drugs can also enter pleural, peritoneal, synovial, and sinus fluids; cross the placenta; and enter phagocytic cells. Penetration into the CSF is poor and increases only minimally in the setting of meningeal inflammation; however, minocycline achieves therapeutic concentrations in brain tissue.

Tetracyclines do not bind to formed bone but are incorporated into calcifying tissue and into the dentin and enamel of unerupted teeth.

The disposition of the tetracyclines occurs by renal and biliary elimination and by metabolism. Although most of the biliary-eliminated drug is reabsorbed by active transport, some is chelated and excreted in feces. This occurs even for drugs administered parenterally. Renal clearance of these drugs is by glomerular filtration. All tetracyclines, except doxycycline, accumulate in patients with decreased renal function, thus only doxycycline should be given to patients with renal impairment.

Tetracyclines are also metabolized; this is an important mechanism for chlortetracycline but less important for doxycycline and minocycline. Metabolism of doxycycline is increased in patients receiving barbiturates, phenytoin, or carbamazepine because these agents induce the formation of hepatic drug-metabolizing enzymes. The half-life of doxycycline decreases from 16 to 7 hours in such patients. Decreased hepatic function or common bile duct obstruction also prolongs the half-life of tetracyclines because of the reduction in biliary excretion.

Chloramphenicol

Chloramphenicol is well absorbed from the GI tract, with peak plasma concentrations reached about 2 hours after ingestion. It is also available as an inactive palmitate, most of which is hydrolyzed by pancreatic lipases in the duodenum, with subsequent absorption of the active compound. Parenterally administered chloramphenicol is available as a succinate ester, which must be hydrolyzed to the active compound by esterases in the liver, lungs, and kidney. The succinate should not be given IM because the plasma concentrations are unpredictable.

Because it is highly lipid soluble, chloramphenicol is well distributed throughout the body and enters pleural, ascitic, synovial, eye, abscess, and cerebrospinal fluids and lung, liver, and brain tissues. About 90% of a dose of chloramphenicol is conjugated in the liver to an inactive and nontoxic glucuronide that is filtered by the kidney. The normal plasma half-life is prolonged in patients with hepatic disease but not in patients with renal disease.

High concentrations of free drug may accumulate in infants deficient in forming glucuronides. In addition, hydrolysis of the succinate may be depressed in newborns and infants. Thus serum concentrations should be monitored if the drug is used in newborns or infants.

Erythromycin

Erythromycin in its free base form is inactivated by acid. Therefore it is administered orally with an enteric coating that dissolves in the duodenum. Even in the absence of food, which delays absorption, peak plasma concentrations are difficult to predict. Ester forms of erythromycin are available to help overcome this problem. Lactobionate and gluceptate, water-soluble forms of the drug, are available for IV administration.

Erythromycin is well distributed and produces therapeutic concentrations in tonsillar tissue, middle ear fluid, and lung. It enters prostatic fluid, where it reaches concentrations about one third those in plasma. It does not diffuse well into brain or CSF. Erythromycin crosses the placenta and is found in breast milk, with high concentrations also observed in liver and bile. It achieves high concentrations in alveolar macrophages and neutrophils.

The main routes for the disposition of erythromycin are metabolic demethylation by liver and biliary excretion. Inactive metabolites are responsible for causing the gastric intolerance observed. Only a small percentage is excreted unchanged.

Azithromycin

Azithromycin is stable in response to acid, as compared with erythromycin. About 37% of a dose is absorbed, but this is greatly reduced in the presence of food. Serum concentrations are low because of its rapid distribution in tissues. Therapeutic concentrations are reached in lung, genital tissues, and liver. Azithromycin is highly concentrated in phagocytic cells, macrophages, and fibroblasts, from which it is slowly released. The prolonged tissue half-life with azithromycin allows for shorter durations of therapy. The presence of bacteria causes the drug to be released from neutrophils.

Azithromycin is eliminated unchanged in feces and to a lesser extent in urine. Concentrations in the elderly and patients with decreased renal function are increased but are not significantly affected by hepatic disease.

Clarithromycin

Clarithromycin is about 55% absorbed by the oral route and is widely distributed to lung, liver, and soft tissues. Concentrations in phagocytic cells are about ninefold greater than those in serum. The drug is metabolized to a 14-hydroxy derivative, which has antibacterial activity greater than that of the parent compound. About 30% of drug is excreted in the urine and the remainder in feces. The half-lives of clarithromycin and its active metabolite are increased in patients with declining renal function but are not appreciably affected by hepatic disease. Currently, an intravenous preparation of clarithromycin is not available.

Clindamycin

Clindamycin is well absorbed from the GI tract, although absorption is delayed but not decreased in the presence of food. Mean peak plasma concentrations occur within 1 hour. Clindamycin is available as a palmitate ester, which is rapidly hydrolyzed to free drug and also available as a phosphate ester, with the latter used for IM administration.

Distribution is widespread, with clindamycin entering most body compartments and achieving adequate concentrations in lung, liver, bone, and abscesses. It enters CSF and brain tissue, but the concentrations are inadequate to treat meningitis and should not be relied on to treat brain infections except toxoplasmosis. This drug enters polymorphonuclear leukocytes and alveolar macrophages and crosses the placenta.

Clindamycin is metabolized to the bacteriologically active *N*-dimethyl and sulfoxide derivatives, which are excreted in urine and bile. The half-life is prolonged in patients with severe liver disease.

Ketolides

After oral administration, telithromycin is well absorbed; however, 33% undergoes first-pass metabolism in the liver, with 57% reaching the systemic circulation. Absorption is not affected by food. Telithromycin achieves high intracellular concentrations, particularly within neutrophils and alveolar macrophages and has extensive penetration into respiratory and tonsillar tissues. Metabolism occurs in the liver, with elimination primarily in feces, and a smaller portion in urine. Telithromycin inhibits cytochrome P450 activity, which can lead to drug interactions. Dosing does not require modification in patients with hepatic or renal impairment.

Streptogramins

Quinupristin and dalfopristin are water-soluble derivatives of pristinamycin that are only available for parenteral use. After intravenous administration, quinupristin-dalfopristin rapidly achieves a wide tissue distribution, but does not have significant CSF penetration and does not cross the placenta. High concentrations are found in macrophages. Quinupristin-dalfopristin is metabolized in the liver and eliminated primarily through biliary excretion into feces. In addition, a small fraction is excreted by the urinary system unchanged. Dose adjustment is not required for either hepatic or renal impairment.

Oxazolidinones

Linezolid undergoes rapid and complete absorption after oral administration, and although this is slower when taken with food, overall bioavailability is not affected. Linezolid penetrates into muscle, bone, alveolar cells, and CSF; in a small number of patients with gram-positive bone and joint infections, intra-bone tissue concentrations of linezolid were found to be below the MIC_{90} for the tested pathogens, while joint and periarticular tissue concentrations were twice the MIC_{90}. Additional studies are needed to fully define linezolid tissue distribution. Metabolism of linezolid occurs by non-enzymatic oxidation throughout the body, with the majority of unchanged linezolid and its primary metabolites eliminated by urinary excretion. Dose adjustment is not required for either mild or moderate hepatic impairment or for renal insufficiency. Accumulation of metabolites does occur in renal insufficiency, but the clinical significance is unknown.

Relation of mechanisms of action to clinical response

Aminoglycosides

The aminoglycosides are effective primarily against **aerobic gram-negative** bacilli such as Enterobacteriaceae or *Pseudomonas aeruginosa* and have little effect on anaerobic species. Most staphylococci are inhibited.

Aminoglycosides should be reserved for the treatment of **serious** infections for which other agents such as penicillins or cephalosporins are not suitable. Aminoglycosides have no role as initial therapy of gram-positive infections. They must be given **in combination** with penicillins or glycopeptides to treat endocarditis resulting from enterococci, viridans streptococci, or coagulase-negative staphylococci. Gentamicin is the preferred agent, however, because streptomycin resistance is common.

The initial treatment of suspected sepsis has consisted of an aminoglycoside such as gentamicin or tobramycin in combination with a penicillin or cephalosporin, but newer cephalosporins and other β-lactams such as aztreonam or imipenem have lower toxicity and are being used with increased frequency in this setting. Local antimicrobial resistance patterns should be used to help define empiric therapies for sepsis.

Aminoglycosides are particularly effective in treatment of urinary tract infections, probably because of their elevated concentrations in the kidney. However, many other agents are available for this purpose, particularly orally administered quinolones. Hospital-acquired pneumonia has been treated with aminoglycosides; an aminoglycoside in combination with an antipseudomonal penicillin, cephalosporin, or monobactam is usually selected for the treatment of serious respiratory tract infections resulting from *P. aeruginosa.*

In the past, aminoglycosides combined with either clindamycin or metronidazole were used in the treatment of community-acquired intraabdominal infections. However, given the availability of equally efficacious and less-toxic alternatives, aminoglycosides are no longer recommended for routine treatment of these infections. However, aminoglycosides may be indicated in combination treatment regimens for intraabdominal infections acquired in the hospital where the potential for serious *Pseudomonas* and *Enterobacter* infections exists. Additionally, the combination of an aminoglycoside with clindamycin can be used to treat gynecological infections, including pelvic inflammatory disease.

Although aminoglycosides have been used to treat aerobic gram-negative osteomyelitis and septic arthritis, other agents of the β-lactam or quinolone classes are preferred. Gram-negative meningitis is more appropriately treated with third-generation cephalosporins, though rarely the intraventricular instillation of an aminoglycoside may be necessary for the management of selected *Pseudomonas* or *Acinetobacter* meningitis or ventriculitis. Serious endophthalmitis can be treated with gentamicin instilled intravenously.

Aminoglycosides are used in combination with an antipseudomonal β-lactam to treat suspected sepsis in febrile neutropenic patients. Choice of the particular agent depends on local susceptibility patterns. In general, gentamicin is the first agent to use, with tobramycin reserved for *Pseudomonas* infections and netilmicin or amikacin used in the event of resistance. Alternatives should be used in treatment of neutropenic fever when patients have received prior nephrotoxic chemotherapy.

Streptomycin is used primarily to treat uncommon infections such as those caused by *Francisella tularensis, Brucella* species, *Yersinia pestis* and resistant tuberculosis strains or infections in patients allergic to the usual antituberculosis drugs (see Chapter 49). Amikacin is also used to treat multidrug resistant tuberculosis.

Spectinomycin

Although spectinomycin inhibits many gram-negative bacteria, it is used as an alternative agent for gonococcal infections when the drugs of choice (cephalosporin or quinolone) cannot be used. It is ineffective for the treatment of pharyngeal gonorrhea.

Tetracyclines

Tetracyclines are **broad-spectrum** agents that inhibit a wide variety of aerobic and anaerobic gram-positive and gram-negative bacteria and other microorganisms such as rickettsiae, *Ehrlichia,* mycoplasmas, chlamydiae, and some mycobacterial species. The tetracyclines have many clinical uses, but because of increasing bacterial resistance and development of other drugs, they are no longer as widely used. For example, some *S. pneumoniae, S. pyogenes,* and staphylococci are resistant to them. Among the Enterobacteriaceae, resistance has increased greatly in recent years, such that many *E. coli* and *Shigella* species and virtually all *P. aeruginosa* are resistant. However, tetracyclines inhibit *Pasteurella multocida, F. tularensis, Yersinia pestis, Vibrio* species and *Brucella* organisms. Doxycycline inhibits *Bacteroides fragilis,* but most *Bacteroides* species are resistant to the other tetracyclines. Other anaerobic species such as *Fusobacterium* and *Actinomyces* are inhibited, as are *Borrelia burgdorferi* (the cause of Lyme disease) and others. *Mycobacterium marinum* is inhibited, and some activity is observed against *Plasmodium* species.

Tetracyclines are the preferred agents for the treatment of rickettsial diseases such as Rocky Mountain spotted fever, typhus, scrub typhus, rickettsial pox, and Q fever (see Box 46-1). Doxycycline is the drug of choice for the treatment of ehrlichiosis and is used to treat Lyme disease and relapsing fever caused by *Borrelia* species. Atypical respiratory pathogens including *Mycoplasma pneumoniae, Chlamydia pneumoniae,* and *Chlamydia psittaci* respond to tetracyclines, which may be better tolerated by adults than erythromycin. Systemic *Vibrio* infections and peptic ulcer disease associated with *Helicobacter pylori* may also be treated with tetracyclines. Chlamydial infections of a sexual origin, such as nongonococcal urethritis, salpingitis, cervicitis, and lymphogranuloma venereum are effectively treated with doxycycline. Tetracyclines are also effective for the treatment of inclusion conjunctivitis and trachoma caused by chlamydiae. For penicillin-allergic patients, tetracycline or doxycycline represent important alternative treatments for some forms of syphilis. Additionally, doxycycline is a recommended treatment for granuloma inguinale.

Tetracyclines are no longer used for treating urinary tract infections, because of increased resistance and availability of better drugs. They have no role in treatment of pharyngitis, and other drugs are preferred for treatment of staphylococcal infections. In general, other agents should be used to treat osteomyelitis, endocarditis, meningitis, and life-threatening gram-negative infections. Minocycline inhibits some methicillin-resistant staphylococci and has been used to treat these infections; vancomycin remains the drug of choice, however. Doxycycline represents an important option for prophylaxis against *Plasmodium falciparum* for travelers to regions where malaria is endemic, particularly those with mefloquine-resistant species.

Chloramphenicol

Chloramphenicol has an extremely **broad spectrum** of antimicrobial activity, inhibiting aerobic and anaerobic gram-positive and gram-negative bacteria, chlamydiae, rickettsiae, and mycoplasmas. It is particularly active against *B. fragilis.* Although it is bacteriostatic for Enterobacteriaceae, staphylococci, and streptococci, it is bactericidal for *Haemophilus influenzae, Neisseria meningitidis,* and many *S. pneumoniae.*

Because of the serious diverse side effects associated with its use, chloramphenicol should be used only when no other drug is suitable. In the U.S., chloramphenicol is used mainly as an alternative therapy for patients with bacterial meningitis who have a severe penicillin allergy that precludes treatment with a β-lactam. However, clinical failures have been observed with chloramphenicol when used to treat meningitis caused by penicillin-resistant *Streptococcus pneumoniae.* Chloramphenicol also represents an alternative therapy for patients with rickettsial diseases who cannot be treated with a tetracycline. In certain parts of the world, chloramphenicol continues to be widely used to treat typhoid fever given its low cost and availability. Unfortunately, chloramphenicol-resistant *Salmonella typhi* are becoming increasingly problematic.

Erythromycin, Azithromycin, Clarithromycin, and Dirithromycin

The macrolides, erythromycin, azithromycin, clarithromycin, and dirithromycin, are active primarily against gram-positive species such as staphylococci and streptococci but also inhibit some gram-positive bacilli (see Box 46-2). Chlamydiae, *M. pneumoniae, Ureaplasma urealyticum, Legionella, Corynebacterium diphtheriae, Bordetella* species, *Campylobacter jejuni,* and most oral anaerobic species are inhibited. Most aerobic gram-negative bacilli are resistant, though azithromycin inhibits *Salmonella.*

Both azithromycin and clarithromycin inhibit *Haemophilus influenzae,* but of all the macrolides, azithromycin is most effective. Azithromycin and clarithromycin both have activity against *Mycobacterium avium complex* and *Mycobacterium chelonae,* although clarithromycin is more active against the latter. Both agents also have important activity against *Helicobacter pylori.*

Dirithromycin, the macrolide most recently approved for use in the United States, is generally similar to erythromycin in its spectrum of antibacterial activity.

Erythromycin and other macrolides are used as an alternative to penicillin, particularly in children and especially in those with streptococcal pharyngitis, erysipelas, scarlet fever, cutaneous streptococcal infections, and pneumococcal pneumonia. However, levels of macrolide resistance in *S. pneumoniae* and *S. pyogenes* continue to increase making therapy with macrolides increasingly problematic. Despite increasing resistance, macrolides continue to be used widely in combination with β-lactams in treatment of community-acquired pneumonia because of their excellent activity against atypical respiratory pathogens. Although macrolides can cure *S. aureus* infections, the high frequency of resistance does not make them an initial choice for therapy. Azithromycin is useful for treating sexually transmitted diseases, including ones caused by chlamydiae (potential for treatment with a single 1-gram dose that significantly increases compliance), and erythromycin can be used to treat chlamydial pneumonia of the newborn. Trachoma can be effectively treated with a single dose of azithromycin. Recent data also support the use of azithromycin for the treatment of traveler's diarrhea. Erythromycin is also useful for eradicating the carrier state of diphtheria and may shorten the course of pertussis if administered early. Clarithromycin and azithromycin are useful in both preventing and treating *M. avium complex* infections in patients with the acquired immunodeficiency syndrome (AIDS). Bacillary angiomatosis in patients with AIDS has also been successfully treated with erythromycin.

Erythromycin can be used to prevent bacterial endocarditis in penicillin-allergic patients with rheumatic fever.

Clindamycin

Clindamycin inhibits **many anaerobes** and most **gram-positive cocci** but not enterococci or the aerobic gram-negative bacteria *Haemophilus, Mycoplasma,* and *Chlamydia.* The occurrence of serious diarrhea, including pseudomembranous colitis from *Clostridium difficile,* in patients taking clindamycin limits its use to specific indications. Clindamycin is useful for anaerobic pleuropulmonary and odontogenic infections. It is appropriate therapy for intraabdominal or gynecological infections in which *Bacteroides* organisms are likely pathogens, although increased levels of clindamycin resistance in *Bacteroides* species are increasingly common. Clindamycin should not be used for brain abscesses if anaerobic species are anticipated.

Clindamycin is an alternative to penicillin and may be preferable in certain situations in which β-lactamase–producing *Bacteroides* organisms are present. Clindamycin is also an alternative to penicillinase-resistant penicillins in the treatment of staphylococcal infections but is usually not preferred to a cephalosporin or vancomycin and should not be used for treatment of endocarditis. Clindamycin may be useful for some methicillin-resistant *S. aureus* infections, but inducible clindamycin resistance may occur in isolates resistant to erythromycin. For severe group A streptococcal infections or toxic shock syndrome, clindamycin is often used in combination with penicillin to limit bacterial growth and reduce toxin production.

In AIDS patients with sulfonamide allergy or intolerance, clindamycin represents an important component of alternative combination treatments for central nervous system toxoplasmosis or *Pneumocystis carinii* pneumonia.

Ketolides

Telithromycin displays excellent activity against most of the **pathogens causing community-acquired pneumonia,** including atypical intracellular pathogens. Potent in vitro activity against *S. pneumoniae, H. influenzae, Moraxella catarrhalis, Mycoplasma pneumoniae, Chlamydia pneumoniae,* and *Legionella pneumophila* has been demonstrated. As noted previously, telithromycin **retains** activity against most penicillin-resistant and macrolide-resistant *S. pneumoniae* regardless of macrolide resistance phenotype. Clinically, telithromycin represents an additional treatment option for community-acquired pneumonia, acute exacerbations of chronic bronchitis, and acute sinusitis. Given its activity against drug-resistant pneumococci, telithromycin may prove to be useful in the treatment of community-acquired pneumonia in areas with high levels of penicillin and macrolide resistance. Efforts to limit overuse will be important to prevent development of telithromycin resistance.

Streptogramins

Quinupristin-dalfopristin primarily inhibits the growth of **gram-positive** organisms and has limited activity against gram-negative respiratory pathogens; Enterobacteriaceae, *Acinetobacter,* and *Pseudomonas* are inherently resistant to quinupristin-dalfopristin. Activity is demonstrated against methicillin-susceptible and methicillin-resistant *S. aureus,* coagulase-negative staphylococci, vancomycin-susceptible and resistant *E. faecium,* penicillin-resistant *S. pneumoniae,* viridans streptococci, and *S. pyogenes.* Of note, quinupristin-dalfopristin has extremely limited activity against *E. faecalis* because of an intrinsic efflux pump.

In the United States, quinupristin-dalfopristin is approved for use in the treatment of adults with serious **vancomycin-resistant *E. faecium*** infections and for skin and soft tissue infections caused by methicillin-susceptible *S. aureus* or *S. pyogenes.* It has activity against MRSA and has been used on a limited basis for treatment of MRSA infections that are poorly responsive to glycopeptides; however, treatment of MRSA infections with quinupristin-dalfopristin is not an FDA-approved indication.

Oxazolidinones

Oxazolidinones display activity against many **gram-positive** pathogens, including those resistant to standardly used antibiotics; these include methicillin-susceptible and methicillin-resistant *S. aureus,* penicillin, and macrolide-susceptible or macrolide-resistant *S. pneumoniae, S. pyogenes,* and vancomycin-susceptible or vancomycin-resistant *E. faecium* and *E. faecalis.* Activity against aerobic gram-negative organisms is limited. Linezolid also has activity against mycobacteria, including *Mycobacterium tuberculosis, M. avium complex,* and rapidly growing mycobacteria.

Clinical indications approved for use in the U.S. include treatment of **vancomycin-resistant enterococcal infections,** complicated or uncomplicated skin and soft tissue infections caused by *S. aureus* or streptococci, and hospital- or community-acquired pneumonia caused by *S. aureus* or *S. pneumoniae.* Since linezolid is bacteriostatic, its use for *S. aureus* infections associated with bacteremia should be avoided unless alternative agents for treatment are not available or additional data become available to support its use in this setting. Currently, the primary role for linezolid is in the treatment of VRE infections, in step-down to oral therapy for MRSA skin and soft tissue infections, and for treatment of MRSA infections in patients with glycopeptide intolerance or allergy; linezolid may also be useful for treating *S. aureus* infections caused by isolates with reduced glycopeptide susceptibility if the isolates are linezolid susceptible. Prudent use of linezolid should be emphasized to avoid development of resistance; routine use for infections caused by pathogens susceptible to other available antibiotics should be avoided.

Given its activity against *M. tuberculosis,* linezolid may prove effective as an adjunctive therapy in the treatment of multi-drug resistant tuberculosis. However, further study is needed to better define the role and efficacy of linezolid in this setting.

Side effects, clinical problems, and toxicity

The major clinical problems associated with these drugs are summarized in the Clinical Problems box.

Aminoglycosides

Aminoglycosides can produce serious side effects, with vestibular, cochlear, and renal toxicities the most important and most common.

Renal toxicity Reversible renal impairment develops in 5% to 25% of patients receiving an aminoglycoside for more than 3 days. The impairment can progress to severe **renal insufficiency** in a small number of patients, but it is usually reversible. In the renal cortex, aminoglycosides are transported across the luminal brush border of proximal tubular cells by binding to phosphatidylinositol in the cytoplasmic membrane and undergo internalization by pinocytosis. The agents fuse with and ultimately are trapped in the lysosomes.

Multilamellar structures, called *myeloid bodies,* also accumulate in the lysosomes and phosphatidylinositol-specific phospholipases are then inhibited (Fig. 46-7). These enzymes are important in prostaglandin synthesis, and the initial decrease in glomerular filtration that occurs in response to aminoglycoside toxicity may result from inhibition of vasodilatory prostaglandins. Aminoglycosides also inhibit sphingomyelinases and adenosine triphosphatases and alter mitochondria and ribosomes in proximal tubular cells.

The initial manifestation of aminoglycoside renal toxicity is an increased excretion of brush border enzymes such as β-D-glucosaminidase, alanine aminopeptidase, and alkaline phosphatase. However, it is not clinically useful to monitor excretion of these enzymes, because fever and other factors cause similar

CLINICAL PROBLEMS

Aminoglycosides

Nephrotoxicity
Ototoxicity
Vestibular toxicity
Neuromuscular blockade (infrequent)

Tetracyclines

Binding to bone and teeth: can be serious in infants or children under 8 years of age and during pregnancy
Gastrointestinal tract upsets
Hepatic and renal dysfunction
Vaginal candidiasis
Vertigo (minocycline)
Photosensitivity

Other drugs

Chloramphenicol: major hematological effects can be fatal (aplastic anemia, bone marrow suppression); gray baby syndrome if glucuronidation process not well developed (for chloramphenicol elimination); drug interactions with other agents that are metabolized; optic neuritis may result
Erythromycin: relatively safe; mild gastrointestinal tract disturbances; infrequent hepatotoxicity; drug interaction with theophylline (metabolism); deafness with high doses
Clindamycin: pseudomembranous colitis; serious rash (rare)
Telithromycin: well-tolerated, inhibits cytochrome P450 with potential for drug interactions
Quinupristin-dalfopristin: venous irritation when given by peripheral vein, myalgias and arthralgias; inhibits cytochrome P450 with potential for drug interactions
Linezolid: well-tolerated; gastrointestinal complaints; thrombocytopenia; peripheral neuropathy

changes. Of greater clinical significance is the decrease in renal concentrating ability, proteinuria, and the appearance of casts in the urine, followed by a reduction in the glomerular filtration rate and a **rise in the serum creatinine concentration.**

The risk factors for renal toxicity are not completely understood despite extensive study. Toxicity correlates with the amount of drug given and duration of administration, but older age, female sex, concomitant liver disease, and concomitant hypotension appear to favor the development of toxicity. Coadministration of aminoglycosides with vancomycin, cisplatin, cyclosporin, or amphotericin B is associated with increased renal toxicity, as is volume depletion. Additionally, the risk of nephrotoxicity is higher when aminoglycosides are administered in two or three divided doses compared to a single daily dose.

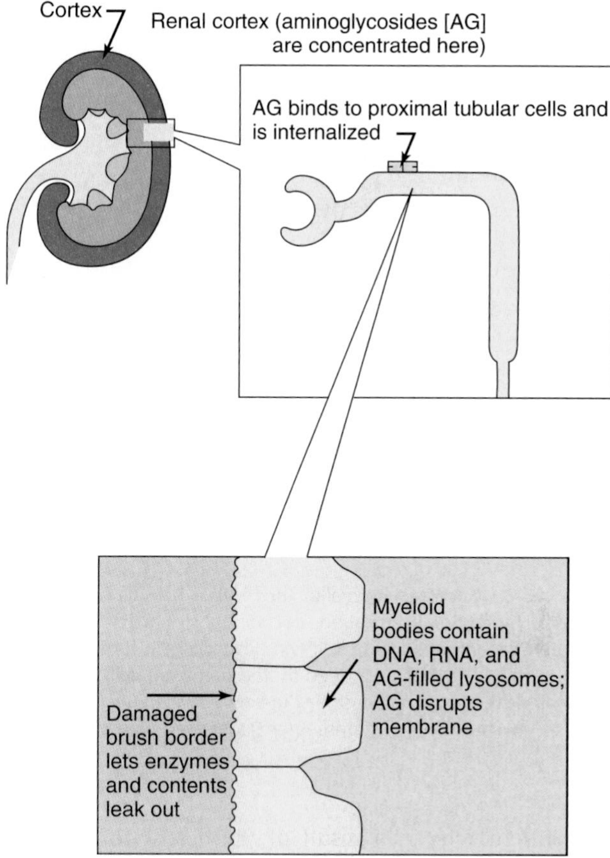

Figure 46-7 Steps leading to nephrotoxicity caused by aminoglycosides.

Aminoglycosides themselves differ in their nephrotoxic potential. Neomycin is the most nephrotoxic, and streptomycin is the least. However, clinical trials comparing the nephrotoxicity of the other agents have yielded contradictory results.

Because tubules can regenerate, renal function usually returns to normal after the drug is cleared. A few patients whose renal function does not return to pretreatment values require dialysis.

Ototoxicity Aminoglycosides can damage either or both the **cochlear** and **vestibular** systems. Aminoglycoside-induced ototoxicity is usually irreversible. Although the exact frequency is unknown, some damage probably occurs in 5% to 25% of patients, depending on the underlying auditory status and duration of therapy.

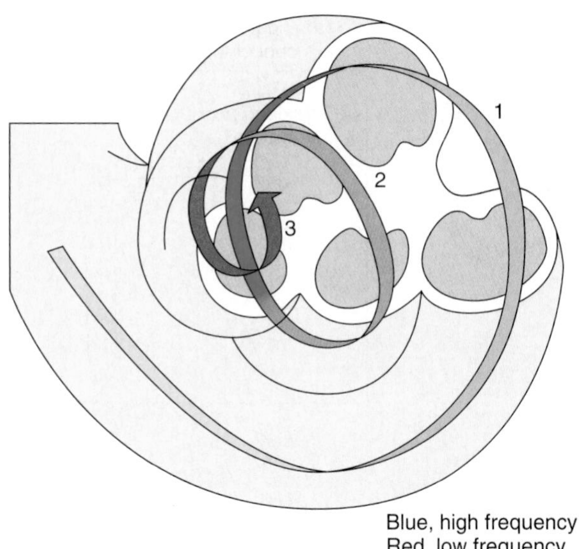

Figure 46-8 Cochlea, normally lined with hair cells, that are destroyed by high concentrations of aminoglycosides. Aminoglycosides produce damage to the hair cells, especially in turn No. *1* and part of turn No. *2*. Hairs are shed by the damaged cells to cause a loss of high-frequency response first (associated with turn No. 1) and a loss of low-frequency response later (associated with turn No. *3*).

Cochlear toxicity is a result of the destruction of hair cells of the organ of Corti, particularly the outer hair cells in the basal turn (Fig. 46-8), accompanied by subsequent retrograde degeneration of the auditory nerves. Aminoglycosides also damage hair cells of the ampullar cristae, leading to vestibular dysfunction and vertigo. In addition, aminoglycosides accumulate in perilymph and endolymph and inhibit ionic transport, the cause of cochlear cell damage. The drug accumulates when plasma concentrations are high for prolonged periods, and ototoxicity is probably enhanced by persistently elevated plasma concentrations. Single daily high-dose therapy produces less ototoxicity.

The amount of auditory or vestibular function loss correlates with the amount of hair cell damage. Repeated courses of therapy continue to cause damage to more hair cells. Concomitant use of loop diuretics, such as furosemide, is thought to increase the risk of ototoxicity. The incidence of vestibular toxicity is highest for patients who receive 4 weeks of therapy or longer.

Clinical signs of auditory problems such as tinnitus or a sensation of fullness in the ears are not reliable predictors of this toxicity. The initial hearing loss is of high frequencies outside the voice range; thus toxicity will not be recognized unless hearing tests are performed. Eventually the loss of hearing may progress into the auditory range. For patients receiving prolonged courses of aminoglycosides, serial high-frequency audiometric testing should be undertaken.

Vestibular toxicity is usually preceded by headache, nausea, emesis, and vertigo, so patients who are ill often have difficulty identifying the onset of vestibular toxicity. These patients may go through a series of stages from acute to chronic symptoms that are apparent only on standing, or the patients may achieve a compensatory state in which they use visual cues to adjust for the loss of vestibular function.

Neuromuscular blockade Neuromuscular paralysis is rare but appears to result from the inhibition of presynaptic release of acetylcholine and from postsynaptic receptor blockade. Aminoglycosides inhibit internalization of calcium at the presynaptic nerve terminal, thus blocking release of acetylcholine. Presynaptic blockade is more readily caused by neomycin and tobramycin than by streptomycin, whereas the opposite is true for the postsynaptic effects. Neuromuscular paralysis is most likely to occur during surgery when anesthesia and neuromuscular blockers such as succinylcholine are used but can also occur in patients with myasthenia gravis.

Tetracyclines

Although usually well tolerated, tetracyclines may produce adverse effects ranging from minor to life-threatening. Allergy to a tetracycline precludes its further use. **Photosensitization** with a rash is a toxic rather than an allergic effect and is most often seen in patients receiving demeclocycline or doxycycline.

Effects on **bone and teeth** preclude the use of tetracycline in children less than 8 years of age, because a permanent brown-yellow discoloration of teeth will develop in 80%. The effect is permanent and the enamel is hypoplastic. The effects on bone and teeth may also result from maternal use of tetracyclines during pregnancy. Thus, pregnant women should not take tetracyclines. Tetracyclines cause dose-dependent GI tract disturbances, including epigastric burning, nausea, and vomiting. Esophageal ulcers have also been reported. Pancreatitis is rarely observed.

Hepatic toxicity is encountered most often in conjunction with parenteral use but can also occur with oral administration. Tetracyclines also aggravate existing renal dysfunction.

Demeclocycline can cause nephrogenic diabetes insipidus, leading to its use for the treatment of chronic inappropriate antidiuretic hormone secretion. Other side effects include minocycline-produced vertigo, particularly in women. Superinfection caused by an overgrowth of other bacteria, particularly oral and vaginal candidiasis, frequently occurs after the use of tetracyclines.

Chloramphenicol

Chloramphenicol produces serious side effects attributed to its action on mitochondrial membrane enzymes, cytochrome oxidases, and adenosine triphosphatases. Because of these adverse effects, chloramphenicol has limited clinical uses, primarily when no alternative treatment is suitable.

Its hematological effects are the most important, and regular monitoring of complete blood count should be performed in patients receiving chloramphenicol. **Aplastic anemia** occurs in 1:25,000 to 1:40,000 patients, with a high death rate in those in whom an aplastic state develops or who progress to acute leukemia. Aplastic anemia is usually not dose dependent and most often occurs weeks to months after therapy is completed but can occur concurrently with therapy.

A second important hematological side effect is **reversible bone marrow suppression.** This form of toxicity usually develops during therapy, is dose dependent, and is reversible. It is manifested by either anemia, thrombocytopenia and leukopenia, or a combination of these.

A complication known as the *gray baby syndrome* also is encountered in infants given chloramphenicol. This syndrome of pallor, cyanosis, abdominal distention, vomiting, and circulatory collapse, resulting in approximately a 50% mortality rate, develops in neonates with excessively high plasma concentrations of drug. High concentrations result from inadequate glucuronidation and failure to excrete the drug by the kidneys. Children less than 1 month of age should receive only low doses of chloramphenicol, though in overdose situations excess drug can be removed by hemoperfusion over a bed of charcoal. Chloramphenicol also can produce optic neuritis in children; gastrointestinal side effects including nausea, vomiting, and diarrhea; and hypersensitivity rashes.

Chloramphenicol inhibits hepatic cytochrome P450 enzymes, thereby prolonging the half-life of phenytoin, tolbutamide, and other drugs; barbiturates, on the other hand, decrease the half-life of chloramphenicol.

Macrolides

Erythromycin is one of the safest antibiotics, with GI side effects characterized by epigastric pain, abdominal cramps, nausea, and emesis representing the most common side effects. Intravenous administration may be associated with thrombophlebitis. Cholestatic hepatitis may occur in patients receiving estolate preparations of erythromycin, usually beginning 10 to 20 days into treatment and characterized by jaundice, fever, leukocytosis, and eosinophilia. The problem rapidly abates once drug administration is stopped. Erythromycin at high doses can cause reversible transient deafness. Rarely, erythromycin use has been associated with polymorphic ventricular tachycardia (torsade de pointes). Erythromycin stimulates GI motility by acting as a motilin receptor agonist leading to enhanced gastric emptying. Thus, erythromycin can be used to improve gastric motility in patients with gastroparesis.

Erythromycin also inhibits the cytochrome P450 system, which can lead to significant drug-drug interactions. Erythromycin prolongs the half-life of theophylline, and this can lead to theophylline toxicity. It also inhibits the metabolism of carbamazepine, cyclosporine, corticosteroids, warfarin, and digoxin.

Azithromycin is generally well tolerated and has fewer GI side effects than erythromycin. Because it does not interfere with cytochrome P450 enzymes, it does not have the same drug-drug interactions.

Clarithromycin is similarly well tolerated, although the incidence of intolerance caused by GI side effects is greater than for azithromycin but less than for erythromycin. Clarithromycin also inhibits cytochrome P450 and may cause increased serum concentrations of other drugs.

Like erythromycin, dirithromycin can also cause GI side effects. It does not interfere with cytochrome P450 metabolism.

Clindamycin

Diarrhea may occur in up to 20% of patients treated with clindamycin. The most important adverse effect of clindamycin is **pseudomembranous enterocolitis,** estimated to occur in 3% to 5% of patients. Pseudomembranous colitis is caused by the toxin produced by ***Clostridium difficile***. It is characterized by diarrhea, abdominal pain, and fever, with diarrhea beginning either during or after drug therapy. Orally administered vancomycin or metronidazole may be needed.

Ketolides

Overall, ketolides are well-tolerated, with diarrhea and nausea being the most commonly reported side effects. Like erythromycin, telithromycin inhibits cytochrome P450 activity but does not form complexes with cytochrome P450, which may lead to fewer drug-drug interactions. Concomitant administration of telithromycin with drugs known to prolong the QT_c interval, such as midazolam or class IA or IIIA antiarrhythmics, should be avoided. The potential for increased levels of cyclosporine exists requiring diligent monitoring of cyclosporine levels.

Streptogramins

Local inflammation, pain, edema, and thrombophlebitis at the infusion site may occur with quinupristin-dalfopristin administration, particularly when infused via a peripheral vein. Therefore, administration usually requires central venous access. In noncomparative trials, myalgia and arthralgia were encountered in up to 13% of patients administered quinupristin-dalfopristin, but these occurred with lower frequency in comparative trials.

Quinupristin-dalfopristin inhibits cytochrome P450 activity creating the potential for significant drug-drug interactions. Concomitant use of quinupristin-dalfopristin and drugs known to prolong the QT_c interval should be avoided.

Oxazolidinones

Linezolid is generally well tolerated, with the most common side effects related to GI complaints, including nausea and diarrhea. Headache, rash, and altered taste may also occur. **Thrombocytopenia,** often occurring with therapy duration greater than 2 weeks, is the most problematic side effect. The mechanism may be related in part to reversible myelosuppression. Platelet counts usually normalize after linezolid is discontinued. Linezolid use may also be associated with anemia. Complete blood counts should be monitored at least weekly in patients receiving linezolid. Additionally, peripheral neuropathy may develop, necessitating discontinuation of therapy.

Linezolid may interact with serotonergic agents, resulting in an increased risk of serotonin syndrome when administered with serotonergic agents (see Chapter 23). Weak and reversible inhibition of monoamine oxidase occurs with linezolid use. Therefore, patients taking linezolid should avoid eating large quantities of food with high tyramine content.

TRADE NAMES

In addition to generic and fixed-combination preparations and the drugs listed in the Major Drugs box, the following trade-named materials are some of the important compounds available in the United States.

Aminoglycosides

Amikacin sulfate (Amikin)
Gentamicin sulfate (Garamycin, G-Myticin)
Kanamycin sulfate (Kantrex)
Netilmicin sulfate (Netromycin)
Tobramycin sulfate (Nebcin)

Tetracyclines

Doxycycline (Doryx)
Doxycycline calcium (Vibramycin calcium)
Minocycline HCl (Minocin)
Oxytetracycline or salt (Terramycin, Urobiotic)
Tetracycline (Achromycin, Sumycin)

Other drugs

Azithromycin (Zithromax)
Clarithromycin (Biaxin)
Dirithromycin (Dynabac)
Erythromycin (ERYC, Erycette, EryDerm, Erygel, Ilotycin)
Erythromycin ethylsuccinate (contains sulfisoxazole) (Pediamycin, Eryzole, Wyamycin)
Erythromycin estolate (Ilosone)
Linezolid (Zyvox)
Quinupristin-dalfopristin (Synercid)
Telithromycin (Ketek)

New horizons

Emerging antimicrobial resistance continues to be problematic, and the need for agents active against drug-resistant organisms is expanding. Development of new inhibitors of bacterial ribosomes may provide additional options. Currently, the glycylcyclines represent a promising new agent within the tetracycline class. Glycylcyclines have an expanded spectrum of activity, with *in vitro* activity against methicillin-resistant *S. aureus,* vancomycin-resistant enterococci, and penicillin-resistant *S. pneumoniae* and may be active against some resistant gram-negative organisms. Furthermore, additional ketolides and oxazolidinone derivatives under investigation may expand the possibilities for treating infections caused by drug-resistant organisms.

FURTHER READING

Ackermann G, Rodloff AC. Drugs of the 21st century: telithromycin (HMR 3647)—the first ketolide. *J Antimicro Chemotherapy* 2003; 51:497-511.

Diekema DJ, Jones RN. Oxazolidinone antibiotics. *Lancet* 2001; 358:1975-82.

Eliopoulos GM. Quinupristin-dalfopristin and linezolid. Evidence and opinion. *Clin Infect Dis* 2003; 36:473-81.

Gilbert DN. Aminoglycosides. In Mandell GL, Bennett JE, Dolin R, editors: *Principles and practices of infectious diseases.* Philadelphia, Churchill Livingstone, 2000.

Kasten MJ. Clindamycin, metronidazole, and chloramphenicol. *Mayo Clin Proc* 1999; 74:825-833.

Self-assessment questions

1. Mupirocin inhibits which of the following organisms?

a. *Bacteroides fragilis*
b. *Staphylococcus aureus*
c. *Pseudomonas aeruginosa*
d. *Candida albicans*

2. Spectinomycin is used to treat infection caused by which of the following?

a. *Streptococcus pyogenes*
b. *Escherichia coli*
c. *Klebsiella pneumoniae*
d. *Neisseria gonorrhoeae*

3. Which of the following is used as prophylaxis for meningococcal meningitis?

a. Rifampin
b. Gentamicin
c. Erythromycin
d. Chloramphenicol
e. Clindamycin

4. Which of the following chemotherapeutic agents does not achieve adequate concentrations within phagocytic cells to kill intracellular pathogens?

a. Gentamicin
b. Telithromycin
c. Clarithromycin
d. Azithromycin

5. Which of the following are toxic effects of the aminoglycoside antibiotic amikacin?

a. Hearing impairment resulting from toxic effect on hair cells of the cochlea
b. Nephrotoxicity caused by damage to proximal renal tubular cells
c. Production of neuromuscular blockade
d. All of the above
e. None of the above

6. Chloramphenicol is inactivated by which of the following mechanisms?

a. Oxidation to 1-oxo derivatives
b. Glucuronidation
c. *N*-Acetylation
d. Phosphorylation
e. Excretion by tubular secretion

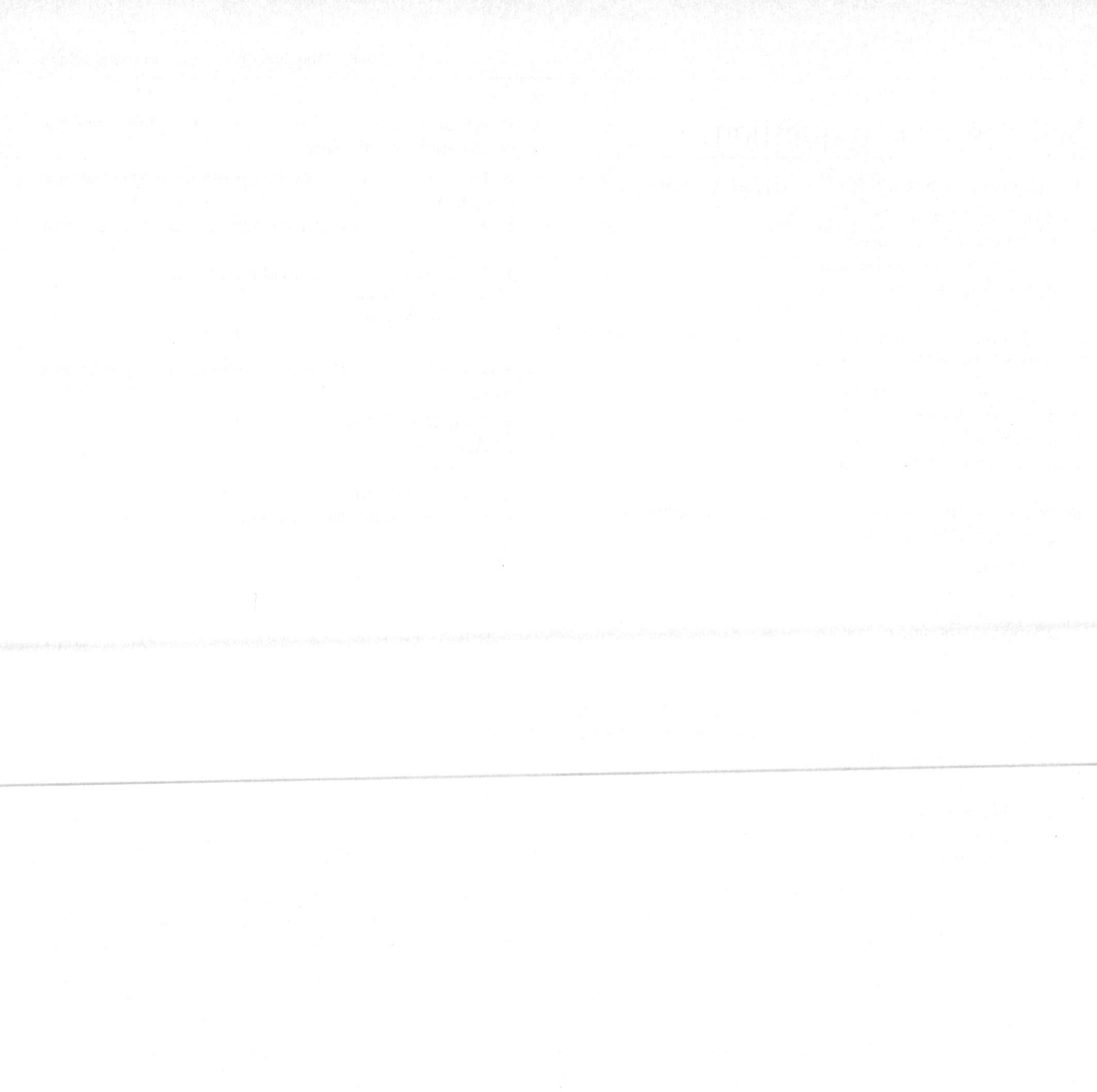

CHAPTER 47

Bacterial folate antagonists, fluoroquinolones, and other antibacterial agents

Susan M. Ray

Major Drugs	
Ciprofloxacin (Cipro)	Polymyxin B (Aerosporin)
Gatifloxacin (Tequin)	Sulfamethoxazole (Gantanol)
Levofloxacin (Levaquin)	Trimethoprim (Proloprim, Trimpex)
Moxifloxacin (Avelox)	Trimethoprim-sulfamethoxazole (Bactrim, Septra)
Nitrofurantoin (Furadantin, Macrodantin)	
Norfloxacin (Noroxin)	

Therapeutic overview

The sulfonamides, such as sulfamethoxazole (SMX), and trimethoprim (TMP) act by inhibiting synthesis of folic acid in bacteria. Most bacteria must synthesize folic acid derivatives, whereas humans can rely on dietary sources. Thus inhibition of folate synthesis constitutes a route for selective antibiotic development. Many sulfonamide derivatives have been synthesized and tested in humans, but only a few are still in clinical use, because resistance to these drugs has become widespread. Sulfonamides are useful in treatment of nocardiosis (usually administered in the combination form of TMP-SMX) and are also administered topically to burn wounds. Sulfadiazine is used in combination with the antimalarial drug pyrimethamine to treat toxoplasmosis. The TMP-SMX combination has many therapeutic applications, which are summarized in the Therapeutic Overview box.

Several other types of antimicrobial agents act by inhibiting or damaging bacterial DNA (fluoroquinolones and nitrofurans) or by disrupting bacterial cell membranes (polymyxins). Quinolones were first developed in the 1960s and can be classified into generations based on antimicrobial activity. Fluoroquinolones (second and third generation) are the only quinolones in current use. Norfloxacin (an older second-generation fluoroquinolone) and the nitrofurans are not effective for systemic infections and are used primarily to treat urinary tract infections. Another second-generation fluoroquinolone, ciprofloxacin, is also effective against gonorrhea, diarrhea, prostatitis, and osteomyelitis. Ciprofloxacin is the fluoroquinolone with the most activity against *Pseudomonas aeruginosa*. The third-generation fluoroquinolones have increased activity against gram-positive pathogens including the important respiratory pathogen *S. pneumoniae*. Most fluoroquinolones are available in both oral and IV formulations and can be used to treat a broad range of serious infections. Polymyxin B is an old agent that is being used with some frequency in the last few years for treatment of multidrug-resistant gram-negative infections.

Abbreviations	
CSF	cerebrospinal fluid
GI	gastrointestinal
IV	intravenous
SMX	sulfamethoxazole
TMP	trimethoprim

THERAPEUTIC OVERVIEW

Sulfonamides

Effective for treatment of nocardiosis and toxoplasmosis
Topical agents for burn wounds

Trimethoprim-sulfamethoxazole combination

No longer drugs of choice for upper respiratory tract infections
Effective for urinary tract infections
 Resistant bacteria
Effective for treatment of *Pneumocystis carinii* and prevention of *Pneumocystis carinii* infections and *Toxoplasma gondii* encephalitis in AIDS patients
 Significant side effects
Prevention of spontaneous bacterial peritonitis in patients with cirrhosis

Fluoroquinolones

Urinary tract infections
Prostatitis
Sexually transmitted diseases
 Increasing resistance in *N. gonorrhea*
Bacterial diarrheal infections
Community-acquired pneumonia
 Third-generation agents only
Osteomyelitis
Agents of biowarfare
Mycobacterial infections

Nitrofurans

Urinary tract infections

Polymyxins

Mainly topical uses
IV treatment only therapeutic alternative for serious nosocomial infections caused by multiresistant gram-negative organisms

Mechanisms of action

Folic acid synthesis and regeneration

The bacterial synthesis of folic acid involves a multistep enzyme-catalyzed reaction sequence (Fig. 47-1). Tetrahydrofolic acid is the physiologically active form of folic acid and required as a cofactor in synthesis of thymidine, purines, and bacterial DNA. Sulfonamides are structural analogues of para-aminobenzoic acid and competitively inhibit dihydropteroate synthase. TMP blocks the production of tetrahydrofolate from dihydrofolate by reversibly inhibiting the required enzyme, dihydrofolate reductase. Thus these two drugs block the synthesis of tetrahydrofolate at different steps in the synthetic pathway and result in a bactericidal action. (see Fig. 47-1).

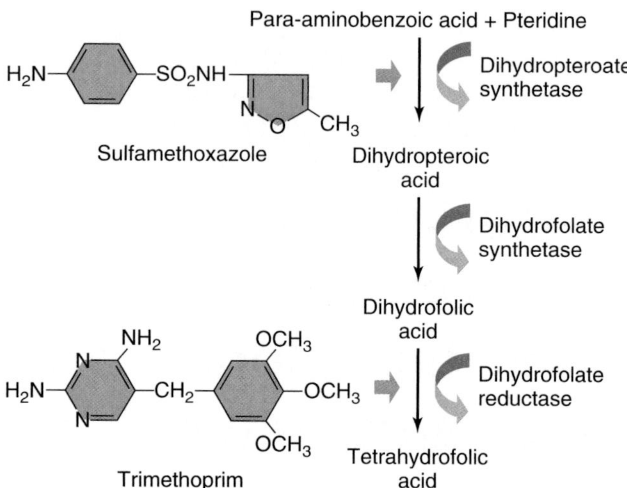

Figure 47-1 Folate synthesis pathway and sites of action of trimethoprim and sulfamethoxazole. (From Masters PA, et al: Trimethoprim-sulfamethoxazole revisited, *Arch Intern Med* 2003; 163:402. Copyright 2003 American Medical Association. All rights reserved.)

Sulfonamides

The sulfonamides are bacteriostatic, since microorganisms must synthesize their own folic acid while mammalian cells do not. When folate synthesis is inhibited, bacterial cell growth is halted. This inhibition can be reversed by addition of purines, thymidine, methionine, and serine. Resistance to sulfonamides is widespread, and its incidence continues to increase among all major bacterial pathogens. Reduced cellular uptake of the drug, which can be chromosomal or plasmid in origin, is one mechanism. Another is an altered dihydropteroate synthetase, which can result from a point mutation or the presence of a plasmid that causes synthesis of a new enzyme. Replacement of a single amino acid in the enzyme alters its affinity for sulfonamides. In enteric species, plasmid-propagated resistance is the common form. A final mechanism of resistance is the production of increased amounts of *p*-aminobenzoic acid. This mechanism is exhibited by some staphylococci but is not common. Resistance stemming from an altered enzyme can develop during therapy.

Trimethoprim

TMP was initially used as an antimalarial drug but has been replaced by pyrimethamine, which acts by a similar mechanism. The antimalarial and antibacterial actions of TMP stem from its high affinity for bacterial dihydrofolate reductase. TMP binds competitively and inhibits this enzyme in bacterial and mammalian cells. About 100,000 times higher concentrations of drug are needed to inhibit the human enzyme as compared with the bacterial enzymes. This enzyme is also inhibited by methotrexate, discussed in Chapter 42. TMP thus prevents conversion of dihydrofolate to tetrahydrofolate and blocks formation of thymidine, some purines, methionine, and glycine in the bacteria, leading to rapid death of the microorganisms.

TMP and SMX are used effectively in combination to achieve synergistic effects, which they accomplish by blocking different steps in folic acid synthesis. Moreover, sulfonamide potentiates the action of TMP by reducing the dihydrofolate competing with TMP for binding to dihydrofolate reductase. The combination of the two drugs is bactericidal.

Resistance to TMP and to the combination of TMP-SMX stems from permeability changes and from the presence of an altered dihydrofolate reductase. Production of this enzyme can be modified by a chromosomal mutation or by a plasmid. There is an increasing incidence of resistance to TMP-SMX mediated by the plasmid mechanism. A mutation to thymine dependence has also been found, as has an overproduction of dihydrofolate reductase.

Fluoroquinolones

The fluoroquinolones include norfloxacin, ciprofloxacin, levofloxacin, gatifloxacin, and moxifloxacin (see Fig. 47-2 for basic structure). Fluoroquinolones all have a fluorine at position 6 in the 2 ring structure.

The fluoroquinolones act by inhibiting type 2 bacterial DNA topoisomerases, DNA gyrase and topoisomerase IV. These topoisomerases are enzymes that consist of α- and β-subunits (encoded for by *gyr*A and *gyr*B or *par*C and *par*E respectively) and catalyze the direction and extent of supercoiling and other topological reactions of DNA chains. Fluoroquinolones act by binding to and trapping the enzyme-DNA complex. This trapped complex blocks DNA synthesis and cell growth and ultimately has a lethal effect on the cell, possibly by releasing lethal double-strand DNA breaks from the complex. The primary target for the quinolone is determined by the differing sensitivities of DNA gyrase and topoisomerase IV to the particular quinolone in each organism (Fig. 47-3).

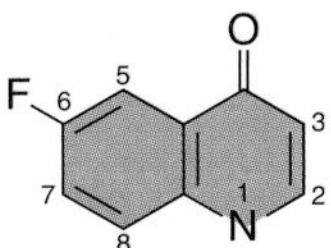

Figure 47-2 Basic 2-ring structure of fluoroquinolones. All fluoroquinolones have a fluorine at position 6 in the 2 ring structure. Other substitutions at positions 1-5 and 7-8 are associated with changes in antibacterial spectrum and pharmacokinetics.

Bacterial resistance is the most common and serious problem confronting the clinical use of fluoroquinolones. Mutations in the type 2 topoisomerases DNA gyrase or topoisomerase IV account for most bacterial resistance to fluoroquinolones. Stepwise increases in resistance are associated with sequential mutations in *gyr*A (or *gyr*B) and *par*C (or *par*E). Decreased permeability, active efflux, and plasmid-mediated resistance have also been described. Fluoroquinolone resistance of clinical significance occurs in *Staphylococcus aureus, Pseudomonas aeruginosa, Campylobacter* spp., *E. coli* and other Enterobacteriaceae, *N. gonorrhea* and, more recently, *Streptococcus pneumoniae.* Higher rates of fluoroquinolone resistance in a population are often associated with high rates of fluoroquinolone use, implicating selection of spontaneous mutants. However, community spread of single clones of fluoroquinolone-resistant *S. pneumoniae* has recently been observed.

Nitrofurans

Nitrofurantoin is a member of a group of synthetic nitrofuran compounds that also includes nitrofurazone. The precise mechanism of action of the nitrofurans is not established. They inhibit many bacterial enzyme systems, most probably through DNA damage. A nitroreductase bacterial enzyme converts the compounds to short-lived intermediates, including oxygen free radicals, which interact with DNA to cause strand breakage and bacterial damage.

Resistance develops infrequently. It is not plasmid mediated but appears to result from a mutation associated with a loss of bacterial nitroreductase activity.

Polymyxins

The polymyxins are branched-chain cyclic decapeptides. They are basically bactericidal cationic detergents with both lipophilic and lipophobic groups that interact with phospholipids and disrupt bacterial cell membranes. The initial damage is to the cell wall, with a subsequent loss of periplasmic enzymes. The divalent cationic sites on the lipopolysaccharide component of the outer membrane of gram-negative organisms

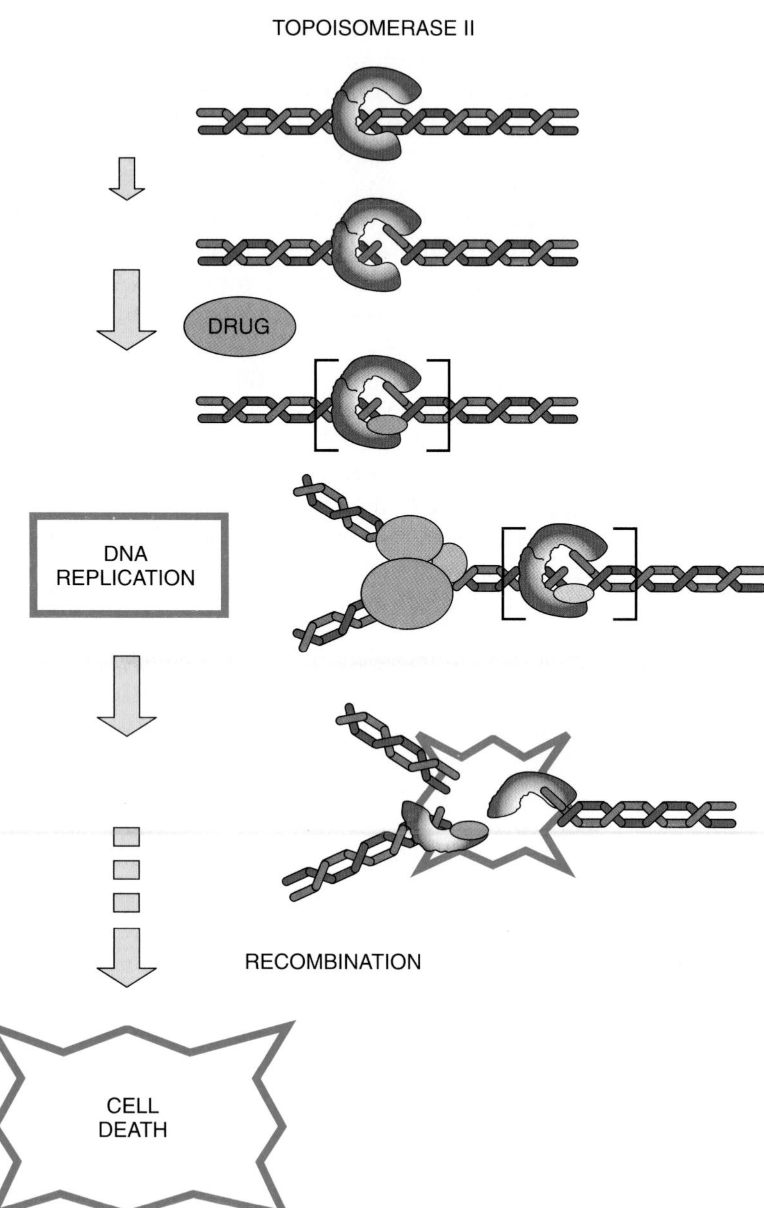

Figure 47-3 Mechanism of cytotoxicity by quinolones. Topoisomerases bind to DNA in a noncovalent fashion followed by formation of transient cleavage complexes. In these complexes, type 2 topoisomerase (DNA gyrase or topoisomerase IV) creates double-stranded breaks. In the presence of quinolones, levels of cleavage complexes (shown in *brackets*) increase dramatically. Following traversal by replication complexes or helicases, transient topoisomerase-mediated breaks become permanent double-stranded fractures, triggering events that ultimately culminate in cell death. (Adapted from Froelich-Ammon SJ, Osheroff N. *J Biological Chem* 1995; 270:21429.)

interact with the amino groups of the cyclic polymyxin peptide. The fatty acid tail portion of the drug molecule penetrates into the hydrophobic areas of the outer wall to produce holes in the membrane through which intracellular constituents leak out of the bacteria (Fig. 47-4). A bacterium is rendered susceptible to the agent as a result of phospholipids in the bacteria cell wall interacting with the drug. The cell walls of resistant bacteria restrict the transport of polymyxin and prevent access of the drug to the cell membrane. Elevated concentrations of calcium or magnesium reduce the activity of the polymyxins.

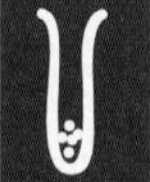

Pharmacokinetics

Relevant pharmacokinetic parameters are summarized in Tables 47-1 and 47-2.

Sulfonamides

Sulfonamides are generally well absorbed from the gastrointestinal (GI) tract, with most absorption occurring in the small intestine. There is minimal absorption from topical application.

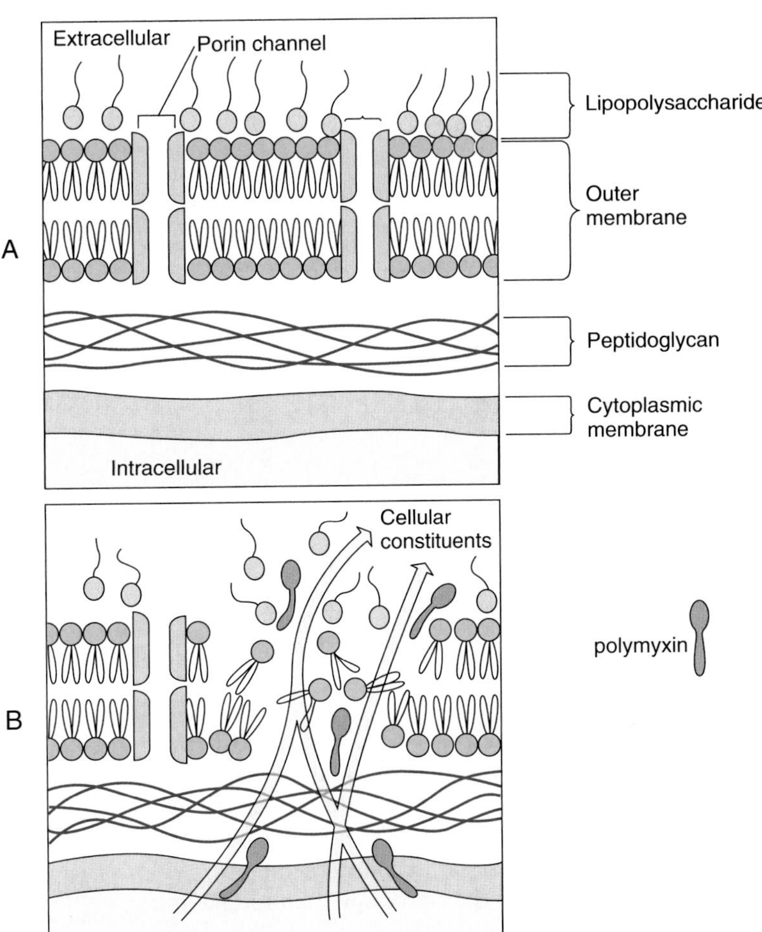

Figure 47-4 Mechanism of action of polymyxins. Microbial cell in absence **(A)** and presence **(B)** of polymyxin.

Table 47-1 Pharmacokinetic properties for sulfonamides and trimethoprim

Drug	Route of Administration	Half-Life (hrs)	Disposition	Plasma Protein Bound (%)
Sulfacetamide	Topical	—	—	—
Sulfisoxazole	Oral	6	R, M	90
Sulfamethoxazole	Oral/IV	11	R, M	70
Sulfadiazine	Oral/IV	17	M, R	45
Sulfadoxine	Oral	120-200	R, M	98
Sulfasalazine	Oral	6-10	R, M	99
Trimethoprim	Oral	11	R (60%)	70

M, Metabolized; *R*, renal excretion as unchanged drug.

Sulfonamides differ in their protein-binding capacity, from a low of 35% to 50% for sulfadiazine to 80% to 99% for sulfisoxazole or sulfasalazine, with less protein binding occurring in renal failure. The drugs enter most body compartments, including ocular, pleural, peritoneal, synovial, and cerebrospinal fluid (CSF). Highest concentrations in the CSF are achieved with sulfadiazine, reaching 30% to 80% of simultaneous plasma concentrations. Sulfonamides cross the placenta and enter the fetal circulation.

Acetylation in liver is a major mechanism of inactivation of sulfonamides. These compounds are also metabolized by glucuronidation. All metabolites are excreted in the urine. Renal elimination is by filtration, with some tubular reabsorption but only slight tubular secretion. Some sulfonamides are poorly soluble and precipitate in acidic urine.

Rapid-acting sulfonamides—including sulfisoxazole, SMX, and sulfadiazine—are rapidly absorbed and eliminated. Sulfadoxine is well absorbed and highly

Table 47-2 Pharmacokinetic properties of fluoroquinolones, nitrofurantoins, and polymyxins

Agent	Administration	Absorption	Half-Life (hrs)	Disposition
Norfloxacin	Oral	50%	4 (8 in anuria)	M (20%) R (27%)
Ciprofloxacin	Oral, IV	75%	4 (10 in anuria)	R (50%) M
Levofloxacin	Oral, IV	98%	7	R (80%)
Gatifloxacin	Oral, IV	96%	7-8	R (70%)
Moxifloxacin	Oral, IV	89%	10-14	R (20%) M (25%) (in liver)
Nitrofurantoin	Oral	Adequate	0.6-1.2	R, M (in tissue)
Polymyxin B	Topical, oral, IV	Not absorbed in adults; absorbed in children	6 by IV	R

M, Metabolized; *R*, renal excretion as unchanged drug.

bound to plasma proteins, with an extraordinarily long half-life of 10 to 17 days. It is combined with pyrimethamine in treatment of falciparum malaria (see Chapter 49).

Sulfasalazine is poorly absorbed from the GI tract and therefore can be used to treat GI infections. It is metabolized by intestinal bacteria to sulfapyridine, which is absorbed from the intestine and excreted in the urine, and in turn to a second metabolite, 5-aminosalicylate, which is the active agent. Sulfasalazine can produce all the toxic reactions of the other sulfonamides.

Trimethoprim

TMP is well absorbed from the GI tract, with peak plasma concentrations reached in about 2 hours. Absorption is not influenced by SMX.

TMP is rapidly and widely distributed to body tissues and compartments, entering pleural, peritoneal, and synovial fluids, as well as the aqueous fluid of the eye, the CSF, and brain. Because of its high lipid solubility, TMP crosses biological membranes and enters bronchial secretions, prostate and vaginal fluids, and bile. TMP and SMX cross the placenta.

Only 10% to 20% of TMP is metabolized by oxidation and conjugation to inactive oxide and hydroxyl derivatives. It is excreted in urine, with 60% of the dose excreted in 24 hours in patients with normal renal function and a linear relationship between the serum creatinine concentration and the half-life of TMP. The half-life of 11 hours in normal adults and children is shortened to approximately 6 hours in young children. Urinary concentrations of TMP are high, even in the presence of decreased renal function, and a small amount of TMP is excreted in bile.

Fluoroquinolones

Fluoroquinolones are well-absorbed from the upper GI tract, with absorption decreased in the presence of magnesium, aluminum, calcium, zinc, or iron. The fluoroquinolones have good tissue penetration with levels in prostate, stool, bile, lung, and neutrophils exceeding serum concentration. Urine and kidney tissue concentrations are also usually high when renal elimination is high. Concentrations of fluoroquinolones in bone are usually lower than serum but still adequate for treatment of osteomyelitis. CSF penetration is not usually sufficient for treatment of meningitis.

The half-lives of norfloxacin and ciprofloxacin require twice-a-day dosing, but levofloxacin, gatifloxacin, and moxifloxacin can be given once daily. Renal elimination is the principle route of elimination for most of these agents, and dose adjustments are required for patients with compromised renal function; moxifloxacin is excreted hepatically.

Nitrofurans

Nitrofurantoin is well absorbed from the GI tract, and absorption is not altered in the presence of food. No drug accumulation occurs except in urine and bile. The drug is excreted into bile, after which it is reabsorbed and eliminated through glomerular filtration and tubular secretion to yield a brown urine. It has a short half-life of 0.6 to 1.2 hours in normal people as the result of rapid excretion and metabolism in tissues. Less drug enters the urine in patients with declining renal function, and treatment of urinary tract infections is ineffective in patients with creatinine clearances of less than 40 ml/min. The drug accumulates and can cause neurotoxicity in patients with severely depressed renal function.

Polymyxins

Polymyxins are not well absorbed after oral or topical administration. Polymyxin B has been given by oral, topical, endobronchial, intramuscular, and IV routes. Colistin, an analog with a structure similar to that of polymyxin E, is given by the IV and oral routes. The drug may be found in urine for up to 3 days after an IV dose. Polymyxins are distributed poorly to tissues and do not enter the CSF. They are excreted by glomerular filtration and accumulate to toxic concentrations in anuric patients.

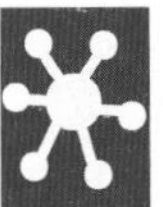

Relation of mechanisms of action to clinical response

Sulfonamides

Sulfonamides have activity against a broad range of gram-positive and -negative bacteria as well as parasites (plasmodia and toxoplasma). However, resistance to sulfonamides has limited their use considerably in the past decade. The sulfonamides are grouped into rapid-acting, intermediate-acting, long-acting, poorly absorbed, and topical agents (see Table 47-1).

Sulfadiazine achieves highest concentrations in CSF and brain. However, when it is used, fluid intake must be high or sodium bicarbonate must be administered to alkalinize the urine and reduce the risk of renal crystalluria. The only long-acting sulfonamide used today is sulfadoxine, which is available in combination with pyrimethamine to treat malaria.

Of the poorly absorbed sulfonamides, sulfasalazine is minimally absorbed from the GI tract and is used to treat ulcerative colitis and regional enteritis. It has no effect on intestinal flora.

Sulfacetamide, a topical agent, is used in ophthalmic preparations because it penetrates into ocular tissues and fluids. Allergic reactions are rare, although it should not be used in patients with a known sulfonamide allergy.

Both silver sulfadiazine and mafenide are active against many bacterial species, including *Pseudomonas aeruginosa* and are used topically in burn patients to reduce the bacterial population in the burn eschar to concentrations low enough to prevent wound sepsis and hasten healing. The activity of silver sulfadiazine probably results from slow release of silver into the surrounding medium. Mafenide is absorbed and converted to *p*-carboxybenzene sulfonamide. Mafenide and its breakdown products are carbonic anhydrase inhibitors, which can cause metabolic acidosis.

Therapeutic uses There are few indications for the use of sulfonamides because of the many other agents available with fewer side effects or better therapeutic profiles. Sulfadiazine is used for treatment of CNS toxoplasmosis (an opportunistic infection in AIDS) in combination with pyrimethamine. Sulfadoxine is given in combination with pyrimethamine in the treatment of malaria. Sulfonamides are drugs of choice for the treatment of nocardiosis, but clinicians usually prefer to give treatment in the form of TMP-SMX combination. The use of sulfasalazine in inflammatory bowel disease and topical sulfonamides are discussed above. Most sulfonamide use is in the form of TMP-SMX (see below).

Trimethoprim

TMP inhibits many different bacteria, and in combination with SMX, several parasites. Because of increasing resistance and the availability of alternative agents, TMP is rarely used alone to treat infection.

TMP-SMX inhibits many *Staphylococcus aureus* (most methicillin-susceptible *S. aureus* and some methicillin-resistant *S. aureus,* especially community-acquired strains); coagulase-negative staphylococci, including *Staphylococcus saprophyticus;* hemolytic streptococci; some *S. pneumoniae, H. influenzae; N. meningitidis; N. gonorrhoeae; Listeria monocytogenes;* aerobic gram-negative bacteria such as *E. coli* and *Klebsiella;* and some more difficult species to inhibit such as *Enterobacter, Citrobacter, Serratia and Stenotrophomonas. Salmonella, Shigella, Aeromonas,* and *Yersinia* species may be susceptible, but enterococci and *Campylobacter* species are resistant.

TMP-SMX inhibits *P. carinii* and *Isospora belli,* the parasitic organisms in immunocompromised patients that cause some pneumonias and diarrhea, respectively.

Therapeutic uses TMP-SMX is active against many Enterobacteriaceae and has been the drug of choice in the U.S. for the treatment of uncomplicated urinary tract infections. The prevalence of resistance in *E. coli* now threatens the empiric use of TMP-SMX. Recent guidelines recommend that once the local prevalence of *E. coli* resistant to TMP-SMX exceeds 20%, quinolones replace TMP-SMX for empiric treatment of urinary tract infections. TMP-SMX is considered an alternative to quinolones for prostatitis resulting from Enterobacteriaceae.

TMP-SMX has been used in treatment of upper and lower respiratory tract infections because of its activity against *H. influenzae, Moraxella* species, and *S. pneumoniae.* Emerging resistance among *S. pneumoniae* and also *H. flu* and *Moraxella* in the U.S., Canada, and Europe have changed recommendations for use in these settings. TMP-SMX is considered an alternative to high-dose amoxicillin in patients allergic to β-lactam antibiotics (adults and children) for treatment of mild acute bacterial sinusitis. TMP-SMX is no longer recommended as an empiric therapy for community-acquired pneumonia.

TMP-SMX is no longer recommended for treatment of traveler's diarrhea or for most identified bacterial diarrhea because of the high prevalence of resistance in *Shigella* and enterotoxigenic *E. coli.*

High-dose TMP-SMX is the treatment of choice for *Pneumocystis* pneumonia in immunocompromised patients. An oral regimen of TMP in combination with dapsone is one of several alternatives to oral high dose TMP-SMX in mild to moderate *P. carinii* pneumonia.

TMP-SMX provides effective prophylaxis against *P. carinii* pneumonia in patients with cell-mediated immune defects, such as those seen in patients with acquired immunodeficiency syndrome and in some solid organ transplant recipients. This combination has also proved useful in preventing spontaneous bacterial peritonitis in patients with underlying cirrhosis. TMP-SMX is also used for the treatment of Whipple's disease caused by *Tropheryma whippleii.*

Fluoroquinolones

Fluoroquinolones are broadly active against aerobic gram-negative bacilli including *Pseudomonas aeruginosa.* Third-generation quinolones have increased activity against gram-positive pathogens including *S. pneumoniae.* Fluoroquinolones are also active against many agents causing zoonotic infection and against mycobacteria.

Therapeutic uses Fluoroquinolones are effective for treatment of uncomplicated and complicated urinary tract infections caused by Enterobacteriaceae and have become drugs of choice in areas where the prevalence of TMP-SMX resistance is over 20% (Table 47-3). Because of activity against *N. gonorrhea* and *C. trachomatis* as well as Enterobacteriaceae, fluoroquinolones are drugs of choice for both acute and chronic prostatitis.

In treating sexually transmitted diseases, fluoroquinolones in a single dose are considered possible alternatives to ceftriaxone for gonorrhea in patients with β-lactam allergy and in multi-day dosing as alternative agents to azithromycin (single dose) or doxycycline (multi-day dosing) for chlamydia treatment. Fluoroquinolones are used in combination with other agents in treatment of pelvic inflammatory disease. Fluoroquinolone-resistant *N. gonorrhea* limits the efficacy of these drugs in Asia, the Pacific (including Hawaii) and more recently, California. Resistance of *N. gonorrhea* to fluoroquinolones is expected to spread, and resistance testing should be pursued when gonorrhea is diagnosed.

Table 47-3 Clinical uses of fluoroquinolones

Disease	Recommendations
RESPIRATORY TRACT INFECTIONS	
Pharyngitis, otitis media	Not appropriate
Necrotizing otitis	Ciprofloxacin for *Pseudomonas aeruginosa*
Sinusitis	Third-generation fluoroquinolone
Community-acquired pneumonia	Third-generation fluoroquinolone
Hospital-acquired pneumonia	Ciprofloxacin, for susceptible gram-negative pathogens
URINARY TRACT INFECTIONS	
Cystitis, uncomplicated	All effective (second generation most appropriate)
Pyelonephritis	All effective (second generation most appropriate)
Prostatitis	All effective
SKIN STRUCTURE INFECTIONS	
Primary cellulitis	Not appropriate as first line therapy
Anaerobic soft-tissue infections	Not appropriate
OSTEOMYELITIS	
Gram-negative bacterial infections	Ciprofloxacin
BACTERIAL DIARRHEAL DISEASES	Ciprofloxacin used most commonly; all considered likely to be effective
SEXUALLY TRANSMITTED DISEASES	
Gonorrhea	Resistance testing required
Chlamydia	Ofloxacin, levofloxacin
Chancroid	All likely to be effective
Mycoplasma	Ofloxacin, levofloxacin
Syphilis	Not appropriate
MYCOBACTERIAL DISEASES	
Disseminated *M. avium* complex	Ciprofloxacin, ofloxacin as fourth agent if needed
M. tuberculosis	Ofloxacin, levofloxacin for drug-resistance or intolerance to first-line agents

Modified from Neu HC. The crisis in antibiotic resistance. *Science* 1992; 257:1054.

Fluoroquinolones are efficacious for treating diarrhea caused by *Shigella* organisms, toxigenic *E. coli, Campylobacter, Salmonella,* and typhoid and are drugs of choice in the empiric treatment of traveler's diarrhea.

Fluoroquinolones are useful in treatment of osteomyelitis, and in particular, ciprofloxacin is effective therapy for susceptible *Pseudomonas* osteomyelitis. The potential for rapid development of quinolone resistance in Staphylococci during quinolone therapy limits the role of fluoroquinolones in the treatment of skin and soft tissue infections, especially if *S. aureus* is suspected. In combination with a gram-positive agent such as clindamycin, fluoroquinolones may be used for the treatment of complicated diabetic foot infections.

A single dose of ciprofloxacin constitutes an alternative to rifampin for eradication of *Neisseria Meningitidis* in asymptomatic carriers.

Because of their enhanced activity against gram-positive organisms, including pneumococci (both penicillin-susceptible and penicillin-resistant *S. pneumoniae*), levofloxacin, moxifloxacin, and gatifloxacin are drugs of choice for treating community-acquired pneumonia. They, like other fluoroquinolones, are also active against atypical causes of pneumonia, such as *Chlamydia* species, *Mycoplasma pneumoniae,* and *Legionella pneumophila.* Ciprofloxacin is effective in treatment of susceptible *Pseudomonas* respiratory infections in cystic fibrosis.

Fluoroquinolones are drugs of choice for treatment of and postexposure prophylaxis against several agents that could be used in biowarfare. Fluoroquinolones are recommended for treatment of anthrax, cholera, plague, brucellosis, and tularemia.

Fluoroquinolones are useful in the treatment of mycobacterial infections. Multi-drug treatment of *Mycobacterium avium* complex infections may include a fluoroquinolone as a third or fourth agent. Ofloxacin and levofloxacin are commonly used in the treatment of multi-drug resistant tuberculosis and for tuberculosis patients intolerant to first-line therapies. Moxifloxacin pharmacokinetics and potency predict that it may be useful as an additional first-line therapy for tuberculosis.

Nitrofurans

Nitrofurans are used to treat urinary tract infections, while nitrofurazone is used only for topical applications. Both inhibit a variety of gram-positive and gram-negative bacteria, including most *E. coli,* staphylococci, many *Klebsiella* species, enterococci, neisseriae, salmonellae, *Shigella* organisms, and *Proteus* bacteria.

Polymyxins

The polymyxins are used *topically* as a single agent to treat *Pseudomonas* infections of the mucous membranes, eye, and ear and also in combination with other antimicrobials (commonly neomycin and bacitracin) for minor skin, ear, and eye infections. Gram-positive and anaerobic organisms generally are resistant to polymyxins. However, *E. coli, Klebsiella, Enterobacter, Shigella, Pseudomonas,* and *Acinetobacter* are susceptible. In recent years, systemic IV Polymyxin B has been used to treat serious infections caused by multi-drug resistant gram-negative bacilli with over 85% efficacy and a 14% rate of nephrotoxicity (lower than reported in the older literature).

Side effects, clinical problems, and toxicity

The major clinical problems for these drugs are summarized in the Clinical Problems box.

Sulfonamides

Sulfonamides cause many adverse effects, the most important of which are hypersensitivity reactions. Aller-

CLINICAL PROBLEMS

Trimethoprim-sulfamethoxazole

Numerous side effects
- Hypersensitivity: rashes, fever
- Stevens-Johnson syndrome (with long-acting agents)
- Hematological reactions

Increased serum creatinine concentration (Trimethoprim)

Drug interactions
- Protein binding displacement
- Competition for metabolizing enzymes

Fluoroquinolones

Gastrointestinal effects
Central nervous system agitation (rarely seizures)
Damage to growing cartilage (not recommended for use in children)
Theophylline interaction (with ciprofloxacin)

Nitrofurans

Gastrointestinal effects
Hypersensitivity
Cutaneous reactions
Pulmonary reactions

Polymyxins

Nephrotoxicity and neurotoxicity

gic rashes are frequent, occurring in approximately 2% to 3% of patients receiving these drugs. Rashes may be maculopapular, urticarial, or, rarely, exfoliative, as in the Stevens-Johnson syndrome. Most rashes occur after 1 week of therapy but can occur earlier in previously sensitized people. A serum sickness–like illness also is seen, with fever, joint pains, and rash, which can be of the erythema nodosum type. Drug fever occurs in about 3% of patients given sulfonamides. Arteritis of a periarteritis, or a systemic lupus erythematosus type, has also been reported.

Several hematological toxicities are seen with sulfonamides. These include agranulocytosis, megaloblastic anemia, aplastic anemia, hemolytic anemia, and thrombocytopenia. Hemolytic anemia can occur in patients deficient in glucose-6-phosphate dehydrogenase, in whom the sulfonamide serves as an oxidant. Hemolysis can also occur in patients who have normal glucose-6-phosphate dehydrogenase concentrations.

Hepatotoxicity occurs in less than 0.1% of patients receiving sulfonamides, and renal damage is rare in patients receiving the newer sulfonamides, but sulfadiazine can precipitate in the kidneys, ureters, and bladder and lead to renal failure.

Drug interactions include potentiation of the action of sulfonylurea hypoglycemic agents, orally administered anticoagulants, phenytoin, and methotrexate. Mechanisms include displacement of albumin-bound drug and competition for drug-metabolizing enzymes.

Trimethoprim

TMP alone can cause nausea, vomiting, and diarrhea but rarely causes a rash. TMP can increase creatinine concentrations, because both compounds compete for the same renal clearance pathways. Hyperkalemia has been associated with the use of high-dose TMP-SMX and is now known to result from a TMP-induced decrease in potassium secretion in the distal tubule.

TMP-SMX is associated with all the complications of both agents. Hematological toxicity in the form of megaloblastic anemia, thrombocytopenia, and leukopenia occurs more often in patients receiving the combination than in those receiving single agents and can be dose related. Other toxicity-related conditions include glossitis, stomatitis, and occasional pseudomembranous enterocolitis. Central nervous system effects include headache, depression, and hallucinations.

The incidence of rash and neutropenia is greater in patients with acquired immune deficiency syndrome than in other patients treated with TMP-SMX. The importance of TMP-SMX in the prevention of *P. carinii* pneumonia has prompted investigation of ways to manage allergic reactions to TMP-SMX in patients with acquired immune deficiency. Both symptomatic treatment (antihistamines or steroids) of the effect and oral desensitization have been effective.

Fluoroquinolones

Fluoroquinolones can cause GI reactions such as nausea, vomiting, and abdominal pain. Outbreaks of pseudomembranous colitis have been reported in hospitals following the introduction of a third generation fluoroquinolone on the formulary. Central nervous system effects—dizziness, headache, restlessness, depression, and insomnia—are infrequent but more common in the elderly and may be potentiated by the concomitant use of nonsteroidal antiinflammatory drugs. Seizures are a rare problem. Dermatologic reactions including rash, photosensitivity reactions, and pruritus are not uncommon. Hepatotoxicity can occur occasionally in association with these agents; high rates of these adverse events observed in post-marketing surveillance have caused several other fluoroquinolones to be removed from the market.

Quinolones produce damage to cartilage in immature animals and are not recommended for use in children, and quinolone therapy has been associated with multiple reports of tendon rupture (usually the Achilles tendon). Theophylline concentrations become elevated in patients treated with ciprofloxacin.

Nitrofurans

The most common adverse reactions to the nitrofurans are GI in nature, with anorexia, nausea, and vomiting the most prevalent. Hypersensitivity reactions involving the skin, lungs, liver, or blood also occur and are often associated with fever and chills. Cutaneous effects include maculopapular, erythematous, urticarial, and pruritic reactions.

Two major types of pulmonary reactions occur in patients receiving nitrofuran. An acute immunologically mediated reaction, characterized by fever, cough, and dyspnea, begins about 10 days into treatment. A second form occurs in patients receiving long-term therapy. The onset is insidious, with patients exhibiting cough, shortness of breath, and radiological signs of interstitial fibrosis. Patients' conditions improve when the drug is stopped, but many have residual effects, which are believed to be caused by peroxidative destruction of pulmonary membrane lipids. These arise from the reactive oxygen derivatives produced by the action of reductase on the nitrofurans.

The nitrofurans also cause cholestatic and hepatocellular liver disease and granulomatous hepatitis.

Hematological reactions include granulocytopenia, leukopenia, and megaloblastic anemia, with acute hemolytic anemia occurring in patients deficient in glucose-6-phosphate dehydrogenase. Several neurological reactions including headache, drowsiness, dizziness, nystagmus, and peripheral neuropathy of an ascending sensorimotor type are also observed.

Polymyxins

The polymyxins have few adverse effects when used topically. IV administration of polymyxins can cause nephrotoxicity and neurotoxicity, but recent experience suggests that the incidence of these side effects is not high enough to prohibit use when clinically indicated (serious infection with a polymyxin susceptible organism and no alternative therapy). The mechanism of polymyxin-induced nephrotoxicity is not established but appears to result from polymyxin binding to renal tubule cell membranes. This produces proteinuria, casts, and a loss of brush border enzymes and can progress to renal failure. Renal function usually returns when the drug is discontinued.

The polymyxins may damage some mammalian cell membranes and can cause neuromuscular blockade and respiratory paralysis. They can also produce persistent blockade of the action of acetylcholine at the neuromuscular junction, which is not reversed by neostigmine.

New horizons

Sulfonamides and trimethoprim have been mainstays of antibiotic therapy for years. The fluoroquinolones have proven very useful in treatment of a variety of other diseases, but bacterial resistance has become an increasing problem. The search for new antibiotics to replace the older compounds to which bacteria have become increasingly resistant has become a matter of grave concern. Fortunately, with the newfound ability to rapidly sequence and compare genomes of specific bacteria, new targets for antibiotics are rapidly emerging. Hopefully, development of such new compounds will be successful before a crisis occurs in which strains of bacteria emerge that are resistant to all known antibiotics.

TRADE NAMES

In addition to generic and fixed-combination preparations and the drugs listed in the Major Drugs box, the following trade-named materials are some of the important compounds available in the United States.

Mafenide (Sulfamylon)
Nitrofurazone (Furacin)
Ofloxacin (Floxin)
Pyrimethamine-sulfadoxine (Fansidar)
Silver sulfadiazine (Silvadene)
Sulfisoxazole (Gantrisin)
Sulfacetamide (Sulamyd)
Sulfadiazine (generic only)
Sulfadoxine (Fansidar)
Sulfasalazine (Azulfidine)

FURTHER READING

Kovacs JA, Gill VJ, Meshnick S, et al. New insights into transmission, diagnosis, and drug treatment of Pneumocystis carinii pneumonia. *JAMA* 2001; 286:2450.

Masters PA, O'Bryan TA, Zurlo J, et al. Trimethoprim-sulfamethoxazole revisited. *Arch Intern Med* 2003; 163:402.

Oliphant CM. Quinolones: a comprehensive review. *Am Fam Physician* 2002; 65(3):455.

Self-assessment questions

1. The activity of which of the following is antagonized by *para*-aminobenzoic acid?
   a. Trimethoprim
   b. Sulfamethoxazole
   c. Metronidazole
   d. Norfloxacin
   e. Polymyxin B

2. Trimethoprim alters the excretion of:
   a. Penicillins.
   b. Creatinine.
   c. Aminoglycosides.
   d. Uric acid.

3. Which of the following organisms is routinely resistant to trimethoprim-sulfamethoxazole?

a. *Escherichia coli*
b. *Nocardia asteroides*
c. *Toxoplasma gondii*
d. *Candida albicans*

4. Which is the mechanism of action of levofloxacin?

a. It interferes with peptidoglycan synthesis.
b. It damages membranes, with loss of K.
c. It inhibits DNA gyrase and topoisomerase IV.
d. It inhibits peptidyl transfer on ribosomes.
e. It inhibits DNA-directed RNA polymerase.

5. Polymyxins inhibit bacteria by which of the following mechanisms?

a. Interfere with cell wall synthesis
b. Inhibit DNA gyrase β
c. Inhibit protein synthesis
d. Damage cytoplasmic membrane by interacting with phospholipids

6. Second-generation fluoroquinolones, ciprofloxacin, and ofloxacin, inhibit which of the following?

a. *E. coli*
b. *Bacteroides fragilis*
c. *Streptococcus pneumoniae*
d. *Staphylococcus aureus*

CHAPTER 48

Selection of an antibacterial agent

James P. Steinberg

The basic principles that should be considered when selecting an antibiotic to treat a specific patient are described in Chapter 44, and specific agents are discussed in Chapters 45 through 47. The extensive variety of pathogenic bacteria, the numerous antibiotics available, and the significant list of factors to be considered in rationally selecting antibiotic therapy can be confusing for the student or even the nonspecialist in infectious diseases. In this chapter, the complexities of antimicrobial therapy are reduced to tables, which, at risk of oversimplification, should help provide an overview of the clinical utility of specific agents in treatment of common pathogens and clinical syndromes.

The following considerations are critical:

- Which bacteria are inhibited by each drug type and subtype
- Which bacteria are most commonly associated with infections at different anatomical sites
- The antibiotics that do or do not attain high enough concentrations at specific anatomical sites of infections for effective therapy
- Trends in antibiotic resistance.

Antibiotic activity

The major classes of antibiotics are listed in Table 48-1, along with the types of bacteria that they inhibit. The classifications are a simplification. For example, not all cephalosporins are active against all gram-positive or gram-negative bacteria, and several gram-negative species are not inhibited by any of the cephalosporins. The relative activities of some representative antibiotics against individual microbial species are given in greater detail in Table 48-2. Because of variable rates of antibiotic resistance, the relative activities are approximate and subject to change.

Bacteria and anatomical sites

It is estimated that initial antimicrobial therapy is started in 75% of bacterial infections before the pathogenic microorganisms have been identified and that the specific organisms are never identified in approximately 50% of treated infections. It is important to know the bacterial strains that may be present at selected anatomical sites, because this may be the only meaningful way of guiding the selection of an antibiotic when the locus of infection is known. Table 48-3 lists the common organisms that infect specific anatomical sites, and Table 48-4 groups organisms with the anatomical locations of the infection and the drugs often used for treatment.

Most infections can be treated successfully with different antibiotics, so there may be more than one correct therapy. Local antibiotic resistance rates should be taken into consideration when choosing a regimen.

Table 48-1 Overview of antibacterial activity of major antibiotics

Antibiotics	Effective Against
Penicillins	Many gram-positive cocci, some gram negative
Penicillin/β-lactamase inhibitor	More gram positive, gram negative, anaerobes
Cephalosporins	
First generation	Gram positive, some gram negative
Second generation	More gram negative, similar gram positive
Third generation	More gram negative, less gram positive; some inhibit *Pseudomonas*
Fourth generation	Better gram positive; more gram negative (more β-lactamase stable), inhibit *Pseudomonas*
Carbapenems	Broad gram positive, gram negative, anaerobes
Aztreonam	Aerobic gram negative only
Vancomycin	Gram positive only
Quinolones	Variable gram positive, most gram negative, *Mycoplasma, Chlamydia, Legionella*
Aminoglycosides	Aerobic gram-negative bacilli
Tetracyclines	Aerobic and anaerobic gram-positive and gram-negative *Mycoplasma, Chlamydia*
Macrolides	Gram positive, *Mycoplasma, Chlamydia, Legionella*
Clindamycin	Many gram-positive cocci, many anaerobes
Sulfonamides	Some gram positive and gram negative
Rifampin	Gram positive (in combination with other agents)
Streptogramins	Gram positive
Oxazolidinones	Gram positive
Metronidazole	Anaerobes

Table 48-2 Susceptibility of common bacteria to antibiotics*

Organisms	A	B	C	D	E	F	G	H	I	J	K	L	M	N	O	P	Q
GRAM POSITIVE																	
Streptococcus pyogenes	4	4	4	4	4	4	4	3	4	0	0	3	3	4	4	2	4
Streptococcus pneumoniae	3	3	3	3	3	3	3	2	3	0	0	3	2	3	4	2	4
Staphylococcus aureus	0	0	0	2	2	2	2	1	2	1	2	2	2	2	4	1	2
Enterococcus faecalis	2	3	3	3	0	0	0	0	2	0†	0	0	1	0	3	1	1
GRAM NEGATIVE																	
E. coli	0	2	2	4	3	3	4	4	4	3	4	2	0	0	0	3	3
Klebsiella spp.	0	0	2	3	3	3	3	3	4	3	4	2	0	0	0	3	3
Enterobacter spp.	0	0	2	2	0	1	2	2	4	3	4	2	0	0	0	4	4
Pseudomonas aeruginosa	0	0	3	3	0	0	0	3	3	2	3	0	0	0	0	2	2
Haemophilus influenzae	1	2	2	4	2	4	4	4	4	3	3	2	1	0	0	4	4
Neisseria gonorrhoeae	2	2	2	4	2	4	4	4	4	0	3	3	0	0	0	3	3
ANAEROBES																	
Clostridium spp.	4	4	4	4	2	3	3	1	4	0	0	3	2	3	4	0	1
Bacteroides spp.	1	1	2	4	0	0	1	0	4	0	0	1	1	3	0	1	2

A, Penicillin G; *B,* ampicillin; *C,* piperacillin; *D,* piperacillin/tazobactam; *E,* cefazolin (first); *F,* cefuroxime (second); *G,* cefotaxime, ceftriaxone, ceftizoxime (third); *H,* ceftazidime; *I,* Imipenem; *J,* gentamicin; *K,* amikacin; *L,* doxycycline; *M,* erythromycin; *N,* clindamycin; *O,* vancomycin: *P,* ciprofloxacin; *Q,* levofloxacin.

*Ratings based on tissue or plasma concentration expected for normal dosing schedule; *4,* resistance uncommon; *3,* clinically useful but not predictably active; *2,* variably active; *1,* limited activity or resistance widespread; *0,* inactive.

†Has activity when combined with a cell wall active drug such as ampicillin.

Table 48-3 Common microorganisms causing infections

OTITIS MEDIA	**INTRAABDOMINAL SEPSIS**
Streptococcus pneumoniae	*E. coli*
Haemophilus influenzae	*Klebsiella*
Moraxella catarrhalis	*Enterobacter*
Viral	*Proteus*
SINUSITIS	Enterococci
S. pneumoniae	*Bacteroides*
H. influenzae	Anaerobic streptococci
Streptococci	*Clostridium* sp.
Staphylococcus aureus	**GYNECOLOGIC**
Anaerobes (chronic sinusitis)	Gonococci
Viral	*Chlamydia*
PNEUMONIA	*E. coli*
S. pneumoniae	*Klebsiella*
H. influenzae	Streptococci
Mycoplasma pneumoniae	*Bacteroides*
Chlamydia pneumoniae	**URINARY TRACT INFECTION**
Legionella pneumophila	*E. coli*
Klebsiella pneumoniae	*Klebsiella*
S. aureus	*Proteus*
Other gram negative bacilli	Enterococci
Mixed anaerobes	*Staph saprophyticus*
Tuberculosis	*Pseudomonas*
Viral	**SKIN**
MENINGITIS	Group A streptococci
Cryptococcus neoformans	*S. aureus*
Group B streptococci	Other streptococci
Listeria	Gram-negative rods (rarer)
H. influenzae	**ENDOCARDITIS**
Meningococci	*Strep viridans*
S. pneumoniae	*S. aureus*
DIARRHEA	Enterococci
Salmonella	Coagulase negative staph
Shigella	Gram-negative bacilli
Campylobacter	*Bartonella*
E. coli	
Vibrio	
Yersinia	
C. difficile	
Viral	

Table 48-4 Organisms with common infection sites and drugs of choice for treatment

Bacteria	Infection	First Choice	Alternatives
GRAM POSITIVE			
Staphylococcus aureus	Abscess, cellulitis, bacteremia, pneumonia, endocarditis	Nafcillin, cefazolin Vancomycin, if methicillin resistant	Clindamycin TMP-SMX, linezolid, daptomycin
Streptococcus pyogenes (group A)	Pharyngitis	Penicillin V	1-Cephalosporin
	Cellulitis		Clindamycin, macrolide
Streptococcus (group B)	Meningitis	Penicillin G	Cefotaxime
	Cellulitis, sepsis	Penicillin G or ampicillin	1-Cephalosporin
Enterococcus	Bacteremia	Ampicillin	Vancomycin Linezolid if vancomycin resistant
	Endocarditis	Ampicillin/gentamicin	Vancomycin/gentamicin
	Urinary tract	Ampicillin	Fluoroquinolone, nitrofurantoin
Streptococcus (viridans group)	Endocarditis	Penicillin/gentamicin	Cephalosporin, vancomycin
Streptococcus pneumoniae	Pneumonia	Penicillin G, ceftriaxone	Fluoroquinolone, vancomycin
	Otitis, sinusitis	Amoxicillin	Erythromycin
	Meningitis	Penicillin G (or, for penicillin-resistant strains, vancomycin)	Cefotaxime, ceftriaxone
Listeria monocytogenes	Bacteremia, meningitis, endocarditis	Ampicillin	TMP-SMX
GRAM NEGATIVE			
Escherichia coli	Urinary tract	TMP-SMX, fluoroquinolone	Cephalosporin
	Bacteremia	3-Cephalosporin	TMP-SMX, fluoroquinolone
Klebsiella pneumoniae	Urinary tract	Fluoroquinolone	Cephalosporin, TMP-SMX
	Pneumonia, bacteremia	3-Cephalosporin	Imipenem, aztreonam, fluoroquinolone
Proteus mirabilis	Urinary tract	Ampicillin	TMP-SMX
Haemophilus influenzae	Otitis, sinusitis, bronchitis	Amoxicillin-clavulanate	2-3-Cephalosporin, TMP-SMX, azithromycin
	Epiglottitis	Cefotaxime, ceftriaxone	Cefuroxime
Pseudomonas aeruginosa	Urinary tract	Fluoroquinolone	Antipseudomonal penicillin ceftazidime, aminoglycoside
	Pneumonia, bacteremia	Antipseudomonal penicillin, ceftazidime	Aztreonam, aminoglycoside, quinolones, carbapenem
Moraxella catarrhalis	Otitis, sinusitis	Amoxicillin-clavulanate	TMP-SMX, macrolide
Neisseria gonorrhoeae	Genital	Ceftriaxone	Fluoroquinolone
ANAEROBES			
Bacteroides spp.	Abdominal infections, abscesses	Metronidazole	Penicillin/β-lactamase inhibitor combinations, carbapenems, clindamycin
Clostridium perfringens	Abscesses, gangrene	Penicillin G	Metronidazole
Clostridium difficile	Diarrhea	Metronidazole	Vancomycin
OTHER			
Legionella spp.	Pulmonary	Azithromycin, fluoroquinolone	Erythromycin, doxycycline (±rifampin)
Mycoplasma pneumoniae	Pulmonary	Azithromycin, doxycycline	Ciprofloxacin, levofloxacin, clarithromycin
Chlamydia pneumoniae	Pulmonary	Doxycycline, azithromycin	Clarithromycin, fluoroquinolone
Chlamydia trachomatis	Genital	Azithromycin, doxycycline	Levofloxacin
Rickettsia	Rocky Mountain spotted fever	Doxycycline	Chloramphenicol
Ehrlichia spp.	Ehrlichiosis	Doxycycline	Chloramphenicol

TMP-SMX, Trimethoprim-sulfamethoxazole; *1-Cephalosporin,* first-generation cephalosporin; *2-Cephalosporin,* second-generation cephalosporin; *3-Cephalosporin,* third-generation cephalosporin.

FURTHER READING

The choice of antibacterial drugs. *Med Lett* 2001; 43:69-78.

Virk A, Steckelberg JM. Clinical aspects of antimicrobial resistance. *Mayo Clinic Proceedings* 2000; 75:200-214.

Self-assessment questions

1. Which of the following is not appropriate to treat *Legionella* pneumonia?

a. Erythromycin
b. Rifampin
c. Gentamicin
d. Ciprofloxacin

2. A 32-year-old pregnant woman develops a fever and sore throat. Culture confirms streptococcal pharyngitis. Which antibiotic would be the best choice?

a. Doxycycline
b. Levofloxacin
c. Trimethoprim-sulfamethoxazole
d. Penicillin V

3. Which of the following is appropriate to treat meningitis caused by *Listeria monocytogenes?*

a. Cefotaxime
b. Ampicillin
c. Ceftriaxone
d. Erythromycin

4. Tetracyclines are not used in the treatment of:

a. Ehrlichiosis.
b. Rocky Mountain spotted fever.
c. *Mycoplasma pneumonia.*
d. *Chlamydia salpingitis.*
e. *Streptococcus viridans* endocarditis in a penicillin-allergic patient.

5. Which of the following is used to treat *Clostridium difficile* colitis?

a. Rifampin
b. Amphotericin B
c. Erythromycin
d. Metronidazole
e. Clindamycin

6. Which one of the following statements is *incorrect?*

a. Ceftriaxone is a good choice to treat pneumococcal pneumonia but it is not useful against "atypical" pneumonia pathogens such as *Mycoplasma pneumonia*.
b. β-Lactamase inhibitor combinations and imipenem have excellent activity against anaerobes
c. Vancomycin has broad activity against gram positive and gram negative organisms
d. Aztreonam is active against gram negative aerobic organisms only.
e. Nafcillin is no longer predictably active against *Staphylococcus aureus*.

CHAPTER 49

Antimycobacterial agents

Henry M. Blumberg

Major Drugs

First-Line Drugs for Tuberculosis
Isoniazid (INH, Laniazid)
Rifampin (Rimactane)
Rifabutin (Mycobutin)
Rifapentine (Priftin)
Pyrazinamide (PZA)
Ethambutol (Myambutol)

Second-Line Drugs for Tuberculosis
Fluoroquinolones
Streptomycin
Kanamycin (Kantrex)
Amikacin (Amikin)
Capreomycin (Capastat)
Ethionamide (Trecator-SC)
p-Aminosalicylic acid (PAS)
Cycloserine (Seromycin)

Other Drugs
Dapsone
Clofazimine (Lamprene)
Minocycline (Dynacin, Minocin)
Azithromycin (Zithromax)
Clarithromycin (Biaxin)

Therapeutic overview

The genus *Mycobacterium* consists of relatively slow-growing, obligate **aerobic** bacilli with a unique lipid-rich cell wall that allows these organisms to take up basic dyes and resist decolorization with acid-alcohol ("acid-fast" organisms). The acid fast cell wall of *Mycobacterium* contains a large amount of glycolipids. A waxy lipid called **mycolic acid** makes up approximately 60% of the cell wall and makes it relatively impermeable. *M. tuberculosis* and *M. leprae* are virulent and the major human mycobacterial pathogens, while most mycobacteria inhabit soil and water and occasionally cause human disease. For example, *M. avium* complex (MAC) causes infections among highly immunocompromised patients with HIV infection (CD4 T lymphocyte counts of <75/μl) and in persons with abnormal lung anatomy or physiology. More rapidly growing non-tuberculous mycobacteria can cause skin and soft tissue infection after trauma or surgery (e.g., *M. chelonae* or *M. fortuitum*) or after exposure to salt water (*M. marinum*). This chapter focuses on agents used to treat *M. tuberculosis*, *M. leprae*, and *M. avium* complex.

Tuberculosis (TB) is transmitted person to person by airborne droplet nuclei, which are small particles (1-5 micron diameter). TB classically is a pulmonary disease, but disseminated and extrapulmonary disease, especially among immunocompromised persons, also occurs.

TB has emerged as a global public health **epidemic** and is the second leading cause of death worldwide caused by an infectious disease. In 2004, the World Health Organization estimates that there will be more than 8 million persons who develop active disease and more than 2 million deaths, mostly in resource-poor countries. In the United States, there was a resurgence of TB between 1985 and 1992, largely because of under-

Abbreviations

AIDS	acquired immunodeficiency syndrome
CNS	central nervous system
CSF	cerebral spinal fluid
DOT	directly observed therapy
GI	gastrointestinal
HIV	human immunodeficiency virus
INH	isoniazid (isonicotinic acid hydrazide)
LTBI	latent tuberculosis infection
MAC	*Mycobacterium avium* complex
MDR	multidrug resistant
PAS	*p*-aminosalicylic acid
PZA	pyrazinamide
TB	tuberculosis

funding and decline of the public health infrastructure. With increased attention and funding, since 1992 there has been a decline in the number of TB cases in the U.S. to 14,871 TB cases in 2003 (5.1 per 100,000 population). The global epidemic of TB has impacted the United States, where the majority of cases now occur among foreign-born persons. There are great racial/ethnic disparities among case rates. In 2003, the rate among U.S.-born African-Americans was almost 8 times that of Caucasians.

Treatment of TB is much different than treatment of other diseases because of its public health implications. The provider has the responsibility for prescribing an appropriate regimen *and* ensuring that treatment is completed. **Directly observed therapy** (DOT) is recommended for all patients with active TB disease and can help ensure higher completion rates (Fig. 49-1), decrease risk for emergence of resistance, and enhance TB control. DOT is generally provided by public health agencies. Active TB should never be treated with a single drug because of the risk of emergence of resistance; multidrug therapy is required. The minimum length of therapy is 6 to 9 months. Patients with drug resistance, especially multidrug resistance (MDR) (i.e., resistance to at least isoniazid and rifampin) require longer therapy. MDR-TB is associated with much higher morbidity and mortality. Drug resistance is an important factor in determining the appropriate therapeutic regimen. Patients who are infected with *M. tuberculosis* (latent TB infection or LTBI) are at risk for progressing to active disease. This can be greatly reduced by treating persons with LTBI who are at high or increased risk for progression to active disease (e.g., HIV-infection, other illnesses that increase risk of progression, recent infection, recent immigration from high TB endemic area).

Leprosy is rare in the U.S. and Canada but is not uncommon in developing countries (620,000 cases in 2002). India, Brazil, and Nepal have the highest prevalence; the largest number of cases is in Southeast Asia. Transmission is thought to occur by the respiratory route, since the nasal discharge from patients with untreated multibacillary leprosy often contains large numbers of bacilli. Transmission may occasionally occur through direct skin contact. In the United States, leprosy is seen primarily among immigrants, although small pockets occur in Texas, Hawaii, and Louisiana. *M. leprae* is the causative organism, which multiplies very slowly with a generation time of 12.5 days and an incubation period of years. Clinical manifestations depend on the infected person's immune response to *M. leprae.* Skin and peripheral nerves in cooler areas of the body are most commonly affected. Prompt recognition is key to limiting morbidity caused by irreversible nerve damage. The disease is curable with multidrug therapy.

THERAPEUTIC OVERVIEW

Tuberculosis

Tuberculosis is a huge global health problem; the second leading cause of death due to an infectious disease worldwide.

More than 8 million new cases and two million deaths occur annually.

M. tuberculosis is an aerobic organism.

M. tuberculosis can cause latent infection as well as active pulmonary or extrapulmonary disease.

Combinations of drugs are used for active disease; a single drug can be used for latent infection.

Long-term treatment is needed (at least 6-9 months).

Bacterial resistance is of growing importance.

Multidrug resistant tuberculosis is associated with increased morbidity and mortality.

Directly observed therapy is an important component in treatment.

Leprosy (Hansen's disease)

Leprosy is caused by *M. leprae,* an aerobic acid-fast bacillus organism.

M. leprae grows extremely slowly with a long incubation period (average 2-4 years).

It is a chronic disease; clinical manifestations depend upon immune responses.

Long-term treatment is needed, usually with multi-drug therapy.

Leprosy "reactions" can result from immunologically mediated acute inflammatory responses.

Mycobacterium avium complex (MAC) disease

Disseminated MAC most commonly occurs in patients with advanced HIV/AIDS.

Pulmonary infections are also seen in HIV-seronegative individuals, particularly with underlying or chronic pulmonary disease.

Treatment requires a multidrug regimen for prolonged periods.

Prophylaxis is indicated in patients with advanced HIV infection.

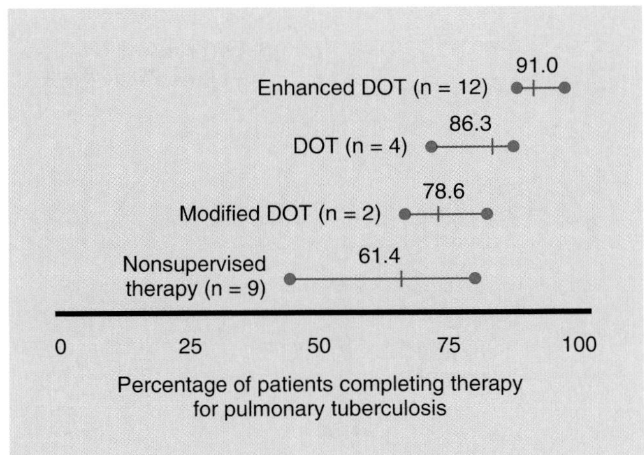

Figure 49-1 Impact of Directly observed therapy (DOT) on completion rates of antituberculosis therapy. Range and median treatment completion rates classified by treatment intervention for pulmonary tuberculosis. (Adapted from Chaulk CP, Kazdanjian VA. *J Am Med Assoc* 1998; 279:943-948.)

The incidence of invasive (i.e., disseminated) MAC disease among HIV-infected persons in the United States has decreased markedly in recent years because of the use of highly active antiretroviral therapy and MAC prophylaxis. In immunocompetent individuals, MAC most commonly causes pulmonary disease among those with underlying or chronic lung disease.

Mechanisms of action

Anti-tuberculosis drugs

Anti-TB drugs can be categorized on the basis of whether they are first- or second-line drugs (see Major Drugs box). They are divided into 3 groups based on their mechanism of action.

Inhibition of protein synthesis The **rifamycins** (rifampin, rifabutin, rifapentine) are bactericidal and inhibit DNA-dependent RNA polymerase of mycobacteria (but not mammals). This enzyme is composed of four subunits; rifamycins bind to the β-subunit, which results in blocking of the growing RNA chain (Fig. 49-2). Resistance is conferred by single mutations that tend to occur (>95%) in an 81-base pair region of the *rpo*B gene that codes for the β-subunit. The **aminoglycosides** streptomycin, kanamycin, and amikacin act by inhibiting protein synthesis and are described in Chapter 46. Capreomycin, a macrocyclic polypeptide antibiotic, has similar activity and toxicities as aminoglycosides.

Inhibition of cell wall synthesis Isoniazid (INH) is a bactericidal agent that is thought to inhibit mycolic acid synthesis. Mycolic acids are a major constituent of mycobacterial cell walls (along with arabinogalactan and peptidoglycan). The mode of action of INH is complex and a current model is shown in Figure 49-3. INH is a prodrug that has to be activated by the *M. tuberculosis* catalase-peroxidase enzyme encoded by the *kat*G gene. Deletions or mutations in this gene may account for 40% to 50% of clinical INH-resistant isolates. Other mechanisms of resistance may include mutations in three other genes. *inh*A and *kas*A code for mycolic acid biosynthetic enzymes and mutations are found in some INH-resistant isolates. *ahp*C has also been associated with some INH resistance strains, but its role is unclear.

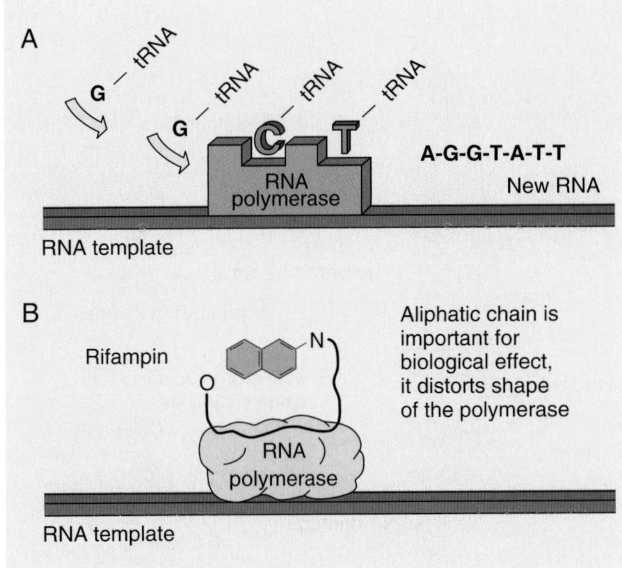

Figure 49-2 Mechanism of rifampin action. The drug binds to the β-subunit of DNA-dependent RNA polymerase and inhibits RNA synthesis. **A,** Drug is absent. **B,** Drug is bound to the polymerase and distorts the conformation of the enzyme so that it cannot initiate a new chain.

Pyrazinamide (PZA) is active only against *M. tuberculosis* and *M. africanum*; it is inactive against *M. bovis* and nontuberculous mycobacteria. PZA is active at a low pH (e.g., pH 5), is bactericidal, and has excellent sterilizing activity against semidormant bacteria. PZA is thought to enter *M. tuberculosis* by passive diffusion and is converted to pyrazinoic acid (POA), its active metabolite, by nicotinamidase/pyrazinamidase (PZase). The target of POA may involve fatty acid synthase I and disruption of mycobacterial membranes by acid (Fig. 49-4). Selected mutations in the PZase gene (*pnc*A) are associated with PZA resistance in *M. tuberculosis*.

The mechanism of action of **ethambutol** is not well understood. It is thought to interfere with mycobacter-

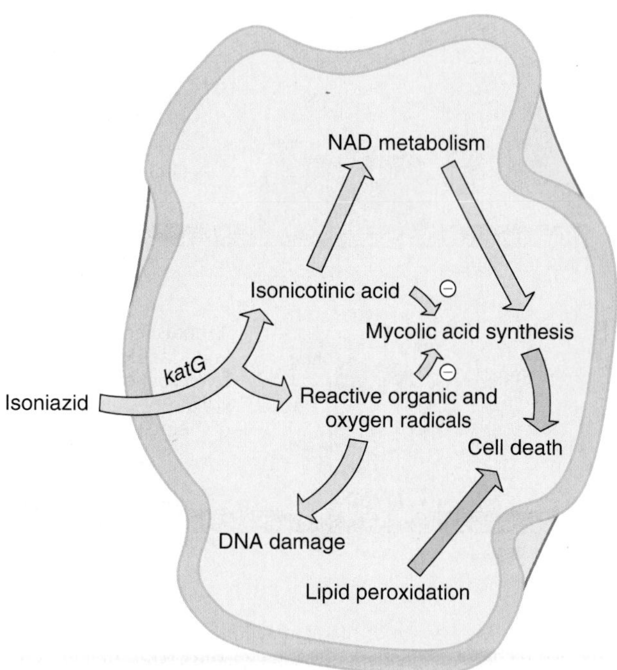

Figure 49-3 Mechanism by which isoniazid kills tubercle bacilli. INH enters by passive diffusion and is activated by *katG* to a range of reactive species or radicals and isonicotinic acid. These attack multiple targets, including mycolic acid synthesis, lipid peroxidation, DNA damage, and NAD metabolism. Deficient efflux and insufficient antagonism of INH-derived radicals, such as defective antioxidative defense may underlie the unique susceptibility of *M. tuberculosis* to INH.

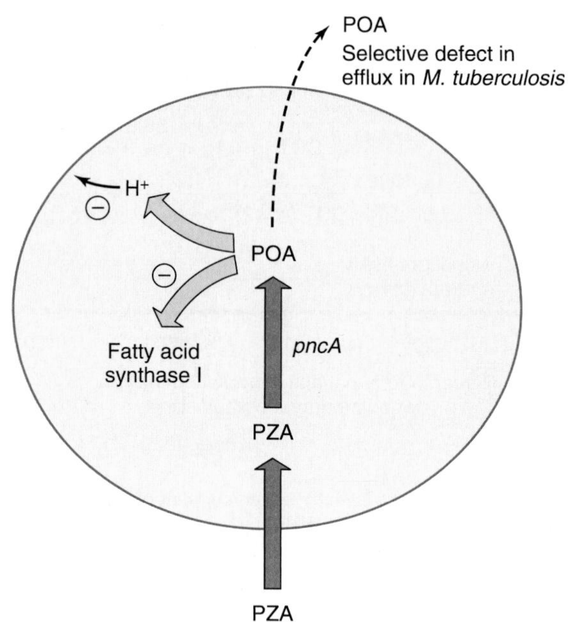

Figure 49-4 Proposed mechanism of action of pyrazinamide *(PZA)*. PZA is converted to pyrazinoic acid *(POA)* by the enzyme encoded by *pncA*. Its ability to kill *M. tuberculosis* and not other *Mycobacteria* species may be due to a selective defect in POA efflux in *M. tuberculosis.* Proposed targets include the mycobacterial fatty acid synthase 1 and disruption of mycobacterial membranes by acidic action. (Adapted from Chan ED, Chatterjee D, Iseman MD, et al. Pyrazinamide, ethambutol, ethionamide, and aminoglycosides. In Rom WN, Garay SM, eds.: *Tuberculosis*, 2nd ed. Philadelphia, Lippincott, Williams & Wilkins, 2004.)

ial cell wall synthesis, by inhibiting synthesis of polysaccharides and transfer of mycolic acids to the cell wall. The target is thought to be encoded by a three gene operon (*emb*C, *emb*A, *emb*B) that produces arabinosyl transferases that mediate polymerization of arabinose into arabinogalactan, particularly *embB.* Resistance to ethambutol is most common among *M. tuberculosis* isolates that are also resistant to INH and rifampin (i.e., MDR strains), probably because of mutations in *emb*B. Ethambutol is effective only on actively dividing mycobacteria.

Other mechanisms p-Aminosalicylic acid (PAS) acts as a competitive inhibitor of *p*-aminobenzoic acid in folate synthesis. Because PAS inhibits only this step in *M. tuberculosis,* and sulfonamides do not generally inhibit mycobacteria, the enzyme in tubercle bacilli is thought to be distinct.

Other agents used in treatment of mycobacterial diseases include the **fluoroquinolones** (e.g., levofloxacin, gatifloxacin, moxifloxacin), which have emerged as important second-line drugs used in the treatment of drug-resistant TB. They are discussed in Chapter 47.

Anti-leprosy drugs

Drugs for treatment of leprosy include rifampin, dapsone, clofazimine, ofloxacin, and minocycline. **Rifampin** is highly bactericidal against *M. leprae* and is discussed above. Its mechanism of action is presumed to be inhibition of *M. leprae* DNA-dependent RNA polymerase. Similar to sulfonamides, **dapsone** acts as an inhibitor of dihydropteroate synthetase in folate synthesis to produce a bacteriostatic effect. **Clofazimine** is active against *M. leprae* (weakly bactericidal), but its mechanism of action is unknown. **Ofloxacin,** a fluoroquinolone, is discussed in Chapter 47, and **minocycline** is discussed in Chapter 46.

Anti–*M. avium* complex drugs

Clarithromycin and **azithromycin** have excellent activity against *M. avium* complex (MAC), and these macrolides are the cornerstone of therapy. They can be used in both prevention and treatment (see Chapter 46). Ethambutol is usually combined with clarithromycin (or azithromycin) for treatment of MAC infections, especially among HIV-infected patients with disseminated MAC. **Rifabutin** can also be used to prevent MAC in HIV-infected patients who are unable to take macrolide drugs and can be used in combination with other agents. **Fluoroquinolones** and **amikacin** also have activity against MAC and are discussed in Chapters 46 and 47.

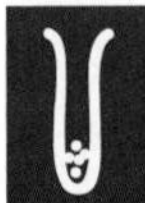

Pharmacokinetics

Key pharmacokinetic parameters are summarized in Table 49-1 and in Chapters 46 and 47.

Anti-tuberculosis drugs

First line INH is well absorbed orally and widely distributed, with peak concentrations achieved in pleural, peritoneal, and synovial fluids. Cerebrospinal fluid (CSF) concentrations are about 20% of plasma levels but can increase to 100% with meningeal inflammation. INH is **metabolized** by a liver *N*-acetyltransferase. The rate of acetylation determines its concentration in plasma and its half-life. As discussed in Chapter 3, slow acetylation is inherited as an autosomal recessive trait. The average plasma concentration of drug in rapid acetylators is half of that in slow acetylators. However, there is no evidence that these differences are therapeutically important if INH is administered once daily, because plasma levels are well above inhibitory concentrations.

Rifampin is well absorbed orally and widely distributed, achieving therapeutic concentrations in lung, liver, bile, bone, and urine and entering pleural, peritoneal, and synovial fluids and CSF, tears, and saliva. Its high lipid solubility enhances its entrance into phagocytic cells, where it kills intracellular bacteria. Rifampin is metabolized in liver to a desacetyl derivative that is biologically active. Unmetabolized drug is excreted in bile and reabsorbed from the gastrointestinal (GI) tract into the enterohepatic circulation; the deacetylated metabolite is poorly reabsorbed with eventual elimination in urine and from the GI tract. Rifampin induces its own metabolism by inducing cytochrome P-450 expression, resulting in increased biliary excretion with continued therapy. Induction of metabolism results in reduction of the plasma life by 20% to 40% after 7 to 10 days of therapy. Patients with severe liver disease may require dose reduction, but dose adjustment is not necessary in renal failure. Oral bioavailability of **rifabutin** is less than rifampin, and the plasma half-life is about 10 times greater. Rifabutin is more lipid soluble than rifampin and is extensively distributed. Rifabutin also induces its own metabolism but has less of an effect on cytochrome P450. **Rifapentine** is used once weekly in the continuation phase of highly selected patients with TB. It is metabolized in a similar manner but does not significantly induce its own metabolism.

Rifamycins are among the most-potent known inducers of hepatic cytochrome P-450 oxidative enzymes and the P-glycoprotein transport system and have a large number of drug interactions. This greatly impacts clinical care as discussed below.

PZA is well absorbed orally and widely distributed, readily penetrating cells and the walls of cavities. It enters the CSF if meninges are inflamed. PZA is metabolized by the liver. Its metabolic products are excreted mainly by the kidneys, and dose modifications are necessary in renal failure.

Approximately 75% to 80% of **ethambutol** is orally absorbed and widely distributed. Normally, little ethambutol penetrates into the CSF; however, CSF concentrations are 10% to 50% of plasma values with meningeal

Table 49-1 Selected pharmacokinetic properties

Drug	Administered	Half-life (hrs)	Average C_{max} (µg/ml)	Elimination
Isoniazid	Oral, IV	<2-4	2-8	M
Rifampin	Oral, IV	2-4	4-12	M
Rifabutin	Oral	32-67	0.2-0.6	M
Rifapentine	Oral	14-18	10-20	M
Pyrizinamide	Oral	2-10	30-60	M
Ethambutol	Oral	2-4	1-4	R
Capreomycin	IV, IM	4-6	20-45	R
Cycloserine	Oral	10	15-25	R, M
PAS	Oral	1	20	R, M
Ethionamide	Oral	3	1.5	M

M, Metabolized; *R*, renal excretion; C_{max}, peak plasma levels.

inflammation. It crosses the placenta. Ethambutol is mainly excreted unchanged by the kidneys, and dose adjustments are necessary in renal failure. It can be removed from the body by peritoneal dialysis or hemodialysis.

Second line The **fluoroquinolones** are discussed in Chapter 47 and the **aminoglycosides** in Chapter 46.

Capreomycin is administered IM or IV and is eliminated by the kidneys. It enters the CSF poorly and accumulates during renal dysfunction.

Ethionamide is well absorbed orally and widely distributed, entering the CSF and reaching concentrations equal to those in plasma. It is metabolized in the liver, with metabolites renally excreted. Ethionamide interferes with INH acetylation.

Cycloserine is rapidly absorbed orally and widely distributed, with CSF concentrations equal to those in plasma. About 35% is metabolized; the remainder is excreted by glomerular filtration. It accumulates in renal failure but can be removed by hemodialysis. *PAS* is available in the United States as granules in 4-gram packets; a solution for IV administration is available in Europe. PAS is well absorbed orally and enters lung tissue and pleural fluid. It is metabolized in the liver by an acetylase different from that acting on isoniazid. Most of the absorbed dose is excreted in the urine as metabolites.

Anti-leprosy drugs

Rifampin is discussed above. Ofloxacin, a fluoroquinolone, is discussed in Chapter 47; minocycline, a tetracycline, is discussed in Chapter 46.

Dapsone is well absorbed from the upper GI tract, is distributed to all body tissues, and achieves therapeutic concentrations in skin. It is about 70% bound to plasma proteins, excreted in bile, and reabsorbed via the enterohepatic circulation. It is acetylated in liver by the same enzyme that acetylates isoniazid, but the acetylation phenotype does not affect its half-life. Dapsone is excreted as glucuronide and sulfate conjugates in urine. It has a plasma half-life of 25 hours, which is reduced in patients receiving rifampin. Dosage should be reduced in renal failure.

Clofazimine pharmacokinetics are complex. Clofazimine is variably absorbed from the GI tract and distributed in a complex pattern, with high concentrations reached in subcutaneous fat and the reticuloendothelial system. It is not metabolized but is excreted slowly by the biliary route. It is estimated to have a half-life of 70 days.

Anti–*M. avium* complex drugs

Most of the drugs used to treat MAC infections (e.g., macrolides, ethambutol, rifamycins, fluoroquinolones) are described earlier or in Chapters 46 or 47.

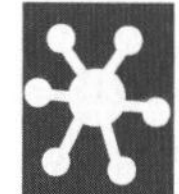

Relation of mechanisms of action to clinical response

Anti-tuberculosis drugs

The goals of anti-TB therapy are to kill tubercle bacilli rapidly, minimize or prevent development of drug resistance, and eliminate persistent organisms from the host's tissue to prevent relapse. **Multidrug therapy** is required for prolonged periods (at least 6-9 months for susceptible disease), and ensuring adherence to therapy (through use of DOT) is an important component of treatment. **INH** and **rifampin** are the two most important anti-TB drugs and the cornerstones of therapy. Resistance to both (MDR-TB) is associated with much higher morbidity and mortality. **PZA** is an important first-line drug that is a necessary component for "short course" therapy (6-9 months). **Ethambutol** is also a first line drug included in the initial four-drug regimen.

It is believed that there are three separate subpopulations of *M. tuberculosis* in the host with TB disease. The first and largest consists of rapidly growing extracellular organisms that mainly reside in well-oxygenated cavities (abscesses) containing 10^7 to 10^8 organisms. The second subpopulation consists of poorly oxygenated closed solid caseous lesions (e.g., non-caseating granulomas) containing 10^4 to 10^5 organisms. These organisms are considered semi-dormant and undergo only intermittent bursts of metabolic activity. The third subpopulation consists of a small number of organisms (less than 10^4 to 10^5) believed to be semidormant within acidic environments—both intracellular (e.g. in macrophages) or extracellular within areas of active inflammation and recent necrosis. INH is most potent in killing rapidly multiplying *M. tuberculosis* (the first subpopulation) during the initial part of therapy (early bactericidal activity). Rifampin and ethambutol have less early bactericidal activity than INH but considerably more than PZA, which has weak early bactericidal activity during the first 2 weeks of treatment. Drugs with potent early bactericidal activity reduce the chance of resistance emerging. Multidrug therapy is required to prevent development of resistance as a consequence of the selection pressure from administration of a single agent.

The rapidly dividing population of bacilli (first subpopulation) is eliminated early in effective therapy and by 2 months of treatment about 80% of patients are culture negative. The remaining (second and third) subpopulations account for treatment failures and relapses and are the reason prolonged therapy is required. The **sterilizing activity** of a drug is defined by its ability to kill bacilli mainly in the second and third subpopulations that persist beyond the early months of therapy, thus decreasing the risk of relapse. The use of drugs with good sterilizing activity is essential for short course therapy (e.g., 6 months). Rifampin and PZA have the greatest sterilizing activity, followed by INH and streptomycin. The sterilizing activity of rifampin persists throughout the course of therapy; however, that of PZA is mainly seen during the initial 2 months.

There are two phases of treatment of patients with TB disease—the **initiation** phase (bactericidal or intensive phase) and the **continuation** phase (subsequent sterilizing phase). Patients with TB, or a high clinical suspicion for TB, should be initiated on a **four-drug regimen** consisting of INH, rifampin, PZA, and ethambutol. It is important to obtain appropriate specimens for acid-fast bacilli smear and culture to try to establish a definitive diagnosis so that a positive culture for *M. tuberculosis* can be obtained. All initial isolates should undergo susceptibility testing, which is essential in providing appropriate drug therapy. For patients with drug-susceptible disease, PZA and ethambutol can be discontinued after 2 months of therapy. INH and rifampin are continued in the continuation phase (4 more months). Patients at high risk for relapse include those with cavitary pulmonary disease who remain culture positive after 2 months therapy. Such patients should have the continuation phase extended 3 more months (to complete 9 months total therapy).

Several different regimens are available for treatment of drug susceptible disease. In addition to the total duration of therapy, the number of completed doses should be counted and tracked to ensure the proper amount of therapy is given. **Nonadherence** is the most common cause of treatment failure, relapse, and emergence of resistance. DOT has been proven to improve completion rates and outcomes and is recommended for all patients with TB. Administration of anti-TB therapy on an intermittent basis is possible (especially in the continuation phase) for patients with drug susceptible disease and facilitates supervision of therapy. Intermittent therapy (e.g., twice or thrice weekly) should only be given by DOT to patients with drug susceptible disease. Specific regimens for treatment of active TB disease have been developed (e.g., see Fig. 49-5) but are beyond the scope of this text.

HIV serologic testing should be offered to all patients with TB. Treatment in patients with HIV is similar to that in other patients, with two major exceptions. The first is that HIV co-infected patients should not be treated with a once-weekly INH-rifapentine regimen in the continuation phase (which is reserved for highly selected HIV seronegative patients without cavitary disease) and HIV-infected patients with CD4 lymphocyte counts of <100/µl should not receive twice-weekly intermittent regimens (e.g., INH-rifampin or INH-rifabutin) because of increased risk of relapse resulting in rifamycin resistance. As discussed below, there are many **drug interactions** between rifamycins and other drugs, including antiretroviral agents. Paradoxical or immune reconstitution reactions are more common among HIV-infected patients with TB who are started on antiretroviral therapy early in the course of TB treatment. Therefore, some have recommended a delay of initiation of antiretroviral therapy in HIV-infected patients if possible until after 1 to 2 months of TB disease therapy. However, data are lacking, and recommendations on the use of antiretroviral therapies in HIV infected patients with TB continue to evolve. They are available from the Centers for Disease Control and Prevention at www.cdc.gov/nchstp/tb/.

Treatment of drug-resistant TB, especially MDR-TB, is quite challenging and should be done by, or in close consultation with, an expert. Treatment of INH monoresistance can be accomplished with a daily regimen of rifampin, PZA, and ethambutol for 6 months. Treatment of isolated rifampin-resistant disease requires a minimum of 12 months (e.g., INH, PZA, ethambutol and a fluoroquinolone). Treatment of MDR-TB (resistance to both INH and rifampin) requires 18 to 24 months depending on the resistance pattern and is associated with higher morbidity and mortality rates. Specific treatment regimens are available elsewhere and must be individualized based on the drug-susceptibility pattern.

Therapy for **LTBI** can markedly reduce the risk of progression to active disease and is recommended in those infected with *M. tuberculosis* who are at increased risk. The tuberculin skin test is the most common diagnostic test, but there is hope that improved tests will become available. The risk of progression from infection to active disease can range from a 5% to 10% lifetime risk in immunocompetent persons, to 10% per year in HIV infected persons with LTBI. HIV/AIDS is clearly the greatest risk factor. Others include recent infection, as well as LTBI among injection drug users and those with silicosis, diabetes mellitus, renal failure, certain malignancies, gastrectomy or jejunoileal bypass, solid organ transplantation, or use of immunosuppressive drugs. Others at increased risk include immigrants who have arrived in the United States within 5 years from areas with a high incidence of TB, racial/ethnic minorities, children 4 years of age or less with LTBI, and children and adolescents exposed to high-risk adults. All persons with suspected LTBI should have a chest radiograph performed to exclude active disease. Those with LTBI and risk factors for progression should be encouraged to take LTBI therapy, which generally involves a 9-month course of INH. A course of 6 months of INH is an alternative in HIV-seronegative adults. Rifampin

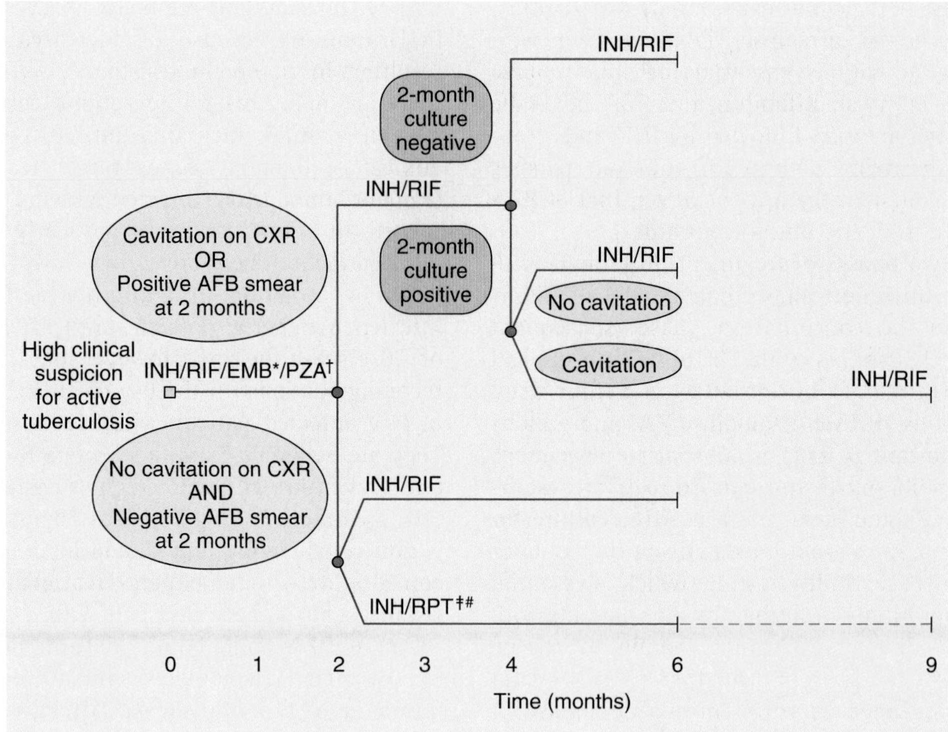

Figure 49-5 Treatment algorithm for tuberculosis. Patients in whom tuberculosis is proven or strongly suspected should have treatment with isoniazid *(INH)*, rifampin *(RIF)*, pyrazinamide *(PZA)*, and ethambutol *(EMB)* for an initial 2 months. A repeat smear and culture should be performed at that time. If cavities were seen on chest radiograph *(CXR)* or the acid fast bacillus *(AFB)* smear is positive after 2 months, the continuation phase should consist of INH and RIF daily or twice weekly for 4 months to complete a total of 6 months of treatment. If cavitation was present on the initial CXR and the culture at the time of completion of 2 months of therapy is positive, the continuation phase should be lengthened to 7 months (total 9 months). If no cavitation was seen on CXR and negative AFB smears at completion of 2 months of treatment, the continuation phase may consist of either once weekly INH and rifapentine *(RPT)*, or daily or twice weekly INH and RIF, to complete a total of 6 months *(bottom)*. Patients receiving INH and RPT, and whose 2 month cultures are positive, should have treatment extended by an additional 3 months. (Adapted from Blumberg H, Burman WJ, Chaisson RE, et al. *Am J Respir Crit Care Med* 2003; 167:603-662.)

*EMB may be discontinued when results of drug susceptibility testing indicate no resistance.
†PZA may be discontinued after 2 months.
‡RPT should not be used in HIV-infected patients with TB or in patients with extrapulmonary TB.
#Therapy should be extended to 9 months if 2 month culture is positive.

for 4 months is an alternative therapy for adults or those suspected of being infected with an INH resistant strain of *M. tuberculosis.* A 2-month short course of rifampin plus PZA for treatment of LTBI is *not* recommended because of a high rate of hepatotoxicity (although these drugs remain important in multidrug regimens for active TB).

Anti-leprosy drugs

Recommended therapy for leprosy is based on the classification of disease and includes **multidrug therapy.** Rifampin, dapsone, and clofazimine are included in the recommended regimens. **Rifampin** is the most effective agent; it is bactericidal against *M. leprae* and a single dose kills 99.99% of organisms, rendering patients with lepromatous leprosy non-infectious within days. Patients with paucibacillary disease receive rifampin (via supervised therapy) once monthly plus dapsone on a daily basis (self administered) for 6 months. Dapsone is a slow-acting bacteriostatic drug. It was formerly used as monotherapy, which led to emergence of resistance (up to 40%). Patients with single lesion paucibacillary disease can be treated with single-dose multidrug therapy (rifampin, ofloxacin, and minocycline). Patients with multibacillary disease require a minimum of 12 months of triple drug therapy (i.e., rifampin plus dapsone monthly by supervised therapy plus clofazimine either monthly or daily), although they are frequently treated for 24 months. Long-term follow-up (5-10 years) has been suggested, because relapses generally occur late. Treatment can be complicated by immune reactions that can be severe and cause significant morbidity because of nerve damage, described below. Chemoprophylaxis with rifampin or dapsone for high-risk contacts of leprosy patients has proven unsuccessful.

Anti–*M. avium* complex drugs

In AIDS patients with disseminated MAC disease, a regimen combining clarithromycin (or azithromycin) (see Chapter 46) with ethambutol is recommended. Some add rifabutin as a third drug, although data on whether this improves outcome is conflicting. The addition of clofazimine to a multidrug anti-MAC regimen is contraindicated because it was found to be associated with a worse outcome and higher mortality in HIV-seropositive patients. In treatment of MAC infections in HIV-seronegative immunocompetent patients (e.g., pulmonary MAC), treatment regimens generally include clarithromycin, ethambutol, and rifabutin (or rifampin). Rifabutin is preferred by some because it decreases the serum levels of clarithromycin less than rifampin and may be more active in vitro against MAC. Treatment of MAC disease requires long-term therapy (at least 12 months). Adult and adolescent HIV-infected patients with disseminated MAC should receive lifelong therapy unless immune reconstitution occurs as a consequence of highly active antiretroviral therapy. Among immunocompetent patients with pulmonary MAC, treatment is often recommended for 12 months after sputum conversion.

HIV-infected individuals should receive prophylaxis against disseminated MAC disease if they have a $CD4^+$ T lymphocyte count of <50 cells/μl. Clarithromycin or azithromycin are preferred. If they cannot be tolerated, rifabutin is an alternative, although its drug interactions can make its use difficult. MAC prophylaxis is indefinite unless immune reconstitution occurs. Patients with an increase in $CD4^+$ T lymphocyte counts to >100 cells/μl for >3 months can safely discontinue prophylaxis.

Side effects, clinical problems, and toxicity

The main adverse effects of these drugs are outlined in Clinical Problems box.

CLINICAL PROBLEMS

Anti-tuberculosis drugs

Isoniazid	Hepatoxicity, peripheral neuropathy, CNS effects
Rifampin	Orange discoloration of secretions, GI upset, hepatoxicity, hypersensitivity reactions, many drug interactions, rash
Pyrazinamide	GI upset, hepatitis, hyperuricemia, arthralgias
Ethambutol	Optic neuritis
Capreomycin	Ototoxicity, renal toxicity
Ethionamide	GI upset, hepatoxicity
Cycloserine	Psychosis, seizures, headache, depression, other CNS effects
PAS	GI upset, hypersensitivity, hepatoxicity, drug interactions

Anti-leprosy drugs

Dapsone	Hemolytic anemia, methemoglobinemia
Clofazimine	GI upset, changes in skin pigmentation

Immune reactions in leprosy

Type I	Skin lesions, inflammation of nerve trunk
Type II	Skin lesions, fever, arthralgia, neuritis, vasculitis, adenopathy, iridocyclitis, orchitis, and dactylitis

Anti-tuberculosis drugs

First line Although adverse reactions to INH are not common, a few are serious. **Hepatotoxicity** is the most potentially serious side effect, although recent data suggest the incidence is lower than previously thought (0.1% to 0.15%). The risk of hepatotoxicity is age related, is rare in persons less than 20 years old, but may be about 2% in people aged 50 to 64. The risk of hepatitis is higher when INH is administered with other potentially hepatotoxic drugs such as PZA or rifampin. The risk may also increase with underlying liver disease, a history of heavy alcohol consumption, or in the postpartum period (especially among Hispanics). Asymptomatic elevation of aminotransferases, which are generally transient, can occur in 10% to 20% of those taking INH for LTBI. The risk of fatal hepatitis caused by INH is very low. The drug should be discontinued when aminotransferases are increased by more than five-fold normal in asymptomatic patients or more than three-fold in symptomatic patients. Patients should be advised to discontinue INH at the onset of symptoms consistent with hepatitis such as nausea, loss of appetite, and dull midabdominal pain. Routine laboratory monitoring is recommended for persons at increased risk of toxicity. Liver function tests should be obtained on any patient who develops symptoms that could suggest hepatitis.

Other side effects of INH include peripheral neuropathy; it occurs more commonly in those with a nutritional deficiency, diabetes, HIV infection, renal failure, alcoholism, and pregnant and breast-feeding women. Pyridoxine is recommended for all patients with these risk factors to help prevent neuropathy. INH-induced CNS toxicity includes dysarthria, irritability, psychosis, seizures, dysphoria, and inability to concentrate, but the prevalence is not well quantified. Other side effects include rare hypersensitivity reactions such as fever, rash, hemolytic anemia, and vasculitis. A lupus-like syndrome is rare (<1%) although about 20% of patients develop anti-nuclear antibodies.

Rifampin is generally well tolerated. Patients should be advised that it will result in an orange discoloration of sputum, urine, sweat, and tears. Soft contact lenses may become stained. Rifampin can cause nausea and vomiting in 1% to 2% of patients, but they are rarely severe enough to warrant discontinuation. The major toxicity is **hepatitis.** Transient asymptomatic hyperbilirubinemia may occur in up to 0.6% of patients. More severe hepatitis that has a cholestatic pattern may also occur. It is more common when the drug is given in combination with INH (2.7%) than when given alone or in combination with other drugs (1.1%). Severe hepatic toxicity has been reported when rifampin is used in combination with PZA for short course (2 month) therapy for treatment of LTBI, and the risk of death has been estimated to be as high as 0.09%. This combination is no longer recommended for LTBI, but both drugs remain important components of multidrug regimens described above.

Hypersensitivity reactions are uncommon but include thrombocytopenia, hemolysis, transient leukopenia, and/or renal failure caused by interstitial nephritis. A flu-like syndrome with fever, chills, muscle aches, headache, and dizziness may occur on a biweekly, but not daily, regimen.

Rifampin **interacts** with many other drugs, usually resulting in increased metabolism and enhanced clearance. It is a potent inducer of cytochrome P450 enzymes, and Box 49-1 lists a number of clinically significant drug-drug interactions involving the rifamycins. The concomitant use of anti-TB drugs, including rifampin, and antiretroviral drugs is complex.

Box 49-1 Examples of drugs with reduced half-lives caused by concomitant administration of rifampin

Barbiturates	Metoprolol
Chloramphenicol	Methadone
Cimetidine	Phenytoin
Clarithromycin	Prednisone
Clofibrate	Propranolol
Contraceptives (oral)	Quinidine
Cyclosporin	Protease inhibitors
Dapsone	Ritonavir
Digitoxin	Sulfonylureas
Digoxin	Tacrolimus
Efavirenz	Theophylline
Estrogens	Thyroxine
Fluconazole	Verapamil
Itraconazole	Warfarin
Ketoconazole	

Rifampin cannot be used with protease inhibitors, although it can be used with nucleoside and some non-nucleoside reverse transcriptase inhibitors. Rifabutin has less of an effect on P450 than rifampin and can be used with several protease inhibitors. It is substituted for rifampin when treating HIV-infected patients taking protease inhibitors. The Centers for Disease Control and Prevention has established a Web site that provides updated information on TB/HIV drug interactions at http://www.cdc.gov/nchstp/tb/tb_hiv_drugs/toc.htm.

Women of child-bearing age should be advised to use alternative contraceptive methods while on rifampin because oral contraceptives will not be effective.

Adverse effects of **rifabutin** are similar to those of rifampin. In addition, neutropenia has been described, especially among persons with advanced HIV/AIDS. Rifabutin can also cause uveitis, and the risk is increased with higher doses or when used in combination with macrolide antibiotics that reduce its clearance. It may also occur with other drugs that reduce clearance, such as protease inhibitors and azole antifungal drugs. Although drug interactions are less problematic with rifabutin than with rifampin, they still occur, and close monitoring is required.

Adverse effects of **rifapentine** are similar to those of rifampin. Monitoring is also similar.

Hepatotoxicity is the most serious adverse effect of PZA, and elevation of liver aminotransferase concentration is the first sign. The effect is less frequent in patients who receive the lower doses currently used than in earlier trials. Mild anorexia and nausea are common, but severe nausea and vomiting are rare. PZA causes hyperuricemia by inhibiting renal excretion of urate.

Clinical gout caused by PZA is rare, although nongouty polyarthralgia can occur in up to 40% of patients. As mentioned above, severe hepatoxicity has been reported among patients taking rifampin and PZA for short course therapy for LTBI, and liver function should be carefully monitored.

The most important toxicity of **ethambutol** is a dose-related retrobulbar (optic) neuritis. This is manifest as decreased visual acuity or decreased red-green color discrimination. Patients should have baseline visual acuity and color discrimination monitored and be questioned about possible visual disturbances. Monthly testing is recommended for patients taking doses greater than 15 mg/kg/day, receiving the drug for longer than 2 months, or with renal insufficiency.

Second line Most second-line drugs have less activity against *M. tuberculosis* and significantly greater toxicity. They are generally used in treatment of drug-resistant TB (including MDR-TB) and should be used only in consultation with an expert.

Adverse effects of the aminoglycosides and fluoroquinolones are discussed in Chapters 46 and 47. Adverse effects of **capreomycin** are similar to those of aminoglycosides and include nephrotoxicity and ototoxicity. Close monitoring of renal function is required.

CNS effects are most important for **cycloserine** and are not uncommon. They range from mild reactions, such as headache or restlessness, to severe reactions including depression, psychosis, and seizures. Cycloserine may exacerbate underlying seizure disorders or mental illness. Pyridoxine may help prevent and treat these side effects. Rarely cycloserine can cause peripheral neuropathy.

Ethionamide frequently causes significant GI reactions, and many patients cannot tolerate elevated doses. Nausea; vomiting; abdominal pain; diarrhea; a metallic taste in the mouth; and many CNS complaints including depression, headache, and feelings of restlessness are typical. Endocrine disturbances including gynecomastia, alopecia, hypothyroidism, and impotence have been described. Diabetes may be more difficult to manage. Ethionamide is similar in structure to INH and may cause similar side effects, including hepatitis (about 2%). Liver function tests should be monitored if there is underlying liver disease and if symptoms develop. Thyroid hormone levels should also be monitored.

The most common side effects of **PAS** include nausea, vomiting, abdominal pain, and diarrhea. The incidence of GI side effects is lower with the granular formulation, the only formulation available in the United States. A malabsorption syndrome has been described, and hypothyroidism is not uncommon, especially among those taking PAS and ethionamide. Hepatitis is uncommon. With prolonged therapy, thyroid function should be monitored.

Anti-leprosy drugs

Adverse effects of rifampin are discussed above, and fluoroquinolones are discussed in Chapter 47.

Hemolytic anemia and **methemoglobinemia** are the common adverse effects of **dapsone.** Hemolysis is greatly enhanced in patients with glucose-6-phosphate dehydrogenase deficiency. Methemoglobinemia is caused by a dapsone *N*-oxidation product, is usually asymptomatic, but may become important if the patient develops hypoxemia from lung disease. Although bone marrow suppression is rare, agranulocytosis and aplastic anemia may occur. GI intolerance including anorexia, nausea, and vomiting can occur, as well as hematuria, fever, pruritus, and rash.

The most common adverse effects of **clofazimine** are GI intolerance, including anorexia, diarrhea, and abdominal pain. Skin pigmentation resulting from drug accumulation and producing red-brown to black discoloration is common, especially in dark-skinned persons.

Chemotherapy-associated reactions in leprosy Patients with leprosy can experience episodic immunologically mediated acute inflammatory responses termed "reactions," which can cause nerve damage. These reactions can be characterized by swelling and edema in pre-existing skin lesions or peripheral neuropathy/neuritis, which can cause pain, tenderness, and loss of function. They occur in up to one third of patients with leprosy and can, if not recognized and treated aggressively, lead to irreversible nerve damage and limb deformity. There are two common types: type I, or reversal, reactions characterized by cellular hypersensitivity; and type 2, or erythema nodosum leprosum, characterized by a systemic inflammatory response to immune complex deposition. In-depth characterization and treatment of these two types of reactions are beyond the scope of this chapter. However, the reversal reactions typically occur after initiation of treatment (especially with dapsone and rifampin) but can occur spontaneously before therapy or after multidrug therapy. A decline in type 2 has been observed since introduction of multidrug therapy and is thought to be due in part to the anti-inflammatory effects of daily clofazimine treatment. Recurrences of both types of reactions are common and can result in prolonged use of steroids for suppression.

Anti–*M. avium* complex drugs

The main problems posed by most anti-MAC drugs (macrolides, ethambutol) are noted earlier in this chapter and Chapter 46. **Rifabutin** is generally well tolerated at the lower doses used for prophylaxis against MAC infections, although serious side effects such as uveitis have been reported.

New horizons

Worldwide TB control will probably require development of an effective vaccine. The World Health Organization recommended DOT short course program has made important contributions to control, and the number of countries implementing it has increased markedly over the past several years. However, most people with TB do not receive such treatment. Furthermore, the impact of HIV on the TB epidemic will necessitate new strategies and technologies for the dream of TB elimination to be realized.

Even if an effective vaccine is developed, there is still a critical need for new anti-TB drugs because of the large number of people currently developing active disease and the very large numbers of persons with LTBI at risk for progressing to active disease. New drugs are needed in order to:

- Shorten the length of therapy for drug susceptible disease
- To improve treatment options and outcomes for patients with MDR-TB
- To provide more effective and shorter regimens for treatment of LTBI.

MDR-TB is emerging as a serious global problem, especially in republics of the former Soviet Union.

No novel compounds likely to have a significant impact on TB treatment are currently available. After decades of neglect, there is some hope for new anti-TB drug development, given the formation of the Global Alliance for TB Drug Development. This includes public-private partnerships whose objective is development of new, affordable, faster-acting anti-TB drugs.

Global eradication of leprosy is proposed by the World Health Organization. The total number of cases of leprosy has decreased and research has declined, but case detection is largely passive, even in countries of hyperendemicity. Public health programs have historically focused on education and then relied on patients to present themselves once they become symptomatic. Multidrug therapy has reduced the prevalence of leprosy, but the incidence rate has remained relatively stable because such therapy has little effect on transmission within households. Effective chemoprophylaxis would be welcome for high-risk contacts, but use of rifampin and dapsone have unfortunately been unsuccessful. The only prophylactic measure with any degree of success has been vaccination with bacille Camille-Guérin, with one dose conferring approximately 50% protection. An effective vaccine would be highly desirable, and development of such a vaccine may benefit from the high priority of developing an effective vaccine for TB.

Further understanding of the immunology of leprosy is needed. It is hoped the sequencing of the *M. leprae* genome will help identify protective genomic DNA sequences and that there will be a continuing commitment to research. Since leprosy will persist in many countries, the unprecedented mobility of people around the globe suggests that cases of imported leprosy are likely to continue to occur in the United States. Clinicians must therefore be aware of the signs and symptoms so patients may be appropriately managed and treated.

TRADE NAMES

All of the important compounds available in the United States are listed in the Major Drugs box.

FURTHER READING

Blumberg HM, Burman WJ, Chaisson RE, et al. American Thoracic Society/Centers for Disease Control and Prevention/ Infectious Diseases Society of America: treatment of tuberculosis. *Am J Respir Crit Care Med* 2003;167:603-62. (Also published as: Centers for Disease Control and Prevention. Treatment of Tuberculosis, American Thoracic Society, CDC, and Infectious Diseases Society of America. *MMWR* 2003; 52(No. RR-11):1-77.)

Benson CA, Williams PL, Currier JS, et al. AIDS Clinical Trials Group 223 Protocol Team. A prospective, randomized trial examining the efficacy and safety of clarithromycin in combination with ethambutol, rifabutin, or both for the treatment of disseminated *Mycobacterium avium* complex disease in persons with acquired immunodeficiency syndrome. *Clin Infect Dis* 2003; 37:1234-1243.

Boggild AK, Keystone JS, Kain KC. Leprosy: a primer for Canadian physicians. *CMAJ* 2004; 170:71-78.

Neurmberger E, Grassert J: Pharmacokinetics and pharmacodynamic issues in the treatment of mycobacterial infections. *Eur J Clin Microbiol Infect Dis* 2004; 23:243-255.

Self-assessment questions

1. Which of the following statements about rifampin is *false?*
   a. Its mechanism of action involves interfering with bacterial cell wall synthesis.
   b. Its mechanism of action involves inhibiting DNA-dependent RNA polymerase.
   c. Resistance to rifampin is due to mutations that occur in a highly restricted 81 base pair region of the *rpoB* gene.
   d. It is a potent inducer of the hepatic cytochrome P-450 system and this leads to a number of clinically important drug interactions.

2. Which of the following statements about isoniazid (INH) is *true?*
   a. INH is poorly absorbed orally and not available in an parenteral preparation for administration.
   b. INH is metabolized by a liver *N*-acetyltransferase.
   c. Slow acetylators of INH are less likely to respond to tuberculosis treatment with this drug.
   d. INH does not effect mycolic acid synthesis.

3. Which statement about pyrazinamide (PZA) is *true?*
   a. PZA can cause optic neuritis.
   b. PZA is a common cause of gout and routine monitoring of uric acid is indicated.
   c. PZA is converted to pyrazinoic acid (POA) by nicotinamidase/pyrazinamidase (PZase). POA is believed be the active metabolite.
   d. PZA has excellent early bactericidal activity and poor sterilizing activity against semidormant bacteria.

4. Multidrug therapy is required for the treatment of all of the following *except:*
   a. Tuberculosis disease.
   b. Leprosy.
   c. Disseminated *M. avium* complex infections.
   d. Latent tuberculosis infection (LTBI).

5. Isoniazid (INH) can produce all of the following adverse effects *except:*
   a. Anemia.
   b. Hepatitis.
   c. Peripheral neuropathy.
   d. Positive antinuclear antibody.
   e. Hypersensitivity reactions.

6. Ethambutol produces which of the following adverse reactions?
   a. Deafness
   b. Optic neuritis
   c. Vestibular toxicity
   d. Renal insufficiency

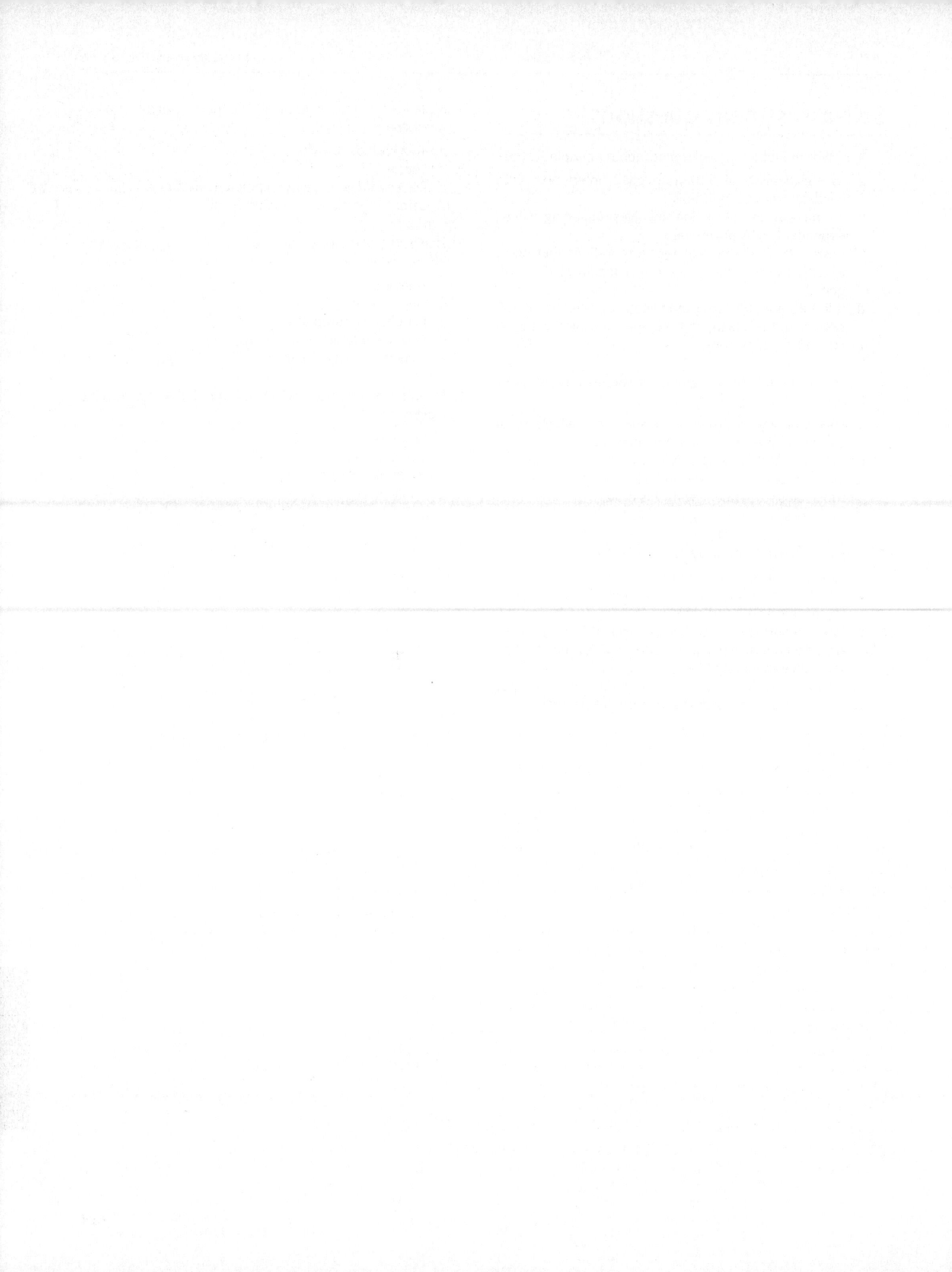

CHAPTER 50

Antifungal agents

Brian Wispelwey
Christopher H. Parsons

Major Drugs

Amphotericin B (Fungizone)
Fluconazole (Diflucan)
Itraconazole (Sporanox)
Caspofungin (Cancidas)

Therapeutic overview

Fungal infections (mycoses) are less frequent than bacterial or viral infections but may be prevalent in some locations that favor growth of specific pathogenic strains. However, serious infections have become increasingly common in the hospital setting. A person must almost always have a predisposing condition that disables one or more **host defense mechanisms** for a fungal infection to develop. Fungal infections are facilitated by a loss of mechanical barriers (burns, major surgery, intravascular catheters), the presence of immunodeficiency conditions (malignancies and their treatments, organ transplantation and anti-rejection therapy, acquired immunodeficiency syndrome [AIDS]) or metabolic derangements (diabetes mellitus), and suppression of competing microorganisms (excessive broad-spectrum antibacterial agent use). Many fungal infections are superficial and primarily annoying. Others are **systemic** and can be **life-threatening**, particularly in patients with compromised defenses, such as those receiving immunosuppressive drugs. The toxicity of many antifungal drugs limits their use, and unfortunately there are few agents useful in treating systemic fungal infections.

Fungi are more complex than bacteria or viruses. They have different ribosomes and cell wall components and possess a discrete nuclear membrane, and antibacterial antibiotics are not effective against pathogenic fungi. The major classes of fungal infections and examples of prevalent species that are often causative organisms are summarized in the Therapeutic Overview box.

THERAPEUTIC OVERVIEW

Cutaneous and subcutaneous mycoses

Epidermophyton species
Microspora species
Sporothrix species
Trichophyton species
Treat with dermatological preparations, occasionally systemic agents

Systemic mycoses

Aspergillus species
Candida species
Blastomyces dermatitidis
Cryptococcus neoformans
Coccidioides immitis
Fusarium species
Histoplasma capsulatum
Paracoccidioides brasiliensis
Mucormycosis
Difficult to treat; available drugs often cause deleterious side effects; often need long-term therapy

Abbreviations

ABLC	amphotericin B lipid complex
AIDS	acquired immunodeficiency syndrome
CSF	cerebrospinal fluid
GI	gastrointestinal
IV	intravenous

Mechanisms of action

The principal antifungal drugs are polyenes, flucytosine, azoles, allylamines, and griseofulvin. The sites of action are shown in Figure 50-1.

Polyenes

The polyene (i.e., multiple double bonds) antibiotics are macrocyclic lactones that contain a hydrophilic hydroxylated portion and a hydrophobic conjugated double-bond portion. The structure of amphotericin B, the most widely used antifungal drug, is shown in Figure 50-2.

Polyenes act by **binding to sterols** in the cell membrane and forming channels, allowing K^+ and Mg^{2+} to leak out. The polyenes become integrated into the membrane to form a ring with a pore in the center about 0.8 nm in diameter. K^+ leaks out through these pores, followed by Mg^{2+}, and with the loss of K^+, cellular metabolism becomes deranged (Fig. 50-3). It is thought that derangement of the membrane alters activity of membrane enzymes. The principal sterol in fungal membranes, **ergosterol**, has a higher affinity for polyenes than does cholesterol, the principal sterol of mammalian cell membranes. Therefore the polyenes show greater activity against fungal cells than mammalian cells, and fungi that lack ergosterol are not susceptible to amphotericin B.

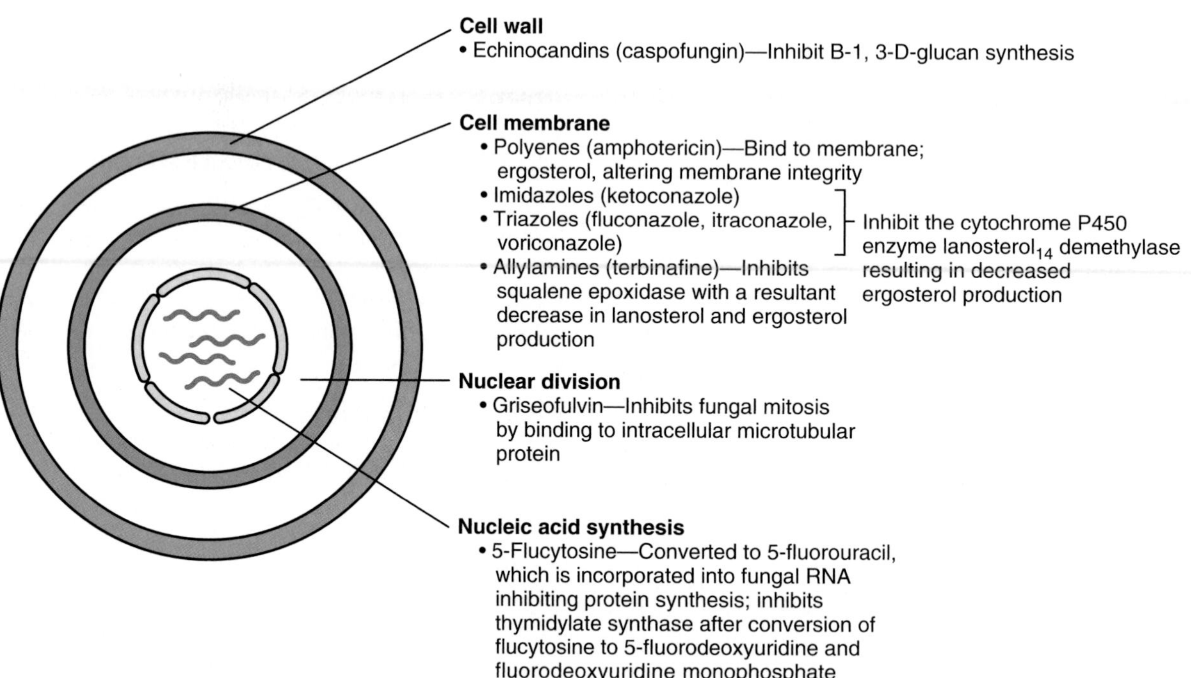

Figure 50-1 Mechanism of action of antifungal agents.

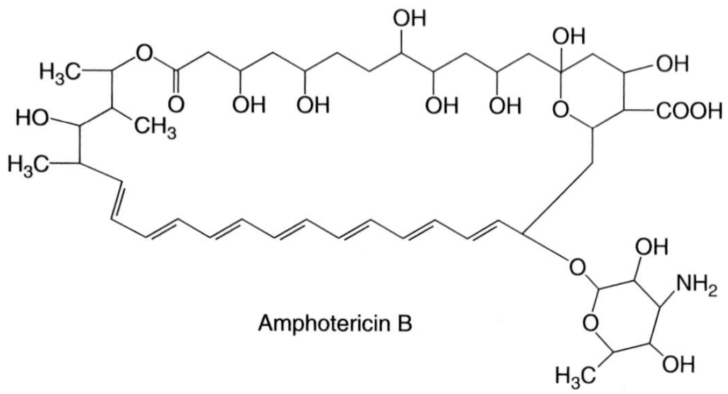

Amphotericin B

Figure 50-2 Structure of amphotericin B.

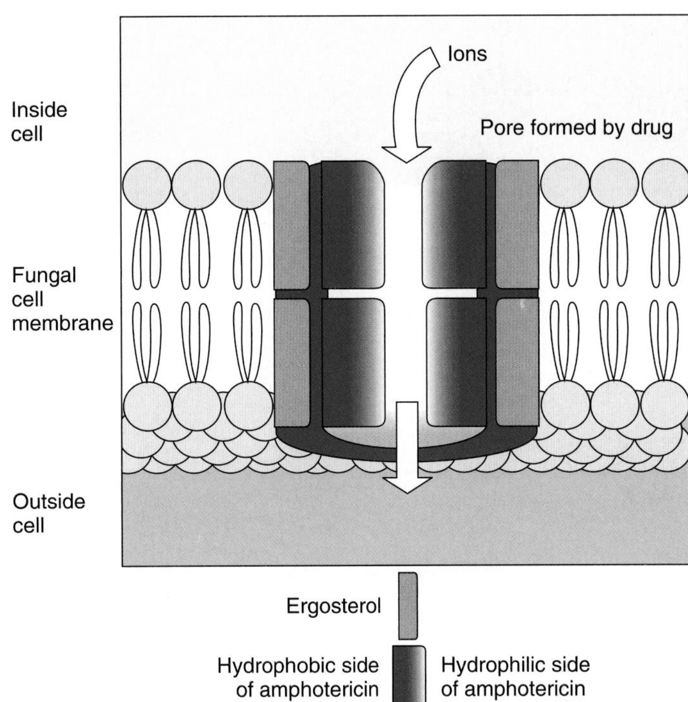

Figure 50-3 Action of polyene agents to form pores in the fungal cell membrane through which K^+ and Mg^{2+} can leak out of the cell.

Amphotericin B lipid complex (ABLC) and liposomal amphotericin are among the first amphotericin-lipid formulations to receive approval for use in the U.S. ABLC is an amphotericin B–non-liposomal formulation that complexes with two phospholipids. Liposomal amphotericin incorporates the drug into small unilamellar lipid vesicles. It is postulated that by incorporating amphotericin B into these lipid moieties, active drug can be selectively transferred to ergosterol-containing fungal membranes without interfering with the cholesterol-containing human membrane, thereby resulting in decreased toxicity.

Flucytosine

Flucytosine, also called *5-fluorocytosine,* is an **antimetabolite** that undergoes intracellular metabolism to an active form, which leads to inhibition of DNA synthesis.

Flucytosine is transported into susceptible fungi by a **permease** system for purines. The drug is then deaminated by cytosine deaminase to 5-fluorouracil. Because cytosine deaminase is not present in mammalian cells, the drug is not activated in humans. Fluorouracil in turn is converted by uridine phosphate pyrophosphorylase and other enzymes to 5-fluoro-2′-deoxyuridine 5′-monophosphate, which inhibits thymidylate synthase and interferes with DNA synthesis (Chapter 42).

Fungi can be resistant to flucytosine because they lack a permease, have a defective **cytosine deaminase,** or have a low concentration of the uridine monophosphate pyrophosphorylase. Whether the faulty RNA produced by incorporation of fluorouracil contributes to its action is unclear.

Azoles

The structures of some of the principal azole antifungal agents are shown in Figure 50-4. Ketoconazole, miconazole, clotrimazole, and econazole are available, as are the new agents fluconazole, itraconazole, and voriconazole.

Depending on drug concentration, azoles can have **fungistatic** or **fungicidal** effects. In actively growing fungi, azoles inhibit synthesis of membrane sterols by inhibiting incorporation or **synthesis of ergosterol.** These agents interact with cytochrome P450–dependent 14-α-demethylase, and ergosterol is not produced as a result. At high concentrations, azoles cause K^+ and other components to leak from the fungal cell, an action that may involve inhibition of plasma membrane ATPase. Because azoles inhibit fungal respiration under aerobic conditions, an alternative mechanism may be blockade of respiratory-chain electron transport.

Griseofulvin

Whether griseofulvin is fungicidal or fungistatic is not established. It enters susceptible fungi by an energy-dependent transport system and **inhibits mitosis.** It binds to the **microtubules** that form the mitotic spindle and blocks the polymerization of tubulin into microtubules. It also binds to a microtubule-associated

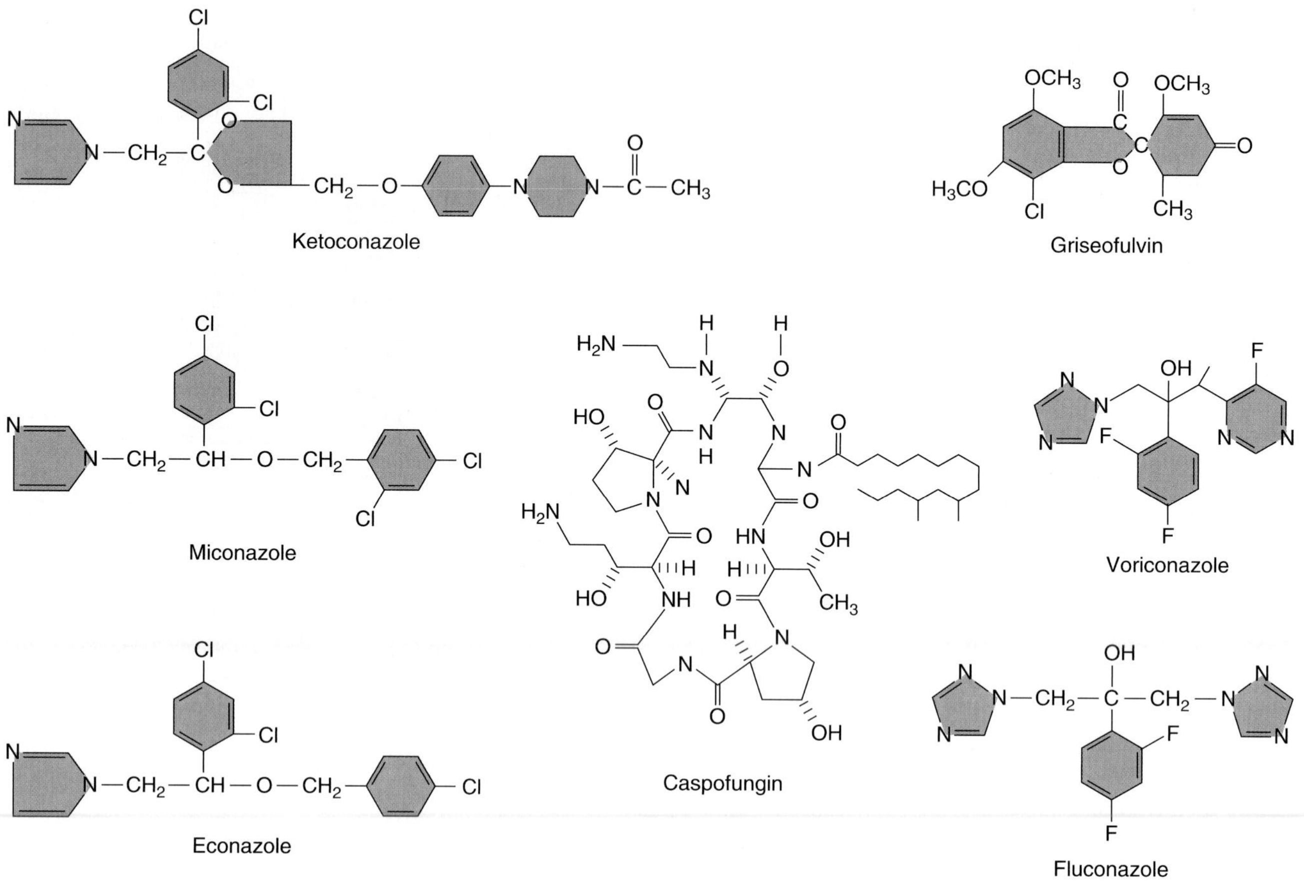

Ketoconazole

Griseofulvin

Miconazole

Caspofungin

Voriconazole

Econazole

Fluconazole

Figure 50-4 Structures of selected antifungal drugs.

protein, although the role of this protein is not known. The binding site for griseofulvin on **tubulin** differs from that of colchicine and the plant alkaloids. This effect on microtubule assembly probably explains the morphological changes, such as curling, that are observed in the fungi. Mechanisms of resistance are unknown but may stem from decreased uptake of the drug. The structure of griseofulvin is shown in Figure 50-4.

Allylamines

Terbinafine is the first allylamine available for systemic use. It selectively inhibits fungal cell squalene epoxidase, the enzyme that converts squalene to squalene epoxide. This interferes with biosynthesis of ergosterol at an earlier step than do the azoles. Squalene epoxide inhibition results in a fungicidal intracellular accumulation of squalene and a fungistatic depletion of ergosterol.

Echinocandins

Caspofungin is the first echinocandin compound to gain approval for use in the United States. It **blocks production of B-1,3-D-glucans,** the major structural component of the fungal cell wall, by inhibition of glucan synthesis. Fungi have been shown to develop *in vitro* resistance to echinocandins through mutations in genes coding for the target enzymes.

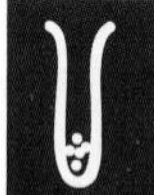

Pharmacokinetics

Pharmacokinetic parameters for the antifungal drugs are summarized in Table 50-1.

Polyenes

Amphotericin B is insoluble in water, has a large lipophilic domain in its structure, and is not absorbed from the gastrointestinal (GI) tract. It is administered orally only to treat fungal infections of the GI tract, which sometimes develop after depletion of bacterial microflora following administration of broad-spectrum antibacterial drugs. For parenteral use, amphotericin B

Table 50-1 Pharmacokinetic parameter values for antifungal drugs

Drug	Administration	Absorption	Half-Life (hrs)	Urine Concentration	Disposition	Plasma Protein Bound (%)
POLYENES						
Amphotericin B	IV, topical, oral	No	24 (15 days)*	Good	B (some) ?(main)	>90
ABLC	IV	No	24 (15 days)*	Poor	—	—
Liposomal amphotericin	IV	No	24 (15 days)*	Poor	—	—
Nystatin	Topical	No	—	—	—	>90
ANTIMETABOLITES						
Flucytosine	Oral	Good	3-6	Good	R (85%)	<10
AZOLES						
Ketoconazole	Oral, topical	75%[†]	8	Poor	M (95%) R (3%)	99
Miconazole	Topical, IV	Poor	0.5	—	M (95%)	90
Econazole	Topical	<1%	—	—	M (95%)	—
Clotrimazole	Topical	<1%	—	—	M (95%)	—
Fluconazole	IV, oral	85%	25-30	Good	R (main), M	12
Itraconazole	Oral	99% (40%[‡])	17	Poor	M	99
Voriconazole	Oral, IV	>90% (fasting)	6	Poor	M	58
GRISEOFULVIN						
Griseofulvin	Oral, topical	Poor[§]	20	—	M (main)	—
ALLYLAMINES						
Terbinafine	Oral, topical	>70%	16 (16 days)*	Poor	M (main)	99%
ECHINOCANDINS						
Caspofungin	IV	Poor	9-11	Poor	M (>98%)	>97%

M, Metabolism; *R*, renal; *B*, biliary.
*Terminal elimination phase.
†Needs acidic pH to be absorbed.
‡Less well-absorbed during fasting.
§Particles taken up by unknown process.

is combined with the detergent deoxycholate to form a colloidal suspension.

Amphotericin B enters pleural, peritoneal, and synovial fluids, where it reaches a concentration about half that in serum. It crosses the placenta and is found in cord blood and amniotic fluid and also enters the aqueous but not the vitreous humor of the eye. Cerebrospinal fluid (CSF) concentrations reach one third to one half those in serum. Most amphotericin B in the body probably is bound to cholesterol-containing membranes in tissues.

The principal pathway for amphotericin B disposition is not known. Some is excreted by the biliary route, and only 3% is eliminated in urine. Renal dysfunction does not affect plasma concentrations, and amphotericin B is not removed by hemodialysis.

The pharmacokinetics of ABLC and liposomal amphotericin, and their relation to clinical efficacy, are less clear. ABLC is taken up rapidly by the reticuloendothelial system and achieves high concentrations in the lung, liver, and spleen. As a result, the elimination phase is much longer than with amphotericin B. Liposomal amphotericin, at similar recommended doses, achieves higher serum levels and improved penetration of the central nervous system as well as more-rapid plasma clearance than amphotericin B or ABLC.

Flucytosine

Flucytosine is well absorbed from the GI tract and is widely distributed in the body, with CSF concentrations 70% to 85% of those in plasma. It enters the peritoneum, synovial fluid, bronchial secretions, saliva, and bone.

Approximately 85% to 95% is excreted unchanged by glomerular filtration, with a normal half-life of 3 to 6 hours, which increases greatly as creatinine clearance diminishes. For special conditions, the drug can be removed by hemodialysis and peritoneal dialysis. A small fraction of the dose may be converted by intestinal bacteria to 5-fluorouracil and lead to hematological toxicity.

Azoles

Ketoconazole is administered orally and its absorption is favored at an acidic pH. Therefore coadministration of antacids, H_2 receptor antagonists, or proton pump inhibitors reduces absorption. The effects of food on absorption of this agent have been inconsistent, and plasma concentrations vary widely among patients receiving the same dose.

Ketoconazole is distributed in saliva, skin, bone, and pleural, peritoneal, synovial, and aqueous humor fluids. It penetrates very poorly into the CSF (~5% of plasma concentration). The plasma concentration declines biexponentially, with a distribution half-life of about 2 hours followed by an elimination half-life of 8 hours.

Ketoconazole is extensively metabolized by hydroxylation and oxidative *N*-dealkylation. It does not induce its own metabolism, as clotrimazole does. However, rifampin induces the release of microsomal enzymes that increase ketoconazole oxidation. Only 2% to 4% of a dose is excreted in urine unchanged, and renal insufficiency does not affect plasma concentrations or half-life, although half-life is prolonged in patients with hepatic insufficiency.

Miconazole is now used topically and rarely IV. It is minimally water soluble and not adequately absorbed from the GI tract. Its half-life is only 30 minutes, and it is metabolized by *O*-dealkylation and oxidative *N*-dealkylation but does not induce its own metabolism. Only 1% is excreted in the urine unchanged. Penetration of into CSF and sputum is poor, but penetration into joint fluid is good.

Fluconazole is water soluble and rapidly absorbed after oral administration, with about a 90% bioavailability and a half-life of 25 to 30 hours. Fluconazole does not require an acidic environment for absorption. Although it does not induce metabolism of most other drugs, it does alter metabolism of orally administered hypoglycemic agents. About 70% is eliminated unchanged through the kidneys, with small amounts of metabolites present in urine and feces. Fluconazole is widely distributed, with therapeutic concentrations attained in CSF, lung, and many other areas of the body.

Voriconazole is also rapidly absorbed, with greater than 90% bioavailability that decreases when the drug is taken with food. More than 95% of this drug is metabolized by P450s to inactive compounds in the liver, with only a small amount excreted unchanged in the urine. This can cause interactions with other drugs. Dosage is adjusted in patients with liver disease, or in patients with kidney disease receiving the IV formulation, due to its administration with a cyclodextrin carrier that accumulates with lower renal clearance rates.

Griseofulvin

Griseofulvin is insoluble; however, about half of an oral dose passes from the GI tract into the circulation. This uptake is related to particle size and is increased when the drug is ingested with a full meal. Whether it diffuses through the intestinal wall or is taken up as micelles is not clear. When applied topically, griseofulvin penetrates the stratum corneum, but this does not result in effective local concentrations.

Griseofulvin is widely distributed and becomes concentrated in fat, liver, and muscle. It is deposited in the keratin layer of the skin; becomes concentrated in keratin precursor cells in the stratum corneum of the skin, nails, and hair; and is secreted in perspiration. New keratin formed during treatment with griseofulvin is resistant to fungus, but griseofulvin does not destroy fungi in previously infected outer layers of skin. Thus a dermatophyte infection can be cured only when infected skin, nails, or hair is shed and the new keratin containing the griseofulvin replaces all the old keratin. Skin and hair infections require 4 to 6 weeks of therapy, fingernails require up to 6 months, and toenails require up to a year.

Most absorbed griseofulvin is metabolized in the liver by dealkylation, and the inactive metabolite is excreted in the urine as a glucuronide.

Allylamines

Terbinafine is well absorbed from the GI tract, has an initial distribution half-life of about 1.1 hours, and an elimination half-life of about 16 hours. Similar to the polyenes, it has a prolonged terminal half-life of about 16 days. Terbinafine is highly lipophilic and keratophilic, resulting in high concentrations in the stratum corneum, sebum, hair, and nails. The drug may be detected in nails for up to 90 days after treatment is discontinued. It is extensively metabolized by the liver and excreted in the urine and feces as inactive metabolites. Clearance is decreased in patients with renal or hepatic impairment. It is currently used for treating fungal infections of the nails, and prolonged courses lasting 6 to 12 weeks are necessary to effect cure.

Echinocandins

Caspofungin is rapidly distributed to tissues after intravenous administration with extensive binding to plasma serum albumin. It is metabolized by hydrolysis and *N*-acetylation in the liver to inactive metabolites that are excreted in both bile and urine. Dose adjustment is required for patients with impaired hepatic function, and there are important drug interactions with certain immunosuppressive agents that require careful monitoring.

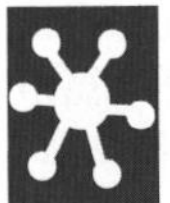

Relation of mechanisms of action to clinical response

Polyenes

Amphotericin B inhibits most fungi listed in Table 50-2. *Candida* and *Aspergillus* are likely to be a cause of a systemic mycosis, as are *Mucor, Rhizopus,* and *Absidia* species, which are often present as opportunistic pathogens in debilitated patients. Amphotericin B also inhibits *Sporothrix,* as well as some ameboflagellates and the freshwater ameba *Acanthamoeba.* It has variable activity against *Trichosporon* species, and treatment failures have been reported. A few fungal species, such as *Pseudallescheria boydii* and *Fusarium* species, show resistance. Amphotericin B acts synergistically with flucytosine against *Candida* organisms and cryptococci. Synergy of amphotericin B with other agents, such as rifampin and tetracyclines, can be demonstrated *in vitro,* but there are no clinical studies to support this.

The lipid formulations of amphotericin are active against a spectrum of fungi similar to that of amphotericin B. It is unclear whether lipid formulations results in improved activity against fungal pathogens broadly, but limited clinical data suggest that they may show improved efficacy for select fungi, including *Histoplasma capsulatum, Cryptococcus neoformans,* and *Aspergillus fumigatus.* Also, the lipid formulations may be superior to amphotericin B in certain clinical scenarios, including fungal infections of the central nervous system (due to better penetration) and those occurring in patients with a low neutrophil count. Recent data suggest a possible synergistic role for treatment of *Aspergillus* species with amphotericin lipid formulations and newer antifungal agents, particularly caspofungin.

Nystatin has a mode of action and antifungal spectrum of activity similar to those of amphotericin B. It is too toxic for parenteral administration and is only used topically.

Flucytosine

Flucytosine inhibits *Cryptococcus neoformans,* many strains of *Candida albicans,* and *Cladosporium* and *Phialophora* species, which cause chromoblastomycosis. Resistance of *Candida* species to this drug is extremely variable. Flucytosine does not inhibit *Aspergillus* and *Sporothrix* organisms, *Blastomyces dermatitidis, Histoplasma capsulatum,* or *Coccidioides immitis.* This drug acts synergistically with amphotericin B against *Cryptococcus* organisms.

Azoles

The azoles inhibit many dermatophytes, yeasts, dimorphic fungi, and some phycomycetes. Interpretative standards for the *in vitro* inhibition of several fungi by these drugs is now available, although more data is needed to confidently correlate these cutoffs with *in vivo* responses.

Ketoconazole inhibits most of the common dermatophytes and many of the fungi that cause the systemic mycoses listed in Table 50-2. However, it is not

Table 50-2 Activity of various antifungal agents against systemic fungal pathogens

Agent	*Aspergillus*	*Blastomyces dermatitidis*	*Candida albicans*	*Candida, other*	*Chromoblastomycosis agents*	*Cryptococcus neoformans*	*Coccidioides immitis*	*Fusarium*	*Histoplasma capsulatum*	*Mucormycosis agents*	*Paracoccidioides brasiliensis*	*Pseudoallescheria*	*Sporothrix*
Amphotericin B	+	+	+	+	–	+	+	±	+	+	+	–	+
Flucytosine	±	–	+	+	+	+	–	–	–	–	–	–	–
Miconazole	–	NA	+	±	+	+	+	–	+	–	+	+	+
Ketoconazole	–	+	+	±	–	+	+	±	+	–	+	–	+
Fluconazole	–	+	+	±	–	+	+	±	+	–	+	–	+
Itraconazole	+	+	+	±	+	+	+	±	+	–	+	–	+
Voriconazole	+	+	+	+	NA	+	+	+	+	–	NA	+	±
Caspofungin	+	±	+	+	–	–	–	–	±	–	±	–	–

active against *Aspergillus* organisms or Phycomycetes such as *Mucor* species. The membrane actions of ketoconazole also block the formation of branching hyphae, which may aid in white blood cell attack on the fungi.

Since ketoconazole interferes with synthesis of ergosterol, it probably should not be used with amphotericin B because it would antagonize its effect. This has been demonstrated *in vitro* and in an animal model of *Cryptococcus* infection.

Miconazole, econazole, and clotrimazole have activity similar to that of ketoconazole, but miconazole also inhibits *P. boydii*.

Voriconazole has a higher affinity for the 14-α-demethylase enzyme than other azoles and also inhibits both 24-methylene dehydrolanosterol demethylation and formation of conidial structures by certain molds. As a result, the drug has improved activity compared with other azoles, including fluconazole, for *Candida* and *Aspergillus* species, *Pseudoallescheria boydii,* and *Fusarium.* Furthermore, data suggest synergy with other antifungal agents, including caspofungin, for treatment of *Aspergillus* species.

Griseofulvin

Griseofulvin inhibits dermatophytes of *Microsporum, Trichophyton,* and *Epidermophyton* species. It has no effect on filamentous fungi such as *Aspergillus,* yeasts such as *Candida* organisms, or dimorphoric species such as *Histoplasma.*

Allylamines

Terbinafine is highly active *in vitro* against all dermatophytes of the *Trichophyton, Epidermophyton,* and *Microsporum* genera, showing greater activity than itraconazole. Moreover, some isolates of *Aspergillus* species, *Candida* species, *Sporothrix schenckii,* and *Malassezia furfur* are inhibited by achievable concentrations.

Echinocandins

Caspofungin inhibits *Candida* and *Aspergillus* species and exhibits dose-dependent fungicidal activity, although the drug is fungistatic for *Aspergillus* species. *Cryptococcus neoformans* and other molds show reduced sensitivity to caspofungin possibly related to either reduced amounts of β-glucans in the cell wall of these fungi or alterations in cell wall binding of the drug.

Therapeutic Use

Amphotericin remains the treatment of choice for most serious mold infections and most endemic fungal infections. Disseminated cryptococcal infection, including meningitis, is treated either with amphotericin B alone or in combination with flucytosine. Severe cases involving the endemic fungi, including *Histoplasma capsulatum, Blastomyces dermatitidis,* and *Coccidioides immitis,* should be treated with amphotericin B. This is also the drug of choice for Zygomycetes infections. In addition to these fungi, amphotericin remains active against the majority of other fungi that cause severe illness, with notable exceptions including *P. boydii, Fusarium* species, *Candida lusitaniae* and *Aspergillus terreus.* Lipid formulations of amphotericin are indicated for patients who are failing therapy with amphotericin B or who suffer unacceptable toxicity. They may also be indicated as first-line therapy for specific fungal infections as more data become available, including endemic fungi.

Fluconazole remains an effective treatment for serious *Candida* infections, including candidemia, esophagitis, and peritonitis. Furthermore, fluconazole is effective for preventing serious fungal infections in select hosts, including liver transplant patients. Some *Candida* species are less susceptible to fluconazole, including *Candida krusei.* Fluconazole is also active against *Cryptococcus neoformans* and used for maintenance therapy following initial amphotericin therapy.

Voriconazole is more active against certain molds than amphotericin B, including *Aspergillus, Fusarium,* and *P. boydii* and should be used as first-line therapy for these infections. Because of data suggesting synergy, it is also used in combination with caspofungin for treatment of severe infections with *Aspergillus fumigatus.* Voriconazole is likely also effective for the majority of *Candida* isolates that are resistant to fluconazole.

Nystatin is used to treat *Candida* infections of the skin, mucous membranes, and intestinal tract. It is effective for oral candidiasis, vaginal candidiasis, and *Candida* esophagitis. Although it is used prophylactically in neutropenic patients, it is ineffective except at very large daily doses.

Ketoconazole is effective for treatment of cutaneous mycoses and oral and esophageal candidiasis in immunocompromised patients. However, it is less effective than fluconazole. The only systemic infection for which miconazole IV is appropriate is that caused by *P. boydii.* Administered topically, it is comparable to clotrimazole in the management of cutaneous candidiasis, ringworm, and pityriasis versicolor. Econazole is used topically because it can penetrate the stratum corneum.

Itraconazole is effective therapy for histoplasmosis, paracoccidioidomycosis, blastomycosis, coccidioidomycosis, and sporotrichosis. It is approved for treatment of fungal nail infections.

Clotrimazole is available only for topical use because it is poorly absorbed and induces the release of microsomal enzymes, which inactivate it. It is used topically for *Candida* infection and superficial dermatophyte (ringworm) infections. It is also effective prophylactically for oral *Candida* colonization and infection in neutropenic patients.

Caspofungin is indicated for treatment of serious *Candida* infections, particularly those involving azole-resistant *Candida*. Caspofungin is also used in combination with voriconazole or amphotericin for treatment of *Aspergillus* infection because of its fungistatic and apparently synergistic effects.

Griseofulvin is used to treat only dermatophyte infections of the skin, nails, or hair, with mild forms effectively handled topically.

Tolnaftate is a topical antifungal that inhibits dermatophytes such as *Trichophyton* and *Microsporum* species but not *Candida*. Its mechanism of action is unknown. It is less effective on hyperkeratotic lesions, and scalp lesions respond poorly. It has no effect on onychomycosis. Tolnaftate has no known toxic reactions.

Haloprogin is a fungicidal agent that is effective against some *Epidermophyton*, *Microsporum*, and *Trichophyton* species and inhibits *Candida* organisms. Its mechanism of action is unknown. Burning sensations and peeling of the skin are the main side effects. It is used primarily to treat tinea pedis.

Terbinafine is approved only for the treatment of fungal nail infections.

Side effects, clinical problems, and toxicity

The clinical problems and major side effects encountered with the antifungal agents are summarized in the Clinical Problems box.

CLINICAL PROBLEMS

Drug	Adverse Effects
Polyenes	
Amphotericin B	Nephrotoxicity; fever, chills; phlebitis; hypokalemia; anemia; GI disturbance
Fluorinated pyrimidines	
Flucytosine	Bone marrow suppression; hepatotoxicity; GI disturbance
Azoles	
Imidazoles	
Miconazole	Headache; pruritus; thrombophlebitis; hepatotoxicity; autoinduction of hepatic metabolizing enzymes
Ketoconazole	GI disturbance; hepatotoxicity
Triazoles	
Itraconazole	GI disturbance; rare hepatotoxicity
Fluconazole	GI disturbance; rare hepatotoxicity; rare Stevens-Johnson syndrome
Voriconazole	Reversible photopsia, mild rash, Stevens-Johnson syndrome, toxic epidermal hepatotoxicity, necrolysis, visual hallucinations
Echinocandins	
Caspofungin	Fever, thrombophlebitis, rare hepatotoxicity

Polyenes

Amphotericin B IV administration of amphotericin B causes many adverse effects. The initial reactions, usually fever to as high as 40° C, chills, headache, malaise, nausea, and occasionally hypotension, can be controlled by antipyretics, antihistamines, antiemetics, and adrenocorticoids.

Some degree of renal toxicity develops in most patients treated with amphotericin B. This is manifested by an early decrease in glomerular filtration rate resulting from vasoconstrictive actions on afferent arterioles. It may also have an effect on the distal renal tubule, leading to K^+ loss, hypomagnesemia caused by failure to reabsorb Mg^{2+}, or tubular acidosis. Drug-induced changes in the kidney include damage to the glomerular basement membrane, hypercellularity, fibrosis, and hyalinization of glomeruli with nephrocalcinosis. The extent of renal damage is related to the total dose of drug, and although most renal function recovers even if therapy is continued, some residual damage occurs. Hydration may reduce the degree of toxicity, but mannitol infusions have not been of benefit. Pentoxifylline may reduce the degree of renal toxicity.

A normochromic, normocytic anemia with hematocrits of 22% to 35% develops in most patients who receive a normal course of therapy. This is the result of reduced erythropoiesis due to inhibition of erythropoietin production. Red blood cell production returns to normal after therapy is stopped.

Other toxicities include neurotoxicity (rare), cardiac dysrhythmias, pulmonary infiltrates, rash, and anaphylaxis. Hepatotoxicity has been reported.

Lipid formulations of amphotericin B are better tolerated with fewer infusion-related effects and considerably less nephrotoxicity than amphotericin B. As a result, these agents are preferred in situations where significant renal toxicity is likely or has developed, or in patients who cannot tolerate the infusion-related effects of amphotericin B.

Nystatin Nystatin has minimal side effects, except for a bad taste when taken as an oral suspension, which in large doses can produce nausea. It is not allergenic on the skin.

Flucytosine

Occasionally patients taking flucytosine experience nausea, vomiting, and diarrhea. Serious side effects are hematological and include anemia, leukopenia, and thrombocytopenia. Because this drug is usually coadministered with amphotericin B, there may be reduced renal clearance. Toxicity is attributable to the metabolite 5-fluorouracil. Some cases of transient hepatotoxicity have been reported.

Azoles

Common side effects of ketoconazole, which occur in 3% to 20% of those treated, are nausea and vomiting, though the severity of nausea can be reduced if the drug is taken with food. The most serious toxicity is hepatic, which is seen as transient elevations of serum aminotransferase and alkaline phosphatase concentrations and occurs in 5% to 10% of patients. Fulminant hepatic damage is uncommon, with an incidence of 1 in 12,000, although jaundice, fever, liver failure, and even death occur in a few patients. Thus the seriousness of the infection must be weighed against the risk of liver damage produced by ketoconazole.

Ketoconazole can cause transient gynecomastia and breast tenderness by blocking testosterone synthesis. High doses can lead to azoospermia and impotence and may block cortisol secretion and suppress adrenal responses to adrenocorticotropic hormone.

In a principal drug-drug interaction, ketoconazole interferes with metabolism of cyclosporin, which can lead to nephrotoxicity. In contrast, warfarin metabolism is not changed.

IV infusion of miconazole produces nausea and vomiting in 25% of patients. It may also cause chills, malaise, tremors, confusion, dizziness, or seizures.

Fluconazole absorption is decreased 15% to 20% by cimetidine, and warfarin-adjusted prothrombin times are altered by fluconazole.

Voriconazole causes transient visual disturbances in about 40% of patients that are reversible upon discontinuation of the drug. Rash and hepatotoxicity occur at rates similar to those with other triazoles. Severe dermatological manifestations are rare.

Griseofulvin

Many patients receiving griseofulvin initially complain of headaches, but the symptoms may disappear as therapy continues. Other CNS side effects include lethargy, confusion, memory lapses, and impaired judgment. Nausea, vomiting, bad taste, occasionally leukopenia or neutropenia, hepatotoxicity, skin rashes, and photosensitivity also may occur. Although renal function is not decreased, albuminuria has developed. Griseofulvin administered in very large doses is teratogenic and carcinogenic in animals. Although no similar reports in humans are available, griseofulvin should not be given to pregnant women.

Griseofulvin may interact and increase the metabolism of warfarin by inducing the release of microsomal enzymes.

Allylamines

The most commonly reported adverse effects of terbinafine are headache, diarrhea, dyspepsia, and abdominal pain. Some patients experience disturbances in taste, which may persist for several weeks after discontinuing the drug. Rashes, including toxic epidermal necrolysis, have been described. Increases in liver transaminase concentrations occur in less than 5% of patients, but rare cases of severe hepatoxicity have been reported. Finally, anaphylaxis, pancytopenia, and agranulocytosis have rarely been reported.

Echinocandins

The most common adverse effects for caspofungin include fever and thrombophlebitis. Hepatoxicity also occurs, although serious liver damage appears less common than what has been reported with other antifungals, including triazoles.

New horizons

At least two new azoles (posaconazole, ravuconazole) and echinocandins (micafungin, anidulafungin) are scheduled for release by early 2005. Posaconazole is of particular interest because it is the first imidazole with significant activity versus agents of Zygomycosis. In addition, multiple studies are in progress evaluating combinations of agents (azoles and polyenes, azoles and echinocandins) and appear promising in the treatment of select serious fungal infections (e.g., aspergillosis).

TRADE NAMES

In addition to generic and fixed-combination preparations and the drugs listed in the Major Drugs box, the following trade-named materials are some of the important compounds available in the United States.

Amphotericin B lipid complex (Abelcet)
Clotrimazole (Lotrimin, Mycelex)
Econazole nitrate (Spectazole)
Flucytosine (Ancobon)
Griseofulvin (Grifulvin)
Haloprogrin (Halotex)
Ketoconazole (Nizoral)
Liposomal amphotericin (AmBisome)
Miconazole (Monistat)
Nystatin (Mycostatin, Nystex, Nilstat)
Terbinafine (Lamisil)
Tolnaftate (Tolnate)
Voriconazole (Vfend)

FURTHER READING

Steinbach WJ, Stevens DA. Review of newer antifungal and immunomodulatory strategies for invasive aspergillosis. *Clin Infect Dis* 2003; 37 (suppl 3):S157-187.

Johnson MD, Perfect JR. Caspofungin: first approved agent in a new class of antifungals. *Expert Opin Pharmacother* 2003; 4:1-17.

Self-assessment questions

1. The absorption of which of the following is greatly decreased in the absence of gastric acidity?

a. Flucytosine
b. Fluconazole
c. Nystatin
d. Ketoconazole

2. Which of the following enters the CSF in adequate concentrations to treat cryptococcal meningitis in HIV-infected patients?

a. Miconazole
b. Ketoconazole
c. Fluconazole
d. Clotrimazole

3. Amphotericin B produces which of the following adverse effects?

a. Leukopenia
b. Decrease in glomerular filtration rate
c. Vestibular toxicity
d. Rash

4. Which agent is used to treat cryptococcal meningitis?

a. Bacitracin
b. Neomycin
c. Griseofulvin
d. Nystatin
e. Amphotericin B

5. Which of the following could be used to treat an *Aspergillus* infection of the lung?

a. Griseofulvin
b. Ketoconazole
c. Nystatin
d. Amphotericin B

6. Which antifungal agent is effective in the treatment of ringworm of the skin and nails?

a. Bacitracin
b. Neomycin
c. Griseofulvin
d. Nystatin
e. Amphotericin B

CHAPTER 51

Antiviral agents

Daniel H. Havlichek, Jr.

Major Drugs

Amantadine (Symmetrel)	Lamivudine (Epivir)
Acyclovir (Zovirax)	Nevirapine (Viramune)
Didanosine (Videx)	Ribavirin (Virazole)
Foscarnet (Foscavir)	Ritonavir (Norvir)
Idoxuridine (Stoxil, Herplex)	Tenofovir (Viread)
	Trifluridine (Viroptic)
Indinavir (Crixivan)	Zalcitabine (Hivid)
Immunoglobulins	Zanamivir (Relenza)
Interferons	Zidovudine (Retrovir)

Therapeutic overview

Viruses are responsible for significant morbidity and mortality in populations worldwide. These infectious agents consist of a core genome of nucleic acid (nucleoid) contained in a protein shell (capsid) and sometimes surrounded by a lipoprotein membrane (envelope) (Fig. 51-1). Viruses cannot replicate independently. They must instead enter cells and use the energy-generating, DNA- or RNA-replicating, and protein-synthesizing pathways of the host cell to replicate. Some viruses can integrate a copy of their genetic material into host chromosomes, achieving viral latency, in which clinical illness can recur without reexposure to the virus.

Some genera of viruses that cause human infections are listed in Table 51-1. Also listed is information about which genomic material—RNA or DNA—is present and examples of clinically important diseases attributed to each virus.

The way antiviral agents act is not always known. Most currently available antiviral drugs interfere with viral **nucleic acid synthesis** and/or **regulation**; however, some agents work by interfering with virus **cell binding**, interrupting viral **uncoating**, or stimulating the host **immune system.** Because viruses generally take over host cell nucleic acid and protein replication pathways before clinical infection is discovered, antiviral drugs often must penetrate cells that are already infected to produce a response. Side effects to healthy cells can occur when the drug penetrates into them and disrupts normal nucleic acid or protein synthesis. This toxicity limits clinical utility of many drugs.

In vitro susceptibility testing of antiviral compounds differs significantly from that done for antibacterial agents, because viruses require host cells to replicate. Generally greater than a 50% reduction in plaque forming units at an achievable serum concentration qualifies a drug to be classified as active against a given virus. In recent years, the polymerase chain reaction has provided the technology to allow detection of individual virus mutations, allowing physicians to predict viral susceptibility to many antiviral agents.

Many antiviral agents inhibit single steps in the viral replication cycle. They are considered virustatic and do not destroy a given virus but only temporarily halt replication. For an antiviral agent to be optimally effective, the patient must have a competent host

Abbreviations

AIDS	acquired immunodeficiency syndrome
CMV	cytomegalovirus
CSF	cerebrospinal fluid
HIV	human immunodeficiency virus
NNRTIs	non-nucleoside reverse transcriptase inhibitors
NRTIs	nucleoside reverse transcriptase inhibitors

Table 51-1 Virus groups of clinical importance

Virus Genera or Groupings	Nucleic Acid	Clinical Examples of Illnesses
Adenovirus	DNA	Upper respiratory tract and eye infections
Hepadnaviridae	DNA	Hepatitis B, cancer (?)
Herpesvirus	DNA	Genital herpes, varicella, meningoencephalitis, mononucleosis, retinitis
Papillomavirus	DNA	Papillomas (warts), cancer (?)
Parvovirus	DNA	Erythema infectiosum
Arenavirus	RNA	Lymphocytic choriomeningitis
Bunyavirus	RNA	Encephalitis
Coronavirus	RNA	Upper respiratory tract infections
Influenzavirus	RNA	Influenza
Paramyxovirus	RNA	Measles, upper respiratory tract infections
Picornavirus	RNA	Poliomyelitis, diarrhea, upper respiratory tract infections
Retrovirus	RNA	Leukemia, AIDS
Rhabdovirus	RNA	Rabies
Togavirus	RNA	Rubella, yellow fever

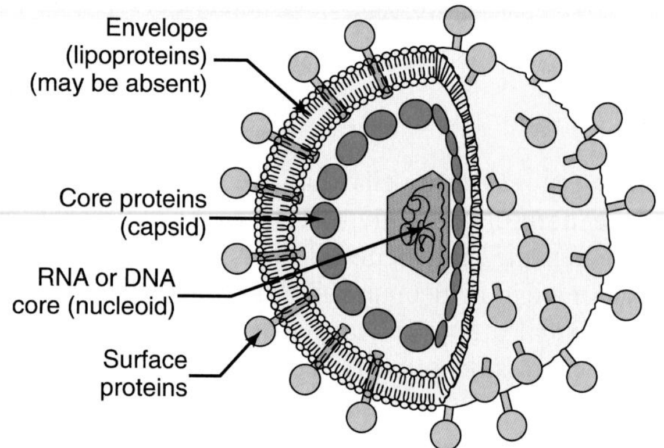

Figure 51-1 Basic components of virus particles.

immune system that can eliminate or effectively halt virus replication. Patients with immunosuppressive conditions are prone to frequent and often severe viral infections that may recur when antiviral drugs are stopped.

Prolonged suppressive therapy is often necessary. Currently there is no antiviral agent that eliminates viral latency. Strains of viruses resistant to specific drugs can also develop.

Several agents are converted in the body to active compounds (acyclovir, ganciclovir) or must be present continuously to have an antiviral effect (amantadine). Other important considerations include drug distribution, duration of infection, and difficulty of administration. Approaches to the treatment of viral infections with drugs are summarized in the Therapeutic Overview box.

THERAPEUTIC OVERVIEW FOR TREATMENT OF VIRAL INFECTIONS

Block viral attachment to cells
Block uncoating of virus
Inhibit viral DNA/RNA synthesis
Inhibit viral protein synthesis
Inhibit specific viral enzymes
Inhibit viral assembly
Inhibit viral release
Stimulate host immune system

Mechanisms of action

Viral replication cycle

A virus binds to an appropriate host cell to initiate an infection. The virus penetrates the cell and promotes the synthesis of viral components by controlling host protein and nucleic acid synthesis. Virions are then formed and released to infect other cells (Fig. 51-2 shows the replication cycle of the AIDS virus in some detail). In the situation of human immunodeficiency virus (HIV) infection, infectious virions bind to appropriate host cell receptors. The viral genome crosses into the cell, uncoats, and disassembles. An HIV-specific **reverse transcriptase** converts viral RNA into DNA, and an **integrase** incorporates the DNA into the cell's chromosomes. The host cell then produces a copy of the HIV genome for packaging into new virions and viral messenger RNA, which is the template for protein

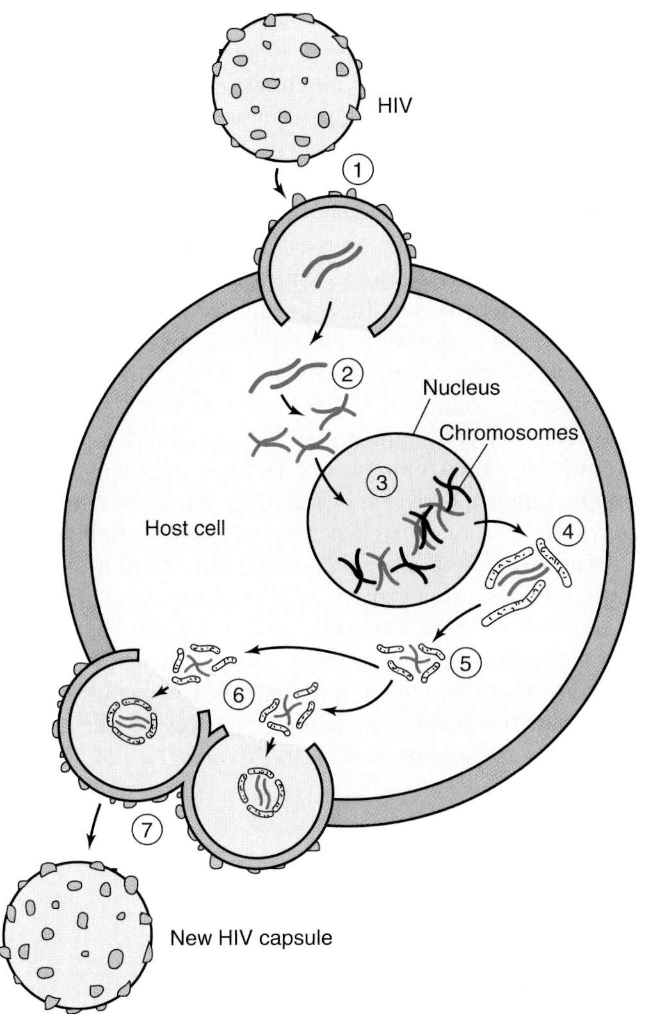

Figure 51-2 Replication of the AIDS virus.

synthesis. An HIV-specific **protease** hydrolyzes a viral polyprotein into smaller subunits, which then assemble to form mature infectious virions.

Four classes of compounds have been used to interfere with the HIV reproductive cycle. These include fusion inhibitors, nucleoside reverse transcriptase inhibitors (NRTIs), non-nucleoside reverse transcriptase inhibitors (NNRTIs), and protease inhibitors. Anti-HIV therapy with multiple agents has been very effective in limiting the progression to AIDS in persons carrying HIV.

Other viruses also contain unique enzymes or metabolic pathways that make them susceptible to certain drugs. For example, herpes simplex virus encodes a **thymidine kinase** that monophosphorylates acyclovir significantly better than does the host cell enzyme. Because acyclovir monophosphate is trapped in cells, it becomes highly concentrated there. This causes significant inhibition of viral growth with few side effects on cells that do not contain the herpes simplex thymidine kinase. Because CMV (another herpes family virus) does not encode such a thymidine kinase, it is inhibited only by concentrations of acyclovir that are not tolerated clinically and is therefore not effective in treating CMV.

Inhibitors of cell penetration

Enfuvirtide HIV entry into cells is accomplished by a complex series of virus host interactions. Initially, virus approximates the CD4 cell by interactions of HIV surface protein and the host CD4 receptor. Following approximation, host co-receptors interact with HIV surface proteins, resulting in folding of the HIV protein gp41. This folding results in fusion of the HIV membrane with the host cell membrane and insertion of the HIV nucleoid into the cell. Enfuvirtide prevents entry of HIV into cells by lying along the gp41 coils causing steric hindrance of protein folding. Resistance occurs when mutations of gp41 occur that alter conformation and folding.

Inhibitors of viral uncoating

Amantadine and rimantadine The mechanism of action of amantadine (Fig. 51-3) is not fully established but appears to involve blocking the ion channel activity of the M_2 protein, thereby inhibiting late-stage uncoating of influenza A virions. This drug is not effective against influenza B, which lacks the M_2 protein. A single amino acid change in the M_2 protein results in amantadine resistance. Resistant virus is virulent and causes disease in exposed people. Rimantadine is a related compound with similar actions but an improved side effect profile.

Inhibitors of viral DNA and RNA synthesis

Acyclovir Acyclovir (see Fig. 51-3) is a synthetic guanosine analog and is the prototypical agent for this group of anti-herpesvirus drugs. The group includes the related drugs valacyclovir and famciclovir, a prodrug for penciclovir. All of these drugs must be **phosphorylated** to be active and are initially monophosphorylated by viral **thymidine kinase.** Because the thymidine kinases of herpes simplex virus types 1 and 2 are many times more active on acyclovir than host thymidine kinase, high concentrations of acyclovir monophosphate accumulate in infected cells. This is then further phosphorylated to the active compound acyclovir triphosphate. The triphosphate cannot cross cell membranes and accumulates further. The resulting concentration of acyclovir triphosphate is 50 to 100 times greater in infected cells than in uninfected cells.

Acyclovir triphosphate inhibits virus growth in three ways. First, it competitively inhibits **DNA polymerases,** with human DNA polymerases being significantly less susceptible to it than viral enzymes. Second, it **terminates DNA elongation.** Third, it produces **irreversible binding** between viral DNA polymerase and the interrupted chain, causing permanent inactivation.

The result is a several hundred-fold inhibition of herpes simplex virus growth with minimal toxic effects on uninfected cells. However, herpes simplex viruses with altered thymidine kinase (acyclovir-penciclovir resistant) have developed, although they occur primarily in patients receiving multiple courses of therapy. These mutants are susceptible to foscarnet. Changes in

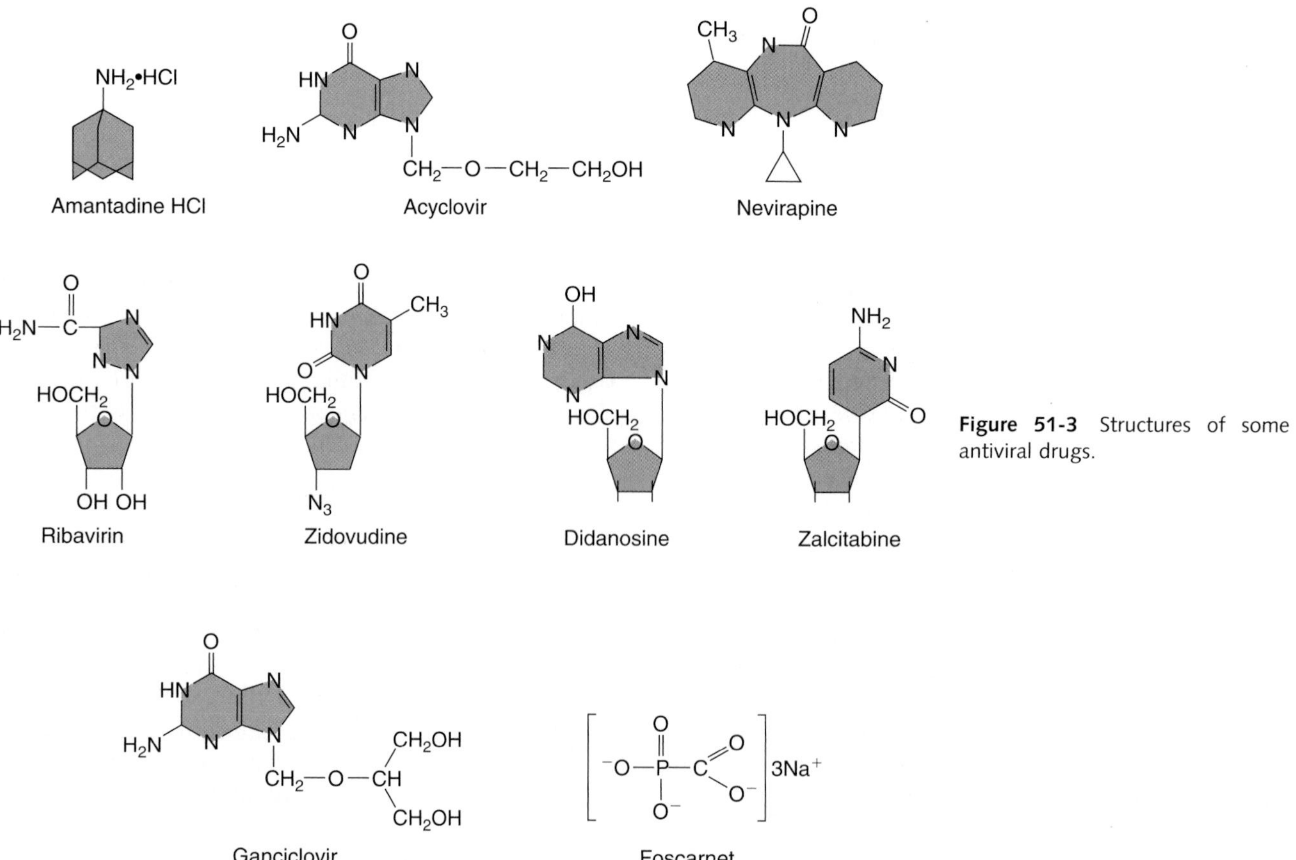

Figure 51-3 Structures of some antiviral drugs.

viral DNA polymerase structures can also mediate resistance to acyclovir.

Ganciclovir The structure of ganciclovir is shown in Figure 51-3. It is also a synthetic guanosine analog active against many herpes viruses and must also be **phosphorylated** to be active. Infection-induced kinases, viral thymidine kinase, or deoxyguanosine kinase of various herpes viruses can catalyze this reaction. After monophosphorylation, cellular enzymes convert ganciclovir to the triphosphorylated form, and the triphosphate inhibits viral DNA polymerase rather than cellular DNA polymerase. Ganciclovir triphosphate competitively inhibits the incorporation of guanosine triphosphate into DNA. Because of its toxicity and the availability of acyclovir for treatment of many herpesvirus infections, its use is currently restricted to treatment of CMV retinitis.

Foscarnet Foscarnet inhibits DNA polymerases, RNA polymerases, and reverse transcriptases (see Fig. 51-3). *In vitro* it is active against herpesviruses, influenza virus, and HIV. Foscarnet is used primarily in treatment of CMV retinitis. Viral resistance is attributable to structural alterations in CMV DNA polymerase. Foscarnet inhibits CMV herpesviruses that are resistant to acyclovir and ganciclovir.

Ribavirin Ribavirin is a synthetic purine nucleoside active against many viruses, including respiratory syncytial virus, Lassa fever virus, and influenza viruses (see Fig. 51-3). Ribavirin appears to be phosphorylated in host cells by host **adenosine kinase.** The 5′-monophosphate subsequently inhibits cellular inosine monophosphate formation, resulting in depletion of intracellular guanosine triphosphate. In some situations, ribavirin triphosphate suppresses guanosine triphosphate–dependent capping of messenger RNA, thereby inhibiting viral protein synthesis. It also acts by suppressing the initiation or elongation of viral messenger RNA. Exogenous guanosine can reverse the antiviral effects of ribavirin with some viruses.

Box 51-1 Mechanism of action of antiviral agents

Drug inhibition of specific viral enzymes

HUMAN IMMUNODEFICIENCY VIRUS

Reverse Transcriptase

Zidovudine
Abacavir
Lamivudine
Zalcitabine
Didanosine
Stavudine
Tenofovir
Nevirapine
Efavirenz
Delavirdine

HIV Protease

Ritonavir
Saquinavir
Nelfinavir
Lopinavir/Ritonavir
Amprenavir
Zanamivir

INFLUENZA A AND B

Neuraminidase Inhibitors

Oseltamivir
Zanamivir

Nucleoside reverse transcriptase inhibitors and nucleotides

These drugs include zidovudine, didanosine, lamivudine, stavudine, and others (Box 51-1), and all work through a similar mechanism. Zidovudine (AZT) is the prototype for use in HIV infection. It is a thymidine analog that is phosphorylated to monophosphate, diphosphate, and triphosphate forms by cellular kinases in infected and uninfected cells. NRTIs have two primary methods of action: First, the triphosphate form acts as a competitive inhibitor of **HIV reverse transcriptase.** Second, after the nucleoside is incorporated into the elongating DNA chain, the forming sugar phosphate backbone of the DNA is blocked from further elongation by substitution at the 3 position. This results in **chain termination.** In the case of zidovudine, this substitution is an azido (N3) group. Zidovudine inhibits HIV reverse transcriptase at much lower concentrations than those needed to inhibit cellular DNA polymerases, leading to a more targeted effect against HIV.

Tenofovir is the only nucleotide currently available for use. It is a monophosphate derivative of adenosine that is administered as the disoproxil salt. Following ingestion, it is converted to triphosphates by cellular enzymes. Tenofovir acts as an adenosine analog to inhibit HIV reverse transcriptase and cause chain termination.

Differences in NRTIs and investigational nucleotides are primarily based on which nucleic acid is employed and the type of substitution that causes chain termination. NRTIs have been produced for each of the 4 nucleic acids. Neither NRTIs nor nucleotides should be used as monotherapy.

Non-nucleoside reverse transcriptase inhibitors

Nevirapine, delavirdine, efavirenz As a class, NNRTIs bind to HIV reverse transcriptase at a site distant from the catalytic site. This binding causes a conformational change in the enzyme disrupting enzyme activity. Because NRTIs and NNRTIs do not bind at the same site, they can be used effectively as combination therapy with significant inhibition of HIV reverse transcriptase. When resistance to NNRTIs occurs, all drugs currently available are affected, and this class of drugs is unavailable for therapy.

HIV protease inhibitors

Saquinavir, ritonavir, indinavir Protease inhibitors inhibit an HIV-specific proteolytic enzyme necessary for the production of infectious HIV virions. Currently available protease inhibitors **inhibit cleavage of the gag/pol HIV polyprotein** and act synergistically with NRTIs. Resistance to protease inhibitors can occur within weeks when they are used as single agents or intermittently. These drugs are therefore usually given in combination with other anti-HIV therapies. The possibility of cross-resistance between these agents is being investigated.

Inhibitors of influenza neuraminidase

Oseltamivir and zanamivir Influenza A and B possess a unique neuraminidase enzyme that is highly conserved in both viruses. The enzyme catalyzes removal of terminal **sialic acid residues** that are linked to glycoproteins and glycolipids. Oseltamivir and zanamivir are analogs of sialic acid and prevent release of new viruses. Proper neuraminidase activity seems to be necessary for such release.

Other antiviral agents

Idoxuridine Idoxuridine is an iodinated thymidine nucleoside analog that is incorporated into DNA in place of thymidine and blocks further DNA chain elongation. In vitro it inhibits many DNA viruses, and exogenous thymidine eliminates its antiviral effect. Idoxuridine affects mammalian cells, and its teratogenic, mutagenic, and immunosuppressive effects limit its use to topical preparations. It is used especially for the treatment of herpes simplex infections of the cornea. Herpesviruses resistant to idoxuridine do occur and generally have decreased thymidine kinase activity.

Trifluridine Trifluridine, or trifluorothymidine, is a pyrimidine analog that inhibits viral DNA synthesis by being incorporated into viral DNA. It does not require thymidine kinase for it to become active and is active against thymidine kinase–deficient mutants of herpes simplex virus that are resistant to acyclovir or idoxuridine, or both. It can only be administered topically.

Fluorouracil Fluorouracil is an anticancer drug that blocks production of thymidylate and interrupts normal cellular DNA and RNA synthesis. Its primary action may be to cause **thiamine deficiency** and resultant cell death. The effect of fluorouracil is most pronounced on rapidly growing cells. Its antiviral activity stems primarily from its ability to kill cells infected with papillomavirus (warts), and it is applied topically for this purpose.

Interferons Interferons are naturally occurring glycoproteins produced by lymphocytes, macrophages, fibroblasts, and other human cells. There are three distinct classes: α, β, and γ. They act as antiviral agents by inhibiting viral protein synthesis or assembly or by stimulating the immune system. Interferons bind specific cell receptors and produce rapid changes in RNA. These effects may result in inhibition of viral penetration; uncoating, synthesis, or methylation of mRNA; translation of viral proteins; or assembly and release of virus. A 2′,5′-oligoadenylate synthetase and a protein kinase are usually produced that inhibit protein synthesis in the presence of double-stranded RNA. Interferons can also protect uninfected cells from infection by mechanisms that are as yet unclear. Interferons are used for the treatment of hepatitis B and C and papillomavirus infections.

Immunoglobulins Immunoglobulins are used as antiviral agents, primarily to prevent infections. Some immunoglobulin preparations with high titers against specific viruses (e.g., hepatitis B, rabies) may be used for treatment or prophylaxis. Standard human immune globulin is used to prevent hepatitis A infection.

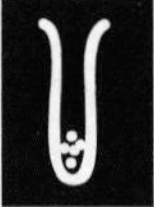

Pharmacokinetics

For most antiviral agents to be active they must become concentrated within cells. Many compounds are nucleoside analogs and are rapidly metabolized to inactive compounds, which are then eliminated from the body. This necessitates frequent dosing to maintain adequate intracellular drug concentrations. Because of severe systemic toxicity, some agents can be applied only topically to treat certain viral infections.

Because these compounds often interfere with human DNA or RNA synthesis, any antiviral agent should be used with the utmost caution in pregnancy and only when the potential benefits of treatment clearly outweigh the potential risks. The pharmacoki-

Table 51-2 Pharmacokinetic parameters of some commonly used drugs

Drug	Routes of Administration	Peak Serum Concentrations (µg/ml)	Half-Life (hrs)	Disposition
Amantadine	Oral	0.3-0.7	12-18 (doubles in elderly)	R (90%), M (9%)
Rimantadine	Oral	0.2-0.3	24-36	M (90%), R (10%)
Acyclovir	Topical, oral, IV	0.6-10.0	3-4	R (80%), M (20%)
Valacyclovir	Oral	3.0 (ACV)	3-4	R (80%), M (20%)
Famciclovir	Oral	4.0 (PCV)	2-3 (PCV serum)	R (90%)
Ganciclovir	IV, oral	4-6	3-4	R (90%)
Foscarnet	IV	30	3	R (80%)
Ribavirin	Aerosol, oral	0.8-3.5	9	M (60%), R (30%)
Zidovudine	Oral, IV	0.05-1.5	0.8-2	M (75%), R (15%)
Didanosine	Oral	1.5	0.5	R (50%), M (50%)
Zalcitabine	Oral	0.01	2	R (70%)
Stavudine	Oral	1-2	1-2	M (60%), R (40%)
Lamivudine	Oral	2-3	5-7	R (70%), M (30%)
Nevirapine	Oral	5-10	25-50	M (80%), R (10%)
Saquinavir	Oral	0.2	1-2	M (80%), R (20%)
Indinavir	Oral	5-10	1-2	M (80%), R (20%)
Ritonavir	Oral	10-15	3-5	M (80%), R (20%)
Idoxuridine	Topical	—	—	M
Trifluridine	Topical	—	—	—
Fluorouracil	Topical	—	—	—

R, Renal; *M*, metabolic; *ACV*, acyclovir; *PCV*, penciclovir.

netic parameters for some antiviral drugs are listed in Table 51-2.

Inhibitors of viral uncoating

Amantadine is completely but slowly absorbed from the gastrointestinal tract, is 65% protein bound, and is distributed well throughout the body. Serum drug concentrations vary widely with the age of the patient, although peak drug concentrations occur 2 to 4 hours after ingestion. The plasma half-life of amantadine doubles in the elderly, necessitating dosage reductions. Amantadine is eliminated by kidney glomerular filtration and tubular secretion but is also metabolized to at least eight different compounds, although the biological activity of these metabolites is unknown.

Inhibitors of viral DNA and RNA synthesis

Acyclovir can be administered topically, orally, or IV; valacyclovir and famciclovir are only available orally. Valacyclovir has a higher bioavailability than acyclovir. Acyclovir is minimally protein bound and well distributed throughout the body. Percutaneous absorption of topical acyclovir is very low. Because of poor absorption and the need for higher drug concentrations in the treatment of shingles, different dosage formulations of oral acyclovir are available.

Valacyclovir is rapidly metabolized in the liver to acyclovir. Because valacyclovir is better absorbed than acyclovir, serum concentrations of acyclovir are three to five times higher after valacyclovir administration. Famciclovir is also metabolized in the liver to its active compound, penciclovir. Most acyclovir is excreted unchanged. As a result, acyclovir may interfere with the renal excretion of drugs, such as methotrexate, that are eliminated through the renal tubules. Probenecid significantly decreases renal excretion of acyclovir. Penciclovir is eliminated in the same way as acyclovir.

Ganciclovir is primarily eliminated unchanged in urine, and therefore the plasma half-life can increase substantially in patients with severe renal insufficiency. It can also be administered intravitreally, in which setting it has a half-life of 50 hours.

Foscarnet has a low bioavailability and is only administered IV at this time. Because foscarnet can bind calcium and other divalent cations, it accumulates in bone and may be detectable for many months after treatment. It is mainly excreted unchanged in the urine, and therefore dosage must be adjusted for impaired renal function.

Ribavirin is about 45% bioavailable. Peak concentrations after IV administration are tenfold greater than those after oral administration. Ribavirin is administered by aerosol in treatment of severe respiratory syncytial virus infections. About 3% of ribavirin accumulates in red blood cells in the form of ribavirin triphosphate, to give a prolonged serum half-life of 40 days, during which the compound is slowly eliminated. Hepatic metabolism is the main route of elimination.

HIV fusion inhibitors

Enfuvirtide is a 36 amino acid polypeptide that is available only for subcutaneous injection. Peak concentrations of 5 μg/ml occur 4 to 6 hours after injection. Enfuvirtide is poorly water-soluble and is highly protein bound. Elimination of enfuvirtide is thought to be by catabolism of the polypeptide to constituent amino acids by a variety of tissue enzymes.

Nucleoside reverse transcriptase inhibitors and nucleotides

NRTIs and nucleotides are available for oral administration. Zidovudine is the only drug in this class available IV and can be helpful in managing pregnant women during labor. Peak serum concentrations for NRTIs and nucleotides generally occur within 30 to 90 minutes. Importantly, the intracellular half-life of the phosphorylated compounds is many hours. This can allow once or twice daily dosing for many agents improving compliance and decreasing toxicity.

Drug absorption is unique for each of the drugs in this class, and food or stomach pH can affect absorption for some of these agents. Didanosine and tenofovir are most affected in this regard. Didanosine is extremely acid labile and is formulated with a buffer to neutralize stomach acid and maximize absorption. Food significantly improves tenofovir absorption. CSF penetration varies widely for the drugs. NRTIs and nucleotides are eliminated by a combination of renal excretion and glucuronidation. Drugs that can interfere with hepatic glucuronidation (e.g., acetaminophen) or renal tubular transport (e.g., probenecid) may inhibit elimination of some agents and should be used with caution. Also, patients with renal insufficiency may need dosage adjustments. The improved dosing pattern of NRTIs and the need to use multiple NRTIs in management of HIV disease has allowed manufacture of fixed drug combinations, further improving patient compliance.

Non-nucleoside reverse transcriptase inhibitors

Bioavailability of NNRTIs is generally high. They are rapidly absorbed, with half-lives of 6 to 40 hours. No dietary restrictions are necessary for this class of drugs. Nevirapine induces and is extensively metabolized by the cytochrome P450 system, necessitating a modification in the doses of other drugs metabolized by this route. Efavirenz possesses the longest half-life and can be given once daily.

HIV protease inhibitors

Several protease inhibitors are now available for use. The absorption of these medications is usually improved with food, however indinavir absorption is decreased with food. Peak serum concentrations of protease inhibitors are reached 1 to 3 hours after ingestion and are eliminated primarily by metabolism through cytochrome P450 3A4. Inhibition of the P450 system can cause significant interactions with other medications. The elimination of protease inhibitors can be preferentially decreased by low-dose ritonavir, causing higher serum levels for longer periods of time. Lopinavir and ritonavir are available as a fixed drug combination utilizing this effect. Patients with liver disease who need protease inhibitor therapy need to be monitored carefully.

Other antiviral agents

Idoxuridine is used only topically, and systemic absorption is minimal. The small amount that is absorbed is metabolized to uracil and iodouracil. In vitro, resistance to idoxuridine develops easily, and resistant clinical isolates have been described that may be a source of treatment failure.

Trifluridine is available for topical use only, especially as an ophthalmic preparation. Minimal drug absorption occurs; no trifluridine has been detected in serum or aqueous humor from treated patients. Fluorouracil is also available as a topical preparation.

Because interferons are glycoproteins, their pharmacokinetics are difficult to assess. Simple detection of circulating interferon may not approximate clinical activity, because cellular binding is necessary and an intact immune system is important to achieve a maximal response. Also, the biological activity may last days, even though the compound has been cleared from serum (see Chapter 53).

Interferons are administered IM or SC. Serum concentrations peak in 4 to 8 hours and decline steadily over 1 to 2 days. Biological activity of interferons begins within an hour of injection, peaks at 24 hours, and decreases over 4 to 6 days. Interferons are distributed throughout the body and are detectable in brain and CSF. The elimination of exogenous interferon is complex. Liver, lung, kidney, heart, and skeletal muscle are capable of inactivating the compounds. Negligible amounts are found in urine. Polyethylene glycol has been attached to some interferons, resulting in slower subcutaneous rates of absorption, longer serum half-lives, less-frequent dosing, and more-sustained antiviral activity. Interferons are injected three times per week in management of chronic hepatitis while pegylated interferon is injected once per week. Interferons are also effective when injected directly into condylomas or given SC or IM in management of papillomavirus infections.

As antiviral therapies, immunoglobulins are given SC, IM, and IV. They are distributed throughout the body. After IM injection, immunoglobulin serum concentrations peak in 4 to 6 days and then decline, with half-lives of 20 to 30 days. Repeat immunization every 3 to 6 months is often recommended for people who are continually exposed to infectious agents such as hepatitis A. After exposure to rabies, it is recommended that the wound be infiltrated with high-titer immunoglobulin to neutralize virus, with the remaining immunoglobulin administered IM. IV gamma globulin is administered every 3 to 4 weeks to agammaglobulinemic patients. Clearance of immunoglobulins is variable, with a mean half-life of 20 days.

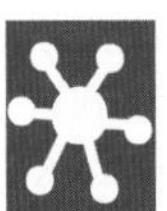

Relation of mechanisms of action to clinical response

Many of the most effective antiviral agents target **unique viral enzymes** or **life cycle pathways**. Such specific inhibition is beneficial because uninfected cells experience minimal toxicity. As a result, many antiviral drugs only inhibit replication of specific viruses and are not useful against other viruses. Because antiviral drugs are used primarily after infection has occurred, they are most effective when given early. Viruses with latent characteristics may need chronic suppression. Many agents are limited in their use by their toxic effects on uninfected cells. Such compounds are primarily used topically.

Immunoglobulins and interferons have **wide antiviral activity** based on their mechanism of action. Interferons interfere with the replication of a large number of viruses (hence the origin of their name). They also broadly stimulate the immune system, further enhancing antiviral activity. Immune globulin has the ability to neutralize some viruses. The spectrum of immune globulin activity is dependent on neutralizing antibody being present and the capacity of the virus to be neutralized by antibody. Hepatitis C and HIV are not neutralized by currently available immune globulin preparations, so administration is not recommended following exposure to these viruses. All agents are significantly less effective in immunosuppressed patients.

Amantadine Amantadine and rimantadine are both used for treatment and prophylaxis of influenza A infections but are ineffective against influenza B. They are most effective when given before exposure or within 48 hours of development of symptoms. It has been estimated that these drugs are 50% effective in protecting against infection and 60% to 70% effective in protecting against illness. Medications do not inhibit antibody responses to influenza, and immunity develops during therapy in both immunized and infected patients. Protective effects of medications are lost approximately 48 hours after therapy is stopped. Specific patients targeted for drug therapy include those who are unvaccinated and have greatest risk for complications of influenza infection. Such people should also be vaccinated, because resistant mutants may develop during therapy. The major advantage of rimantadine is that it carries a lower risk for causing CNS effects.

Zanamivir and oseltamivir are inhibitors of influenza A and B viral neuraminidase. Both agents effectively stop the release of virus and subsequent spread to healthy cells. These compounds improve symptoms and decrease duration of illness when started within 48 hours of symptoms. Zanamivir is administered via inhalation.

Acyclovir Systemic acyclovir is effective in reducing viral shedding, alleviating local symptoms, and decreasing the severity and duration of herpes simplex infections. Recurrences after termination of therapy are common because of viral latency. Acyclovir decreases mortality in patients with herpes encephalitis to approximately 20%. About 50% of acyclovir-treated patients return to normal life. High-dose acyclovir is needed to treat encephalitis to improve penetration across the blood brain barrier. Acyclovir should be administered as soon as possible after encephalitis is diagnosed to lessen patient morbidity and mortality.

IV or oral acyclovir should be used to treat primary genital herpes simplex infection. Both treatments decrease viral shedding, local and systemic symptoms, and time to resolution. Neither form of therapy decreases the rate or severity of recurrences. Recurrent genital herpes is managed with orally administered acyclovir. Treatments begun when the first prodrome of clinical recurrence is noted to demonstrate decreased symptoms and viral shedding. Patients with four to six recurrences of genital herpes infection per year are often given suppressive therapy. Approximately 75% of patients taking suppressive acyclovir will have no recurrences for 12 months, and the total number of recurrences decreases by 90%. After discontinuation of acyclovir, recurrence rates generally return to near pretreatment levels. Resistance has been noted in people with active lesions taking suppressive therapy. Patients taking acyclovir may shed virus even if no lesions are visible.

Oral acyclovir can be effective in suppressing recurrences of mucocutaneous herpes simplex infections in immunosuppressed patients, and it is sometimes given after chemotherapy. It can also be used prophylactically in bone marrow and other transplant patients to prevent herpes recurrence. Therapy is most effective when begun before transplantation and continued for many weeks.

Acyclovir is effective in the management of acute varicella. Acyclovir, valacyclovir, and famciclovir are effective in the treatment of herpes zoster (shingles). Patients whose treatment is begun within 72 hours of the onset of symptoms show decreased viral shedding and more-rapid healing. The total duration of illness is decreased by 2 days in healthy children with varicella who receive acyclovir.

Acyclovir is not effective in treating CMV pneumonia or visceral disease, Epstein-Barr virus, mononucleosis, or chronic fatigue syndrome. However, a condition in AIDS patients known as hairy leukoplakia (a proliferation of oral epithelium related to Epstein-Barr virus infection) is responsive to oral acyclovir.

Idoxuridine and trifluridine can be used topically to treat herpes simplex keratitis. Toxicity prevents systemic use of these agents.

Ganciclovir Ganciclovir and valganciclovir are used in management of CMV disease in AIDS and transplant patients. In situations of CMV retinitis, ganciclovir implants or other ocular injections may be necessary. Retinitis recurs in patients when therapy is stopped. About 65% of AIDS patients with visceral CMV infection have significant virological responses, but clinical improvement in response to ganciclovir is not as significant. Bone marrow transplant patients with CMV pneumonia also show virological responses, but there are no differences in overall mortality in patients receiving this antiviral agent.

Foscarnet Foscarnet is approved only for IV administration in the treatment of CMV retinitis. It is equally as effective as ganciclovir; however, drug-related toxicity is more common.

Ribavirin Ribavirin alters intracellular GTP concentrations and has activity against respiratory syncytial virus and Lassa fever virus and is synergistic with interferon in treatment of chronic hepatitis C infection. When administered as an aerosol, special generators are required to generate the necessary particle sizes.

HIV

Initial studies with zidovudine monotherapy demonstrated that inhibition of HIV reverse transcriptase improved CD4 counts and clinical outcomes in patients. The effect was not sustained as reverse transcriptase mutations developed, viral replication progressed, CD4 counts fell, and clinical illnesses recurred. Other NRTIs were initially used as salvage therapy, and then in combination in an attempt to halt HIV replication. Since NRTIs all work in the same way at the same active site, inhibitors of other stages of the HIV replication cycle were actively sought.

NNRTIs and HIV protease inhibitors provided other mechanisms to inhibit viral replication (highly active antiretroviral therapy). With the agents currently available it has become clear that HIV resistance occurs rapidly when medications are used as single agents or irregularly. Therefore, medication compliance is crucial in achieving the best outcomes, which occur when viral replication is low. Improved understanding of cellular metabolism of NRTIs has shown intracellular half-lives to be significantly longer than serum half-lives, allowing less-frequent dosing of many medications and improving patient compliance. A further advance in management of HIV disease is the development of fusion inhibitors, which are still under active investigation.

The numerous agents currently available make good clinical outcomes possible for the majority of HIV-infected patients when seen early in the disease process.

Papillomavirus

Fluorouracil Fluorouracil has been used topically to treat condylomas (warts) caused by human papillomaviruses. It acts primarily as an ablative agent, destroying infected and uninfected cells, and can therefore be used only externally over relatively small areas.

Nonspecific viral inhibitors

Interferons All three classes of human interferons (α, β, γ) are nonspecific immune stimulators that also have significant antiviral activity. As an antiviral agent, interferon is approved for the treatment of condyloma acuminata and chronic hepatitis B or C (often in combination with ribavirin). Adding polyethylene glycol to interferon has improved outcomes in chronic hepatitis C, presumably from more-sustained blood levels of interferon.

Immunoglobulins Some human immunoglobulins have high titers against specific viruses such as hepatitis B and rabies and are more efficacious against these viruses than nonspecific immunoglobulins are. Some viral infections amenable to immunoglobulin therapy

Box 51-2 Viral infections amenable to immunoglobulin treatment

Cytomegalovirus	Rabies
Hepatitis A	Varicella*
Hepatitis B	Measles*

*Immunoglobulin treatment reserved for patients at high risk for complications.

are listed in Box 51-2. Immunoglobulins are usually given IM, as close as possible to the time of exposure to the virus. In some circumstances, an immunoglobulin should also be given very close to the lesion (as in rabies) to provide high concentrations to lymphatic tissues. In most situations, IM injection provides systemic immunoglobulin concentrations adequate to prevent the development of clinical infection. However, because immunoglobulins do not confer long-term immunity, they must often be given in a series of injections, together with vaccine therapy.

CLINICAL PROBLEMS

Amantadine	GI upset, CNS effects (nervousness, insomnia), anticholinergic effects
Rimantadine	GI upset, CNS effects
Acyclovir, valacyclovir, famciclovir	CNS effects (nervousness, headache), decreased renal function
Ganciclovir	Bone marrow suppression, CNS effects, rash, fever
Ribavirin	Headache, GI upset, dyspnea, teratogenic
Zidovudine	Bone marrow suppression, granulocytopenia, myositis
Didanosine	Pancreatitis, neuropathy
Zalcitabine	Neuropathy
Lamivudine	Bone marrow suppression, neuropathy, malaise
Stavudine	Neuropathy, GI upset
Nevirapine	Rash
Saquinavir	Drug-drug interactions
Indinavir	Renal stones, drug-drug interactions
Ritonavir	Drug-drug interactions

Side effects, clinical problems, and toxicity

Because many antiviral drugs are derivatives of nucleic acids, significant toxicities to uninfected cells can occur. Most toxicity involves bone marrow suppression with a loss of granulocytes, platelets, and erythrocytes. In many instances, systemic toxicities are so severe that the drug can only be administered topically. Several of the clinical problems are summarized in the Clinical Problems box.

Amantadine and rimantadine

The most common side effects of amantadine therapy are GI upsets and CNS side effects such as nervousness, insomnia, and headache. These develop within the first week of therapy and decrease with time, despite continued treatment. Side effects are reversible after discontinuation of the drug and are less frequent in patients receiving lower doses. Adverse effects occur in 5% to 33% of persons taking amantadine for influenza prophylaxis.

Amantadine also has anticholinergic properties that can cause urinary retention, ventricular arrhythmias, pupillary dilatation, and psychosis in some patients. The anticholinergic effects of amantadine are enhanced by antihistamines and anticholinergic drugs. Because its safety in pregnant and breast-feeding women is not established, caution should be exercised. Physostigmine given every 1 to 2 hours in adults may temporarily reverse serious neurological reactions. Rimantadine is better tolerated than amantadine.

Oseltamivir and zanamivir

Side effects of oseltamivir include nausea, vomiting, and diarrhea, which occur in about 15% of patients. Zanamivir is administered by a disk inhalation device, and patients need to be instructed about proper use of the inhaler. Absorption of parent medication is minimal, and side effects in persons without underlying lung disease are less than 5%. Patients with a history of bronchospasm or sensitive airways should not receive zanamivir.

Acyclovir

Acyclovir is well tolerated with few side effects. Because the pH of IV-administered acyclovir is 9 to 11, phlebitis is the most-common side effect, occurring in 15% of patients. Acyclovir is excreted renally, and crystalline nephropathy can occur. Transient elevated creatinine concentrations are more common in patients receiving rapid infusions, especially in those who are dehydrated. About 1% of patients experience CNS effects sometimes associated with significant confusion. If probenecid is co-administered with the acyclovir, this can reduce renal clearance and prolong serum half-life. Valacyclovir and famciclovir are also well tolerated.

Acyclovir has not shown increased teratogenicity in animal models, but mutagenicity has been observed at extremely high doses. Because its safety in pregnancy is unknown, acyclovir should be given only after its potential benefits and risks are carefully evaluated. To date no congenital syndromes have been identified in children of women who received acyclovir.

Ganciclovir

Most clinical experience with ganciclovir has been gained in the treatment of CMV retinitis in AIDS patients, in whom the most-common side effects are bone marrow suppression (up to 40%) and CNS abnormalities (up to 15%). Neutropenia and thrombocytopenia are the most-common manifestations of bone marrow suppression, usually observed in the second week of therapy. Effects are usually reversible, but significant infections during granulocytopenia can occur. Concurrent use of NRTIs increases bone marrow toxicity. About 33% of AIDS patients developed CNS or bone marrow toxicities significant enough to interrupt therapy. AIDS patients who have received long-term ganciclovir therapy have significant increases in their follicle-stimulating hormone, luteinizing hormone, and testosterone concentrations. Side effects of oral therapy are less frequent. Because of significant side effects, some patients with CMV retinitis receive intraocular ganciclovir implants. Ganciclovir has proved to be teratogenic and mutagenic in several different experimental systems.

Foscarnet

Foscarnet is a strongly anionic compound and can chelate divalent cations. This has resulted in hypocalcemia and hypomagnesemia in up to 20% of patients receiving the drug. Seizures and cardiac dysrhythmias may occur, presumably secondary to hypocalcemia. Foscarnet causes renal insufficiency, and dosages must be adjusted in patients with decreased creatinine clearance. Up to 30% of AIDS patients receiving foscarnet therapy for CMV retinitis have increases in their serum creatinine. Foscarnet is less myelosuppressive than ganciclovir.

Ribavirin

Aerosolized ribavirin is generally well tolerated, but bronchospasm may occur. In adults with chronic obstructive pulmonary disease and asthmatics receiving aerosol therapy, significant deterioration of pulmonary function has been reported. Ribavirin may be passively absorbed by employees working with patients treated with aerosols. Pregnant women should not be exposed to the aerosol. The primary toxicity of oral ribavirin is that of hemolytic anemia and dyspnea. This occurs in about 10% of recipients and often begins 1 to 2 weeks after starting therapy. Patients should have serial measurement of hemoglobin while on ribavirin. Ribavirin is teratogenic or embryolethal at doses that are 5% of the recommended human dose. It should never be started in women until a negative pregnancy test is obtained. Also, couples must use two effective forms of contraception while ribavirin is being given and for 6 months after the drug is discontinued.

Fusion inhibitors

The main side effect issue with enfuvirtide is reactions at the injection site and possible hypersensitivity reactions. Patients need to rotate injection sites to allow resolution of the problem. Analgesics are sometimes necessary. Hypersensitivity reactions have been rarely reported, but clinical experience with enfuvirtide has been limited to date. As the medication is more widely used, physicians need to be aware of the possibility of immune complex disease or acute hypersensitivity reactions, especially on reexposure to drug.

Nucleoside reverse transcriptase inhibitors and nucleotides

Side effects of NRTIs and nucleotides vary with clinical stage of HIV disease. Persons with CD4 counts above 200 generally tolerate these medications very well. The most-common side effects in this group are gastrointestinal upset, nausea, and headache. These effects occur in about 5% of patients and may decrease with time. Lamivudine is generally the best-tolerated NRTI. Patients with more-advanced HIV disease often experience more-frequent and more-significant side effects to NRTIs and nucleotides. Bone marrow suppression and granulocytopenia have developed in up to 50% of NRTI recipients whose initial absolute CD4 count was less than 100 cells/mm^3 but only 20% of recipients whose initial CD4 count was greater than that. Megaloblastic erythrocyte changes occur within 2 weeks in most patients on zidovudine therapy. Black nail pigmentation may occur during therapy but is more common in people of African descent. All NRTIs and nucleotides inhibit mitochondrial DNA formation. Severe lactic acidosis and hepatic steatosis may occur. NRTIs have also been associated with lipodystrophy. The teratogenicity and mutagenicity of NRTIs has not been completely evaluated; however, zidovudine use in pregnancy to date has not been associated with abnormal birth patterns.

Didanosine's major side effects are pancreatitis and peripheral neuropathy. Pancreatitis has been observed in 5 to 10% of all didanosine recipients. Peripheral neuropathy has been reported to occur in about 10 to 30% of patients on NRTIs and often improves upon discontinuation of the drug. Because didanosine is acid labile, stomach acid must be neutralized for proper absorption. In some situations buffer can interfere with the absorption of other medications. The main side effect of stavudine is peripheral neuropathy, which occurs in up to 20% of patients.

Non-nucleoside reverse transcriptase inhibitors

NNRTIs, although a single class of drugs, have widely varying side effects and treatment issues. One of the most significant side effects is rash. One third of patients taking nevirapine can develop significant rash, with life-threatening reactions occurring. Patients who experience the rash should not be rechallenged. Rash is less common in patients taking the other NRTIs. Efavirenz use can be associated with severe depression and sleep disturbances. A history of clinically significant depression is a relative contraindication for efavirenz use. Delavirdine appears to be the best-tolerated NNRTI. All NNRTIs can cause lipodystrophy.

Protease inhibitors

Protease inhibitors are primarily metabolized by the P450 system, and the metabolism of other drugs can be altered in patients taking them. Ritonavir has the greatest capacity for drug-drug interactions, although this may occur with any protease inhibitor. Patients on protease inhibitor therapy need their medications routinely reviewed to check for significant drug-drug reactions. Lipodystrophy is common with all protease inhibitors, and glucose intolerance, dyslipidemia, may also occur. Patients on protease inhibitors have an increased risk of myocardial infarctions. Indinavir may precipitate in renal tubules and create clinically significant kidney stones. Adequate hydration is required for patients receiving indinavir. Other common side effects for PIs include gastrointestinal upset and diarrhea.

Interferon

Systemic interferon use is associated with significant and frequent side effects. Common problems include severe malaise, myelosuppression, depression, and thyroid abnormalities. Patients on systemic interferon need to be closely monitored for signs of toxicity. Intralesional interferons produce pain at the injection site. Leukopenia, malaise, and fever also occur. The side effects are severe enough in about 10% to 20% of patients to warrant discontinuing therapy.

Immunoglobulins

Immunoglobulins are well tolerated, with pain at the injection site and brief low-grade fever the most commonly reported side effects. True allergic reactions with urticaria or angioedema rarely occur, but IV gamma globulin can activate the alternative complement pathway, producing an anaphylactoid reaction.

Others

Topical antivirals (idoxuridine, trifluorothymidine, trifluridine) are generally well tolerated. The most-common side effects include mild local irritation, headaches, and nausea. Some topical agents include glucocorticoids to lessen this inflammation. The most-common side effects of topical fluorouracil therapy are local pain, pruritus, and irritation. Contact dermatitis with scarring has also been reported.

New horizons

Available antiviral agents have significantly increased since 1995. Research has been accelerated in large part by the need for effective therapies against HIV. Our ability to find, test, and produce new antivirals has been aided by our ability to clone specific viral enzymes and use computer-aided drug design to map possible target sites. Much work still needs to be done to optimize antiviral therapy in both HIV and other chronic viral infections such as hepatitis. The utility of using mismatched RNA to inhibit viral growth is also being evaluated (see Chapter 5). Management of CMV infections in the immunocompromised patient continues to be problematic, and agents more effective against this infection are being sought.

TRADE NAMES

In addition to generic and fixed-combination preparations and the drugs listed in the Major Drugs box, the following trade-named materials are some of the important compounds available in the United States.

Delavirdine (Rescriptor)
Efavirenz (Sustiva)
Enfuvirtide (Fuzeon)
Famciclovir (Famvir)
Ganciclovir (Cytovene)
Immunoglobulins (H-Big, HyperHep, Hyperab, VZIG)
Interferon (Actimmune, IntronA, Alferon)
Lopinavir/ritonavir (Kaletra)
Oseltamivir (Tamiflu)
Rimantadine (Flumadine)
Saquinavir (Invirase)
Stavudine (Zerit)
Valacyclovir (Valtrex)

FURTHER READING

Collier AC, Coombs RW, Schoenfeld DA, et al. Treatment of human immunodeficiency virus infection with saquinavir, zidovudine, and zalcitabine. *N Engl J Med* 1996; 334:1011-1017.

Drugs for HIV Infection: Treatment guidelines. *Med Lett* 2004; 2:17.

Drugs for non-HIV viral infections. *Med Lett* 2002; 44:1123.

Self-assessment questions

1. Which of the following is not at least partly responsible for the increasing concentration of acyclovir in infected cells compared with uninfected cells?

a. Monophosphorylation of acyclovir by viral thymidine kinase
b. Triphosphorylation of acyclovir monophosphate by cellular kinases
c. Amination of acyclovir to the active compound by adenosine deaminase
d. Alterations in acyclovir that prevent the movement of activated drug extracellularly

2. Which of the following drugs does not require modification to become active?

a. Amantadine
b. Acyclovir
c. Ganciclovir
d. Zidovudine

3. Which of the following drugs is not an HIV reverse transcriptase inhibitor and a DNA chain terminator?

a. Zidovudine
b. Didanosine
c. Lamivudine
d. Nevirapine

4. Which of the following drugs has the greatest potential for drug-drug interactions?

a. Ritonavir
b. Stavudine
c. Zalcitabine
d. Saquinavir

5. Which of the following drugs is administered as treatment of chronic hepatitis C infection?

a. Amantadine
b. Interferon
c. Idoxuridine
d. Foscarnet

6. Immunoglobulins have been shown to be effective in modifying the following viral diseases *except:*

a. Rabies.
b. Hepatitis A.
c. Hepatitis B.
d. Condyloma acuminatum.

CHAPTER 52

Drugs to treat parasitic infections

Richard D. Pearson
Erik L. Hewlett

Major Drugs

Treatment of nematode infections

Albendazole (Albenza)
Pyrantel pamoate (Antiminth)
Diethylcarbamazine (Hetrazan)
Mebendazole (Vermox)
Ivermectin (Stromectol)

Treatment of cestode and trematode infections

Praziquantel (Biltricide)
Bithionol (Bitin)
Niclosamide (Yomesan)

Treatment of intestinal and vaginal protozoa

Diloxanide furoate (Furamide)
Furazolidone (Furoxone)
Iodoquinol (Yodoxin)
Metronidazole (Flagyl)
Tinidazole (Tindamax)
Nitazoxanide (Alinia)
Paromomycin (Humatin)

Treatment of malaria

Quinine
Chloroquine (Aralen)
Atovaquone and proguanil (Malarone)
Mefloquine (Lariam)
Primaquine
Doxycycline (Vibramycin)

Treatment of kinetoplastides

Amphotericin B (lipid associated)
Melarsoprol (Arsobal)
Pentamidine isethionate (Pentam 300)
Eflornithine (Ornidyl)
Nifurtimox (Lampit)
Stibogluconate sodium (Pentostam)

Treatment of systemic protozoal pathogens

Pentamidine isethionate (Pentam 300)
Pyrimethamine (Daraprim)
Sulfonamides
Trimethoprim-sulfamethoxazole (Bactrim, others)

Abbreviations

AIDS	acquired immunodeficiency syndrome
GI	gastrointestinal

Therapeutic overview

Parasitic infections are an important cause of morbidity throughout the world. Enteric parasites are prevalent in developing areas where sanitation and public health measures are poor. They intermittently cause epidemics in industrialized countries when they gain access to water or food supplies. An estimated 1.2 billion people, for example, are infected with *Ascaris lumbricoides* worldwide, and hookworms are the leading cause of iron deficiency anemia in many areas. Arthropod-borne parasites are endemic in the tropics. Malaria poses a major health problem for residents of many tropical areas and for international travelers. More than 1 million deaths are attributed annually to malaria in sub-Saharan Africa alone. *Trichomonas vaginalis* is a common cause of vaginitis. Of the Kinetoplastida, *Trypanosoma cruzi,* the cause of Chagas' disease, is endemic in Latin America; *Trypanosoma brucei gambiense* and *Trypanosoma brucei rhodesiense* cause sleeping sickness in Africa; and *Leishmania* species are present in widely scattered areas on every continent except Australia and Antarctica. *Toxoplasma gondii* is endemic worldwide. In industrialized countries parasitic diseases most commonly affect refugees, immigrants, military personnel, returning international travelers, and occasionally residents who have not traveled. Several protozoa have emerged as important opportunistic pathogens in patients with acquired immunodeficiency syndrome (AIDS).

THERAPEUTIC OVERVIEW

Prevention strategies

Control disease vectors or reduce contact with them
Improve hygiene and sanitation
Vaccine development
Drugs

Transmission of protozoal infection

Malaria—mosquitoes
Leishmaniasis—sand flies
African trypanosomiasis—tsetse flies
Chagas' disease—reduviid bugs
Amebiasis—food, water
Giardiasis—food, water
Toxoplasmosis—cats, undercooked meats

Classification of major parasitic groups

There are two major groups of parasites:

- Multicellular helminths (or worms)
- Single-celled protozoa.

Helminths

Helminths have sophisticated organ systems and many have complex life cycles. Clinical manifestations of helminthic diseases are usually proportionate to the worm burden. Infections with light worm burdens are often asymptomatic, whereas heavy worm burdens can result in life-threatening disease. Exceptions occur when one or more helminths gain access to a critical organ such as the brain or an eye, or when an adult worm migrates into and obstructs the common bile duct, such as with *A. lumbricoides*. Helminths have finite life spans. Infestations resolve over time, unless there is autoinfection as in the case of *Strongyloides stercoralis* or *Hymenolepis nana*, or the parasite has an extremely long life span as in the case of *Clonorchis sinensis*. Eosinophilia is common when helminths migrate through tissue but may be absent after intestinal helminths have reached maturity in the bowel lumen.

Morphologically, helminths are composed of nematodes (roundworms) and platyhelminths (flatworms). Some roundworm species reside as adults in the human GI tract, whereas others invade the body and migrate to specific organs. The platyhelminths include cestodes (tapeworms) and trematodes (flukes). Considering helminths in this manner is helpful clinically because species in these groups frequently have similar life cycles, metabolic pathways, and susceptibilities to anthelmintic (or antihelminthic) medications.

Nematodes Intestinal nematodes include *A. lumbricoides;* the hookworms, *Ancylostoma duodenale* and *Necator americanus; Trichuris trichiura; S. stercoralis;* and other species spread through feces. They are prevalent among persons living in conditions of poor hygiene. Such individuals, particularly children, are frequently infected with more than one species and often have high parasite burdens. *Enterobius vermicularis,* which is common in industrialized countries, is spread among children after the mature female worm migrates from the rectum and deposits ova in the perianal area.

A number of nematode species reside outside the GI tract. The filariae *Wuchereria bancrofti, Brugia malayi,* and *Loa loa,* are transmitted by mosquitoes, and *Onchocerca volvulus* is transmitted by black flies. Acute infections with *W. bancrofti* or *B. malayi* may be associated with lymphangitis, epididymitis, and fever. Chronic infections result in elephantiasis among residents of endemic areas. Adult *O. volvulus* produce microfilariae that cause inflammation in the skin and eyes. Other filariae that cause human disease include *L. loa* and *M. perstans.* Animal ascarids such as *Toxocara* species can produce visceral larva migrans, and animal hookworm species cause cutaneous larva migrans.

Platyhelminths The cestodes, or tapeworms, live as adults in the GI tract of their definitive hosts and in cystic forms in organs of their intermediate hosts. Humans infected with *Taenia saginata,* the beef tapeworm; *Taenia solium,* the pork tapeworm; and *Diphyllobothrium latum,* the fish tapeworm, have ingested inadequately cooked infected meat or fish. With the exception of *D. latum,* which can compete with its host for vitamin B_{12} and on rare occasions results in symptomatic vitamin B_{12} deficiency, patients with adult tapeworms are asymptomatic or experience mild symptoms. Ova and proglottids are excreted in human feces.

Trematodes, or flukes, have complex life cycles involving snails. In the case of *Schistosoma* species, cercariae are released from snails into fresh water and enter humans through direct penetration of the skin after contact with infested fresh water. *Schistosoma mansoni, Schistosoma japonicum,* and *Schistosoma mekongi* undergo further development and reside as adults in venules of the GI tract, producing disease in the intestine and liver, whereas *Schistosoma haematobium* resides in venules of the urinary tract, resulting in damage to the ureters and bladder. Other trematode species encyst in secondary intermediate hosts such as fish or freshwater crustaceans, or on water plants. After they are ingested, trematodes excyst and develop in specific organs. Adult *Paragonimus westermani* reside in the lungs; *C. sinensis, Opisthorchis viverrini,* and *Fasciola hepatica* exist in the liver; and *Fasciolopsis buski, Heterophyes heterophyes, Metagonimus yokogawai,* and *Nanophyetus salmincola* are found in the intestine.

Protozoa

Protozoa are composed of a single cell and can multiply in their human hosts. Theoretically, infection with only one cell can result in overwhelming disease. Protozoal species differ widely in their sensitivity to antiparasitic drugs as summarized in the Major Drugs box.

Enteric pathogens are spread in fecally contaminated food and water. *T. vaginalis* is spread by intimate personal contact. In contrast, *Plasmodium* species, which cause malaria, are transmitted by anopheline mosquitoes, whose life cycle is depicted in Figure 52-1. Sporozoites are inoculated when an infected female attempts to take a blood meal, travel to the liver through the circulation, invade hepatocytes, and develop within liver cells in 1 to 3 weeks. The erythrocytic stage, which is the only symptomatic stage, begins when merozoites are released from the liver and invade red blood cells. *Plasmodium vivax* and *Plasmodium ovale,* in contrast, can persist for months in the liver as hypnozoites before completing development and initiating symptomatic malaria.

The Kinetoplastida also are transmitted by arthropod vectors; *T. cruzi* by reduviid bugs that live in adobe dwellings in Latin America; *T. brucei gambiense* and *T. brucei rhodesiense* by tsetse flies in Africa; and *Leishmania* species by sand flies. They contain a unique mitochondrial structure, the kinetoplast.

Other diverse protozoa also produce human disease. *T. gondii* is spread in the feces of infected cats and in inadequately cooked, contaminated meat. Infection is often asymptomatic but can cause a mononucleosis-like syndrome; in utero infection resulting in birth defects or chorioretinitis; or encephalitis, particularly in persons with AIDS or other immune defects. Based on conserved structural proteins, *Pneumocystis jiroveci* is more closely related to fungi than protozoa, but its treatment is discussed here. The infection is ubiquitous and apparently spread by inhalation. *P. jiroveci* has emerged as an important cause of pneumonitis in persons with AIDS and occurs occasionally in others with abnormal T-cell mediated immunity.

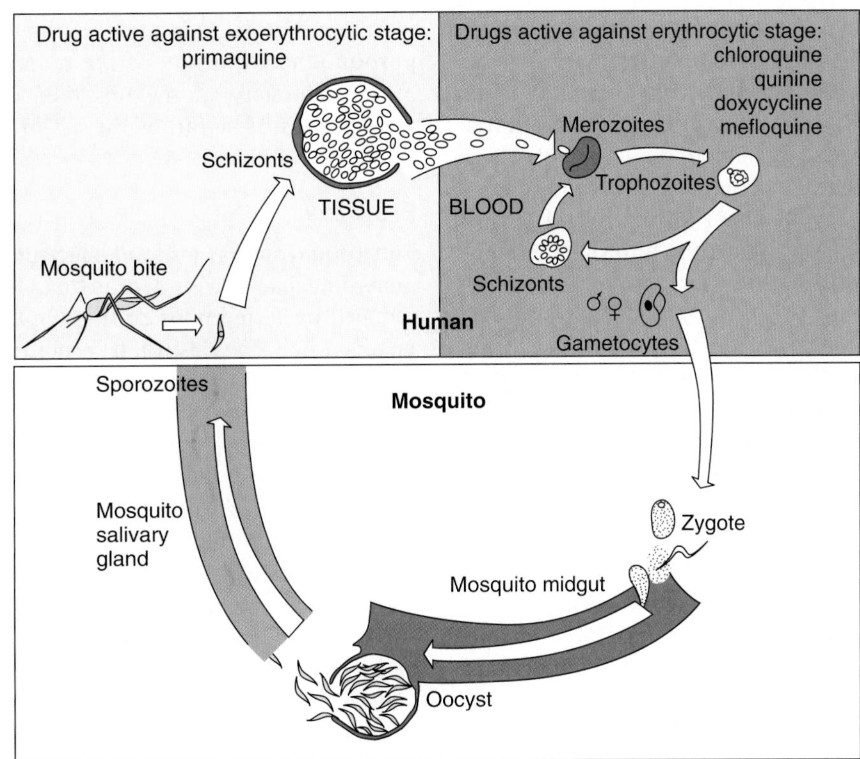

Figure 52-1 The life cycle of *Plasmodium* species. Drugs used to treat infections are effective against erythrocytic or exoerythrocytic stages of the parasite.

Mechanisms of action

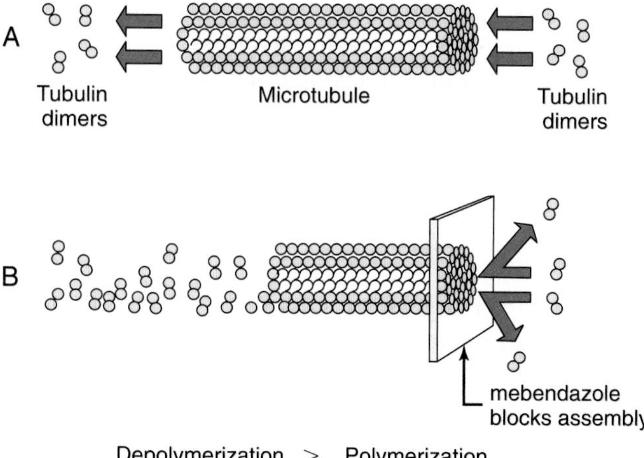

Figure 52-2 **A,** Under normal conditions, tubulin dimers are continually being polymerized and depolymerized from the ends of the microtubule. **B,** Albendazole and mebendazole can bind to β-tubulin and prevent polymerization, resulting in breakdown of microtubules.

Helminths

Albendazole sulfoxide, the primary metabolite of albendazole, and **mebendazole** bind to β-tubulin in susceptible nematodes and inhibit microtubule assembly, leading to disruption of microtubules and selective and irreversible inhibition of glucose uptake (Fig. 52-2). This results in depletion of the parasite's glycogen stores, reduced formation of adenosine triphosphate, disruption of metabolic pathways and, ultimately parasitic death. Serum glucose concentrations are not affected in the human host.

Pyrantel pamoate, which is also active against several intestinal nematodes, acts as an agonist at nicotinic cholinergic receptors. Muscles of susceptible nematodes undergo depolarization and an increase in spike discharge frequency, leading to a short period of calcium-dependent stimulation, resulting in irreversible paralysis. Pyrantel pamoate is also an acetylcholinesterase inhibitor. Affected helminths are unable to maintain their attachment in the intestinal lumen and are expelled from the body in the feces. Piperazine, an antihelminthic drug used to treat *A. lumbricoides,* paralyzes worms by hyperpolarization and is therefore a mutual antagonist of pyrantel pamoate; the two drugs should not be administered concurrently.

Diethylcarbamazine is a piperazine derivative. The basis for its activity is uncertain, although microfilaria are paralyzed, perhaps by hyperpolarizing of their musculature. Diethylcarbamazine also alters the microfilarial surface and may facilitate killing by the host's immune responses. It also affects the parasite's arachidonic acid metabolism and disrupts microtubule formation.

Ivermectin is a macrocyclic lactone produced by *Streptomyces avermitilis.* It activates the opening of voltage-gated chloride channels that are found only in helminths and arthropods. The result is an influx of chloride ions and paralysis of the pharyngeal pumping motion in helminths.

Praziquantel is a heterocyclic pyrazine-isoquinoline derivative. It is rapidly taken up by tapeworms and flukes, but its precise mechanism of action is not known. Studies of the tapeworm *Hymenolepis diminuta* indicate that praziquantel releases calcium from endogenous stores, resulting in contraction and subsequent expulsion of the worm from the GI tract. In the schistosomes, praziquantel damages the tegument, causing intense vacuolation, exposure of sequestered schistosomal antigens, and increased permeability to calcium, causing tetanic contraction and paralysis. Adult schistosomes are then swept back through the portal circulation to the liver, where they are destroyed by phagocytes. Figure 52-3 depicts the marked alterations in the schistosomal surface after drug exposure.

Niclosamide appears to uncouple oxidative phosphorylation in adult cestodes. The result is death of the worm, partial disintegration of the scolex and proximal portion, and expulsion of the remainder in the feces.

A summary of the observed effects and possible mechanisms of action of the major antihelmintic drugs is found in Table 52-1.

Protozoa

Metronidazole has a broad spectrum of activity against anaerobic bacteria and protozoa. It is activated when reduced by ferredoxins or their equivalents in protozoa or bacteria. The resultant products react with DNA and other intracellular parasite constituents, causing damage and death. **Tinidazole** has a similar mechanism of action. **Paromomycin,** an aminoglycoside antibiotic (see Chapter 46), inhibits protein synthesis. **Iodoquinol** acts against *E. histolytica* cysts and, to a lesser extent, trophozoites by an unknown mechanism. **Diloxanide furoate** is directly amebicidal, and little is known about its mechanism of action also. **Nitazoxanide** has a broad spectrum of activity against protozoa and helminths and was recently approved for giardiasis and cryptosporidiosis. The mechanism involves inhibition of electron transport reactions essential to metabolism of anaerobic organisms. **Furazolidone** interferes with several bacterial enzyme systems, but its mechanism of action against *G. lamblia* is uncertain.

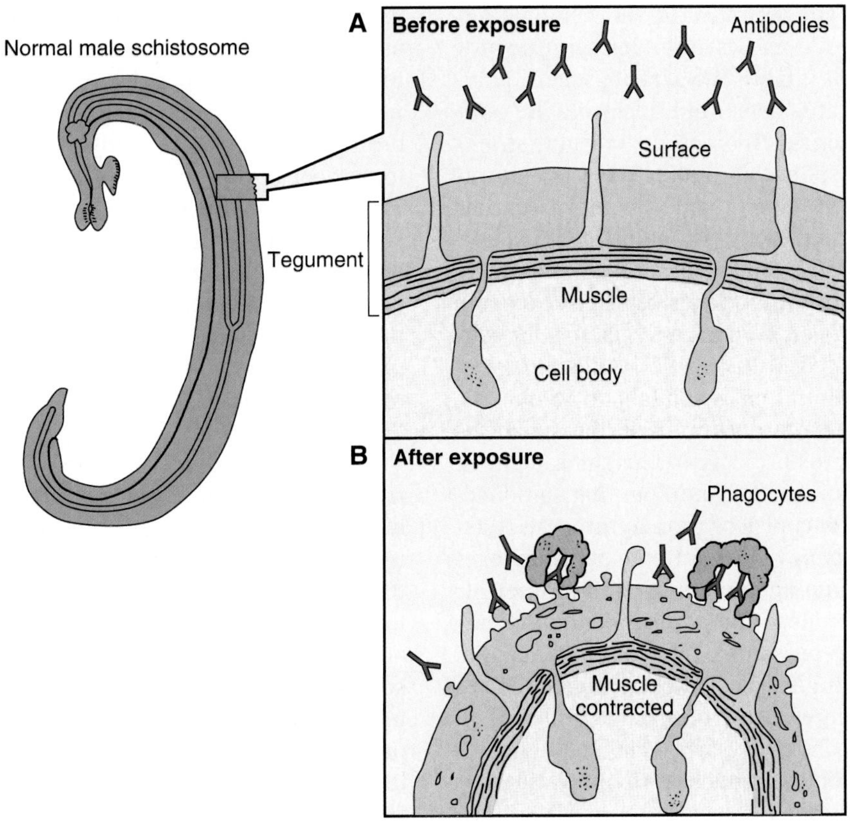

Figure 52-3 Before exposure to praziquantel, the schistosome is capable of avoiding antibodies directed toward surface and internally located antigens. **A,** Cross-section of the surface of a normal schistosome. After exposure to praziquantel, the muscles of the schistosome contract because of drug-induced influx of Ca^{2+}. **B,** Changes in the schistosome tegument include small holes and balloonlike structures and exposure of hidden parasite antigens, resulting in the binding of antibodies and phagocytes.

Table 52-1 Observed effects and possible mechanisms of action of the major anthelmintic drugs

Drug	Observed Effects on Helminths	Possible Mechanism of Action
Albendazole	Inhibition of glucose transport; depletion of glycogen stores, inhibition of fumarate reductase	Binding to β-tubulin, prevents microtubule polymerization
Mebendazole	Inhibition of glucose transport; depletion of glycogen stores	Binding to β-tubulin
Pyrantel pamoate	Muscles depolarize, increased spike wave activity, spastic paralysis	Depolarizing neuromuscular blockade
Diethylcarbamazine	Hyperpolarization and paralysis of worm's musculature; exposure of antigens, leading to antibody binding and attack by phagocytes	Hyperpolarization and neuromuscular blockade
Ivermectin	Alters chloride currents, resulting in death of microfilariae	Altered chloride channel function
Praziquantel	Depolarization of muscles, increased intracellular calcium, displacement of schistosomes to the human liver, exposure of surface antigens, binding by antibody and phagocytes, tegument disruption	Uncertain
Niclosamide	Uncouples phosphorylation; may inhibit anaerobic metabolism	Uncertain

Chloroquine is concentrated in the hemoglobin-containing digestive vesicles of intraerythrocytic *Plasmodium* species. It inhibits the parasite's heme polymerase that incorporates heme into an insoluble, nontoxic crystalline material. Chloroquine-resistant strains of *P. falciparum* transport chloroquine out of the intraparasitic compartment more rapidly than susceptible strains. **Primaquine** has activity against the exoerythrocytic stage of *P. vivax* and *P. ovale,* and may interfere with electron transport or generate reactive oxygen species. **Quinine** has been used to treat malaria for centuries. It is concentrated in the acidic food vacuoles of intracellular plasmodium and is thought to inhibit the activity of heme polymerase. **Quinidine,** the stereoisomer of quinine, presumably acts in the same manner. **Mefloquine** is an analog of quinine that produces swelling in the food vacuoles of intraerythrocytic plasmodium. Mefloquine may also form toxic complexes with heme. **Atovaquone-proguanil (Malarone)** is formulated as a fixed dose for prophylaxis and treatment of chloroquine-resistant *P. falciparum* malaria. Proguanil acts synergistically with atovaquone to inhibit mitochondrial electron transport, resulting in collapse of the mitochondrial membrane potential. It also inhibits dihydrofolate reductase-thymidylate synthase in *Plasmodium* ssp.

Atovaquone has activity against *Plasmodium* spp., *Babesia* spp., *P. jiroveci* and *T. gondii.* It selectively inhibits electron transport, resulting in collapse of the mitochondrial membrane potential. It also inhibits pyrimidine biosynthesis, which is obligatorily coupled to electron transport in *Plasmodium* spp. **Pyrimethamine** binds to and irreversibly inhibits dihydrofolate reductase. It is approximately 1000-fold more active against plasmodium dihydrofolate reductase-thymidylate synthetase than against human dihydrofolate reductase. Pyrimethamine is often used with one of the sulfonamides to inhibit sequential steps in folate metabolism. **Trimethoprim** inhibits the dihydrofolate reductase of many bacteria and some protozoa and is frequently administered with **sulfamethoxazole** (see Chapter 47). **Proguanil** is metabolized to an active cyclic triazine metabolite that selectively inhibits plasmodium dihydrofolate reductase-thymidylate synthetase. **Nifurtimox** undergoes partial reduction followed by autooxidation, forming superoxide anion, hydrogen peroxide, and hydroxyl radicals that damage cell membranes and DNA. **Eflornithine** is an irreversible inhibitor of ornithine decarboxylase, the enzyme that catalyzes the rate-limiting step in polyamine synthesis. Although polyamines are essential for growth and differentiation of all cells, eflornithine has clinical activity only against *T. brucei gambiense.*

Pentamidine isethionate also has an unknown mechanism of action but may interfere with polyamine biosynthesis and inhibit topoisomerase II. **Melarsoprol** is an arsenical and reacts with sulfhydryl groups on proteins and inhibits many enzymes, including trypanothione. *T. brucei rhodesiense* and *T. brucei gambiense* have an unusual purine transporter that concentrates melarsoprol in the organisms. **Sodium stibogluconate** and **meglumine antimonate** are dosed on the basis of their pentavalent antimony content. They appear to affect bioenergetics in leishmania, inhibiting glycolysis and fatty acid β-oxidation.

A number of the antibiotics discussed in previous chapters have activity against some protozoa. Tetracycline, doxycycline, and clindamycin inhibit protein synthesis, and sulfonamides inhibit dihydropteroate synthetase and para-aminobenzoic acid binding to it. Amphotericin B is thought to act on leishmania as it does on susceptible fungi by disrupting membranes (see Chapter 50). In addition, liposomal and lipid-associated amphotericin is selectively targeted to macrophages, the cells in which this parasite resides.

A summary of the possible mechanisms of action of the major antiprotozoal drugs is found in Table 52-2.

Table 52-2 Possible mechanisms of action of major antiprotozoal drugs

Drug	Possible Mechanism of Action
Metronidazole	Activated when reduced by ferredoxins, reacts with DNA and other parasite constituents
Paromomycin	Inhibits protein synthesis
Nitazoxanide	Inhibition of electron transfer reactions essential to the metabolism of anaerobic organisms
Chloroquine	Concentrated in hemoglobin-containing digestive vesicles, inhibits heme polymerase
Quinine	Concentrated in food vacuoles, probably inhibits heme polymerase
Mefloquine	Concentrated in food vacuoles, may form toxic complexes with heme
Pyrimethamine	Inhibits dihydrofolate reductase
Sulfonamides	Inhibit binding of *p*-aminobenzoic acid to dihydropteroate synthetase
Nifurtimox	Forms reactive oxygen species that damage cell membranes and DNA
Eflornithine	Irreversibly inhibits ornithine decarboxylase, inhibits polyamine synthesis
Melarsoprol	Reacts with sulfhydryl groups, inhibits proteins

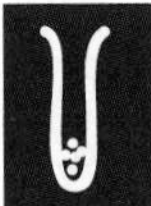

Pharmacokinetics

Pharmacokinetic parameters for selected antiparasitic drugs are listed in Table 52-3.

Helminths

Albendazole is easily absorbed when taken with a fatty meal. It undergoes extensive first-pass metabolism, and only albendazole sulfoxide, which is responsible for systemic anthelmintic activity, is detectable in the serum. Sulfoxidation also occurs in the intestinal tract, and there is evidence of hepatobiliary recirculation. Albendazole sulfoxide reaches peak serum concentrations in 2 to 3 hours. CNS concentrations are 40% of those in serum; concurrent administration of dexamethasone increases the serum concentration by about half, which is advantageous for treatment of neurocysticercosis. The concentration of albendazole sulfoxide in echinococcal cysts is approximately 25% of that in serum. Elimination of albendazole and its metabolites is accomplished primarily by renal excretion. **Mebendazole** is only slightly soluble in water and is poorly absorbed from the GI tract. These properties contribute to its low incidence of side effects but limit its effectiveness against tissue-dwelling helminths. Peak serum concentrations occur in 2 to 5 hours. Up to 10% of an orally administered dose is absorbed, metabolized, and excreted in the urine within 48 hours; the remainder is excreted unchanged in the feces. **Pyrantel pamoate** is poorly absorbed and therefore acts effectively in the lumen of the bowel. The bulk of the drug is found in the feces. **Diethylcarbamazine** is well absorbed after oral ingestion and reaches peak serum concentrations in 1 to 2 hours. It is primarily excreted in the urine, unchanged or as a metabolite. **Ivermectin** is rapidly absorbed after oral ingestion and reaches a serum peak after 4 to 5 hours. It is highly protein bound and has a half-life of 12 hours. It is eliminated by biliary excretion with enterohepatic circulation and tends to accumulate in adipose and hepatic tissues. **Praziquantel** is well absorbed orally and reaches peak serum concentrations in 1 to 3 hours. There is extensive first-pass metabolism, generating metabolites that are inactive and excreted primarily in the urine. Concentration of praziquantel in cerebrospinal fluid is 15% to 20% of that of the serum. Serum concentrations of praziquantel are increased in patients with moderate to severe liver impairment. **Niclosamide** is poorly absorbed and therefore selectively active against susceptible helminths in the lumen of the GI tract. It is ineffective in treating systemic infections.

Table 52-3 Pharmacokinetic parameters of selected antiparasitic drugs

Drug	Administration	Absorption	Half-Life	Disposition
HELMINTHS				
Albendazole	Oral	Good with fatty meal; poorly soluble in water	Extensive first-pass metabolism to sulfoxide, 8-9 hrs	M, R
Mebendazole	Oral	Poor (5%-10%)	2.5-5.5 hrs	F
Pyrantel pamoate	Oral	Very little	—	F
Diethylcarbamazine	Oral	Good	8 hrs	M, R
Ivermectin	Oral	Good	12 hrs	R
Praziquantel	Oral	Good	0.8-1.5 hrs	M
Niclosamide	Oral	Very little	—	F
PROTOZOA				
Metronidazole	Oral, IV	Good	8 hrs	M, R
Paromomycin	Oral	Poor		R
Furazolidone	Oral (liquid)	Good		M, R
Nitazoxanide	Oral (liquid)	Good		M (active)
Chloroquine	Oral	Good	4 days	R, M
Mefloquine	Oral	Good	6-23 days	M
Primaquine	Oral	Good	24 hrs (major metabolite)	M
Pyrimethamine	Oral	Good	3-4 days	R
Quinine	Oral, IV	Good	16-18 hrs	M, R
Atovaquone/proguanil	Oral	Adequate/good	12-60 hrs	R
Eflornithine	Oral, IV	Good	3-4 hrs	R
Pentamidine	IV or IM	—	IV 6 hrs, IM 9-13 hrs	R
Sodium stibogluconate	IM or IV	—	Variable	R

M, Metabolized; *R*, renal excretion; *F*, fecal; *IV*, intravenous; *IM*, intramuscular.

Protozoa

Metronidazole is rapidly and completely absorbed after oral administration and reaches peak plasma concentrations in 1 hour. More than half is metabolized in the liver, and the parent drug and metabolites are excreted in the urine. **Paromomycin** is poorly absorbed after oral administration and achieves high concentrations in the intestine. **Iodoquinol** is variably absorbed after oral administration. **Diloxanide furoate** is hydrolyzed in the intestine and well absorbed. Up to 90% of an oral dose is excreted in the urine within 24 hours. **Nitazoxanide** is well absorbed orally and rapidly hydrolyzed to its active metabolite, tizoxanide, which undergoes conjugation to glucuronide. Maximal concentrations of these two metabolites are found within to 1 to 4 hours. Tizoxanide is highly protein bound and is excreted in urine, bile, and feces, while the glucuronide is excreted in urine and bile. **Furazolidone** is well absorbed after oral administration and extensively metabolized, and more than 60% is excreted in the urine.

Chloroquine phosphate is well absorbed when taken orally, with peak serum concentrations reached in 3.5 hours. It is eliminated slowly after treatment is terminated. Approximately 50% of the drug is excreted unchanged in the urine, and the rest is metabolized in the liver. **Primaquine phosphate** is well absorbed after oral administration, and peak plasma concentrations occur in 3 hours. The drug is rapidly metabolized. **Quinine sulfate** is rapidly absorbed after oral administration and reaches peak serum concentrations in 3 hours. Quinine is metabolized in the liver. **Quinidine gluconate** is administered intravenously to patients with acute malaria who are unable to take oral medications. **Mefloquine** is slowly and incompletely absorbed after oral administration with peak serum concentrations after 7 to 24 hours. The drug is highly protein bound with a long half-life. **Pyrimethamine** is absorbed slowly but completely after oral administration, with a time to peak plasma concentration of 4 to 6 hours. It is eliminated through the kidney. **Proguanil** is slowly but well absorbed after oral administration, with peak serum levels reached in 5 hours and an elimination half-life of 12 to 21 hours. The concentration in erythrocytes is approximately 6 times that in plasma. **Atovaquone** is highly lipophilic, and administration with food enhances absorption by two-fold. Plasma concentrations do not correlate with dose, and it is highly protein bound with a half-life exceeding 60 hours. This is due to enterohepatic recycling with eventual fecal elimination. There is little excretion in urine. **Atovaquone-proguanil (Malarone)** combinations have pharmacokinetics as described for the individual drugs.

Nifurtimox is well absorbed when taken orally, with a peak serum concentration observed in about 3.5 hours. It is rapidly metabolized. **Eflornithine** can be administered orally or intravenously. Peak plasma concentrations are reached approximately 4 hours after oral administration. It is widely distributed in the body, including the CNS, with the bulk of drug excreted in the urine. **Pentamidine isethionate** is administered intramuscularly or intravenously and has a plasma half-life of about 6 hours and a terminal elimination phase of approximately 12 days. It accumulates in tissue and is only slowly eliminated by the kidney. **Melarsoprol** is administered intravenously, and a small but therapeutically significant amount enters the CNS. It is rapidly excreted in the feces. **Sodium stibogluconate** and **meglumine antimonate** are administered intramuscularly or intravenously daily for a period of 3 to 4 weeks. They have biphasic kinetics, with a short first-phase half-life of 2 hours and a second-phase half-life of 1 to 3 days. Most is excreted in the urine.

Doxycycline, tetracycline, ciprofloxacin, and sulfonamides are well absorbed when taken orally. Their pharmacokinetics are discussed in detail in Chapters 46 and 47. Amphotericin B is discussed in Chapter 50.

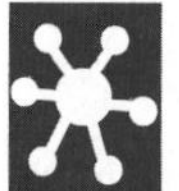

Relation of mechanisms of action to clinical response

Helminths

Albendazole and **mebendazole** are active against the common intestinal nematodes—*A. lumbricoides,* the hookworms, *T. trichiura,* and *E. vermicularis.* The advantage of albendazole is that it can be administered as a single dose for these helminths, whereas mebendazole is given twice daily for 3 days. In persons with heavy *T. trichiura* infection, albendazole is administered daily for 3 days. Single-dose albendazole has been used successfully in mass treatment programs in developing areas, resulting in enhanced growth and development of children infected with intestinal helminths, but treatment must be repeated at intervals of approximately 4 months because of re-infection. Albendazole can be used to treat cutaneous larva migrans.

Mebendazole is recommended for patients with *Trichinella spiralis, Trichostrongylus* species, and *Capillaria philippinensis.* Albendazole may be effective for these infections, but clinical experience is limited. Steroids are administered concurrently to patients with trichinosis who experience severe symptoms. Neither single-dose albendazole nor mebendazole is reliably effective against *S. stercoralis*, but albendazole twice a day for 2 or more days can be used. Thiabendazole, a related benzimidazole, was the treatment of choice. Recent studies indicate that ivermectin is equally effective and better tolerated, and it is now the treatment of choice. Thiabendazole is no longer available in the United States.

Albendazole and praziquantel are recommended for the treatment of neurocysticercosis caused by the larvae of *T. solium*. Albendazole alone, with percutaneous aspiration and installation of a scolicidal agent followed by re-aspiration or with surgical resection, is used for patients with echinococcosis.

Pyrantel pamoate is effective for treatment of *E. vermicularis* and *Trichostrongylus* species. It also has activity against hookworms and *A. lumbricoides*.

Diethylcarbamazine has long been recommended for treatment of *W. bancrofti, B. malayi, L. loa,* and tropical pulmonary eosinophilia. Acute allergic reactions after release of microfilarial antigens, especially severe and including life-threatening encephalopathy in heavy *L. loa* infection, can be reduced by use of antihistamines or corticosteroids. Reactions to released microfilorid antigens are often severe in patients with onchocerciasis treated with this drug; therefore ivermectin is the drug of choice.

Ivermectin has an expanding spectrum of clinical applications in humans. Although widely used for veterinary parasitic diseases, currently its use in humans is in treatment of onchocerciasis and strongyloidiasis. Ivermectin is recommended for *Onchocerca volvulus,* which causes river blindness, because in killing the microfilariae in the skin and eye it elicits a less-severe inflammatory response than does diethylcarbamazine. Because ivermectin appears to have no effect on the viability or fecundity of adult worms, the patient may require additional treatment at 6- to 12-month intervals. Ivermectin can also be used to treat cutaneous larva migrans.

Praziquantel is active against all *Schistosoma* species and all but one of the human flukes, *F. hepatica,* for which treatment with triclabendazole or bithionol is effective. Both praziquantel and niclosamide are effective against adult *T. saginata, T. solium, D. latum,* and *H. nana* in the human GI tract. Praziquantel is preferable for the treatment of *T. solium* because it is active against larvae and adults and may prevent internal autoinfection, a theoretical possibility after niclosamide treatment. In the case of *H. nana,* praziquantel is effective as a single dose because it kills cysticerci in the wall of the intestine and kills adult worms, whereas niclosamide kills only adult worms and must be administered for 7 days.

In most cases the chemotherapy of helminthic infections is effective and reasonably well tolerated. Drug resistance among the helminths has been reported but is infrequent. Some anthelmintics are available through pharmacies in the United States, whereas others must be obtained from the manufacturer or the Drug Service at the Centers for Disease Control and Prevention in Atlanta, Georgia. A number of other anthelmintic compounds, which are more toxic or less effective, can be obtained abroad.

Protozoa

Intestinal and vaginal protozoa *G. lamblia, E. histolytica* (major causes of diarrhea), and *T. vaginalis* live in anaerobic environments and are susceptible to **metronidazole** and **tinidazole**. Because these drugs are effective against *E. histolytica* trophozoites but do not eradicate cysts, a second "luminal" agent—such as **paromomycin, iodoquinol,** or **diloxanide furoate**—is administered concomitantly in the treatment of persons with symptomatic amebic infections. A luminal agent is used alone for the treatment of asymptomatic *E. histolytica* infection. **Furazolidone** or **nitazoxanide** are available in liquid formulations and often used for the treatment of giardiasis in children.

Two other enteric protozoal pathogens, *Cyclospora* species and *Isospora belli,* are susceptible to **trimethoprim-sulfamethoxazole.** *Cryptosporidium* infections are usually self-limiting in immunocompetent persons but may be persistent and severe in those with AIDS. Treatment with **nitazoxanide** has been of benefit in immunocompetent patients with cryptosporidiosis and has been approved for use in children.

Prevention and treatment of malaria Efforts to prevent malaria focus on minimizing mosquito contact and the use of chemoprophylaxis as discussed in the Therapeutic Overview section. Persons traveling to areas where *Plasmodium* species remain chloroquine sensitive should take **chloroquine** weekly, and people with intense or prolonged exposure to *P. vivax* or *P. ovale* should receive a course of **primaquine** after leaving the endemic area. For travelers to chloroquine-resistant areas, there are three choices of comparable efficacy: **doxycycline, Malarone,** and **mefloquine.** Doxycycline is least expensive but can cause untoward effects. It is administered daily starting 2 days prior to travel and continued for 4 weeks after exposure to kill parasites released into the blood after completing their incubation in the liver. Malarone is the most expensive but also the best tolerated. It is also administered 2 days before travel and for 1 week after leaving the endemic area. Mefloquine has the advantage of being used weekly but has neuropsychiatric effects in some individuals. It is started 1 to 2 weeks before departure and continued for 4 weeks after leaving the endemic area. Recent data suggest that primaquine taken daily can be used for prophylaxis, but recipients must be screened to ensure that they are not G6PD deficient. Neither doxycycline, Malarone, or primaquine can be used during pregnancy.

Chloroquine is recommended for treatment of acute infections with *P. ovale, Plasmodium malariae,* and chloroquine-sensitive strains of *P. vivax* and *P. falciparum*. Primaquine is administered to patients with *P. vivax* and *P. ovale* to prevent relapses. Oral **Malarone** or **quinine** plus **doxycycline** or **tetracycline** is used for treatment of chloroquine-resistant *P. falciparum* malaria. Clindamycin is used in place of doxycycline with quinine in children or pregnant women. Mefloquine used at full treatment doses is effective but has frequent side effects. **Halofantrine** is used in Europe and Africa to treat persons with chloroquine-resistant *P. falciparum,* but it has potentially serious side effects, including sudden death.

The recommendations for prophylaxis and treatment of malaria are reviewed regularly and are available from the Centers for Disease Control and Prevention (www.cdc.gov/travel) and in The Medical Letter on Drugs and Therapeutics (www.medicalletter.org).

Kinetoplastida The drug currently recommended for the treatment of Chagas' disease, **nifurtimox**, is administrated over long periods of time and has substantial toxicity. Benznidazole is used in Latin America. They are not effective in patients with chronic chagasic cardiomyopathy, megaesophagus, or megacolon. **Pentamidine isethionate** is used for treatment of patients with the hemolymphatic stage of *T. brucei gambiense,* and suramin is used for *T. brucei rhodesiense.* **Melarsoprol** is used in patients with CNS disease but is highly toxic. **Eflornithine,** also known as the resurrection drug, is effective for the treatment of *T. brucei gambiense* in both the hemolymphatic and later CNS stages of infection, but supplies are very limited. Liposomal **amphotericin** B is the only drug approved for treatment of visceral leishmaniasis in the United States. The pentavalent antimonials **sodium stibogluconate,** and **meglumine antimoniate** have historically been used for treatment of visceral and cutaneous leishmaniasis around the world, but resistance is increasing. **Miltefosine,** an orally administered drug, is now considered the treatment of choice for visceral leishmaniasis in India. Amphotericin B deoxycholate and pentamidine isethionate are more-toxic alternatives for leishmaniasis.

Other protozoal diseases Treatment of symptomatic toxoplasmosis consists of pyrimethamine and a short-acting sulfonamide, such as sulfadiazine. **Leucovorin** is administered concurrently to prevent bone marrow suppression. The combination of pyrimethamine and clindamycin is also effective and frequently used in patients with AIDS. The macrolide **spiramycin** has been used to treat women infected with *T. gondii* during pregnancy.

The drug of choice for *P. jerovici* is **trimethoprim-sulfamethoxazole.** There is, however, a very high incidence of adverse reactions to sulfonamides in patients with AIDS, and it is often necessary to use alternatives, such as pentamidine isethionate, trimethoprim plus dapsone, atovaquone, or primaquine plus clindamycin. Prophylactic administration of trimethoprim-sulfamethoxazole, dapsone, atovaquone, or pentamidine aerosol is effective in reducing recurrences and preventing disease in AIDS patients with low $CD4^+$ counts.

Side effects, clinical problems, and toxicity

Helminths

Albendazole is usually well tolerated when given as a single dose for treatment of intestinal helminthic infections. Diarrhea, abdominal discomfort, and drug-elicited migration of *A. lumbricoides* occur in a few cases. High-dose, prolonged therapy for echinococcal infections is occasionally complicated by alopecia, hepatocellular injury, or reversible bone marrow suppression. **Mebendazole** is well tolerated when used to treat intestinal nematodes. When administered at high doses for prolonged periods as in the treatment of echinococcal liver cysts, it can produce alopecia, dizziness, transient bone marrow suppression with neutropenia, and hepatocellular injury. **Pyrantel pamoate** has minimal toxicity at the recommended dose. **Diethylcarbamazine** may cause headache, malaise, dizziness, nausea, and vomiting. Acute psychotic events have been reported. Of greater concern is the Mazzotti reaction, resulting from lysis of *O. volvulus* microfilariae and release of their antigens. The manifestations can include pruritus, fever, wheezing, tachycardia, and hypotension. For these reasons, ivermectin is the drug of choice for persons with onchocerciasis. Ocular sequelae include chorioretinitis and uveitis. Encephalopathy has been noted in patients with heavy *L. loa* infections treated with ivermectin or diethylcarbamazine. In patients with *W. bancrofti* or *B. malayi,* localized swelling or nodules can develop along lymphatics, and transient lymphedema or a hydrocele may be observed after diethylcarbamazine treatment. **Ivermectin** is generally well tolerated but on occasion may also trigger an inflammatory or Mazzotti-type reaction, resulting from the release of onchocercal antigens. Toxicity may include fever, pruritus, tender lymph nodes, headache, and arthralgias. Hypotension has been reported on rare occasions. **Praziquantel** is frequently also associated with side effects such as dizziness, headache, lassitude, nausea, vomiting, and abdominal pain, but side effects are usually mild and transient. Allergic reactions can occur and are usually attributed to release of worm antigens. Urticarial reactions have been associated with the treatment of *P. westermani*. Increased intracranial pressure has been observed among some patients treated for neurocysticercosis. Praziquantel and albendazole are contraindicated in persons with ocular cysticercosis or cysticerci in the spinal cord because destruction of the cysticercus can result in irreparable inflammatory damage. **Niclosamide** is well tolerated except for occasional side effects of dizziness, lightheadedness, abdominal pain, loss of appetite, diarrhea, and nausea.

Protozoa

Metronidazole administration is commonly associated with GI complaints such as nausea, vomiting, diarrhea, and a metallic taste. Neurotoxicity including dizziness, vertigo, and numbness is rare but is a basis for discontinuation of treatment. Metronidazole has a disulfiram-like effect, and patients undergoing treatment should abstain from alcohol while taking this drug. Tinidazole has a similar spectrum of untoward effects but is generally better tolerated. **Paromomycin's** side effects consist of GI disturbances and diarrhea. The small percentage of paromomycin that is absorbed can produce ototoxicity and renal toxicity, particularly in persons with preexisting renal disease. **Iodoquinol** is contraindicated in persons sensitive to iodine. It occasionally causes rash, anal pruritus, acne, slight enlargement of the thyroid gland, nausea, and diarrhea. **Diloxanide furoate** administration is occasionally associated with mild side effects of nausea, vomiting, diarrhea, flatulence, pruritus, and urticaria. **Nitazoxanide** is very well tolerated. On rare occasions, the eyes may appear yellow, and the urine may be similarly discolored.

Chloroquine is relatively well tolerated when used for malaria treatment or prophylaxis. The side effects are dose related and reversible and include headache, nausea, vomiting, blurred vision, dizziness, and fatigue. When high doses are used, as in the treatment of rheumatologic diseases, serious and permanent retinal damage may occur, and chloroquine is contraindicated in persons with retinal disease, psoriasis, or porphyria. Children are especially sensitive to chloroquine, and cardiopulmonary arrest has occurred after accidental overdoses and in adults attempting suicide. **Primaquine** is also relatively well tolerated, although abdominal discomfort and nausea occur in some persons. The major toxicity is hemolysis in persons with glucose-6-phosphate dehydrogenase (G6PD) deficiency. Primaquine is contraindicated during pregnancy because intrauterine hemolysis can occur in a G6PD-deficient fetus. Neutropenia, GI disturbances, and methemoglobinemia have been reported. **Quinine** has the poorest therapeutic index among antimalarial drugs. Common side effects include tinnitus, decreased hearing, headache, dysphoria, nausea, vomiting, and mild visual disturbances. Quinine therapy has been associated with severe hypoglycemia in persons with heavy *P. falciparum* infections as a result of the parasite's use of glucose and the quinine-mediated release of insulin from the pancreas, which responds to intravenous administration of glucose. Rare complications include allergic skin rashes, pruritus, agranulocytosis, hepatitis, and massive hemolysis in patients with *P. falciparum* malaria, which has been termed "blackwater fever." Quinine causes respiratory paralysis in persons with myasthenia gravis, stimulates uterine contractions, and may produce abortion, but has been used successfully to treat serious cases of malaria during pregnancy. **Quinidine gluconate** decreases ventricular ectopy, affects cardiac conduction, and prolongs the QT_c interval. Life-threatening dysrhythmias can occur but are rare. Hypotension may result if the drug is administered too rapidly. **Mefloquine** is relatively well tolerated when used for prophylaxis, but CNS side effects have limited its use. Side effects are more frequent and severe in patients receiving higher doses. Neuropsychiatric reactions such as seizures, acute psychosis, anxiety neurosis, and other disturbances occur in a small percentage of individuals but can be severe, and mefloquine should not be used in persons with a history of epilepsy or psychiatric disturbances. **Pyrimethamine** is generally well tolerated. Blood dyscrasias, rash, vomiting, and seizures are rare side effects. Bone marrow suppression sometimes occurs when high doses are used, but it can be prevented by concurrent administration of folinic acid. **Proguanil** can cause GI signs and symptoms with occasional nausea, diarrhea, urticaria, or oral ulceration when administered in low doses. **Atovaquone** is generally well tolerated but has been associated with GI side effects including nausea, vomiting, and diarrhea. It has also been reported to cause skin rash and pruritus. **Malarone** is the best tolerated of all medications available for prophylaxis against chloroquine-resistant *P. falciparum*. Side effects include those of both proguanil and atovaquone. Asymptomatic transient elevations in liver enzymes have also been reported.

Nifurtimox is often toxic. Side effects include anorexia, vomiting, weight loss, memory loss, sleep disorders, tremor, paresthesias, weakness, and polyneuritis. **Pentamidine isethionate** toxicity is common, including GI complaints, dizziness, flushing, hypotension, renal damage, and blood dyscrasias. A major adverse reaction is hypoglycemia caused by acute damage to β-cells of the pancreatic islets, resulting in insulin release and the long-term consequence of insulin-dependent diabetes mellitus. **Melarsoprol** is extremely toxic, which limits its use to patients with CNS involvement by *T. brucei rhodesiense*. Myocardial toxicity, albuminuria, hypertension, abdominal pain, vomiting, and peripheral neuropathy are all side effects. Approximately 10% of recipients develop allergic encephalitis, which may be fatal. **Eflornithine** is tolerated much better than other antitrypanosomal medications. Its side effects include flatulence, nausea, vomiting, diarrhea, anemia, leukopenia, and thrombocytopenia. On rare occasions diplopia, dizziness, cutaneous hypersensitivity reactions, hearing loss, or seizures may occur. **Sodium stibogluconate** and **meglumine antimonate** have frequent side effects, but they usually do not prevent completion of therapy. Chemical pancreatitis is common, and recipients also frequently experience myalgias, arthralgias, fatigue, and nausea. Nonspecific ST-T wave changes are observed on the electrocardiogram. Untoward effects are more common in persons with renal failure. Side effects of antibiotics and amphotericin B are discussed in Chapters 45 through 47 and 50 (see Clinical Problems box).

CLINICAL PROBLEMS

Anti-helminthic drugs

Albendazole and Mebendazole	GI discomfort, alopecia, bone marrow suppression, hepatic injury
Diethylcarbamazine	Central and GI effects, Mazzotti reaction
Ivermectin	Inflammatory reactions
Praziquantel	GI side effects, allergic reactions due to release helminthic antigens

Anti-protozoal drugs

Metronidazole	GI side effects, neurotoxicity, alcohol intolerance
Paromomycin	GI side effects, ototoxicity, renal toxicity
Chloroquine	Headache, nausea, vomiting, blurred vision, retinal damage
Primaquine	GI side effects, hemolysis in people with glucose-6-phosphate deficiency
Quinine	Tinnitus, decreased hearing, headache, dysphoria, GI side effects, visual disturbances
Mefloquine	Neuropsychiatric reactions
Pyrimethamine	Rare blood dyscrasias, rash, vomiting, seizures, shock

New horizons

Helminths

Ivermectin has emerged as the treatment of choice for onchocerciasis and *S. stercoralis*. Ivermectin also has activity against *A. lumbricoides, T. trichiura*, and *E. vermicularis*. However, it has only limited activity against the hookworm *N. americanus*. Its effectiveness against some ectoparasites also has been documented, and its clinical indications are likely to expand in the future.

Malaria

The emergence of multidrug-resistant *P. falciparum* has stimulated the search for new forms of treatment and prophylaxis for malaria. Among the exciting new compounds are the **artemisinin** derivatives, which include **artesunate.** These were identified in studies of quinghaosu, the Chinese herbal treatment for malaria derived from the wormwood plant *Artemisia annua*. Artemisinin and other artemisinin relatives are endoperoxide-containing compounds. In the presence of intraparasitic iron these drugs may be converted into free radicals and other intermediates that alkylate specific malaria proteins. Artesunate and its derivatives have been used successfully to treat acute *P. falciparum* malaria in areas where mefloquine- and quinine-resistant strains are endemic. In many instances artemisinin derivatives are used concurrently with mefloquine or another antimalarial drug. Currently available artemisinin derivatives are not useful prophylactically because of their short half-lives and concern about neurotoxicity with long-term use. Other antimalarials are being studied in combinations to determine their additive or synergistic effects and whether they may be useful against drug-resistant isolates.

Kinetoplastida

Drugs used to treat Chagas' disease are toxic and variably effective in eradicating *T. cruzi.* Better drugs are needed. With respect to African sleeping sickness, eflornithine is effective and reasonably well tolerated in treatment of *T. brucei gambiense,* but economic and logistical factors have limited its production and supplies are very limited. Drugs recommended for treatment of the hemolymphatic and CNS stages of *T. brucei rhodesiense* have substantial, at times life-threatening toxicity.

Pentavalent antimonials remain the treatment of choice for leishmaniasis in many areas despite their toxicity and reports of clinical failures and resistance. Liposomal and lipid-associated amphotericin preparations are effective for visceral leishmaniasis. They are theoretically attractive because they target macrophages, the only cells infected by *Leishmania* species. Unfortunately, these preparations are expensive and must be given parenterally. The most exciting recent advance in this area has been the development of **miltefosine,** a phosphocholine analog that is administered orally. It is currently the drug of choice for treating visceral leishmaniasis in India where resistance to stibogluconate sodium is common. Although it has GI and liver side effects, these are seldom severe enough to require discontinuation of therapy. In time, this drug may become more widely used.

TRADE NAMES

In addition to generic and fixed-combination preparations and the drugs listed in the Major Drugs box, the following trade-named materials are some of the other compounds used for parasitic diseases around the world.

Atovaquone (Mepron)
Halofantrine (Halfan)
Meglumine antimonate (Glucantime)
Miltefosine (Miltex)
Proguanil (Paludrine)
Pyrimethamine (Daraprim)
Quinidine (Quinaglute)
Spiramycin (Rovamycine)

FURTHER READING

Drugs for parasitic infections. *Med Lett Drugs Ther* August 2004.

Pearson RD. Antiparasitic drugs. In Mandell GL, Bennett JE, Dolin R, editors: *Principles and practice of infectious diseases,* ed 5, Philadelphia, 2005, Churchill Livingstone.

Centers for Disease Control and Prevention: *Health information for international travel*: 2003-2004, US Department of Health and Human Resources, Public Health Service, www.cdc.gov/travel.

Self-assessment questions

1. Which of the following drugs is administered as a single dose in mass treatment programs for persons in developing areas infected with one or more of the following intestinal nematodes: *A. lumbricoides,* hookworms, and *T. trichiura?*

a. Albendazole
b. Pyrantel pamoate
c. Metronidazole
d. Diethylcarbamazine
e. Ivermectin

2. Which of the following drugs is effective for the treatment of the *Schistosoma* species that infect humans?

a. Albendazole
b. Mebendazole
c. Praziquantel
d. Ivermectin
e. Niclosamide

3. *O. volvulus,* the cause of river blindness, should be treated with which of the following drugs?

a. Albendazole
b. Mebendazole
c. Niclosamide
d. Diethylcarbamazine
e. Ivermectin

4. Which of the following drugs is well absorbed, subject to extensive sulfoxidation, and has a major metabolite with anthelmintic activity against the larval forms of cestodes in tissue?

a. Albendazole
b. Mebendazole
c. Praziquantel
d. Diethylcarbamazine
e. Ivermectin

5. Which of the following drugs has a major side effect of hemolysis in persons with glucose-6-phosphate dehydrogenase deficiency?
   a. Chloroquine
   b. Primaquine
   c. Mefloquine
   d. Pyrimethamine
   e. Doxycycline

6. Which of the following drugs is used to kill hypnozoites in the liver of a person infected with *P. vivax?*
   a. Chloroquine
   b. Mefloquine
   c. Pyrimethamine
   d. Quinine
   e. Primaquine

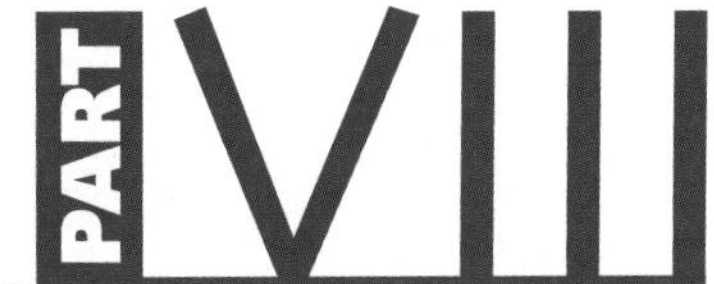

Special topics

CERTAIN TYPES OF DRUGS that do not easily fit in other sections are covered in Part VIII. The increasing role of the use of antibodies and other biological compounds is discussed extensively in Chapter 53. Although the administration and use of these compounds pose special challenges and problems, they are an increasingly important part of the modern pharmacological armamentarium for treating many important diseases. Histamine and antihistamines are dealt with in Chapter 54, with Chapter 55 devoted to a discussion of the therapy of gastrointestinal disorders. Basic immune mechanisms underlying the release of histamine, its actions on cells and organs, and the mechanisms of action of antihistamines are described in Chapter 54. A knowledge of histamine's effects on the immune, gastrointestinal, respiratory, cardiovascular, and central nervous systems is important to understand the therapeutic applications of these agents.

Advances in the treatment of gastrointestinal diseases, including ulcers and gastroesophageal reflux disease, are detailed in Chapter 55. Other important agents discussed include prokinetic drugs that enhance gastrointestinal emptying, laxatives, and antidiarrheal drugs, all of which are of practical importance in managing disease, particularly in the hospital setting.

On the other side of the coin, Chapter 56 deals with toxicology, specifically that resulting from industrial pollutants including metals, organic solvents, toxic gases, and other toxic chemicals. Included in the discussion are the mechanisms of toxicity and counteractive antidote therapy. Teratogenic and carcinogenic toxic agents are also discussed, particularly as they relate to environmental toxicology.

CHAPTER 53

Immunopharmacology

Thomas T. Kawabata
James B. Chung

Major Drugs

Immunosuppressive/antiinflammatory drugs
Cyclophosphamide (Cytoxan)
Mycophenolate mofetil (CellCept)
Azathioprine (Imuran)
Cyclosporine (Sandimmune, Neoral)
Monoclonal antibodies
Interferons
Interleukins

Immunostimulatory drugs
Interleukins
Colony stimulating factors
Interferons

Therapeutic overview

The immune system protects the host from invading organisms and growing neoplastic cells through interaction of a wide variety of cell types and secreted factors while sparing host cells. Alterations to this highly regulated system can tip the delicate balance of host defense toward immune reactions against self-proteins and generation of **autoimmune diseases.** Robust immune reactions against foreign antigens may also lead to **hypersensitivity** (allergic) reactions. There are now many agents with different mechanisms of actions, targets, and side-effect profiles that can be used for treatment. These drugs can be split into two general categories:

- **Immunosuppressive/antiinflammatory**
- **Immunostimulatory**

The goal for these drugs has intended to increase specificity for the immune system and minimize toxicity toward other organs. Another goal has been to minimize non-specific immune suppression or enhance select components to obtain the desired effect while avoiding decreases in host resistance or autoimmune diseases.

Suppression of the immune response has been the primary target of most drugs to date. Most of them were originally developed as anticancer drugs to inhibit cell proliferation, such as **azathioprine, cyclophosphamide,** and **methotrexate.** Development of **corticosteroids** enhanced the ability to suppress the immune response and inhibit inflammatory processes; however, none of these drug classes are particularly selective for the immune system, and they all produce significant toxicity.

Increased selectivity for the immune system was achieved with development of **cyclosporine,** and sub-

Abbreviations

APC	antigen presenting cell
CNS	central nervous system
CSF	colony-stimulating factor
CTL	cytolytic T lymphocytes
GA	glatiramer acetate
G-CSF	granulocyte colony–stimulating factor
GM-CSF	granulocyte-macrophage colony–stimulating factor
IFN	interferon
Ig	immunoglobulin
IL	interleukin
IV	intravenous
M-CSF	macrophage colony–stimulating factor
MHC	major histocompatibility complex
MMF	mycophenolate mofetil
MS	multiple sclerosis
NFAT	nuclear factor for activated T cells
Th	T-helper cells
TNF	tumor necrosis factor

sequently **tacrolimus** and **rapamycin. Mycophenolate mofetil** was found to have greater selectivity on lymphocyte proliferation than other antiproliferative immunosuppressive agents. To achieve immunosuppression and minimize adverse effects, treatment regimens with various combinations of these drugs were developed. More recently, **biological compounds** such as recombinant cytokines or receptors or monoclonal antibodies against cytokines, receptors, and specific immune cell antigens have provided greater selectivity and less toxicity. These drugs have made important contributions to treatment of autoimmune diseases such multiple sclerosis (MS) and rheumatoid arthritis.

Although the immune system has redundant processes for host resistance, current immunosuppressive/antiinflammatory therapy is still limited by an increased risk of opportunistic infections and tumors. The goal is to suppress the immune response against a specific antigen without compromising the response to other antigens (e.g., bacterial, viral proteins). **Glatiramer** acetate utilizes this approach to downregulate the specific immune response in the MS disease process. Many other drugs with an antigen-specific target are being explored and developed.

Immunostimulatory drugs currently approved are primarily human recombinant **cytokines** for treatment of viral infections and cancer. Cytokines such as interferon-γ (IFN-γ), IFN-α, and interleukin-2 (IL-2) stimulate the immune system to kill bacteria, virally infected cells, and tumor cells. The cytokines granulocyte colony-stimulating factor (G-CSF), granulocyte-macrophage colony-stimulating factor (GM-CSF), and IL-11 stimulate growth of hematopoietic cells from bone marrow.

The benefits of these different categories of agents are shown in the Therapeutic Overview box.

THERAPEUTIC OVERVIEW

Immunosuppressive/antiinflammatory drugs

Prevents or modulates immune-mediated organ/tissue transplantation rejection

Inhibits initiation and/or progression of autoimmune diseases

Immunostimulatory drugs

Enhances immune responses against infectious disease (viral, bacterial, fungal)

Enhances immune responses against neoplastic cells

Stimulates development of immunocompetent cells from bone marrow

Mechanisms of action

Immune response

The role of the immune system is to recognize and remove invading microorganisms and tumor cells, while ignoring host cells, through innate and acquired immune responses. When exposed to an invading organism, nonspecific **innate** immunity, comprising the first line of defense, is immediately called into action. The antigen-specific responses of **acquired** immunity also develop in tandem to more effectively remove the organism. When reexposed to the invading organism, antigen-specific cells of the acquired immune response are called back into action for a more rapid and effective response. This "memory" and the ability to specifically recognize antigens differentiates acquired from innate immunity. Key differences between innate and acquired immune responses are listed in Table 53-1.

Innate immunity

With bacterial infections, complement and phagocytic cells (macrophages and neutrophils) play a vital role in producing a local inflammatory response that leads to killing and removal of the invading microbes. Complement can be activated by antigen-antibody complexes or by natural substances such as bacterial cell wall components to produce split products that activate and recruit macrophages and neutrophils. The two pathways converge on a single final pathway in which complement components assemble into a pore-forming membrane attack complex that can directly lyse invading cells. Macrophages are activated and phagocytize the microbes, producing a variety of cytokines and chemoattractants (chemokines). The cytokines activate neighboring cells and recruit neutrophils that kill and remove the invading microbe. For viral infections, IFN is immediately produced by fibroblasts and macrophages. IFNs directly inhibit viral replication and activate natural killer cells to lyse virally infected cells.

Acquired immunity

Acquired immunity is commonly divided into **humoral** and **cell-mediated** responses. Initiation of acquired immunity first involves antigen-specific activation of naive T cells ($CD4^+$, T-helper cells). This requires participation of antigen presenting cells (APC) (dendritic cells, macrophages, and B cells) that take up and process antigens into peptide fragments. Peptides bind to major histocompatibility complex (MHC) Class II molecules

Table 53-1 Characteristics of innate and acquired immune responses

Characteristic	Innate Immunity	Acquired Immunity
Onset of action	Immediate	Days to weeks
Mechanism of antigen recognition	Receptors that recognize common molecules on microbes and viruses	Unique antigen specific receptors (T-cell receptor, B cell receptor)
Cell types/factors	Macrophages, neutrophils, mast cells, natural killer cells, complement, interferon	Antigen presenting cells, T-lymphocytes, B-lymphocytes

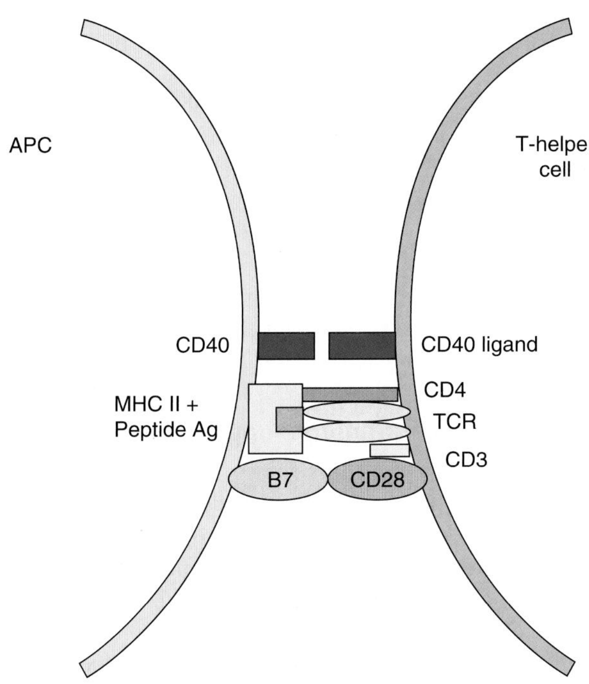

Figure 53-1 Molecular interactions between antigen presenting cells (APC) and T cells. The T-cell receptor (TCR) and CD4 complex on T-helper cells act as co-receptors for the immunogenic peptide associated with the MHC class II molecule. The TCR and CD8 molecules on cytotoxic T lymphocytes act as co-receptors for the immunogenic peptide associated with the MHC Class I molecule (not shown). T cells require two signals to become activated. The first signal involves the binding of the T-cell receptor and CD4 or CD8 with antigen–MHC complex. This binding results in the transduction of a signal via the CD3 molecule. The second signal is mediated by co-stimulatory molecules CD28 and B7. The stimulated T cell will in turn stimulate the APC via CD40 ligand–CD40 interactions. MHC class II antigens are found on dendritic cells, macrophages, B cells, and other specialized APCs. MHC class I antigens are present on all somatic cells.

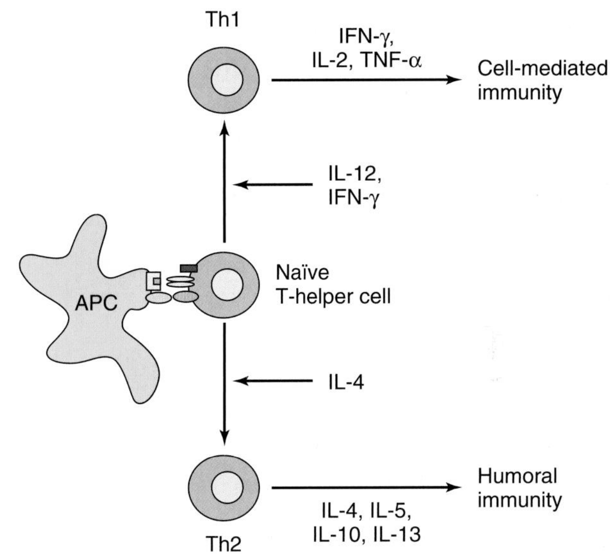

Figure 53-2 Generation of effector Th1 and Th2 Cells. APCs take up, process, and present peptide antigen to naïve $CD4^+$ T-helper cells. The interaction between APC and T-helper cells results in activation and proliferation of effector Th1 or Th2 cells. Cytokines IFN-γ and IL-12 stimulate the formation of Th1 cells, while IL-4 drives the formation of Th2 cells. Th1 cells secrete IFN-γ, TNF-α, and IL-2, which result in the activation of macrophages and CTL generation. Th2 cells secrete IL-4, IL-5, and IL-10 that drives the generation of an antibody response. Th1 and Th2 cells can also secrete the same cytokines. The distinctions between these cell types are not always clear in certain human diseases.

within the APC and are presented to $CD4^+$ T cells that possess a T-cell receptor specific for the peptide-MHC complex. The naïve T cell requires **two signals** to be fully activated. The first is provided by the peptide binding to the T-cell receptor, and the second comes from interaction of costimulatory molecules of the APC and the T cell (Fig. 53-1). "Signal One" in the absence of "Signal Two" leads to tolerance, or functional silencing, of the T cell. Fully activated T cells proliferate and differentiate into effector T-helper cells that produce cytokines, such as ILs. In general, there are two types of effector T-helper (Th) cells: Th1 and Th2 cells. The type of cytokines produced by each Th cell determines its function. Cytokines produced by Th1 cells (IFN-γ, IL-2, tumor necrosis factor (TNF)-α) stimulate generation of cell-mediated immune responses (Fig. 53-2), whereas Th2 cells produce cytokines (IL-4, IL-5, IL-10, IL-13) that drive formation of an antibody response (humoral immunity).

Cell-mediated immunity Cell-mediated immune responses involve Th1-mediated activation of macrophages (type IV hypersensitivity) and generation of $CD8^+$ cytotoxic T-lymphocytes (CTLs). Th1 cells secrete cytokines, which recruit and activate macrophages. Macrophages are then capable of killing intracellular bacteria and produce a localized inflammatory response. This also occurs with chemicals such as urushiol from poison ivy (contact hypersensitivity).

CTLs mediate antigen-specific lysis of tumor cells, virally infected cells, and graft/transplant cells. Generation of CTLs for all three functions generally involve similar mechanisms (Fig. 53-3). Naïve, precursor CTLs (pCTLs) require activation by two signals, as described for T-helper cells. The first is delivered by binding of peptide antigens associated with MHC Class I molecules on APC to the T-cell receptor on $CD8^+$ pCTLs. The second is provided by receptor-ligand interaction of costimulatory molecules. Th1 cells produce cytokines that stimulate dendritic cells to upregulate a costimulatory molecule that will activate antigen-stimulated $CD8^+$ cells. Activated CTLs produce IL-2, which stimulates it own proliferation and differentiation. In certain situations, APC cells that contain high levels of costimulatory molecules are able to activate $CD8^+$ CTLs without the help of Th1 cells. Antigen recognition and binding of activated CTLs to antigen on cells result in cell lysis.

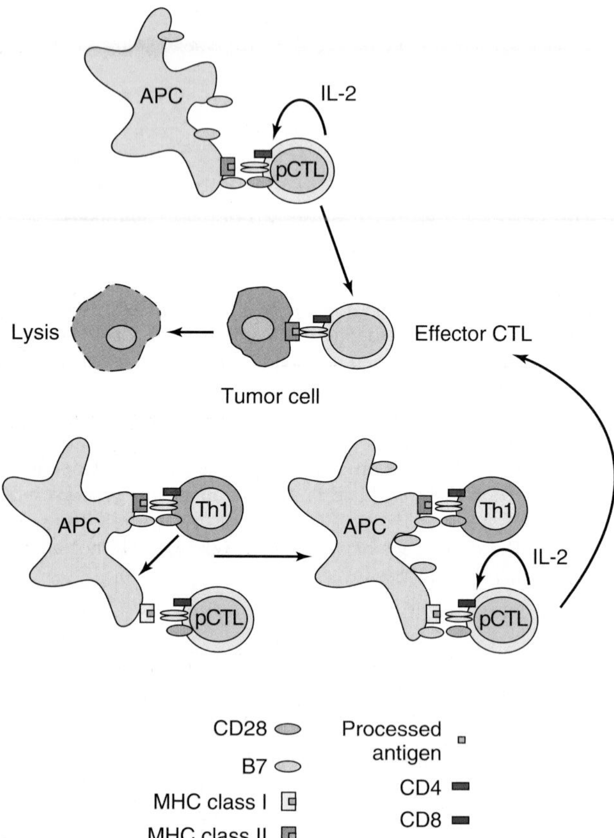

Figure 53-3 Cytolytic T-lymphocyte (CTL) generation against tumor cells. CTLs may be generated with or without support from Th1 cells. Tumor antigens are taken up by APCs, processed, and presented with MHC class II molecules to $CD4^+$ T-helper cells. This leads to the generation of effector Th1 cells. Activated Th1 cells stimulate the upregulation of co-stimulatory molecules (B7) on APC and provide the second signal to antigen-activated precursor CTLs (pCTL). Activated CTLs secrete IL-2 and stimulate their own proliferation and differentiation to effector CTLs. Tumor cells are then recognized and lysed by effector CTLs.

Humoral immunity Th2 cells secrete cytokines that stimulate proliferation and differentiation of B cells to antibody-secreting plasma cells or to long-lived memory cells (Fig. 53-4). Specific antibodies can remove harmful foreign antigens (e.g., bacterial toxins) by binding to and neutralizing their effects. Antigen-antibody immune complexes can activate complement to elicit a local inflammatory reaction for further antigen removal by phagocytes. Once bound to foreign protein or bacteria, the Fc region of antibodies can bind to receptors on phagocytic cells, leading to internalization of the invading pathogens.

Pharmacological immunosuppression

Pharmacological approaches to immunosuppressive therapy may involve selective eradication of immune-competent cells, similar to the selective killing of tumor cells by antineoplastic drugs (see Chapter 42) or down-regulation of the immune response without deleting the target cell. In both cases, the goal is to balance the activity and selectivity of the drug to optimize clinical efficacy while preventing adverse effects. The principal drugs currently used to obtain immunosuppression include corticosteroids, cytotoxic agents, calcineurin inhibitors, and biologicals. Most of these compounds are highly effective in inhibiting the immune response. However, their usefulness is limited by their **severe toxicities.** Therefore the different drugs are used in **combination** at lower doses to obtain a synergistic effect on immune responses while minimizing adverse effects. Immunosuppressive drugs are used primarily to prevent transplant rejection and treat autoimmune diseases.

Corticosteroids The actions of the corticosteroids are discussed in Chapter 33. Glucocorticoids are effective in treating autoimmune diseases and preventing graft rejection because of their immunosuppressive and antiinflammatory effects. When glucocorticoids are administered, the numbers of circulating lymphocytes, basophils, and eosinophils decrease over a 24-hour period, whereas the number of neutrophils increases. In addition, changes in corticosteroid concentrations during the normal diurnal cycle and in stressful situations correlate with decreases in circulating lymphocytes. Lymphopenia is attributed to migration of cells

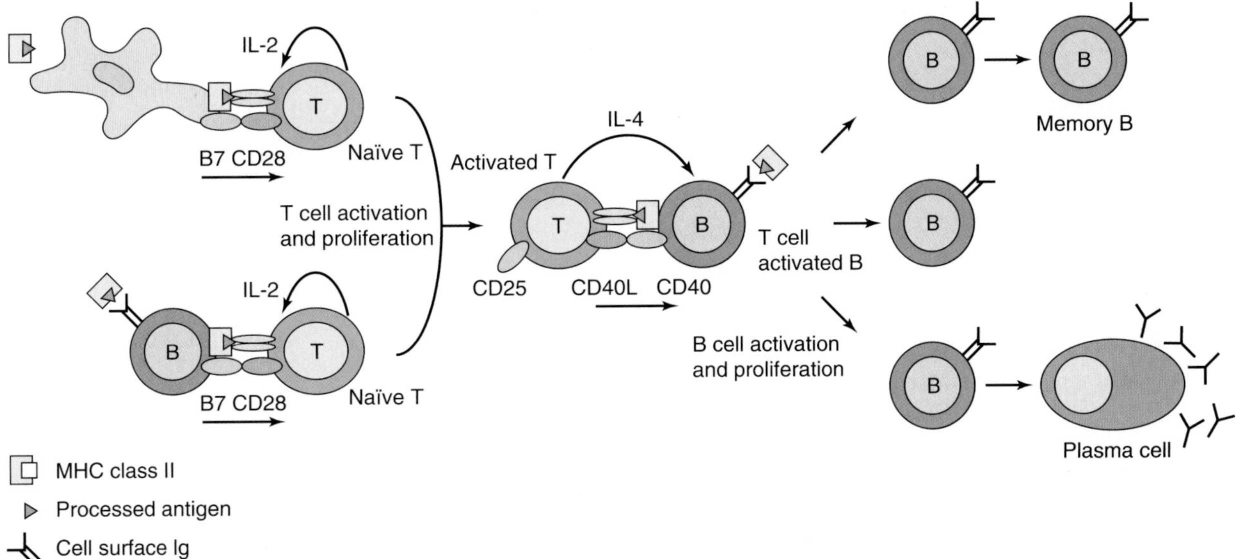

Figure 53-4 Generation of a humoral immune response. APCs internalize antigen through phagocytosis or antibody-mediated endocytosis (B cells). The antigen is processed, and the resulting peptides are presented on the surface to naïve T cells in the setting of MHC class II molecules. The interaction of the specific TCR: peptide/MHC pair and the co-stimulatory molecules B7/CD28 are necessary for full activation. The activated T cell produces IL-2, which leads to its proliferation and upregulation of CD25, a component of the IL-2 receptor. CD40L is also upregulated. In the lymphoid organs such as the lymph nodes or the spleen, the activated T cell interacts with a B cell that is specific for the same antigen and provides "help" to the B cell through interaction of CD40L and CD40 and by producing cytokines such as IL-4 that lead to B cell activation and proliferation. The activated B cells can differentiate into antibody-producing plasma cells or into memory cells.

into extravascular spaces, with more T cells than B cells or monocytes migrating. Most cells migrate to bone marrow. High-dose glucocorticoid therapy is also known to reduce the size of lymphoid organs.

Although corticosteroid-induced lymphopenia is well documented, its importance in immunosuppression is not clear. It is known, however, that corticosteroids alter the immune response by directly changing immune cell function, and the macrophage is a primary target. Exposure of macrophages to corticosteroids results in decreased IL-1 production; decreased expression of MHC class II antigens; and decreased phagocytosis of virus-infected cells, tumor cells, bacteria, and fungi. T and B cells are also directly affected, with T-cell–mediated responses affected to a greater extent.

Cytotoxic agents This class of drugs acts predominantly by deleting proliferating cells. Proliferation is a key step in the immune response and therefore a primary target. Although many cytotoxic agents have been used in treating cancer, a relatively small number of drugs are used in treating immune diseases. The main categories are **alkylating agents**, such as cyclophosphamide, and **antimetabolites,** such as azathioprine and methotrexate.

The structure of **cyclophosphamide,** its activation to phosphoramide mustard and acrolein, and its antitumor actions are discussed in Chapter 42. The ways in which the active metabolites phosphoramide mustard and acrolein alter the immune response are unclear. The mustard is believed to alkylate DNA and mediate the antiproliferative and immunosuppressive effects. This is consistent with the hypothesis that selective cytotoxic effects on B cells are attributable to a greater proliferation rate. However, the highly reactive, sulfhydryl-binding acrolein may also play an important role in the drug's action.

The structure of **azathioprine** is shown in Figure 53-5. This drug is metabolized to the antiproliferative drug 6-mercaptopurine (see Chapter 42), which is further metabolized to the active antitumor and immunosuppressive thioinosinic acid. This inhibits hypoxanthine-guanine phosphoribosyltransferase, which catalyzes conversion of purines to the corresponding phosphoribosyl-5' phosphates and the conversion of hypoxanthine to inosinic acid. This leads to the inhibition of cellular proliferation. Azathioprine's immunosuppressive effects stem from its antiproliferative actions.

The immunosuppressive effects of **mycophenolate mofetil** (MMF) are mediated by inhibiting T and B lymphocyte proliferation through inhibition of purine synthesis. Purine nucleotides are synthesized in most cell types by the de novo or salvage pathways. MMF selec-

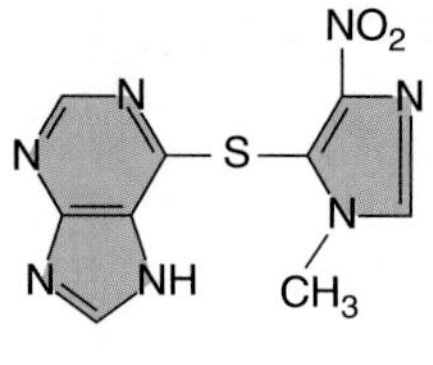

Azathioprine

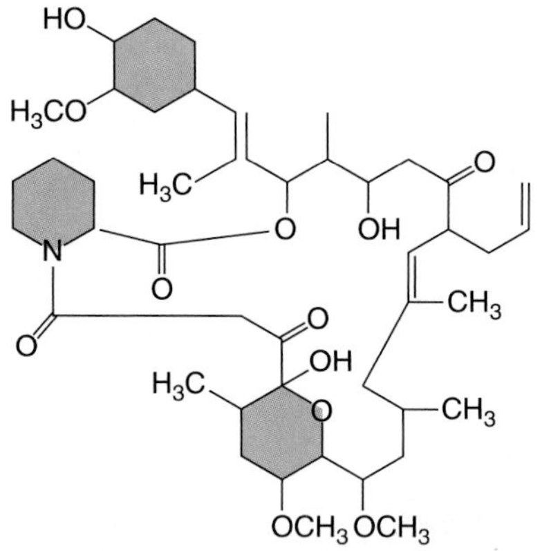

Tacrolimus

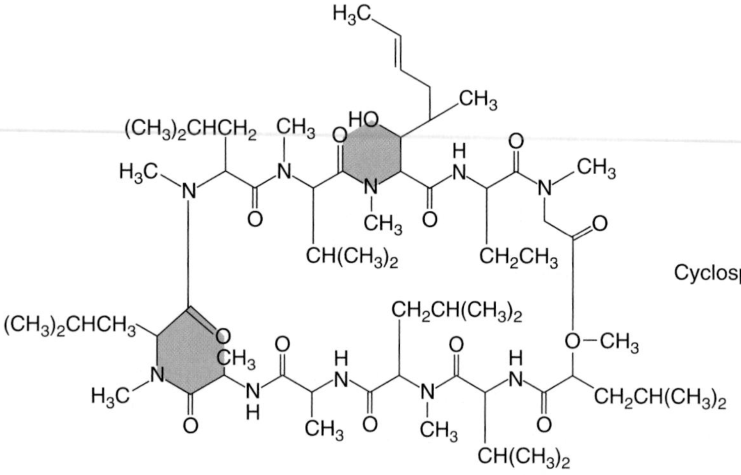

Cyclosporin A

Figure 53-5 Structures of several immunosuppressants.

tively inhibits inosine monophosphate dehydrogenase, blocking de novo synthesis of purines. Lymphocytes, unlike other rapidly dividing cell types, depend entirely on the de novo pathway for purine synthesis, thus explaining MMF's selectivity for lymphocytes. MMF is an antimetabolite like azathioprine and is reported to have greater selectivity for T and B lymphocytes than for neutrophils and platelets. MMF inhibits the generation of CTLs and antibody-producing cells by inhibiting the proliferation of T and B lymphocytes. It also affects expression of adhesion molecules on lymphocytes, thereby inhibiting their binding to vascular endothelial cells, which is necessary for migration from the circulation to tissues.

Methotrexate was originally developed as an anticancer drug (see Chapter 42) but is now being widely used at lower doses in several inflammatory diseases, including rheumatoid arthritis. The immunological and antitumor mechanisms are similar. An antimetabolite, methotrexate binds and inactivates dihydrofolate reductase, leading to inhibition of the synthesis of thymidylate, inosinic acid, and other purine metabolites. Methotrexate also stimulates the release of adenosine, which inhibits stimulated neutrophil function and has potent antiinflammatory properties.

Calcineurin inhibitors/immunophilin binding agents

Calcineurin inhibitors downregulate immune responses by inhibiting production of IL-2 in activated T cells. IL-2 is a key driver of many immune responses and especially important in mediating organ transplant rejection. The two calcineurin inhibitors **cyclosporin**

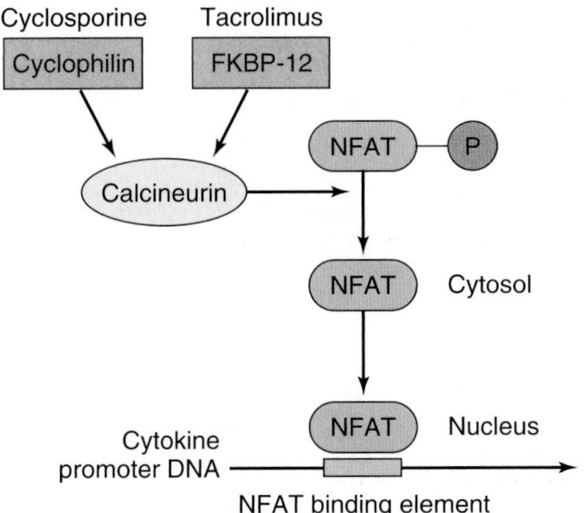

Figure 53-6 Mechanism of action of cyclosporine and tacrolimus. Transcription of various cytokines requires the transcription factor NFAT. Removal of a phosphate group from NFAT by the Ca^{2+}/calmodulin–dependent calcineurin phosphatase results in translocation of NFAT to the nucleus, where it binds to the NFAT binding element of the promoter region of cytokine genes (IL-2, IL-3, IL-4, GM-CSF, TNF-α, IFN-γ). This results in activation of cytokine transcription. Cyclosporine and tacrolimus bind to cyclophilin and FKBP-12 (known as immunophilins), respectively. These complexes inhibit calcineurin activity and inhibit NFAT dephosphorylation.

and **tacrolimus** bind to cyclophilin and FK binding protein, respectively, and the drug-immunophilin complex binds to calcineurin. This leads to dephosphorylation of nuclear factor for activated T cells (NFAT) and prevention of its translocation to the nucleus, causing downregulation of cytokine transcription (Fig. 53-6).

Cyclosporine is a cyclic endecapeptide purified from fungi (see Fig. 53-5). Cyclosporine primarily affects T-cell–mediated responses, whereas most humoral immune responses not requiring T cells are spared. The effectiveness of cyclosporine stems from its selective inhibition of Th cell activation. Its major effect on Th cells is inhibition of cytokine production. Decreased IL-2 production in turn leads to a decrease in IL-2 receptors and in a lack of responsiveness of CTL precursor cells. Because there is positive feedback through IL-2 production and IL-2 receptors, the decreased IL-2 production of Th cells also leads to decreased IL-2 receptors. Cyclosporine does not, however, affect the proliferative response of activated CTLs to IL-2 or the lytic activity of CTLs. Consistent with this is the observation that cyclosporine is effective only during the very early stages of antigen activation of Th cells. There is also evidence for inhibition of macrophage antigen presentation and IL-1 production by macrophages.

The cytoplasmic receptor for cyclosporine is cyclophilin, a propyl cis-trans isomerase involved in protein folding. Although cyclosporine is known to inhibit isomerase activity, that mechanism does not appear to be important in its immunosuppressive effects. Instead, the cyclosporine-cyclophilin drug complex binds to and inhibits calcineurin and inhibits translocation of the transcription factor NFAT as described above.

The structure of **tacrolimus** (formerly known as FK506) is shown in Figure 53-5. Its mechanism of action is similar to that of cyclosporine (see Fig. 53-6) in that it inhibits synthesis of cytokines. Tacrolimus also binds to a cytosolic receptor known as FK506–binding protein, which is also a peptidylpropyl cis-trans isomerase but is distinct from cyclophilin. Like cyclosporine, the tacrolimus-FK506 binding protein complex also binds and inhibits calcineurin. The major effects of these immunosuppressive actions are summarized in Figure 53-7.

Rapamycin (sirolimus) is structurally similar to tacrolimus and also binds to the FK506-binding protein. Unlike the calcineurin inhibitors, it blocks B and T cell activation at a later stage. It blocks signal transduction in T cells and inhibits cell-cycle progression from G1 to S phase. Rapamycin and cyclosporine appear to act synergistically to inhibit lymphocyte proliferation.

Biologicals Advances in biotechnology and understanding of the mechanisms underlying immunologic diseases have resulted in many novel biological agents. "Biologicals" refers to a diverse group of naturally occurring compounds that are primarily manufactured by advanced biotechnology techniques and includes recombinant vaccines, blood products, cytokines, growth factors, and monoclonal antibodies. Antibodies and cytokine antagonists designed to bind to soluble proteins and surface receptors that mediate inflammatory processes and drive the immune response have demonstrated clinical efficacy in a variety of neoplastic and immune disorders. Monoclonal antibodies exert their effects through one or more of the following ways (Fig. 53-8):

- Blocking the function of the target protein
- Altering the function of the target cell
- Direct induction of cytotoxicity
- Immune-mediated removal of target cells through complement-dependent cytotoxicity, antibody-dependent cellular cytotoxicity, or phagocytosis

Biologicals targeting lymphocytes **Anti-thymocyte globulin** is purified IgG obtained from rabbits immunized with human thymocytes. IV administration of these polyclonal antibodies leads to rapid and profound depletion of peripheral lymphocytes and is used to

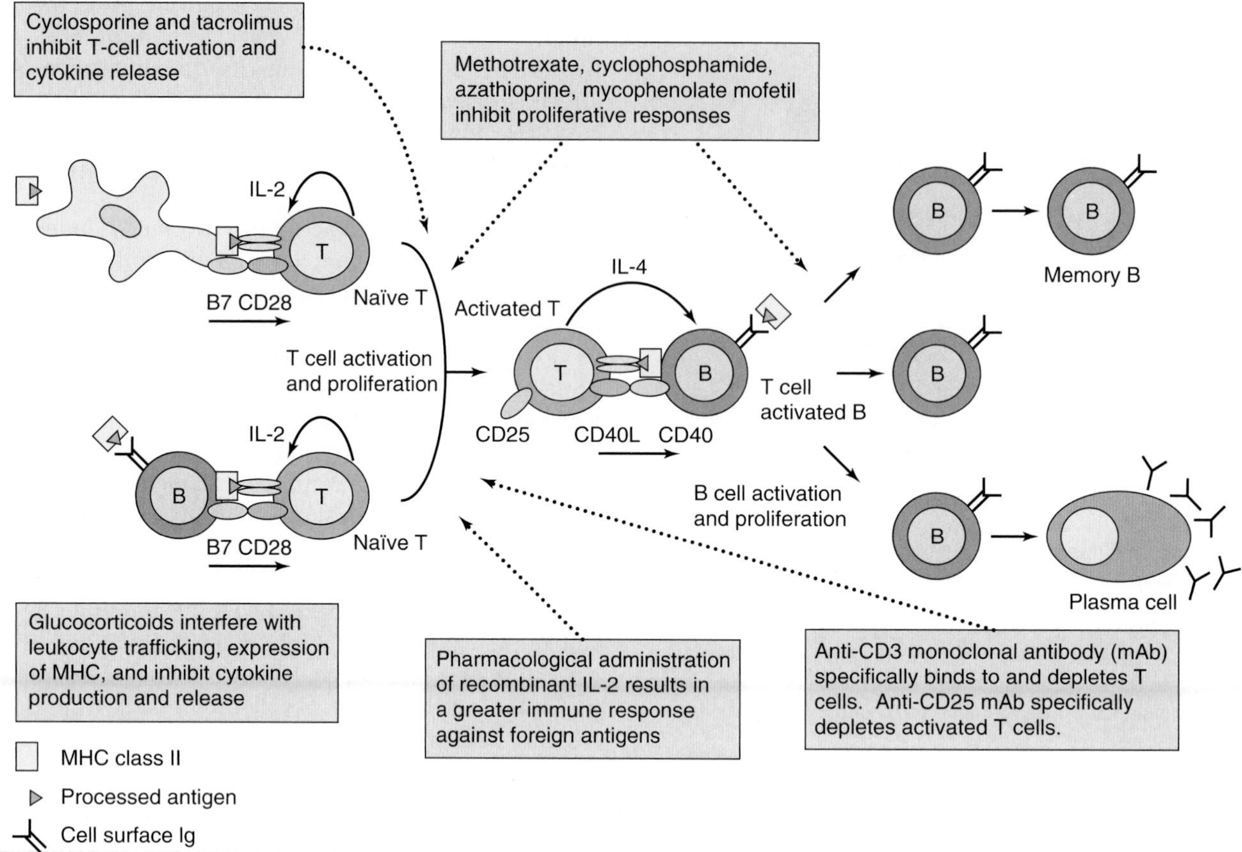

Figure 53-7 Primary mechanisms of action of immunosuppressive drugs. The antibody response shown in Figure 53-4 is used as an example to demonstrate the primary targets and mechanisms of action of immunosuppressive drugs.

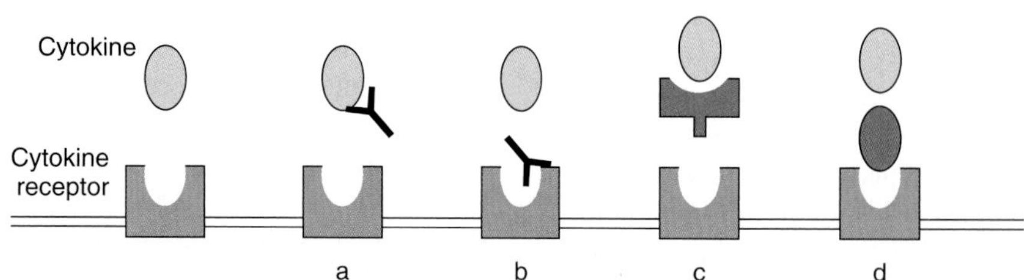

Figure 53-8 Strategies to inhibit cytokine action. Cytokines exert their effects through binding to cell surface receptors. Monoclonal antibodies may be developed to bind to the cytokine *(a)*, or to the receptor *(b)*. A soluble receptor may be employed to bind to the cytokine *(c)* as well. A soluble receptor antagonist *(d)* that binds specifically to the receptor without activating it may be used to compete against the activating cytokine.

prevent graft rejection. Severe side effects limit the use of these antibodies to second-line status behind calcineurin inhibitors. In addition, because of the nature of its production, there is poor standardization between batches. Monoclonal antibodies, on the other hand, are well standardized. **OKT3 (muromonab)** is a monoclonal antibody directed against the CD3 molecule on the membrane of T cells. CD3 is associated with the T-cell antigen receptor complex involved in signal transduction to the T cell after binding of antigen (see Figure 53-1). Muromonab is approved for treatment of acute rejection of renal transplants. It also has severe side effects and is generally reserved for patients resistant to first-line therapies.

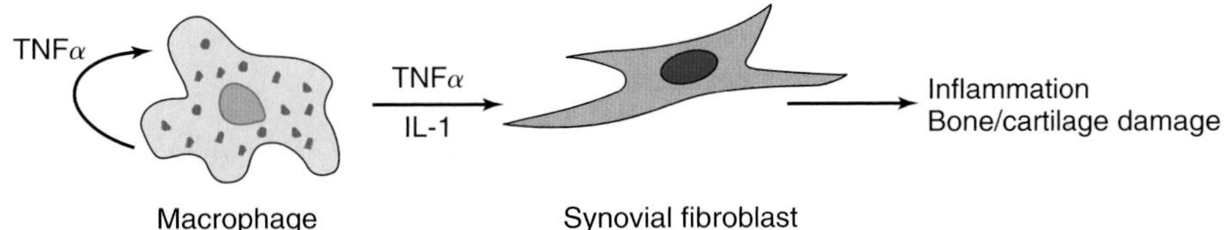

Figure 53-9 TNF-α and IL-1 play a central role in rheumatoid arthritis. Although the inciting factors are unknown, activated macrophages produce TNF-α and IL-1, which activate synovial fibroblasts in the synovium of affected joints. This in turn leads to recruitment of other inflammatory cells to the joint and to release of metalloproteinases that results in bone and cartilage degradation characteristic of the disease. TNF-α also acts in an autocrine fashion to perpetuate the inflammatory pathway. Other cytokines such as IL-6 also play important pro-inflammatory roles.

Biologicals targeting cytokines TNFα and IL-1β are proinflammatory cytokines implicated in the pathogenesis of inflammatory disorders such as rheumatoid arthritis (Fig. 53-9) and Crohn's disease (see Chapter 55). They are involved in activation and proliferation of synovial cells, inducing the production of collagenases and other cytokines that lead to continued inflammation and bone resorption. **Infliximab** and **adalimumab** are antibodies that bind to soluble TNFα and lower its level in blood. The former is a murine/human chimeric antibody and the latter is a recombinant humanized monoclonal antibody. **Etanercept** is a dimeric fusion protein combining the p75 TNF receptor with the Fc portion of human IgG1.

IL-1 receptor antagonist (IL-1ra) is a naturally occurring antagonist of IL-1. IL-1ra binds to the two receptor forms of IL-1 (Type I and II) and inhibits binding of both IL-1α and IL-1β without stimulating the cells. **Anakinra** is a recombinant IL-1ra that is used for treatment of rheumatoid arthritis.

IL-2 receptor antagonists prevent IL-2 from binding to activated T lymphocytes. Unlike muromonab which targets both resting and activated lymphocytes, IL-2 receptor antagonists target actively dividing cells by binding to the α chain of the trimolecular IL-2 receptor (CD25), which is transiently expressed only on antigen-activated T cells. There are two currently available monoclonal antibodies directed against IL-2 receptor α, **basiliximab** and **daclizumab.** Early clinical studies demonstrate efficacy in combination with calcineurin inhibitors. Although long-term data are lacking, they appear to be well tolerated.

Cytokine biologicals The IFNs comprise a family of cytokines produced by many cell types that produce antiproliferative, antiviral, and immunomodulatory effects. They were originally named for their ability to interfere with viral RNA and protein synthesis. IFNs are categorized as either type I (α and β) or type II (γ). The α and β forms are similar in structure and bind to the same receptors. There is little sequence homology between the γ and the other two types. Upon viral stimulation, the α form is primarily synthesized in macrophages and the β form in macrophages and fibroblasts. Type I IFNs are known to both stimulate the immune response (see below) and mediate antiinflammatory actions (treatment of MS). MS is mediated by myelin-reactive Th1 cells that migrate into the central nervous system (CNS) and produce an inflammatory reaction. Although the exact mechanism for the effect of IFN-β on MS is not known, data indicate that it inhibits T cell migration by suppressing synthesis of chemokines and adhesion proteins. The γ form is primarily produced in T lymphocytes after stimulation with antigen or mitogens (see below).

Biologicals targeting hypersensitivity mediators Allergen binding and cross-linking of specific-IgE bound to mast cells leads to mast cell degranulation and release of various mediators (histamine, leukotrienes) involved in asthma (see Chapter 34). A monoclonal antibody specific for IgE (**omalizumab**) is approved for allergic asthma. Omalizumab inhibits binding of IgE to the IgE Fc receptor on mast cells, preventing antigen-induced mediator release.

Antigen-specific immunomodulation Glatiramer acetate (GA) is a drug that was specifically designed for treatment of MS with a mechanism of action different from that of IFN-β. MS is an autoimmune disease in which an immune response against myelin proteins is believed to result in a localized inflammatory response to the cells of the CNS. GA is a synthetic copolymer composed of four amino acids that range from 40 to 90 amino acids in length and has a structure similar to myelin basic protein. GA administration results in the generation of GA-specific Th2 cells, which are recruited into the CNS, activated by myelin proteins, and produce various cytokines (e.g., IL-10) that depress immune responses to MBP. Thus GA has a unique mechanism of action in that it is antigen specific.

Pharmacological immunostimulation

Immunostimulatory drugs mediate their effects by directly activating, or stimulating growth of, immuno-

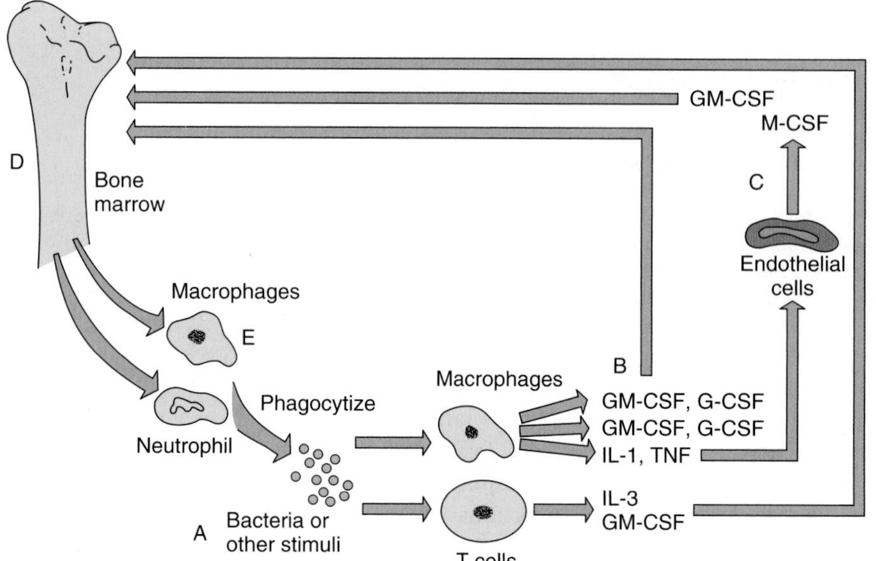

Figure 53-10 Secretion of colony-stimulating factors (CSFs) in response to immune stimulation. Bacteria or other stimuli *(A)* activate macrophages and T cells to produce a variety of CSFs *(B)*, which also stimulate endothelial cells to produce CSFs *(C)*. CSFs stimulate production of macrophages and neutrophils from bone marrow *(D)*. These cells are then able to phagocytose the bacteria *(E)*.

competent cells. Given the benefits of stimulating the immune response against tumor cells or pathogens, there have been many attempts to develop immunostimulant drugs. However, only a few are efficacious without overriding toxicities. The available compounds are primarily human recombinant cytokines (excluding vaccine adjuvants).

IL-2 is secreted by helper CD4$^+$ T-lymphocytes, and its primary effect is autocrine stimulation of T-lymphocyte proliferation. This results in a greater immune response against a variety of antigens. Recombinant human IL-2 has been found to be effective in treatment of certain types of cancer. The exact mechanism is not known.

CSFs comprise a group of cytokines named for their ability to induce formation of certain types of colonies from bone marrow cells in soft agar cultures. They affect bone marrow cells at different stages of maturity. Multi-CSF (IL-3) stimulates the primitive progenitor cells that give rise to granulocytes, megakaryocytes, mast cells, macrophages, and erythrocytes. In contrast, more-differentiated progenitor cells are stimulated by G-CSF and M-CSF to proliferate and differentiate into granulocytes and macrophages, respectively. Both of these cell lineages are stimulated by GM-CSF. As cells of certain lineages mature from progenitors to more-committed states, however, they become refractory to certain CSFs and sensitive to others. With exposure to a pathogen (e.g., bacteria, virus-infected cells), T cells activate and produce IL-3 and GM-CSF, whereas activated macrophages produce M-CSF, G-CSF, and GM-CSF. Activated macrophages also produce IL-1 and TNF, which stimulate production of GM-CSF, G-CSF, and M-CSF by endothelial and mesenchymal cells. In this manner, the host produces more granulocytes and macrophages to combat the invading organism (Fig. 53-10).

IFN-α is used in treatment of viral infections (α2b, α2a, αcon1, αn3) and treatment of tumors (α2b, α2a). These actions are attributed to direct inhibition of viral replication in host cells and inhibition of tumor cell proliferation. Inhibition of viral replication may result from induction of an enzyme that inhibits viral replication by catalyzing the breakdown of viral RNA. Anti-tumor actions appear to result from reduced oncogene expression. Both anti-viral and anti-tumor actions may also be indirectly attributed to effects on innate and acquired immune responses. IFN-α activates natural killer cells to kill viral-infected and tumor cells and stimulates upregulation of MHC Class I expression. Class I MHCs present antigen to CD8$^+$ cytotoxic T cells that will also kill viral-infected cells and tumor cells.

IFN-γ stimulates the immune response by induction of MHC expression on dendritic cells, macrophages, and B cells, resulting in an increased ability to present antigen. Macrophages are activated by IFN-γ to increase hydrogen peroxide production, phagocytosis, and expression of Fc receptors and thereby enhance their cytocidal action. These effects are greater than those obtainable with IFN-β or IFN-α. IFN-γ also activates natural killer cells to destroy virus-infected and neoplastic cells. Thus, in contrast to type I IFNs, IFN-γ is a pro-inflammatory cytokine that helps drive cell-mediated immune responses.

A summary of selected biologicals and their targets, actions, and indications are listed in Table 53-2.

Table 53-2 Selected biologicals

Category	Generic Name	Compound Type	Target/Factor	Action	Approved Indications
IMMUNOSUPPRESSIVE	muromonab-CD3	Mab (murine)	CD3 receptor	Depletes T lymphocytes	Organ transplantation
	basiliximab	Mab (chimeric)	IL-2 receptor α chain (CD25)	Blocks IL-2 binding to receptor	Organ transplantation
	daclizumab	Mab (human)	IL-2 receptor α chain (CD25)	Blocks IL-2 binding to receptor	Organ transplantation
	anti-thymocyte globulin	rabbit anti-sera	T cell antigens	Depletes T lymphocytes	Organ transplantation
	alefacept	dimeric fusion protein	CD2/LFA3 interaction	Inhibits lymphocyte activation	Psoriasis
IMMUNOSUPPRESSIVE/ ANTIINFLAMMATORY	etanercept	dimeric fusion protein	TNF-α, TNF-β	Binds circulating TNF	Rheumatoid arthritis Psoriatic arthritis Ankylosing spondylitis
	infliximab	Mab (chimeric)	TNF-α	Binds circulating TNF	Rheumatoid arthritis Crohn's disease
	adalimumab	Mab (human)	TNF-α	Binds circulating TNF	Rheumatoid arthritis
	anakinra	recombinant receptor antagonist	IL-1 receptor antagonist	Competitively inhibits IL-1 binding to IL-1 receptor	Rheumatoid arthritis
ANTI-ALLERGY	omalizumab	Mab (human)	IgE	Binds circulating IgE	Asthma
IMMUNOMODULATORY/ IMMUNOSUPPRESSIVE	interferon-β1a	recombinant cytokine	IFNβ1a	Unclear immunomodulation mechanisms	Multiple sclerosis
	interferon-β1b	recombinant cytokine	IFNβ1b	Unclear immunomodulation mechanisms	Multiple sclerosis
IMMUNOSTIMULATORY	aldesleukin	recombinant cytokine	IL-2	Enhanced immune function and killing of tumor cells	Renal cell carcinoma Melanoma
	interferon-α2b	recombinant cytokine	IFNα2b	Immunomodulation, direct antiproliferative (certain tumors), antiviral	Hairy cell leukemia Melanoma Follicular lymphoma Condylomata acuminata Kaposi's sarcoma Chronic hepatitis C and B
	interferon-α2A	recombinant cytokine	IFNα2a	Immunomodulation, direct antiproliferative (certain tumors), antiviral	Hairy cell leukemia Kaposi's sarcoma, Chronic hepatitis C
	interferon-αcon-1	recombinant cytokine	IFNα	Antiviral, antiproliferative, and immunomodulatory	Chronic hepatitis C
	interferon-αn3	purified cytokine	IFNα	Antiviral, antiproliferative, and immunomodulatory	Condylomata acuminata
	interferon-γ1B	recombinant cytokine	IFNγ	Phagocyte activation	Chronic granulomatous disease Malignant osteopetrosis

Continued

Table 53-2 Selected biologicals—cont'd

Category	Generic Name	Compound Type	Target/Factor	Action	Approved Indications
GROWTH FACTORS	sargramostim	recombinant cytokine	GM-CSF	Induces proliferation and differentiation of progenitor cells in the granulocyte-macrophage pathways	Bone marrow transplantation
	filgrastim	recombinant cytokine	G-CSF	Regulate production and function of neutrophils in the bone marrow	Cancer patients receiving chemotherapy
	pegfilgrastim	pegylated recombinant cytokine	G-CSF	Regulate production and function of neutrophils in the bone marrow	To decrease infection associated with chemotherapy
	oprelvekin	recombinant cytokine	interleukin-11	Stimulation of megakaryocytopoiesis and thrombopoiesis	Prevention of chemotherapy associated thrombocytopenia

Mab, Monoclonal antibody.

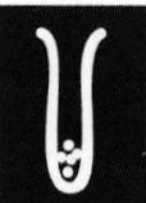

Pharmacokinetics

Many immunopharmacological agents have relatively narrow therapeutic indices and are often used in combination. Therefore the combined toxicity and the effect of drug-drug interactions must be considered in choosing a safe and effective dosing regimen. In addition, biologicals have unique pharmacokinetics that greatly affect their use. Pharmacokinetic parameters for selected drugs are shown in Table 53-3. Because of their unique properties, little information is available about many biologicals.

Table 53-3 Selected pharmacokinetic parameters

Drug	Route	Half-Life (hrs)	Disposition
LOW MOLECULAR WEIGHT DRUGS			
Azathioprine	IV, oral	5-6 hrs	M*
Mycophenolate mofetil	IV, oral	17 hrs	M*
Cyclosporine	IV, oral	10-40 hrs	M
Tacrolimus	IV, oral	12 hrs	M
ANTIBODIES			
Basiliximab	IV	7-13 days	
Daclizumab	IV	11-38 days	
Infliximab	IV	8-10 days	
Adalimumab	SC	12-13 days	

M, Metabolized.
*Active metabolite.

Low molecular weight drugs

Glucocorticoids are summarized in Chapter 33, while cyclophosphamide and methotrexate are discussed in Chapter 42. Methotrexate is used at low oral doses to treat chronic autoimmune diseases. Azathioprine is usually given IV as a loading dose on the day of transplantation, with subsequent oral maintenance doses. It is rapidly absorbed and converted to 6-mercaptopurine, which is the active drug. Most metabolites are excreted in urine. One pathway of metabolism of 6-mercaptopurine involves oxidation by xanthine oxidase, which is inhibited by allopurinol. Therefore, coadministration of these drugs requires a dose adjustment.

Mycophenolate mofetil is rapidly metabolized to the active metabolite, mycophenolic acid. The mofetil moiety dramatically increases bioavailability. Most plasma mycophenolic acid is bound to serum albumin and is primarily excreted in the kidney as the glucuronide conjugate.

Cyclosporine is poorly absorbed from the small intestine (bioavailability of ~30%) and is dependent on biliary flow for absorption. It is metabolized by cytochrome P450 3A, which may cause drug interactions (see Chapter 3). A major constraint in dosing is nephrotoxicity, and owing to high variability in absorption and metabolism, levels fluctuate. Tacrolimus is 10 to 100 times more potent than cyclosporine and does not rely on bile for absorption. It is also metabolized by cytochrome P450 3A, and nephrotoxicity occurs with similar frequencies as with cyclosporine. Blood concentrations for these drugs are monitored to optimize their effects.

Biologicals

Biologicals, such as monoclonal antibodies and cytokines, are administered only by parenteral routes (IV, SC, or IM). The half-life of the compound will depend on its stability and clearance mechanisms. The primary clearance mechanism of proteins less than 70 kilodaltons is via filtration through the kidneys. Larger proteins are cleared by proteases and liver uptake. For human monoclonal antibodies, the half-life is similar to that of normal immunoglobulin (up to 3 weeks).

Since biologicals can be recognized as foreign, an antibody response can develop. This can lead to development of anti-cytokine and anti-monoclonal antibodies that could bind the compound, neutralize its activity, and enhance its clearance by immune complex uptake by the reticuloendothelial system. Given the significance of immune responses on efficacy, pharmacokinetics, and safety, all package inserts of biologicals include a section on drug immunogenicity.

Early monoclonal antibodies were entirely rodent in origin, and immune responses in humans were very robust. The presence of human anti-mouse antibodies led to rapid clearance, resulting in decreased efficacy. Muromonab administration is associated with 80% human anti-mouse antibody formation with a resulting decrease in exposure and efficacy. Simultaneous use of low-dose cyclosporine reduces the frequency to 15%. Chimeric antibodies are produced by combining the human heavy chain constant region sequences to the mouse variable region. Basiliximab is a chimeric antibody with 25% murine content, and daclizumab has a murine content of 10%. The "humanization" of these antibodies results in prolongation of serum half-life. Monoclonal antibodies against TNF-α also induce antibody formation. Infliximab, a chimeric monoclonal antibody, is administered with low-dose methotrexate to decrease antibody formation. More recently, monoclonal antibodies have been designed with almost all or entirely human sequences. However, antibodies can still develop against the variable domain of the human monoclonal antibody. For example, the humanized adalimumab is associated with immune responses.

To increase the half-life of biologicals, polyethylene glycol has been added. Conjugation with polyethylene glycol increases the size and modifies the overall charge to decrease glomerular filtration. In addition, it is thought to decrease immunogenicity by masking antigenic sites. IFN-α2b (peginterferon α2b) and G-CSF (pegfilgrastim) have been conjugated to enhance pharmacokinetic properties. For example, the serum half-life of IFN-α2b is increased from 7 to 9 hours to 40 hours after conjugation with polyethylene glycol.

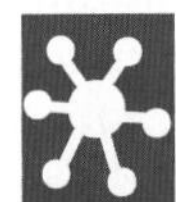

Relation of mechanisms of action to clinical response

Immunosuppression

Graft rejection Genetically coded antigens are the determining factor in rejection of a graft by the host. Most human studies of transplant rejection involve renal allografts. Rejection processes can be classified according to how quickly they occur. **Hyperacute** rejection can occur within minutes and is mediated by cytotoxic antibodies already circulating in the host because of prior exposure to graft antigens. Cytotoxic antibodies to type ABO blood group antigens may mediate rejection in a mismatch. **Accelerated** rejection occurs in 2 to 5 days, with the mechanism being an accelerated form of the acute process, again mediated by prior exposure to graft antigens (secondary immune response). **Acute** rejection occurs over 7 to 21 days and is mediated by a primary response that requires effector cells to be generated. **Chronic** rejection occurs after about 3 months. The immune process of graft rejection is divided into afferent and efferent stages.

In the **afferent stage** the response is initiated by graft cells possessing MHC class II antigens (bone marrow–derived dendritic cells, Langerhans cells, certain endothelial cells) that are incompatible with the host. These cells, termed passenger cells, drain into the host lymphatics and directly stimulate T cells without the need for host APCs. Contact between circulating T cells and special antigens may also occur in the graft. It is known that tissues containing a greater burden of passenger cells are more likely to be rejected (e.g., skin and bone marrow). In addition, removal of passenger cells before transplantation dramatically decreases rejection.

The **efferent stage** involves activation of macrophages and T cells by various effector mechanisms to destroy the graft: antibody, CTLs, and delayed hypersensitivity. Common to all three responses is the involvement of Th cells. Special antigens on the graft can activate Th cells and the production of cytokines, which stimulate activation, proliferation, and growth of T and B lymphocytes and macrophages. In the delayed-type hypersensitivity response, Th cell–produced cytokines activate and recruit monocytes to the graft. These activated macrophages nonspecifically destroy surrounding tissue.

Autoimmune diseases The immune system selectively destroys infectious microbes and tumor cells through its ability to mount a response to foreign antigens while ignoring self-antigens. It is thought that the deletion or deactivation of autoreactive lymphocytes occurs during their early development in the bone marrow or thymus, or that they are functionally silenced in the circulation by regulatory cells or other external factors. If this finely regulated system malfunctions, an immune response against one's own tissue, or an **autoimmune disease**, may develop. Autoimmune diseases may be broadly categorized as either organ specific or systemic. In **organ-specific** diseases, immune responses are mounted against antigens specific to a certain organ, with manifestations specific to that organ. Examples of organ-specific diseases and the possible targets of the immune response include Hashimoto's thyroiditis (thyroid antigens), myasthenia gravis (acetylcholine receptor), Graves' disease (thyroid-stimulating hormone receptor), and insulin-dependent diabetes mellitus (pancreatic β cells). In contrast, in **systemic** autoimmunity, immune responses are mounted against tissue components in most cell types (e.g., DNA, cytoskeletal proteins). Systemic lupus erythematosus and rheumatoid arthritis are two examples. The association of several autoimmune disorders in the same individual or in related family members points to common pathogenic mechanisms that may underlie both types of autoimmunity.

The cause of autoimmunity remains unknown, but intrinsic signaling defects in the activated lymphocytes, abnormal presentation of self-antigens, or dysregulation of the immune response by regulatory cells may all be involved. In addition, there is a striking increased susceptibility of most autoimmune diseases in women, suggesting a role for hormonal factors. Despite the different mechanisms, common pathways and cell types involved in the immune response has led to the use of immunosuppressive drugs for treatment.

Immunosuppressive drugs

Glucocorticoids Many synthetic glucocorticoid derivatives (see Chapter 33) are used as immunosuppressive agents. Glucocorticoids are often administered at high doses during acute exacerbations of disease for rapid control, followed by a slow tapering and maintenance on the lowest efficacious dose to minimize toxicity. Glucocorticoids are usually administered with other immunosuppressive agents to treat graft rejection and autoimmune diseases. Many of these combinations result in a synergistic effect. This allows doses of glucocorticoids to be decreased, decreasing the risk of toxicity. Because of their anti-inflammatory actions, glucocorticoids are effective in treatment of immunological problems exacerbated by inflammatory reactions. This is especially evident for topical use of these agents for treatment of dermatological problems such as contact hypersensitivity to poison ivy and atopic dermatitis and in treatment of asthma (see Chapter 34).

Cyclophosphamide is often administered in cases of severe manifestations of autoimmune disease such as lupus nephritis and systemic vasculitides. However, since the discovery of cyclosporine, it is now used much less to prevent rejection of grafts. As with other immunosuppressive drugs, cyclophosphamide is often given in combination with corticosteroids. Because life-threatening toxicities may occur with cyclophosphamide, extreme care should be taken to administer only the minimal dose necessary. Humoral immune responses are more sensitive to cyclophosphamide than are cell-mediated responses. However, at high doses, both arms of the immune response are affected.

Azathioprine is approved for prevention of acute rejection of kidney transplants. Azathioprine is ineffective alone in solid organ transplantation and is commonly used with corticosteroids and cyclosporine in triple-combination therapy. It is also often used in treatment of moderate to severe manifestations of systemic lupus erythematosus and is indicated for rheumatoid arthritis, although not as a first-line treatment. The primary targets of azathioprine are cell-mediated immune responses. Inhibition of the *in vitro* immune responses is maximal during initiation of the response. This time-dependent action is consistent with clinical observations that azathioprine is ineffective against ongoing graft rejection. Additional *in vitro* investigations have revealed that azathioprine primarily affects antigen-stimulated lymphocytes, whereas unstimulated spleen cells are unaffected. Primary immune responses are suppressed by azathioprine, whereas secondary responses are not.

MMF is indicated for prophylaxis against renal transplant rejection and is used in combination with corticosteroids. Like azathioprine, it does not inhibit cytokine production but does inhibit lymphocyte proliferation. It is also gaining wider use in the treatment of systemic lupus erythematosus, given its favorable side effect profile relative to cyclophosphamide.

Although **methotrexate** is a potent immunosuppressive agent, its numerous adverse effects (see Chapter 42) have limited its widespread use in treatment of immune-associated diseases. However, low-dose, weekly administered oral methotrexate is widely used to treat rheumatoid arthritis. It is also used for psoriasis, as well as to reduce required doses of glucocorticoids in chronic vasculitis or conditions that require prolonged periods of immunosuppression.

The objective of immunosuppressive therapy is to specifically inhibit the immune response against the graft or autoantigen. However, drugs that also affect proliferating cell populations such as cyclophosphamide, azathioprine, and methotrexate may produce life-threatening bone marrow suppression. Until the early 1980s, the use of these drugs in combination with corticosteroids was the preferred therapy. They have now been largely supplanted by **cyclosporine,** which usually is effective in preventing acute graft rejection (during the first 3 weeks), generally without bone marrow toxicity. Cyclosporine is also used in patients with rheumatoid arthritis unresponsive to other therapies, as well as certain types of lupus nephritis.

Tacrolimus is indicated for prevention of acute rejection of liver transplants. Although tacrolimus and cyclosporine have similar mechanisms of action, tacrolimus has been found effective in reversing liver transplant rejection resistant to cyclosporine. It is recommended that corticosteroids be given with tacrolimus.

Rapamycin is indicated for prevention of acute organ rejection in combination with the calcineurin inhibitors. Its main role may be to allow for lower doses of cyclosporine or tacrolimus to be used to decrease toxicity.

Muromonab is used to reverse acute allograft rejection in patients receiving other immunosuppressive drugs (rescue therapy) and to prevent acute graft rejections (induction therapy). Because of its relatively greater toxicity, and because it has not demonstrated significant benefits relative to calcineurin inhibitors as induction therapy, it is usually reserved for patients with severe steroid-resistant rejection. Rescue therapy is followed by administration of other immunosuppressants. Its usefulness in rescue therapy stems from its ability to immediately reduce the number of circulating T lymphocytes. Because it is a murine monoclonal antibody, neutralizing antibodies usually develop in patients after 10 days. However, this rarely results in allergic or anaphylactic reactions. When it is given with prednisone and azathioprine, the development of neutralizing antibodies is reduced.

IL-2 receptor antagonists such as **basiliximab** and **daclizumab** are indicated for prevention of acute organ rejection in patients receiving renal transplants. They have demonstrated efficacy when used in combination with cyclosporine and corticosteroids. Although long-term studies are not yet available, they should allow less-toxic doses to be used.

The relative safety, early onset of symptom relief, and efficacy in rheumatoid arthritis patients who fail to respond to methotrexate have made **anti-TNF biologicals** an increasingly valuable class of agents for several autoimmune diseases. **Etanercept** is indicated for treatment of rheumatoid arthritis as well as psoriatic arthritis and ankylosing spondylitis. **Infliximab** was first approved for Crohn's disease and is also indicated for rheumatoid arthritis. **Adalimumab,** the most recently approved anti-TNF monoclonal antibody, is indicated for rheumatoid arthritis.

IFN-α and IFN-β were originally proposed as therapeutics for MS, based on the belief that viral infections and low interferon production contribute to its pathogenesis. Through many years of clinical study, β-IFNs (β1a and 1b) were found to be efficacious and are marketed for treatment of relapsing forms of MS to decrease the frequency of clinical exacerbations and delay physical disability.

Omalizumab is used for treatment of patients with asthma that are not adequately controlled by inhaled corticosteroids and with demonstrated sensitivity to aeroallergens. GA is approved for use in the reduction of the frequency of relapses in patients with relapsing-remitting multiple sclerosis.

Immunostimulant drugs

IL-2 is approved for metastatic renal carcinoma and melanoma. The mechanism of action may be related to increased killing of tumor cells by immune-mediated mechanisms.

Sargramostim, a recombinant human GM-CSF, is used to stimulate bone marrow growth in patients undergoing bone marrow transplantation. **Filgrastim** is a recombinant human G-CSF used in patients undergoing myelosuppressive chemotherapy. G-CSF conjugated to polyethylene glycol (**pegfilgrastim**) is approved for the same indications as filgrastim but has a longer half-life and requires less-frequent administration. Human recombinant IL-11 (**oprelvekin**) is also available for treatment of severe thrombocytopenia produced by myelosuppressive therapy of non-myeloid malignancies. IL-11 works in concert with IL-4 and IL-3 to stimulate hematopoiesis. Therapy with CSFs has been found to be useful in dramatically increasing levels of neutrophils, eosinophils, and monocytes with minimal side effects. It also decreases the time it takes for engraftment to occur, the need for antibiotics, and the incidence of infections in bone marrow transplant recipients.

Recombinant human IFN-α (2a or 2b) is marketed for treatment of hepatitis C, hairy cell leukemia, and

AIDS-related Kaposi's sarcoma. IFN-α2b is also indicated for chronic hepatitis B, malignant melanoma, follicular lymphoma, and condylomata acuminata (genital warts associated with human papilloma virus). Two additional α IFNs are also marketed, IFN-αcon1 (for chronic hepatitis C) and -αn3 (for condylomata acuminata). The antitumor and antiviral effects are mediated through a direct effect on tumor and viral infected cells and through stimulation of immune responses. A polyethylene glycol conjugate of IFN-α2a (peginterferon α2a) was also developed to increase its half-life.

IFN-γ is approved for treatment and prophylaxis of infections associated with chronic granulomatous diseases and severe malignant osteopetrosis. Chronic granulomatous disease is an inherited deficiency in oxidative metabolism by phagocytes that limits their ability to kill intracellular bacterial infections. Osteopetrosis is an inherited disease in which osteoclasts are unable to resorb bone, resulting in abnormal bone accumulation. IFN-γ activates macrophages and osteoclasts to increase superoxide production, leading to killing of intracellular bacteria and decreased rates of infections and reduced trabecular bone volume.

Side effects, clinical problems, and toxicity

Clinical problems associated with the use of these agents are summarized in the Clinical Problems box.

Side effects common to immunosuppressive therapy

Cytotoxic and antimetabolite drugs that inhibit proliferating cells can lead to clinically significant myelosuppression, and severe or prolonged suppression of bone marrow function may predispose a patient to opportunistic infections. Prophylactic therapy with antibacterial and antifungal drugs is therefore commonly instituted in patients receiving cytotoxic agents. Also, anti-CD3 therapy has been found to increase the incidence of cytomegalovirus infections in organ transplant patients, and anti-TNF-α biologicals have been associated with an increased risk of tuberculosis.

Prolonged immunosuppression is associated with an increased risk of lymphoproliferative diseases (e.g.,

CLINICAL PROBLEMS

- Problems common to most immunosuppressive/antiinflammatory agents
  - Increased risk of infections
  - Increased risk of malignancies
- Problems common to many biologicals
  - Flu-like symptoms
  - Immunogenicity/hypersensitivity reactions
  - Injection site reactions
- Cyclophosphamide
  - Myelosuppression
  - Hemorrhagic cystitis
- Methotrexate
  - Liver function abnormalities
  - Bone marrow suppression
  - Nausea
- Azathioprine
  - Bone marrow suppression
- Mycophenolate mofetil
  - Neutropenia
- Cyclosporine
  - Nephrotoxicity (reduced glomerular filtration)
  - Hypertension
  - Hepatotoxicity (cholestasis)
  - Neurotoxicity
  - Hypersensitivity to vehicle
- Tacrolimus
  - Nephrotoxicity
  - Hepatotoxicity
  - Neurotoxicity
- Muromonab
  - Cytokine release syndrome
  - Fluid retention
- Interleukin (IL-2)
  - Capillary leak syndrome
- Interferons (α and β)
  - Depression
  - Suicide ideation
- Filgrastim and pegfilgrastim
  - Spleen rupture
  - Acute respiratory distress syndrome
- Oprelvekin
  - Fluid retention
  - Pulmonary edema

non-Hodgkin's lymphoma) that are associated with Epstein-Barr virus–infected B cells. The mechanism involved is not known.

The side effects of corticosteroids are discussed in Chapter 33 and those of cyclophosphamide and methotrexate in Chapter 42.

Side effects common to cyclosporine and tacrolimus

One of the major advantages of cyclosporine and tacrolimus is their relatively selective effect on Th cells and the absence of myelotoxicity. However, their use is limited by other toxicities. Nephrotoxicity with reduced glomerular filtration is a common and dose-limiting side effect for both agents, with the mechanism unknown. Moderate hypertension is common. Incidences of hepatotoxicity with cholestasis and hyperbilirubinemia are increased in patients receiving cyclosporine. Neurotoxicity, including tremors, is increased in patients taking tacrolimus. Its use has also been associated with post-transplant insulin-dependent diabetes mellitus.

Side effects associated with biologicals

Several biologicals produce acute systemic clinical syndromes ranging from mild "flu-like" symptoms (fever, chills, myalgia, fatigue, headaches) to severe, life-threatening shock-like reactions that occur minutes to hours after exposure. Although the symptoms are similar, the mechanisms are poorly understood and are likely to be variable and related to the cytokine release syndrome (see below) or hypersensitivity reactions.

Cytokine release syndrome is one of the primary adverse effects with muromonab therapy and includes a wide spectrum of symptoms such as fever, chills, dyspnea, nausea, and vomiting. It is caused by rapid release of TNF-α and IFN-γ into the systemic circulation followed by IL-6 release. This can lead to pulmonary edema and cardiovascular collapse. Although some symptoms may be similar to those observed with anaphylactic reactions, and it may be difficult to differentiate, anaphylactic reactions occur within seconds to minutes, whereas cytokine release syndrome occurs 30 to 60 minutes following infusion. Other biologicals such as anti-thymocyte antibodies, which lead to rapid lysis of immune competent cells, are also associated with this syndrome.

Vascular leak syndrome involves vascular leakage that may lead to serious hypotension and reduced vascular perfusion. This is one of the most serious adverse effects with aldesleukin administration and may be related to endothelial cell activation. Other biologicals have been associated with this syndrome but to a much lesser degree.

Hypersensitivity and **anaphylactic reactions** are issues with all biologicals since there is a potential to induce an immune response. The relative immunogenicity of biologicals varies significantly between drugs and subjects. Although antibody responses may occur in many individuals, they may have no clinical impact. However, rare cases in which specific IgE antibodies are generated may lead to type 1 hypersensitivity reactions. Symptoms of these reactions can range from urticaria and angioedema to severe anaphylaxis. In addition, in individuals with a high anti-biological antibody titer, the rapid administration of biologicals may lead to immune complex formation, complement activation, and systemic cytokine release. Some of the flu-like symptoms discussed above may be attributed to such antibodies. With IV administration, a systemic serum sickness reaction may occur, or a local arthus reaction may occur with SC or IM administration (type 3 hypersensitivity reaction).

Local irritation/inflammation at the site of injection (IM or SC) is common for most biologicals.

Other serious side effects with specific biologicals

IFN-α and IFN-β are known to increase psychiatric disorders such as depression and suicidal ideation, although the mechanism is unknown. Fluid retention and cardiovascular problems have been observed with oprelvekin treatment. With alefacept treatment, dramatic decreases in T cell numbers can be a serious problem. Filgrastim and pegfilgrastim have been associated with adult respiratory distress syndrome and potential spleen rupture.

New horizons

A primary focus of research is to develop drugs that are more **selective** for specific components of the immune system, thereby preventing general immunosuppression and effects on other tissues. Given the severity and frequency of adverse effects associated with current immunosuppressive drugs, there is significant room for improvement, particularly for chronic diseases (e.g., autoimmunity).

Increased understanding of the mechanisms involved in normal and aberrant immune responses, the availability of animal models of immunological diseases, and advances in biotechnology have resulted in development of many new agents. Many are monoclonal antibodies, which exploit their exquisite specificity to deliver clinical efficacy. Some promising approaches include the interruption of CD28/B7 co-stimulatory interactions and inhibition of the action of adhesion molecules. Monoclonal antibodies directed against inflammatory cytokine responses are also showing promise.

A more-selective approach to immunomodulation in the future will involve altering **antigen-specific interactions.** In this manner, immune responses to other antigens will not be compromised. For example, oral administration of autoantigens or foreign-graft antigens has been shown to produce immunological tolerance to those antigens and decrease autoimmune and graft-rejection responses. In the treatment of cancer, tumor-antigen vaccines are being developed as a potential method to stimulate a selective immune response. These approaches will be more difficult to develop but may be more efficacious. Solving problems associated with the delivery, metabolism, and toxicity of these proteins will greatly enhance the potential usefulness of this approach.

The difficulties of manufacturing biologicals and their complex nature have raised concerns about cost, convenience in delivery, and immunogenicity. Traditional small molecule drugs do not typically face such issues, and ongoing research and development is directed at small molecules that interact with extracellular targets such as cytokine receptors and activated complement components as well as intracellular targets such as kinases and caspases.

TRADE NAMES

In addition to generic and fixed-combination preparations and the drugs listed in the Major Drugs box, the following trade-named materials are some of the important compounds available in the United States.

Low molecular weight drugs

Tacrolimus (Prograf)
Sirolimus (rapamycin, Rapamune)

Biologicals

Adalimumab (Humira)
Aldesleukin (IL-2, Proleukin)
Alefacept (Amevive)
Anakinra (Kineret)
Anti-thymocyte globulin (ATG, Thymoglobulin)
Basiliximab (Simulect)
Daclizumab (Zenapax)
Etanercept (Enbrel)
Filgrastim (G-CSF, Neupogen)
Glatiramer acetate (Copaxone)
Infliximab (Remicade)
IFN-α2a (Roferon-A)
IFN-α2b (Intron A)
IFN-αn3 (Alferon N)
IFN-αcon-1 (Infergen)
IFN-β1a (Avonex, Rebif)
IFN-β1b (Betaseron)
IFN-γ1b (Actimmune)
Omalizumab (Xolair)
Muromonab-CD3 (anti-CD3, Orthoclone OKT3)
Oprelvekin (IL-11, Neumega)
Pegfilgrastim (G-CSF, Neulasta)
Sargramostim (GM-CSF, Leukine)

FURTHER READING

Loertscher R. The utility of monoclonal antibody therapy in renal transplantation. *Transplant Proceed* 2002; 34:797-800.

Janeway CA Jr, Travers P, Walport M, et al. *Immunobiology. The immune system in health and disease,* ed 5, New York, Garland Publishing, 2001.

Noseworthy JH, Lucchinetti C, Rodriguez M, et al. Multiple sclerosis. *N Engl J Med* 2000; 343:938-952.

Self-assessment questions

1. Corticosteroids are utilized extensively in the treatment of autoimmune disease and in the prevention of graft rejection for the following reason or reasons:

a. Corticosteroids alkylate DNA and inhibit the proliferation of B cells.
b. Corticosteroids are also effective antiinflammatory agents.
c. Corticosteroids stimulate cytokine production.
d. Corticosteroids inhibit purine biosynthesis.
e. b and c

2. Cyclosporine is considered one of the more selective immunosuppressive agents for the following reason:

a. It alkylates DNA and inhibits B-cell proliferation.
b. It specifically inactivates lymphocytes by binding to CD3 surface antigens on T cells.
c. It specifically inhibits hypoxanthine-guanine phosphoribosyltransferase activity in T cells.
d. It specifically inhibits production of cytokines by T lymphocytes.
e. It specifically inhibits production of IL-1.

3. Which of the following immunosuppressive drugs is *not* correctly matched to its toxicity?

a. Anti-CD3 monoclonal antibodies: flu-like symptoms
b. Cyclosporine: bone marrow depression
c. Corticosteroids: electrolyte imbalance
d. Azathioprine: predisposition to opportunistic infections
e. Cyclophosphamide: myelosuppression

4. Cyclosporine prevents graft rejection by:

a. Selectively enhancing B-lymphocyte production of antibody.
b. Inhibiting cytotoxic T-lymphocyte responses.
c. Inhibiting graft cell proliferation.
d. Inhibiting innate immune responses.
e. Selectively depleting CD3-bearing T lymphocytes.

CHAPTER 54

Histamine and antihistamines

Jeffrey R. Martens

Major Drugs

First-generation (sedating)	Second-generation (non-sedating)
Chlorpheniramine (Chlor-Trimeton, Teldrin)	Cetirizine (Zyrtec)
Diphenhydramine (Benadryl)	Desloratadine (Clarinex)
Promethazine (Phenameth, Phenergan)	Fexofenadine (Allegra)
	Loratadine (Claritin)

Therapeutic overview

Histamine is synthesized, stored, and released primarily by **mast cells** and has profound effects on many organs. It is an important mediator of immediate **hypersensitivity reactions** and acute **inflammatory responses** and is a primary stimulator of **gastric acid secretion.** It is also an important neurotransmitter in the central nervous system (CNS) (see Chapter 20).

Histamine's many undesirable effects preclude its use as a drug. However, drugs that block histamine receptors or prevent its release from mast cells have important clinical uses.

The administration of histamine to humans produces many effects, primarily on heart, vascular, and nonvascular smooth muscle and on the secretion of gastric acid. These actions are mediated by at least three distinct receptors: H_1, H_2, and H_3. A fourth histamine receptor (H_4) was identified following the sequencing of the human genome, but as yet little is known about it.

H_1 and H_2 receptors have been most widely characterized and mediate well-defined responses in humans, as summarized in Table 54-1. Most responses are mediated by H_1 receptors, such as bronchoconstriction, and are selectively antagonized by classical **antihistamines.** These are more accurately described as selective H_1-receptor blocking drugs such as **diphenhydramine.** Antihistamines are widely used to treat allergic reactions, motion sickness, and emesis and as over-the-counter sleeping aids. H_2-mediated responses such as gastric acid secretion are selectively antagonized by specific H_2-receptor blocking drugs such as **cimetidine.** The H_2-receptor antagonists are discussed extensively in Chapter 55; this chapter focuses on histamine and H_1-receptor blockers.

H_3 receptors have so far been studied mainly in animals, where they are found on nerve endings and mediate the inhibition of transmitter release. This receptor remains an attractive target for drug development, as discussed below.

Clinical uses of histamine and its antagonists are summarized in the Therapeutic Overview box.

Abbreviations

CNS	central nervous system
IgE	immunoglobulin E

Table 54-1 Histamine receptor subtypes mediating selected responses in humans

Subtype	Responses
H_1 only	Basilar, pulmonary, coronary artery constriction; increased permeability of postcapillary venules; contraction of bronchiolar smooth muscle; stimulation of vagal sensory nerve endings promoting bronchospasm and coughing; gastrointestinal smooth muscle relaxation and contraction; epinephrine release from adrenal medulla
H_2 only	Acid and pepsin secretion from oxyntic mucosa; facial cutaneous vasodilation; pulmonary and carotid artery relaxation; increased rate and force of cardiac contraction; relaxation of bronchial smooth muscle; inhibition of IgE dependent degranulation of basophils
H_1 and H_2 (?)	Decreased total peripheral resistance; increased forearm blood flow; increased cardiac atrial and ventricular automaticity; stimulation of cutaneous nerve endings causing pain and itching

THERAPEUTIC OVERVIEW

Histamine and histamine receptor agonists

No significant clinical uses

Antihistamines (H_1-receptor antagonists)

Allergic reactions
Motion sickness
Insomnia
Nausea and vomiting

H_2-receptor antagonists

Peptic ulcers and gastroesophageal reflux disease (Chapter 55)

Mechanisms of action

Synthesis and metabolism of histamine

Histamine is synthesized by decarboxylation of the amino acid L-histidine by histidine decarboxylase (Fig. 54-1). Most histamine is stored in an inert form at its site of synthesis, and very little exists in a freely diffusible form. Following synthesis and release from its storage sites, histamine acts at its targets and is rapidly metabolized through two primary pathways (see Fig. 54-1). Oxidative deamination leads to formation of imidazole acetic acid, while methylation, which predominates in the brain, is mediated by histamine-*N*-methyltransferase. Both metabolites are inactive and subject to further biotransformation (see Fig. 54-1).

Storage and release of histamine by mast cells and basophils

Histamine is stored and released primarily by mast cells. Although basophils and central neurons also contribute, their role is not fully understood. Histamine is widely distributed, with the highest concentrations in the skin, lungs, and gastrointestinal tract mucosa, consistent with mast cell densities in these tissues.

Mast cells and basophils have high-affinity **IgE-binding sites** on their surface membranes and store histamine in secretory granules. Different types of mast cells can be classified by their staining properties, anatomical locations, or susceptibility to degranulation by polyamines. Anatomically, mast cells are classified as being of mucosal or connective tissue origin. However, there are mixed populations in both tissues and additional heterogeneity within these two classes. Human mast cells differ with respect to their proteoglycan structure and content, the types of serine proteases in their storage granules, the eicosanoids synthesized and released on degranulation, and the extent to which degranulation is inhibited by cromolyn sodium.

Histamine in mast cell granules exists as an **ionic complex** with a proteoglycan, chiefly **heparin** sulfate, but also chondroitin sulfate E. Histamine in basophils is also stored in granules as an ionic complex, predominantly with proteoglycans. The release of histamine and other mediators from mast cells and basophils is common during allergic reactions but also can be induced by drugs and endogenous compounds to produce pseudoallergic, anaphylactoid reactions as shown in Figure 54-2. The role of mast cells in immediate and delayed hypersensitivity reactions and nonallergic disorders explains the therapeutic utility of antihistamines and degranulation inhibitors.

Histamine is released by noncytolytic or cytolytic **degranulation. Cytolytic** release occurs when the membrane is damaged, does not require energy or intracellular Ca^{2+}, and is accompanied by leakage of cytoplasmic contents. Cytolytic release can be induced by drugs such as phenothiazines, H_1-receptor antagonists, and opioids (see Chapter 31). However, the concentrations required are usually greater than therapeutic concentrations.

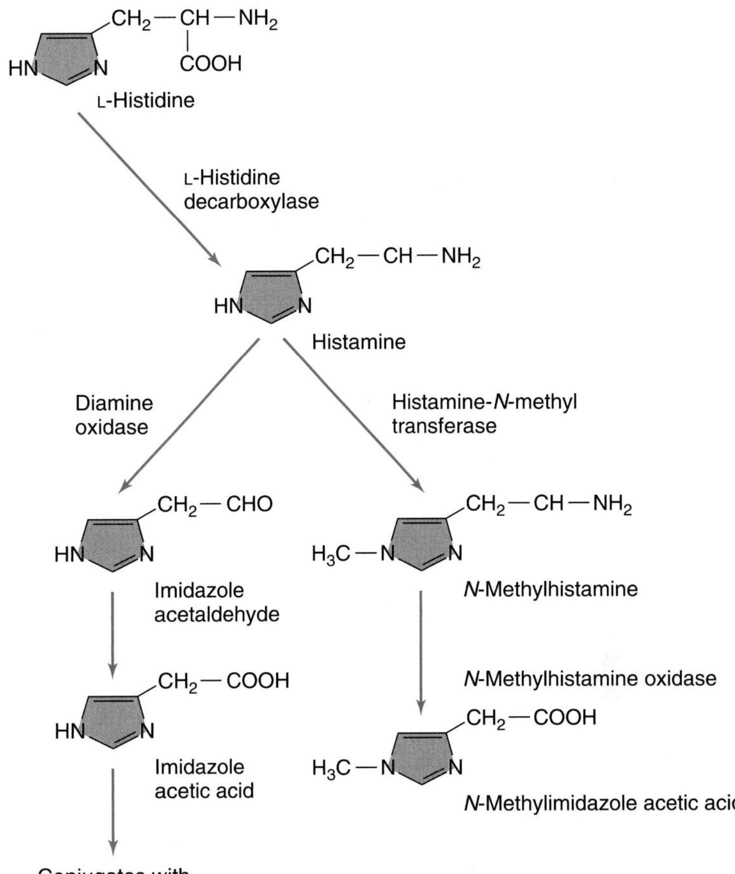

Figure 54-1 Synthesis and metabolism of histamine.

Noncytolytic release is evoked by binding of a specific ligand to a receptor in the plasma membrane, resulting in **exocytosis** of secretory granules. Noncytolytic release requires energy, depends on intracellular Ca^{2+}, and is not accompanied by leakage of cytoplasmic contents. A classic example is degranulation of sensitized mast cells or basophils induced by cross-bridging of adjacent IgE molecules on the cell surface. This involves activation of various phospholipases, fusion of secretory granules with the plasma membrane, and extrusion of their contents. Such exocytosis results in the release of histamine, heparin, eosinophil, and neutrophil chemotactic factors; neutral proteases; and other enzymes. The release of other mediators, such as eicosanoids and platelet-activating factor, can also occur.

Noncytolytic release can also be produced by other mechanisms, often by highly basic substances. These include the polyamine compound 48/80, polypeptides such as bradykinin, substance P, formylmethionylleucinylphenylalanine, protamine, anaphylatoxins, and a protein present in bee venom. With the exception of **protamine**, a heparin antagonist, none of these agents has any therapeutic use, but they are probably important in pathological responses.

Noncytolytic degranulation can also be induced by several drugs, including D-tubocurarine, succinylcholine, morphine, codeine, doxorubicin, and vancomycin (see Chapters 29, 31, 42, and 45). Histamine release in vivo may also be produced by some plasma expanders, notably those based on cross-linked gelatin, and by radiocontrast media, especially those of high osmotic strength. Intravenous administration of these compounds is most likely to result in histamine release. Life-threatening reactions are rare but occur occasionally.

The most acute and potentially severe allergic reaction is **anaphylaxis.** In both animals and humans, parenterally administered histamine triggers responses that mimic the early responses of anaphylaxis, including hypotension, vasodilation, myocardial depression, dysrhythmias, urticaria, angioedema, and bronchospasm. These can be partially reversed by H_1 and H_2 antagonists; however they are most effective when administered prophylactically rather than after an acute reaction has begun. Histamine is only one of many

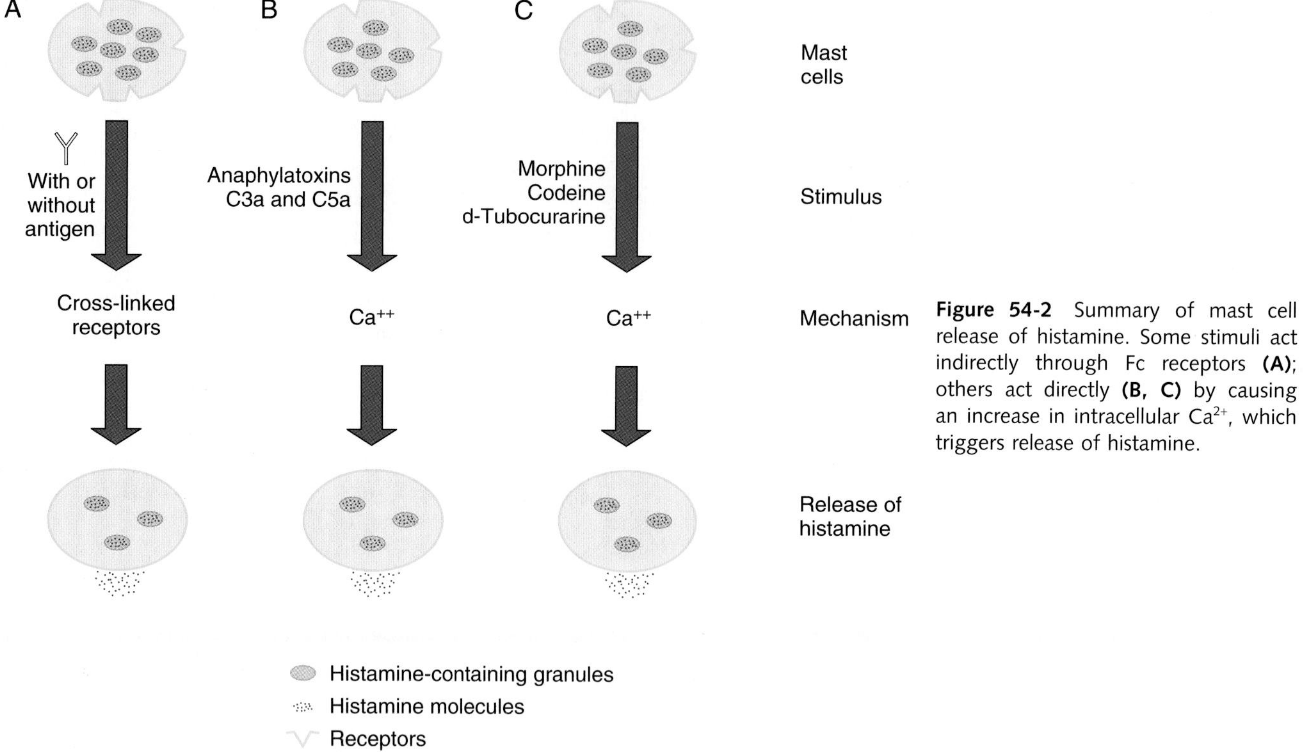

Figure 54-2 Summary of mast cell release of histamine. Some stimuli act indirectly through Fc receptors **(A)**; others act directly **(B, C)** by causing an increase in intracellular Ca^{2+}, which triggers release of histamine.

anaphylactic mediators, but it has important effects on the production and effectiveness of others.

Noncytolytic degranulation of mast cells results in both anaphylactic and anaphylactoid reactions. Many substances can release histamine independently of IgE. However, the clinical signs and symptoms are indistinguishable from those of true anaphylaxis, because the same mediators are involved. The term **anaphylactoid** is used to refer to a clinical syndrome indistinguishable from anaphylaxis but caused by something other than an immune response.

Many of the solutions and drugs used in **general anesthesia** can produce mast cell degranulation, especially if administered intravenously. However, skeletal muscle paralysis, the effects of other drugs, and mechanical ventilation can mask signs of histamine release. Cardiac dysrhythmias or hypotension without flush, rashes, or angioedema may be seen. Indeed, most patients undergoing general anesthesia have elevated histamine levels but are relatively asymptomatic. Preoperative prophylaxis with H_1 and H_2 receptor antagonists remains controversial but is used for certain patients at risk (atopic patients and patients with previous reactions).

A summary of agents that release histamine is presented in Table 54-2. Histamine concentrations of 0.2 to 1.0 ng/ml in humans produce mild signs and symptoms, including metallic taste, headache, and nasal congestion. Concentrations exceeding 1 ng/ml produce moderate effects, including skin reactions, cramping, diarrhea, flushing, tachycardia, cardiac dysrhythmias, and hypotension. Life-threatening hypotension, ventricular fibrillation, and bronchospasm leading to

Table 54-2 Common causal factors involved in anaphylactic and anaphylactoid reactions

IgE-Mediated Anaphylaxis	Non–IgE-Mediated Anaphylactoid Reactions
FOOD	**DRUGS**
Peanuts, seafood, eggs, milk products, grains	Anesthesia related: neuromuscular blocking agents, opioids, plasma expanders
DRUGS	Antibiotics: vancomycin
Antibiotics: penicillins, cephalosporins, sulfonamides	Others: protamine
VENOMS	**DYES**
Hymenoptera, fire ants, snakes	Radiocontrast media, fluorescein
FOREIGN PROTEINS	**OTHER IDIOPATHIC REACTIONS**
Nonhuman insulin, corticotropin, serum proteins, seminal proteins, vaccines, antivenoms	Some cases of exercise-induced bronchospasm
ENZYMES	Urticaria related to cold, heat, sunlight, and other physical factors
Chymopapain	
OTHER	
Some cases of exercise-induced bronchospasm	

cardiopulmonary arrest can occur when concentrations approach 12 ng/ml.

Inhibitors of degranulation and histamine release

Because many mediators are released from mast cells and basophils during noncytolytic degranulation, agents that can prevent this reaction are of therapeutic value. **Cromolyn sodium** is used to treat asthma and bronchospastic diseases and is discussed in Chapter 34.

H_1 receptor antagonists

Antihistamines are selective H_1 receptor antagonists. Before the development of antihistamines, histamine was thought to be the primary mediator of immediate hypersensitivity reactions. Although early H_1 antagonists could reverse histamine-induced hypotension and bronchoconstriction, they were not very effective in the management of global anaphylaxis, probably because of the involvement of other mediators. Also, the inability of H_1 antagonists to block the effects of histamine on cardiovascular H_2 receptors limited their effectiveness.

H_1 antagonists have little structural resemblance to histamine (Figs. 54-1 and 54-3). A common feature, however, is a substituted ethylamine containing a nitrogen atom in an alkyl chain or ring. H_1 antagonists are classified by the chemical group containing the substituted ethylamine.

All currently available antihistamines share the common property of **competitively blocking** H_1 receptors. Terfenadine and astemizole are exceptions but were withdrawn from the U.S. market because of serious side effects. Differences between the many available compounds are due to their pharmacokinetic properties and specific adverse reactions. Since a major clinical problem with the use of early antihistamines was their marked sedative effects, many compounds were subsequently developed that did not easily enter the brain. Differences in their abilities to cross the blood-brain barrier are the basis for classification as **first-generation** (sedating) or **second-generation** (nonsedating) drugs.

Other antiallergic properties of antihistamines

Antihistamines also have important actions at receptors other than H_1 receptors. Many first-generation antihistamines also block muscarinic cholinergic, dopamine, α_1-adrenergic, and serotonin receptors. For example, azatadine is a fairly potent antagonist of serotonin, and promethazine exhibits weak α_1-adrenergic and moderate D_2 receptor blocking activity. Antihistamines also inhibit mediator release, basophil migration, and eosinophil recruitment, which can contribute to their antiallergy effects through poorly understood mechanisms.

Other effects have also been observed for second-generation antihistamines, including inhibition of allergen-induced migration of eosinophils, basophils, and neutrophils and an inhibition of platelet-activating factor–induced eosinophil accumulation in skin. The clinical significance of these effects remains to be established.

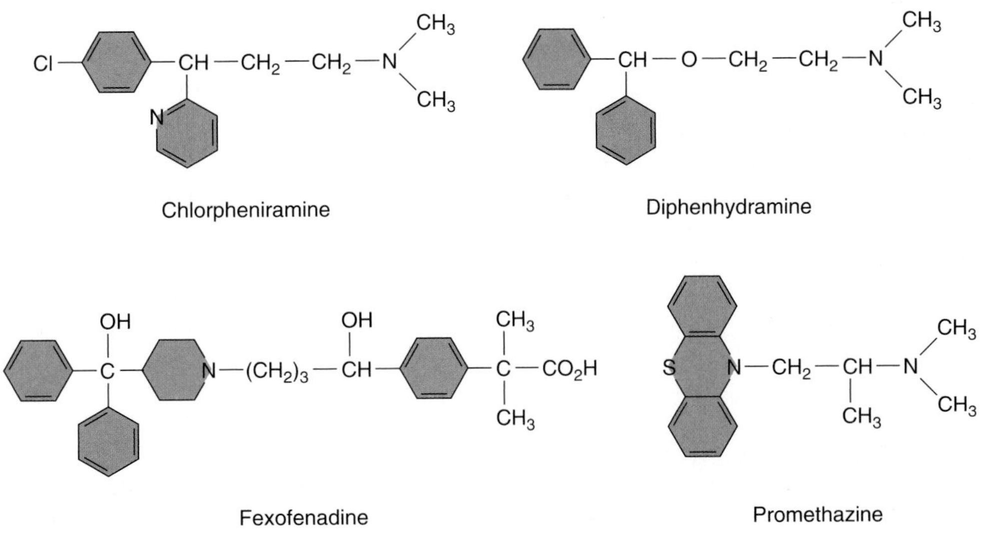

Chlorpheniramine

Diphenhydramine

Fexofenadine

Promethazine

Figure 54-3 Structures of selected H_1 receptor antagonists.

Pharmacokinetics

The pharmacokinetic parameters of selected H_1 receptor antagonists are given in Table 54-3. Those of cromolyn are presented in Chapter 34, and those of H_2 receptor antagonists are presented in Chapter 55.

H_1 antagonists are all well absorbed after oral administration and have onsets of action of about 30 to 60 minutes. All have good bioavailability, and most have a duration of action between 3 and 6 hours; however, several others have much longer durations of action. In terms of distribution, first-generation antihistamines distribute throughout the body and readily penetrate the CNS. By design, second-generation antihistamines—such as fexofenadine, loratadine, and desloratadine—do not readily penetrate the CNS and are much less sedative.

All antihistamines are extensively metabolized by the liver, and metabolites are eliminated by renal excretion. Some are substrates for monoamine oxidase. They often induce hepatic cytochrome P450 enzymes and may facilitate their own metabolism or that of other drugs. Their actions and/or toxicities can be enhanced in patients with hepatic failure.

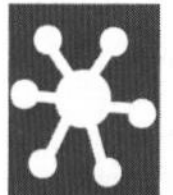

Relation of mechanisms of action to clinical response

Actions of histamine

Vascular system The effects of histamine on the systemic vasculature are complex, and different vascular beds show different responses (see Table 54-1). The predominant action is vasodilation resulting from relaxation of arteriolar smooth muscle, precapillary sphincters, and muscular venules mediated by H_1 and H_2 receptors. Vasodilation produced by H_1 receptors occurs at lower doses and is transient, while that caused by H_2 receptors occurs at higher doses and is sustained. Both H_1 and H_2 antagonists are required to completely block the hypotensive response.

Histamine also acts at H_1 receptors on endothelial cells in postcapillary venules to cause endothelial cells to contract and expose permeable basement membranes. This results in edema from the buildup of fluid and plasma protein in the surrounding tissue.

A summary of the actions of histamine on the vasculature is seen in the **triple response of Lewis** that occurs after intradermal injection. Initially a small red spot is produced at the site of injection that then is slowly surrounded by a flushed area. In a few minutes a wheal appears at the site of the original red spot. The red spot and the erythema are caused by vasodilation, with the red spot resulting from the direct actions of histamine on the cutaneous vasculature and the erythema from axon reflexes that produce vasodilation. These responses are mediated by H_1 and H_2 receptors, with H_1 receptors predominating. The wheal results from edema. Intradermal histamine also stimulates nerve endings to produce pain and itching. These local reactions represent a microcosm of the systemic effects of large doses of histamine that cause cardiovascular shock.

Heart Histamine exerts direct and indirect actions on the human heart. Indirectly it accelerates rate and increases force of contraction because of a baroreceptor-mediated increase in sympathetic tone in response to systemic vasodilation. Direct actions on the heart are mediated primarily by H_2 receptors and include increases in rate, atrial and ventricular automaticity, and contractile force. Modest tachycardia occurs at doses of histamine that produce little change in systemic pressure, while low doses cause primarily indirect actions that are due to systemic vasodilation.

Respiratory system Histamine causes bronchoconstriction in humans following inhalation or intravenous injection through activation of H_1 receptors. Normally, histamine is not especially potent; however, patients with asthma are often hyperreactive and therefore aerosolized histamine has been used as a provocative test for bronchial reactivity.

Histamine may also produce a modest relaxation of contracted bronchial smooth muscle through H_2 receptors, although this is not usually clinically significant. Histamine also acts on H_1 receptors to increase

Table 54-3 Pharmacokinetic parameters of selected H_1 receptor antagonists

Drug	Administered	Half-Life (hrs)	Disposition
Cetirizine	Oral	7-9	R, N
Chlorpheniramine	Oral	~20	M
Desloratadine	Oral	~27	M, N
Diphenhydramine	Oral	4-8	M
Fexofenadine	Oral	14	R, N
Loratadine	Oral	2-15	M, A, N
Promethazine	Oral	7-15	M

M, Metabolism; *A*, Active metabolite that contributes to therapeutic effect; *N*, Non-sedating; *R*, Renal elimination.

secretion of airway fluid and electrolytes, which may produce pulmonary edema and contribute to bronchial obstruction in patients with extrinsic asthma (Chapter 34).

Gastrointestinal system An important physiological function of histamine is its role as a primary mediator in the secretion of gastric acid, discussed in Chapter 55.

Other actions Headaches, nausea, and vomiting have also been observed in human volunteers receiving histamine. In high doses, histamine stimulates catecholamine release from the adrenal medulla, an effect particularly pronounced in patients with pheochromocytoma.

CNS The role of histamine in the brain is largely inferred from results of studies in experimental animals. Postulated roles include the regulation of temperature, water balance, nociception, blood pressure, and arousal. The role(s) of individual receptor subtypes remain unclear.

Anaphylaxis and anaphylactoid reactions

Histamine is an early mediator in anaphylactoid reactions and probably has a permissive effect on the release of other mediators, since antihistamines are far more effective prophylactically than after an inflammatory reaction has begun. Anaphylaxis can result in death from cardiovascular collapse or respiratory obstruction and must be treated immediately.

Diagnosis of anaphylaxis

When possible, the causative agent in anaphylaxis should be identified and histamine concentrations monitored. Serum histamine concentrations begin to rise 5 to 10 minutes after exposure to the causative agent and may remain elevated for up to 60 minutes. Urinary histamine and its metabolites may stay elevated longer and can be valuable in diagnosis. Serum tryptase is released almost exclusively from mast cells in parallel with release of histamine. Its concentrations increase 1 to 1.5 hours after the onset of symptoms, may stay elevated for 4 to 5 hours, and have been used to diagnose anaphylaxis postmortem. The clinical severity of rechallenge with Hymenoptera venom correlates with the extent to which serum histamine and tryptase concentrations increase, although there is sometimes a curious dysjunction between the two. This relationship may depend on the nature of the triggering agent or be due to individual variations; thus both should be measured.

Histamine agonists

Several histamine agonists are available but are rarely used clinically. The H_2-selective agonist betazole is used occasionally as a gastric secretagogue in diagnostic tests for acid secretion. However, pentagastrin is preferred because it produces fewer systemic effects.

Inhibitors of mast cell degranulation

Cromolyn sodium inhibits the degranulation of mast cells and activation of inflammatory cells. It is used in treatment of asthma and bronchospastic disorders (see Chapter 34).

H_1 antagonists

All H_1 antagonists are useful in treating allergic reactions. They also have varying degrees of sedative, antiemetic, anti-motion sickness, antiparkinsonian, antitussive, and local anesthetic actions. Certain antihistamines are used exclusively for one or another of these properties rather than in treatment of allergic reactions.

The effectiveness of H_1 antagonists in the treatment of motion sickness and extrapyramidal symptoms may result from their **antimuscarinic actions.** They may promote sleep by blocking central H_1 receptors as well as muscarinic receptors. The drugs with antiemetic activity are largely those in the phenothiazine class, and they may work through the blockade of D_2 dopamine receptors. Local anesthetic actions result from the blockade of sodium channels. Thus the actions of antihistamines at sites other than H_1 receptors are the source of both therapeutic and adverse effects. Pharmacological properties of representative H_1 antagonists are summarized in Table 54-4.

The release of histamine from mast cells and basophils is accompanied by the release of many other mediators of the immediate hypersensitivity response. Drugs that antagonize H_1 receptors are useful as monotherapy in mild pseudoallergic or true allergic reactions and as adjunct agents in the treatment of severe reactions. The treatment of severe allergic reactions requires the use of a physiological antagonist such as epinephrine (see Chapter 10) that will reverse the hypotension, laryngeal edema, and bronchoconstriction produced by mast cell mediators.

The effectiveness of antihistamines in the treatment and prevention of allergic disorders is limited to symptoms resulting mainly from the actions of histamine. Allergic reactions that respond best to treatment with H_1 antagonists are seasonal ones, but perennial allergic rhinitis, conjunctivitis, and itching associated with acute and chronic urticaria may also respond. Antihistamines are also of some value in the treatment of atopic and contact dermatitis. The choice of a nonsedating or sedating compound depends on whether sedation is desirable, although tolerance to sedative properties may develop within a few days.

Table 54-4 Properties of H_1 receptor antagonist classes

Chemical Class/Agents	Comments
ALKYLAMINES	
Brompheniramine Chlorpheniramine Triprolidine	Moderately sedating in usual doses, moderate antimuscarinic activity, no antiemetic or antimotion sickness actions
ETHANOLAMINES	
Clemastine Carbinoxamine Dimenhydrinate Diphenhydramine	Significant sedative actions, marked antimuscarinic and antimotion sickness actions; diphenhydramine is in many over-the-counter preparations; dimenhydrinate contains diphenhydramine as the 8-chlorotheophyllinate salt
ETHYLENEDIAMINES	
Pyrilamine Tripelennamine	Low to moderate sedative actions, very little antimuscarinic actions, no antimotion sickness activity in usual doses
PIPERIZINES	
Cetirizine Hydroxyzine Meclizine Cyclizine	Varying degrees of antimuscarinic, antimotion sickness, and sedative actions; meclizine is less sedating than hydroxyzine, used primarily in treatment of motion sickness and vertigo; hydroxyzine has marked sedative and antimuscarinic actions, used as an antiemetic, sedative, and mild anxiolytic agent; cetirizine, a carboxy metabolite of hydroxyzine, is nonsedating
PIPERIDINES	
Azatadine Fexofenadine Desloratadine Loratadine Phenindamine	Fexofenadine, loratadine, and desloratadine are non-sedating and have little or no antimuscarinic activity; azatadine has low to moderate sedative and antimuscarinic actions, marked antiserotonin activity; phenindamine is more likely to produce stimulation
PHENOTHIAZINES	
Methdilazine Promethazine Trimeprazine	Marked antimuscarinic, antiemetic, antimotion sickness activities; α_1-adrenergic receptor–blocking activity can cause orthostatic hypotension; sedation is common, especially with promethazine

H_1 antagonists are not primary drugs for treating bronchial asthma (see Chapter 34) but may be useful in asthmatics who require therapy for allergic rhinitis, allergic dermatoses, and/or urticaria.

Tolerance to antihistamines often occurs. Frequently the desired therapeutic effects can be restored by switching a patient to a drug from a different chemical class. The mechanisms involved are not well understood.

Antihistamines that enter the CNS are used in prophylaxis of motion sickness. Promethazine and diphenhydramine are most potent but are also associated with a high incidence of sedation. Promethazine is an effective antiemetic that can reduce vomiting stemming from a variety of causes. Meclizine,* cyclizine, and dimenhydrinate (a salt of diphenhydramine) are used in over-the-counter preparations for the prevention of motion sickness. However, none is as effective as scopolamine (see Chapter 9). These agents also are used in symptomatic treatment of vertigo.

H_2 antagonists

The H_2 antagonists are discussed in Chapter 55.

Combination of H_1 and H_2 antagonists

Combinations of H_1 and H_2 antagonists are used in the prophylaxis and treatment of severe allergic reactions. Such a combination is more effective than either antagonist alone in reducing histamine-induced vasodilatation, hypotension, mucus secretion, decrease in diastolic blood pressure, and widening of pulse pressure that occur in this setting. Because many mediators are involved, other antiallergic agents are often required, including corticosteroids (see Chapter 33).

Side effects, clinical problems, and toxicity

Clinical problems with the H_1 antagonists are listed in the Clinical Problems box. Problems associated with H_2 antagonists are covered in Chapter 55 and those with cromolyn are covered in Chapter 34.

CLINICAL PROBLEMS

H_1-receptor antagonists

- Antimuscarinic actions
- Sedative effects
- CNS depression
- Paradoxical excitation in children
- Topical use leading to allergic reactions
- Antimuscarinic and CNS effects are minimal for second-generation agents

*In the UK the drug name is meclozine.

H_1 antagonists

Most adverse effects of H_1 antagonists stem from their antimuscarinic and sedative actions. CNS depression is common with the older agents and occurs in 25% to 50% of patients. Antihistamines with antimuscarinic activity may cause dry mouth, blurred vision, urinary retention, constipation, and other symptoms typical of muscarinic receptor blockade (see Chapter 9). Additional effects include insomnia, nervousness, tremors, and euphoria. Appetite stimulation and weight gain have been reported for some drugs. Paradoxical excitation can occur in children; nausea, vomiting, diarrhea, and epigastric distress are also reported.

The main signs of acute overdose of most first-generation antihistamines are similar to those of antimuscarinic drugs. Overdose can result in a rare but potentially hazardous quinidine-like effect, resulting in prolongation of the QT interval and development of torsades de pointes, a prefibrillatory ventricular dysrhythmia. Such dysrhythmias are reported for both first- and second-generation antihistamines. The possibility of serious adverse effects is increased if hepatic metabolism is reduced, when adverse effects can occur at usual therapeutic doses. No such effects have been reported for cetirizine, fexofenadine, loratadine, or desloratadine.

The incidence of CNS depression and antimuscarinic effects are less in patients receiving second-generation agents and are comparable to those produced by placebo. The incidence of true allergic responses is low for drugs administered systemically. However, allergic responses are relatively common after repeated topical use; therefore, such use is discouraged. Teratogenic effects of piperazine derivatives are observed in experimental animals, and although there is no evidence of this in humans, antihistamines are not recommended during pregnancy.

The centrally acting H_1 antihistamines can potentiate the actions of other CNS depressants, including sedative hypnotics, narcotic analgesics, general anesthetics, and alcohol.

New horizons

Much effort is now focused on developing and characterizing drugs that act on H_3 receptors. H_3 agonists, which inhibit transmitter release, may be useful in the treatment of asthma by virtue of their ability to inhibit neurogenically evoked bronchospasm. Similarly, such agents may provide a novel means of reducing gastric acid secretion and reducing intestinal hypermotility. Actions of H_3 antagonists may prove useful in increasing alertness, and the possibility that they could be used for attention deficit hyperactivity disorder is currently causing much excitement.

The development of new orally effective agents that exhibit both antihistamine and cromolyn-like activity is also an area of current research. Agents in clinical trials or in preclinical tests that may possess such actions include azelastine, ketotifen, and epinastine.

TRADE NAMES

In addition to generic and fixed-combination preparations and the compounds listed in the Major Drugs box, the following trade-named materials are some of the important compounds available in the United States.

H_1 antagonists

Azatadine (Optimine)
Brompheniramine (Atrohist, Bromarest, Bromfed, Dimetane)
Clemastine (Tavist)
Cyclizine (Marezine)
Dexchlorpheniramine (Dexchlor, Poladex, Polaramine)
Dimenhydrinate (Dimetabs, Dramamine, Marmine)
Meclizine (Antivert, Bonine)
Methdilazine (Tacaryl)
Phenindamine (Nolamine, Nolahist)
Trimeprazine (Temaril)
Tripelennamine (PBZ)
Triprolidine (Actidil)

FURTHER READING

Gelfand EW, Appajosyula S, Meeves S. Anti-inflammatory activity of H1-receptor antagonists: review of recent experimental research. *Curr Med Res Opin* 2004; 20(1):73–81.

Nielsen LP, Dahl R. Comparison of intranasal corticosteroids and antihistamines in allergic rhinitis: a review of randomized, controlled trials. *Am J Respir Med* 2003; 2(1):55–65.

Self-assessment questions

1. First-generation antihistamines differ from second-generation antihistamines in that the latter generally show:
   a. Greater affinities for H_1 receptors.
   b. Partial agonist activity.
   c. Greater antimuscarinic activity.
   d. Fewer sedative effects.

2. Vasodilatation produced by high doses of histamine can be antagonized fully by:
   a. H_1 antagonists.
   b. H_2 antagonists.
   c. H_3 antagonists.
   d. A combination of both a and b.

3. Responses mediated by H_2 receptors include:
   a. Bronchoconstriction.
   b. Gastric acid secretion.
   c. Decreased force of ventricular contraction.
   d. Stimulation of basophil degranulation.
   e. Inhibition of norepinephrine release.

4. Sedating actions of first-generation H_1 antagonists can be caused by:
   a. Blockade of brain H_3 receptors.
   b. Blockade of brain muscarinic cholinergic receptors.
   c. Blockade of brain H_1 receptors.
   d. Either b or c.

CHAPTER 55

Gastrointestinal drugs

Rosemary R. Berardi

Major Drugs

Antacids	Laxatives
Aminosalicylates	Promotility agents
Antidiarrheal agents	Prostaglandins
Anticholinergic agents	Mucosal protectants
H_2 histamine-receptor antagonists	Proton pump inhibitors

Therapeutic overview

The gastrointestinal (GI) tract stores, digests, and absorbs nutrients and eliminates wastes. Regulation of the GI organs is mediated by intrinsic nerves of the enteric nervous system, neural activity in the central nervous system (CNS), and an array of hormones. These processes are summarized in Figure 55-1.

Pharmacologically treatable GI disorders include:

- Peptic ulcer disease (PUD)
- Gastroesophageal reflux disease (GERD)
- Gastroparesis (delayed gastric emptying)
- Constipation
- Diarrhea
- Irritable bowel syndrome (IBS)
- Inflammatory bowel disease (IBD)

In each case, the potential beneficial effects of drugs must be carefully considered against their potential adverse effects.

Peptic ulcers occur primarily in the stomach and duodenum at a site where the mucosal epithelium is exposed to acid and pepsin. There is a constant confrontation in the stomach and upper small bowel between acid-pepsin aggression and mucosal defense. Usually the mucosa can withstand the acid-pepsin attack and remain healthy; that is, a mucosal "barrier" to back-diffusion of acid is maintained. However, an excess of acid production or an intrinsic defect in the barrier functions of the mucosa can cause defense mechanisms to fail and ulcers to form. Although most patients with duodenal ulcers have an increase in acid secretion, patients with gastric ulcers often have normal or low rates of acid secretion. The role of pepsin in the development of PUD is not known, despite the name of the disease.

Most peptic ulcers are associated with either a gram-negative bacillus, *Helicobacter pylori* (*H. pylori*), or chronic use of nonsteroidal antiinflammatory drugs (NSAIDs). Chronic colonization of the gastric and

Abbreviations

5-ASA	5-aminosalicylic acid
5-HT	serotonin
CNS	central nervous system
COX	cyclooxygenase
GERD	gastroesophageal reflux disease
GI	gastrointestinal
H. pylori	*Helicobacter pylori*
IBD	inflammatory bowel disease
IBS	irritable bowel syndrome
NSAID	nonsteroidal antiinflammatory drug
PPIs	proton pump inhibitors
PUD	peptic ulcer disease

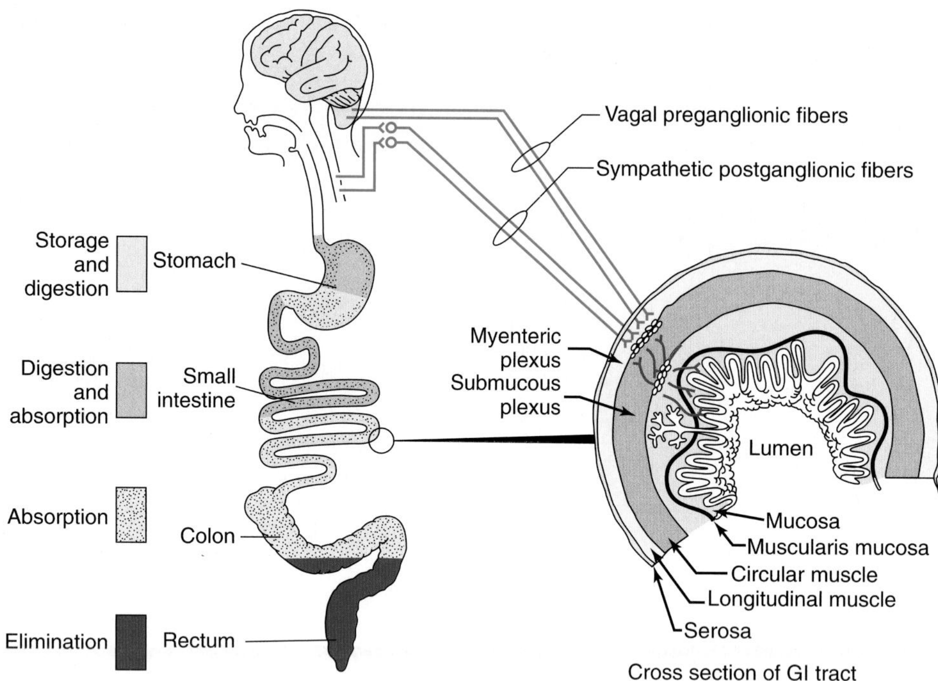

Figure 55-1 Overall regulation and functions of the GI tract, depicting the extrinsic and intrinsic autonomic efferent innervation of the wall of the intestine. The enteric nervous system of the GI tract innervates smooth muscle and mucosa. Efferent and afferent neurons are organized in intramural plexuses; the most prominent plexuses are the myenteric plexus between the longitudinal and circular muscle coats and the submucosal plexus between the circular muscle and the muscularis mucosa.

duodenal mucosae with *H. pylori* is causally associated with PUD. *H. pylori* infection produces inflammatory changes in the mucosa, impairs mucosal defense mechanisms (barrier function), and increases acid secretion. Although H_2-histamine receptor antagonists, proton pump inhibitors (PPIs), and sucralfate heal peptic ulcers in *H. pylori*-positive patients, there is a high rate of ulcer recurrence upon discontinuing drug treatment. Continuous low-dose maintenance therapy reduces the risk of ulcer recurrence but does not cure the disease, because the organism has not been eliminated. Eradication of *H. pylori* cures the disease and in most patients eliminates the need for continuous antisecretory maintenance therapy.

Nonselective NSAIDs, including aspirin, damage the gastric mucosa by a direct topical effect or by systemic inhibition of endogenous mucosal prostaglandin synthesis. The initial topical injury is caused by the acidic property of the NSAID, but inhibition of protective prostaglandins is the primary cause of the ulcer. Nonselective NSAIDs inhibit cyclooxygenase (COX), which is the rate-limiting enzyme in the conversion of arachidonic acid to GI mucosal prostaglandins (see Chapter 17). Two isoforms of COX exist:

- COX-1, which produces protective prostaglandins that maintain mucosal integrity
- COX-2, which is expressed during inflammation and produces prostaglandins involved with fever and pain

Nonselective NSAIDs (e.g., aspirin, ibuprofen) inhibit both COX-1 and COX-2 to varying degrees, but selective COX-2 inhibitors (e.g., celecoxib) spare the protective prostaglandins and are associated with a decrease in ulcers. The concomitant use of a PPI or misoprostol with a nonselective NSAID can also reduce the risk of ulcers and their complications.

Patients with Zollinger-Ellison syndrome have a hypersecretion of gastric acid caused by a gastrin-secreting tumor (gastrinoma). The excess acid overwhelms the mucosal barrier and results in severe and multiple duodenal ulcers. PPIs are the drugs of choice for treating patients with such hypersecretory disorders.

GERD is most often associated with inappropriate relaxation of the lower esophageal sphincter, which allows the acidic gastric contents to flow into the esophagus. The most common symptom of GERD is heartburn, but some patients also develop inflammation, erosions of the esophageal mucosa (esophagitis), and extraesophageal (atypical) manifestations (e.g., chronic asthma, cough, laryngitis). GERD is treated by using drugs that decrease gastric acidity or increase the tone of the lower esophageal sphincter. Although the H_2-histamine receptor antagonists and PPIs effectively relieve GERD symptoms, the PPIs are the treatments of choice for patients with esophagitis. Over-the-counter H_2 antagonists and PPIs are available for treatment and prevention of acid indigestion and heartburn.

Gastroparesis is a delay in gastric emptying stemming from diabetes or other diseases that damage gastric nerves or smooth muscle. Gastric emptying can be improved by using promotility agents, which act by increasing the propulsive contractions of the stomach.

Constipation is a common symptom associated with hard or infrequent stools (fewer than three bowel movements a week), excessive straining, and a sense of incomplete evacuation. Constipation can arise from low-fiber diets, decreased mobility, treatment with certain drugs (narcotics, aluminum-containing antacids, iron) and certain GI, metabolic, or neurologic disorders. Constipation in pregnancy is associated with a decrease in motilin and pressure from the gravid uterus. Excessive use of laxatives may lead to a reliance on laxatives for bowel movements. Dietary changes alone may be sufficient to restore normal bowel habits. However, treatment with a laxative may be indicated in patients with intermittent or chronic constipation.

Diarrhea results from the presence of excessive fluid in the intestinal lumen; this generates rapid, high-volume flow and overwhelms the absorptive capacity of the colon. In most diarrheas, fluid and electrolyte absorption occur at an essentially normal rate. However, diarrhea increases fluid secretion into the lumen to a rate that exceeds its absorptive capacity, thus leading to a net accumulation of luminal fluid. Diarrhea can be acute, secondary to an enteric bacterial or viral infection, or chronic, secondary to inflammatory or functional bowel disease. The most effective way to manage diarrhea is to eliminate the infection, remove the secretagogue-producing tumor, or cure the inflammation. The major hazard associated with diarrhea is loss of fluid and electrolytes. Serious sequelae of diarrhea can generally be prevented by replacement of fluid and electrolytes. However, many patients with serious acute or chronic diarrhea require antidiarrheal therapy.

IBS is characterized by abdominal discomfort or pain and bloating associated with a change in bowel habit (constipation or diarrhea). For years, treatment was largely ineffective and aimed at single symptom relief (e.g., altered bowel habit, abdominal pain, or bloating). Because serotonin and its receptors (primarily 5-HT_3 and 5-HT_4) play a major role in gut function and the physiologic abnormalities in IBS, drugs such as alosetron and tegaserod target these receptors and provide relief of symptoms.

IBD describes two nonspecific inflammatory disorders of the GI tract, ulcerative colitis and Crohn's disease. These are characterized by recurrent acute inflammatory episodes of diarrhea, abdominal pain, and GI bleeding and periods of remission. Although the exact cause of IBD remains unknown, both disorders appear to be immunologically mediated and influenced by genetics and environment. Treatment includes antidiarrheals, antispasmodics, and analgesics; aminosalicylates; and glucocorticoids, antibiotics, and immunomodulators. The aminosalicylates are the cornerstones of drug therapy.

Drugs used to treat diseases or disturbances of the GI tract are summarized in the Therapeutic Overview box.

THERAPEUTIC OVERVIEW

Problem	Treatment
Peptic ulcer disease	H_2 receptor antagonists, proton pump inhibitors, sucralfate, misoprostol, antibiotics to eradicate *Helicobacter pylori*
Gastroesophageal reflux disease	Antacids, H_2 receptor antagonists, proton pump inhibitors
Delayed gastric emptying	Promotility agents
Constipation	Laxatives
Diarrhea	Antidiarrheals
Irritable bowel syndrome	5-HT_3 antagonists, 5-HT_4 agonists
Inflammatory bowel disease	Aminosalicylates

Mechanisms of action

Antisecretory drugs, antacids, protectants, and prostaglandins

The secretion of gastric acid by gastric parietal cells is regulated by histamine, acetylcholine, and gastrin (Fig. 55-2). Psychic stimuli (sight and smell of food) and the presence of food in the mouth or stomach stimulate vagally mediated acid secretion, which results from the action of acetylcholine on parietal and paracrine cells. Acetylcholine acts at parietal cell muscarinic cholinergic receptors (M_3 in Fig. 55-2) coupled to Ca^{2+} channels that increase Ca^{2+} concentrations in the parietal cell. When food is present in the stomach, the antral pH is raised, causing gastrin to be released from the mucosa. Gastrin then circulates through the blood to act at gastrin receptors on parietal and paracrine cells. Activation of gastrin receptors is believed to mobilize intracellular Ca^{2+} in the parietal cell. Histamine is released from nearby paracrine cells to act at parietal cell H_2-histamine receptors. These receptors increase intracellular cyclic adenosine monophosphate. This ultimately

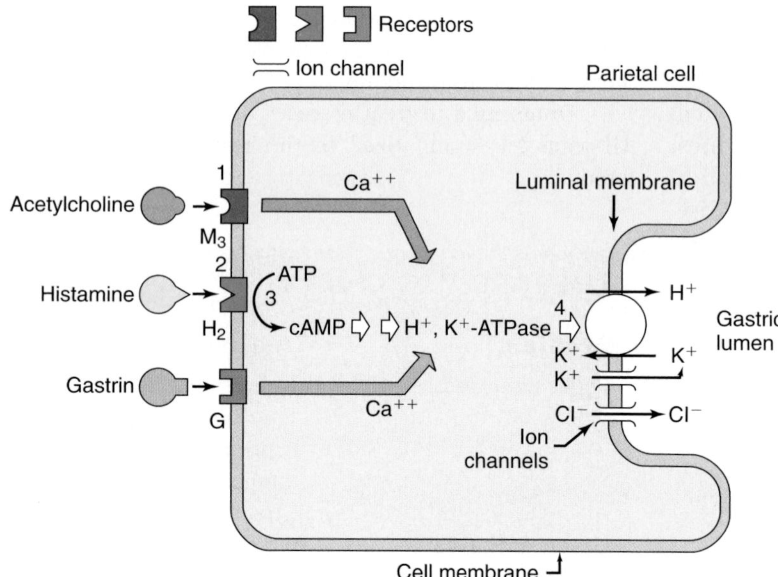

Figure 55-2 Mechanisms regulating secretion of HCl by gastric parietal cell. Receptors for acetylcholine, histamine, and gastrin interact when activated by agonists to increase the availability of Ca^{2+} and stimulate the H^+,K^+-ATPase of the luminal membrane. Acid secretion can be decreased pharmacologically by blockade of acetylcholine M_3 receptors *(1)*, H_2 receptors *(2)*, intracellular cyclic AMP *(3)*, or the H^+,K^+-ATPase *(4)*.

activates a H^+,K^+-ATPase at the luminal border of the parietal cell. The H_2, muscarinic, cholinergic, and gastrin receptors interact to augment acid secretion. However, histamine is considered the most important of the three and may serve as the final common pathway in the regulation of gastric acid secretion.

Neurally secreted acetylcholine and circulating gastrin may exert two distinct types of stimulatory effects (one indirect and one direct) on gastric parietal cells. The more important indirect effect is exerted at small histamine-containing paracrine cells located near parietal cells in oxyntic glands. Acetylcholine released from secretomotor terminals of the vagus nerve acts at M_1 receptors on histamine paracrine cells to cause the release of histamine, which acts at parietal cell H_2 receptors to stimulate acid secretion. Acetylcholine also acts directly at parietal cell M_3 receptors to stimulate acid production. Similarly, circulating gastrin released from G cells of the antral mucosa acts at gastrin receptors on paracrine cells to cause the release of histamine and also may act directly at gastrin receptors on parietal cells to stimulate acid production. Thus histamine release constitutes the major event in the stimulation of acid production by acetylcholine and gastrin, and they in turn also act directly on parietal cells to augment the actions of histamine. Activation of any of the three types of parietal cell receptors increases the activity of a protein kinase that activates the H^+,K^+-ATPase located at the luminal membrane of the parietal cell. This H^+,K^+-ATPase serves as the so-called proton pump that secretes H^+ into the gastric lumen.

Histamine and antihistamines are discussed in detail in Chapter 54 but are briefly discussed here as they relate to gastric acid secretion. H_2 histamine receptors on parietal cells mediate the stimulatory effect of histamine on acid secretion and augment the secretory actions of gastrin and acetylcholine. The only important role of peripheral H_2 histamine receptors in humans appears to be in the regulation of acid secretion.

Drugs can decrease gastric secretion (see Fig. 55-2) by blocking H_2 receptors, blocking M_1 or M_3 receptors, or by inhibiting the activity of the H^+,K^+-ATPase in the parietal cell.

The **H_2-histamine receptor antagonists** cimetidine, famotidine, nizatidine, and ranitidine competitively and reversibly block H_2 receptors on parietal cells, diminishing basal, nocturnal, and food-stimulated gastric acid secretion (Table 55-1). Although relative antisecretory potencies vary from cimetidine, the least potent, to famotidine, the most potent, increased potency does not confer greater efficacy if the drugs are given in an equipotent antisecretory dose.

The **PPIs**—omeprazole, esomeprazole (the S-enantiomer of omeprazole), lansoprazole, pantoprazole, and rabeprazole—share a common mechanism of action. The PPIs irreversibly inhibit parietal cell H^+,K^+-ATPase, decreasing basal, nocturnal, and food-stimulated gastric acid secretion. The parent drug is inactive, but under highly acidic conditions in the parietal cell, it is protonated and converted to an active compound that reacts covalently with cysteine residues in the H^+,K^+-ATPase. This inactivates the pump and prevents the transport of H^+ into the stomach lumen (see Figure 55-2). Because all secretory stimuli ultimately cause acid production by augmenting the activity of the H^+,K^+-ATPase transporter, irreversible blockade of this enzyme inhibits the final step and is the most effective way to diminish acid secretion.

Table 55-1 Summary of action of the antisecretory drugs, antacids, protectants, and prostaglandins

Category	Prototype	Mechanism of Action
Antacids	Magnesium oxide and magnesium hydroxide	Neutralize secreted acid
Anticholinergics	Propantheline	Block muscarinic receptors, decrease acid secretion
Bismuth salts	Bismuth subsalicylate	Topical antibacterial activity
H_2 receptor antagonists	Cimetidine	Block H_2 receptors, decrease acid secretion
Prostaglandins	Misoprostol	Inhibit mucosal prostaglandins, decrease acid secretion
Mucosal protectants	Sucralfate	Protect mucosal barrier
Proton pump inhibitors	Omeprazole	Inhibit H^+,K^+-ATPase, decrease acid secretion

(1) $Al(OH)_3 + 3HCl \rightleftharpoons AlCl_3 + 3H_2O$

(2) $Mg(OH)_2 + 2HCl \rightleftharpoons MgCl_2 + 2H_2O$

(3) $MgCl_2 + Na_2CO_3 \rightleftharpoons MgCO_3\,(PPT) + 2NaCl$

(4) $MgCl_2 + 2R\text{–}COONa \rightleftharpoons Mg(R\text{–}COO)_2\,(PPT) + 2NaCl$

Figure 55-3 Intragastric and intestinal interactions of prototype antacids. *(1)* Interaction of aluminum hydroxide with gastric acid to form soluble aluminum chloride. *(2)* Interaction of magnesium hydroxide with gastric acid. *(3)* Soluble magnesium chloride interaction with sodium carbonate in the lumen of the intestine to form insoluble magnesium carbonate. *(4)* Interaction of soluble magnesium chloride with fatty acid salts in the lumen of the intestine to form an insoluble magnesium soap. *PPT,* Precipitate.

Table 55-2 Drugs used for eradication of *H. pylori*–associated ulcers

Therapeutic Category	Drug Choices
Antisecretory	Proton pump inhibitor or H_2 receptor antagonist
Bismuth salt	Bismuth subsalicylate
Nitroimidazole	Metronidazole
Antibiotic	Clarithromycin, amoxicillin, or tetracycline

Anticholinergic agents (see Chapter 9) block M_1 muscarinic receptors on histamine-containing paracrine cells in the oxyntic mucosa to inhibit acetylcholine-induced release of histamine. These agents also block M_3 muscarinic receptors on parietal cells to inhibit acetylcholine-induced acid secretion.

Antacids are weak bases that act primarily by neutralizing intragastric hydrochloric acid. They do not decrease acid secretion. The cations (sodium, calcium, magnesium, aluminum) initially form soluble chloride salts (Fig. 55-3). NaCl can be absorbed from the small intestine, but the divalent ions subsequently form poorly soluble bicarbonates and carbonates, which precipitate and remain in the bowel to be excreted in the feces. The acid neutralizing effects in the stomach lumen decrease total acid load to the duodenum and inhibit pepsin activity at an intragastric pH of 5 or above. Antacids also bind bile salts, and aluminum-containing antacids may enhance mucosal prostaglandins.

Mucosal protectants such as sucralfate, an aluminum salt of sucrose octasulfate, bind electrostatically to positively charged tissue proteins and mucin within the ulcer crater to form a viscous barrier and protect the ulcer from gastric acid. Sucralfate also inhibits pepsin, binds bile salts, and stimulates mucosal prostaglandins. Unlike H_2 receptor antagonists and PPIs, sucralfate has no important effect on gastric acid secretion.

In parietal cells, many **prostaglandins** (see Chapter 17) inhibit histamine-stimulated acid secretion. Misoprostol, a synthetic prostaglandin E1 analog, modestly inhibits the concentration and total amount of acid in the gastric lumen, resulting in a reduction of basal, nocturnal, and food-stimulated acid secretion. Misoprostol also increases mucus, mucosal bicarbonate secretion, and mucosal blood flow and inhibits mucosal cell turnover, all of which enhance mucosal defense.

Eradication of *H. pylori* Single antimicrobial agents are not effective in eradicating *H. pylori.* Therefore a combination of antibiotics and an antisecretory drug must be employed for effective eradication. A typical regimen for eradication of *H. pylori* includes two antibiotics (usually clarithromycin and amoxicillin or metronidazole) and an antisecretory drug (usually a PPI). Other regimens include bismuth subsalicylate, metronidazole, tetracycline, and either a proton pump inhibitor or an H_2 receptor antagonist (Table 55-2).

Promotility agents

Promotility agents increase GI tract contractions and propulsion by increasing cholinergic stimuli at smooth muscle M_3 receptors (Fig. 55-4). Cholinergic stimulation

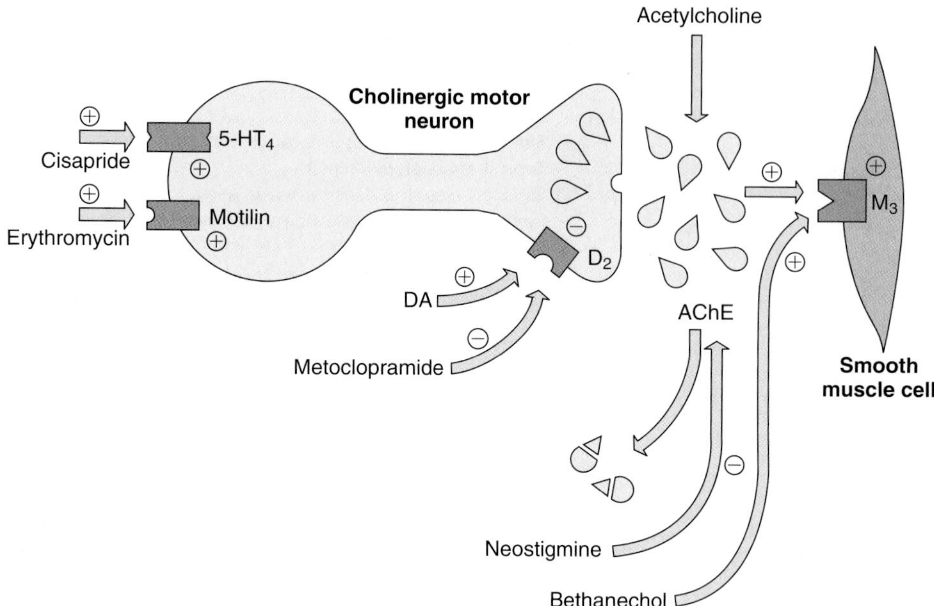

Figure 55-4 Mechanisms of promotility drugs. These agents directly or indirectly increase agonist activity at smooth muscle M_3-receptors. Erythromycin is an agonist (+) at excitatory (+) motilin receptors. Cisapride is an agonist (+) at excitatory (+) neural 5-HT_4 receptors on enteric nervous system cholinergic motor neurons. Metoclopramide is an antagonist (–) at dopamine (DA) receptors (D_2) that inhibit (–) the release of acetylcholine. Neostigmine inhibits (–) hydrolysis of acetylcholine by acetylcholinesterase (AChE). Bethanechol acts directly as an agonist (+) at excitatory (+) M_3 smooth muscle receptors.

Table 55-3 Summary of action of promotility drugs

Mechanism	Category	Prototype	Mechanism of Action
1	Muscarinic agonists	Bethanechol	Increase contraction of GI smooth muscle
2	Acetylcholinesterase inhibitors	Neostigmine	Block destruction of acetylcholine
3	Dopamine inhibitors	Metoclopramide	Block inhibitory presynaptic D_2 receptors
4	5-HT_4 agonists	Cisapride	Activate excitatory neuronal 5HT_4 receptors
5	Motilin agonists	Erythromycin	Activate neural and smooth muscle motilin receptors

can be accomplished by five different mechanisms, which are summarized in Table 55-3.

The most useful mechanisms, in terms of therapeutic benefit-risk ratios, involve agonist activity at 5-HT_4 (mechanism 4) or motilin receptors (mechanism 5). Mechanisms 1 and 2, seen for cholinergic drugs, lead to significant side effects stemming from excessive secretory activity. Cholinergic agonists and cholinesterase inhibitors increase cholinergic stimuli at salivary, gastric, pancreatic, and intestinal secretory cells in addition to smooth muscle cells. Moreover, the cholinergic drugs fail to produce the types of closely coordinated contractions between the antrum of the stomach and the duodenum required for effective gastric emptying.

Dopamine D_2 antagonists (mechanism 3) increase the tone of the lower esophageal sphincter (important in the therapy of GERD), increase the force of gastric contractions, improve the coordination of gastroduodenal contractions, and enhance gastric emptying. Some drugs are highly effective as antiemetic agents, an action attributable to their blockade of central dopamine receptors in the chemoreceptor trigger zone and other sites controlling emesis.

5-HT_4 agonists increase the tone of the lower esophageal sphincter and the force of gastric contractions and improve gastroduodenal coordination. Cisapride and tegaserod also stimulate colonic motility and enhance transit through the proximal colon. Several chemically related drugs such as alosetron, ondansetron, and granisetron are antagonists at the 5-HT_3 receptor. Alosetron acts primarily to decrease intestinal motility, but ondansetron and granisetron have a greater antiemetic effect as they act on vagal afferent nerves that activate CNS emetic mechanisms.

Motilin is a GI tract hormone that participates in the initiation of migrating motor complexes that characterize the fasting motility pattern of the stomach and small intestine. Erythromycin and several analogs bind to nerve and muscle motilin receptors to enhance GI tract contractions and increase gastric emptying. This promotility effect is not related to the antimicrobial activity of these drugs.

Laxatives

There are several categories of laxatives (sometimes called evacuants, cathartics, or purgatives) including:

- Fiber supplements (bulk-forming)
- Emollients (stool softeners)
- Lubricants
- Saline
- Hyperosmolar agents
- Stimulants

A summary of the action of laxatives is presented in Table 55-4.

Fiber supplements (bulk-forming) are non-absorbable cellulose fibers that, when taken with water, become hydrated in the intestine, swell, and form a large mass that activates the defecation reflex. Intestinal transit time is reduced as a result of the increased water content and bulk. Natural fiber supplements (e.g., psyllium) undergo bacterial degradation in the colon, which contributes to bloating and flatulence. Semisynthetic (e.g., methylcellulose) and synthetic (e.g., polycarbophil) fibers are more resistant to bacterial degradation.

Emollients are ionic detergents that soften feces and permit easier defecation by lowering the surface tension and permitting water to interact more effectively with the solid stool.

Lubricants (e.g., mineral oil) are oral non-absorbable laxatives that act by lubricating the stool to facilitate passage. Malabsorption of fat-soluble vitamins may occur with long-term use.

Hyperosmolar agents act by increasing stool osmolarity, leading to accumulation of fluid in the colon. Lactulose and sorbitol are poorly absorbed from the small intestine but undergo bacterial fermentation in the colon to organic acids and CO_2. Abdominal bloating and flatulence are common side effects. Polyethylene glycol is poorly absorbed but is not metabolized by colonic bacteria. Solutions with electrolytes are used for bowel cleansing prior to colonoscopy. A formulation without electrolytes may be used daily.

Saline laxatives are inorganic salts, with one or both poorly absorbed cations (e.g., magnesium) or anions (e.g., sulfate or phosphate). They draw water into the intestine by osmotic means, resulting in increased gut propulsion and evacuation. Because appreciable amounts of magnesium may be absorbed, these should be avoided in patients with renal insufficiency.

Stimulant laxatives include anthraquinones (e.g., senna), diphenylmethanes (e.g., bisacodyl), and castor oil. The anthraquinones are converted by colonic bacteria to their pharmacologically active form, which increases fluid accumulation in the distal ileum and colon. Bisacodyl has a similar action. Castor oil is hydrolyzed by lipase in the small intestine to ricinoleic acid, which increases intestinal secretion, decreases glucose absorption, and stimulates colonic motor function through the release of neurotransmitters from mucosal enterochromaffin cells.

Antidiarrheal drugs

Transport of fluid and electrolytes by the intestinal mucosa is regulated by neurons of the enteric nervous system and by the composition of the luminal contents. It is believed that neurons of the submucosal plexus of the intestine terminate near mucosal epithelial cells and act to increase or decrease absorption by villus cells and secretion by crypt cells. A summary of the action of antidiarrheal drugs is presented in Table 55-5.

Opioids act on enteric neurons to decrease secretion and promote mucosal transport from the lumen. In addition, opioids act in the CNS to alter extrinsic neural influences on the intestine and promote a net absorption of fluid and electrolytes. Opioids also convert propulsive patterns of motility to segmenting patterns, thereby increasing resistance to flow. These actions result in slowed transit through the GI tract, allowing time for more-complete fluid absorption and leading to an increased viscosity of the luminal content. Morphine and codeine effectively cross the blood-brain barrier

Table 55-4 Summary of actions of laxatives

Category	Prototype	Mechanism of Action
Fiber supplements	Psyllium	Increases colonic residue, stimulating peristalsis
Emollients	Docusate sodium	Lowers surface tension allowing water to interact with stool
Lubricants	Mineral oil	Lubricates the stool
Hyperosmolar agents	Lactulose	Increases stool osmolarity
Saline laxatives	Magnesium hydroxide	Draws water into the intestine along osmotic gradient
Stimulant laxatives	Senna	Stimulates intestinal secretion and motility

Table 55-5 Summary of action of antidiarrheal drugs

Category	Prototypes	Mechanism of Action
Opioids	Loperamide, diphenoxylate	Increase resistance to flow, decrease propulsion, decrease net fluid secretion
Antisecretory agents	Bismuth subsalicylate	Decrease net fluid secretion
Gel-forming adsorbents	Hydrated aluminum silicate, pectin, kaolin	Increase resistance to flow, increase formed stools
Ion-exchange resins	Cholestyramine	Bind water and bile salts

Table 55-6 Selected pharmacokinetic parameters

Drug	Route of Administration	Absorption (%)	Half-Life (hrs)	Disposition
H_2 RECEPTOR ANTAGONISTS				
Cimetidine	Oral, IV	60	2	R (Main), M
Nizatidine	Oral	90	1.5	R (Main), M
Ranitidine	Oral, IV	50	3	R (Main), M
Famotidine	Oral, IV	45	3	R (Main), M
PROTON PUMP INHIBITORS				
Omeprazole	Oral	40	1	M
Lansoprazole	Oral, IV	85	1.5	M
Rabeprazole	Oral	50	1-2	M
PROMOTILITY AGENTS				
Metoclopramide	Oral, IV, IM	80	2	R (Main), M
Ondansetron	Oral, IV	60	3.5	M
Granisetron	Oral, IV	60	6.2	M
OTHERS				
Sucralfate	Oral	Poor	—	
Diphenoxylate	Oral	90	12	M (Main), B, R
Loperamide	Oral	Poor	11	B (Main), R

M, Metabolized; *R*, renal excretion as unchanged drug; *B*, biliary excretion.

and act in the brain and spinal cord to decrease transit and fluid accumulation in the intestinal lumen. Loperamide and diphenoxylate, which cannot effectively cross the blood-brain barrier, act locally at neural and smooth muscle sites, primarily in the submucosal plexus, to increase segmenting contractions. The increased segmenting contractions in the proximal duodenum decrease the gastroduodenal pressure gradient and delay gastric emptying.

Bismuth subsalicylate contains topical antibacterial properties and inhibits the formation of diarrhea-producing prostaglandins.

Aminosalicylates

Sulfasalazine, the prototype aminosalicylate, is a conjugate of 5-aminosalicylic acid (5-ASA) and sulfapyridine linked by a diazo bond. The parent drug passes into the colon unchanged, where colonic bacteria cleave the diazo bond to form 5-ASA (the active moiety) and sulfapyridine. 5-ASA acts locally to interfere with arachidonic acid metabolism which, by an unknown mechanism, has a beneficial effect in IBD. Newer oral preparations include coupling 5-ASA with agents other than sulfapyridine (e.g., balsalazide). Delayed release pH-dependent enteric-coated tablets and time-dependent enteric-coated granules release 5-ASA proximal to the colon.

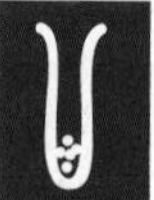

Pharmacokinetics

Pharmacokinetic parameters for selected drugs are given in Table 55-6.

H_2-receptor antagonists are available orally and parenterally. H_2-receptor antagonists are well absorbed when given orally, but bioavailability is variable. Onset of acid inhibition occurs within 1 hour, and lasts from 4 to 12 hours, and is dose-dependent. These drugs are excreted primarily unchanged in the urine; therefore dosage reduction is recommended in patients with renal insufficiency.

PPIs are also available orally and parenterally. Omeprazole has a low and variable bioavailability that increases with repeated daily dosing, reaching a plateau after 3 to 4 days. The bioavailability of other PPIs is less sensitive to repeated dosing. Because PPIs bind irreversibly to parietal cell H^+,K^+-ATPase, they suppress gastric acid far longer than expected from their short plasma elimination half-lives. Onset of acid inhibition occurs within 1 hour but lasts from 14 to 20 hours and is dose-dependent. All PPIs undergo hepatic metabolism, and a dosage reduction is unnecessary in renal insufficiency but should be considered in patients with severe liver disease.

Antacids have a rapid onset of action but a neutralizing capacity that lasts about 30 minutes on an empty (fasted) stomach. If an antacid is taken after a meal, food delays gastric emptying and prolongs the antacid neutralizing effect for up to 2 to 3 hours.

Sucralfate is available orally and for treatment of PUD. Only a small amount is absorbed, as the majority is excreted in the feces.

Sulfasalazine is available orally. Some drug is absorbed and excreted in the bile. The remainder passes unchanged into the colon to form 5-ASA and sulfapyridine. Most of the 5-ASA is excreted in the feces. Sulfapyridine is absorbed, metabolized in the liver, and excreted in the urine. When given as a pH-dependent enteric-coated tablet or as time-dependent granules, some 5-ASA is released in the small intestine and absorption is increased. Topical 5-ASA exerts a local antiinflammatory effect and is available as a rectal enema.

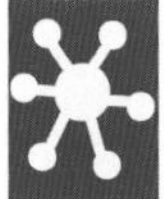

Relation of mechanisms of action to clinical response

Antisecretory drugs, antacids, protectants, and prostaglandins

H_2-receptor antagonists Cimetidine, famotidine, nizatidine, and ranitidine provide similar antisecretory effects. They all relieve PUD symptoms (e.g., epigastric pain) and GERD symptoms (e.g., heartburn) and promote ulcer and esophageal healing. When used as continuous maintenance therapy, they also maintain ulcer and esophageal healing. Tolerance to the gastric antisecretory effect may develop with continuous dosing and may be responsible for diminished efficacy.

PPIs All of the PPIs provide similar antisecretory effects. Because of their potent suppression of gastric acid, PPIs provide more-rapid relief of epigastric pain and heartburn and more-rapid and effective ulcer and esophageal healing than the H_2 receptor antagonists. They are also effective as single agents when used to maintain ulcer and esophageal healing. The PPIs are the drugs of choice for the treatment of Zollinger-Ellison syndrome. Tolerance to the antisecretory effect of a PPI has not been reported. Rebound hypersecretion of gastric acid has been reported, but data are conflicting.

Eradication of *H. pylori* Treatment of *H. pylori* is susceptible to many antimicrobial agents in vitro, but it has proved difficult to eradicate the infection with single agents in humans. The PPI-based three- and four-drug regimens (see Table 55-2) are successful in about 80 to 90% of patients. *H. pylori* organisms have been shown to develop resistance to nitroimidazoles (e.g., metronidazole) and macrolides (e.g., clarithromycin), but resistance to tetracycline and amoxicillin is uncommon. Therefore, eradication regimens should contain at least two antimicrobial agents.

Anticholinergics Anticholinergics are effective in reducing gastric acid secretion, but high dosages are required to heal peptic ulcers, resulting in adverse side effects.

Antacids Antacid neutralization provides almost immediate relief of symptoms, but large volumes and frequent dosing are necessary for mucosal healing. The neutralizing effects occur for as long as the antacids are present in the stomach. Because of their side effects, disagreeable taste, and poor compliance, antacids are not used as single agents to heal peptic ulcers or esophagitis. Today they are used primarily for the occasional relief of acid indigestion, epigastric pain, and heartburn.

Mucosal protectants Sucralfate heals peptic ulcers as effectively as the H_2 receptor antagonists with a minimum of adverse side effects. Because sucralfate has no important effect on intragastric pH, it is not very effective in relieving acid-related symptoms or in healing esophagitis. The use of sucralfate has decreased with the introduction of more-effective drugs such as the PPIs.

Prostaglandins Misoprostol exerts both a gastric antisecretory effect and a protective effect on the gastric and duodenal mucosa. Its primary therapeutic effect, however, is thought to be related to stimulation of mucosal defense mechanisms. Misoprostol is effective in reducing the risk of NSAID-induced peptic ulcers, but adverse side effects limit its use.

Promotility drugs

Promotility drugs are used to increase gastric emptying in the treatment of diabetic gastroparesis and to increase the tone of the lower esophageal sphincter in the management of GERD. Some, such as metoclopramide, also exhibit significant antiemetic activity and are used in patients receiving antineoplastic drugs (see Chapter 42). Tolerance to the promotility effects of metoclopramide may develop and render the drug ineffective. Promotility agents devoid of dopamine antagonist activity produce antiemetic effects by exerting an antagonist action at 5-HT_3 receptors, indicating that local gastric effects may be important in the suppression of emesis. Ondansetron and granisetron are more effective than other promotility drugs in decreasing the nausea and vomiting associated with antineoplastic agents. Cisapride and erythromycin have little antiemetic activity but are effective promotility drugs.

Laxatives

Fiber supplements soften feces and are effective for treating mild constipation. Beneficial effects usually take about 1 week. Emollients also soften feces and permit easier defecation but are not very effective laxatives. The hyperosmolar agents, lubricants, and saline laxatives usually work within a day. Stimulant laxatives usually work within hours but may cause abdominal cramping.

Antidiarrheal drugs

Opioids The opioid antidiarrheal drugs are remarkably effective in the management of acute diarrhea. Those with CNS activity should be used cautiously for acute diarrhea and should not be used for management of chronic diarrhea. The most-effective antidiarrheal drugs are morphine, codeine, loperamide, and diphenoxylate. Loperamide is effective for control of diarrhea secondary to IBS or IBD. Opioid antidiarrheal agents should not be employed in the symptomatic treatment of diarrhea caused by enteric infections, especially those caused by *Shigella* or *Salmonella.*

Bismuth subsalicylate Bismuth subsalicylate is an effective antidiarrheal agent especially useful against enterotoxigenic strains of *E. coli.* It is sometimes included for its antimicrobial properties in therapy directed against *H. pylori.*

Gel-forming substances Substances that form semisolid gels within the intestinal lumen increase resistance to flow and also increase the firmness of stools. Typical gel substances include kaolin and pectin, which form clay-like gels when hydrated. They do not, however, reduce the volume of fluid excreted and thus have little therapeutic benefit.

Serotonin 5-HT_3 antagonists and 5-HT_4 agonists

Serotonin 5-HT_4 agonists, such as tegaserod, increase the frequency of bowel movements and improve stool consistency. Abdominal pain and bloating is also reduced in patients with IBS. 5-HT_3 antagonists, such as alosetron, decrease the frequency of bowel movements and improve stool consistency. Abdominal pain and bloating are also reduced in patients with IBS.

Aminosalicylates

Sulfasalazine and the newer aminosalicylate forms are effective in treating mild to moderate ulcerative colitis and Crohn's disease. The forms that release 5-ASA in the small intestine are more likely to be effective in patients with ileal involvement. Symptomatic improvement in abdominal pain and diarrhea is seen in about 3 weeks. Lower daily dosages are effective in maintaining remission. Topical 5-ASA rectal enemas are effective in treating ulcerative proctitis and proctosigmoiditis.

Side effects, clinical problems, and toxicity

The clinical problems associated with the drugs used for the treatment of ulcers are summarized in the Clinical Problems box.

Antisecretory drugs, antacids, protectants, and prostaglandins

H_2-receptor antagonists The H_2 receptor antagonists a have a low incidence of side effects, which are unrelated to their blockade of the H_2 receptors. The most-common side effects are similar for all H_2 antagonists and include headache, diarrhea, constipation, flatulence, and nausea. Dizziness, somnolence, lethargy, agitation, and confusion occur occasionally and have been reported with all of these drugs. Risk factors include renal impairment and advanced age. Transient skin rashes have been observed in a small number of patients. Thrombocytopenia and neutropenia are uncommon. Most side effects disappear with continued treatment or upon discontinuation of the drug. Cimetidine—but not famotidine, nizatidine, or ranitidine—binds to testosterone receptors and exerts antiandrogenic effects, resulting in decreased libido, decreased

CLINICAL PROBLEMS

Antacids

Aluminum salts
- Constipation

Magnesium salts
- Diarrhea
- Magnesium absorption

Sodium salts
- Increased plasma sodium concentration

Bismuth subsalicylate

Black tongue and stool
Tinnitus

H_2 antagonists

Cimetidine
- Interference with metabolism of many drugs
- Antiandrogenic effect, e.g., gynecomastia, impotence, decreased sperm count

Laxatives

Saline
- Magnesium absorption

Lubricants (mineral oil)
- Decreased absorption of fat-soluble vitamins
- Pulmonary aspiration

Stimulants
- Abdominal cramping
- Watery diarrhea

Proton pump inhibitors

Gastric mucosal hyperplasia

Prokinetic drugs

Bethanechol, neostigmine
- Excess GI secretions, cramps, cholinergic stimulation

Metoclopramide
- Extrapyramidal effects
- Hyperprolactinemia

Prostaglandins

Misoprostol
- Diarrhea
- Uterine stimulation

sperm count, impotence, and gynecomastia in men. The antiandrogenic effects are associated with high doses and long-term use. Cimetidine also interferes with drugs metabolized by hepatic cytochrome P450 enzymes. Thus the use of cimetidine in conjunction with drugs metabolized by this system can lead to elevated plasma concentrations and toxic responses to these other drugs. Because famotidine, nizatidine, and ranitidine do not bind substantially to cytochrome P450 isoenzymes, they do not have this problem. All H_2 antagonists increase intragastric pH and may decrease the bioavailability of drugs that require gastric acidity for absorption (e.g., ketoconazole).

PPIs The PPIs are well tolerated and have a low incidence of side effects. The most-common side effects are similar to those observed with the H_2 receptor antagonists. Diarrhea has been reported more frequently with lansoprazole and omeprazole and appears to be dose-related. Most antisecretory drugs increase fasting and postprandial serum gastrin as a function of their acid-inhibiting effect. The profound effects on acid secretion and the resultant hypergastrinemia in patients taking PPIs have raised concern regarding their long-term use and the potential for causing gastric mucosal hyperplasia and cancer. However, significant hyperplasia or gastric cancer has not been observed in humans taking PPIs for as long as 15 years. Omeprazole and esomeprazole may interfere with drugs metabolized by hepatic cytochrome P450 subfamily IIC (e.g., warfarin, phenytoin, diazepam), but toxicities are uncommon. All PPIs increase intragastric pH and may also decrease the bioavailability of drugs that require gastric acidity for absorption.

Antacids The most-common problems encountered in patients taking antacids are constipation (with aluminum-containing antacids) and diarrhea (with magnesium-containing antacids). An acceptable balance in stool frequency and consistency can be achieved by using agents that include mixtures of magnesium and aluminum salts or by alternating doses of magnesium- or aluminum-containing antacids. Calcium, magnesium, and aluminum are usually poorly absorbed but in patients with renal insufficiency can exert systemic toxicity. Calcium salts can produce systemic hypercalcemia, with the resultant formation of calculi (milk alkali syndrome). Aluminum can bind phosphate in the gut lumen and reduce the absorption of phosphate, leading to phosphate deficiency with muscle weakness and reabsorption of bone. Most antacids have been reformulated to contain little or no sodium. All antacids increase intragastric pH and may decrease the bioavailability of drugs that require gastric acidity for absorption. Aluminum-containing antacids may inhibit the absorption of tetracycline and iron supplements. Systemic antacids (e.g., sodium bicarbonate) are absorbed into the blood and have the potential to increase blood pH and alkalinize urine.

Mucosal protectants Sucralfate is virtually devoid of systemic side effects because it not readily absorbed. Constipation occurs in a small number of patients and is related to the aluminum salt. Aluminum may also bind dietary phosphate, leading to a phosphate deficiency. Sucralfate may bind to drugs such as the quinolone antibiotics, warfarin, and phenytoin and limit their absorption.

Prostaglandins Prostaglandins, such as misoprostol, induce diarrhea by promoting secretion of fluid and electrolytes into the bowel lumen and by inhibiting the intestinal segmenting contractions that retard the flow of luminal contents. Prostaglandins also increase intestinal secretion, leading to a net luminal fluid accumulation. Diarrhea occurs frequently, is dose-related, and often limits use of the drug. Misoprostol also stimulates uterine contractions and may endanger pregnancy and should be used with caution in women of child-bearing age. It is contraindicated in pregnancy.

Bismuth subsalicylate Bismuth subsalicylate temporarily turns the tongue and stool black and can cause tinnitus, especially when taken with other salicylate-containing drugs (e.g., aspirin, 5-ASA).

Promotility agents

Cholinergic agonists produce a variety of side effects typically associated with cholinergic stimulation (see Chapter 9). Because of its activity as a dopamine receptor antagonist, metoclopramide can induce dystonia or parkinsonian side effects. Dopamine antagonists also can induce symptoms of hyperprolactinemia consisting of gynecomastia, galactorrhea, and breast tenderness. Metoclopramide also often induces sedation. More recently developed promotility drugs such as cisapride do not block dopamine receptors and do not produce extrapyramidal side effects. However, cisapride is metabolized by *CYP*3A4, as are ketoconazole, fluconazole, miconazole, erythromycin, clarithromycin, and many other drugs, raising the potential for drug interactions. Because of these concerns, the Food and Drug Administration removed cisapride from the market, reclassified it as an investigational drug, and imposed severe restrictions on its use.

Laxatives

Fiber supplements (especially the natural fibers such as psyllium) and lactulose may cause abdominal fullness, bloating, and flatulence. Stimulant and saline laxatives may cause abdominal cramping, watery stools, dehydration, and fluid and electrolyte imbalances. In patients with renal insufficiency or cardiac dysfunction, saline laxatives may cause electrolyte and volume overload. A brown-black pigment (melanosis coli) may develop in the colon of patients taking anthraquinones but does not lead to the development of colon cancer. Laxatives should never be prescribed for patients with undiagnosed abdominal pain or intestinal obstruction. Because castor oil causes severe intestinal cramping and diarrhea, its use should be avoided.

Antidiarrheals

The side effects of the natural opioids such as morphine and codeine and the synthetic opioids such as loperamide and diphenoxylate are discussed in Chapter 31. Diphenoxylate crosses the blood-brain barrier poorly, and in usual therapeutic doses it does not produce CNS side effects. However, in an overdose, it can cause respiratory depression, which can be reversed by naloxone. Diphenoxylate is available in combination with atropine, the latter added to deter abuse. Loperamide poorly traverses the blood-brain barrier and therefore has virtually no CNS effects and a low abuse potential.

Serotonin 5-HT$_3$ antagonists and 5-HT$_4$ agonists

The most-common side effect associated with alosetron is constipation, whereas diarrhea occurs most frequently in patients taking tegaserod.

Aminosalicylates

The side effects associated with sulfasalazine may be dose-dependent or dose-independent. Dose-dependent effects correlate with sulfapyridine in the blood and include nausea, loss of appetite, headache, malaise, and diarrhea. Dose-independent effects include hypersensitivity reactions typical of sulfonamides. Skin rashes occur occasionally and require that the drug be withdrawn. Fever, hemolytic anemia, pulmonary complications, hepatitis, and pancreatitis have been reported. A hypersensitivity reaction has been reported in patients taking 5-ASA dosage forms. Patients allergic to aspirin should not take 5-ASA. The potential for renal damage exists in patients taking high doses of 5-ASA.

New horizons

Eradication of *H pylori* has changed the way PUD is treated. Although significant progress has been made, there is no ideal treatment, and development of antibiotic-resistant strains remains a major concern. Future research should provide less-complex and more-effective drug regimens. Co-therapy with misoprostol or a PPI, or switching to a COX-2 inhibitor, reduces the risk of NSAID-induced ulcers, and newer NSAIDs that spare the GI tract are under investigation.

Better drugs that alter GI motility for treating gastroparesis, GERD, and chronic constipation are needed. At present there is considerable interest in novel pharmacologic approaches to correct the motor abnormalities associated with these disorders. Of interest is a macrolide motilin agonist with minimal antibiotic activity and predictable pharmacokinetic characteristics that is devoid of tolerance.

Future therapies for IBS will be aimed at understanding the mechanisms involved in GI motility and sensation. Novel agents under investigation include cholecystokinin-A receptor antagonists, neurokinin-1 and neurokinin-3 receptor antagonists, κ (peripheral) opiate receptor agonists, α_2-adrenergic receptor agonists, M_3-selective muscarinic receptor antagonists, and probiotics. Antidiarrheal drugs that are free of constipating properties are also needed. Among candidates under investigation are enkephalinase inhibitors and calmodulin antagonists. Ulcerative colitis and Crohn's disease are serious IBDs that cannot be adequately managed by using existing drugs. Promising new agents include drugs that reduce the formation of inflammatory mediators (e.g., interleukins and other cytokines) or that can block their receptors.

TRADE NAMES

In addition to generic and fixed-combination preparations, the following trade-named materials are some of the important compounds available in the United States.

Aminosalicylates

Balsalazide disodium (Colazal)
Mesalamine (Asacol, Pentasa)
Sulfasalazine (Azulfidine)

Antacids

Aluminum hydroxide (AlternaGEL, Amphojel)
Aluminum hydroxide/magnesium hydroxide/ simethicone (Mylanta)
Calcium carbonate (Tums)
Magaldrate (Riopan)
Magnesium hydroxide (Milk of Magnesia)
Simethicone (Mylicon)

Antidiarrheal drugs

Diphenoxylate/atropine (Lomotil)
Loperamide (Imodium)

Bismuth salts

Bismuth subsalicylate (Pepto-Bismol)

H_2 receptor antagonists

Cimetidine (Tagamet)
Famotidine (Pepcid)
Nizatidine (Axid)
Ranitidine (Zantac)

Laxatives

Castor oil (Neoloid)
Lactulose (Chronulac)
Methylcellulose (Citrucel)
Polycarbophil (Fibercon)
Psyllium (Metamucil)

Proton pump inhibitors

Esomeprazole (Nexium)
Lansoprazole (Prevacid)
Omeprazole (Prilosec)
Pantoprazole (Protonix)
Rabeprazole (Aciphex)

Mucosal protectant

Sucralfate (Carafate)

Prostaglandin

Misoprostol (Cytotec)

Promotility and antiemetic agents

Erythromycin (E-Mycin)
Granisetron (Kytril)
Metoclopramide (Reglan)

Serotonin 5-HT_3 antagonist

Alosetron (Lotronex)
Granisetron (Kytril)
Ondansetron (Zofran)

Serotonin 5-HT_4 agonist

Tegaserod (Zelnorm)

FURTHER READING

Chan FKL, Leung WK. Peptic ulcer disease. *Lancet* 2002; 360:933-941.

Lembo A, Camilleri M. Chronic constipation. *N Engl J Med* 2003; 349:1360-1368.

Richardson P, Hawkey CJ, Stack WA. Proton pump inhibitors: pharmacology and rationale for use in gastrointestinal disorders. *Drugs* 1998; 56:307-335.

Self-assessment questions

1. Cimetidine and related antisecretory drugs act as antagonists at parietal cell:

a. M_3 receptors.
b. Prostaglandin receptors.
c. H_2 receptors.
d. H_1 receptors.
e. Gastrin receptors.

2. Metoclopramide produces promotility and antiemetic effects primarily because it acts as an:

a. Antagonist at M_2 receptors.
b. Agonist at 5-HT_4 receptors.
c. Inhibitor of acetylcholinesterase.
d. Agonist at motilin receptors.
e. Antagonist at D_2 receptors.

3. Which one of the following is most likely to interfere with cytochrome P450 drug metabolism?

a. Cimetidine
b. Ranitidine
c. Pantoprazole
d. Sucralfate
e. Metoclopramide

4. Which one of the following is most likely to induce parkinsonism-like extrapyramidal symptoms?

a. Sulfasalazine
b. Ranitidine
c. Omeprazole
d. Sucralfate
e. Metoclopramide

5. Major serious side effects associated with the long-term use of an aluminum-containing antacid include:

a. Diarrhea.
b. Systemic alkalosis.
c. Phosphate depletion.
d. Kidney stones.
e. Dementia.

6. Dry mouth, visual disturbance, constipation, and difficulty in urination are side effects commonly associated with use of:

a. Muscarinic receptor antagonists.
b. H_2 receptor antagonists.
c. D_2 receptor antagonists.
d. 5-HT_3 receptor antagonists.
e. Gastrin receptor antagonists.

CHAPTER 56

Toxicology

I. Glenn Sipes
Richard C. Dart
Lawrence J. Fischer

Major Chemicals

Acetaminophen (Tylenol)	Heavy metals
Aromatic amines	Lead
Carbon monoxide	Organophosphate insecticides
Cyanide	
Halogenated benzenes	

What is toxicology?

Industrial chemical and pharmaceutical development, environmental contamination, and illicit drug use present significant health hazards to the general population. It is estimated that each year in the United States approximately 8 million people suffer acute poisoning. In addition, about 20,000 persons die from illicit drug overdose per year. Acute toxicity from drug or poison ingestion accounts for as much as 10% to 20% of hospital admissions. A more-difficult challenge to health care providers is the identification of health effects resulting from long-term exposure to very low doses of environmental or occupational chemicals. In these cases, adverse effects may take years to develop.

Principles of toxicology

Any substance injurious to humans may be classified as a poison. Sodium chloride, oxygen, and many other substances generally considered nontoxic can be dangerous under certain conditions. The most important axiom of toxicology is that "the dose makes the poison," since any chemical can be toxic if the dose or exposure is high enough. Similarly, the degree of injury increases as dose increases.

The terms *poison, toxic substance, toxic chemical,* and *toxicant* are synonymous. Toxicity refers to the adverse effects manifested by an organism in response to a substance.

The dose of a chemical that kills 50% of animals receiving it (LD_{50}) is a common test that was originally developed to quantify lethality. However, LD_{50} is obviously inappropriate in the assessment of toxicity in humans, and it is more important to understand how the dose of a chemical alters biochemical and physiological processes and if they produce toxicity. Also, findings in one species cannot always be reliably extrapolated to another species. The ultimate determinant is the effect on humans.

The time between ingestion of or exposure to a chemical and the onset of its deleterious effects can vary considerably. Generally, if a toxic response results from a single dose or exposure, it is considered **acute toxicity. Subacute** or **subchronic** toxicity usually refers to that occurring after several weeks to months of exposure, and **chronic** toxicity refers to that occurring after months to years. Most acutely toxic agents rapidly

Abbreviations

ARDS	adult respiratory distress syndrome
CNS	central nervous system
CO	carbon monoxide
EDTA	ethylenediaminetetraacetic acid
GI	gastrointestinal
IgG, IgM	immunoglobulins

interfere with critical cellular processes. For example, cyanide causes immediate injury by inhibiting cellular respiration. Acetaminophen is another example of an agent that causes acute injury if a single large dose is ingested. Hepatic necrosis, however, may not be evident for 1 to 3 days after ingestion. Acetaminophen produces reactive intermediates that injure liver cells within a few hours but takes time (2 to 3 days) to become clinically apparent. Organophosphate insecticides cause an early cholinergic syndrome, which resolves before the peripheral neuropathy develops several days later.

A chemical causing **direct** toxicity injures a cell after coming in direct contact with it. Chemicals causing **indirect** toxicity do so by injuring one group of cells, which precipitates injury in others. Interference with normal physiological processes may injure cells dependent on that process, while other processes are able to repair tissues damaged by toxicants.

Some substances, such as strong acids or bases, act locally. Most other toxic substances produce systemic effects or a combination of local and systemic effects. For example, hydrofluoric acid, a common industrial chemical, produces an extremely painful local penetrating injury at the site of skin exposure. In larger exposures, enough fluoride ions enter the blood to bind Ca^{2+} and produce hypocalcemia.

Target organ toxicity

Many toxic substances are known to affect a specific target organ, such as the liver, nervous system, kidneys, or lungs. Because of a dual blood supply from the hepatic artery and the portal vein, the **liver** may be exposed to toxicants entering from the systemic circulation (e.g., via inhalation) or from the splanchnic circulation (absorbed from the gastrointestinal [GI] tract). The leaky capillary system of the hepatic sinusoids promotes the extraction of toxicants from the blood into the liver. The liver contains enzymes that metabolize many endogenous and exogenous chemicals (see Chapter 3). In some cases, chemical modification produced by biotransformation results in **bioactivation** (production of toxic-reactive metabolites). Figure 56-1 presents a schematic for bioactivation of chloroform to phosgene. Factors that enhance the activity of *CYP*2E1 (enzyme-inducing agents) or reduce the hepatic concentration of glutathione can exacerbate chloroform-induced liver injury. The popular over-the-counter-analgesic acetaminophen also causes hepatic injury. The liver is a target because it is rich in cytochrome P450s, which metabolize acetaminophen to a reactive metabolite. At therapeutic doses, little if any of this metabolite is formed. However, at high doses, the rate of formation of this metabolite exceeds detoxification capacity, causing hepatotoxicity. Other compounds that can cause liver injury after metabolism include solvents (carbon tetrachloride, halogenated benzenes), therapeutic drugs (isoniazid), and carcinogens (aflatoxin B, aromatic amines).

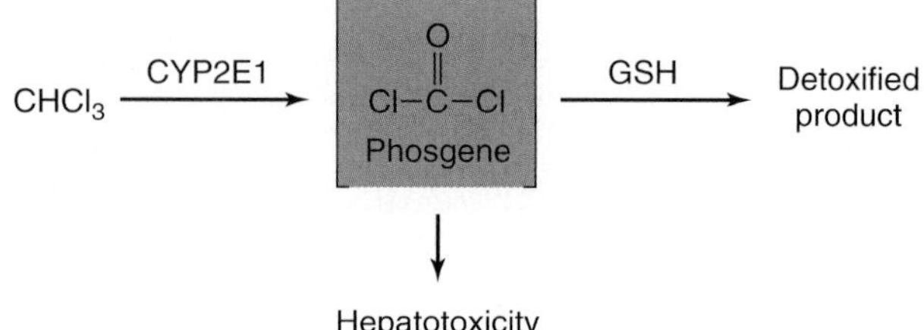

Figure 56-1 *CYP2E1* converts chloroform to phosgene within the hepatocyte. Phosgene is highly reactive and has been used as a chemical warfare agent. *GSH* (glutathione) can conjugate with and detoxify phosgene. The liver is protected until the rate of formation of phosgene exceeds the rate of detoxification.

Because of the integrative role of the nervous system, toxic injury to one part can result in adverse effects in other sites. Similarly, toxic injury in other organs can result in neuronal lesions. For example, chemicals that cause severe hypotension or hypoglycemia may result in neuronal cell death and central nervous system (CNS) damage, since neurons have a high metabolic rate that requires a sustained delivery of oxygen and nutrients. Similarly, chemicals that interfere with oxidative metabolism (i.e., cyanide or dinitrophenol) can also compromise neuronal viability.

Neurons are unique because the cell body must provide support for dendrites and axons. The axon is devoid of metabolic functions (i.e., protein synthesis) and must rely on the transport of materials, often over long distances, from the cell body to the distal axon. Acrylamide and n-hexane produce peripheral neuropathies by interfering with axonal transport. Diketone metabolites of n-hexane can derivatize and cross-link neurofilaments. As these cross-links accumulate with repeated exposure, axonal transport is retarded, ultimately causing axonal atrophy.

Mature neurons also lack regenerative repair mechanisms; therefore cumulative damage can occur within the nervous system (Fig. 56-2). However, such neurotoxicity is often delayed such that repeated chemical exposures are required to reach a critical concentration. There is also a normal, **age-related attrition** of neurons. Chemical exposure to neurotoxicants may reduce the age at which neurological and behavioral deficits appear. If exposure to the chemical occurred in the remote past, a causal relationship between exposure and neurotoxicity will not always be apparent.

Pulmonary toxicity primarily results from respiratory exposure, although blood-borne toxicants may also

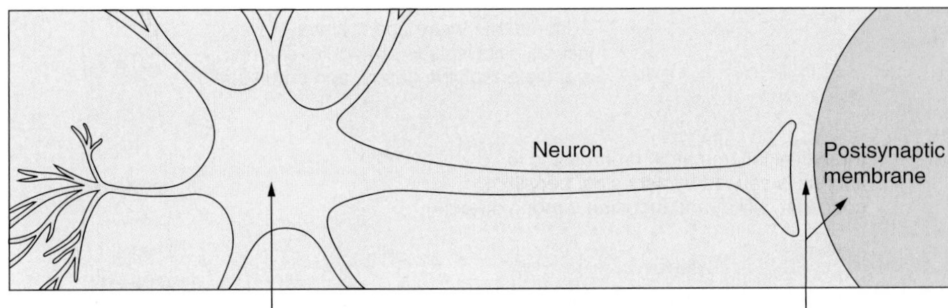

Figure 56-2 Summary of some toxicant actions on central and peripheral neuronal cells.

contribute. The pulmonary system is composed of the nasopharyngeal and tracheobronchial airways and the pulmonary parenchyma (alveoli). Airways are directly exposed to many gaseous or particulate toxicants. Gases may react with airway mucosal cells or penetrate to the alveoli. For example, chlorine gas reacts with upper airway fluids and produces hydrochloric acid, causing mucosal injury. Cyanide and chloroform penetrate to the alveoli, are well absorbed, and cause systemic, not pulmonary, toxicity. Particulates can also become impacted in the airway or, if small enough (less than 5 μm), can reach the alveoli. If trapped in the airway, they may be cleared by the mucociliary apparatus. Substances reaching the alveoli can be eliminated only by absorption into the blood, by macrophage phagocytosis, or by biotransformation. Macrophages phagocytose toxicants in particulate form and then enzymatically degrade them or simply carry them out of the alveolus. If asbestos is the toxicant involved, this function may actually produce toxicity because macrophages engulf but cannot degrade asbestos particles. When the macrophages ultimately die, they release degradative enzymes into the interstitium, which damage adjacent cells. Repetition of this process eventually leads to progressive fibrosis and restrictive respiratory dysfunction. The pulmonary biotransformation of chemicals may also lead to toxicity. The **Clara cells,** located in terminal bronchioles, and the alveolar type II cells possess cytochrome P450, which can produce toxic metabolites of certain chemicals. Inhalation of benzo[a]pyrene and other polycyclic aromatic hydrocarbons causes lung cancer by this mechanism.

The blood can be the route of exposure of the lung in the case of paraquat, a herbicide taken up by type II pneumocytes. Biotransformation in the lung yields a reactive intermediate that undergoes redox cycling, which produces reactive oxygen species that injure the cell. Although exposure to paraquat usually occurs after ingestion or skin contamination, death results from pulmonary injury. Similarly, certain pyrrolidine alkaloids are metabolized in the liver to metabolites that circulate in the blood and produce toxicity in the lung (Fig. 56-3).

The kidney is also susceptible to toxicants. The mechanisms of **renal injury** are similar to those in other organs but also include unique mechanisms. Delivery of blood-borne toxicants to the kidney is high, because (1) the kidney receives 25% of cardiac output and (2) its functions include filtering, concentrating, and eliminating toxicants. As water is reabsorbed, the concentration of chemicals in the tubule can increase to toxic levels. In some cases, the concentration may exceed the solubility of a chemical and lead to precipitation and obstruction of the affected area (Fig. 56-4).

The kidney also biotransforms chemicals, although to a lesser extent than the liver. Cytochrome P450 is located in the proximal tubule, which may explain the susceptibility of this region to chemical injury. For example, carbon tetrachloride and chloroform, two halogenated hydrocarbons that injure the proximal tubule, must be biotransformed by the cytochrome P450 system to be toxic. In addition, many heavy metals damage the proximal tubules. Because they are not metabolized by cytochrome P450, other mechanisms must be involved. Heavy metals may concentrate in renal tubular cells and may also injure blood vessels supplying the proximal tubule cells, a combination of direct and indirect toxicity.

The kidney can compensate for excessive chemical exposure since, like many organs, it has a reserve mass. Thus tissue injury equal to one entire kidney must occur before loss of function is clinically apparent. The kidney also replaces lost functional capacity by hypertrophy. In

Figure 56-3 Summary of some toxicant actions on pulmonary tissues.

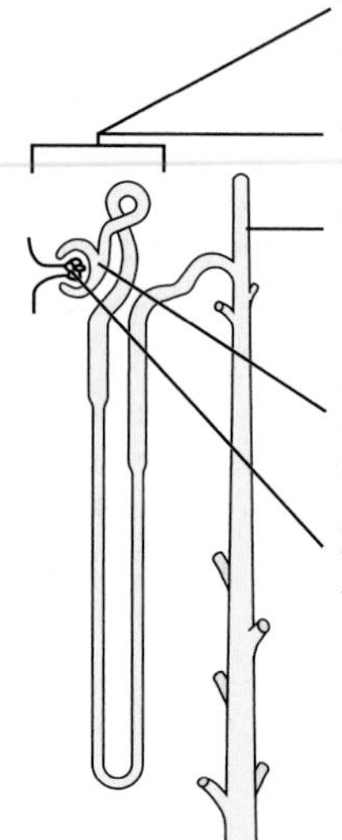

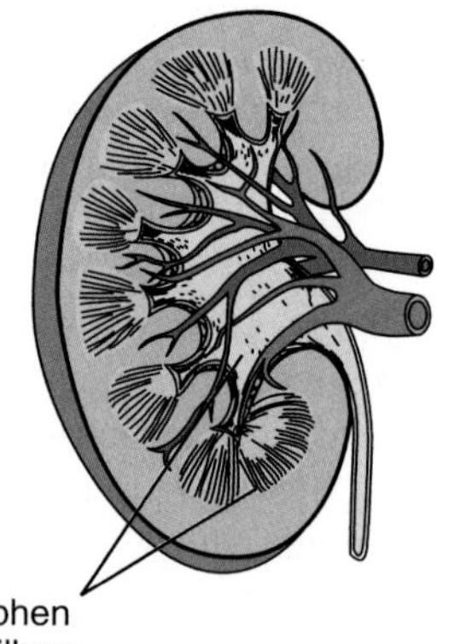

Figure 56-4 Summary of some toxicant actions on the kidney.

addition, the kidney has developed binding proteins to remove heavy metals. For example, metallothioneins avidly bind cadmium, protecting the kidney and other organs from toxicity. However, renal toxicity will develop if exposure exceeds the binding capacity or if a large amount of the cadmium-metallothionein complex accumulates.

Although certain anatomical or functional characteristics may predispose organs to injury, designation of chemicals as specific organ toxicants (e.g., neurotoxic, cardiotoxic) is misleading, for several reasons. First, toxic substances may have adverse effects throughout the body. Although a chemical may primarily affect one organ, other organs probably also incur less-notable injury. Second, a toxic response in one tissue will undoubtedly have serious consequences for other tissues. The intensity depends on the characteristics of the chemical (physical state, site of exposure, dose, and duration of exposure) and of the patient (general health, nutritional state, age, sex, enzyme induction, immune response, antioxidant concentrations). Thus a minor insult to a compromised organ may cause unexpected injury to that organ and may also affect other organs.

Determinants of the toxic response

Generally the means by which a toxicant reaches its target organ is governed by the same pharmacokinetic principles that govern the actions of therapeutic drugs (see Chapter 4). These principles also provide the basis for methods to reduce, reverse, or prevent toxicity of many substances.

Chemicals may be absorbed by dermal, GI, and/or pulmonary routes, and measures to prevent absorption may reduce the concentration of a toxicant at its site of action. Washing the skin, stomach lavage, and oral administration of charcoal are examples of ways to reduce dermal or GI absorption of toxicants. After absorption, toxic substances are distributed to tissues through the blood, and in some cases it is possible to intercept the toxicant before it reaches its target. This can be accomplished by the following mechanisms:

- Hemodialysis, which can remove the toxic compound by filtration
- Hemoperfusion, which can remove toxicants from blood by circulating blood through an activated charcoal filter
- Binding of a toxicant by a chemical or antibody before it reaches the site of toxicity

It is generally too late to prevent cell or organ damage after the toxicant reaches its target, although the effects of many toxicants may still be minimized at this stage. Compounds metabolized to reactive intermediates are good examples. An antidote that prevents biotransformation can minimize injury produced by a reactive intermediate. The competitive antagonism of methanol by ethanol is based on this principle (see Chapter 25). Similarly, drugs that inhibit certain cytochrome P450 isozymes can reduce biotransformation of some toxicants, either reducing or enhancing their effects.

Toxic metabolites produced by biotransformation may injure the cell in which they are produced, or they may diffuse in the blood and affect other areas. For a few substances, this offers a final opportunity to eliminate toxic metabolites by using hemodialysis to clear the blood.

Another strategy for reducing cellular injury is to prevent the reactive intermediate from interacting with important cell constituents (e.g., enzymes, DNA). The treatment of acetaminophen toxicity with *N*-acetylcysteine is based on this principle (see Chapter 31). Other interventions will be developed as the sequence of events involved in the progression of chemical-induced tissue injury becomes better understood. For example, agents that can consume reactive oxygen species or downregulate an inflammatory response may be effective if administered up to several hours after a drug overdose or chemical exposure.

The immune system

The immune system can be affected by a wide variety of toxicants. These agents often cause immunosuppression by interfering with cell growth or proliferation, resulting in a reduction of capacity. Other compounds may directly destroy immune system components. Some chemicals distort normal signaling mechanisms that ultimately reduce the immune response. For example, benzene causes lymphocytopenia but also affects other bone marrow elements. The functional result is a deficiency in cell-mediated immunity. Workers exposed to benzene show decreased humoral immunity, as evidenced by depressed complement and immunoglobulin concentrations.

In humans, immunosuppression may lead to an increased incidence of bacterial, viral, and parasitic infections. Theoretically, immunosuppression may also interfere with the immune system's surveillance function, resulting in an increased incidence of cancer, although this is still being investigated.

It is becoming increasingly apparent that activation and recruitment of phagocytic cells to sites of chemical-induced injury play a major role in the progression of tissue injury. Therapeutic interventions that could minimize the effects of these activated phagocytic cells include preventing the adhesion of phagocytic cells at the site of injury, reducing the release of cytotoxic factors, or inactivating these cytotoxic factors.

In addition to being a target for chemical-mediated injury, the immune system may mediate injury by producing hypersensitivity reactions (see Chapter 53). Such reactions are adverse events caused by an immune response to foreign antigens. A type I hypersensitivity reaction (anaphylaxis) is an immediate reaction mediated by IgG bound to mast cells and basophils. The binding of antigen causes the release of histamine and other mediators. Acute life-threatening responses to penicillin are examples of anaphylaxis. Type II (cytolytic) reactions involve IgG or IgM produced against a foreign compound. In some cases these immunoglobulins bind to other cells and cause destruction by stimulation of complement-mediated or other cytotoxic mechanisms. Several drugs including penicillins, sulfonamides, and quinine stimulate antibody formation, producing red blood cell hemolysis mediated by a type II mechanism. Type III (serum sickness) reactions involve a deposition of antibody-antigen complexes in skin and membranes. An immune reaction to these complexes causes inflammation of the skin, joints, kidney, and other organs. Serum sickness after antivenom administration is an example of this type of drug toxicity. Finally, type IV (cell-mediated) hypersensitivity is caused by T lymphocytes. T lymphocytes recognize antigens and recruit other cells to mount an inflammatory response. Contact dermatitis to nickel, several industrial chemicals, and poison ivy is caused by this mechanism.

Teratogenesis

A teratogen is a drug or other agent that causes abnormal fetal development. Thalidomide is a notorious example. However, the toxicity caused by teratogens is only one form of toxicity occurring in utero. Any known toxic effect that can occur in adults can also occur in the fetus, although there are certain special considerations.

Carcinogenesis

Cancer cells are cells that escape from the control mechanisms that govern growth, development, and division of normal cells (see Chapter 42). Some human cancers are of environmental origin, caused by radiation, viral infection, or chemical exposure.

Because cancer often develops in rats and mice exposed to extremely large doses of chemicals for long periods, many people believe that synthetic chemicals such as drugs, pesticides, or industrial agents are a primary cause of cancer. In fact, however, most chemicals that produce cancer in laboratory animals after large doses do not produce cancer in humans. Exceptions are vinyl chloride, benzene, and naphthylamine, which can cause cancer in humans after prolonged occupational exposure. Also, lifestyle choices result in significant exposure to chemical carcinogens. For example, cigarette smoke contains many potent cancer-causing chemicals and is a causative factor of lung cancer. Similarly, chronic ethanol consumption is associated with an increased risk of esophageal and liver cancer. Charcoal broiling contaminates food with polycyclic aromatic hydrocarbons, which are the same as those in coal tars and soot. It is possible that many human cancers could be prevented or delayed by "lifestyle" changes.

Duration, dose, and frequency of exposure are important variables in chemical-induced cancers. Because cancer may take 20 or more years to develop, cause-and-effect relationships are difficult to establish. The induction of cancer by chemicals is divided into three major steps:

1. Initiation
2. Promotion
3. Progression

Initiation consists of the conversion of a normal cell into a neoplastic cell. Chemicals that cause this conversion are called initiating agents, which target DNA.

Advances in our understanding of chemical carcinogenesis have led to the development of systems to test for the carcinogenic potential of chemicals. Such tests include a structural comparison to known carcinogens, *in vitro* mutagenesis and cell transformation assays, and cancer bioassays in rodents. Some chemicals interact directly and covalently with DNA, but many must be metabolically transformed before they can do so. If cell division occurs before enzymatic repair of the damaged DNA, a permanent mutation is encoded in the genome. Because cellular damage undoubtedly kills some cells in the target tissue, the stimulus for division of adjacent cells is high. The result is a new cell type with altered genotypic and phenotypic properties. Additional mutational events can then convert transformed cells to malignant cells.

In animal studies, some chemicals, referred to as **promoters,** have been observed to increase the incidence of cancers or decrease the latency period for tumor development without interacting with DNA or producing mutations. These chemicals are effective only when administered repeatedly after an initial insult. For example, a cytosolic receptor in animals that promotes liver carcinogenesis in the presence of the environmental chemical tetrachlorodibenzo-p-dioxin has been identified. This triggers a pleiotropic response that results in enhanced gene expression, cell proliferation, and clonal expansion into phenotypically altered foci, nodules, or papillomas. Endogenous substances such as **growth factors** and **hormones** may also act as promoters. For example, follicle-stimulating hormone and leuteinizing hormone may promote chemical-induced ovarian cancers as a result of their tropic effect on the ovary. Certain carcinogens that are initiating agents also can act as promoters, which create an environment conducive to the proliferation of initiated cells or produce other changes supporting autonomous division and tumor growth.

Toxic gases

Among the most-toxic gases are carbon monoxide (CO) and volatile cyanides. Both are toxic because they deprive the cell of energy. Other gases such as ozone, nitrogen oxides (NO, NO_2), and phosgene are toxic because of their chemical reactivity. They are irritating to mucous membranes and may trigger asthma-like symptoms in susceptible people.

Carbon monoxide

CO is the leading cause of death by poisoning. It also inflicts sublethal injuries, including myocardial infarction and cerebral atrophy.

CO primarily acts by displacing oxygen from hemoglobin and impairing oxygen release from hemoglobin. CO displaces oxygen from hemoglobin because it has more than 200 times higher affinity for hemoglobin than oxygen. Even at a concentration in air of only 0.5%, CO displaces oxygen to produce 50% carboxyhemoglobin. However, CO produces more injury than that predicted on the basis of the simple replacement of oxygen. This is explained by the fact that normal hemoglobin binding of oxygen shows **cooperativity.** Binding of one oxygen molecule promotes binding of subsequent molecules, and hemoglobin also shows cooperativity in releasing oxygen. However, carboxyhemoglobin does not release oxygen normally. CO therefore shifts the oxyhemoglobin dissociation curve to the left and reduces oxygen release, causing enhanced anaerobic metabolism and cell death if not reversed.

The symptoms of CO poisoning reflect the effects of oxygen deprivation. Early symptoms of nervous system dysfunction resemble those of the flu and include nausea, headache, malaise, light-headedness, and dizziness. Later signs and symptoms are more ominous, including depressed sensorium, loss of consciousness, seizures, and death.

The heart is particularly susceptible to CO poisoning. It has high oxygen requirements, and because it normally extracts more oxygen from the blood than other organs, it compensates poorly for decreased delivery. When CO decreases oxygen delivery, severe **myocardial ischemia** may develop.

As CO dissociates from the hemoglobin, it is expired. However, this is a slow process because of its high affinity for hemoglobin. The half-life of carboxyhemoglobin without treatment is 3 to 4 hours, depending on the patient's ventilation. Administration of 100% oxygen by face mask shortens the time to 90 minutes. Hyperbaric oxygen reduces the half-life to 20 minutes. The patient's outcome depends on the duration and severity of the hypoxic episode.

Cyanide

Exposure to cyanide commonly occurs through the inhalation of smoke produced by the burning of plastics. Certain paints may also contribute. Other potential sources are fruit seeds (e.g., apricots and cherries), which contain toxic amounts of soluble cyanide that must be metabolized by intestinal bacteria to release it. Salts of cyanide have been used in suicide or homicide poisoning.

Cyanide produces toxicity by binding avidly to ferric iron (Fe^{3+}), which prevents its reduction to the ferrous form (Fe^{2+}) involved in the **cytochrome oxidase** electron-transport system. Transfer of electrons from cytochromes to molecular oxygen is prevented, which in turn inhibits adenosine triphosphate production and forces the cell to produce energy by anaerobic metabolism. As in all cases of hypoxia, anaerobic glycolysis produces only small amounts of ATP and large quantities of lactic acid.

Thus victims of cyanide poisoning show symptoms of hypoxia. Similar to CO toxicity, cyanide toxicity first affects organs that have a large oxygen requirement. However, onset is often faster but depends on route of exposure. Inhalation may produce a rapid demise, whereas symptoms may be delayed for 30 minutes or more if the cyanide is ingested orally. CNS dysfunction causes loss of consciousness and respiratory arrest.

Treatment is focused on preventing cyanide from reaching its target, cytochrome oxidase. Because cyanide has a high affinity for ferric iron, ferric iron in the form of oxidized hemoglobin can be provided by administration of **sodium nitrite.** This converts hemoglobin to methemoglobin, the ferric form, which effectively competes with cyanide for cytochrome a_3, forming cyanmethemoglobin. Cyanide is removed from the body after being converted to thiocyanate by the enzyme rhodanese and is ultimately excreted in the urine. **Sodium thiosulfate** is administered to facilitate thiocyanate formation. An alternative is to administer hydroxocobalamin, which reacts with cyanide to produce cyanocobalamin. Because hydroxocobalamin and cyanocobalamin have little toxicity, they hold promise for the treatment of cyanide poisoning.

Heavy metals

The widespread occurrence of metals in the environment and their numerous industrial and medical uses make them important potential toxicants.

The rate at which heavy metals are absorbed depends on their physical state. Metals may exist in their elemental state or bound to inorganic or organic ligands. The elemental and inorganic forms of metals may be well absorbed because of their physical similarity to nutritionally essential metals. For example, lead is absorbed by the normal transport protein for iron located in the GI tract mucosa. Organs containing these transport systems are prone to injury from these metals. Commonly injured organs include liver, kidney, and GI tract mucosa. Organic forms of metals are more lipid soluble than inorganic forms and may be well absorbed without specific transport systems.

The state of the metals also affects their distribution, and lipid-soluble forms reach higher concentrations in areas such as the brain. Inorganic and elemental forms of mercury primarily injure the kidney, whereas organic forms such as methylmercury injure the brain.

The body has developed specific defense mechanisms against certain metals. For example, as noted earlier, the kidney has a binding protein for cadmium called **metallothionein,** which strongly binds cadmium, concentrates it in the kidney, and reduces its excretion. The binding prevents toxicity until the protein is saturated, at which time additional cadmium accumulation causes injury.

Mechanisms involved in heavy metal toxicity are poorly understood. Many metals function as essential enzyme cofactors. Substitution by a similar but toxic metal may produce enzymatic dysfunction. Metals are generally very reactive and may bind key sulfhydryl groups in active centers of enzymes. Besides causing direct metal toxicity, metals can also produce hypersensitivity reactions. Nickel, chromium, gold, and others cause cell-mediated (type IV) hypersensitivity reactions (Table 56-1).

Table 56-1 Mechanisms of heavy metal toxicity

Metal	Mechanism	Target Organs
Arsenic	Reacts with sulfhydryl groups Interferes with oxidative phosphorylation	Peripheral neurons GI tract Liver Cardiovascular system
Lead	Reacts with sulfhydryl groups Interferes with heme synthesis Direct toxic effect on CNS	Hematopoietic system Central and peripheral nervous system Kidney
Mercury	Reacts with sulfhydryl groups Some forms have direct cytotoxic effect	Central and peripheral nervous system Kidney GI tract Respiratory tract

Table 56-2 Metals chelated by therapeutic agents

Chelator	Metal
Succimer	Lead, arsenic, mercury
Deferoxamine	Iron
EDTA	Lead
Penicillamine	Copper, lead
British anti-Lewisite	Lead, arsenic, mercury

Metal chelation

Treatment for metal toxicity focuses on increasing excretion of the metal from the body. Chelator drugs bind the metal between two or more functional groups to form a complex that is excreted in urine. Specific chelators work best in the removal of certain metals. The uses of chelators are summarized in Table 56-2.

Lead

Lead is one of the oldest known poisons but continues to pose a significant health problem. Industrialization, mining, and leaded gasoline have dramatically increased the amount of lead in the environment and consequently in humans. However, the switch to unleaded gasoline has resulted in decreases in environmental lead contamination. Lead is also present in some ceramic glazes and paints. In older homes, paint containing lead flakes off or is present in dust and may be ingested or inhaled by children, producing toxicity. Adults are exposed to toxic concentrations in certain work environments.

Lead binds to sulfhydryl and other active sites in many enzymes, leading to inactivation. Although its effects are diffuse, certain manifestations predominate. Two enzymes in the heme biosynthetic pathway are inhibited by lead, and inhibition of heme synthesis can result in anemia.

Lead is particularly toxic to the **nervous system,** especially in children. Early signs and symptoms include anorexia, colicky abdominal pain, lethargy, and vomiting. If lead exposure continues, children are more likely than adults to develop encephalopathy, manifested by irritability progressing to seizures and coma. Approximately 30% will develop permanent neurological sequelae.

Low-concentration lead exposure may pose special risks for children. Subtle neurological injuries including depressed IQ scores and learning disorders have been reported. This may be due to enhanced accumulation in the immature nervous system. Lead may cross the blood-brain barrier more easily in children, and their CNS may also be less capable of removing it. Children with blood lead concentrations exceeding 10 μg/dl are considered to be at risk.

Vague complaints of headache and light-headedness develop in adults exposed to lead. With increased exposure, a peripheral neuropathy develops.

The whole-blood lead concentration is the best indicator of exposure in the patient with lead-poisoning signs and symptoms. As the concentrations increase, the danger of encephalopathy increases, al though overt signs and symptoms do not usually occur until lead concentrations approach 50 μg/dl.

Lead is slowly excreted from the body. The primary treatment of lead poisoning is removal from the source. Excretion may be hastened by the use of chelators such as British anti-Lewisite.

Other toxicants

Toxicities resulting from organophosphates or drugs of abuse are described in Chapters 9 and 32, respectively.

Interactive toxicology

It is important to understand how exposure to one or more chemicals affects the toxic potential of another chemical, an area referred to as *interactive toxicology*. The scope of interactive toxicology is large, because there are many opportunities for multiple chemical exposures (environmental/occupational/drug) and for exposure to complex mixtures of undefined chemicals (cigarette smoke, hazardous waste). Interactions can result in additive, synergistic, or antagonistic events. Synergistic interactions are of greatest concern, because the toxicological outcome is more than additive and often unpredictable. Two major mechanisms are involved. The first are toxicokinetic interactions, which occur when the amount of toxicants at the target site is increased or decreased because of chemical-induced changes in absorption, distribution, metabolism, or excretion of the toxicant, or some combination of these. The second are toxicodynamic interactions, which occur when the sensitivity of the target tissue to the toxicant is altered. Mechanisms include the upregulation or downregulation of receptors, an altered inflammatory response, an inhibition of tissue repair capacity, and others.

Environmental toxicology

Chemical exposure and health outcomes

Chemical contaminants in the environment (soil, water, food, indoor/outdoor air) are a hazard to human health. Petroleum mixtures contains benzene, a known human carcinogen commonly found in air and water. Agricultural chemicals, industrial waste, and incineration by-products also contribute pollutants such as pesticides, polychlorinated biphenyls, dioxins, and polyaromatic hydrocarbons. Naturally occurring chemicals such as arsenic (found in drinking water), methylmercury (found in fish), and aflatoxin B (produced by a fungus that grows on corn and peanuts) are examples. Chronic exposure of humans to high doses over a lifetime is likely to produce adverse health effects.

Exposure may occur in several ways and under different circumstances. Catastrophic accidents producing immediate morbidity and mortality are infrequent. In 1984 an explosion in a pesticide factory produced over 2000 deaths and 10,000 injuries in Bhopal, India. High concentrations of methylisocyanate, a chemically reactive gas, were released in an urban setting and caused immediate lung damage and death in both workers and residents of the city.

Continual exposure over a long period of time can also result in accumulation of chemicals to toxic levels. Accumulation may result from slow elimination of the harmful chemical and/or a lack of cellular repair mechanisms. This can contribute to chronic diseases such as cancer, heart disease, and neurodegenerative disorders. Well-documented examples include the multiple health threats from tobacco use and exposure to second-hand smoke, the development of rare hepatic angiosarcomas in factory workers exposed to vinyl chloride, mesothelioma as a result of asbestos exposure, and male infertility caused by occupational exposure to the fumigant 1,2-dibromo-3-chloropropane. The current incidence of these cases is relatively low due to environmental advocacy, governmental regulation, and improved manufacturing and waste-handling processes.

Associating chemical exposure with a particular disease or set of symptoms is problematic. The low-dose environmental exposure situation often creates a dilemma because a causal relationship often cannot be made with adequate certainty, confounding diagnosis, treatment, and subsequent remedial action to inhibit further exposure.

Estimation of health risks

A lower incidence or even an absence of harmful effects from hazardous chemicals is expected if exposure is low enough. Strategies for prevention of toxic effects require knowledge of the threshold dose above which chemical toxicity will likely occur. Unfortunately, there are severe difficulties involved in determining the toxicological threshold exposure for a particular chemical in humans. Data from laboratory animal studies are usually available, but species differences make extrapolation of results to humans uncertain. Differences among individuals (age, health status, genetics) also makes selection of a single threshold value questionable. Epidemiology studies in exposed and control human populations can yield useful information, but such studies are rarely available.

Government agencies, particularly the United States Environmental Protection Agency, are mandated to develop regulatory controls to limit exposure of human and wildlife populations to harmful chemicals. This is accomplished by selecting a threshold value of daily exposure above which the risk of toxicity from a particular chemical is unacceptable. Because these are rarely clearly established, safety factors are applied to lower the threshold exposure value to an **acceptable** or **tolerable daily intake.** This value, smaller by 10-fold to 1000-fold (depending on the adequacy of the data), is adopted to protect the health of individuals with extreme sensitivity to the chemical (e.g. infants, aged, diseased). The adjusted value is used to calculate how much of a chemical can be released into the environment or to select an allowed concentration in drinking water, air, or food. The public and health professionals must realize that these regulatory procedures, known as "**risk assessment,**" do not provide values that can be equated with actual risk to a single individual. Instead they are used to ensure that public health, as it relates to exposure to toxic chemicals in the environment, will be maintained with a high margin of safety.

Clinical management of toxic patients

Clinical diagnosis and management of patients suffering from chemical toxicity is beyond the scope of this book. However, a summary of the variety of signs and symptoms (Table 56-3), the main contraindications and problems associated with emesis and gastric lavage (Box 56-1), and antidotes for common types of chemical toxicants (Table 56-4) is provided.

Table 56-3 Physical findings with exposure to toxic agents

Agent	Signs of Toxicity
Narcotic	Miotic pupils, CNS and respiratory depression, hypotension; may have needle-track marks
Anticholinergic	Dry, flushed appearance; mydriasis; decreased bowel motility, tachycardia, hallucinations
Cholinergic	Muscarinic—salivation, lacrimation, urination, defecation Nicotinic—muscle fasciculations, weakness, paralysis
Stimulants (cocaine, amphetamines)	Tachycardia, hypertension, hyperthermia, mydriasis, agitation, psychosis
Tricyclic antidepressants	Anticholinergic findings and electrocardiogram abnormalities (QRS widening, QT prolongation)

New horizons

Elucidation of mechanistic and receptor-mediated chemical toxicity has led to the development of specific antidotes. One such agent, flumazenil, a potent benzodiazepine antagonist, is used for benzodiazepine overdose (see Chapter 24). New antidotes for toxic alcohols, cyanide, venoms, and tricyclic antidepressants are on the horizon.

Prevention is becoming an important part of toxicology. Genotyping may make it possible to identify people particularly susceptible to the effects of a given toxicant. However, most exposures involve multiple chemicals, which may not be accurately predicted by this approach. Hazardous waste sites, for example, may contain pesticides, heavy metals, and a variety of industrial byproducts. Predicting the toxicological profiles of such mixtures is an important challenge.

The increasing sensitivity of analytic methodologies has shown that chemicals once believed to be safe are increasingly found to cause toxicity at levels present in the environment. For example, many children are exposed to concentrations of lead once predicted to be safe but now known to cause injury. The near future will find governments attempting to cope with enormous costs to make older housing safe and to treat these children with toxic lead levels. As research progresses, other chemicals may be found to pose similar problems.

Table 56-4 Common antidotes

Toxicant	Antidote	Mechanism
Venoms—snake, black widow	Antivenom	Immunological binding to toxicant
Cholinesterase inhibitors	Atropine	Blocks muscarinic receptors
Cyanide	Cyanide kit (Na nitrite, Na thiosulfate)	Induction of methemoglobinemia; cyanide binds preferentially to methemoglobin
Digoxin	Digoxin antibodies	Immunological binding to toxicant
Metals	Chelators	Binding of metal with subsequent urinary excretion
Methanol, ethylene glycol	Ethanol	Competition for alcohol dehydrogenase
Acetaminophen	*N*-Acetylcysteine	Provides sulfhydryl groups to detoxify reactive metabolite
Opiates	Naloxone	Blockade of opiate receptors
Carbon monoxide	Oxygen	Displaces CO molecules from carboxyhemoglobin
Isoniazid	Pyridoxine HCl	Provides substitute for pyridoxine kinase
Benzodiazepines	Flumazenil	Blockade of benzodiazepine receptor

Box 56-1 Contraindications and complications of emesis and gastric lavage

Contraindications

Emesis

Conditions in which the gag reflex is reduced or absent
Age less than 6 months
Inability to protect airway
Ingestion of agents causing rapid deterioration of mental status:
- Convulsants
- Tricyclic antidepressants
- Camphor

Ingestion of:
- Acid
- Alkali
- Hydrocarbons

Sharp objects
Pregnancy

Gastric Lavage

Strong acid or alkali ingestion
Petroleum product ingestion
Unconscious patients without endotracheal intubation

Complications

Emesis

Aspiration
Prolonged vomiting
Esophageal tearing

Gastric Lavage

Aspiration
Esophageal perforation
Intratracheal insertion

FURTHER READING

Dart RC, editor. *Medical toxicology.* 3rd ed. Lippincott, Williams and Wilkins, Philadelphia, 2004.

Klaassen CD, editor. *Casarett and Doull's Toxicology: the basic science of poisons*, 6th ed. McGraw Hill, New York, 2001.

Sipes IG, McQueen CA, Gandolfi AJ, editors. *Comprehensive Toxicology*, volumes 1-12, Pergamon/Elsevier, New York, 1997.

Self-assessment questions

1. Which of the following statements is *correct?*

a. Narcotic syndrome consists of dry, flushed appearance with mydriatic pupils, tachycardia, and hallucinations.
b. The anticholinergic syndrome includes miotic pupils, respiratory depression, hypotension, and depression of mental activities.
c. The cholinergic syndrome includes salivation, lacrimation, urination, diarrhea, muscle weakness, and fasciculation.
d. Stimulants cause the skin to be dry and flushed, and this is accompanied by tachycardia, hallucinations, and mydriatic pupils.

2. Which of the following statements regarding the site of injury produced by pulmonary toxicants is *correct?*

a. Toxic substances in the form of small particulates (less than 5 μm in diameter) may penetrate and be deposited in the alveoli.
b. Water-soluble chemicals are primarily absorbed in the alveoli.
c. The route of exposure of all pulmonary toxicants is through respiration.
d. Cyanide causes tissue hypoxia because it produces bronchoconstriction.

3. The kidney is a common target of toxic injury. Which of the following statements concerning the renal injury caused by toxic substances is *correct?*
   a. The kidney does not possess enzymes that can detoxify chemicals.
   b. Because of the concentrating capacity, kidney cells can be exposed to high levels of toxicants.
   c. Renal metallothionein metabolizes organic solvents to toxic metabolites.
   d. The blood supply of the kidney exposes it directly to chemicals absorbed from the small intestine.

4. Which of the following statements concerning lead toxicity in the United States today is *correct?*
   a. Low-level lead exposure has been shown to be safe for adults and children.
   b. A typical adult with lead poisoning will complain of abdominal pain, headache, and vomiting.
   c. The blood lead concentration is useful in the assessment of lead poisoning.
   d. Lead is an endogenous trace metal with important biological functions.

APPENDIX

Answers to self-assessment questions

Chapter 1

1. b. Pharmacodynamics is what a drug does to the body.
2. d. The proprietary name is the trade name patented by the manufacturer but is not necessarily related to its pharmacology or structure.
3. b. Pharmacokinetics refers to the time course of action.
4. e. Any of these variables could be involved in drug and dosage selection.

Chapter 2

1. b. Binding usually involves multiple weak bonds. It is rarely covalent, is usually stereoselective, and may or may not occur with a high affinity (K_D).
2. a. Chronic antagonist exposure will often increase receptor sensitivity. The other answers all decrease receptor sensitivity.
3. b. The affinity of drugs for receptors vary by many orders of magnitude. All other answers are correct.
4. e. Hormone receptor signaling can occur through any of the mechanisms listed.
5. b. Based on the information given, one can conclude only that the potencies are different. No conclusions can be made about structure, types of receptors involved, whether they are directly acting agonists, or whether they cause the same extent of relaxation.
6. d. The affinity constant is the concentration of a drug that occupies half of available receptor sites, is the ratio of the rate constants, and is important in determining fractional occupancy.

Chapter 3

1. d. There is no DNA in cell membranes.
2. b. Renal tubular reabsorption *increases* plasma drug concentrations.
3. d. $pH - pK_a = \log [A^-]/[HA] = 7.4 - 5.4 = 2$. Therefore the antilog of 2 is 100 and [HA] is 1%.
4. e. Highly polar and quaternary nitrogen compounds do not easily diffuse across cell membranes.
5. d. All of the answers listed are involved except esterases.
6. e. Conjugation reactions require drug-metabolizing enzymes and activation by high-energy phosphates, can occur with a variety of amino acids, and can also involve acids and weak bases.

Chapter 4

1. e. See equation 7.
2. a. Clearance is an independent pharmacokinetic parameter.

3. e. See discussion on protein binding.

4. d. Glomerular filtration rate (GFR) may slow, which alters the clearance of drugs.

5. d. Phase two drug metabolism such as glucuronidation does not change significantly with aging.

Chapter 5

1. d. A non-mutant gene is added to the cell in so-called complementation therapy. Optimized, this strategy is more efficient than adding RNA or protein to the cell. Current technology does not permit efficient repair of mutant DNA.

2. b. Transfer of genes in human gene therapy must be safe and non-toxic. Delivery of foreign DNA in a plasmid or viral vector may induce an immune response, which should be monitored. The success of gene transfer should be determined by evaluating the expression of the added DNA. The target cell for gene delivery should be a somatic cell, since transfer to germ cells is not ethical.

3. b. Microsomes (phospholipids) have not been used for gene transfer in clinical trials. Lipids in the form of liposomes are widely used. Many other viral and non-viral vehicles have been used.

4. c. Oligonucleotide antisense therapy depends on complementary binding of the delivered oligonucleotide and mRNA. RNaseH attacks this heteroduplex to degrade the mRNA. The effect is transient and depends on continued availability of antisense. Antisense oligonucleotides can be generated by a viral vector, but production of new mRNA is not the therapeutic mechanism.

Chapter 6

1. d. The FDA restricts only drugs that are Schedule 1. It does not restrict how it is used or whether or not a generic form exists.

2. c. Safe dosage on a small number of human volunteers and pharmacokinetics of the drug are determined by Phase I studies.

3. a. See Table 6-3.

4. b. q.i.d. means four times a day.

5. d. 1 grain equals about 65 mg, so 5 grains is about 325 mg.

Chapter 7

1. b. Randomized controlled clinical trials provide the most-solid evidence.

2. b. The Dietary Supplement Health Education Act (DHSEA) provides the regulatory framework for herbal and dietary supplements.

3. c. Echinacea is used to modulate immune function.

4. d. St. John's wort is used as an antidepressant.

5. c. No claims about efficacy can be made without sufficient scientific evidence.

6. a. Middle-aged people are most likely to use dietary supplements.

Chapter 8

1. c. Postganglionic parasympathetic neurons are short and unmyelinated.

2. a. Cell bodies for preganglionic sympathetic neurons originate in the intermediolateral cell column of the spinal cord.

3. e. β_1-Adrenergic receptors activate adenylate cyclase, whereas α_2-adrenergic receptors and some muscarinic receptor subtypes inhibit adenylate cyclase.

4. d. The stimulation by NE or another agonist of prejunctional α_2-adrenergic receptors on postganglionic sympathetic neurons results in inhibition of NE release. Acetylcholine is not released from most postganglionic sympathetic neurons.

5. e. Some muscarinic receptor subtypes (M_2 and M_4) inhibit adenylate cyclase, whereas other muscarinic receptor subtypes (M_1, M_3, and M_5) activate phospholipase C.

6. c. Activation of the parasympathetic system results in constriction of airway smooth muscle.

Chapter 9

1. b. Acetylcholine activates muscarinic receptors in the circular muscle of the iris (iris sphincter) to cause constriction (i.e., miosis). Acetylcholine activates muscarinic receptors in the lacrimal glands to increase secretion and in the longitudinal ciliary muscle to increase drainage of aqueous humor.

2. e. The muscarinic agonist pilocarpine contracts the longitudinal ciliary muscle to stretch open the trabecular meshwork and decrease intraocular pressure. Pilocarpine contracts the ciliary muscles, causes a spasm of accommodation through contraction of the circular

ciliary muscle, contracts the iris sphincter, and has no effect on the production of aqueous humor by the ciliary epithelium.

3. a. The patient exhibits typical parasympathetic symptoms with little neuromuscular involvement; consequently the muscarinic antagonist atropine is administered to antagonize the actions of the anticholinesterase insecticide. Atropine is preferred over the quaternary ammonium muscarinic antagonist propantheline, which does not enter the brain. In the presence of more-neuromuscular symptoms, atropine plus pralidoxime would be the appropriate treatment. The reversible carbamate cholinesterase inhibitor physostigmine is sometimes administered as an antidote to organophosphorus cholinesterase poisoning; however, this treatment is not as effective as pralidoxime. The short-acting competitive inhibitor of cholinesterase, edrophonium, has no use in treatment of cholinesterase poisoning.

4. d. The cause of death from anticholinesterase poisoning is usually respiratory failure, resulting from bronchoconstriction, excessive bronchial secretions, and paralysis of the diaphragm. Cholinesterase inhibitors do not cause hypertension or congestive heart failure. Although cholinesterase inhibitors cause hypotension, it usually is not the cause of death.

5. b. The mechanism of action of botulinus toxin is inhibition of vesicular release of acetylcholine. It does not block nicotinic receptors or peristalsis, nor does it stimulate the vagus nerve or cause circulatory collapse.

6. e. Bethanechol activates muscarinic receptors, causing a decrease in heart rate, peripheral vasodilation, and constriction in the airways of the lung. Bethanechol does not activate nicotinic receptors at the neuromuscular junction.

Chapter 10

1. b. Metoprolol is a relatively selective β_1-adrenergic receptor antagonist; the other responses to Epi are mediated by different adrenergic receptor subtypes (a, α_2; c, β_2; d, α_1; and e, α_1).

2. c. Labetalol has α_1-adrenergic receptor antagonist properties in addition to its β-receptor blocking actions. Propranolol and nadolol are β-receptor antagonists that lack α_1-blocking properties. Dobutamine and methoxamine are β_1- and α_1-agonists, respectively, and do not reduce sympathetic output to the vascular system.

3. e. Nadolol is more effective in blocking β_2-adrenergic receptors on bronchial smooth muscle than atenolol, which tends to be more specific in blocking β_1-adrenergic receptors. The other three drugs are β_2-agonists that would reduce airway resistance.

4. c. Phenylephrine, by activating α_1-adrenergic receptors, increases blood pressure, resulting in reflex bradycardia. The other drugs would be expected to have little effect or increase heart rate by acting directly on the heart (a and e) or by causing reflex tachycardia (b and d).

5. a. Terbutaline is a β_2-adrenergic receptor agonist, and all effects are produced by activation of β_2-receptors (reflex tachycardia) except mydriasis, which can be caused by activating α_1-adrenergic receptors on the radial smooth muscle of the iris.

6. c. After blockade of α_1- and α_2-adrenergic receptors by phentolamine, epinephrine activates β_1- and β_2-adrenergic receptors and thus most closely resembles the β_1/β_2-agonist isoproterenol. The other drugs have α- (a and e), α/β_1- (norepinephrine), or β_2-(b) agonist properties.

Chapter 11

1. e. Activation of the sympathetic nervous system causes all of the effects listed.

2. b. Skin is the tissue that is least influenced by the baroreceptor reflex, because it is relatively unimportant in such critical physiological processes as maintaining an upright posture.

3. c. Cyclic guanosine monophosphate is the only substance that is not increased by exocytotic release of norepinephrine. All other answers are correct.

4. d. A decrease in arterial blood pressure will DECREASE vagal discharge as a mechanism to promote the dominant sympathetic control.

Chapter 12

1. c. Thiazide diuretics have no direct action on the sympathetic nervous system. All of the statements about thiazide diuretics are correct.

2. b. Minoxidil produces marked arterial dilation, reduction in blood pressure, and significant side effects. For these reasons, it is recommended for use only in cases of severe hypertension, or when hypertension is resistant to other drug treatments. All of the other statements about minoxidil are correct.

3. b. The directly acting vasodilator drugs produce rapid and marked reduction in arterial pressure that engages the baroreceptor reflex to produce sympathetically mediated tachycardia and renin release. This would not occur with the other drug types listed because they all reduce sympathetic nervous system function and/or activation of β-adrenergic receptors.

4. a. Dihydropyridine-type drugs are Ca^{2+}-channel blocking drugs. They have no action at α-adrenergic receptors. All of the other statements about dihydropyridines are true.

5. b. Only clonidine acts on the central nervous system to produce sedation.

6. d. Reflex bradycardia can occur only if blood pressure increases. Since ACE inhibitors lower blood pressure, they cannot produce reflex bradycardia. All of the other statements about ACE inhibitors are true.

Chapter 13

1. a. Loop diuretics such as furosemide or bumetanide inhibit the Na^+-K^+-2Cl cotransporter present in the apical cell membrane of the ascending limb of the loop of Henle.

2. d. Transepithelial Na^+ transport involves two steps: (1) Active extrusion (ATP dependent) of Na^+ from the cell interior to the interstitial fluid across the basolateral membrane mediated by the Na^+,K^+-ATPase. (2) The activity of this pump provides the electrochemical gradient for apical Na^+ entry across the apical membrane.

3. e. Spironolactone blocks aldosterone receptors. Aldosterone increases Na^+ conductance in the apical membrane of principal cells of the late distal tubule and collecting tubule and increases Na^-,K^+-ATPase activity. The net result is an increase in the electrochemical gradient for K^+ secretion. By blocking aldosterone receptors, spironolactone abolishes the effect of aldosterone on K^+ secretion.

4. a. Hypokalemia, hyperglycemia, and hyperlipidemia are known consequences of thiazide use.

Chapter 14

1. c. Amiodarone is a Class III antiarrhythmic.

2. c. The plateau of action potential of a nonpacemaker cardiac cell is characterized by a low-conductance state in which Ca^{2+} influx is balanced by K^+ efflux.

3. c. Lidocaine is the only agent listed that is not orally active, which is a result of extensive first-pass hepatic metabolism.

4. e. Propranolol has negative inotropic effects and slows conduction, which can be detrimental to patients with congestive heart failure or AV conduction disturbances. Because propranolol lacks cardioselectivity, it also blocks β_2-adrenergic receptors on bronchi and bronchioles, thereby increasing airway resistance.

5. c. Depression is the only side effect listed that has not been associated with chronic amiodarone therapy.

6. d. Ibutilide is the only agent listed likely to precipitate this effect.

Chapter 15

1. b. Digitalis glycosides bind directly to the Na^+,K^+-ATPase and inhibit its electrogenic function.

2. d. Both nitrovasodilators and loop diuretics will decrease preload.

3. b. An ACE inhibitor, such as captopril, is most likely to reduce afterload.

4. f. Digoxin and milrinone act through mechanisms that do not involve β-adrenergic receptor activation, while dobutamine and isoproterenol stimulate these receptors. Thus the effects of the latter two will be blocked by a β-blocker.

5. c. Milrinone is a type III phosphodiesterase inhibitor; the other drugs act by different mechanisms.

6. b. Eplerenone is an aldosterone antagonist.

Chapter 16

1. d. This is a class of diseases characterized by skin lesions; it is an adverse side effect of hydralazine therapy. All of the other side effects are related to nitrovasodilator therapy.

2. e. This drug inhibits angiotensin converting enzyme, thereby reducing blood levels of angiotensin II, which causes both arteriolar and venous constriction. Hydralazine and minoxidil act on arteriolar vessels, whereas nitroglycerin acts on venous vessels.

3. e. Activator Ca^{2+} for contraction of smooth muscle can either enter through voltage-operated channels or be released from intracellular sites by IP_3. Ca^{2+} combines with calmodulin to activate myosin light chain kinase and promote cross-bridge formation leading to vascular contraction.

4. a. Nitrovasodilators act by mechanisms similar to that of endothelium-derived relaxing factor or nitric oxide. They stimulate soluble guanylate cyclase, causing an increase in cyclic GMP in smooth muscle cells. Phosphodiesterase inhibition is a potential area for the development of new vasodilators.

5. c. Vasodilators used to treat chronic congestive heart failure influence preload, afterload, or both. Minoxidil is generally not very effective when used alone.

6. c. NO synthesis in the endothelium is due to activation of a constitutive form of the enzyme. The constitutive form of the enzyme is dependent upon the concentration of the Ca^{2+}-calmodulin complex in the endothelial cell.

Chapter 17

1. b. Eicosanoids do not all contain a pentane ring. Thromboxane A_2 contains a six-membered oxane ring.

2. d. Prostaglandins can act to stimulate or inhibit adenylyl cyclase or to activate phospholipase C.

3. b. PGI_2 possesses vasodilator activity.

4. c. TxA_2 is a very unstable metabolite of arachidonic acid with a short chemical half-life of less than 1 minute at body temperature.

5. b. Hypertension. Most prostaglandins cause vasoconstriction.

6. c. A leukotriene receptor antagonist such as montelukast or zafirlukast.

Chapter 18

1. b. LDL cholesterol is formed primarily in blood. All other statements are true.

2. a. Statins do not always reduce cholesterol.

3. c. Cholesterol absorption blockers reduce HDL concentrations.

4. d. All of the statements are correct.

Chapter 19

1. c. In contrast to warfarin, heparin must be given by injection, has a short half-life, and may cause platelet aggregation and thrombocytopenia. It acts by binding to antithrombin, thereby increasing the activity of this serine protease inhibitor.

2. d. Warfarin, which can be taken orally, acts by inhibiting vitamin K regeneration, thus preventing the posttranslational modification of clotting factors. Warfarin metabolism is accelerated by barbiturates and other drugs that stimulate the activity of cytochrome P450.

3. b. Aspirin and other drugs that inhibit platelet function increase the risk of bleeding in patients receiving other types of anticoagulants.

4. d. Aspirin and clopidogrel increase the antithrombotic effect by inhibiting platelet aggregation; chloral hydrate does so by displacing warfarin from binding sites on plasma albumin, and heparin does so by increasing antithrombin activity. Cholestyramine decreases warfarin absorption.

5. a. Aspirin inhibits platelet cyclooxygenase, thereby preventing the formation of TXA_2, a powerful platelet-aggregating agent. Inhibition of platelet aggregation lengthens the bleeding time without affecting the coagulation mechanism.

Chapter 20

1. a. ACh is the only neurotransmitter whose action is terminated by hydrolysis via the action of acetylcholinesterase; the actions of all the other amine neurotransmitters listed are terminated by reuptake.

2. a. All of the biogenic amine neurotransmitters are synthesized in nerve terminals and transported into vesicles by an active process; their concentration in vesicles is 10-100 times that in the cytosol.

3. c. The long-term administration of agonists leads to a downregulation of receptors in the postsynaptic cell membrane.

4. c. Dopaminergic neurons originate in the substantia nigra and hypothalamus; the other types of neurons listed originate in other brain regions.

5. b. A high degree of lipophilicity will facilitate the ability of drugs to cross the blood-brain barrier; the other choices would hinder it.

6. c. Ethanol, a CNS depressant, produces an initial stage of excitation by reducing the activity of tonically active inhibitory brain systems. It has none of the other effects listed.

Chapter 21

1. b. Bromocriptine is the only DA agonist listed. Administration of any of the other drugs results in an *indirect* activation of D_2 receptors: L-DOPA enhances DA synthesis and release; amantadine facilitates DA release; selegiline enhances DA action by preventing its metabolism.

2. d. A cardinal sign of Parkinson's disease is tremor at rest, often consisting of a "pill-rolling" tremor. This should be distinguished from essential tremor, which occurs with the use of a limb. Tremor at rest is often treated with antimuscarinic agents.

3. b. Carbidopa is an inhibitor of aromatic L-amino acid decarboxylase and does not cross the BBB; thus, carbidopa does not influence l-DOPA metabolism in the brain.

4. a. Peripheral cholinergic effects are common with the use of these compounds.

4. b. Imipramine, diazepam, and buspirone are not used to treat mania, and renal disease is a contraindication for the use of lithium.

5. b. Mirtazapine is the only drug that enhances noradrenergic and serotonergic neurotransmission in the brain by blocking α_2-adrenergic receptors.

Chapter 22

1. c. Neuroleptic malignant syndrome is a life-threatening complication associated with antipsychotic drug treatment. It involves a near-complete collapse of the autonomic nervous system. Immediate hospitalization is required.

2. e. The efficacy of typical antipsychotic drugs is essentially the same. The potency of these agents differs and is correlated with their affinity for the D_2-receptor. Acute (but not chronic) treatment with antipsychotic drugs increases the firing rate of dopamine neurons. Chronic treatment results in an upregulation or supersensitivity of D_2 dopamine receptors.

3. a. The actions of antipsychotics include production of depolarization blockade and some anticholinergic effects, but these are unrelated to tardive dyskinesia. Tardive dyskinesia is a late-onset movement disorder that is thought to be related to the delayed induction of D_2-receptor supersensitivity that occurs with chronic antipsychotic drug treatment.

4. d. Clozapine, the prototypic atypical antipsychotic, is characterized by its *failure* to produce parkinsonian symptoms, tardive dyskinesia, or hyperprolactinemia. It does produce the potentially fatal complication of agranulocytosis.

5. e. The pharmacological profile of newer antipsychotic drugs is that they are relatively weak antagonists of dopamine at D_2-receptors. Consequently they have less propensity to produce extrapyramidal symptoms and hyperprolactinemia. For unknown reasons these agents appear to selectively affect limbic dopamine neurons.

Chapter 23

1. e. All other side effects are due to blockade of the receptors listed, and the increase in intraventricular conduction time is not.

2. b. Fluoxetine is about 15-fold more potent in blocking the uptake of serotonin than norepinephrine and has negligible effects on the other neurotransmitters.

3. e. Fluoxetine does not cause the side effects listed.

Chapter 24

1. c. Benzodiazepines act indirectly on chloride-inhibitory mechanisms through modulating $GABA_A$-receptor activity.

2. e. Buspirone's mechanism of action as a partial $5\text{-}HT_{1A}$-agonist is least likely to induce sedation of the choices listed.

3. c. Buspirone is a partial agonist at brain $5\text{-}HT_{1A}$-receptors.

4. d. General CNS depressant drugs have common mechanisms of action to a considerable extent.

5. a. Of those effects listed, only the anxiolytic effects persist over long periods of treatment with minimum development of tolerance.

Chapter 25

1. e. Cardiac toxicity, increased caloric intake, and disturbed lipid metabolism caused by alcohol use contribute to cardiovascular disease. Ethanol is metabolized in the liver, and this leads to a myriad of biochemical disturbances via increased NADP and acetaldehyde concentrations. Alcohol is associated with cancer of the larynx and pharynx. Fetal alcohol syndrome (intake of ethanol by the mother during pregnancy) is the leading preventable cause of mental retardation.

2. a. Obstructed hepatic venous return causes increased venous pressure and leakage of fluid. B is incorrect because this would decrease ascites, and just the opposite happens because of decreased serum protein synthesis by the liver. The other answers are unrelated.

3. b. However, recent evidence indicates that the genetic risk for women is greater than first thought. Also, these altered genes may be protective, if anything. Dopamine is important to the rewarding effects of ethanol, but there is no evidence that increased concentrations are responsible.

4. d. The interaction of estrogens may be responsible for the nearly twofold increase in the risk of liver damage in women compared with men.

5. d. Disulfiram (via a metabolic product) inhibits high K_m ALDH enzymes in the liver. The mitochondrial enzyme (low K_m enzyme) is inactive in some Asians because of a genetic abnormality. The end result in either case is increased acetaldehyde concentrations in the liver and blood, and a flushing reaction results.

6. e. Induction of cytochrome P450 2E1 is independent of ethanol oxidation. When it is present with other substrates for the enzyme, it competes with them for the enzyme, thus inhibiting their metabolism. When ethanol is absent, the increased enzyme content and activity lead to increased metabolic activity.

Chapter 26

1. c. Orlistat is the one agent for the treatment of obesity that has no cardiovascular side effects. Since the patient has a history of hypertension and angina, this would be the preferred treatment. Fluoxetine has not been shown to benefit obese individuals.

2. a. Underweight patients are extremely sensitive to cardiovascular side effects of drugs. Of the agents listed, fluoxetine is an selective serotonin reuptake inhibitor which has minimal risk of these adverse effects. All of the other drugs are tricyclic antidepressants.

3. d. Orlistat acts locally within the intestines to reduce the absorption of dietary fat via inhibition of intestinal lipase, which decreases the production of free fatty acids from triglycerides.

4. e. The presence of the active metabolites of sibutramine make it effective with once daily dosing.

Chapter 27

1. e. The 3-per-second spike and wave activity on the EEG and the clinical presentation are classic for absence seizures. The drug of choice for absence seizures is ethosuximide. Valproic acid also can be used but is not listed as a choice.

2. b. Phenytoin is one of few drugs that convert from first-order kinetics to zero-order kinetics in the therapeutic dose range. Therefore it is impossible to estimate a serum concentration based on a direct relationship to dose. When phenytoin becomes zero-order, the serum concentration will be higher than predicted from the dose.

3. c. This patient should be treated with antiepileptic drugs because she is having repeated (daily) seizures. The choice of drug is based on her generalized tonic-clonic seizures. The first-line drugs for generalized tonic-clonic seizures are phenytoin and carbamazepine. Phenytoin has side effects of hirsutism and coarsening of facial features, and many clinicians would not use it in young girls. Therefore the best choice for this patient is carbamazepine.

4. c. All the choices listed would be good characteristics of a new antiepileptic drug. However, a specific feature of generalized tonic-clonic seizures are repetitive action potentials in the cortex. Therefore the most desirable characteristic for treatment of generalized tonic-clonic seizures would be the ability to block repetitive action potentials.

5. d. Carbamazepine causes autoinduction of its own metabolism over the first several weeks of treatment. As the patient continues to take the same dose, the half-life shortens and the average plasma concentration falls, possibly below the therapeutic level.

6. d. Many insults to the brain can cause seizures, including metabolic derangements, tumors, and drug use and abuse. Mental retardation does not cause seizures.

Chapter 28

1. b. None of the other drugs reduce cardiac output significantly at doses usually used, and effects on blood pressure are small compared with those of halothane. Ketamine often *increases* blood pressure.

2. e. All volatile anesthetics and morphine-like opioids decrease the sensitivity of chemoreceptors in the respiratory centers of the brainstem to carbon dioxide, thus blunting the ventilatory response to increases in carbon dioxide tension in blood and cerebrospinal fluid.

3. c. As an ED50, MAC is unaffected by the size of the patient (although it takes longer to anesthetize a large patient than it does a smaller one) the patient's gender, or the length of time over which the anesthetic is administered. Morphine depresses the CNS so that *less* anesthetic is required (i.e., the MAC is lowered). Probably because of their high basal metabolism, infants have a higher anesthetic requirement than do older patients.

4. d. Inhalational anesthetics do not act at specific cell-surface receptors. The other three drugs act at different sites on the GABA-receptor complex; antagonists have been developed for only the benzodiazepine recognition site, which is where midazolam acts.

5. e. All morphine-like opioids, including fentanyl, have similar spectra of pharmacological activity; most differences of clinical significance are due to pharmacokinetic characteristics.

6. a. The answer is self-explanatory.

Chapter 29

1. d. Metocurine and tubocurarine cause noncytotoxic degranulation of mast cells, which induces release of histamine.

2. e. Although competitive nicotinic receptor blockers such as doxacurium *may* affect other targets, at therapeutic concentrations their predominant action is to cause a nondepolarizing block of the acetylcholine receptor.

3. c. Succinylcholine has the fastest onset and the shortest duration of action of any of the agents listed.

4. a. Gallamine is the only drug listed that is cleared from the body by renal filtration.

5. e. Common therapeutic uses of neuromuscular blockers are to relax the muscles to allow for controlled ventilation and to allow insertion of endotracheal tubes during surgery. Neuromuscular blockers also have been used to confirm the diagnosis of myasthenia gravis. This entails use of a low dose of d-tubocurarine (such as 0.5 mg), which can elicit muscle weakness in a patient with myasthenia gravis. However, this test is potentially hazardous and generally is not used.

Chapter 30

1. e. Local anesthetics block nerve impulses through their reversible binding to voltage-dependent Na^+ channels. Binding occurs at a site accessible from the intracellular surface. The affinity for local anesthetics depends on the conformation or the "state" of the channel (i.e., whether it is closed, open, or inactivated at rest).

2. e. Local anesthetics are weak bases (p*K*a ~8 to 9), thus existing primarily in the protonated, cationic form in solutions at physiological pH (~7.4). Whereas the protonated species blocks Na^+ channels with higher affinity, the neutral species passes more readily across the membrane to reach its site of action.

3. e. Local anesthetic molecules contain both hydrophobic (i.e., substituted aromatic) groups and hydrophilic (i.e., amine) groups, the latter of which combine with acids (e.g., HCl) to form salts (e.g., lidocaine HCl). The duration of nerve block depends on whether local hydrolysis occurs because ester-linked (but not amide-linked) drugs are cleaved by tissue-associated cholinesterases and on the vascular supply because both types of drugs can be rapidly reabsorbed by the local circulation.

4. e. Systemically circulating local anesthetics first cause CNS seizure activity, then CNS depression, and cardiac dysrhythmias. In some individuals certain local anesthetics, usually the ester-linked forms, can provoke allergic reactions (hypersensitivity).

Chapter 31

1. d. Naloxone is a short-acting antagonist that is selective for opioid receptors. It does not antagonize the effects of nonopioid drugs such as barbiturates. As a "pure" antagonist it has no intrinsic efficacy. It does not activate opioid receptors and produces no effects by itself.

2. e. All opioid analgesics decrease the sensitivity of chemoreceptors in the brainstem to CO_2, which is a stimulant of respiration. After an analgesic dose of any opioid, the ventilatory response to CO_2 is blunted and respiration is depressed, albeit not to a clinically significant extent in a patient with otherwise normal pulmonary function.

3. a. Butorphanol is a low-efficacy agonist at the μ-opioid receptor, which mediates the effects of morphine-like opioids, including analgesia, respiratory depression, and physical dependence. It is a higher-efficacy agonist at the κ-opioid receptor, which also mediates analgesia, particularly in the spinal cord. This profile of activity results in analgesic efficacy that is roughly comparable to that of morphine and a ceiling on those side effects that result primarily from activation of the μ-opioid receptor. Naloxone has a lower affinity for the κ-opioid receptor than it does for the μ-opioid receptors and therefore is less potent in reversing effects mediated by the μ-opioid receptor.

4. e. Surmountable tolerance develops to the analgesic effect of all morphine-like opioids such as methadone and meperidine, and there is cross-tolerance to this effect among all drugs of this group. However, tolerance does not develop to the same extent to every effect of these drugs. For example, little or no tolerance develops to their constipating effect and their effect on pupil size.

5. e. Aspirin decreases body temperature, should not be used in children due to the possibility of Reye's syndrome; it does not affect PG receptors in the hypothalamus.

6. c. All the drugs listed, with the exception of codeine, work by inhibiting COX; one can only achieve a greater effect by using drugs with different mechanisms.

Chapter 32

1. c. The ability of one drug to completely prevent the onset of withdrawal signs and symptoms during abstinence from another drug is evidence of cross-dependence between them.

2. b. The withdrawal syndrome from depressant drugs such as alcohol and barbiturates may include severe tremors and convulsions.

3. b. There is a very large therapeutic index for benzodiazepines, and they can be administered quite safely over a very wide range of doses. This is not true for barbiturates.

4. a. Convulsions are signs of withdrawal from barbiturates and other depressant drugs, not from opiates.

5. c. Cocaine is a psychomotor stimulant with actions similar to amphetamines. Their patterns of abuse are also very similar.

6. e. Alcohol, barbiturates, and benzodiazepines belong to the CNS depressant class. They produce a similar withdrawal syndrome after chronic use, which reflects CNS hyperexcitability. They show cross-dependence to each other. Because benzodiazepines have a long duration of action, the withdrawal syndrome after their discontinuation is generally milder than that seen in alcoholics and barbiturate abusers.

Chapter 33

1. e. The best way to assess recovery of the hypothalamic-pituitary-adrenal axis is the short ACTH stimulation test, in which ACTH is given intravenously and plasma cortisol is measured 30 and 60 minutes later. If the adrenal gland has not atrophied or has recovered in the presence of endogenous ACTH, a bolus of ACTH should increase serum cortisol to 20 μg/dl or better.

2. b. The hydroxyl group at carbon 11 confers glucocorticoid activity to the corticoid molecule.

3. c. Alternate-day glucocorticoid therapy can be beneficial in minimizing the suppressive effect on the hypothalamic-pituitary-adrenal axis; however, this approach may not be optimal for the patient with adrenocortical insufficiency for two reasons. First, the antiinflammatory effect may be insufficient. Second, some patients may begin to suffer from effects of clinical hypercortisolism, particularly if an abrupt switch from constant to alternate-day therapy is made.

4. c. Mineralocorticoid treatment is used only rarely but can be valuable in any case in which endogenous aldosterone concentration or activity is very low (primary adrenal insufficiency, etc.). This therapy is of no benefit in an autoimmune disease when the target organ (kidney) itself is damaged.

5. c. Although all answers can in some cases cause clinical cortisol excess, the most common cause is administration of excess exogenous glucocorticoids to treat other clinical conditions such as inflammation.

Chapter 34

1. b. The cromes are recommended for *prevention* of exercise-induced bronchospasm, and have an onset of action of 10-15 minutes. None of the other agents listed are indicated as preventive therapy for exercise induced bronchospasm.

2. a. The bronchoconstrictive component of COPD has been shown to respond better to antimuscarinic agents than β_2-adrenergic selective agonists.

3. b. The only drugs shown to reduce recruitment of eosinophils are the glucocorticoids. They decrease bone marrow production of eosinophils and enhance their removal from the circulation.

4. c. Of the β_2 selective agonists, salmeterol has the longest duration of action, approximately 12 hours, which reduces the risk of desensitization.

Chapter 35

1. c. Aromatase is the enzyme that is specifically targeted by both anastrozole and aminoglutethimide.

2. c. Levonorgestrel is a synthetic progestin.

3. b. Estrogens alone increase the risk of endometrial cancer, thromboembolic disorders, and gallbladder disease but do not alter the risk of breast cancer.

4. b. Estrogen plus progestin for postmenopausal replacement therapy causes a significantly increased risk of stroke, thromboembolic disorders, breast cancer and myocardial infarction, but not endometrial cancer.

5. d. The purpose of the ethinyl group is to decrease metabolism so these compounds can be taken orally.

Chapter 36

1. c. Finasteride blocks the conversion of testosterone to dihydrotestosterone, but because it does not bind to androgen receptors, it does not block the suppressive effect of testosterone on breast growth or increase plasma estradiol concentrations. Thus gynecomastia does not occur.

2. d. HDL cholesterol concentrations are reduced by androgens, especially nonaromatized androgen derivatives.

3. c. Cimetidine is a weak androgen antagonist with no effect on testosterone biosynthesis.

4. b. Testosterone cypionate is a long-acting ester suitable for androgen-replacement therapy in hypogonadal men.

5. e. Danazol is a steroidal antiandrogen with progestational activity. Because of the latter property, it reduces gonadotropin secretion in women.

6. b. The concentration of dihydrotestosterone in an adult man's plasma is about 10% of the value for testosterone.

Chapter 37

1. d. All answers are possible. Generic preparations of T_4 do not always have equivalent bioavailability. Calcium and iron can cause malabsorption. Finally, as a patient with Hashimoto's thyroiditis progresses, its contribution to circulating T_4 is lost.

2. b. T_4 must be converted to T_3 for its clinical effects to occur, thus providing the body with some control over regulation of the hormonal effect. All other statements are incorrect.

3. e. β-Adrenergic receptor blockers control only some clinical features, and control is not permanent.

Chapter 38

1. e. Insulin decreases gluconeogenesis.

2. c. Lente insulin does not contain protamine, but is a mixture of precipitated forms of insulin that are generated when insulin is mixed under the appropriate conditions with Zn^{2+}.

3. d. Glimepiride is a sulfonylurea which depolarizes the β cell plasma membrane.

4. a. Metformin is a biguanide that is used to treat type 2 diabetes.

5. c. Glucose entry into hepatocytes is mediated by GLUT-2, which is different than GLUT-4 and is not insulin sensitive.

Chapter 39

1. c. OT acts through Gq mediated phospholipase C activation, initiating a series of changes in Ca^{2+} handling. It does not activate adenylyl cyclase.

2. d. Misoprostol causes uterine stimulation; the other choices are relaxants.

3. b. Indomethacin is an NSAID, which inhibits formation of PG synthesis by blocking cyclooxygenase.

4. a. β-Adrenergic receptor agonists cause hypotension, not hypertension. The other effects listed are common with tocolytic therapy with this class of drugs.

5. d. A combination of the two treatments, with an appropriate interval to prevent adverse effects, is preferred.

6. c. OT is a peptide with a very short half-life. It does not easily cross the placenta, is not indicated for cervical ripening, has an increased sensitivity in *late* pregnancy, and cannot be administered orally.

Chapter 40

1. f. AVP is synthesized by and secreted from the posterior pituitary which is not under hypothalamic control; all the others listed are secreted from the anterior pituitary.

2. c. Both arginine vasopressin and arginine vasopressin tannate have significantly greater pressor effects than does desmopressin.

3. b. Of patients, 18% develop sludge in the gallbladder or stones; not all are symptomatic.

4. g. Children must be GH-deficient. Short stature may be genetic. GH is now approved for use by adults.

Chapter 41

1. d. Approximately 10 g of Ca^{2+} is filtered per day with 99% of that is reabsorbed; Furosemide and ethacrynic acid inhibit Na^{+}-linked calcium reabsorption; Thiazide diuretics can prevent nephrolithiasis by decreasing calcium excretion; low phosphate stimulates the renal 25-hydroxyvitamin D1-α-hydroxylase.

2. d. PTH acts through a G-protein coupled receptor; PTH stimulates vitamin D activation through an effect on the renal 25-hydroxylase-vitaminD-1-α-hydroxylase; PTH stimulates bone resorption; PTH increases intestinal Ca^{2+} absorption.

3. d. Vitamin D stimulates the synthesis of an intestinal Ca^{2+}-binding protein; active vitamin D metabolites promote cell differentiation; Vitamin D inhibits parathyroid hormone secretion; Ultraviolet light activates the vitamin D precursor in the skin by cleaving the B ring.

4. d. Raloxifene.

Chapter 42

1. a. Cisplatin does not resemble any endogenous amino acid, nucleotide, or vitamin and thus is not an antimetabolite. After spontaneous activation it reacts covalently with nuclear DNA, forming interstrand and intrastrand cross-links.

2. d. Bleomycin damages endothelial and epithelial cells in the lungs, which leads to a progressive loss of lung function from the deposition of extracellular matrix in the interstitial space of the alveolar sacs.

3. b. Anticancer drugs kill a fixed fraction of the total cell population, and thus the toxicity-versus-dose curve is best described by a first-order equation.

4. d. Topoisomerase II is a common target for compounds derived from natural sources such as etoposide, doxorubicin, and daunorubicin. It functions normally to relieve torsional strain on DNA that occurs during replication. Many compounds block or poison the enzyme activity and produce frank DNA breaks that lead to cell death.

5. b. Ribonucleotide reductase is an essential enzyme for reduction of ribonucleoside diphosphates to deoxyribonucleoside diphosphates needed for DNA synthesis. Hydroxyurea inhibits ribonucleotide reductase by destroying a tyrosyl free radical that is formed in the catalytic center of the enzyme.

6. c. Antimetabolites mimic endogenous substances that are involved in DNA and either block or disrupt DNA synthesis. Consequently, cell death occurs in the phase of the cell cycle dedicated to DNA synthesis, namely S phase.

Chapter 43

1. b. Hodgkin's disease is curable with chemotherapy even in situations in which the liver and lung are involved by metastatic disease. Breast, colon, lung, and stomach cancer are curable only with surgery.

2. c. Both MOPP and ABVD are effective regimens for Hodgkin's disease. Because MOPP includes procarbazine, which is an alkylating agent, it has a significant rate of secondary leukemia. CMF and CAF are used for breast cancer, and BIP is used for cervical cancer.

3. d. Cisplatin is associated with significant nausea and vomiting. Tamoxifen is associated with hot flashes and rarely alopecia. Methotrexate and 5 FU are both associated with stomatitis, diarrhea, and bone marrow suppression. Vincristine is associated with peripheral neuropathy.

4. c. Renal cell carcinoma is highly resistant to all known chemotherapeutic agents. Recently interleukin-2 has produced some complete responses in patients with metastatic renal cell cancer. The remainder of the cancers, including AML, lymphoma, small cell carcinoma of the lung, and seminoma, are all very sensitive to chemotherapy. All these diseases are potentially curable even when metastasized.

5. e. Generally, when patients fail to respond to first-line chemotherapy the chances of a meaningful response to second-line drugs are small, particularly for solid tumors, for all of the reasons indicated. The higher the performance status of a patient, the greater the likelihood of an objective response to chemotherapy.

Chapter 44

1. c. Meningitis requires killing the bacteria.

2. b. Tetracycline should be avoided in pregnant women.

3. b. The two agents work by different mechanisms and cause synergistic effects.

4. a. Prophylaxis should be started prior to surgery.

5. d. Fluoroquinolones cause DNA damage.

6. c. Vancomycin is not enzymatically inactivated but resistance develops through production of an altered target.

Chapter 45

1. c. β-Lactam agents and vancomycin both prevent cross-linking of the peptidoglycan matrix of bacterial cell walls, but by different mechanisms. The β-lactams inhibit transpeptidase enzymes which react with the D-Ala-D-Ala terminus of the pentapeptide, whereas vancomycin binds to the terminal D-Ala-D-Ala itself, preventing cross-linking.

2. b. Nafcillin is a semisynthetic β-lactamase-resistant penicillin which is highly effective against most penicillinase-producing strains of *S. aureus* but not methicillin-resistant *S. aureus* (MRSA) which has low affinity penicillin-binding proteins. It is more effective against sensitive *S. aureus* strains than vancomycin. Nafcillin is not useful for treating gram-negative bacteria and should not be used in persons with immediate hypersensitivity reactions to penicillins.

3. c. Resistance to vancomycin is mediated by the production of altered cell wall precursors with different termini (D-Ala-D-Ala changed to D-Ala-D-Lac, for example) that have low affinity for vancomycin, thus allowing synthesis of the cell wall in the presence of vancomycin.

4. c. Penicillin G is rapidly eliminated from the body, primarily through the kidneys. About 10% is removed by glomerular filtration and 90% by tubular secretion.

5. c. The use of imipenem does not eliminate the need for specimen collection for culture. Although it is highly resistant to hydrolysis by most β-lactamases, resistance to imipenem by other mechanisms is increasingly a problem, particularly in nosocomial gram-negative organisms such as *Pseudomonas aeruginosa* and *Acinetobacter.* Other organisms, including MRSA, vancomycin-resistant enterococci (VRE) and *Stenotrophomonas,* are also most often resistant.

6. c. Aztreonam is a monocyclic β-lactam (monobactam) active against most aerobic gram-negative bacteria. Because of its structural difference, there is no clinically significant immune cross-reactivity between aztreonam and the penicillins. For cephalosporins, there is a 3% to 7% cross-reactivity rate with penicillins, so a cephalosporin should not be administered to patients with a history of severe (IgE-mediated) penicillin allergy. There is a high degree of immune cross-reactivity between imipenem and the penicillins.

Chapter 46

1. b. Mupirocin, a topical agent, inhibits primarily gram-positive organisms such as *S. aureus.*

2. d. The only clinical use for spectinomycin is as an alternative regiment for treating *N. gonorrhoeae* infections in patients unable to take cephalosporins or quinolones.

3. a. Rifampin is highly active against meningococci, and effective in preventing secondary cases of meningococcal meningitis.

4. a. Because of their high polarity, aminoglycosides such as gentamicin do not enter phagocytic (or other) cells and therefore cannot kill intracellular pathogens.

5. d. All side effects listed can occur.

6. b. Chloramphenicol is metabolized in the liver by conjugation to an inactive and nontoxic glucuronide that is subsequently filtered by the kidney.

Chapter 47

1. b. Sulfonamides, such as sulfamethoxazole, primarily exert their antibacterial activity through competitive inhibition of p-aminobenzoic acid incorporation, an essential precursor for normal bacterial synthesis of folate. One mechanism of resistance to sulfonamides is increased bacterial production of p-aminobenzoic acid.

2. b. Trimethoprim and creatinine are excreted via the same renal clearance pathways. Hence trimethoprim can cause an increase in creatinine concentrations.

3. d. Trimethoprim-sulfamethoxazole has proven useful against a wide range of organisms, including bacteria (such as *E. coli*), higher bacteria (such as *N. asteroides*), and parasites (such as *T. gondii*), but has no useful clinical activity against fungi, including *C. albicans.*

4. c. Levofloxacin inhibits DNA gyrase and topoisomerase IV.

5. d. Polymyxins function essentially as cationic detergents. Both lipophilic and lipophobic domains interact with membrane phospholipids to disrupt bacterial cell membranes.

6. a. Second generation fluoroquinolones are broadly active against gram-negative bacteria such as *E. coli,* but in general do not have clinically useful activity against gram-positive organisms or anaerobes.

Chapter 48

1. c. Erythromycin (in combination with rifampin in severe cases) is the therapy of choice for *Legionella* species pneumonia. Ciprofloxacin also has activity against *Legionella* species and may be used when treatment with macrolides is not possible. Gentamicin is not effective against *Legionella* species.

2. d. Penicillin V is effective against streptococcal pharyngitis.

3. b. Ampicillin in high doses is the treatment of choice for *Listeria* species meningitis. Penicillin is also effective. Many isolates are sensitive to tetracycline, erythromycin, chloramphenicol, TMP/SMX, vancomycin, and cephalothin. In some cases gentamicin is added to ampicillin for synergy.

4. e. Tetracyclines are not useful in treating *S. viridans* endocarditis because these agents are bacteriostatic rather than bactericidal. For infections in sites relatively protected from host defenses (such as endocarditic vegetations), bacteriostatic antibiotics are generally not effective.

5. d. For most cases of *C. difficile* colitis, metronidazole is the therapy of choice. Although oral vancomycin is equally effective, it is much more expensive and predisposes to colonization with vancomycin-resistant enterococci. None of the other agents listed are effective for *C. difficile* disease.

6. c. Vancomycin does not have broad activity against both gram positive and gram negative organisms.

Chapter 49

1. a. Rifampin does not block cell wall synthesis, but inhibits RNA polymerase.
2. b. INH is metabolized by a liver *N*-acetyltransferase.
3. c. PZA is converted to an active metabolite.
4. d. LTBI does not require multidrug therapy.
5. a. Isoniazid does not cause anemia but does cause the other symptoms listed.
6. b. Ethambutol causes optic neuritis.

Chapter 50

1. d. Ketoconazole and itraconazole both require gastric acid for maximum bioavailability, and therefore coadministration with H_2-blockers or other antacids may interfere with their absorption and efficacy.
2. c. Fluconazole is the only azole that attains adequate concentrations in the CSF and urine.
3. b. The major toxicity of amphotericin B is nephrotoxicity. Bone marrow suppression may occur, but this is largely manifested by anemia.
4. e. Amphotericin B remains the drug of choice for cryptococcal meningitis; however, fluconazole is now indicated for the condition as well. Fluconazole does not sterilize the CSF as rapidly, but has proven superior to amphotericin B for chronic maintenance therapy in patients with AIDS and cryptococcal meningitis.
5. d. Amphotericin B and amphotericin B lipid complex are the drugs of choice for invasive *Aspergillus* organism infections. Itraconazole is currently the only azole with activity, and in one uncontrolled study it had an efficacy approaching amphotericin B.
6. c. Griseofulvin has historically been the agent of choice for fungal infections of the nails. Recently, itraconazole and terbinafine have been approved for this indication, and in general they require shorter durations of therapy, largely supplanting the griseofulvin for this indication.

Chapter 51

1. c. Amination of acyclovir to the active compound does not occur.
2. a. Acyclovir, ganciclovir, and zidovudine require phosphorylation to become active.
3. d. Zidovudine, didanosine, and lamivudine work at the same active site of HIV reverse transcriptase. Nevirapine works at a different active site on the same enzyme.
4. a. All protease inhibitors exhibit significant metabolism in the liver, affecting the metabolism of other drugs. The largest interactions occur with ritonavir.
5. b. Interferon is used for hepatitis C, often in conjunction with ribavirin.
6. d. Immunoglobulins may modify illness occurring after an individual has been exposed to infectious virus particles. There is no evidence that condyloma acuminatum (papillomavirus infection) is responsive to immunoglobulin therapy.

Chapter 52

1. a. Albendazole has been used effectively in mass treatment programs for persons with common intestinal roundworms (nematodes), *A. lumbricoides;* hookworms; and *T. trichiura.*
2. c. Praziquantel is effective for the treatment of all forms of schistosomiasis. Albendazole, mebendazole, ivermectin, and niclosamide are not active against *Schistosoma* species.
3. e. The drug of choice for onchocerciasis is ivermectin. Albendazole and mebendazole have activity against a broad spectrum of intestinal roundworms, but they are not active against *O. volvulus* and other filariae. Niclosamide has activity against many tapeworm species but not roundworms. Diethylcarbamazine kills microfilariae of *O. volvulus* quickly, but in the process it elicits acute, frequently severe inflammatory reactions. Ivermectin, which kills microfilariae more slowly, produces less severe inflammatory responses and has replaced diethylcarbamazine as the treatment of choice for *O. volvulus.*
4. a. Albendazole is metabolized to albendazole sulfoxide, which is responsible for its activity against helminths in tissue. Mebendazole, praziquantel, diethylcarbamazine, and ivermectin are not metabolized to an active sulfoxide metabolite in humans.
5. b. Primaquine is a well-known cause of hemolysis in persons who have G6PD deficiency. Chloroquine, mefloquine, pyrimethamine, and doxycycline do not cause G6PD deficiency–related hemolysis, although pyrimethamine can cause anemia by inhibiting human dihydrofolate reductase.
6. e. Primaquine is the only drug that is active against hypnozoites of *P. vivax* and *P. ovale* in the liver. Chloroquine, mefloquine, pyrimethamine, and quinine act on the asexual erythrocytic stages of susceptible *Plasmodium* species.

Chapter 53

1. b. Corticosteroids suppress immune and inflammatory responses.
2. d. Cyclosporine is considered to be more selective than the antiproliferative immunosuppressive agents (azathioprine and cyclophosphamide) by inhibiting cytokine synthesis in T-lymphocytes.
3. b. Cyclosporine does not produce bone marrow suppression.
4. b. Cyclosporine prevents graft rejection by inhibiting several T-lymphocyte–dependent immune responses–the cytotoxic T-lymphocyte response, delayed-type hypersensitivity response, and antibody response.

Chapter 54

1. d. Second-generation antihistamines do not penetrate the CNS very well and mainly differ from the first-generation agents by producing much less sedation. Also, currently available second-generation agents have very little antimuscarinic activity. None have partial agonist activity.
2. d. Both histamine H_1 and H_2 receptors mediate vasodilation. At high doses of histamine, both receptors are activated, and full antagonism requires the use of a combination of H_1 and H_2 antagonists.
3. b. Histamine-induced bronchoconstriction is mediated by H_1 receptors. The inhibition of norepinephrine release can be mediated by H_3 receptors. Neither a stimulation of basophil degranulation nor a decreased inotropy is an action of histamine.
4. d. Arousal is mediated by the activation of central histamine H_1 or muscarinic receptors. Sedation can be caused by drugs that block either receptor, such as first-generation antihistamines. Blockade of H_3 receptors on histaminergic terminals enhances transmitter release and might cause arousal.

Chapter 55

1. c. Cimetidine is one of four currently marketed H_2 antagonists that inhibit histamine-stimulated secretion of acid. Because of the important role of histamine in the regulation of acid secretion, H_2 antagonists are highly effective inhibitors of gastric secretion.
2. e. The prokinetic effects of metoclopramide seem to result from antagonism at D_2 receptors and from agonist actions at 5-HT_4 receptors on neurons in the enteric nervous system. Metoclopramide's pronounced antiemetic actions, however, clearly result from D_2 receptor antagonism in the brainstem.
3. a. Although not extensively metabolized itself, cimetidine binds to certain isoforms of cytochrome P450 and can decrease activity of the enzyme in the metabolism of several other drugs.
4. e. Metoclopramide, because it is a D_2 receptor antagonist and crosses the blood-brain barrier, can act in brain nigrostriatal pathways to induce extrapyramidal motor dysfunction characteristic of Parkinson's disease.
5. c. Aluminum ions avidly bind phosphate, and chronic use of aluminum salts as antacids can diminish absorption of phosphate from the small intestine, thus depleting phosphate from the body. Bone resorption can result.
6. a. Muscarinic receptor antagonists are notorious for producing these and other side effects because acetylcholine, acting at muscarinic receptors, is the principal neurotransmitter at many different sites. It is hoped that improved definitions of multiple subtypes of muscarinic receptors will lead to more selective and thus more specific drugs.

Chapter 56

1. c. The cholinergic syndrome includes salivation, lacrimation, urination, diarrhea, muscle weakness, and fasciculation. The cholinergic syndrome is caused by increased acetylcholine at the synapse. This results in overstimulation of muscarinic and nicotinic acetylcholine receptors, which produces the SLUDGE (*s*alivation, *l*acrimation, *u*rination, *d*efecation, *g*astroenteritis, *e*mesis) syndrome.
2. a. Only extremely small particulates remain airborne and penetrate all the way to the alveolus.
3. b. A major function of the kidney is water reabsorption and concentration. As stated in the text, high concentrations of chemicals can occur. The kidney can metabolize (activate and detoxify) certain chemicals but does not use metallothionein to catalyze such reactions.
4. c. Lead tends to concentrate on the red cell, and the blood lead concentration is an index of the degree of lead exposure.

Index

Page numbers followed by f refer to figures, t refer to tables, and b refer to boxes.